FUNDAMENTALS OF
BASIC EMERGENCY CARE

SECOND EDITION

FUNDAMENTALS OF
BASIC EMERGENCY CARE

SECOND EDITION

Richard W. O. Beebe, MEd, RN, NREMT-P

Program Director
Bassett Healthcare
Center for Rural Emergency Medical Services Education
Cooperstown, New York

Adjunct Faculty
Herkimer County Community College
Herkimer, New York

Deborah L. Funk, MD, FACEP, NREMT-P

Assistant Professor
Emergency Medicine
Albany Medical College
Albany, New York

Attending Physician
Emergency Department
Albany Medical Center Hospital
Albany, New York

THOMSON

DELMAR LEARNING

Australia   Canada   Mexico   Singapore   Spain   United Kingdom   United States

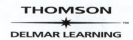

THOMSON
———★———™
DELMAR LEARNING

Fundamentals of Basic Emergency Care, Second Edition
by Richard W. O. Beebe and Deborah L. Funk

Vice President, Health Care Business Unit:
William Brottmiller

Editorial Director:
Cathy L. Esperti

Acquisitions Editor:
Maureen Rosener

Senior Developmental Editor:
Darcy M. Scelsi

Editorial Assistant:
Elizabeth Howe

Marketing Director:
Jennifer McAvey

Marketing Coordinator:
Christopher Manion

Art and Design Specialist:
Jack Pendleton

Production Coordinator:
Anne Sherman

Project Editor:
David Buddle

Library of Congress Cataloging-in-Publication Data
Beebe, Richard W. O.
  Fundamentals of emergency care / Richard W. O. Beebe, Deborah L. Funk. — 2nd ed.
    p. cm.
  Rev. ed. of: Fundamentals of emergency care.
  Includes bibliographical references and index.
ISBN 1-4018-7933-0
1. Emergency medicine.
[DNLM: 1. Emergency Medical Services—methods. 2. Emergencies. 3. Emergency Medical Technicians. 4. Emergency Treatment. 5. Wounds and Injuries—therapy. WX 215 B414f 2005] I. Funk, Deborah L. II. Beebe, Richard W. O. Fundamentals of emergency care. III. Title. RC86.7 .B44 2005 616.02'5--dc22
                                    2004023024

NOTICE TO THE READER

There are countless people who have contributed significantly to my career as an EMS physician, but none who have stood by me as consistently and tirelessly as my family, most of all my husband, Tom.

I would like to dedicate this book to the EMTs who continue to motivate me every day and to my husband, without whom I am sure I would not have been able to devote time to this text.

D.F.

Without the love and support of our families, none of us could achieve our aspirations and dreams. I would like to thank my wife, Laura, for her boundless love and support, as well as my daughters, Heather and Amanda, for their inspiration.

I would like to dedicate this book to my students, past, present, and future, who challenge me every day to be the best educator I can be, and to the Western Turnpike Rescue Squad, my home away from home for more than 15 years.

R.W.O.B.

Brief Contents

Contents

Case Studies

SKILLS

EMS in Action Contributors

About the Authors

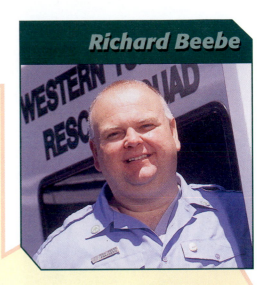

Richard Beebe

Richard Beebe has been an EMT for more than 30 years and an EMS educator for the past 20 years. Beebe started his EMS career as a volunteer EMT-firefighter with the Moyers Corners Fire Department in Upstate New York in 1974 and has continuously maintained his status as an EMT ever since.

In 1983, Beebe became a registered nurse and practiced in the intensive care unit and the emergency department of St. Peter's Hospital, Albany, New York. It was during this time that Beebe became a paramedic. He left nursing to become a full-time EMS educator in 1989.

Beebe is currently the program director for Bassett Healthcare's Center for Rural EMS Education in Cooperstown, New York. He is also an adjunct faculty member at Herkimer County Community College. Beebe remains active in the field as a paramedic for the Town of Guilderland EMS and as a volunteer EMT with the Western Turnpike Rescue Squad.

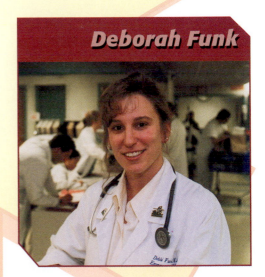

Deborah Funk

Deborah Funk has been an EMT since 1988 and an EMS educator for 15 years. After Funk completed her paramedic education, she went on to medical school. Throughout medical school, she continued to practice as a paramedic and as an EMS educator.

She completed an EMS fellowship and remains active both locally and nationally as an EMS physician. Funk has received state and national recognition for her work in EMS and her contributions to EMS research. In 1999, Funk was recognized as the Emergency Physician of the Year by the New York State Department of Health.

Currently, Funk is a practicing emergency physician and provides physician oversight to several EMS agencies, both ground and air, as well as BLS and ALS. As an educator, she teaches EMTs and paramedics as well as medical students and emergency medicine residents.

Foreword to the Second Edition

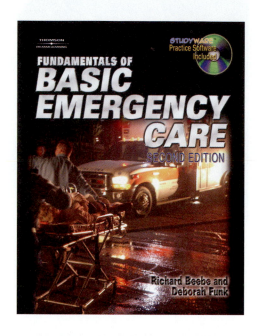

EMS is a practice of medicine, and a very unique practice at that. In today's complex world, an EMT is usually the first health care provider our communities encounter when they experience sudden illness or injury. Our ability to rapidly evaluate and treat our patients often has a direct impact on their eventual morbidity and mortality. Our presence alone is calming and reassuring to those who have suddenly suffered an event that may be painful or confusing. Our experience and knowledge provide the information they need to make difficult decisions about themselves or their loved ones in very chaotic times.

As we understand more about the amazing science of the human body and how it behaves when it's "broken," we appreciate that the best approach to management of illness and injury requires more than just memorizing facts. It requires us to put together everything we know, use all our available resources, and develop a plan of action that incorporates clinical care, different modes of transport, and different receiving facilities. For example, how quickly we get our seriously injured patients to an appropriate trauma facility often has as much impact on outcome as the medical care we provide in the streets.

The devastating and unfortunate events of September 11, 2001, have focused the U.S. public's attention on the importance of emergency medical care and the value of having EMS providers with the knowledge and ability to deal with an entire spectrum of out-of-hospital problems, ranging from the simple to the unimaginable. As emergency care providers ourselves, we learned the importance of always being ready, whether that readiness is the proper working equipment or the clinical skills and knowledge to take care of our patients.

EMS has also become the safety net for many communities suffering from inadequate health care resources. Regardless of the number of facilities, patients still get sick. While the situation increases our obligation and workload, we should be very proud of our collective ability to care for our fellow human beings regardless of their ability to afford it or our community's ability to provide it.

In short, contemporary EMS providers have become an extremely valuable and respected group of dedicated professionals that the public depends on to *take care of them*, regardless of the particular situation, time of day, weather, location, ability to pay, or just about any other imaginable variable. We should be *very, very* proud of that.

We owe our patients the best science has to offer when we care for them. And, we should always provide that care in a compassionate, understanding way. Richard Beebe, Deborah Funk, and their colleagues have done a spectacular job of giving us the tools to do just that. *Fundamentals of Basic Emergency Care* is more than a textbook. It's part of a comprehensive learning system.

Throughout this textbook, you will find a variety of innovative and informative ways to help you develop your skills as an emergency medical technician. The StudyWare CD-ROM that accompanies the book provides a variety of activities to review the concepts discussed in each chapter. There are a variety of practice question types (multiple choice, true/false, fill-in-the-blank, matching, and image labeling) to use in self-assessment. The CD-ROM also provides animation to increase your comprehension of critical concepts, video clips of skills demonstrated step-by-step, and valuable links to Web sites with related content for more information. Icons throughout the book alert you to additional content on the StudyWare CD-ROM.

As the scientific evidence in medicine continues to change practice, you will find expanded and comprehensive discussions of management of stroke patients, acute coronary syndromes, and commonly encountered medical problems. The textbook has the most comprehensive coverage of anatomy and physiology of any EMT–Basic text available. New and expanded areas also include information on organizations that provide a voice in the provision of EMS, such as the National Registry of EMTs, the International Association of Fire Fighters, and the American Ambulance Association. There are discussions on the often-difficult-to-interpret implications of federal laws such as HIPAA and EMTALA for EMS Providers. Finally, you will find a powerful emphasis on one of the most important principles in emergency care: *Looking out for number 1.* The authors discuss emerging concepts in management of acute and chronic stress in EMS, infection control, and the important ergonomic factors in our daily care of patients.

As with any educational tool, the more attractive and interesting a textbook is, the more likely we are to spend time in it. *Fundamentals of Basic Emergency Care* has done a great job of providing illustrations, listing Internet resources at the end of each chapter on specific topics and providing **EMS in Action** boxes throughout the text that highlight our colleagues in EMS and the lessons learned from their experiences. **Ask the Doc** boxes throughout provide relevant scientific information, contemporary research, and position papers from the National Association of EMS Physicians.

I have had the privilege over the years of working with amazing professionals who have dedicated their lives to caring for others in the toughest of circumstances. There is no more honorable, more rewarding profession on the planet than caring for our fellow human beings when they need it most. Beebe, Funk, and their colleagues have given us the tools to do it right and have presented it in a way that makes it educationally sound and easy to digest.

Be proud of what you do. Be good at what you do. And always remember how important your knowledge, skills, and compassion are for those at the other end of the 9-1-1 call.

Edward M. Racht, MD
Austin, Texas

Foreword to the First Edition

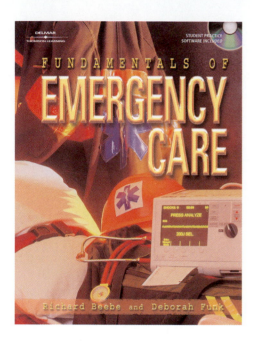

A lifelong student recognizes the importance of the written word in the acquisition of knowledge. Textbooks specifically serve as the nutritional staple for the development or expansion of intellectual capacity. What's different about textbooks related to emergency medical technician education is that they not only serve as the benchmark for standards of care in the street, but they also must allow the written word to be easily translated into patient care.

The textbook that you are about to explore employs perhaps the most successful strategy for facilitating both an in-depth understanding of the subject matter and the translation of the subject matter into clinical practice. The problem-based learning methodology has been developed with the education of out-of-hospital providers in mind. While the successful end result of any educational endeavor is to "pass," the burden for emergency medical technicians is to not only "pass" but to expertly apply the knowledge gained to the care of patients in the field. This textbook accomplishes this through problem-based learning that allows for educational independence, case-based learning, and an analytic approach that builds on each successive subject matter presented.

The requisite topics are covered in great detail with contemporary information. The notable enhancements, however, are the expanded sections on pediatrics and geriatrics. In addition, the trauma management sections present very comprehensive information on thoracoabdominal injuries. Finally, in keeping with the premise that the out-of-hospital clinicians are the most important resource in the health care delivery system, the section on stress management is uniquely suited to the needs of future emergency medical technicians.

Overall, you will be very pleased with the material, the presentation, and the ultimate result from using this textbook. I am confident that the end product, the street savvy emergency medical technician, will be the finest caregiver of basic life support medicine seen in a very long time.

Vince Verdile, MD

Preface

DISCLAIMER

The EMT must be aware of the regional differences that will be encountered in practice. Not all areas of the country provide EMS in the same manner. This book cannot begin to encompass all of the regional differences throughout the United States. *Fundamentals of Basic Emergency Care*, Second Edition, provides learning of the national standard for care. The EMT student should actively seek out the standards set forth in his or her region through contact with instructors, medical directors, and state EMS agencies.

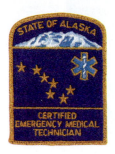

Throughout this text, the EMT student will be encouraged to problem-solve based on case studies within the text. These are simulations and are not based on fact. There may be many solutions to a single case study. It is important for the student to realize that no one case is representative of a single method of assessment and treatment. This text provides concepts for patient care and treatment that are most commonly used. This is not the definitive source for all the answers to every patient encounter. This text provides a means for the EMT student to increase his or her problem-solving abilities to determine the proper course of action when in the field. However, the only definitive source for questions regarding specific patient care is the EMS instructor and the medical director.

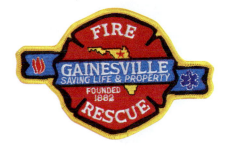

The authors and publisher have made a conscientious effort to ensure that the drug information and recommended dosages in this text are accurate and in accord with accepted standards at the time of publication. However, pharmacology and therapeutics are rapidly changing sciences. Therefore, before administering any drug, students are advised to check the package insert provided by the manufacturer for the recommended dose, for any contraindications for administration, and for any added warnings and precautions.

TO THE STUDENT

Welcome to *Fundamentals of Basic Emergency Care*, Second Edition, a textbook for EMT students using problem-based learning. *Fundamentals of Basic Emergency Care*, Second Edition, is organized logically, beginning with foundational material, followed by a step-by-step approach to emergency calls, and ending with typical emergency situations.

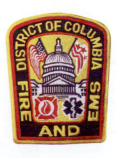

Section 1 is intended as a foundation for EMTs. There is an extensive discussion of the history of EMS, the authors believing that EMTs need to know their roots. It also includes a thorough discussion of medico-legal responsibilities. In these times of increased personal responsibility and accountability, the new EMT must know what his or her vocation requires.

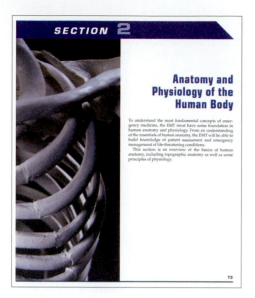

SECTION 2

Anatomy and Physiology of the Human Body

To understand the most fundamental concepts of emergency medicine, the EMT must have some foundation in human anatomy and physiology. From an understanding of the essentials of human anatomy, the EMT will be able to build knowledge of patient assessment and emergency management of life-threatening conditions.

This section is an overview of the basics of human anatomy, including topographic anatomy as well as some principles of physiology.

73

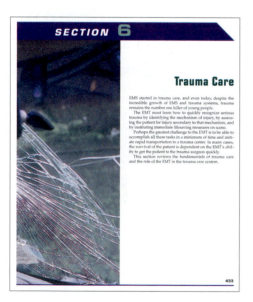

SECTION 6

Trauma Care

EMS started in trauma care, and even today, despite the incredible growth of EMS and trauma systems, trauma remains the number one killer of young people.

The EMT must learn how to quickly recognize serious trauma by identifying the mechanism of injury, by assessing the patient for injury secondary to that mechanism, and by instituting immediate lifesaving measures on scene.

Perhaps the greatest challenge to the EMT is to be able to accomplish all these tasks in a minimum of time and initiate rapid transportation to a trauma center. In many cases, the survival of the patient is dependent on the EMT's ability to get the patient to the trauma surgeon quickly.

This section reviews the fundamentals of trauma care and the role of the EMT in the trauma care system.

433

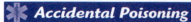

✳ Accidental Poisoning

An elderly woman meets EMS at the door and ushers the two EMTs into her living room. She explains that she called the emergency number after she found her 4-year-old grandson playing with her heart pills.

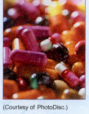

The grandmother explains, "But I only left him for a moment." While EMT Rodriguez attempts to calm the visibly distraught grandmother, EMT Ruoff notes that the child is happily playing on the floor and wonders just how much trouble those pills can cause.

(Courtesy of PhotoDisc.)

- What signs and symptoms should the EMT look for in this child?
- What are the management priorities in the patient after the suspected ingestion of a poison?

The authors purposely expanded the information on anatomy beyond what is typically found in other EMT textbooks. As the EMT student learns about medicine, the need for more information about anatomy grows. Also, many EMTs aspire to become paramedics one day. A solid foundation in anatomy is crucial to a future paramedic student.

Section 3 introduces the EMT to the ABCs of care. This is where the student learns the most essential components of patient care. A sound understanding of these principles is critical to the EMT's success.

Section 4 explores, in a methodical fashion, each of the components of an EMS call, starting with scene safety and ending with the ongoing assessment. Over the years, EMS professionals have shifted to a more cautious, safety-oriented approach. The authors have identified this trend, expanding the section on safety to include both street and house calls. The EMT "basic assessments" are then covered extensively to ensure that the EMT student walks away with a clear understanding of these important skills.

Section 5 introduces the EMT to the "three Rs" of EMS—radio, report, and record. Communication and documentation of each call is addressed.

Sections 6 through 10 develop the EMT's understanding of emergency care from trauma to medical emergencies. The number of deaths from trauma has dropped proportionally, and medical emergencies have become more prominent in EMS in the past 20 years. To reflect these changes in emergency medicine, the authors have purposely chosen to emphasize the medical emergencies an average EMT is likely to encounter. There are also sections on maternity, newborn, pediatric, and geriatric medical emergencies, emphasizing the life span of the person and the unique developmental differences at each stage of life. There is a chapter devoted to advance directives to reflect the changing demographics of the United States. As Americans get older, EMTs will have to become more competent in the care of the elderly patient, and *Fundamentals of Basic Emergency Care*, Second Edition, can help prepare them for the challenges ahead.

Finally, Section 11 discusses operational skills and the special circumstances an EMT may encounter, such as multiple-casualty incidents and hazmat scenes. Although most prehospital care is still provided by EMTs, they are often providing that care in cooperation with advanced providers, such as paramedics. With this in mind, the authors have created an appendix on Advanced Life Support Assist Skills. The EMT who can provide assistance with ALS improves team efficiency and patient care, an important added value to an EMT.

SPECIAL FEATURES

- **Real-Life Scenarios.** Case studies encourage critical thinking and problem solving, allowing the EMT student the ability to take what they learn to the streets.

- **Added Depth to the Curriculum.** There is coverage of the 1994 National Standard Curriculum (NSC) for the EMT–Basic and more. Going beyond the curriculum, this text strives to truly cover all the fundamentals of emergency care, serving as a textbook for EMTs and a resource for EMS professionals.

- **Introduction to Medical Terminology.** EMTs must know certain medical terms and phrases in order to communicate with the hospital staff; however, they must also be able to explain these terms to patients in plain English. *Fundamentals of Basic Emergency Care*, Second Edition, attempts to introduce the medical terms at appropriate times, in a manner that the EMT can understand and could explain to the patient.

- **Photographic Procedures.** Each procedure is accompanied by a colorful photo demonstration of that procedure as well as a skill-teaching sheet (found in the student workbook and instructor manual).

- **Street Smart.** Boxed information found throughout the text highlights the field experience of the authors in providing prehospital emergency care.

- **Cultural Considerations.** America is becoming more ethnically diverse. To help the new EMT meet the challenge of providing appropriate care to an increasingly complex society, the authors have inserted special segments on cultural diversity. These segments are designed to increase the new EMT's awareness of various cultures and enable him or her to better care for these patients.

- **Pediatric Considerations.** A child is not a small adult and should not be treated as such. This feature highlights areas of special consideration for providing appropriate care to children.

- **Geriatric Considerations.** America is aging and the demand on EMS for aid and care of the elderly is increasing. EMTs must be aware of special care considerations in this increasing patient population.

- **Medication Notes.** This feature highlights each of the drugs an EMT must be familiar with.

- **StudyWare.** The CD in the back of the book provides a variety of activities to review the concepts discussed in each chapter. Multiple choice, true/false, fill-in-the-blank, matching, and image labeling question types are provided for practice. New to this edition are word-building exercises to help increase your understanding of medical terminology, animations to increase comprehension of important concepts, and video clips to show you how skills are actually completed in a step-by-step manner. Web links to related areas of content are also provided for those who wish to further their understanding and research of particular topics. Possible solutions to case studies found in the book are also available on the StudyWare CD. An icon throughout the book alerts you when additional content can be found on the StudyWare CD.

NEW TO THIS EDITION

Chapter 1

- Information has been included on organizations providing a voice for EMS such as the American Ambulance Association, the International Association of Fire Fighters, and the National Registry of EMTs.

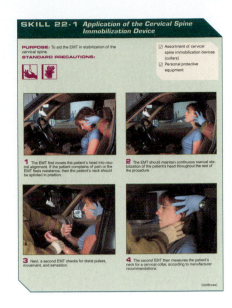

SKILL 22-1 Application of the Cervical Spine Immobilization Device

PURPOSE: To aid the EMT in stabilization of the cervical spine.
STANDARD PRECAUTIONS:

☑ Assortment of cervical spine immobilization devices (collars)
☑ Personal protective equipment

1 The EMT first moves the patient's head into neutral alignment. If the patient complains of pain or the EMT feels resistance, then the patient's neck should be splinted in position.

2 The EMT should maintain continuous manual stabilization of the patient's head throughout the rest of the procedure.

3 Next, a second EMT checks for distal pulses, movement, and sensation.

4 The second EMT then measures the patient's neck for a cervical collar, according to manufacturer recommendations.

(continues)

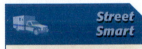

Street Smart

Some EMS calls are also crime scenes. Attention should be paid to the details on scene. Take extreme care to avoid destroying footprints, tire tracks, or broken glass.

Do not touch or move suspected weapons. Call police immediately for assistance, and consider retreating from the scene until they arrive. Always wear gloves whenever handling any object on scene.

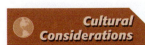

Cultural Considerations

Be sensitive to the patient's right to privacy. Some patients, after having had a seizure, are embarrassed because the seizure occurred in public. In simple-to-understand terms, tell the patient who you are and that he may have just seized. Then tell the patient what you are going to do.

The EMT should cover the patient, if possible. Consider moving the patient to a more private location or the back of the ambulance before proceeding with detailed assessments.

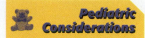

Pediatric Considerations

Children (and some adults) may use a device called a spacer between the inhaler and their mouth to assist in coordination (Figure 26-18). This device reduces the coordination of breathing necessary to effectively administer the medication. The EMT should definitely utilize this device if it is available with the inhaler.

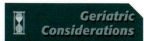

Geriatric Considerations

While an AAA may occur at any age, the majority of patients who require treatment for this condition are over the age of 60. The EMT should keep this life-threatening diagnosis in mind when caring for patients in this age group with complaints of abdominal pain.

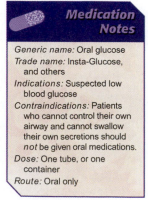

Medication Notes

Generic name: Oral glucose
Trade name: Insta-Glucose, and others
Indications: Suspected low blood glucose
Contraindications: Patients who cannot control their own airway and cannot swallow their own secretions should *not* be given oral medications.
Dose: One tube, or one container
Route: Oral only

- Information on universal access has been updated to the most recent statistics and innovations being made in the public's ability to access the EMS system through 9-1-1 calls and services.

Chapter 2

- Content related to certification and licensure has been expanded.

Chapter 3

- Discussions of the Health Insurance Portability and Accountability Act as well as the Emergency Medical Treatment and Active Labor Act have been added.

Chapter 4

- Discussion of debriefing after stressful incidents on the job has been completely revised and updated based upon the latest research in this area.

Chapter 5

- Content on homeostastis and the lymphatic system have been added.
- This chapter continues to provide the most comprehensive coverage of anatomy and physiology found in any EMT–Basic textbook.

Chapter 6

- Expanded coverage of the Ryan White Comprehensive AIDS Resource Emergency Act.
- This chapter continues to provide the most comprehensive coverage on infection control than any other EMT–Basic textbook.

Chapter 7

- Added content on the use of the cross-finger technique and properly checking the suction tubing prior to a call.

Chapter 8

- This chapter includes expanded coverage on assessing level of consciousness.
- Added content related to providing humidified oxygen.
- Added content on calculating the duration of time an oxygen tank will last.
- Added content on additional types of oxygenation devices such as the Venturi mask and the simple facemask.

Chapter 11

- Expanded content on back exercises that can be done to maintain back health.
- Added content related to moving obese patients.

Chapter 14

- Expanded discussion of when to call for ALS backup.

Chapter 18

- Added discussion of satellite phones.

Chapter 20

- Expanded discussion on uses of abbreviations and symbols when documenting.

The section on trauma care has been moved forward in the text at the request of our market reviewers. Many are teaching this content before the medical content. To accommodate those needs, we have reorganized these sections of the text.

Chapter 23

- Expanded content on signs of abdominal injury.

Chapter 24

- Added information regarding CHEMTREC.

Chapter 26

- Added discussion of the use of aspirin in patients experiencing an acute coronary event.
- Added discussion on the use of glucagos for patients experiencing an acute diabetic event.

Chapter 27

- Added discussion on delivering humidified oxygen in the management of the patient with croup.

Chapter 30

- Added discussion on hyperosmolar hyperglycemic non-ketonic coma.
- Added discussion on fingerstick glucose testing.

Chapter 31

- New chapter to this edition. This chapter deals specifically with the assessment and management of stroke patients.

Chapter 33

- New chapter to this edition. This chapter deals specifically with abdominal pain in the medical patient.

Chapter 41

- Expanded content related to dementia and delirium.
- Added content related to specific effects of trauma and specific medical disorders in the elderly.

Chapter 43

- Added content on the use of LED warning lights.

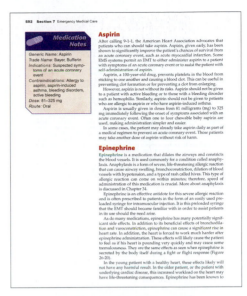

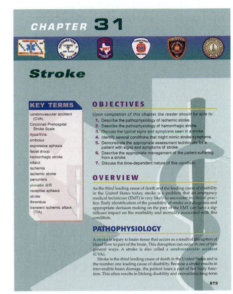

New chapter

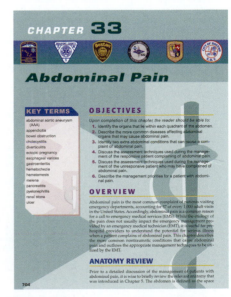

New chapter

INTERNET RESOURCES

For additional information related to chest pain and heart attack, visit these Web sites:

- American Heart Association, http://www.americanheart.org
- Chest Pain Perspectives, http://www.chestpainperspectives.com
- HeartInfo, http://www.heartinfo.org
- HeartPoint, http://www.heartpoint.com

Look for additional research at http://www.emedicine.com and MedLine Plus at http://medlineplus.gov.

Chapter 46

- New chapter to this edition. This chapter deals with the role EMS plays in response to terrorism.

Chapter 47

- New chapter to this edition. This chapter deals with the types of accidents and calls EMS responds to in rural farm areas.

Appendix A

- Added discussion of gastric distension.
- Added discussion of the combitube and laryngeal mask airway devices.

Appendix B

- New content on cardiopulmonary resuscitation has been added.

New Features in this Edition

- **EMS in Action** boxes throughout the text contain stories of actual EMS calls from people around the country. These stories help to apply the importance of what is being learned to what you may actually experience on a call.
- **Ask the Doc** boxes throughout the text highlight relevant information, research, and position papers from the National Association of EMS Physicians.
- **Internet Resources** at the end of chapters allow you to further your studies of specific topics and do some research on your own.
- **Revamped illustrations** provide a fresher look with more depth than illustrations presented in the first edition.

The *Fundamentals of Basic Emergency Care*, Second Edition, is a comprehensive textbook that provides the EMT student with the raw materials needed to form a foundation in EMS. But as medicine and technology change, so does EMS. The EMT student is encouraged to use the information in *Fundamentals of Basic Emergency Care*, Second Edition, in combination with other sources, especially your medical director and your EMS educator.

TO THE EDUCATOR

Have you ever stood on the sideline of an emergency call and watched your students? This can be an eye-opening experience. You may observe the following:

- Inability to think critically
- Inability to problem-solve
- Lack of ability to respond quickly when in a crisis situation

The authors, EMS providers with more than 45 years of street experience between them, noticed this trend among new EMTs and asked, "Why?"

The revision of the EMT-B curriculum to apply an assessment-based approach was certainly a step in the right direction. It narrowed the focus of an EMT's training, allowing educators more time to concentrate on fewer objectives instead of trying to touch on the entire universe of medicine. But something is still missing. The curriculum does not, and cannot, include two very important EMT skills—problem solving and critical thinking. Teaching EMT students these skills is not a function of the curriculum, it is a function of the instructional methodology.

Problem-Based Learning (PBL)

Problem-based learning (PBL) is an educational strategy. PBL involves giving a team of students a puzzling problem and asking the team to resolve the problem. The problem, structured within the context of a real-life scenario, forces students to refer to available resources for facts and to develop content knowledge in the process. Students must then develop a plan of action. This learning process leads to increased problem-solving abilities.

PBL is a student-centered educational strategy. Direct instruction by the educator is minimized. Instead, the student learns to become a self-directed learner, a role that will serve him or her for a lifetime. The educator assumes a role as coach, resource guide, and subject matter expert, not lecturer.

PBL takes advantage of many sources of information other than traditional scholastic materials. Students can refer to senior EMTs for direction, but not instruction, as they try to resolve the problem. These senior EMTs become mentors, as they share their similar experiences, or "war stories," with like problems. Students can also tap into the Internet for more "e-learning" about the problem.

PBL is about more than just accumulating facts to regurgitate at exam time; it is about learning how to learn. The student learns how to obtain information and apply it to an ill-structured problem and to produce a meaningful result. One of the wondrous discoveries often made by EMTs using PBL is that there is more than one approach to resolving a problem.

More information is available on PBL in the Electronic Classroom Manager that accompanies this text. There is also an abundance of information on PBL available on the Internet. Please take a moment to educate yourself about this novel approach to EMS education. Even a small effort at the end of EMT class to try "one problem" can produce remarkable results.

Sick Building

"Paramedic Engine 9, Ambulance 12, and Battalion Chief 2: respond to the Governors Motor Inn. Report of multiple sick persons. Caller claims no smoke, no fire. Time out 8:45 hours." Elisa had just completed the county's terrorism course and her interest was piqued when she heard the report of multiple sick persons. "Could this be a terrorist attack," she thought, "or another 'sick building' from poor ventilation like the last call that came out like this?"

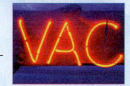

(Courtesy of Morguefile.)

- What information from the dispatch might suggest that this could be a terrorist attack?
- What would be the approach to the scene of a potential terrorist attack?
- What resources might be needed if this EMS call turns out to be a terrorist attack?

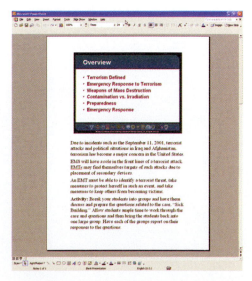

PowerPoint integrates problem-based learning strategies.

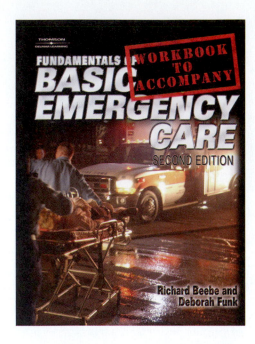

EXTENSIVE TEACHING AND LEARNING PACKAGE

The complete supplements package was developed to achieve two goals:

1. To assist students in learning the essential skills and information needed to secure a career in the area of EMS
2. To assist instructors in planning and implementing their programs for the most efficient use of time and other resources

Student Workbook

ISBN 1-4018-7934-9

An excellent resource to provide additional practice. The workbook includes the following:

- Review of key terms
- Exercises and activities to promote retention of chapter material and further enhance critical-thinking skills
- Skills review checklists
- Correlation to the 1994 National Standard Curriculum

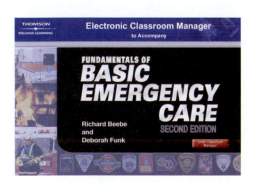

Electronic Classroom Manager

ISBN 1-4018-7936-5

The electronic classroom manager (ECM) helps you, the educator, facilitate student learning. For the educator interested in trying problem-based learning, case studies are provided and may be copied and distributed to the class or to assigned student teams, who are then encouraged to follow through the guiding questions.

Answers to the additional case studies' guiding questions are also provided. The educator is reminded that there may be more correct answers to a problem. However, how the students arrived at their answer is as important as the answer itself. The ECM is intended to be a starting point, not an authoritative source. Educators are encouraged to develop their own personalized problems, using the case studies provided as an example. EMS educators are also encouraged to carefully analyze the student-team responses compared to good EMS practice.

The ECM also includes the following:

- Instructor's Manual with lecture outlines, student outlines, answers to the text questions, additional case studies, skill checklists, a resource list, and student handouts; also available separately (ISBN 1-4018-7935-7)
- PowerPoint presentations correlated to the student outlines
- An image library to enhance the PowerPoint presentations or to create transparencies
- Correlation Guide to the 1994 National Standard Curriculum for the EMT–Basic
- Computerized test bank
- Conversion grids to our competitive texts to allow an easy transition from current product to ours

ADDITIONAL RESOURCES

WebTutor Advantage

Designed to complement *Fundamentals of Basic Emergency Care*, Second Edition, Thomson Delmar Learning WebTutor Advantage on WebCT is a content-rich, Web-based teaching and learning aid that reinforces and clarifies complex concepts and provides an electronic test bank. The WebCT platform also provides communications tools to instructors and students, including a source calendar, chat, e-mail, and threaded discussions.

Fundamentals of Basic Emergency Care, Second Edition, WebTutor Advantage stand-alone, on WebCT Platform
ISBN 1-4018-7937-3

Fundamentals of Basic Emergency Care, Second Edition, hardcover text and WebTutor Advantage bundle on WebCT Platform
ISBN 1-4180-0255-0

Fundamentals of Basic Emergency Care, Second Edition, WebTutor Advantage stand-alone on Blackboard Platform
ISBN 1-4018-7938-1

Fundamentals of Basic Emergency Care, Second Edition, hardcover text and WebTutor Advantage bundle, on Blackboard Platform
ISBN 1-4180-0254-2

Join us on the Web at http://ems.delmar.com.

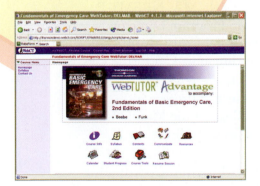

ACKNOWLEDGMENTS

The authors would like to sincerely thank the following individuals and organizations for their contributions to *Fundamentals of Basic Emergency Care*, Second Edition. Without their kind assistance, *Fundamentals of Basic Emergency Care*, Second Edition, would not have become a reality. Each of them can be proud of their contribution, and to the overall success of the book that will surely follow.

Reviewers

The honest input of the reviewers served two purposes for the authors. First, it reminded the authors of the diverse practice of EMS across the United States. Clearly, at times EMS is as much an art as it is a science. In every instance, the authors tried to incorporate their ideas and experiences when they did not violate medical research.

Second, the reviewers' comments periodically forced the authors to review their facts. For this reason, the authors can say we feel strongly that the information in *Fundamentals of Basic Emergency Care*, Second Edition, is factually correct and scientifically supported, in every instance possible, at the time of publication.

We, the authors, sincerely want to thank these reviewers for their time and effort.

Reviewers of the First Edition

Sandy Bagley, RN, EMT-P
    Amarillo College
    Amarillo, Texas

J. Alan Baker
    The Victoria College
    Victoria, Texas

Brenda Beasley, RN, BS, EMT-P
    Calhoun Community College
    Decatur, Alabama

Gloria Bizjak
    Maryland Fire and Rescue Institute
    Berwyn Heights, Maryland

Tom Chartier, EMT-I
    Western Iowa Technical Community College
    Moville, Iowa

Marilyn Collins, RN
    Citrus College
    Glendora, California

Timothy Cooper, EMT-P, IC
Lansing Community College
Lansing, Michigan

Terry Devito, RN, MEd, EMT-P, CEN
Capital Community Technical College
Enfield, Connecticut

Richard Ellis
United States Air Force
Sheppard Air Force Base, Texas

Donna Ferracone, RN, MA, BA
Crafton Hills College
Yocaipa, California

Louann Hall, BS, NREMT, EMS-I, EMT-P
University of Connecticut
Storrs, Connecticut

Rebecca Hill, LPN, Paramedic
DeKalb Technical Institute
Clarkston, Georgia

Tim Murphy
Carl Sandburg College
Galesburg, Illinois

M. Jane Pollock, EMT, CI
East Carolina University
Bethel, North Carolina

Gina Riggs
Kiamichi Technology Center
Poteau, Oklahoma

J. Penny Shutts
Oswego County Health Department
Oswego, New York

Thomas Strange Jr.
Walters State Community College
Morristown, Tennessee

Richard Webb
First Coast Technical Institute
St. Augustine, Florida

Reviewers of the Second Edition

Paul Arens, BS, PS
EMS Program Director
Kirkwood Community College
Cedar Rapids, Iowa

Bruce Bare, BA, EMT-P, PI
Paramedic Science AD Program Chair
Ivy Tech State College
Bloomington, Indiana

Ronald Bowser, MBA, EMT-B
Coordinator

Maryland Fire and Rescue Institute
University of Maryland
College Park, Maryland

Tom Chartier, EMT-I
EMS Instructor
Western Iowa Tech
Woodbury Central High School
Moville, Iowa

Peter Cunnius, MS, NREMT-P
Education Consultant
Drexel University
Philadelphia, Pennsylvania

Ken Davis, NR/CCEMT-P, FP-CI/C
Paramedic Coordinator
Eastern New Mexico University
Roswell, New Mexico

Elaine Dethlefsen, RN, BSN
EMT Program Director
Santa Ana College
Costa Mesa, California

Terry DeVito, RN, EMT-P, MEd, EMS-I
Coordinator
Capital Community College
Hartford, Connecticut

Richard Ellis, SMSgt
Superintendent, Health Services Individual
Reserve Programs
United States Air Force
Denver, Colorado

Lynda Goerish, MA, NREMT-P
EMT Coordinator/Instructor
Century College
White Bear Lake, Minnesota

Arthur Hsieh, MA, NREMT-P
EMS Program Director
Hospital Consortium Education Network
Burlingame, California

Kristine Kern, AAS, LP
Assistant Professor
College of the Mainland
Texas City, Texas

Gregory LaMay, BS, NREMT-P
EMS Program Coordinator
Madison Area Technical College
Reedsburg, Wisconsin

Jeff McDonald LP, NREMT-P
Coordinator, EMS Program
Tarrant County College
Fort Worth, Texas

Jamie Nelson, NREMT-B, CMA
EMS Instructor
Hennepin Technical College
Hopkins, Minnesota

Brian Pio, EMT-P
Prehospital Education Coordinator
Cincinnati Children's Hospital Medical Center
Cincinnati, Ohio

Stephen Smith, MBA, LP
Associate Professor—Health Science
Tarrant County College
Fort Worth, Texas

Debra Southerland, LP
EMS Program Director
Central Texas College
Killeen, Texas

Mark A. Tuttle, EMT-P, CIC
North County Regional EMS Director
State University of New York
Canton, New York

Sandy Waggoner EMT-P, FF, EMSI
Public Safety Coordinator
EHOVE Ghrist Adult Career Center
Milan, Ohio

Kathryn Zepeda, EMT, LP
EMS Degree Program Coordinator
San Antonio College
San Antonio, Texas

Photo Acknowledgments

The authors would like to thank the following organizations and individuals for their support and assistance in the production of *Fundamentals of Basic Emergency Care*, Second Edition.

Organizations

Albany Medical Center Hospital
Department of Emergency Medicine
Albany, New York
Dr. Mara McErlean, Chair

Albany MedFLIGHT
Albany, New York
Dean Dow, RN, Program Director

Bassett Healthcare
Center for Rural EMS Education
Cooperstown, New York
Scott Bonderoff, Administrative Director

Shalom Nursery School
Karen Ekstein, Director

Guilderland Police Department
Guilderland, New York
James Murley, Chief of Police

Guilderland Emergency Medical Services
Guilderland, New York
Thomas Deleon, EMT Director

Watervliet Fire Department
Watervliet, New York
Brian Carroll, Fire Chief

Western Turnpike Rescue Squad
Albany, New York
Scott Bowman, EMT-P, Chief

Individuals

Dr. Michael Dailey, FACEP
Albany Medical Center

Michael Galletelli
Metroland Photo, Inc.
Albany, New York

Geraldine Oakley

Dr. Kevin Reilly, FACEP
Albany Medical Center

David J. Reimer Sr.
Emergency Services Photography
Kutztown, Pennsylvania

Darcy Scelsi

Dr. Ronald Stram, FACEP
Albany Medical Center

Dr. Wayne Triner, FACEP
Albany Medical Center

Technical Advisors

The authors would like to thank the technical advisors for their perseverance and determination to "get the job done." Their valuable contributions to the quality and accuracy of the photographs are clearly evident throughout the book.

Brian Booth, NREMT-P

Western Turnpike Rescue Squad
Albany, New York

Geoff Ekstein, BA, CC-NREMT-P
Guilderland Emergency Medical Services
Guilderland, New York

Thomson Delmar Learning

The authors would also like to extend our sincere appreciation to the entire staff at Thomson Delmar Learning. While the list of individuals at Thomson Delmar Learning who helped this book become a reality is long and distinguished, there are a few individuals that we would like to single out for special recognition.

We would like to first thank Dawn Gerrain, vice president of career education. Dawn saw our vision and agreed to help us achieve our dream, an EMT textbook that was written for the street EMT by a pair of old EMS providers. We would also like to thank Darcy Scelsi, who made our dream into a reality and who has worked tirelessly to see this project completed. We would also like to thank Maureen Rosener, our acquisitions editor, who has been the spark plug, keeping the engine firing on all pistons and running smoothly.

How to Use This Book

OBJECTIVES

Objectives mirror those objectives in the 1994 Department of Transportation EMT–Basic Curriculum. This is the essential knowledge that you must gain upon reading the chapter. Key Terms allow you to become familiar with medical language as well as be able to translate the medical terms into language that your patients will be able to understand.

CASE STUDIES

Real-life case scenarios allow you to problem solve a patient encounter that you may be faced with in the field. The guiding questions prompt you to consider important aspects of the encounter. These case studies will allow you to take what you learn and apply it to the streets, aiding in bridging the gap from student to practitioner.

SKILLS

Pictorial step-by-step skills allow you to see the proper methods used to perform the essential functions of your profession. Use these as a guide to practicing the skills in a lab along with the assessment checklist in your workbook.

Street Smart features allow students to benefit from the authors' years of field experience. It provides insight into handling various situations on scene as well as care of the patient. Safety Tips emphasize the importance of safety on the job and describe methods to maintain safe care of oneself and one's patients.

Highlighted boxed features throughout the reading call your attention to special circumstances to heighten your awareness of special populations, cultural differences, and tips from the professionals.

PEDIATRIC CONSIDERATIONS

Pediatric Considerations highlight areas of special significance to young patients. It brings the student's attention to the variations in presentation, care and management of the pediatric patient.

GERIATRIC CONSIDERATIONS

Geriatric Considerations highlight areas of special significance to elderly patients. It brings the student's attention to the variations in presentation, care and management of the elderly patient.

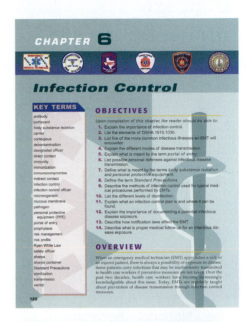

CHAPTER 6

Infection Control

KEY TERMS
antibody
biohazard
body substance isolation
carrier
contagious
decontamination
designated officer
direct contact
immunity
immunization
immunocompromise
indirect contact
infection control
infection control officer
microorganism
mucous membrane
pathogen
personal protective equipment (PPE)
portal of entry
prophylaxis
risk management
risk profile
Ryan White Law
safety officer
sharps
sharps container
Standard Precautions
sterilization
transmission
vector

OBJECTIVES
Upon completion of this chapter, the reader should be able to:
1. Explain the importance of infection control.
2. List the elements of OSHA 1910.1030.
3. List five of the more common infectious illnesses an EMT will encounter.
4. Explain the different modes of disease transmission.
5. Explain what is meant by the term portal of entry.
6. List possible personal defenses against infectious disease transmission.
7. Define what is meant by the terms body substance isolation and personal protective equipment.
8. Define the term Standard Precautions.
9. Describe the methods of infection control used for typical medical procedures performed by EMTs.
10. List the different levels of disinfection.
11. Explain what an infection control plan is and where it can be found.
12. Explain the importance of documenting a potential infectious disease exposure.
13. Describe how notification laws affect the EMT.
14. Describe what is proper medical follow-up for an infectious disease exposure.

OVERVIEW
When an emergency medical technician (EMT) approaches a sick or an injured patient, there is always a possibility of exposure to disease. Some patients carry infections that may be inadvertently transmitted to health care workers if preventive measures are not taken. Over the past two decades, health care workers have become increasingly knowledgeable about this issue. Today, EMTs are regularly taught about prevention of disease transmission through infection control measures.

122

✳ Withdrawal

The war monument was a favorite hangout for the local street alcoholics and a frequent place for EMS calls. Tonight was no different. Joel was usually unkempt, but he normally was not disagreeable. Joel was what people call a "nice drunk."

Today, he was arguing with everybody and telling them all, "I can kick it. I don't need no help from nobody." But he confided in a friend that he did need some help, and that's how EMS appeared at the old war monument.

(Courtesy of PhotoDisc.)

Approaching the scene, careful not to step on the wine bottles strewn about the ground, EMTs Campion and Hilts knelt down and asked Joel what was wrong. Joel reluctantly spoke up and said, "I've got the shakes, man. Can you help me out?"

- What signs and symptoms of substance abuse are evident?
- What past medical history might be important?
- What would be the EMTs' treatment priorities in this case?

SKILL 6-1 Hand Washing

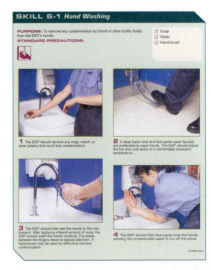

PURPOSE: To remove any contamination by blood or other bodily fluids from the EMT's hands.
STANDARD PRECAUTIONS:
☑ Soap
☑ Water
☑ Hand brush

1 The EMT should remove any rings, watch, or other jewelry that could trap contamination.

2 A deep basin sink and foot-pedal water faucets are preferable to wash hands. The EMT should adjust the hot and cold water to a comfortable lukewarm temperature.

3 The EMT should then wet the hands to the mid-forearm. After applying a liberal amount of soap, the EMT should wash the hands carefully. The area between the fingers deserves special attention. A hand brush may be used for difficult-to-remove contamination.

4 The EMT should then thoroughly rinse the hands, allowing the contaminated water to run off the elbow.

(continued)

CULTURAL CONSIDERATIONS

Cultural Considerations share manners, ways of providing care, communication, and relationships of various cultural and ethnic groups you may encounter in your area of practice.

MEDICATION NOTES

Medication Notes highlight commonly seen and used medications in the field. These are the medications of which the EMT must understand the use and actions.

EMS IN ACTION

These stories from EMS professionals around the country help bridge the gap between book learning and the events that occur on an actual EMS call. This feature highlights how the important concepts found in the book can be applied to the real world.

ASK THE DOC

Ask the Doc boxes highlight information from the National Association of EMS Physicians. These note position papers and research being conducted in the field on emergency services.

INTERNET RESOURCES

At the end of each chapter is a list of Internet resources with some suggestions for searches to perform. This will help you take your education to the next level and allow you to spend some time researching topics on your own. Please share information of interest to others in your class.

How to Use the StudyWare CD-ROM

The StudyWare™ software helps you learn concepts discussed in *Fundamentals of Basic Emergency Care*, Second Edition. As you study each chapter in the text, be sure to explore the activities in the corresponding chapter in the software. CD icons within the text indicate that there is related content on the software. Use StudyWare™ as your own private tutor to help you learn the material in your text.

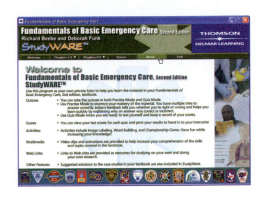

Getting started is easy. Install the software by inserting the CD and following the on-screen instructions. Enter your first and last names so the software can store your quiz results. Then choose a chapter from the menu and take a quiz or explore one of the activities.

Menus. You can access the menus from wherever you are in the program. The menus include Quizzes, Activities, Multimedia, Weblinks, Answers to Cases, and Scores.

Quizzes. Quizzes include multiple choice, true-false, fill-in, and word-building questions. You can take the quizzes in both Practice Mode and Quiz Mode. Use Practice Mode to improve your mastery of the material. You have multiple tries to get the answers correct. Instant feedback tells you whether you're right or wrong and helps you learn quickly by explaining why an answer was correct or incorrect. Use Quiz Mode when you are ready to test yourself and keep a record of your scores. In Quiz Mode, you have one try to get the answers right, but you can take each quiz as many times as you want.

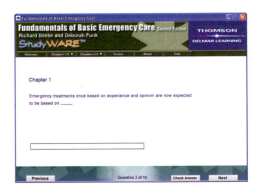

Scores. You can view your last scores for each quiz and print your results to hand to your instructor.

Activities. Activities include image labeling and a "Jeopardy" style championship game. Have fun while increasing your knowledge!

Multimedia. Multimedia consists of animations and video clips related to content you have studied in the text. The animations help you visualize concepts related to physiology and skill practice. The video clips allow you to see skills performed in real-life scenarios.

Weblinks. Weblinks are provided for you to research topics on your own and give you resources for additional information on topics covered in each chapter.

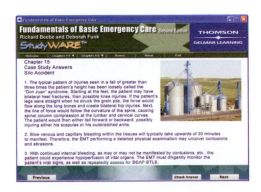

Answers to Cases. Throughout the chapters in your book, cases are presented to help you fine-tune your critical-thinking and problem-solving skills. Possible solutions to the cases can be found here. We encourage you to work on the cases and come up with your own solutions before looking at the potential solutions on the CD. Please also be aware that there is no one right or wrong answer to these cases. Your solution may be valid even if it doesn't match the solution provided. Share your solutions with your instructor and classmates to explore all of the possible answers that may be valid.

FUNDAMENTALS OF
BASIC
EMERGENCY
CARE

SECOND EDITION

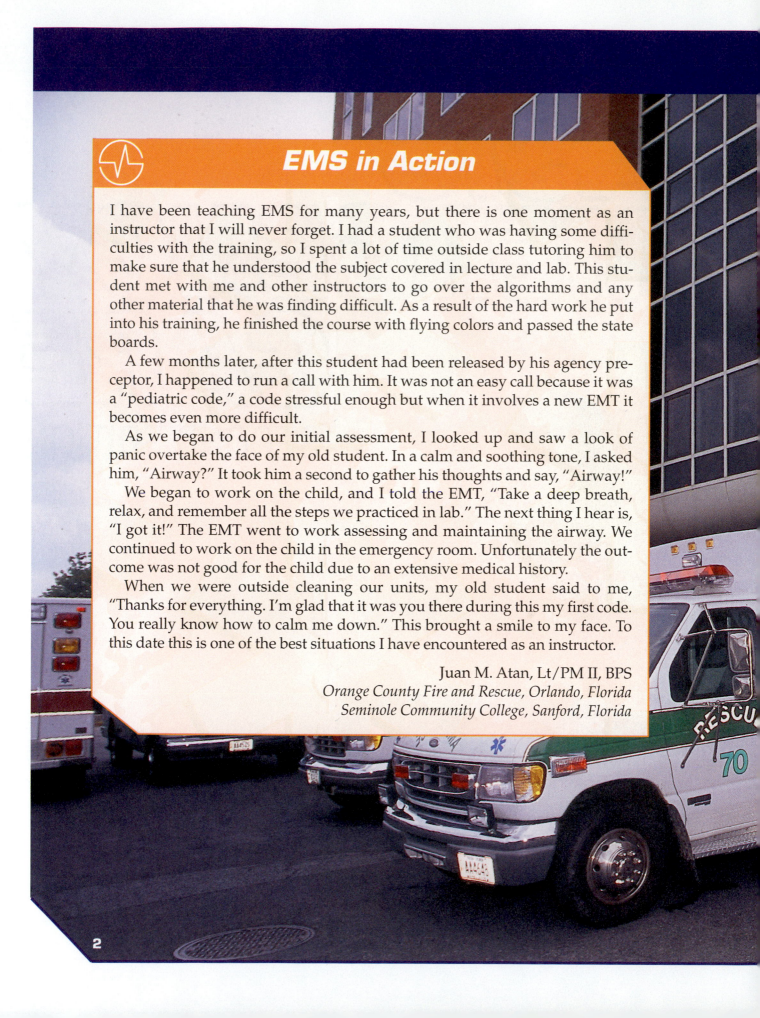

EMS in Action

I have been teaching EMS for many years, but there is one moment as an instructor that I will never forget. I had a student who was having some difficulties with the training, so I spent a lot of time outside class tutoring him to make sure that he understood the subject covered in lecture and lab. This student met with me and other instructors to go over the algorithms and any other material that he was finding difficult. As a result of the hard work he put into his training, he finished the course with flying colors and passed the state boards.

A few months later, after this student had been released by his agency preceptor, I happened to run a call with him. It was not an easy call because it was a "pediatric code," a code stressful enough but when it involves a new EMT it becomes even more difficult.

As we began to do our initial assessment, I looked up and saw a look of panic overtake the face of my old student. In a calm and soothing tone, I asked him, "Airway?" It took him a second to gather his thoughts and say, "Airway!"

We began to work on the child, and I told the EMT, "Take a deep breath, relax, and remember all the steps we practiced in lab." The next thing I hear is, "I got it!" The EMT went to work assessing and maintaining the airway. We continued to work on the child in the emergency room. Unfortunately the outcome was not good for the child due to an extensive medical history.

When we were outside cleaning our units, my old student said to me, "Thanks for everything. I'm glad that it was you there during this my first code. You really know how to calm me down." This brought a smile to my face. To this date this is one of the best situations I have encountered as an instructor.

Juan M. Atan, Lt/PM II, BPS
Orange County Fire and Rescue, Orlando, Florida
Seminole Community College, Sanford, Florida

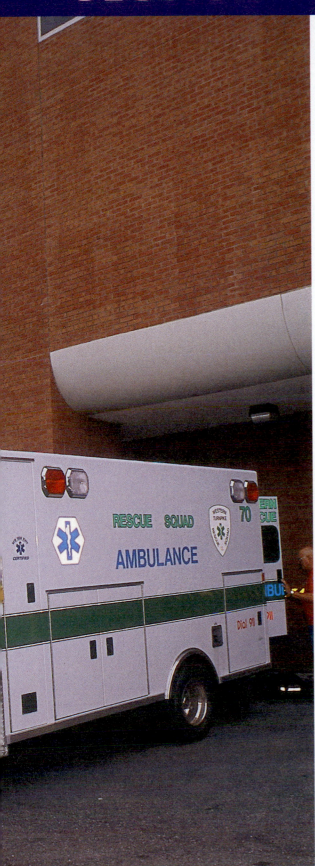

SECTION 1

Emergency Medical Services

Emergency medical services (EMS) has grown from modest beginnings to become one of the fastest growing allied health care professions, and emergency medical technicians (EMTs) are the foundation of that profession.

In many cases, EMTs are the public's first contact with the health care system, and, as a part of the health care team, the EMT is expected to deliver high-quality medical care from the scene, through transport, and until the patient is delivered to the emergency department of the hospital.

This section is an introduction to emergency medicine, as a specialty of medicine; to emergency medical service, as a profession; and to the roles and responsibilities of an EMT.

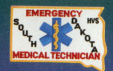

CHAPTER 1

Introduction to Emergency Medical Services

KEY TERMS

9-1-1

ambulances volante

American Ambulance
Association (AAA)

American Red Cross

cardiopulmonary resuscitation
(CPR)

chain of survival

continuous quality
improvement (CQI)

emergency dispatcher

emergency medical dispatch
(EMD)

emergency medical services
(EMS)

Emergency Medical
Technician–Basic (EMT-B)

Emergency Medical
Technician–Intermediate
(EMT-I)

Emergency Medical
Technician–Paramedic
(EMT-P)

emergency physician

first responder

Good Samaritan

International Association of
Fire Fighters (IAFF)

(continues)

OBJECTIVES

Upon completion of this chapter, the reader should be able to:

1. Describe the impact of historical events upon the evolution of EMS.
2. Describe the evolution of emergency health care.
3. Describe the place of modern EMS in the health care system.
4. List key scientific and position papers that directly influenced EMS systems development.
5. Compare the role of the EMT of the 1960s with that of the modern EMT.
6. Identify some organizations that have influenced EMS.
7. List two major professional EMS associations.
8. List the four elements of a good EMS system, as defined by the National Highway Traffic Safety Administration.
9. Compare the evolution of emergency medicine and EMS.
10. Discuss the professional challenges that face the EMT of the future.

OVERVIEW

Welcome to **emergency medical services (EMS)**, a coordinated network of professionals whose function is to provide a variety of medical services to people in need of emergency care (Figure 1-1). You are the newest addition to a long line of proud EMS providers. Although modern EMS has been in existence for only about 35 years, it has grown tremendously since its inception. Many people from across the country and from all walks of life have chosen to become a part of this team.

Historically, EMS can find its roots in the lifesaving missions of fire departments. However, changes in modern health care have transformed EMS providers from "life savers" to the health care system's "medical safety net." As we explore the history of EMS, we will see how changes over time have shaped the system of today.

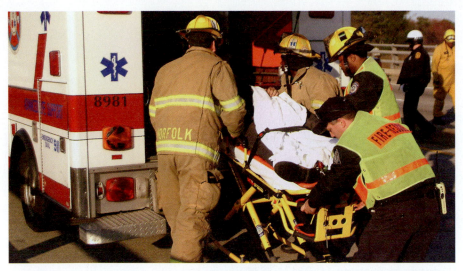

FIGURE 1-1 As part of the public safety team, the emergency medical technician provides care to patients on the scene. (Courtesy of Tod F. Parker/Ayrow Studios.)

KEY TERMS

(continued)

National Association of Emergency Medical Technicians (NAEMT)

National Highway Traffic Safety Administration (NHTSA)

National Registry of EMTs (NREMT)

public safety access point (PSAP)

Star of Life

trauma center

white paper

THE HISTORY OF EMERGENCY MEDICAL SERVICES

In the tradition of the **Good Samaritan**, that ancient wanderer who stopped to help an injured traveler on the roadside, EMS provides aid to the sick and injured, whether the patients are on the streets or in their home, and delivers them to definitive care.

First aid, as a concept, may have been developed by the Roman military who selected soldiers, medical orderlies bearing the title *miles medicus*, to tend to the wounded and excused them from duties, even during combat. As time progressed into the Dark Ages various religious groups, called *apostolic orders*, had members who were active in healing the sick, and generally served their people's needs. That tradition of caring and healing is still carried on today by such religious orders as the Sisters of Mercy.

In many cases emergency medical care grew out of necessity. If drowning was a problem, as it was in was in many seaports, then procedures such as barrel-rolling, rolling the drowning victim over a barrel, would be developed to try to correct the problem. In some cases groups, such as the Royal Society for the Resuscitation of the Apparently Dead, were formed to advance science and to teach others approved lifesaving techniques. This tradition is still continued today by such volunteer organizations as the Red Cross.

The Military and Emergency Medical Services

Historically, no other group had a greater need for methods to care for the ill and injured outside the hospital setting than the military. More deaths resulted from illness, disease, and poor wound care than from combat on the battlefield. Many of the advances made in EMS can be directly related to progress made in military medicine.

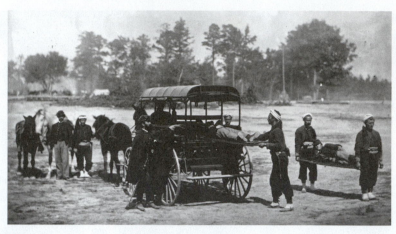

FIGURE 1-2   The Civil War brought about the first use of ambulances in the United States. (Courtesy of the Library of Congress, Selected Civil War Photographs, photo no. LC-B8171-7636.)

The Napoleonic Wars

During the Napoleonic Wars, a French surgeon named Baron Dominique Jean Larrey advanced the concept of the *ambulances volante*, the "flying ambulances." These covered wagons would pick up the wounded on the battlefield and bring them to the army surgeons. These were essentially the first ambulances.

The ideas embodied in that concept live on today. The aim is to quickly send trained personnel to the injured person, treat any life-threatening problems immediately, and transport the person to the nearest appropriate hospital as soon as possible.

The U.S. Civil War

During the Battle of Bull Run, wounded soldiers came into makeshift field hospitals so quickly that surgeons did not have time to wipe the blood off the saws they were using to amputate limbs. Streams of blood ran from under the tent flaps, and soldiers seeing a surgeon coming would draw their pistol to save their limbs from being amputated.

After the chaos that occurred at the Battle of Bull Run, U.S. army surgeons realized that something had to be done to more efficiently treat the large numbers of wounded. Dr. Jonathan Lettermen, under the authority of General McClellan, organized a system of ambulances (similar to Baron Larrey's) to serve the army. The ambulances were specially equipped wagons that were reserved for the treatment and transportation of the wounded (Figure 1-2).

Clara Barton (Figure 1-3), founder of the **American Red Cross** (an organization that trains civilians in first aid and cardiopulmonary resuscitation), aided the wounded in the Civil War and advocated that treatment should begin in the field. The central tenet of her nursing philosophy was to "treat them where they lie." This concept has continued into modern EMS.

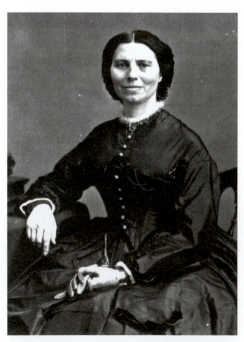

FIGURE 1-3   Clara Barton's motto was "treat them where they lie." Clara Barton treated wounded soldiers in the field during the Civil War. (Courtesy of the National Archives, photo no. 111-B-4246, Brady Collection.)

The World Wars

The two world wars brought about dramatic changes in the care of the wounded. Machine guns, tanks, aerial bombardment, and weapons of mass destruction, including poisonous gases and nuclear bombs, made the efficient care of the wounded more critical than it had ever been.

Soldiers were trained as "first responders," and the combat medic came into being. Systems for trauma care were established that included field hospitals and forward aid stations. The military used ambulances with the characteristic Red Cross emblem on the side, and the era of the "ambulance driver" had arrived.

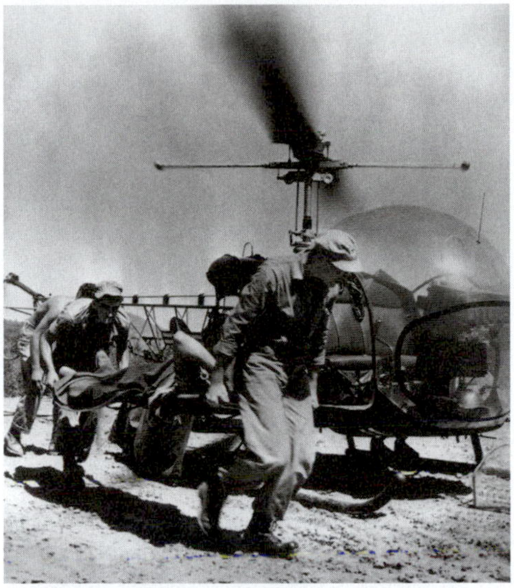

The Korean War

Emergency medical care continued to improve during the Korean War. A significant development was the transportation of wounded soldiers by helicopter to medical units (Figure 1-4). The use of a helicopter for medical evacuation of soldiers in the Korean War was the genesis of modern aeromedical transportation.

The Vietnam War

The use of helicopters for medical transport continued in the Vietnam War. The HU-1, nicknamed the Huey, had a large patient compartment to allow emergency medical care to begin while in flight. Combat field medics were also more highly trained than their predecessors had been, resulting in the lowest rate of combat mortality in U.S. Army history.

The Civilian World

While great strides were being made in field care of wounded soldiers, the civilian sector was lagging far behind. Ambulances used solely for the transport of the sick and injured were rare. In 1966, more than 50% of the ambulances in the United States were owned and operated by morticians. Hearses provided the primary mode of transportation to the hospital simply because they were the only vehicles suited for horizontal transportation.

As veterans returned from war, many became police officers. In the course of their duties, those who were combat-trained medics often put their medical expertise to use. Although sorely needed, the provision of advanced medical care by nonphysicians was fairly new in the United States at the time, but the practices of the veteran medics quickly spread as civilians joined veterans by learning some of the lifesaving techniques that were most useful in the civilian world.

Many rescue squads grew out of existing fire departments; others were independent organizations, such as the Roanoke Life Saving and First Aid Squad (Figure 1-5). This pioneer group, organized in 1928 by Julian Stanley Wise, was the first volunteer rescue squad in the United States. Despite the formation of new emergency squads, training was often poor and equipment scarce.

The American Red Cross

The American Red Cross, whose mission has always been to provide aid to the public, took the lead in providing basic medical training to those who expressed interest. Classes such as Standard and Advanced First Aid quickly became the standard of care for rescue squad members.

FIGURE 1-4 The Korean War saw the advent of aeromedical evacuation. (Courtesy of Bell Helicopter Textron Inc., Fort Worth, TX.)

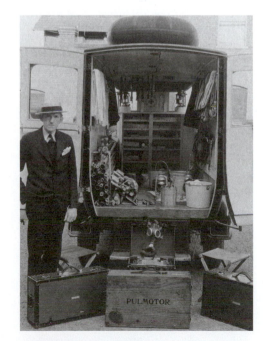

FIGURE 1-5 The Roanoke Life Saving and First Aid Squad was the first volunteer rescue squad in America. (Courtesy of the Julian Stanley Wise Foundation.)

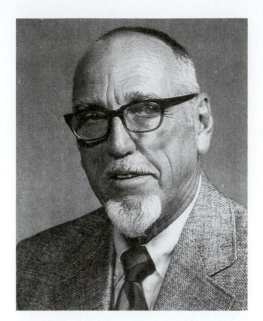

FIGURE 1-6 Dr. J. D. "Deke" Farrington is acknowledged as the father of modern EMS. (From McSwain, N., White, R., Paturas, J., and Metcalf, W. [1997]. *The Basic EMT: Comprehensive prehospital patient care.* St. Louis, MO: Mosby Yearbook.)

In the late 1950s and early 1960s, **cardiopulmonary resuscitation (CPR)** was taught to civilians for the first time. This life-preserving technique involves chest compressions and artificial respiration and can be taught to civilians as well as health care providers. Along with this movement, a large number of civilian ambulances or rescue squads were started.

The Father of EMS

Dr. Joseph D. "Deke" Farrington was particularly concerned about the lack of organized training in prehospital emergency medicine (Figure 1-6). In 1958, he started training the Chicago Fire Department in what was to become the prototype of the EMT-Ambulance course.

Dr. Farrington also took his dilemma to the press. In a 1966 article called "Death in the Ditch," he exposed the poor state of prehospital emergency care at the time.

In 1966, the National Academy of Sciences produced a landmark document titled "Accidental Death and Disability: The Neglected Disease of Modern Society." This **white paper**, an article written by experts for President Kennedy, laid the groundwork for inclusion of EMS in legislation.

The National Highway Safety Act of 1966 encouraged states to begin organized EMS programs. The National Highway Safety Administration (later called the **National Highway Traffic Safety Administration [NHTSA]**), a branch of the U.S. Department of Transportation, was assigned the task of developing standardized training and equipment requirements for EMS.

In 1973, the U.S. Congress passed the Emergency Medical Services System Act, which identified 15 essential components of an EMS system, listed in Table 1-1. In addition, this important legislation allocated federal funding for individual EMS regions to address these components.

Unfortunately, by the late 1970s and early 1980s, federal funding had became more scarce, and many of the newly established EMS regions fell victim to the economy and political bureaucracy of the time. Many EMS programs were relegated to local public safety agencies; others were taken over by private industry. Today, many different models of EMS organizations can be found throughout the country.

Star of Life

In 1973, the **Star of Life** (Figure 1-7) was adopted as the national EMS symbol. Each of its six points represents an aspect of the complete EMS system: detection, reporting, response, on-scene care, care in transit, and transfer to definitive care. The central staff with a serpent wrapped around it represents medicine and healing.

The National Association of Emergency Medical Technicians

As EMS grew and EMTs started to practice emergency medical care, it became apparent that they would need a strong voice to represent them. The fire service had several high-profile national associations,

Detection

Transfer to definitive care

Reporting

Care in transit

Response

On–scene care

FIGURE 1-7 The Star of Life is the national symbol for emergency medical services.

TABLE 1-1

The Elements of an Emergency Medical Services System (EMSS)

1.	Personnel	An adequate number of personnel will be available to respond to calls.
2.	Training	All personnel within the system will be trained at the approptiate level to provide care.
3.	Communications	Ensures that people are able to contact the EMS system and that the appropriate personnel within the system can be called to respond.
4.	Transportation	Appropriate means of transportation can be initiated and called for.
5.	Emergency facilities	Appropriate facilities (emergency and trauma care centers) are available when needed.
6.	Critical care units	Available upon stabilization of the patient for further treatment and care.
7.	Public safety agencies	Cooperation with police and fire departments is critical to the success of the EMS system.
8.	Consumer participation	Working with members of the community helps to meet its needs.
9.	Access to care	Care is provided regardless of the patient's ability to pay.
10.	Patient transfer	If further care is needed after the emergent situation, transfer to rehabilitation or long-term care services is available.
11.	Standardized record keeping	Records from both EMS personnel and the trauma or emergency care centers personnel help to identify needs within the system.
12.	Public information and education	The community needs to know the services that are offered and how to access those services in order for the EMS system to be effective.
13.	System review and evaluation	The system will evaluate and review its operations and work and make adjustments that are necessary to best meet the needs of the community.
14.	Disaster management	The system must be prepared to respond to incidents no matter how great or small.
15.	Mutual aid agreements	The ability to share resources with public and private agencies to meet the needs of the community ensures that the system runs most efficiently.

including the International Association of Fire Chiefs and the International Association of Fire Fighters, to speak on fire-related issues. The **National Association of Emergency Medical Technicians (NAEMT)** was formed in 1975 to meet the needs of all EMTs nationally. This organization continues today to represent EMTs to the public and in the government.

In 1988, the Technical Assistance Program (TAP) of the NHTSA published a list of the elements of a good EMS system: training, communication, trauma systems, and transportation. National standards based upon these elements were established. These standards were crucial in the formation of the current concept of an EMS system.

The Voices of EMS

While the NAEMT is the voice of the EMT, other sectors have developed to represent their constituents' concerns. Perhaps one of the largest groups that speaks on behalf of ambulance service owners is the **American Ambulance Association (AAA)**. The AAA represents the interests of the ambulance service industry; its members provide EMS to 95% of America's urban centers. The AAA is regularly involved in legislature affecting EMS.

More recently the **International Association of Fire Fighters (IAFF)** has lent its voice to EMS. It has been estimated that some 80% of EMS is provided by the fire service. The IAFF, as one of the largest groups representing firefighters, has taken an active role in EMS legislation as well as in community service and is leading EMS in many areas, including emergency response to terrorism, urban search and rescue, and critical incident management.

The **National Registry of EMTs (NREMT)** also speaks loudly for EMS. Through its advocacy and participation in EMS development, witness the EMS blueprint and the EMS agenda for the future, two seminal EMS publications, and its leadership, the NREMT has helped EMS to change the direction of EMS as a system.

Public Perception of EMS

Although EMS had grown rapidly, the public was still largely unaware of its existence or function. That was about to change. Television producer Jack Webb approached a local Los Angeles firefighter named Jim Page and asked for technical assistance in developing a television program called *Emergency*. In the 1970s, firefighter-paramedics John and Roy entered the living rooms of Americans across the country with stories of dramatic rescues and heroism. This television program probably did more to shape the public perception of EMS than anything that had been done before or since.

The impact was dramatic. Victims suddenly became patients, and ambulance drivers were recognized as EMTs and paramedics. Perhaps more important, EMTs were no longer seen as merely giving first aid; instead, they were believed to be capable of providing expert medical care on the scene of an accident.

MODERN EMS

In a modern EMS system, the EMT must appreciate that both the prehospital and hospital care are important parts of a continuum of care. Prehospital care is the first leg of a long journey from illness or injury to recovery and health. As on any journey, a mistake or a misstep made at the beginning costs time, money, and hardship later.

The American Heart Association speaks of the **chain of survival** (Figure 1-8). Although developed to describe the integral nature of the steps necessary to improve the outcome from cardiac arrest, this concept applies as well to all of EMS. Each segment of an EMS system is dependent on a preceding segment and affects the segment that follows it.

Early access to the emergency system is crucial to improving the outcome of time-critical illnesses. In the case of cardiac arrest, early CPR can improve the chance of survival. The sooner defibrillation is performed, the better the outcome is likely to be. Finally, advanced

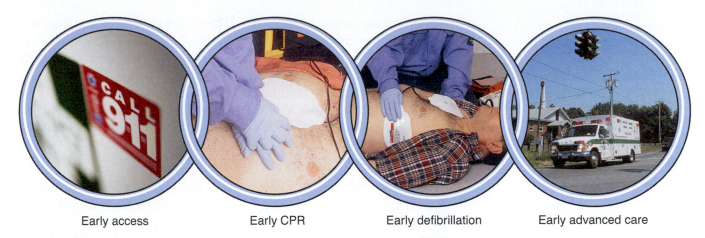

Early access   Early CPR   Early defibrillation   Early advanced care

FIGURE 1-8   The chain of survival illustrates the required interaction between different aspects of the EMS system. (From the American Heart Association.)

care, such as intubation and intravenous medications, should be delivered as soon as possible.

Universal Access

In the past, it was standard across the country to use a seven-digit number to access emergency medical care, police, or fire assistance. Each community had different emergency access numbers, so it was difficult for travelers to obtain help quickly. Even members of the community, who had to find the appropriate number in the phone book, suffered delays because of this system.

The idea of a three-digit universal access number for emergency services was initiated in 1968 by AT&T. Since then, communities across the United States have adopted **9-1-1**. It was hoped that an easily remembered three-digit number (9-1-1) would remedy the problem of difficulty accessing emergency medical services quickly. Today, many 9-1-1 dispatch centers have enhanced capabilities to determine the exact location of the caller through the use of a computerized system that identifies the location of the telephone used to place the phone call. In addition, this computer-aided dispatch (CAD) system identifies the police, fire, and medical units closest to the location. This enhanced 9-1-1 system makes it possible to dispatch emergency response units rapidly and accurately.

The National Emergency Number Association (NENA) reports that, on average, approximately 200 million calls are made a year to a **public safety access point (PSAP)** by citizens using 9-1-1. Answering those calls are call takers in approximately 6,121 primary and secondary regional PSAPs throughout the United States. These regional PSAPs provide 9-1-1 coverage to over 99% of the American population and 96% of the United States landmass. Presently, 9-1-1 service is being expanded to include cellular telephones, using global positioning satellite (GPS) technology to exactly pinpoint the location of the caller.

Emergency Dispatchers

Answering the 9-1-1 call at the PSAP is the **emergency dispatcher**, in some places called the *communication specialist* (COMSPEC) or the *medical communicator* (MEDCOM). These dispatchers would take down the caller information while alerting emergency services such as fire, police, and emergency medical services. Many PSAPs try to have their dispatchers answer the 9-1-1 call within 30 seconds in over 95% of the time and to dispatch appropriate first responding emergency units within 90 seconds from the time the call was received, in accordance with the National Fire Protection Association (NFPA) standards.

Emergency Medical Dispatch

In the past, well-meaning dispatchers would give simple instructions to the injured or ill or to family members waiting for the wail of a distant siren. They would advise the family to turn on the porch light or to roll the unconscious patient onto his or her side. Having a dispatcher give more-extensive instructions to a caller had not yet become routine.

One night in 1976, a paramedic was in the alarm room in Phoenix, Arizona, when a call came in for an infant who was not breathing. The dispatcher, aided by the paramedic, gave the family instructions over the telephone to care for the child until the emergency medical personnel arrived. The baby survived, and EMS saw the birth of **emergency medical dispatch (EMD)**.

EMDs are trained to provide specific medical care instructions to callers while emergency crews respond. These instructions can range from how to control bleeding from a wound to how to deliver a baby to how to perform CPR. Thanks to the pioneering work of Dr. Jeff Clawson of Utah, medical expertise was added to the abilities of the dispatchers. Using these techniques, trained communications specialists will question the caller and give lifesaving instructions while sending the closest and most appropriate aid units to the scene (Figure 1-9), making them the "first first responders."

The practice of evaluating the nature of the illness or injury and assigning it a priority based on strict protocols is an important part of modern dispatch procedures. This practice allows the most appropriate use of sometimes-limited resources within an EMS system. In addition, the type of response by the units assigned to the scene can be prioritized. For example, red lights on the vehicles and sirens are used for only the most serious emergencies. EMD is rapidly becoming the standard of care in EMS and the majority of PSAP (9-1-1) use EMD also.

First Responders

In almost every medical emergency, there is someone standing nearby who could provide assistance. With proper training, these people might have a significant impact on the outcome of an injury or illness. This fact was capitalized upon when the American Red Cross (ARC) and the American Heart Association (AHA) began their programs for training citizens in CPR and first aid.

The first person who arrives at the scene of an injury or illness can be referred to as a **first responder** (FR). Often, first responders were police officers, security guards, or members of the fire department—citizens whose duty it was to help. The classes offered by the ARC and

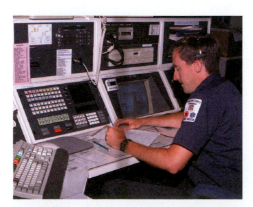

FIGURE 1-9 The communications specialist has a complex job involving protocols, computers, and modern radios.

AHA were useful in providing basic training to these individuals, but a more expanded course in immediate lifesaving techniques was needed. The need for advanced training led to the development of a nationally recognized course in first response. The FR learns basic assessment, simple airway management, oxygen administration, bleeding control, rescuer CPR, as well as defibrillation.

Emergency Medical Technician–Basic

A person who has completed the primary level of training for the pre-hospital care provider is referred to as an **Emergency Medical Technician–Basic (EMT-B)**. All EMT-Bs bring the same skills to a patient's side, whether they work onboard an ambulance, as part of a security detachment at a mall, or in the field as soldiers. The skills an EMT learns include airway maintenance, oxygen administration, bleeding control, CPR, defibrillation, patient assessment, and limited medication administration. The EMT's knowledge covers the basics of many illnesses as well as the proper management of a patient during transport to a hospital. The role of the EMT is discussed in more detail in Chapter 2.

Since the first EMT curriculum in 1969, then called the EMT-Ambulance, the public has recognized this level of training as the minimum standard of care for EMS. This curriculum has undergone changes over time; the most recent, in 1994, brought with it the new title of EMT.

As EMTs advance in the profession, they may aspire to a higher level of training or expertise. After EMT–B, the two most common levels of prehospital provider training are Emergency Medical Technician–Intermediate and Emergency Medical Technician–Paramedic.

Emergency Medical Technician–Intermediate

The next immediate level of EMS provider above the EMT-B is the **Emergency Medical Technician–Intermediate (EMT-I)**. The 1999 National Standard Curriculum for the EMT-I included higher-level patient assessment skills; advanced airway management techniques, including endotracheal intubation; cardiac arrest management skills, such as ECG interpretation and drug administration; venous therapy, including intraosseous infusions; and advanced trauma care.

A description of the role of an EMT-I could be "an EMS provider who can expertly manage the first 10 minutes of any prehospital emergency using advanced skills and specialized equipment often seen in an emergency department."

The skills of an EMT-I are dependent upon a strong foundation in basic emergency care, and in most states one must be an EMT-B for one year before one can apply to become an EMT-I.

Because of the reduced classroom and clinical hours, as compared to an EMT–Paramedic, and the reduced time commitment to maintain skills, many rural and frontier EMS systems elect to maintain their providers at the EMT-I level. These systems, sometimes called intermediate life support, or ILS, are often all that is available in the rural setting because of limited personnel, training opportunities, and financial resources.

Emergency Medical Technician–Paramedic

The highest level of prehospital EMS provider training is the **Emergency Medical Technician–Paramedic (EMT-P)**. Many paramedics are career professionals. Most paramedic education programs are offered at local community colleges or teaching hospitals. The paramedic training program is usually more than 1,000 hours in length and includes expanded training and education in the management of the ill or injured patient. Paramedic skills include comprehensive patient assessment, advanced airway management and intravenous access techniques, expanded medication administration, and cardiac arrest management.

As do the EMT-B and EMT-I, a paramedic works closely with a physician and follows the physician's instructions regarding patient care. These instructions are often in the form of written protocols. Additional training can be obtained to allow some paramedics to function independent of immediate medical supervision.

ACUTE MEDICAL CARE

In the past, a patient brought to the hospital by a family member would be taken to the back door. A nurse would be called down from the hospital floors to the so-called accident room to attend to the patient. In smaller hospitals, the medical residents, doctors in training, would also respond to the emergency. In larger city hospitals, a young and inexperienced doctor who had just started a private practice might work nights "moonlighting" to make extra money. These inexperienced doctors often had no special training in acute medical care.

Emergency Medicine

Inadequately trained physicians and even more poorly equipped emergency rooms became more problematic when the highly mobile U.S. public started to rely less on the family doctor and more on hospitals. As the need for a specialized **emergency physician** was recognized, these physicians banded together to form the American College of Emergency Physicians (ACEP) in 1968. The organization's mission was to advance the cause of emergency medicine as a medical specialty. The belief was that specialized training was necessary for a physician to effectively care for acutely ill and injured patients.

In 1979, emergency medicine was recognized as the 23rd specialty in medicine. Emergency rooms quickly became more appropriately referred to as emergency departments, entities that interacted with both hospital services, such as radiology and cardiology, and prehospital services, such as EMS. The emergency department came to be defined as the emergency medical center for a hospital (Figure 1-10). It is a department to which people with medical emergencies can go, unscheduled, and receive immediate care. By its very definition, the emergency department had to be open 24 hours a day, seven days a week.

Trauma Centers

It was soon recognized that even these newly restructured emergency departments were not able to care for all severely injured patients. Physicians such as R. Adams Crowley of Johns Hopkins researched the factors contributing to trauma death and concluded that trauma patients needed expert surgical care within the first hour of their injury. Proper surgical care within this so-called golden hour is associated with the best chance of survival for a seriously injured patient.

In 1980, the U.S. Department of Health and Human Services released a position paper on trauma centers. It called for the categorization of hospitals and systems of trauma care. Hospitals that were known to have the capability to properly manage trauma patients (persons with severe injuries) were designated as **trauma centers**. Modern patient care protocols call for EMTs to transport certain seriously injured patients to such a designated trauma center.

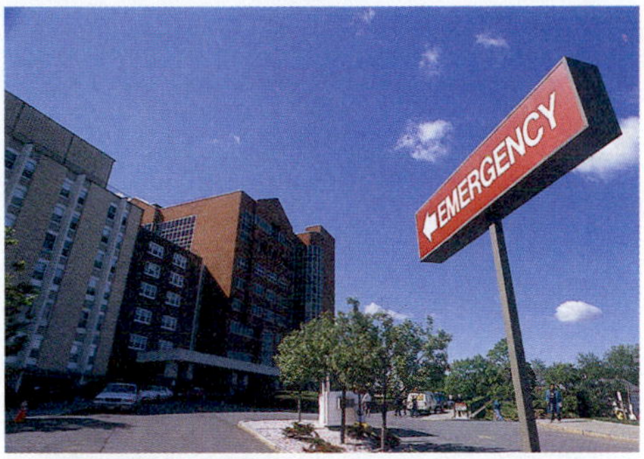

FIGURE 1-10 Emergency departments specialize in the treatment of acute medical emergencies.

Aeromedical Transport

As hospitals have continued to consolidate and specialize and as the health care industry has become increasingly competitive, another need has developed. Health care systems need to be able to transfer patients to the medical centers where specialized services are available. Helicopters and airplanes provide a means of rapid transportation between hospitals (Figure 1-11). Specialized medical crews care for patients during such aeromedical transport.

Today, more than 250 aeromedical services exist in the United States. The missions of these services are a mix of prehospital emergency response and interfacility transport. Because of this mix, many flight teams are made up of a registered nurse and an EMT-P with specialized aeromedical training.

THE FUTURE OF EMS

Although EMS has come a long way in the last 35 years, changes are needed to accommodate the changing needs of the populations it serves and to adjust to new financial and medical developments. Increasing elderly and homeless populations, decreasing health care resources, tightening finances, increasing demands for quality, and a need for organized research all contribute to the challenges that EMS faces today and will face in the future.

Aging Americans

After World War II, there was a population explosion known as the baby boom. Today, these baby-boomers are becoming middle aged or elderly. As people age, they are likely to develop significant health problems. These increasing health problems often lead to an increased use of medical services. Accordingly, the number of EMS calls to the elderly is increasing (Figure 1-12). Older adults have special needs that must be recognized, and treatment of the elderly may differ from treatment of the young. The special needs of the elderly are addressed in Chapter 41.

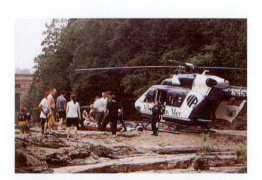

FIGURE 1-11 EMS has seen an increased use of aeromedical services. (Courtesy of Albany MedFlight, Albany, NY.)

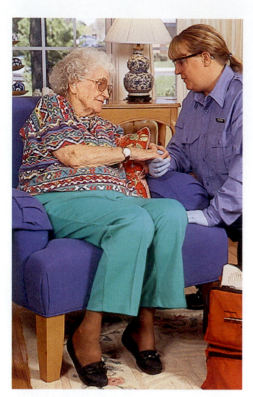

FIGURE 1-12 Increasing numbers of aging Americans will be a challenge for EMTs.

Homelessness

With the increasing use of medications to treat psychiatric illnesses, a large number of psychiatric patients have been released from institutions to live independently. Such deinstitutionalized persons sometimes are unable to properly care for or house themselves. In addition, the nation's changing economy has made it impossible for some Americans to provide food or shelter for themselves or their families. Shelters designed to house such homeless people are usually overcrowded. The social services system often cannot satisfy the needs of all the people in need of help. Because of their lack of regular health care and adequate housing, the homeless have come to rely on the EMS system and emergency departments for treatment and protection.

Human Resources

In many parts of the United States, EMS is largely provided by volunteers. These volunteers provide an invaluable service to their communities. Modern demands have made it difficult for the average citizen to find time to volunteer for EMS. Declining membership is a problem that has been identified by many national EMS groups.

Financial Restrictions

The requirements for equipment, training, insurance, and other costs in today's prehospital health care system can be overwhelming. Small volunteer organizations may find it difficult to fulfill these requirements with the minimal funding that they have at their disposal. The budgets in many municipalities have not increased proportionately to the rising cost of managing an EMS system.

Organizations that represent EMS at a national level are constantly trying to resolve the issues that have forced the closing of volunteer EMS agencies across the country. The EMS community must continue to find ways to better support the mission of emergency care in the field.

Accountability

The competitive marketplace economy of the United States has created questions about the value of certain services, EMS services included. EMS has two customers: the public it serves and the hospitals. Both of these customers demand value. Government regulations also require that EMS be practiced in an environment that is safe to both the patient and the EMT.

EMS has recognized these demands and has responded appropriately. Most EMS agencies are involved in **continuous quality improvement (CQI)** programs, which are designed to find and address areas in need of improvement within the agency. This type of program helps to ensure that a system is in place that will enable quality patient care to be safely delivered. Both state and federal laws are starting to require such programs. For example, to receive accreditation by the Commission for the Accreditation of Ambulance Services

Inc. (CAAS), EMS agencies must demonstrate that they have an active CQI program in place.

EMS Research

For years, the practice of EMS has been based on experience and opinion. Unfortunately, experience and opinion have not always been enough to justify the money needed for EMS. Medicine is a science, and EMS, as a part of that science, could benefit from scientific research.

Increasingly, the practices that have been taken for granted in the past have been examined more carefully. Practices of questionable efficacy or safety have been discarded, and new procedures have been carefully investigated before being implemented. Some of the techniques and practices today's EMT will learn in this text will be different from what may have been previously taught.

For example, it is only recently that EMTs have routinely been taught to defibrillate in cardiac arrest. Research studies have determined that rapid defibrillation is the key to survival from certain types of cardiac arrest. This research has led to the addition of defibrillation to the training and scope of practice of many public safety agencies, including police and fire departments. Training in this skill is now available not only to responding medical providers but also to the general public, with public access defibrillation programs.

Carefully designed scientific research has been rare in the field of EMS, but such research has been gradually increasing since 1990. Although issues such as lack of funding and difficulties in obtaining consent in emergency situations have made conducting quality EMS research difficult, it is by no means impossible. Physicians and prehospital providers have made evidence-based practice a priority. Well-designed studies are being completed every day that help the EMS community shape its practices on the basis of scientific fact rather than popular opinion. Involvement of EMS field providers in such research activities is a necessity for the future.

CONCLUSION

The rich past of EMS is filled with examples of individual heroism and leadership. We share our heritage with other health professions. This association does not diminish EMS; it only amplifies the importance of teamwork.

The future of EMS depends on the assessment and management of many challenges. To face these challenges, the EMT should insist on high-quality EMS and should constantly question, research, and refine practices in order to provide the best quality of patient care in a manner that is safest for the EMS team.

TEST YOUR KNOWLEDGE

1. What historical events had an impact on the evolution of EMS?
2. How have changes in health care affected modern EMS?

3. What is the relationship of EMS to the modern health care system?

4. Name a key paper or piece of legislation that had a noteworthy impact on EMS.

5. How is the EMT of today different from the EMT of the 1960s? How are they the same?

6. What are an EMT's role and responsibilities in the health care system?

7. Name a professional group that represents the interests of EMTs.

8. What are the six elements of an EMS response as represented in the Star of Life?

9. What are some of the challenges that EMTs face in the future?

INTERNET RESOURCES

Accidental Death and Disability: The Neglected Disease of Modern Society can be ordered at the National Academies Press, http://www.nap.edu.

Visit the Web site of the National Highway Traffic Safety Administration at http://www.nhtsa.dot.gov to learn more about its role in EMS.

Visit the Web sites of the following EMS organizations:

- American Ambulance Association, http://www.the-aaa.org
- International Association of Fire Fighters, http://www.iaff.org
- National Association of Emergency Medical Technicians, http://www.naemt.org
- National Registry of Emergency Medical Technicians, http://www.nremt.org

FURTHER STUDY

Barkley, K. T. (1990). *The ambulance: The story of emergency transportation of sick and wounded through the centuries*. Kiamesha Lake, NY: Load N Go Press.

Clawson, J. J., & Dernocoeur, K. B. (1998). *Principles of emergency medical dispatch* (2nd ed.). Salt Lake City, UT: Medical Priority Consultants.

Page, J. O. (1989). A brief history of EMS. *Journal of Emergency Medical Services, 14*, S11.

CHAPTER 2

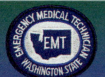

Medical Responsibilities

KEY TERMS

certification

continuing education

lifelong learning

medical direction

medical director

off-line medical control

on-line medical control

personal safety

prehospital health care team

professional conduct

prospective quality assessment

quality improvement

quality management

retrospective quality assessment

OBJECTIVES

Upon completion of this chapter, the reader should be able to:

1. Describe the roles and responsibilities of the EMT–Basic.
2. Differentiate the roles and responsibilities of the EMT–Basic from those of other medical care providers.
3. Describe the roles and responsibilities of the EMT–Basic that are related to personal safety.
4. Discuss the roles and responsibilities of the EMT–Basic toward the safety of the crew, the patient, and bystanders.
5. Describe desirable attributes and conduct of the EMT–Basic.
6. Discuss the EMT Code of Ethics.
7. Define quality improvement and discuss the EMT–Basic's role in the process.
8. Define medical direction and discuss the EMT–Basic's role in the process.

OVERVIEW

The Emergency Medical Technician–Basic (EMT-B) is an important part of the prehospital health care team. Professionalism, training, continuing education, and appropriate medical direction are essential components of an EMT's career. This chapter discusses these issues in detail.

ROLES AND RESPONSIBILITIES OF THE EMT

The EMT-B is an integral part of the **prehospital health care team**. This team is made up of many different members (medical personnel, firefighters, law enforcement officers), all of whom must be thoroughly familiar with their own roles and responsibilities (Figure 2-1).

Anatomy of a Call

"Rescue 50 respond to a Priority One motor vehicle collision at the corner of routes 155 and 20." Deb carefully copied down the information.

Deb and Earl climbed into the ambulance and fastened their seat belts. Deb started the engine, turned on the emergency lights and siren, and proceeded toward the scene of the call.

Upon arrival at the scene, Deb parked the ambulance in a position that was well out of traffic yet still allowed easy access to the rear compartment and would allow for an easy exit from the scene. Deb and Earl donned personal protective equipment and then approached the scene.

Earl quickly scanned the scene and determined that there were three persons involved. One, a young woman, was trapped in her vehicle by damage to the door. He immediately called the dispatcher on the radio and requested additional ambulances to the scene as well as the local fire department for extrication.

Earl and Deb briefly assessed each patient to determine who needed attention first. The woman who was trapped was still seat belted in. Earl assessed her airway and breathing and gave her oxygen. Continuing in his assessment, he found that she had the physical signs of shock. Earl immediately called for assistance in rapidly removing her from the vehicle.

The woman was removed from the vehicle and placed onto a backboard, with the help of several firefighters. Deb maintained spinal immobilization while Earl, with continued assistance from the firefighters, placed the patient onto a stretcher. Then they placed the stretcher into the back of the waiting ambulance.

Deb began driving, using the emergency lights and sirens, toward the regional trauma center while Earl continued to assess the patient in the rear of the ambulance.

As soon as he was able, Earl used the mobile radio to call the trauma center to advise them of the woman's condition and of their impending arrival. Receiving no further orders, Earl continued to provide care for the patient and frequently reassessed her condition.

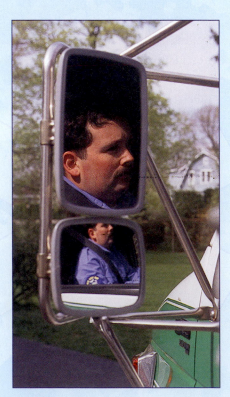

Upon arrival at the hospital, Deb parked the ambulance in the designated ambulance entrance and helped Earl remove the stretcher from the rear of the ambulance. A nurse, who was expecting them, met them at the emergency department's doors.

Earl gave a thorough verbal report of his assessment and treatment as they transferred the woman onto the hospital stretcher. The nurse carefully noted their work.

After quickly cleaning up and placing new sheets on the stretcher, Deb and Earl documented the call and cleaned and restocked the ambulance, in preparation for another call.

- What roles do the EMTs in this case play?
- What are the EMTs' responsibilities in this case?
- What should be included in an EMT's job description?

When all members of the team work together, the common goal will be realized. In this case, the goal is to deliver professional care in a timely manner.

The EMT-B is given the responsibility of bringing quality medical care to patients wherever they may be (Figure 2-2). This care may range from lifesaving procedures to simply comforting the patient. Regardless of the scenario, the EMT is expected to provide a high quality of basic medical care to the patient in a professional manner while maintaining her own safety and the safety of coworkers.

The EMT's responsibility goes beyond medical care. Accurate and thorough patient assessment is necessary to guide appropriate treatment. The EMT must also understand the principles of safe lifting and movement of patients. Decision making is also a key skill. The EMT must be able to quickly and accurately prioritize patients and determine the mode of transport and the appropriate destination hospital.

As in any other health care profession, thorough documentation of all assessment findings and interventions is necessary upon completion of patient care. Both written and verbal reports must be provided to the receiving hospital staff at the time of patient transfer. Written reports must include all necessary data to allow for later review of the details of care and transport. Above all, EMTs must remember that their job is to do what is best for the patient. A certain amount of flexibility is required in order to provide individualized care to each patient.

Job Description

The EMT-B is expected to perform a wide variety of duties in many different circumstances. The National Highway Traffic Safety Administration (NHTSA) has described career requirements for the EMT-B quite specifically.

Procedural Duties

It is important that the EMT work in a manner that reassures both patient and bystanders. A clean, well-stocked ambulance and appropriate training and continuing education help to maintain the professionalism that is crucial for a prehospital health care provider. Table 2-1 shows many of the procedural duties of the EMT.

Patient Care Duties

EMT-Bs may find themselves in many situations that have not been specifically described to them. It is for this reason that EMTs and other EMS team members must be well trained and prepared for a wide variety of situations.

On the basis of assessment findings, an EMT will provide emergency medical care to ill or injured adults, infants, and children. Specific patient care duties are shown in Table 2-2. This text provides detailed discussions of all these duties to assist you in your initial training.

Safety

Safety is very important in many jobs, including that of an EMT. During the course of normal duties, an EMT may be placed in many

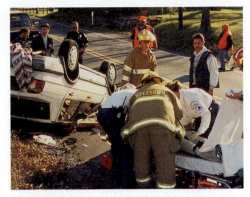

FIGURE 2-1   The EMT is a vital part of the health care team. (Courtesy of David J. Reimer Sr.)

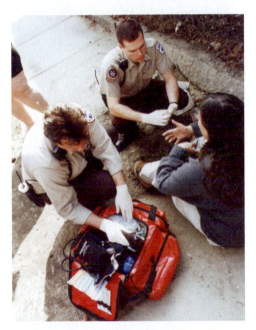

FIGURE 2-2   The EMT brings quality medical care outside of the hospital. (Courtesy of Mark C. Ide.)

TABLE 2-1

Procedural Duties of an EMT

Maintains a clean, fully stocked vehicle

Is able to quickly locate and use any piece of equipment on the vehicle

Receives dispatch information accurately

Drives to the scene quickly but safely, observing all traffic laws

Safely parks the vehicle

Performs a scene assessment to ensure safety and to determine the need for further assistance

Determines the mechanism of injury or the nature of the illness

Assesses the patient and provides appropriate care

Calls for additional help if necessary

Moves the patient to the ambulance

Continues patient care during transport to the hospital

Chooses the appropriate hospital for the patient's needs

Involves medical control when needed

Provides the destination facility with sufficient advance notification

Continually reassesses the patient

Delivers the patient to the hospital

Provides the hospital staff with concise verbal and written reports

Restocks the ambulance and returns to service

TABLE 2-2

Patient Care Duties Performed by an EMT

Airway maintenance

Ventilation of patients

Cardiopulmonary resuscitation (CPR)

Use of automated external defibrillators (AED)

Hemorrhage control

Treatment of hypoperfusion

Bandaging of wounds

Immobilization of painful, swollen, deformed extremities

Assistance in childbirth

Management of respiratory, cardiac, diabetic, allergic, behavioral, suspected poisoning, and environmental emergencies

Assistance with prescribed medications (nitroglycerine, epinephrine, and bronchodilator inhalers)

Administration of oxygen, oral glucose, ipecac, and activated charcoal

difficult-to-control environments. The EMT must learn to control those aspects of the situation that can be controlled and to anticipate any problems that may arise. Considerable time will be spent during EMT training to ensure that the skills and procedures the student learns will be performed in a safe manner.

Personal Safety

The patient's needs are of high priority. However, these needs should not be allowed to place the EMT or other team members in unreasonable danger. The first priority of any prehospital team member must be **personal safety**.

It is senseless for trained medical professionals to allow harm to come to themselves, because they cannot be effective rescuers if they are injured. The EMT must always be aware of potential hazards and take necessary steps to avoid them.

Safety precautions may be simple, such as wearing gloves for protection against potentially infectious bodily fluids, or they may be complicated, such as delaying entry into a possible crime scene until appropriate law enforcement agencies have arrived and determined the safety of the scene. The subject of delaying entry to a crime scene will be dealt with in more detail in Chapter 3.

Crew, Patient, and Bystander Safety

In addition to taking steps to protect themselves, EMTs must be aware of potential danger to the patient, the crew, and bystanders on the scene. If a member of the team is no longer able to perform duties because of an injury, the team is no longer efficient. It is the responsibility of every team member to ensure her own safety and the safety of the other team members.

Some situations may call for the EMT to protect the patient from further harm. If a patient is in a potentially dangerous situation, the EMT must make it a priority to remove the patient from the danger as soon as safety permits.

An EMT must also take the appropriate steps to protect the patient from self-inflicted harm while still maintaining personal safety. To protect the patient while maintaining personal safety, the EMT may have to involve other team members.

Emergencies often draw significant attention from passersby. An EMT must always be aware of potential hazards to private citizens such as bystanders and newspeople. Crowd control may be assigned to another team member, such as a law enforcement officer, but the EMT may need to initiate the call for this assistance (Figure 2-3).

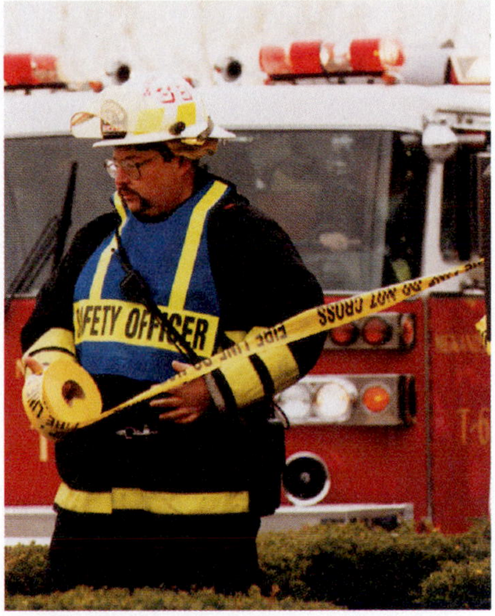

In short, the EMT is responsible for providing medical care to the patient while maintaining personal safety as well as the safety of the crew and bystanders. It is always better to anticipate safety issues and prevent problems than to deal with the results of an unanticipated incident.

FIGURE 2-3 The EMT must also consider potential dangers to the patient, bystanders, and other health care team members.

PROFESSIONAL ATTRIBUTES

As members of the prehospital health care team, EMTs are held to the same standard of professionalism as any other member of the team regardless of level of training, area of practice, or pay scale. Patients who access EMS deserve to receive the same quality of care in their homes as they would receive in a hospital or in their doctor's office.

An EMT must strive to maintain **professional conduct** by demonstrating a caring, confident, and courteous demeanor on the job. The same level of professionalism that is expected of an emergency department physician or nurse is expected of an EMT.

Appearance

It has been said that "a picture speaks a thousand words," and in the case of an EMT's appearance nothing can be truer. A clean uniform that is neatly worn projects a professional attitude (Figure 2-4). An easily identifiable uniform and a name tag help the layperson identify the members of the prehospital medical team. An EMT who takes care in her appearance will likely exercise the same care in managing a patient.

Skill Maintenance

Upon completion of initial training, an EMT will have learned many skills that will be perfected after much practice. As do other skills, these will degenerate if not practiced frequently. It is the responsibility

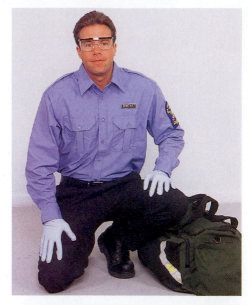

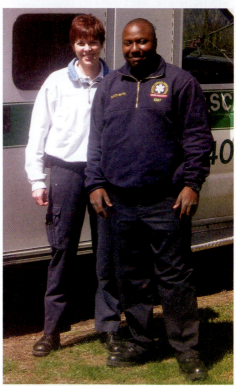

FIGURE 2-4 A neatly dressed EMT with easily recognized identification will instill confidence in patients and their families.

of the EMT to maintain a certain level of proficiency with regard to important skills.

Physical Preparedness

Many of the duties of the EMT will require some physical exertion. The EMT who maintains good physical condition will be best suited to complete these tasks safely. Chapter 4 discusses further benefits physical fitness can have on the EMT's well-being.

Personality Traits

Although anyone can train to become an EMT, there are certain personality traits that are better suited to this role. The EMT should be kind and compassionate, as well as willing to help others regardless of personal considerations.

Training

To provide quality patient care, the EMT must first participate in a basic training course to learn the principles of emergency care (Figure 2-5).

State and federal agencies regulate the initial training courses for the EMT-B. The educational standards are outlined in the U.S. Department of Transportation EMT-B curriculum.

Many national organizations contributed to the preparation of these documents, which are revised regularly to mirror changes in practice and research.

Each state adds to or enriches the curriculum in a way that is felt to be most appropriate for the state's needs. This curriculum serves as a basis upon which training courses are designed.

Because the duties of EMTs will place them in many different situations, their initial training will include different types of learning opportunities. Classroom, or didactic teaching, will be standard to prepare the student with the required cognitive (knowledge-based) objectives. Practical hands-on instruction will enable the student to learn assessment and treatment in a controlled environment. These psychomotor skills are the backbone of an EMT's practice. Clinical requirements may include observation time in the hospital and in the prehospital environment in order to enable the EMT to learn how to put this new knowledge into actual practice.

Certification and Licensure

To reassure the public that the person responding to the emergency is a minimally competent EMT, each state provides for a process of examination that can lead to licensure as an EMT in that state. All EMTs must successfully complete this standardized examination of both skills and knowledge in order to attain this licensure to practice as an EMT.

Once the EMT is licensed, she can practice as an EMT within the scope of practice as defined by state law. Each state has statutes that define the scope of practice of all health care professionals, including the EMT, and they are usually found in the public health law or the medical practice act.

In some cases the state itself provides the certification examination that leads to licensure as an EMT. In those states EMTs are permitted to practice once they are certified by the state.

In other circumstances the state depends on a national examination for certification. A nationally recognized **certification** is recognition of the EMT having attained a certain level of competency as recognized by his or her peers. For EMS, the National Registry of Emergency Medical Technicians (NREMT) certifies EMS providers.

The NREMT has certified over 1 million EMTs in the United States and is used as the certifying examination, at one level of EMS or another, in 44 states (Figure 2-6). The NREMT examination's test plan, called a *test blueprint*, is developed based on the result of the EMT-Basic Practice Analysis conducted in 1995 and again in 1999 and generally is considered to be a very reliable test instrument.

The NREMT's mission statement is to certify and register EMS professionals throughout their careers by a valid and uniform process that assesses their knowledge and skills for competent practice. Many EMS providers take serial examinations as they attain each new level of EMS: EMT-B, EMT-I, and EMT-P.

EMS providers are sometimes confused about the distinction between the terms *certification* and *licensure*. In a legal opinion delivered to the NREMT, and available online, the distinction was made clear. *Certification* is a voluntary process that is completed with a private organization, such as the NREMT, for example. States may elect to use this certification as the basis for their permission for an individual to practice. States may also elect to test the EMT themselves. In those cases the examination, despite the use of the term *certification*, is a licensing examination. The distinction is: whenever the state gives an EMT the right to practice as an EMT, it has licensed that EMT.

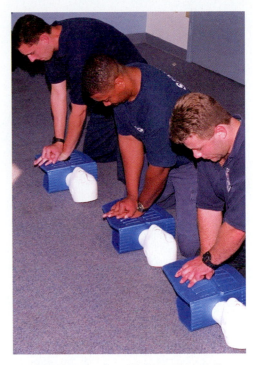

FIGURE 2-5   Practical learning stations are crucial to the initial and continuing training of all members of the health care team.

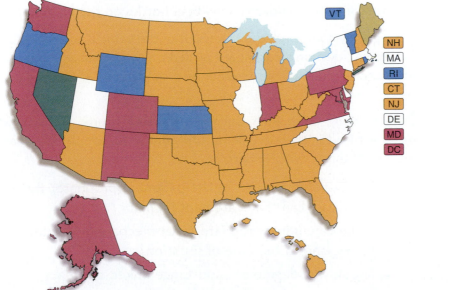

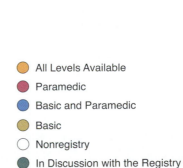

○ All Levels Available
● Paramedic
● Basic and Paramedic
● Basic
○ Nonregistry
● In Discussion with the Registry

FIGURE 2-6   As of 2004, 44 states recognize the NREMT exam as their certifying examination.

Continuing Education–Professional Development

Once initial certification has been achieved, the requirements for education have not ended. All health care professionals must make a commitment to **lifelong learning** through continuing medical education. It is important not only for the EMT to be aware of new information but also to participate in its development and dissemination when possible. As do other areas of medicine, prehospital care continues to change as researchers find new and more efficient ways to provide emergency medical care.

The EMT is responsible for keeping knowledge and skills current by participating in **continuing education** opportunities. This process can be likened to a bucket of water. As time passes, in order to keep

✳ *Fair Treatment*

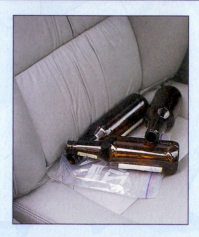

Dave and Rich respond to a motor vehicle collision involving a pick-up truck and a minivan. A mother, the driver of the minivan, was killed instantly, and her three children are seriously injured.

EMS command orders Dave and Rich to care for the driver of the pick-up truck. As Dave and Rich approach the driver, they note the odor of alcohol permeating the air inside the vehicle. Glancing around the interior, they see several dozen empty beer bottles on the front seat.

Dave gruffly commands the driver out of the vehicle and orders him to lie down on a backboard placed on the stretcher. Rich, a little confused, asks Dave whether he should get a cervical collar first.

Dave answers, "Look, Rich, this guy is obviously drunk, and drunks never get hurt in these accidents. Only innocent people, like that mother of three, ever get hurt."

- Was Dave's treatment of the patient appropriate? By what basis can that statement be made?

- If the care is inappropriate, what mechanisms are there to respond to this type of situation?

- Should the degree of importance linked to an act (important, not immediately significant, or critical, for example) affect the reaction of the EMT?

the bucket full, one must periodically dip into the well. The bucket of water is the EMT's fund of knowledge, and the well is the wealth of medical education available. In this way, continuing medical education can be thought of as a lifelong process. To maintain a level of knowledge, an EMT must periodically replenish it with new material. Some states have specific requirements for the continuing education of the EMT-B.

Refresher Training—Competency Assurance

As with any education, after a period of time, some material may be forgotten and may need reviewing. Most states have prescribed time lines with requirements for refresher training. These requirements vary greatly in form but all serve the same purpose: to ensure that the provider has reviewed the core components of the curriculum since initial training.

One requirement may be a refresher course that reviews the core components of the curriculum every 2 or 3 years. Another way of ensuring review is to require participation in a regular continuing education program that covers the core components. Some states require that a test be taken every 2 or 3 years for recertification. Regardless of the form of the review, EMTs must prove regularly that they continue to remain skilled in the procedures and in the assessment and treatment techniques for which they were originally trained.

CODE OF ETHICS

The National Association of Emergency Medical Technicians (NAEMT) is an organization that represents EMS professionals across the United States. Its primary mission is to promote the advancement of EMS as an allied health profession.

An important part of maintaining the necessary professionalism within the group is the ethical principles by which it operates. The EMT Code of Ethics is reproduced in Figure 2-7. The values and principles set forth within the EMT Code of Ethics are crucial in the makeup of the prehospital health care professional.

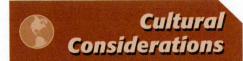

Cultural Considerations

EMTs will often find themselves in highly sensitive situations. Persons who call for emergency assistance from an EMS team deserve to receive compassionate and confidential care regardless of their condition or background. *Remaining nonjudgmental is crucial, although it may sometimes be difficult.*

Professional status as an Emergency Medical Technician and Emergency Medical Technician– Paramedic is maintained and enriched by the willingness of the individual practitioner to accept and fulfill obligations to society, other medical professionals, and the profession of Emergency Medical Technician. As an Emergency Medical Technician–Paramedic, I solemnly pledge myself to the following code of professional ethics:

A fundamental responsibility of the Emergency Medical Technician is to conserve life, to alleviate suffering, to promote health, to do no harm, and to encourage the quality and equal availability of emergency medical care.

The Emergency Medical Technician provides services based on human need, with respect for human dignity, unrestricted by consideration of nationality, race, creed, color, or status.

The Emergency Medical Technician does not use professional knowledge and skills in any enterprise detrimental to the public well-being.

FIGURE 2-7 The EMT Code of Ethics, as adopted by the National Association of EMTs. (continues)

The Emergency Medical Technician respects and holds in confidence all information of a confidential nature obtained in the course of professional work unless required by law to divulge such information.

The Emergency Medical Technician, as a citizen, understands and upholds the law and performs the duties of citizenship; as a professional, the Emergency Medical Technician has the never-ending responsibility to work with concerned citizens and other health care professionals in promoting a high standard of emergency medical care to all people.

The Emergency Medical Technician shall maintain professional competence and demonstrate concern for the competence of other members of the Emergency Medical Services health care team.

An Emergency Medical Technician assumes responsibility in defining and upholding standards of professional practice and education.

The Emergency Medical Technician assumes responsibility for individual professional actions and judgment, both in dependent and independent emergency functions, and knows and upholds the laws which affect the practice of the Emergency Medical Technician.

An Emergency Medical Technician has the responsibility to be aware of and participate in matters of legislation affecting the Emergency Medical Service System.

The Emergency Medical Technician, or groups of Emergency Medical Technicians, who advertise professional service, do so in conformity with the dignity of the profession.

The Emergency Medical Technician has an obligation to protect the public by not delegating to a person less qualified any service which requires the professional competence of an Emergency Medical Technician.

The Emergency Medical Technician will work harmoniously with and sustain confidence in Emergency Medical Technician associates, the nurses, the physicians, and other members of the Emergency Medical Services health care team.

The Emergency Medical Technician refuses to participate in unethical procedures, and assumes the responsibility to expose incompetence or unethical conduct of others to the appropriate authority in a proper and professional manner.

Written by Charles Gillespie M.D. Adopted by The National Association of Emergency Medical Technicians, 1978.

FIGURE 2-7   (continued)

CURRENT AFFAIRS IN EMS

The prehospital health care field of EMS is constantly undergoing change. Many of these changes will affect the everyday practice of the EMT. It is the responsibility of all health care providers to be aware of and to contribute to, as they are able, the changes that their profession undergoes. Professional organizations such as the NAEMT provide the structure for creating change that is beneficial to the EMT and to the ability to provide quality patient care.

The EMT should also be aware of the professional magazines and journals that support the advancement of quality patient care by prehospital providers (Figure 2-8). These journals provide a way to keep up to date on national EMS events and current literature relevant to the practice of medicine by the EMT.

CONTINUOUS QUALITY IMPROVEMENT

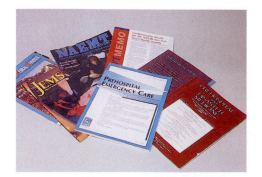

FIGURE 2-8   There are many publications that are geared toward prehospital health care professionals.

The EMS system is an integral part of the emergency management of a sick or an injured patient. The process by which such care is provided needs to be closely examined on a regular basis in order to ensure timely, cost-effective care. This examination can be done through careful quality review and by completing quality research that focuses on prehospital care. It is the responsibility of the EMT to participate in research projects that are designed to examine current practices and that ultimately serve to improve patient care.

Quality Management Roles

The ultimate goal of every EMS team member is to provide quality medical care in a timely manner while maintaining team safety. The recognition of that goal is the first step in quality management within the EMS team. **Quality management** can be thought of as a continual process that involves the planning, execution, assessment, review, and improvement of the overall plan.

Planning

Ensuring that the desired goal is commonly realized by all members of the team requires that a clear system be in place. All members of the team must be familiar with this system in order for it to be effective.

Within EMS, the system is usually organized by protocols and standard operating procedures. These documents provide a plan that, if followed, will lead to the common goal of quality delivery of care. The EMT is responsible for knowing these elements.

Over time, the overall plan may need to be adjusted. It is the responsibility of the EMT to help alter the plan as needed and to adapt to any changes that may be made.

Executing the Plan

The system must be set up in a manner that allows execution of the plan without difficulty. If components of the plan are unreasonable or difficult to accomplish, it is unlikely that the plan will be followed regularly. For example, if the plan includes a response time to emergencies of fewer than 8 minutes but the ambulance station is located more than 8 minutes from a majority of the calls, this response time will not likely be accomplished unless something is changed.

Assessing Quality

To advance, the team must have a method of assessing the quality of the care provided. This assessment is often accomplished by a specific committee of providers that may include administrative personnel, field providers, and the medical director of the organization. This assessment may occur prospectively (before or during a call) or, more commonly, retrospectively (after the call).

Prospective quality assessment is usually accomplished by a member of the assessment team accompanying a crew on an emergency call and observing the care provided. This is useful because it provides a clear picture of the quality of the care given. Such assessment is time and labor intensive and is not always possible, but it should be a part of every quality management program.

Retrospective quality assessment is often accomplished by review of the documentation by the team, with identification of strengths and weaknesses. This review of run reports may be comprehensive, or it may be focused on one particular area during specific audits.

This method of assessment is more easily accomplished than is prospective quality assessment, but it obviously provides a limited view of the actual care provided to the patient. This review can be made more effective by ensuring that the providers use a standard method of documentation and that the method incorporates all of the factors that would be important in determining quality of care.

Many states or regions have produced a standard patient care report (PCR) for use as a documentation tool. This report must be completely filled out in order to be useful in quality assessment.

Another method of retrospective review is to gather feedback. The patients and their families can be surveyed to identify problems or strengths that they may perceive. Other users of the system, such as hospital receiving staff or staff at other frequently visited sites (e.g., local nursing homes, special centers) should also be asked for feedback.

Feedback from patients and facility staff can serve to identify potential problem areas that may need improvement, but it also can identify areas in which the system is highly effective. Being aware of both weaknesses and strengths is important to ensure that the needs of the users are being correctly identified and fulfilled to their satisfaction.

Quality Improvement

Once the assessment has been completed, areas in which the plan was met are identified and reinforced. For example, if part of the plan is to deliver compassionate patient care and a patient writes a letter praising an EMT for her kind and compassionate treatment during a recent event, the EMT should be praised and other members of the team should be made aware of the compliment to the system. Factors that allowed the EMT to deliver this quality of care should be identified and used to improve the entire system.

On the other hand, areas of the plan that clearly were not met should be identified and explored further. The reason for the failure to meet the goal should be determined or that particular goal should be reexamined. For example, if response times are consistently above the recommended time limit, perhaps the time limit is unrealistic for the current situation. Either the limit should be changed or the cause for the extended response time should be determined and corrected.

The findings on quality assessment should be used to improve the ultimate delivery of care. Training can be geared toward areas needing more emphasis. Retraining can be instituted if appropriate. This process is called **quality improvement**.

Once a system is in place that identifies a clear goal and includes a plan for its execution, assessment, and improvement, it should not remain static. As everything in medicine changes with the identification of new means of providing care and current research within the field, this process of quality management must be continuous. The EMT should take responsibility for the level of care practiced and should continually strive for improvement of her own abilities and the improvement of the entire EMS team.

MEDICAL DIRECTION

An essential component of all EMT training is appropriate **medical direction** provided by a higher medical authority. Physicians should be involved in all aspects of EMS training and practice. A **medical director** can serve as a medical expert, consultant, and educator. Physicians can receive specialty training in the field of emergency medical service and can serve as an invaluable resource for all prehospital care providers.

EMS physicians are required to provide medical direction in several areas of prehospital practice. A physician's input is key in establishing treatment protocols and in the preparation of training programs and continuing education events. The ultimate goals of the EMS medical director are to help ensure the safety and well-being of the EMTs; to maintain the delivery of quality patient care; and to assist in the proper education, training, and certification of EMTs (Figure 2-9).

A physician cannot always be present at the bedside when an EMT is caring for a patient, nor is a physician's presence necessary. A physician who has been involved in the training process, the establishment of treatment protocols, and the quality review of calls can be sure that the EMT will provide quality patient care.

This process of preparing protocols and standards of care is referred to as **off-line medical control**. The term indicates that the physician does not have to be physically present while the EMT is caring for a patient but, through protocols and procedures, has control over each patient's care.

If an EMT has a question about the care needed by a patient, or if the issue is not clearly addressed in the protocols, then **on-line medical control** is utilized. This involves communication between the EMT and the physician while care is being rendered in the field. On-line medical control can be established with the system's medical director or, more commonly, with a physician in the local emergency department.

The medical director is ultimately responsible for the medical actions of the EMTs on the team. The EMTs are essentially acting as the physician's designated agents while caring for patients under the physician's direction. It is therefore necessary for the physician to be involved in training, retraining, continuing education, and quality management procedures within the system.

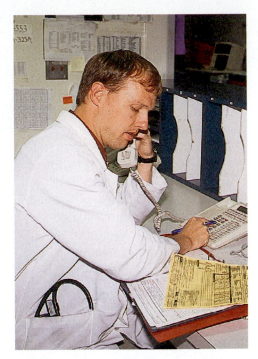

FIGURE 2-9   The physician medical director can be a medical expert, consultant, and educator and is a valuable EMS team member.

? *Ask the Doc*

The National Association of EMS Physicians in its position paper on "Physician Medical Direction in EMS" outlines the essential, desirable, and acceptable qualifications for a medical director as well as the medical director's responsibilities for out-of-hospital care, including communications, field clinical practice, and administration of EMS systems.

CONCLUSION

The EMT is a specially trained health care provider. As a prehospital health care provider, the EMT must be prepared to provide quality care in a multitude of environments and to initiate treatment on the basis of minimal information.

The unique abilities of the EMT to provide calm, compassionate, quality health care in an otherwise chaotic situation is what makes the EMS system successful. The EMT brings to the patient the same quality medical care that would be available from a physician in an office or from staff in a hospital.

Prehospital health care providers must continue to maintain the same level of professionalism that is expected of any other health care provider. This professionalism involves education, ethical care, and quality management, all done with the involvement of a knowledgeable physician.

TEST YOUR KNOWLEDGE

1. What are some of the roles and responsibilities of an EMT?
2. Whose safety is the responsibility of the EMT?
3. Whose safety comes first, and why?
4. Name several attributes of an EMT.
5. What are some elements of the EMT Code of Ethics?
6. What is quality care in EMS?
7. How is quality improved in EMS?
8. What is medical direction?

INTERNET RESOURCES

- Visit the *Occupational Outlook Handbook* and search for information on careers in EMS at http://www.bls.gov/oco
- Visit the Web site of the National Highway and Traffic Safety Administration, http://www.nhtsa.dot.gov, and compare the curriculums for the EMT-B, EMT-I, and EMT-P.
- Visit the Web site of the National Registry of Emergency Medical Technicians, http://www.nremt.org, and look for information on certification and licensure. What do you need to know to successfully complete the test for certification through the registry?
- Visit the Web site of the National Association of Emergency Medical Technicians, http://www.naemt.org.
- Visit the National Association of EMS Physicians Web site at http://www.naemsp.org.
- Do a search for Web sites that provide news services and research updates in the field of EMS.

FURTHER STUDY

Emergency Medical Services: The Journal of Emergency Care, Rescue, and Transportation. Summer Communications, Inc., 7626 Densmore Avenue, Van Nuys, CA 91406-2042, http://www.emsmagazine.com.

Journal of Emergency Medical Services, Jems Communications, PO Box 2789, Carlsbad, CA 92018, http://www.jems.com.

Polsky, S. (1992). *Continuous quality improvement in EMS.* Dallas, TX: American College of Emergency Physicians.

CHAPTER 3

The Legal Responsibilities of the EMT

KEY TERMS

abandonment

advance directive

age of majority

assault

battery

breach of confidentiality

child abuse

competent

consent

domestic violence

do not resuscitate order (DNR)

elder abuse

emancipated minor

emergency doctrine

evidence conscious

express consent

false imprisonment

Good Samaritan laws

guardian

health care proxy

Health Insurance Portability and Accountability Act (HIPAA)

immunity statute

implied consent

in loco parentis

(continues)

OBJECTIVES

Upon completion of this chapter, the reader should be able to:

1. List the legal responsibilities of the EMT.
2. Describe the EMT's duty to act.
3. List some of the elements in the patient's bill of rights.
4. Discuss the patient's right to confidentiality.
5. Explain what is meant by capacity to refuse care.
6. Identify the important components of the EMT's responsibility when a patient refuses care against medical advice.
7. Discuss and define three types of advance directives.
8. Explain how consent is obtained in different circumstances.
9. Discuss the legal importance of documentation.
10. Identify the circumstances under which resuscitation may be withheld.
11. Discuss the EMT's role in reporting suspected abuse.
12. Identify the most common allegations that may be raised against an EMT in a court of law.
13. Discuss the laws that are in place to help protect EMTs from litigation.

OVERVIEW

The EMT has many legal responsibilities. Under certain circumstances the EMT has a legal duty to provide care in a certain manner. The EMT should be familiar with the laws regarding job responsibilities relevant to prehospital patient care.

This chapter discusses the responsibilities of a prehospital health care provider, including issues surrounding a duty to act, patient rights, consent, documentation, resuscitation decisions, collaboration with law enforcement, physical restraint of patients, and the reporting of suspected abuse. In addition, the most common allegations brought against EMTs and the means by which EMTs can protect themselves against lawsuits will be examined.

THE LEGAL RESPONSIBILITIES OF AN EMT

An EMT is viewed by the public and coworkers as a health care professional. The EMT has an association with a physician to provide supervised medical care. An EMT's practice is limited to what that physician will permit. Furthermore, the extent of medical procedures that an EMT can perform is limited by law, the **scope of practice**. Although a physician provides direct authority for the individual procedures that an EMT can perform, the potential group of those skills and procedures is further restricted by law. Those laws that define the scope of practice for an EMT are found in medical practice acts or health regulations, depending on the state. In some cases state laws will refer to those skills and procedures that are contained within the National Standard Curriculum (NSC) for the EMT-B as the limits of an EMT practice. Therefore, a physician could not order an EMT to perform a cesarian section because it is outside the scope of practice for an EMT.

KEY TERMS

(continued)
legal duty to act
liability
living will
mandated reporter
mechanism of injury
medical protocols
negligence
patient's bill of rights
pattern of injury
physical restraint
scope of practice
standard of care

✳ *Consent*

After handcuffing the young shoplifter, Officer Barnes took a moment to catch his breath. He knew that the security cameras had caught all the action on tape. The cameras had recorded the kid picking up the jeans and stuffing them into the shopping bag. The cameras had also recorded him being stopped at the door and asked to open the bag.

Then there was the chase in the parking lot, as he ran from store security, all recorded on tape. The security cameras had recorded him running, slipping on the wet pavement, and falling flat on his face with his hands full of stolen merchandise.

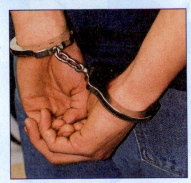

(Courtesy of David J. Reimer Sr.)

The kid's face was a bloody mess, probably from the cut on his forehead and the bloody nose. He looked like he had been beaten. The cameras would prove that the injuries were from the fall.

"Son, how old are you?" asked Officer Barnes, as he used his portable radio to call for EMS. "Sixteen," the teenager replied, "and I don't need EMS."

- Can an adolescent consent to care? Are there any exceptions?
- Who can consent for an adolescent? What if that person is not available?
- What is different about consent in this case?
- Can an adolescent legally refuse care? Are there any exceptions?
- What duties does the EMT have for this teenager?

It is impossible for physicians to attend every patient in the field. Therefore, EMTs tend to patients at the scene of an accident or illness, acting as a physician extender. On the scene, the EMT's practice is limited to lifesaving and immediately needed procedures. Physicians define the limits of an EMT's practice through off-line medical control through the use of written instructions. The most common example of off-line medical control is **medical protocols**, a set of written regulations that specify the proper procedure for implementation of patient care. These medical protocols direct EMTs to which actions they can perform on the scene.

If a patient's needs exceed what is outlined in the EMT's written protocols, the EMT may wish to speak directly to a physician. An EMT who needs advice on how to proceed with a particular situation should consult a physician. This direct contact with a physician during actual patient contact is called on-line medical control.

Physicians who are engaged in a medical relationship with a patient have a duty to care for that patient until the patient no longer wants care or the care has been properly turned over to another health care provider of equal or greater training. This responsibility to patients also pertains to an EMT.

Knowledge of Standard of Care

The emergency nature of many EMS calls requires that the EMT be proficient at certain skills. In addition to performing at a moment's notice, the EMT must always know his role in patient care. The law requires that an EMT act within the guidelines that are recognized as appropriate for others with the same level of training. These guidelines are known as the **standard of care**.

The standard of care is established through a combination of sources such as state statutes, local ordinances, treatment protocols, and textbooks such as this one. It is the responsibility of the EMT to know how he is expected to perform in a medical emergency. Each of these sources should be familiar to every prehospital health care provider.

Clearly, the standard of care is not a single textbook, protocol, or governing law but that expectation, that the public holds regarding how an EMT should behave when caring for a patient. In a court of law, when it might be alleged that an EMT did not provide adequate treatment, the EMT would be held to the standard of what another equally trained EMT would do in the same or similar situation. That decision is based on a reflection of the sum total of all sources of EMS knowledge and its practical application in the field; that is, "standard care." In every instance, if the EMT keeps the patient's best interests as the highest priority then he will be, in large part, performing to the standard of care.

Legal Duty to Act

An EMT who is an employee under contractual obligation to respond to calls has a **legal duty to act**. The EMT who volunteers has the same duty to act during those times that he has agreed to respond to calls. This legal duty to act requires that the EMT treat any patient encountered within the recognized standard of care.

In most states, an EMT does not have a legal duty to act when off duty; there are exceptions. Every EMT should check the local or state regulations. Every EMT should be aware of the state laws regarding off-duty health care providers rendering assistance at the scene of a medical emergency. Many EMTs feel a moral or ethical obligation to render assistance to persons in need regardless of a legal duty.

Once an EMT has initiated patient care, he must continue to care for that patient until care can be relinquished to an equally or higher trained provider. Failure to continue care or to properly turn the patient over to an appropriate provider may constitute patient **abandonment**, a form of EMT misconduct.

Respect for Patients' Rights

Every person in the United States has a right to emergency health care. This health care must be provided within the standard of care and in a confidential manner. Every competent adult has the right to either accept this medical care or refuse it. This ability to accept or refuse medical care is part of the patient's rights. Although at present there is no formal document for the prehospital circumstance, every hospital has a **patient's bill of rights**, which outlines the rights and privileges of a patient. The EMT must be familiar with issues of patient confidentiality, consent, and refusal of care and other patient rights as noted on the patient's bill of rights.

Right to Confidentiality

Historically, patients have enjoyed a sacred trust with their physicians that allows medical information to be kept private. This trust is enforced even in a court of law and cannot be broken without compelling reasons.

The EMT, as an agent of the physician, is usually required to maintain the same confidentiality. The personal details of the patient's health history that an EMT is privy to during the course of an emergency call should be held in the strictest confidence at all times. Information regarding the nature of the care provided should not be shared with anyone who is not involved in the immediate care of the patient. When an EMT turns a patient over to another EMT or other health care provider, it is expected that all pertinent information will be shared. Insurance groups may also have a limited right to patient information for billing purposes.

Patient information must not be disclosed to nonprivileged persons such as family, friends, or the public without the patient's permission. Even law enforcement personnel may not be privy to details of patient care unless written authorization from the patient or a court order is provided. Accordingly, EMTs should be cautioned against discussing details of EMS calls in public places, where they may be overheard by nonprivileged parties.

In some states, EMTs are required to report certain situations to legal authorities, such as suspected child abuse or other violent crimes (this topic is discussed in more detail later). Even if not legally obligated to do so, the EMT may feel morally compelled to report suspicions of such incidents. It is acceptable, and encouraged, for an EMT to report suspicions of abuse or of violent injury to receiving hospital personnel. These physicians and nurses are directly involved in patient care, so they are authorized to be given such information. Licensed health care workers may be mandated by state law to report such incidents. The sharing of such suspicions will assist the hospital providers in protecting the patient.

It is common practice to use details of an incident to illustrate a learning point for other prehospital providers. In those cases, care must be taken to withhold any identifying information in order to protect the confidentiality of the patient involved.

A failure to maintain the confidential nature of detailed patient information is referred to as a **breach of confidentiality** and can have legal implications. These actions are taken very seriously in the legal system. Lives can be seriously affected, and public opinion of EMTs is diminished by such acts. When in doubt, avoid discussing patient information.

Health Insurance Portability and Accountability Act

The **Health Insurance Portability and Accountability Act** of 1996 (HIPAA) was signed into law by President Clinton on August 21, 1996. This law addresses three main issues related to health care. The first seeks to allow insurance portability and continuity. The second requires the standardization of administrative and financial data exchange. Third, and perhaps most relevant to the EMT on a daily basis, relates to the protection of privacy, confidentiality, and security of health care information. While the health insurance reform section of this law has been in effect for some time, the administrative simplification and required privacy protection became enforceable only recently.

On April 14, 2003, the HIPAA privacy rules were enacted, requiring strict confidentiality of all patient information. Additionally, these new standards provide patients with access to their medical records and more control over how their personal information is used and disclosed. HIPAA applies to health care agencies/providers who conduct certain financial and administrative transactions electronically (many EMS agencies fall into this category).

These regulations call for any data that identify a patient and the patient's health status to be kept in strictest confidence. Patient permission is required to share this "protected health information (PHI)" in many circumstances. PHI may be used as necessary for treatment, payment, and health care operations without a patient's specific consent. However, the information that is shared in these circumstances must be limited to what is necessary for the purpose. For example, although quality assurance (QA) records have to contain information about a patient's health and the care provided, the name and other identifiable demographic information are not needed for effective QA. Therefore, the EMS service must take reasonable care to remove such information from QA documents. These regulations are not meant in any way to hinder or limit a provider from freely communicating with other health care staff providing care to the patient, that is, advanced life support (ALS) (i.e., paramedics) providers intercepting with basic life support personnel (i.e., EMT) or hospital staff taking over care of the patient. However, the EMT must take reasonable precautions to maintain the privacy of a patient's PHI.

Further, HIPAA requires that patients be given a notice of privacy practices in use by the agency. Signed acknowledgment of receipt of this notice is also required when it is reasonably obtained. In an emergency situation, the law allows for the EMT to delay the notification and acknowledgment until a more appropriate time.

In summary, the HIPAA regulations are meant to protect patients' privacy while maintaining the health care providers' ability to appropriately manage emergencies. The EMT is encouraged to discuss agency-specific policies regarding HIPAA with the agency's designated privacy officer or corporate compliance officer.

Right to Refuse Care

Any competent adult may refuse medical assistance. Whenever emergency medical care is refused, the EMT must act carefully, balancing the patient's rights against the possible harm that might befall the patient if left untreated.

A patient's refusal of care can be clear and direct, such as "I do not want your help." It can be something as simple as pulling an arm away as the EMT is trying to take a blood pressure. Whatever the patient's action, the EMT cannot use force, or even a threat of force, to gain the patient's agreement.

There are criteria that must be met in order for the EMT to recognize a patient's right to refuse care. First, the patient must be an adult. In legal terms that means the patient must be of the **age of majority** (the age at which a person may act without parental consent and be treated as an adult). In many states, the age of majority is 18 years old.

The patient must also be considered to be **competent**, or able to act in a responsible manner and comprehend the decision at hand. A person who has been determined to be incompetent, or unable to sufficiently comprehend the situation, is not able to consent to medical care. This lack of competence may be due to a permanent medical condition such as mental retardation or dementia. In these circumstances, a **guardian**, an individual given the legal authority to act on behalf of the patient, is usually appointed by the courts to make decisions for the patient.

Other conditions that may render a person temporarily unable to make rational medical decisions include head injury, alcohol or drug intoxication, and mental illness. The EMT must decide whether the patient is capable of making responsible decisions and of understanding the situation. When in doubt as to the patient's competence, the EMT should contact a medical control physician for advice.

Against Medical Advice

With some experience, and the help of local protocols, the EMT may differentiate between a refusal of medical assistance (RMA) and a refusal against medical advice (AMA). In the first case, EMS may have been dispatched to a nonemergency or the situation may be low priority. Nonemergency transport may be appropriate, depending on local protocols. In the case of the AMA, the patient has a potentially life-threatening illness or injury and the refusal of care would likely have an immediate harmful consequence.

Patients who are refusing against medical advice should be approached carefully. The EMT should try to understand why the patient is refusing. Sometimes fear is a greater motivator than the thought of the complications of the injury. Calm and rational explanations of the care being offered must precede any action. Any action permitted, no matter how trivial, may be a step in the right direction. The EMT should start with minimally invasive therapies such as measuring vital signs. If the patient allows vital signs to be taken, then explanations of further treatments can be undertaken. Eventually the patient may trust the EMT enough to allow transportation to the hospital.

If a patient is thought to have the capacity to refuse care, the EMT must then inform the patient of the reasonable and foreseeable consequences of the refusal. For example, it is possible for a patient to die from a minor wound, but it may be considered unlikely. What is more likely is that the wound could become infected and cause the patient pain and even loss of function. The patient must be advised of the potential consequences of lack of evaluation and treatment for the complaint.

The EMT must offer medical care to the limit that the patient will accept. For example, if the patient refuses to go to the hospital in an ambulance for treatment of an injury but will accept a bandage, the EMT must make the bandage available.

The EMT must encourage the patient to seek further medical attention if the problem persists or worsens. Patients should also be reminded that if they desire further treatment or transport later on, they can call EMS back to the scene.

Sometimes, despite the EMT's best efforts, the patient still refuses care and the EMT is forced to leave the patient in a potentially dangerous situation. Whenever possible, the EMT should leave the patient in the care of another competent adult. This person may convince the patient of the need for further medical treatment and can monitor the patient for complications.

In all cases of refusal, the liability for the decision to leave the patient rests with the EMT, the EMT's service, and the service's physician director. In the case of a refusal against medical advice, an EMT should contact medical control, explain the situation calmly and objectively, and let the physician try to convince the patient of the need for further treatment. If the patient does choose to refuse after this process, the EMT must thoroughly document the events. Chapter 20 details the necessary documentation needed in this case.

Advance Directives

Despite advances in medicine, some patients have a terminal disease. Others, having lived a long and full life, do not wish to prolong their life, particularly if living would mean being a burden on their families or would result in prolonged suffering. These patients have a right to self-determination.

Normally, it is safe to assume that an unconscious patient would allow all medical treatment if conscious. However, consistent with their right to refuse treatment, patients can decide in advance of a medical emergency not to accept life support. A number of mechanisms have been developed to facilitate the wishes of such patients. The directions a person leaves for family and caregivers in advance of a life-threatening situation are called **advance directives**. An advance directive may be of several forms. A more detailed discussion of advance directives can be found in Chapter 42.

One such means patients have of conveying their wishes to caregivers is through the use of a **living will**. A document drawn up in private or in consultation with an attorney, a living will simply expresses the patient's wishes regarding specific treatment options in the event of a serious illness or injury. Some states allow prehospital personnel to recognize this document as binding; others do not. The EMT must know the state laws regarding recognition of a living will.

Another form of advance directive is the **do not resuscitate order (DNR)**. This order is written by a physician, after consultation with the person or with the family, if the person is unable to discuss treatment options. The order directs that resuscitative efforts not be initiated in the case of cardiac or respiratory arrest if it has been determined that resuscitation would be futile or would prolong suffering. In some states, only a specific prehospital DNR can be honored by EMTs. In other states, EMTs can honor any type of DNR. Some patients wear a bracelet, necklace, or other indicator that they have a DNR order.

It is important for the EMT to realize that a DNR order applies to the patient who is in cardiac or respiratory arrest. By no means does this order imply that no treatment should be offered to an ill or injured patient. Many times, routine prehospital treatment such as oxygen administration can provide comfort to a terminally ill patient while not contradicting a DNR order. An EMT who is faced with an unclear situation is best advised to begin resuscitation and call medical control for guidance.

A third type of advance directive is the **health care proxy**. The documentation of a health care proxy permits a person previously designated by the patient to make decisions in the event the patient becomes incapacitated. This person, having been chosen by the patient, usually is aware of the patient's beliefs and wishes.

Obtaining Patient Consent

Consent refers to voluntary agreement by a person to allow something to take place. When approaching a patient, an EMT should routinely request permission to care for the patient. Most EMTs do not ask the patient directly, "do you consent to my examination?" Most EMTs approach the patient, identify themselves as an EMT, then ask the patient what the problem is. When the patient engages the EMT in a conversation about the illness or injury, the patient has in essence consented to the assessment. While initiating a physical assessment, the EMT should tell the patient what is being done and the purpose of each action. This explanation will enable the patient to understand and agree with the plan of care.

Once the initial physical assessment has been completed, the EMT must ask permission before initiating any treatments. The EMT

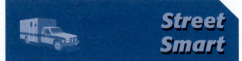

Street Smart

There are situations in which a dying patient needs the comfort and convenience of an ambulance yet does not need emergency medical care. EMS and other hospital systems, such as hospice, should meet and discuss how to best serve such patients before the need arises. This kind of collaborative pre-planning can prevent a lot of uncertainty in the field.

should advise the patient of the treatments that are necessary and explain the need for them in language that the patient will understand. A patient who verbally agrees to such treatment has given **express consent**.

Most patient care is provided after the patient has given express consent. However, it is assumed that an unconscious patient, if conscious, would consent to standard treatment. This type of consent is implied. **Implied consent** is assumed when treating unconscious patients who have potentially life-threatening injuries.

Children and Consent

Children are not legally permitted to give consent for medical treatment. In most situations, the EMT can obtain consent from a parent or from a guardian who has been appointed by a court to make decisions for the child. When a parent or guardian is not immediately available, an adult sibling or close relative can give permission under the doctrine of **in loco parentis**, which literally means the "local parent." Sometimes parents sign permission papers that authorize another individual to consent on their behalf. Coaches of team sports may often be given such permission by parents for use during special activities.

When no parent or legal guardian is immediately available and the child has a life- or limb-threatening injury or illness, an exception to consent must be made. In those emergent cases, the law assumes that the parents would want their seriously ill or injured child to be treated. Such treatment would be possible under implied consent.

As do all rules of law, laws pertaining to children and consent have exceptions. Certain minors are legally entitled to make decisions regarding medical care. These **emancipated minors** are no longer under the control of a parent or guardian and are legally responsible for their own decisions and any consequences that result from those decisions. Laws in different states will grant this privilege for different reasons. Examples of reasons for emancipation of a minor might include marriage, military service, or independent living without parental financial support. The court may provide legal documentation of such a decision to the individual. The EMT should request verification from the patient if any doubt exists.

In some states, a minor can consent to medical treatment in certain special cases. For example, a minor can seek treatment for a sexually transmitted disease without parental permission. In these cases, the courts have decided that the parents' rights are outweighed by the public need to control outbreaks of communicable disease.

Prisoners, Mentally Disturbed Persons, and Consent

Although an individual who is imprisoned does not lose the right to make decisions regarding medical treatment, many states have enacted laws regarding medical treatment of incarcerated individuals. Some states require that prison officials provide consent for medical issues concerning prisoners. EMTs who frequently service prisons should clarify these laws in their state.

The **emergency doctrine** is a legal principle that allows for emergency treatment of prisoners or children if they are incapable of giving consent as a result of injuries or another condition. If treatment will potentially be lifesaving, then the EMT may initiate treatment and transport despite the lack of express consent. If, however, the prisoner refuses treatment, further care may not be provided unless another individual is authorized to consent on the prisoner's behalf.

There are times when a court will authorize specific treatment despite the patient's refusal if it is felt that the patient does not have the capacity to make a reasonable decision and that the treatment is in the patient's best interest. This authorization may be given in the case of a prisoner or in the case of a mentally disturbed person who is in need of medical care. The EMT who is faced with providing care for a patient who is refusing should determine whether such authorization has been given and should request the appropriate legal documentation. The assistance of law enforcement personnel should be obtained if it is necessary for the safety of the medical crew. Medical control should also be consulted if a question arises as to a patient's ability to refuse care.

Often, individual situations require specific responses that can be determined only by collaboration between law enforcement and medical personnel. Experience carries a great deal of weight in resolving such situations positively. Nevertheless, the opinion of the medical director, with counsel from an attorney, about how to handle predictable situations should be sought before such a situation occurs. This kind of preplanning can prevent legal problems later.

Documentation

The EMT is responsible for keeping careful written records of every patient interaction. It is recommended that the record be completed as soon as possible after the patient interaction to avoid any loss of information over time.

The documentation done by an EMT will become a part of the patient's medical record and will be referred to by other health care providers who care for that patient. Accuracy and completeness are essential. Chapter 20 discusses the details of proper prehospital documentation.

Initiating Resuscitation

In general, an absence of pulse and breathing requires that an EMT start CPR unless the patient has a DNR order or if unambiguous signs of death or signs of injury inconsistent with life are present. Most states have clear regulations regarding when it is inappropriate to begin resuscitation. For example, an EMT will not attempt resuscitation if the patient meets any of the conditions listed in Table 3-1. All EMTs must be familiar with the policies regarding initiation of resuscitation in their particular state.

After death, a body begins to cool, and blood pools at the lower, or dependent, parts of the body. The patchy purple mottling seen on the skin is called lividity. After a period of time, the body will become stiff. This condition is called rigor mortis. Rigor mortis starts with the

TABLE 3-1

Unambiguous Signs of Death

Decapitation (separation of the head from the body)

Severe lividity (pooling of blood in the dependent areas of the body)

Rigor mortis (stiffening of the muscles in the body after death)

Decomposition (actual disintegration of skin and muscle)

short muscles, like the jaw, and progresses to the larger muscles. Therefore, if it is difficult to open the airway on a patient who has no pulse, the EMT should suspect rigor mortis. Rigor mortis is usually present within 1 or 2 hours of death under normal temperatures. Lividity and rigor mortis are considered to be signs of death. No amount of resuscitation offered at this point would be effective.

Bodies exhibiting decapitation or decomposition are also considered to be dead and should be left for the police to handle. Other wounds, such as head injuries with large amounts of brain matter exposed, may constitute mortal wounds. The EMT should contact medical control for instructions on cases that are questionable. When in doubt, the EMT should initiate resuscitation, and the medical control physician can decide on the next course of action.

If the decision is not to pursue resuscitation, then it is important to leave the scene as if it were a crime scene. In the event of a death outside of a hospital, law enforcement personnel may want to make a report for future reference.

Collaborating with Law Enforcement

Crime scenes represent a special challenge to EMTs. On the one hand, there is the patient who is hurt and needs help. On the other hand, there has been a crime and there is a criminal who must be caught.

A challenge may exist for an EMT if the patient is also the suspected perpetrator of a crime. The EMT must remember that it is up to the courts to decide the guilt or innocence of an individual. Every EMT must be nonjudgmental and render care without prejudice.

Another challenge faced by EMTs at a crime scene is to provide appropriate care to the patient while trying not to disturb any evidence that the police may find valuable in investigating the crime. Of course, if evidence must be altered in order to care for a patient, the EMT should not hesitate to provide the care that is necessary. In this case, the EMT should take note of the position of any item moved and relay this information to the investigating officer as soon as possible.

Table 3-2 lists some things that an EMT should not do at any potential crime scene. The key problem for an EMT is to know when a scene is a crime scene. Sometimes, police are already on scene; in other cases, the EMT may have a feeling that something is just not right. In fact, many innocent-appearing scenes turn into crime scenes; therefore, the EMT should incorporate these considerations into daily practice.

An EMT who discovers the criminal nature of a scene after the fact may be very helpful to law enforcement by writing down any observations. For example, were there newspapers at the door and was the mail picked up? Upon entering the room, did the EMT notice any unusual smell such as natural gas or cigarette smoke? Were the lights on when the EMT entered the room? Was the television playing, or was a radio on? Were doors open, closed, or locked?

Both EMS and law enforcement have very important jobs. A good working relationship between the agencies can be important in many circumstances. For the EMT, patient care takes priority over evidence collection, but such care can often be given without destroying

---

TABLE 3-2

What Not to Do When Dealing with a Crime Scene

Do *not* allow unneeded personnel on scene.

Do *not* move a deceased patient.

Do *not* cover the body with anything.

Do *not* unnecessarily move objects.

Do *not* touch any weapons (guns, knives, etc.).

Do *not* touch the following objects:

    Telephones

    Answering machines

    Sinks

    Toilets

    Light switches

    Televisions

Do *not* leave waste at the scene (gloves, etc.).

evidence. Attention to a few details can save hundreds of hours of police work, improve the chance of police success in apprehending the criminal, and support a good working relationship between EMS and law enforcement.

Motor Vehicle Collisions

Many communities are viewing motor vehicle collisions that involve serious injury or a drunk driver as criminal acts. Therefore, EMTs are increasingly being asked to testify about the conditions on the scene. EMTs are well advised to consider these scenes as potential crime scenes and to carefully document their observations as soon as possible after patient care responsibilities are over. Table 3-3 lists some of the observations that an EMT might want to make. In every case, the EMT should be **evidence conscious** (aware of the importance of preserving items and conditions that pertain to a crime scene).

Threat of Violence on the Scene

Awareness of the potential for violence against emergency service providers cannot be stressed enough. A source of such violence is gang violence. An EMT responding to a call involving gangs should keep the following in mind.

Always remember that personal safety is the first priority. The EMT should never enter a scene that is potentially unsafe without police assistance. Remember that only law enforcement officers are legally permitted to use force. EMTs should never consider physical force as a viable option.

An EMT who is likely to encounter gang members should become familiar with their rituals and customs. To some gangs, cutting "colors" (cutting clothing that identifies the person as a member of a certain gang) is a sign of disrespect. Local law enforcement agencies will often provide EMS providers with this type of education.

In addition to identifying bodily injuries during a head-to-toe survey, the EMT should note the presence of any weapons or dangerous instruments, such as ice picks, needles, razor blades, and the like, that may be hidden in clothing. It is not safe to allow a patient to have a weapon in the back of an ambulance. Law enforcement personnel should be asked to remove the weapon from the patient before transport.

Physical Restraint of Combative Patients

The first rule of medicine regarding treatment of a combative patient is to assume that the cause of the combativeness is medical until proved otherwise. There are many medical conditions that can cause a patient to be uncooperative, agitated, and even combative. These conditions are discussed in detail in later chapters.

The EMT must remember that only police officers are allowed to use physical force and only under certain conditions. The EMT may use **physical restraint** (a means of restricting freedom of movement) to prevent a patient from hurting herself or others. The police can be very helpful in assisting EMTs with restraining patients because they are usually well trained in techniques of safe physical restraint.

TABLE 3-3
Evidence Worth Noting from a Motor Vehicle Collision

Scene evidence
- Skid marks
- Direction of travel
- Piles of grass or rust debris
- Puddles of fluids
- Downed trees and poles
- Tracks in snow or mud

Vehicle evidence
- "Spidered" or "starred" windshield
- Steering wheel position
- Gear position
- Seat belt position
- Airbag deployment
- Open alcohol bottles
- Drugs in plain view
- Position of patients

 Safety Tip

In some cases, injury of a gang member can result in retaliation and further violence. When this situation is suspected, the patient should be removed as quickly as possible from the scene. This escape from an unsafe situation is similar to the act of quickly rescuing a victim from a burning building.

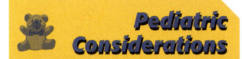

Pediatric Considerations

The EMT should observe the interactions between the child and the parent or caregiver. Does the child appear to be afraid? Does the child recoil when the parent comes close? Is the child ignoring pain that is usually associated with an injury?

These subtle clues are seen only during unguarded moments when the parent and child are out of the public view, such as in the back of the ambulance. Report exactly what is observed to hospital personnel *after* the child's care has been turned over.

Reporting of Abuse

EMTs are in a unique position in that they are invited into people's homes. They have the advantage of being able to observe the patient in home surroundings. Interactions with family members in the home environment are also witnessed. The EMT must observe the situation carefully. Because hospital staff do not have access to a patient's home, they do not have the opportunity to witness the home situation and evaluate its safety.

An EMS crew that finds a patient in a potentially unsafe situation should quickly take the patient away from the situation. Details of the living environment and any suspicions of potentially abusive situations that are noted by the EMTs should be passed along to hospital personnel for further investigation.

Child Abuse

Child abuse is any act of physical, sexual, or psychological maltreatment of a child or the failure of a parent or legal guardian to minimally provide the necessities such as food, clothing, shelter, and medical care.

An EMT has a special role in detecting and reporting child abuse. Emergency department personnel cannot see the scene; they cannot match the **mechanism of injury** (the instrument or event that results in harm) to the **pattern of injury** (injuries characteristic to a particular mechanism). Emergency department personnel depend on the accurate observations of EMTs to help detect child abuse. Child abuse is discussed further in the pediatric section of this text.

A large number of states require that an EMT report any suspicion of child abuse to local authorities, such as child protective services. This requirement makes the EMT a **mandated reporter**. Not only is the EMT obligated, by law, to report suspicious circumstances, but the EMT may even be held criminally responsible for failing to report such suspicions. It is important that every EMT know how local reporting laws affect them.

No matter how obvious the likelihood of abuse may seem, the EMT must not accuse the parents of wrongdoing or make statements that are inflammatory. These types of statements may put the EMT, the EMS crew, and the child in further danger. Care and treatment of the child should be the primary focus.

Domestic Violence

The public is becoming increasingly aware of the prevalence of **domestic violence** (acts of violence against a spouse, partner, or family member) in the United States. Victims of domestic violence may need psychological support and immediate medical attention for potentially life-threatening injuries, in addition to a safe haven from their attackers.

Typically, a victim of abuse is afraid of the abuser. Such fear may prevent the victim from seeking assistance or attempting to leave the situation. Many women are battered or abused during pregnancy, and many do not seek help until the situation is desperate. On average, the battered woman will return home seven times before permanently leaving the situation.

The EMT must remain nonjudgmental and demonstrate empathy toward the patient. It is the job of the police to investigate and arrest the abuser. Compassionate care and nonjudgmental treatment will encourage the abused woman to trust the EMT. This trust will perhaps make her more likely to call again if she needs help. A patient who is treated in a negative manner may lose confidence in EMS as a means of getting help when she is injured. Health care providers must be encouraging and supportive of a woman who has demonstrated the courage to call for help.

Elder Abuse and Neglect

The most likely people to be battered and abused are the vulnerable and the infirm. As do children, the elderly fall into this category.

The patterns of injuries that are seen in **elder abuse** (an act of violence toward or neglect of an elderly person) are similar to the patterns of injuries seen in child abuse. Inconsistent stories, injury patterns that do not match the mechanism of injury, and attempts to hide an injury are typical. This issue is discussed in more detail in later chapters.

Whenever elder abuse is suspected, the first priority is patient care. However, after the call is over, help for the patient and the family is needed. Many EMS agencies have a social services referral system in place that puts the right people in touch with the patient and family.

COMMON ALLEGATIONS AGAINST EMTS

Many members of the EMS community fear litigation. Although the possibility of a lawsuit against you or your service is certainly disconcerting, the reality is that most EMS calls do not result in litigation.

In 1999, C. B. Colwell and colleagues published a study in the *Journal of Emergency Medicine* that examined liability claims made against an urban 9-1-1 ambulance service. This service runs an average of nearly 42,000 calls a year. During the 10-year study period, a total of 82 claims resulted in 11 lawsuits. Motor vehicle collisions involving an ambulance were responsible for 72% of these claims, and 35% were claims of medical negligence. Although not all EMS systems see lawsuits with the same frequency, it is worthwhile for the EMT to be familiar with the most common allegations against EMTs and to learn how to protect against them.

Although mistakes are possible, the EMT will find that the best way to stay out of legal trouble in the workplace is to provide good patient care in a conscientious manner. This type of work ethic will minimize the chances of an EMT's contributing to a situation that may result in legal action.

Ambulance Collisions and Liability

When driving an emergency vehicle, the EMT has a responsibility to the crew, patients, other motorists, and pedestrians to operate in a safe manner. Most state laws require that an emergency vehicle operator

✳ *A Claim of Negligence*

Driving in the early morning, Mr. Miller falls asleep at the wheel and loses control of his truck. The truck runs off the road and crashes into an old oak tree.

Dazed for just a moment, Mr. Miller uses his cell phone to call 9-1-1. After some time Mr. Miller grows tired of waiting for EMS and exits the vehicle. He is intent on walking to the nearest farmhouse for help.

As he stands up, he gets light-headed, his legs buckle under him, and he collapses to the ground. When Mr. Miller regains consciousness, he is no longer able to feel anything below the waist.

On-duty EMTs from the local volunteer rescue squad respond, from their homes, to the EMS call. Upon arrival, they immediately survey the scene, decide that the situation is a trauma, and immediately go about manually stabilizing Mr. Miller's head and neck.

After completing an initial assessment and a rapid trauma assessment, the EMTs correctly conclude that he may have suffered a neck injury. The EMTs carefully apply a cervical collar to protect his cervical spine, and they logroll him onto a backboard. Afterward, they assess his extremities for feeling and motion. The assessment is unchanged from the initial assessment.

After turning Mr. Miller over to the emergency department staff, the rescue squad returns to service. Several months later Mr. Miller's attorney serves the rescue squad with an "intent to sue" notice. In the notice it is alleged that the EMTs were negligent in their treatment and that this negligent treatment caused or aggravated Mr. Miller's condition, resulting in the permanent paralysis of his legs.

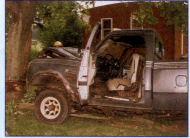

(Courtesy of David J. Reimer Sr.)

- What are the elements of a civil action necessary to prove a case? Are all of those elements here in the case that is presented?

- What is the weakness in the patient's case against the EMTs?

- What should be included in the EMTs' documentation of this call?

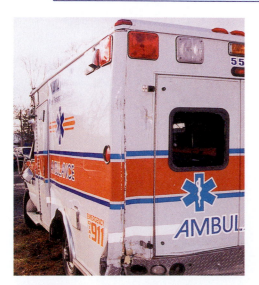

FIGURE 3-1 Emergency vehicles involved in accidents are the number one cause of lawsuits in EMS. (Courtesy of David J. Reimer Sr.)

show due regard for others. The operator can be held responsible for any damages or injuries incurred as a result of lack of due regard. This legal responsibility is known as **liability**.

The most common source of lawsuits against EMTs is emergency vehicle accidents (Figure 3-1). Unfortunately, advances in driver training have not matched advances in attendant training. Driver safety programs such as the Ambulance Accident Prevention Seminar (AAPS) and Emergency Vehicle Operations Course (EVOC) are available but not universally required of emergency vehicle drivers.

In the urban study that was referenced, 59% of the claims related to emergency vehicle accidents involved a vehicle traveling in emergency mode. This fact fits well into the statistics that show that the use of emergency lights and sirens increases the risk of an accident. Emergency vehicle drivers should be familiar with these statistics and should use care when operating in emergency mode. Many EMS systems have begun to limit the number of responses completed with lights and sirens in an effort to decrease this risk. Chapter 43, Emergency Vehicle Operations, provides more information.

Negligence

According to recent literature, claims of negligence in medical care result in the second largest monetary payout for EMS providers, after motor vehicle collisions. Negligence refers to the delivery of care in a manner that is considered to be below the established standard. In EMS, **negligence** can be defined as the failure to provide the care that a reasonably prudent EMT would provide under the same or similar circumstances. The laws regarding negligence provide for compensation to those who have suffered injury as a result of such substandard care.

There are four elements of negligence: duty, breach of duty, causation of injury, and damages. Proving negligence involves showing that all of those four elements has been met.

Duty

Duty is an EMT's legal obligation to conform to a certain standard of care. Duty is the first thing that must be established for negligence to be considered. Responsible vehicle operation, equipment maintenance, and patient care are among an EMT's duties.

As described earlier in the chapter, an EMT's legal duty is somewhat different depending upon whether the EMT is on duty or off duty. It is important for the EMT to know the state's laws regarding duty. When a duty does exist, the EMT may be held liable for failure to act reasonably. If a duty does not exist, the EMT cannot be faulted for failing to perform a task.

Breach of Duty

Breach of duty means a failure to perform in accordance with the standard of conduct that is expected. Once an actual duty has been established, if it is not carried out appropriately, a breach of duty exists. Irresponsible vehicle operation, failure to maintain equipment, or improper care of a patient are examples of breach of duty.

Causation of Injury

The third required element of a negligence claim involves the causation of injury. Because the laws regarding negligence are meant to compensate those who are injured, actual injury is required to claim negligence. Further, it must be shown that the breach of duty directly caused the injury. If injury exists, yet it was not a result of the EMT's breach of duty, then the EMT is not responsible for the compensation. Regardless of duty and breach of duty, if no injury resulted, then there is no negligence.

Damages

Finally, in a claim of negligence, it must be proved that an actual loss or damage has occurred. Such things as lost wages, medical expenses, and property damage are easily quantifiable. Pain and suffering, emotional distress, and the loss of companionship are more difficult to quantify yet are thought to be worthy of compensation. This type of damage allowance is known as compensatory damages.

Another, less common, type of damages that a person found guilty of negligence may be required to pay is known as punitive damages. Such remuneration is meant to punish the defendant and to set an example for others.

Patient Abandonment

An EMT who has established an EMT-patient relationship by beginning emergency medical care for a person has a duty to continue that care until relieved by someone of equal or higher training. This relief usually comes when the patient is delivered to the hospital and the EMT's report is given to the accepting staff.

There are times when a patient is not transported by the first arriving EMT but by another provider. In such a case, the first EMT will give a report to the EMT who is taking over the care of the patient.

There are some circumstances in which the patient does not require further care after initial treatment by the EMT. Each state may have specific regulations regarding this situation. The EMT's documentation of the situation should clearly reflect that both the EMT and the patient find that there is no need for further medical care.

As discussed previously, sometimes a patient will refuse further medical care. If the patient is competent to refuse, then it is the patient who terminated the EMT-patient relationship. The EMT must document the situation carefully to avoid later accusations of inappropriate care.

An EMT who inappropriately leaves a patient without having been relieved of patient care responsibility may be guilty of patient abandonment. This unilateral severance of the EMT-patient relationship is a form of EMT misconduct. If it is found that the EMT intentionally and unjustifiably terminated the EMT-patient relationship, then the EMT can be held responsible for any injuries that resulted.

The Emergency Medical Treatment and Active Labor Act

In 1985, Congress enacted the original Emergency Medical Treatment and Active Labor Act (EMTALA) as a part of a larger law called the Consolidated Omnibus Budget Reconciliation Act (COBRA). This law has also become known as the "antidumping" law and was intended to protect patients whom hospitals might refuse to care for based on financial reasons. Having undergone several revisions, this law requires that any patient who comes to a hospital emergency department requesting care be provided with appropriate emergency treatment within the capabilities of the facility. If a hospital does not have the capability to definitively manage a particular patient, arrangements must be made for an appropriate transfer. There are several conditions that must be met for transfers to occur in emergent situations, and the EMT who will be participating in the interfacility transfer of patients should become knowledgeable regarding the specifics of EMTALA as it relates to the situation.

Breach of Confidentiality

As mentioned previously, an EMT who holds knowledge of private information regarding a patient is expected to keep it in the strictest confidence. Disclosing patient care information to anyone who does not have a right to know can be called a breach of confidentiality. All EMTs must be mindful of who is nearby when patient information is being discussed. *Patient records should always be kept in a confidential manner as specified under HIPAA regulations.*

Assault and Battery

The EMT must remember that every patient who is capable of making decisions has the right to refuse treatment or transport. An EMT who treats or transports a patient without consent or against the patient's will can be held liable.

Charges that may surface regarding the treatment or transport of a patient without consent include assault, battery, and false imprisonment. **Assault** refers to the case in which a patient is afraid that he or she may be touched without having given consent; **battery** refers to the actual touching. The intentional confinement of a patient without the patient's consent and without an appropriate reason is called **false imprisonment**.

Each of those charges can be brought against an EMT, who may then face liability. The EMT should therefore be sure to obtain the appropriate consent before attempting to provide treatment to any person.

PROTECTION AGAINST LAWSUITS

Although most EMTs will never actually be involved in a legal claim, it is certainly helpful for all prehospital health care providers to be familiar with the relevant laws and means of protection. Although there are many means of defending against lawsuits, each state differs significantly in its legislation.

Good Samaritan Laws

With the prevalence of medical lawsuits, health care professionals may be reluctant to help people who suddenly become ill or are injured while in public. In an effort to encourage health care providers to assist such people, the legislatures of many states have enacted laws called **Good Samaritan laws**.

The care provided must be offered freely and given without expectation of compensation. The care rendered must be to the level that another reasonable and prudent caregiver would have provided. Although Good Samaritan laws exist in all 50 states and the District of Columbia, each state has specific conditions that a provider must meet in order to be given protection under these laws. EMTs are well advised to know the laws in their state if they expect to offer care when not on duty.

Immunity Statutes

All states have Good Samaritan laws; some states also have **immunity statutes**. An immunity statute protects a group of people, such as pre-hospital health care providers, from having to pay damages for acts performed as part of the job. Essentially, an immunity statute protects the EMT who is going to be compensated for assisting an injured person. The Good Samaritan laws, which apply specifically to uncompensated performance, generally do not provide this coverage. There are several elements of an immunity statute that must be met for the EMT to qualify for protection, such as maintaining the standard of care. The EMT should be familiar with the state's specific statutes.

Best Practices

The best strategy to avoid being involved in litigation is to use common sense in everyday practice. The EMT who knows and follows protocols and performs his duty in a compassionate manner will be unlikely to be involved in a legal claim.

An EMT who is uncertain as to what treatment to provide should always "err" on the side of the patient. This means to lean more toward providing more treatment as opposed to less. If ever in doubt, the EMT should involve the EMS supervisor or a medical control physician, depending on the nature of the question.

CONCLUSION

This overview of legal concepts is not intended to advise the EMT on how to act in every situation. Rather, it is an overview of the relevant concepts that may be helpful in understanding the legal roles and responsibilities of the EMT.

Specific legal responsibilities vary from state to state, and the EMT should inquire as to the state's laws regarding specific duties and liabilities. The advice of an attorney regarding these matters can be invaluable.

Most EMTs are never required to go to court. Nevertheless, EMTs must do all that they can to protect themselves. The best protection against lawsuits is good patient care provided by a conscientious EMT.

TEST YOUR KNOWLEDGE

1. What are the legal responsibilities of the EMT?
2. What is the EMT's duty to act?
3. What are some of the elements in the patient's bill of rights?
4. What is the patient's right to confidentiality?
5. What is meant by the capacity to refuse care?
6. What are the important components of the EMT's responsibility when a patient refuses care against medical advice?
7. Define three types of advance directives.
8. From whom is consent obtained for
    a. a conscious adult
    b. an unconscious adult
    c. a child
    d. a prisoner

9. What is the legal importance of documentation?

10. Under what circumstances may resuscitation be withheld?

11. What are several situations in which EMTs collaborate closely with law enforcement personnel?

12. What is the EMT's role in reporting suspected abuse?

13. What are the most common allegations that may be raised against an EMT in a court of law?

14. What are some laws that help protect EMTs from litigation?

INTERNET RESOURCES

- To learn more about the latest HIPAA regulations, visit http://www.hipaa.org or http://www.hipaadvisory.com.

- For additional information and resources related to advance directives, visit http://www.partnershipforcaring.org.

- Search for legal cases related to EMS. What did you find?

FURTHER STUDY

Cid, D., & Maniscalco, P. (1999). Integrating criminal investigation into major EMS scenes. *Journal of Emergency Medical Services, 24,* 68–69.

Colwell, C. B., Pons, P., Blanchet, J. H., & Mangino, C. (1999). Claims against a paramedic ambulance service: A ten-year experience. *Journal of Emergency Medicine, 17,* 999–1002.

Hall, S. A. (1998). Potential liabilities of medical directors for actions of EMTs. *Prehospital Emergency Care, 2,* 76–80.

Krebs, D. R., Henry, K. C., & Gabriele, M. B. (1990). *When violence erupts: A survival guide for emergency responders.* Philadelphia: Mosby.

Lazar, R. A. (1989). *EMS law: A guide for EMS professionals.* Rockville, MD: Aspen.

Partridge, R. A., Virk, A., Sayah, A., & Antosia, R. (1998). Field experience with prehospital advance directives. *Annals of Emergency Medicine, 32,* 589–593.

Shanaberger, C. J. (1990, March). Escaping the charge of false imprisonment. *Journal of Emergency Medical Services,* 58–61.

Weaver, J., Brinsfield, K. H., & Dalphond, D. (2000). Prehospital refusal-of-transport policies: Adequate legal protection? *Prehospital Emergency Care, 4,* 53–56.

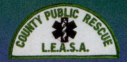

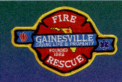

CHAPTER 4

Stress in Emergency Medical Services

KEY TERMS

acute stress

body substance isolation

burnout

chronic stress

diversionary techniques

fight or flight response

healthy lifestyle

multiple casualty incident (MCI)

relaxation exercises

scene survey

stress

stress management program

stressors

unwind time

OBJECTIVES

Upon completion of this chapter, the reader should be able to:

1. Define stress from an EMT's perspective.
2. Identify examples of positive and negative stressors.
3. List several emotions an EMT may experience when exposed to a stressor.
4. List the physical signs and symptoms seen in a stress response.
5. Identify several emotionally charged situations that will likely cause a stress response.
6. Identify several job-specific stressors for EMTs.
7. Identify several home-related stressors for EMTs.
8. List ways an EMT can reduce the effects of stress on the body.
9. Discuss the stress that a patient may perceive.
10. Discuss the possible reactions a patient's family member may exhibit when confronted with illness and injury of a loved one.
11. State the steps an EMT may take to help reduce the stress experienced by patients and their families.
12. Differentiate between an acute stressor and chronic stress.
13. Identify physical, emotional, and behavioral effects of chronic stress.
14. Discuss two general methods for stress management (quantity and quality).
15. Describe a relaxation technique useful for management of an acute stress response.
16. Describe several diversionary activities useful for management of an acute stress response.

OVERVIEW

The EMT will be faced with many situations that may be highly emotionally charged. By the nature of their job, EMS personnel are involved in extreme situations in which the individual is in crisis and overwhelmed. Patients and family members are often unable to cope with the emergency situation or the chaotic environment and may respond very emotionally to the situation. The EMT is susceptible to the same emotional upheaval that the patient and family are experiencing.

These effects should not be denied but, rather, anticipated. If prepared, the EMT may find a way to continue to provide the medical care that she was trained to provide, despite occasional overwhelming emotional stress.

Stress must be recognized and dissipated appropriately. This chapter prepares the student to understand and recognize common stressors within the field and how to handle these issues most effectively.

STRESS DEFINED

Stress is the physical, emotional, and behavioral response of the body to changing conditions in our lives. This response is the body's way of adapting to these changes. Stress is a necessary part of our lives and can provide challenges that keep life interesting.

The events that trigger stress are known as **stressors**. A stressor can occur suddenly, as an acute stimulus, or it may be more prolonged, in the form of multiple smaller events or issues building upon each other. The effects of everyday stress are potentially damaging to our emotional and physical well-being.

Stress can be the result of many types of stressors. Table 4-1 identifies common factors that can cause stress. The way an individual thinks and feels about an event is what causes a stress response. Each person thinks about an event in a different way; therefore, an event that is perceived as stressful to one person may not be at all stressful to another individual.

The Stress Response

Although each individual may react differently to a stressful situation, everyone experiences similar strong emotions and characteristic physical responses. Each person expresses these emotions and physical feelings in a different manner.

Emotional Response

The feelings we experience during a stress response may be very powerful, sometimes even overwhelming. It is important to realize that stressors are not always undesirable. An example of a positive stressor is Dan's waiting to meet a good friend that he hasn't seen in many years. He might be feeling strong emotions such as happiness, excitement, or anticipation, but they are certainly different from the emotions of fear, anxiety, and dread that he felt while enroute to the car accident.

As you can imagine, many different emotions may be experienced during a stress reaction. Table 4-2 lists some of the many emotions an EMT may experience as a response to stress.

Physical Response

Despite the individual factors involved in the perception of stress, the physical response tends to be quite similar among people. When a person is faced with a stressor, the body's physical reaction is to prepare to defend itself either by fighting or running away from the stressor. This is sometimes called the **fight or flight response**.

TABLE 4-1

Common Stressors for an EMT

Type of Stressor	Examples
Physiological	Trauma
	Illness
	Poor nutrition
	Sleep disturbances
	Hunger
	Discomfort
	Pain
Psychological	Worry
	Fear
	Anger
	Happiness
Cognitive	Thoughts
	Perceptions
	Interpretation of events
	Personal significance of events
Environmental	Temperature (weather)
	Air pollution
	Noise pollution
	Crowding
	Time pressures
Sociocultural	Job loss or promotion
	Work situations
	Changes in interpersonal relationships
	Interpersonal conflict

Adapted from DeLaune, S., and Ladner, P. (2002). *Fundamentals of Nursing: Standards & Practice* (2nd ed.). Clifton Park, NY: Thomson Delmar Learning.

TABLE 4-2

Stress-Related Emotions

Anger	Pressure
Anxiety	Distress
Fear	Boredom
Competitiveness	Affection
Embarrassment	Intimacy
Defeat	Love
Confusion	Hopefulness
Jealousy	Superiority
Disappointment	Trust
Regret	Satisfaction
Guilt	Joy
Depression	Happiness
Despair	Exhilaration
Suspicion	Delight
Defensiveness	Silliness
Frustration	Pensiveness
Hurt	Shyness
Inferiority	Thoughtfulness
Rejection	Moodiness
Repulsion	

This response originates in the sympathetic nervous system. The effects on the body include increased heart rate, increased blood pressure, increased respiratory rate, increased use of oxygen and glucose, tensing of muscles, sweating, dilation of pupils, and the shunting away of blood from the skin, toward the muscles and body organs.

The results of these effects are the feeling of a rapid heartbeat, sweatiness, tenseness, cool and clammy skin, and sometimes anxiety. Table 4-3 highlights common physical responses to stress.

Some of the hormones released during this response can last in the body for hours, days, or even weeks. Consequently, the physical effects may continue to be felt for several weeks after the stressful incident (Figure 4-1). EMTs must learn to expect these feelings and cope with them as much as possible to allow continued performance of necessary duties.

TABLE 4-3

Common Responses to Stress

Physiological

Cardiovascular/respiratory
- Increased pulse
- Increased blood pressure
- Rapid, shallow breathing

Neurologic
- Dizziness
- Headache
- Dilated pupils

Endocrine
- Increased blood glucose and cortisol

Gastrointestinal
- Nausea
- Altered appetite
- Diarrhea or constipation

Genitourinary
- Frequent urination

Musculoskeletal
- Tension
- Twitching

Cognitive
- Impaired memory
- Confusion
- Impaired judgment
- Poor decision making
- Delayed response time
- Altered perceptions
- Inability to concentrate

Behavioral
- Pacing
- Sweaty palms
- Rapid speech
- Insomnia
- Withdrawal
- Exaggerated startle reflex

Psychological
- Irritability
- Increased sensitivity
- Sadness, depression
- Feeling "on edge"

Spiritual
- Alienation
- Social isolation
- Feeling of emptiness

Adapted from DeLaune, S., and Ladner, P. (2002). *Fundamentals of Nursing: Standards & Practice* (2nd ed.). Clifton Park, NY: Thomson Delmar Learning.

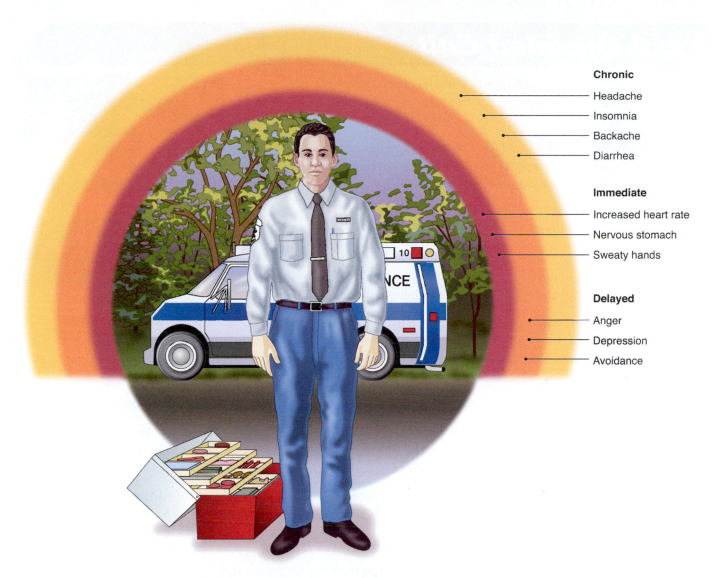

Chronic
- Headache
- Insomnia
- Backache
- Diarrhea

Immediate
- Increased heart rate
- Nervous stomach
- Sweaty hands

Delayed
- Anger
- Depression
- Avoidance

FIGURE 4-1   Stress has numerous physical effects. Some reactions are immediate, whereas others are delayed.

CALL-RELATED STRESS

Several types of circumstance are known to cause stress for most emergency service providers while on the job. These tend to be situations that are highly emotionally charged. A few of them are introduced here to prepare you for what you may see during your job as an EMT. Being prepared for your body's reaction to situations you may encounter will be the first step you take in effectively managing the effects of stress in your life.

Death

Encountering death while on the job is considered to be one of the most stressful events an EMT will experience. Feelings of sadness or grief are expected and are considered healthy for a health care provider when faced with the death of a patient. Feelings of helplessness, despair, or even of failure are also common when an EMT tends to a dying patient.

A Dreaded Call

Just as Dan and Kris sat down to eat, the alert tones sounded. As they hastily departed the restaurant, Dan wondered if he would be likely to eat at all that day.

Dan gingerly slid into the front seat, remembering that his back was still sore from this morning's rescue. He fastened his seat belt and acknowledged the call on the mobile radio.

The dispatcher advised, "Car fire, possible persons trapped, fire-rescue dispatched, corner of Palma Boulevard and Gipp Road, time out 13:40."

This was a call that Dan dreaded. His brother had died from burns due to a fire, and he remembered how much pain his brother had been in before he died. This memory caused his stomach to become instantly queasy.

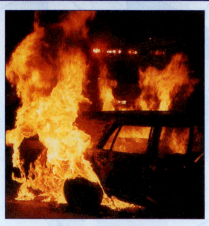

(Courtesy of Craig Smith.)

Attempting to put the painful memory out of his mind, Dan tried to concentrate on the task at hand. "Focus on the basics. Remember, critical trauma patients are extricated in less than 10 minutes; stick to the ABCs." He could almost picture his EMT instructor over his shoulder. His heart was pounding, and his back was getting stiff.

Arriving on scene Dan and Kris found that the car had crashed into the side of a tractor-trailer. The gas tank on the truck had ruptured and caught fire.

The fire was quickly extinguished by fire-rescue, but through the smoke the hands of the driver could be seen thrashing around. Fire-rescue was already busy cutting the car apart as Dan donned his protective gear.

"Will I remember what to do?" Dan thought as he entered the car. The palms of his hands were already slick with sweat as he thought, "Airway. Airway is always first." In the meantime, Kris had climbed into the backseat. She yelled out over the loud din of the power tools, "Hey, do you want me to take head stabilization first?" Frustrated, Dan thought to himself, "I know that I am supposed to take manual stabilization first, how could I forget!" Wondering if Kris could see how red his face was, Dan quickly checked the driver for breathing and a pulse.

- What stressors was Dan experiencing?
- What were Dan's physical and emotional responses to those stressors?
- What triggered Dan's response?

Often in the course of the job an EMT will be faced with a situation in which a life cannot be saved. It is certainly a very powerful situation and would be considered by most to be stressful, whatever the level of experience of the provider.

If a positive aspect of the event is identified, the stress response may be lessened. For example, an EMT may feel sad about the death of a terminally ill patient yet be glad to have been able to comfort the family. The realization that there are positive aspects of most stressors will help EMTs manage the stress in their lives more effectively.

Trauma

Situations involving traumatic injuries may be stressful to EMS providers. Trauma often affects young people and has the potential to devastate many lives (Figure 4-2). The EMT may also be facing a situation in which he experienced a similar incident, as in the case study on page 58. The EMT may experience feelings of fear or anxiety when faced with such a situation.

If prepared, the EMT may be able to quickly dispel those feelings and return to the task of caring for the injured patient. The emotions an EMT may experience at such a scene may be overwhelming. It is sometimes necessary for the EMT to step back from the situation for a moment to clear her thoughts before she can effectively care for the patient. Some specific situations that may evoke particularly powerful emotions include motor vehicle collisions, amputations, shootings, decapitations, and injuries to children.

Family, Friends, and Coworkers As Patients

EMTs will sometimes be required to care for ill or injured family members, friends, or coworkers (Figure 4-3). It is very difficult to have to care for someone with whom you have emotional ties.

The EMT will likely experience overwhelming feelings of fear, anxiety, and frustration when faced with such a situation and may be reminded of her own vulnerability. It is crucial, however, that she be able to continue to work effectively. An EMT who feels that she cannot work effectively should immediately make arrangements for another EMT to take over.

Abuse

Another stressful situation EMTs will likely encounter is that of caring for a potentially abused individual. Whether that patient is an infant, child, adult, or elder, the feelings of suspicion, anger, and perhaps sadness cannot be avoided. It is important for the EMT to withhold blame and treat all involved nonjudgmentally. It is beyond the scope of an EMT's duty to determine the guilt or innocence of a potential abuser.

The responsibility of the EMT is to remove the patient from a potentially harmful environment and care for any injuries. The specifics of how to recognize and report abuse will be discussed in more detail in later chapters. Understanding that a strong emotional reaction is likely will help the EMT to continue to function in such a situation.

Disasters

An incident involving multiple injured patients, or a **multiple casualty incident (MCI)**, is a high-stress situation. These situations are often the result of a natural disaster or an act of terrorism (Figure 4-4). The first arriving teams are often overwhelmed and unable to adequately care for everyone injured.

Special training is also needed to learn to handle such an incident. Handling MCIs is covered in detail in a later chapter. It is important for the EMT to realize that she will not be alone in managing such a scenario.

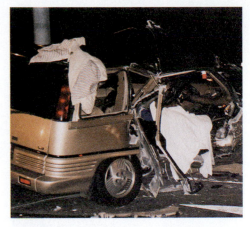

FIGURE 4-2 Terrible suffering can invoke powerful feelings in an EMT. (Courtesy of Craig Smith.)

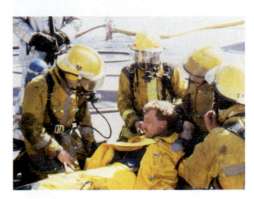

FIGURE 4-3 The death or serious injury of a coworker is a very stressful event for an EMT.

Before the terrorist attacks on the World Trade Center and the Pentagon on September 11, 2001, most EMS providers assumed that terrorism only occurred in other countries and the likelihood of large-scale terrorism occurring in their community was remote. That expectation changed after September 11, and EMS providers must be ever vigilant of the potential for events related to weapons of mass destruction, such as biological, nuclear, incendiary, chemical weapons, and explosives (B-NICE).

Although special training for an emergency response to terrorism can help to mitigate the fear caused by weapons of mass destruction, the addition of another stressor, and the constant attentiveness that it demands, can lead to fatigue and eventual exhaustion.

STRESS RELATED TO JOB DYNAMICS

Several aspects of a job in emergency services are inherently stress producing. The need for constant training, long hours, and relatively low pay add to the stress of recurrent exposure to high-stress events interspersed by sometimes long inactive periods.

The often less-than-ideal working conditions of the EMT certainly do not foster a stress-free work environment. It is important for the EMT to recognize the source of job stressors so that she may identify them and contribute to an effective stress management program.

Training

The training of all health care providers is continuous. Initial training and then continuing education with constant updates are essential to continue to provide quality medical care. This schedule of learning may prove to be stressful for persons who are not comfortable in a classroom environment. Altering the pattern of educational opportunities may reduce the stress brought on by recurrent classroom activities.

Work Hours

In most areas of the United States, EMS providers work 12-hour or 24-hour shifts. This means that they spend long periods of time with coworkers, away from family and friends. In a busy system, such long shifts can be physically and emotionally exhausting.

Pay

In comparison with the important role emergency medical services plays in society, EMTs are compensated rather poorly in many areas of the country. There certainly are exceptions, but for the most part, EMT salaries are on the low end of the pay scale. Because of their low pay, some EMTs have to hold down several jobs or work overtime in order to make ends meet.

Poor Sleeping and Eating Opportunities

During a tour of duty, an EMT must find time to eat and sleep (on longer shifts). This time is often interrupted by emergency calls or

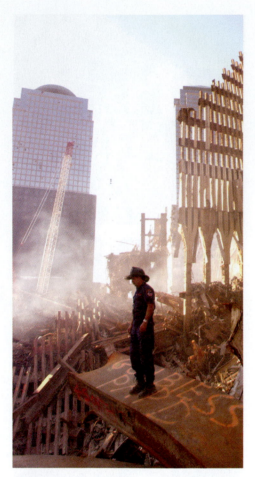

FIGURE 4-4 Terrorist acts, like the September 11 attack on the World Trade Center, are examples of extreme disasters. (Photo by Andrea Booher/FEMA News Photo.)

other job requirements. Lack of adequate time for sleeping and rushed eating habits can cause an EMT to be more susceptible to other stressors (Figure 4-5).

Lack of Formal Rewards

Despite the intense dedication of many EMTs to their work, formal rewards are received infrequently in EMS. The EMT will learn that the most satisfying reward is to be told thank you or to see a patient smile. Regular reward programs can also make a sometimes relatively thankless job more fruitful.

STRESS RELATED TO THE HOME ENVIRONMENT

Many EMTs have significant responsibilities at home as well as at work. Maintaining personal relationships, parenting, caring for elderly parents, and running a household are only some of the key issues many adults face at home.

The family of an EMT may not be able to fully comprehend the daily stressors of a job in emergency services. This lack of understanding may lead the EMT to be reluctant to share with her family the events of her day. This reluctance may cause her family to feel ignored or frustrated. Attempting to relate some of her experiences to her family may provide the EMT with a needed release and will fulfill her family's need to share in her life.

Time Issues

The EMT will often work long hours. A shift is not always over at its scheduled time because of the unexpected nature of emergency calls. Overtime is sometimes required. This type of shift work is often difficult for a family to deal with.

Some EMTs remain "on call" while at home, responding when needed from home. Being on call makes planning difficult for family members. Minimizing changes in work schedules will allow the EMT and her family to become accustomed to a particular schedule and may reduce some of this stress.

It is important for the EMT to keep a significant period of time completely free for family activities (Figure 4-6). This commitment will serve to help the EMT's family avoid feeling ignored.

Social Life

In addition to spending time with family members, it is important for the EMT to find time to spend with friends. It is these social contacts that will provide a necessary break from the stresses of family and work. It is this **unwind time** that can be a means to reduce the effects of daily stress upon the EMT. This time should include participation in hobbies or favorite sports or other forms of exercise (Figure 4-7). The importance of relaxation and of physical exercise is discussed later in this chapter.

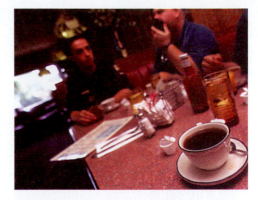

FIGURE 4-5 Poor eating habits can contribute to the body's inability to adequately cope with stressors.

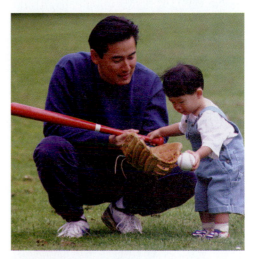

FIGURE 4-6 Family activities may be a useful break from the stress of the job. (Courtesy of PhotoDisc.)

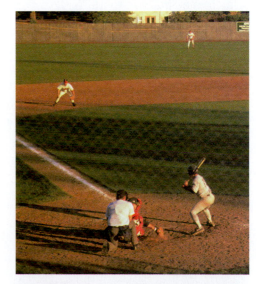

FIGURE 4-7 It is important for an EMT to have some relaxation time. (Courtesy of PhotoDisc.)

TABLE 4-4
Stress-Related Disorders

Respiratory disorders
    Emphysema
    Chronic bronchitis
    Asthma

Cardiovascular disorders
    Hypertension
    Cardiac arrhythmias
    Migraine headaches

Endocrine disorders
    Thyroid problems
    Diabetes
    Excessive weight gain or loss

Musculoskeletal disorders
    Chronic back pain
    Arthritis

Genitourinary disorders
    Loss of bladder control
    Urinary frequency

Sexual and reproductive disorders
    Low libido
    Impotence
    Menstrual irregularities

Gastrointestinal disorders
    Colitis
    Chronic constipation
    Ulcers
    Gastritis

Integumentary disorders
    Eczema
    Hives
    Psoriasis

Adapted from DeLaune, S., and Ladner, P. (2002). *Fundamentals of Nursing: Standards & Practice* (2nd ed.). Clifton Park, NY: Thomson Delmar Learning.

MANAGING PERSONAL STRESS

An EMT will be repeatedly exposed to multiple stressors daily, both at work and at home. It is crucial for the EMT to learn to expect stress and prepare for it as much as possible. There are many actions and techniques an EMT can use to manage the stressors he is exposed to.

Personal Well-Being

Stress can exert an emotional and physical toll on the body. Mental and physical preparations are both key elements in reducing those effects. It is important for the EMT to maintain the best emotional and physical condition he can.

Allowing enough time for nonstressful activities such as hobbies or exercise is crucial. The classic personality of an EMT is often the always-busy, on-the-run type of person. This constant running will allow stress to build up without an avenue for release and can lead to significant health issues.

Persistent stress can actually decrease the body's immune capabilities, leaving the individual susceptible to many infectious diseases. Other physical diseases that have been associated with prolonged stress are high blood pressure, heart disease, migraine headaches, and stomach ulcers. Table 4-4 highlights some common disorders related to stress. The EMT must be aware of these possibilities and take control of her life to prevent such complications.

Healthy Lifestyle

The first step in physical and mental preparation for frequent exposure to stress is to maintain a **healthy lifestyle**. This includes exercise, a balanced diet, and elimination of unhealthy habits such as smoking. If you start with a healthy body, stress will have less of an effect on your physical and mental well-being.

Some form of regular exercise can be helpful in keeping your body in shape and reducing the actual physical effects of a stressor (Figure 4-8). A balanced diet with limited amounts of sugar, caffeine, and alcohol can also prepare your body to respond well to stress.

Tobacco has been shown to negatively affect the body in many ways, one of which is to increase the physical response to stress. It is best not to smoke tobacco products. Maintaining a balance between work, recreation, family, and health is important in preparing yourself to handle a stressful situation most effectively.

Immunizations

Part of advance preparation for a job in health care is to protect your body as much as possible from infectious diseases by staying up to date on recommended immunizations. An EMT will likely be exposed to several disease processes for which vaccines are available to help prevent disease transmission. Hepatitis B, tetanus, measles, mumps, rubella, influenza, and pneumonia are the most common diseases an EMT can be vaccinated against. Regular testing for tuberculosis is also recommended for people in the health care field (Figure 4-9). Other means of effective infection control are addressed in a later chapter.

Stress and Your Health

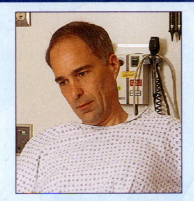

It was the end of another busy night at engine 10. Jim laughed to himself, "Who said EMS means *earn money sleeping*!" Jim had been counting on getting at least a few hours of sleep that night so he could go to his day job and be somewhat productive. He felt exhausted and hadn't been sleeping well lately.

As Jim was changing uniforms, he suddenly had another stomach cramp. The pain was sharp and stabbing. Usually he would have diarrhea afterward. However, this pain was more severe than usual. He called for the supervisor, Nanci, to come into the locker room.

After a quick examination, Nanci advised Jim to go to the hospital, but Jim refused. As a compromise, Jim did allow Nanci to call the company's physician for an appointment later in the day.

At the doctor's office, Jim related that he had been having trouble sleeping, seemed to catch more colds lately, and couldn't sleep, even when he had the chance. Asking to speak to the physician confidentially, he related that he felt he was drinking too much lately and that he was more irritable than usual with both his coworkers and his patients.

- What are Jim's stressors?
- Which of Jim's symptoms could be stress related?
- What can be done to relieve the stress?

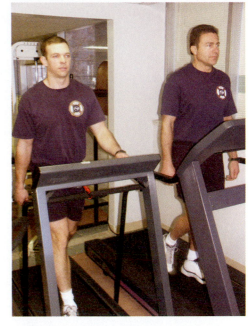

FIGURE 4-8 Exercise is a great way to relieve stress and maintain a healthy body.

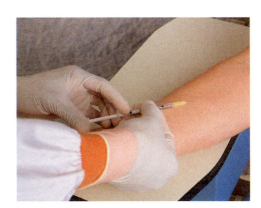

FIGURE 4-9 Health checkups and immunizations are part of an EMT's healthy lifestyle.

Body Substance Isolation

Despite adequate vaccination, it is still crucial for the EMT to take measures to protect himself from infectious diseases such as tuberculosis and hepatitis A, C, and D and from exposure to HIV. Washing our hands frequently and wearing gloves, masks, and gowns when appropriate protect us from potentially infectious body substances. Specifics of such **body substance isolation** are discussed in a later chapter.

Scene Safety

Every emergency scene involves many potential hazards. Potentially infectious body fluids are certainly not to be ignored, but before even coming into contact with the patient, the EMT must address other issues for safety reasons.

The EMT must take every precaution necessary to prevent harm from coming to herself, her crew, the patient, or bystanders. The **scene survey**, discussed in a coming chapter, is the initial evaluation of a situation for potential dangers. It is only by constant vigilance to possible hazards that an EMT will protect herself and remain healthy and able to continue performing her job efficiently.

Stress Relief Techniques

There are several techniques that can be used to help to diffuse or reduce the emotional and physical responses to a highly stressful situation. **Relaxation exercises** can be employed at any time during or after a stressful event. One such technique is the taking of several deep, deliberate breaths while thinking a simple repetitive thought such as "Relax and let go; I am in control." This deep breathing procedure can be initiated when a stress response is first noted and can help the EMT regain focus and decrease or abort the stress response.

Diversionary techniques are also useful for dissipating the effects of an acutely stressful event. Physical exercise such as jogging, swimming, walking, washing the car, or cleaning a room can be useful to release some of the energy and hormones the stressor has created. Other diversionary techniques that can be employed after an event are participation in hobbies or social activities or traveling.

No matter the method used, an EMT should have some form of stress release available at any time. Allowing the effects of stress to build up will only result in a more intensified response to the next stressor.

Recognizing Stress

An EMT's ability to recognize situations that cause a stress response will help her prepare for such an event. Once the cause of the stress is identified, the EMT can find ways to minimize any harmful effects.

Acute Stress

An **acute stress** is a single event that creates a stress response. Once having identified known stressful events, the EMT may attempt to reduce her exposure to them if possible. If the offending stressor consists of being awakened by loud radio tones, the EMT may choose not to work nights or may plan to sleep before and after her shift so that she can stay awake for the duration of the shift. Some stressful events cannot be avoided, but those that can should be avoided when possible.

Chronic Stress

Over a period of time, repeated stressors, resulting in **chronic stress**, can have a significant effect on the EMT's physical and emotional well-being. If not properly managed, these effects can lead to impairment of the EMT's ability to function on the job and even at home.

When an EMT no longer feels able to perform her duties because of the effects of such chronic stress, we describe this condition as **burnout**. If recognized early, burnout can be addressed and managed. If not recognized by the EMT or coworkers, burnout may lead to significant physical and emotional consequences. In some circumstances, formal psychological counseling is required to prevent further deterioration.

Street Smart

One form of relaxation exercise is called guided imagery. The following instructions are a guide to such a technique.

- Assume a comfortable position in a quiet environment.
- Close your eyes and keep them closed until the exercise is completed.
- Breathe in deeply to a count of 4.
- Hold breath for a count of 4.
- Breathe out to a count of 4.
- Continue to breathe slowly and deeply.
- Think of your favorite place and prepare to take an imaginary journey there. Select a place in which you are relaxed and at peace.
- Picture in your mind's eye your favorite place. Look around you and see all the colors, the light and shadows, and all the pleasant sights.
- Listen to all the sounds. Pay attention to what you hear.
- Feel all the physical sensations—the temperature, the textures, the movement of the air.
- As you take in a deep breath, smell the aromas of your favorite place. Savor each aroma fully.
- Focus all your attention totally on your favorite place.
- Breathe in deeply to a count of 4.
- Hold breath for a count of 4.
- Resume your usual breathing pattern.
- Slowly open your eyes and stretch, if desired.

This procedure works best when all five senses are used. Like all other relaxation exercises, guided imagery becomes more effective with repetition. *(Adapted from DeLaune, S., and Ladner, P. [2002]. Fundamentals of Nursing: Standards & Practice (2nd ed). Clifton Park, NY: Thomson Delmar Learning.)*

It is very important that all emergency service providers be aware of the telltale signs and symptoms of chronic stress and burnout. Table 4-5 lists some of the classic warning signs of chronic stress and possible burnout.

If an EMT recognizes these signs and symptoms in herself or a coworker, the situation must be addressed immediately. Most employers have means by which to address such issues.

It is important to take action quickly. The ideal situation is to avoid the cumulative effects of chronic stress by managing issues as they arise. But, if physical and emotional burnout do occur, they should be immediately addressed to return the EMT to her previous level of functioning as well as to equip her with more effective stress management skills.

TABLE 4-5

Physical, Emotional, and Behavioral Signs of Chronic Stress Exposure

Physical
- Increased heart rate
- Gastrointestinal discomfort
- Anxiety
- Headaches
- Insomnia
- Fatigue
- Muscle tension

Emotional
- Feeling on edge
- Depression
- Irritability
- Anger

Behavioral
- Avoidance
- Withdrawal
- Aggression
- Procrastination
- Increased alcohol, tobacco use
- Drug abuse
- Overeating

Stress Management Programs

It is especially important for organizations in high-stress professions, such as EMS, to have a recognized plan to identify and lessen the effects of stress in the workplace. The first step in such a **stress management program** is to realize that prevention is the best option. If stressors can be identified and avoided or minimized, the need for relieving the effects of stress will be lessened.

Many aspects of a job in emergency services will continue to stimulate a stress response. Even though high-stress events are not totally avoidable, an EMT may be able to decrease the number of times she may encounter them.

Even distribution of the stress load among team members should be a goal in every EMS system. In a busy system, the heavier assignments should be rotated. If possible, employees should be cross-trained to allow them to work in several different environments as a way of decreasing exposure to high-stress assignments.

Another way to manage unavoidable stress is to change the way the stimulus is perceived. This can be thought of as changing the quality of the stressor. The EMT should try to think about bothersome situations in a different manner. If a positive aspect of the event can be found, the EMT should focus on that aspect. This positive focus will help to reduce the stress response. For example, if an EMT finds that calls to a local nursing home remind her of her grandmother's death and become quite stressful for her, she should try to focus on a positive aspect of visits to this facility. Perhaps there are interesting paintings on the walls or the nursing staff is particularly helpful. Some aspect of the situation can often be found that will offset the previously unpleasant experience.

Talking about bothersome issues can also help the EMT to lessen the stress response. Coworkers should expect to share such feelings with one another as part of a stress management plan (Figure 4-10).

Comprehensive health and safety programs that are provided by or encouraged by an employer can significantly affect the buildup of stress effects upon employees. Regular physical exercise should be encouraged to help decrease the levels of hormones that are released in a stressful situation. This decrease in stress reactivity can positively affect the EMT. Such an exercise program also will serve to strengthen the body and improve resistance to disease.

Supervisors should be trained to recognize the signs of stress overload and should have feasible options for managing such a situation. Finally, the EMT should not be afraid to speak up and share his thoughts and concerns about the impact of stress upon his life. Once a stressor has been identified, it can be addressed and effectively managed.

Debriefing

After an incident that seems to have had a particularly strong emotional impact on any member of the team, such as those incidents listed in Table 4-6, some form of psychological debriefing may be utilized. In the past, formal debriefing programs such as Critical Incident Stress Debriefing (CISD) or Critical Incident Stress Management (CISM) sessions have been conducted in the immediate post event

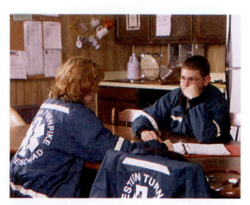

FIGURE 4-10 It is often useful to discuss difficult situations with coworkers as part of stress management.

TABLE 4-6

Incidents That Produce Strong Feelings in Responders

Multiple casualty incident

Death of an infant or a child

Injury or death of an emergency service provider

Severe traumatic injuries

Prolonged response to any situation (e.g., a hostage situation)

Any incident that results in an overwhelming stress response in any of the providers involved period. Programs such as these are structured sessions facilitated by trained personnel meant to review the incident in detail and encourage the involved group of providers to discuss their experience during and after the incident. After these discussions, the group is provided with education regarding stress reactions and stress management techniques. This type of mandatory group debriefing session has been thought to decrease the chance of long-lasting psychological impact of a traumatic event.

The EMS experience with psychological debriefing has increased significantly since the terrorist attacks on the World Trade Center on September 11, 2001. Although most people who have been through a CISD session report that it seemed helpful, long-term studies do not show a clear benefit of CISD in terms of reduction of psychological consequences. Some experts believe that such a process might actually impede the natural recovery that most people experience. Several recent publications report a review of the existing literature, and finding conflicting results. As a result of these newer findings, many professionals are no longer recommending formal CISD sessions. Research on this subject is ongoing. What does seem clear is that in the days following a traumatic event, psychological support, education, and screening to detect those in need of more complex intervention is

EMS in Action

I have worked in EMS for over 20 years and have seen several changes in the field throughout my career. One change I have witnessed is that we have learned it is OK to talk to people about calls or incidents that bother us. In the 1970s, the career expectancy of an EMT or paramedic was 11 months. I am proud to say that now you can have a full career in EMS. It has taken a long time for the field of EMS to get to this point and some good people have suffered before we reached this point.

My partner, also my best friend, was the type of guy who would say after a call, "I don't want to talk about it" and just suck it up. This made it hard to work with him. If you leave things inside too long, you will explode emotionally. One night I was called by my partner's wife. She said he had a gun and was talking about killing himself. I arrived at his home to find him talking about all of the calls that we went on, those calls he could never talk to me about. He was going to kill himself because he just couldn't take it any longer.

I tell you this not to scare you out of the field that I love so much, but to tell you there is always someone to talk to. Many EMS organizations now implement stress management programs. These programs have made the difference in changing the career expectancy from 11 months to a lifelong career.

People may tell you that they could never do your job and the truth is they are right. It takes a person who is well rounded and in good physical and mental shape to do this job. I would encourage you to talk to your partner or to your chief officer. Tell them when you are having problems. Be honest with yourself and with them so that you can better serve others.

This is my career and I welcome you to it. Welcome to my EMS life and have a safe and happy time taking care of yourself and others.

Samuel Yount, EMT-P
Medical Services Officer and Assistant Chief
Pierce County of Washington State (PCFD 17)
Washington State Senior EMS Instructor

appropriate. The presence of severe psychological symptoms one to two weeks after the event may predict the need for individual help. EMS supervisors should be attentive to their staff in this time period and be able to direct individuals toward further treatment when appropriate.

Suicide in EMS

EMTs do not always share their feelings or problems. Some emergency service providers become so overwhelmed by chronic job, home, and social stressors that they take their own life. Suicide is not uncommon in high-stress professions. It is therefore crucial for each provider to be aware not only of her own response to stressors but also of the responses of coworkers.

The EMT must learn to address these issues before friends or coworkers become so overwhelmed that they feel they have no other option but to take their own life. The EMT should know that a job in emergency services is high in stress. Every opportunity must be taken to reduce the effects of this stress and to maintain a constant vigilance to recognize signs of decompensation in others.

MANAGING STRESS OF PATIENTS AND FAMILIES

Understanding the causes of her own stress response is the first step the EMT can take toward understanding and dealing with the emotions experienced by a patient. It is expected that when faced with a painful and frightening experience the average person will feel stressed. Most people have feelings of fear, anxiety, loss of control, and sometimes anger when faced with a personal emergency.

The EMT must remember that despite the seemingly routine nature of a call, the incident is very stressful for the patient. Treating patients with dignity and respect will often gain their confidence. It is crucial that the EMT provide honest explanations and answers to questions.

The EMT must also make every attempt to maintain a patient's privacy and dignity throughout the encounter. Sensitive questions should be asked in a private area, and exposure during examination should be minimized when possible.

Allowing patients to have control over some aspect of their care may help to make them feel more in control. Something as simple as asking whether the patient prefers to sit up or lie down during the transport may return a sense of control and therefore decrease any perceived stress.

Remember that part of the EMT's job is to comfort her patients; things as simple as providing blankets in cold weather, ensuring that the patient's home is secured before leaving, or just holding the patient's hand are very meaningful actions to many patients (Figure 4-11). The EMT can relieve some of a patient's stress by doing any of those things.

A patient's family members will also be experiencing significant stress when their loved one is ill or injured. It falls within the duties of

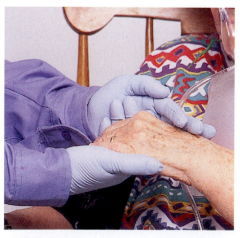

FIGURE 4-11   Simple comforting measures can help to decrease a patient's stress.

the EMT to reassure family members. The family may be experiencing fear, anger, frustration, denial, or depression. Truthful information can be comforting to the family but must be given with regard to a patient's privacy. Listening to a family member's thoughts and fears may provide information useful in the care of the patient and will also reassure the family that the EMT cares about their loved one (Figure 4-12). Providing information and listening to family members will likely help reduce their stress.

CONCLUSION

Stress is the body's emotional, physical, and behavioral response to our changing environment. The EMT should be aware of her own response to stressful situations and should learn to prepare herself in such a way that the consequences of the stressful exposure are minimized.

Because each individual's response to stress is different, the EMT must also be sensitive to the reactions of her coworkers. An effective stress management program will include prevention techniques, relaxation and diversionary techniques, and a comprehensive health and safety program.

Understanding that in the emergency services stress is not entirely avoidable, mechanisms for critical incident stress debriefing must be in place in every EMS system.

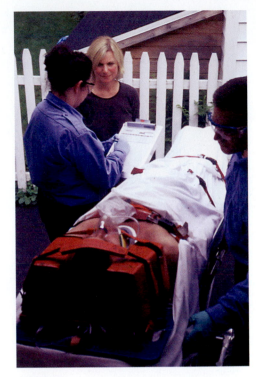

FIGURE 4-12 Taking a moment to reassure a patient's family can go a long way toward decreasing their anxiety.

TEST YOUR KNOWLEDGE

1. What is stress? Is it helpful? Is it harmful?
2. List several personal and EMS-related stresses in your life.
3. What are some of the emotions that an EMT might experience after the death of a baby? Of a partner?
4. What is the fight or flight reaction? What are the physical effects of this reaction? Are these effects seen only with acute stress?
5. What are some positive ways to reduce stress?

INTERNET RESOURCES

For information on dealing with stress in your life, visit the following Web sites:

- The American Institute for Stress, http://www.stress.org
- The Medical Basis of Stress, Depression, Anxiety, Sleep Problems and Drug Use, http://www.teachhealth.com
- Stress Free Net, http://www.stressfree.com

To learn more about dealing with stress related to traumatic events, visit these Web sites:

- National Center for Post-Traumatic Stress Disorder, http://www.ncptsd.org
- International Society for Traumatic Stress, http://www.istss.org

FURTHER STUDY

Angle, J. (1999). *Occupational safety and health.* Clifton Park, NY: Thomson Delmar Learning.

Appelbaum, S. (1981). *Stress management for health care professionals.* Rockville, MD: Aspen.

Bledsoe, B. E. (2003, April–June). Critical incident stress management (CISM): Benefit or risk for emergency services? *Prehospital Emergency Care, 7*(2), 272–279.

Boudreaux, E., Mandry, C., & Brantley, P. J. (1997). Stress, job satisfaction, coping, and psychological distress among emergency medical technicians. *Prehospital Disaster Medicine, 12,* 242–249.

Christie, A. M. (1997). Balancing stress in work and at home. *Emergency Medical Services, 26,* 52–55.

DeLaune, S., & Ladner, P. (2002). *Fundamentals of nursing: standards & practice* (2nd ed.). Clifton Park, NY: Thomson Delmar Learning.

Mitchell, A. M., Sakraida, T. J., & Kameg, K. (2003, April–June). Critical incident stress debriefing: Implications for best practice. *Disaster Management Response, 1*(2), 46–51.

Neely, K. W., & Spitzer, W. J. (1997). A model for a statewide critical incident stress debriefing program for emergency services personnel. *Prehospital Disaster Medicine, 12,* 114–119.

Van Emmerik, A. A., Kamphuis, J. H., Hulsbosch, A. M., & Emmelkamp, P. M. (2002, September). Single session debriefing after psychological trauma: A meta-analysis. *Lancet, 360*(9335), 766–771.

Van Stralen, D., & Perkin, R. M. (1999). Stress reactions: Understand and accept their appearance. *Journal of Emergency Medical Services, 24,* 50–52.

Welser, C. F., & Holmes, J. G. (1997). With'ems: The rest of the story . . . caring for those close to the patient. *Journal of Emergency Medical Services, 22,* 62–63, 65–69.

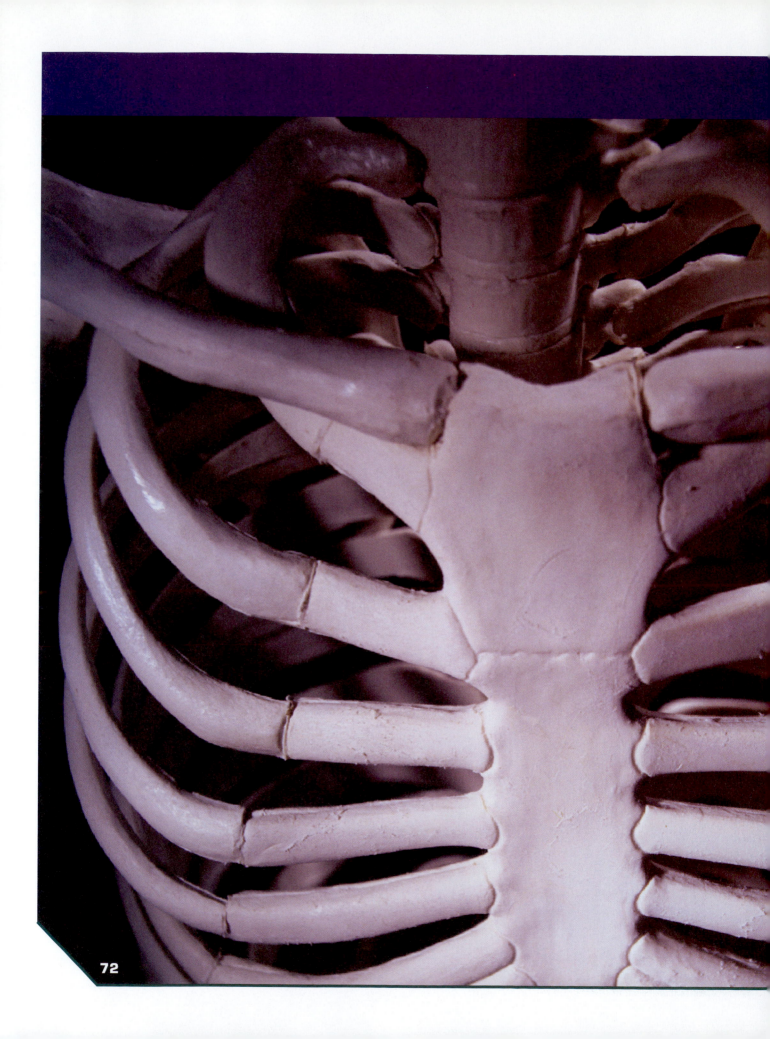

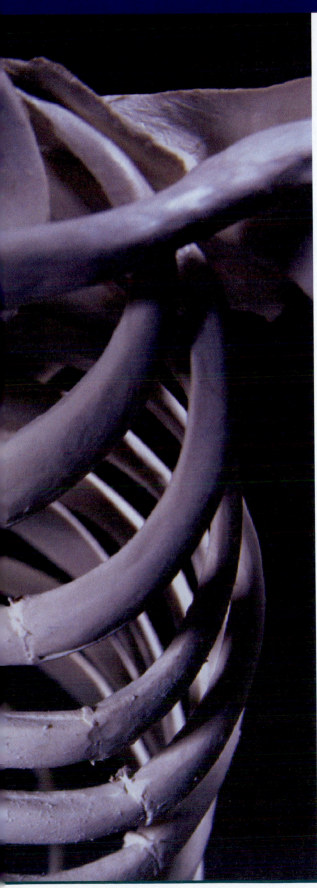

Anatomy and Physiology of the Human Body

To understand the most fundamental concepts of emergency medicine, the EMT must have some foundation in human anatomy and physiology. From an understanding of the essentials of human anatomy, the EMT will be able to build knowledge of patient assessment and emergency management of life-threatening conditions.

This section is an overview of the basics of human anatomy, including topographic anatomy as well as some principles of physiology.

CHAPTER 5

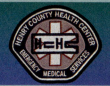 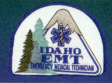 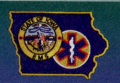

Anatomy and Physiology

KEY TERMS

abdominal cavity
abduction
acetabulum
adduction
alveoli
anatomy
angle of Louis
anterior
anus
aorta
aortic valve
apex
appendicular skeleton
appendix
arachnoid
arteries
atlas
atrioventricular (AV) node
atrium
autonomic nervous system
axial skeleton
axilla
axis
base
biceps muscle
bilateral
bladder
blood
blood vessels

(continues)

OBJECTIVES

Upon completion of this chapter, the reader should be able to:

1. Define the term *anatomy*.
2. Describe and demonstrate the standard anatomical position.
3. List and define the main directional terms.
4. Describe a location of injury using the directional terms.
5. Describe and demonstrate typical patient positions.
6. List the functions of the skin.
7. Describe several important muscles.
8. List the bones in the axial skeleton and describe their function.
9. List the bones of the spinal column and describe their function.
10. List the bones in the appendicular skeleton and describe their function.
11. Describe nervous system function.
12. Describe the physical orientation of the heart.
13. Describe the four chambers of the heart.
14. Describe the heart's conduction system.
15. Compare the locations of the pulmonary and systemic circulation circuits.
16. Define blood and its components.
17. Differentiate between the main types of blood vessels in the body.
18. List the functions of the mucous membranes of the respiratory system.
19. Name the structures of the upper respiratory system.
20. Name the structures of the lower respiratory system.
21. Name the organs of the digestive tract.
22. Describe the location of the major organs within the abdominal cavity.
23. Describe the parts of the urinary system.
24. Name the male and female gonads.

OVERVIEW

To begin to comprehend the nature of a patient's illness, the emergency medical technician (EMT) must have a basic knowledge of human anatomy and physiology. This chapter explores the basic anatomy, anatomical terminology, and concepts of physiology of the human body.

Anatomy refers to the study of the structure of an organism. Physiology refers to the study of the function of the organism. Recognition of signs of disease and the ability to appropriately intervene are dependent upon a basic understanding of normal anatomy and physiology. After learning what is normal, the EMT can begin to recognize abnormalities and learn how to manage them.

This material may seem difficult to understand and the terminology may seem foreign to the EMT student. Nevertheless, it is important that an EMT student learn basic anatomy and physiology in

KEY TERMS

(continued)
brainstem
bronchi
bronchioles
bundle branches
bundle of His
calcaneus
capillaries
carina
carpal bones
central
central nervous system
cerebellum
cerebrospinal fluid (CSF)
cerebrum
cervical spine
cilia
circulation
clavicle
coccyx
costal arch
costovertebral angle
cranium
deep
deltoid muscle

dermis
diaphragm
distal
dorsal
dura mater
endocrine system
epidermis
epiglottis
esophagus
eversion
extension
fallopian tube
false ribs
femur
fibula
flexion
floating ribs
fontanels
foramen magnum
Fowler's position
frontal bone
gallbladder
gastrocnemius muscle
glands
gluteus muscles

goblet cell
gonads
hard palate
heart
hemostasis
high-Fowler's position
homeostasis
hormones
humerus
iliac bones
inferior
insulin
integumentary system
intervertebral disk
inversion
ischium
jugular vein
kidney
knee
large intestine
larynx
lateral
left lateral recumbent position

liver
lower extremities
lumbar vertebrae
lymph
lymph node
lymphatic system
malleolus
mandible
manubrium
mastoid sinus
maxillae
medial
meninges
menstruation
metabolism
metacarpals
midaxillary line
midclavicular lines
midline
mitral valve
modified Trendelenburg position
nasopharynx
nervous system
occipital bone

(continues)

KEY TERMS

(continued)
orbit
oropharynx
ovary
palmar
pancreas
parietal bone
parietal pleura
patella
pectoralis major muscles
penis
perfusion
peripheral
peripheral nervous system
phalanges
physiology
pia mater
plantar
posterior
posterior tibial pulse
pressure points
pronation
prone
prostate gland
proximal
pubis
pulmonary artery
pulmonary circuit
pulmonary valve
pulmonary vein
pulse
Purkinje fibers
quadriceps muscle
radius
recovery position
rectum
red blood cells
respiration
retroperitoneal cavity
rib cage
sacral vertebrae
scapulas

(continues)

order to effectively communicate with other health care professionals. In short, the EMT should be able to "speak the language" of other health care professionals, using correct medical terminology.

TOPOGRAPHIC ANATOMY

All health care providers use standard terminology when referring to different parts of the body. Some of these anatomical terms are based upon the landmarks that exist on every person's body. Other terms use a conceptual framework that is widely accepted among health care professionals. The study of the relationship of one body part to another is called topographic anatomy.

Whenever an EMT describes a patient, he is comparing the patient with a person in the standard anatomical position. As demonstrated in Figure 5-1, the person is facing forward, legs slightly apart, with feet pointing forward, arms straight and extended a few inches away from the side, with palms facing forward.

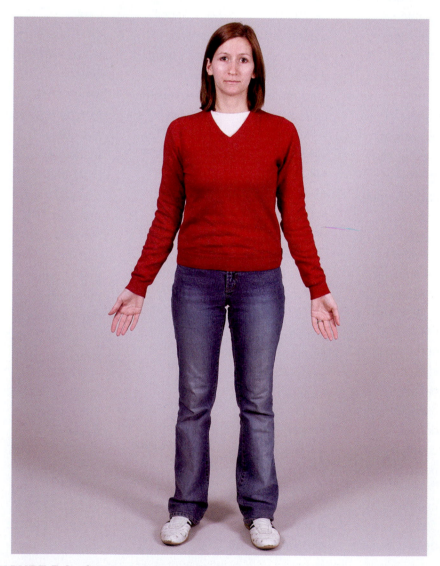

FIGURE 5-1   Standard anatomical position.

Lines of Reference

Imagine the body with several invisible lines across it. These lines of reference can be used when describing an injury. The first line to imagine is the **midline**. The midline runs down the center of the body, equally dividing it into a right half and a left half. To either side of the midline are the right and left **midclavicular lines**. These lines start at the midpoint of each collarbone (**clavicle**) and run parallel to the midline.

Another useful imaginary line is the **midaxillary line**. The midaxillary line runs from the middle of the armpit, or **axilla**, parallel to the midline. These are a few of the more common examples of the lines used in topographic anatomy and are depicted in Figure 5-2.

Directional Terms

With an accepted reference point, the EMT can describe physical findings, such as injuries, in a precise manner. The following describes directional terms, which refer to a landmark or to a line of reference. These terms are illustrated in Figure 5-2. Notice that each term has an opposite.

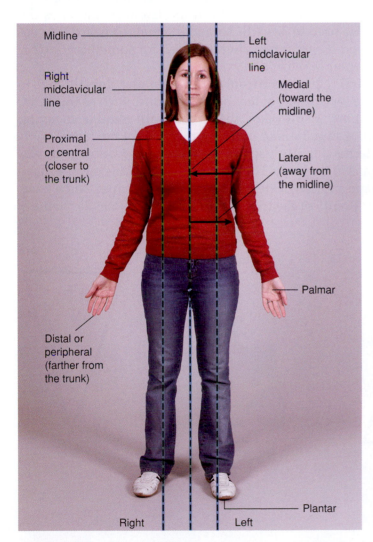

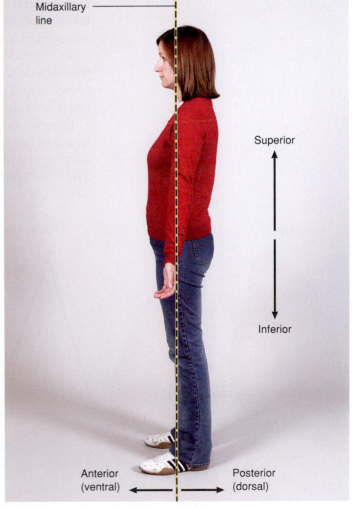

FIGURE 5-2 The standard planes of reference and directional terms.

Any point that is above the reference landmark is considered **superior**. For example, the mouth is superior to the chin. Therefore, any point below the chin must be **inferior** to it. *Superior* and *inferior* can be used to describe any injury or other physical finding provided the reference point is noted, which in this case was the chin.

Similarly, any point that is toward the front of the body is referred to as **anterior**, and any point that is toward the back of the body is called **posterior**.

The patient's flanks (sides) are **lateral** to the umbilicus (belly button). Conversely, the umbilicus is **medial** to the flanks. As can be seen in Figure 5-2, *medial* describes a point closer to the middle of the body, and *lateral* refers to a point farther from the midline.

Many parts of the body are in pairs. For example, ears, eyes, and arms all come in right and left. When describing injury to one but not both, use the term **unilateral**, meaning one side only. Conversely, if both right and left wrists are injured, then say that the patient has **bilateral** injuries.

EMTs often use the terms **proximal** and **distal** to describe a location where an injury exists between two points on an extremity. For example, the cut on the forearm was proximal to the wrist but distal to the elbow. *Proximal* describes something that is closer to the trunk; *distal* describes something that is farther from the trunk. Sometimes the term **central** is also used to describe something that is toward the center of the body, and the term **peripheral** is used for something farther away from the center of the body.

The term **ventral** refers to the front of the body, and **dorsal** refers to the back or to the top surface of any body structure, such as the hand. Other terms that are used to describe position are **plantar**, meaning the sole of the foot, and **palmar**, meaning the palm of the hand.

Directional terms are also used to describe the location and relationship of organs in the body. The heart and lungs, for example, have a triangular shape and can be described as having an **apex** and a **base**. The apex is the "point" of the triangle, and the base is the flat bottom.

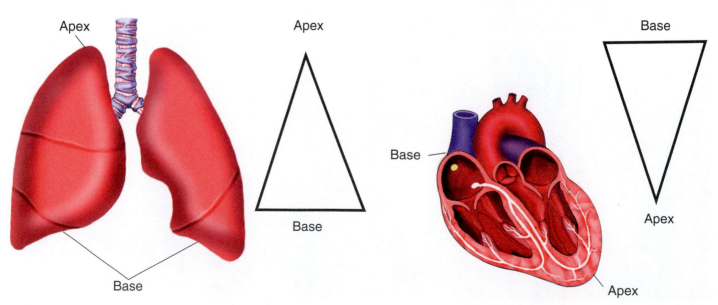

FIGURE 5-3 Apex and base.

The apex of the lungs is at the top, and the apex of the heart is toward the bottom. See Figure 5-3 for an illustration of this concept.

Directional terms are also used to describe the severity of injuries, such as injuries to the skin. The terms **superficial** and **deep** may be used to describe the degree of injury. *Superficial* describes an injury close to the surface, and a superficial injury is less severe than a deep one. See Figure 5-4 for an example of this contrast.

ANATOMIC POSITIONS

The position that a patient is found in or is placed into can also be described using standard terminology. A patient found face down is said to be **prone** (Figure 5-5A). The patient who is placed flat on a backboard facing up with his backbone or spine on the backboard is **supine** (Figure 5-5B).

Some patients may prefer to sit upright. The EMT may place the patient on the stretcher in **Fowler's position** (Figure 5-5C). This is a semisitting position with the head and chest elevated to between 45

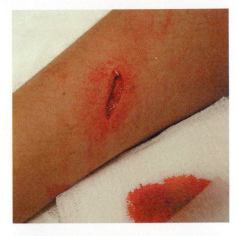
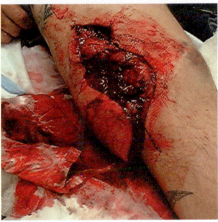

FIGURE 5-4   Superficial and deep injuries. (Courtesy of Deborah Funk, MD, Albany Medical Center, Albany, NY.)

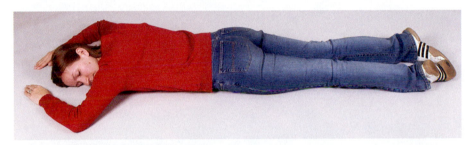

FIGURE 5-5A   Prone position.

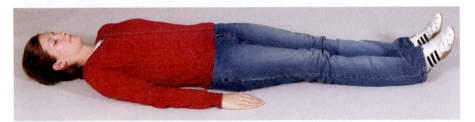

FIGURE 5-5B   Supine position.

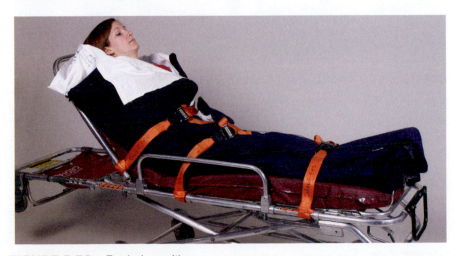

FIGURE 5-5C   Fowler's position.

and 60 degrees. A patient who is sitting bolt upright at 90 degrees is in **high-Fowler's position** (Figure 5-5D).

Patients suffering from shock may be placed in the **modified Trendelenburg**, or **shock position** (Figure 5-5E). In this position, the patient is supine with the legs elevated 12–16 inches. This position is thought to improve blood flow to the brain and other vital organs. Shock and its treatment are discussed in a later chapter. True Trendelenburg position inclines the entire body so that the feet, legs, and abdomen are above the head, but it is often difficult to accomplish in an ambulance.

If a patient is found unconscious but does not appear to have any spinal injury, the EMT may turn the patient toward one side. This position encourages natural drainage of the secretions from the mouth and is referred to loosely as the **recovery position**. In Figure 5-5F, the patient is lying on the left side or is said to be in the **left lateral recumbent position**.

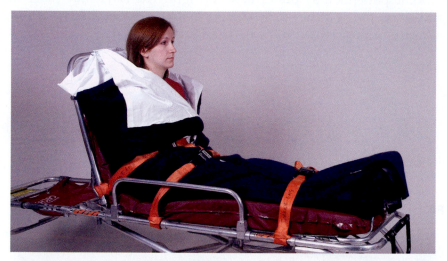

FIGURE 5-5D   High Fowler's position.

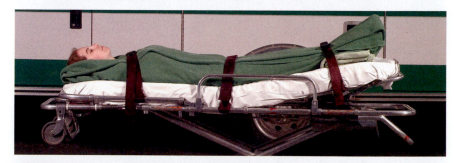

FIGURE 5-5E   Modified Trendelenburg position.

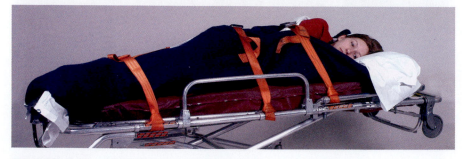

FIGURE 5-5F   Left lateral recumbent position.

RANGE OF MOTION

The ability of arms and legs to move permits walking as well as lifting, carrying, and holding. The arms and legs have a range of motion that enables us to perform these actions. Sometimes injuries limit that range of motion. During a patient assessment, an EMT should note any limitation to the range of motion caused by an injury. Therefore, it is important for an EMT to know the common terminology used to describe motion.

Putting your arm out to shake another person's hand is called **extension**. During extension, the movement widens the angle at the joint between two bones. When a hand is pulled back, with elbow bent, then the arm is in **flexion**. During flexion, the movement narrows the angle at the joint between two bones. Extension and flexion are illustrated in Figure 5-6.

An arm raised straight away from the midline is in **abduction**; when the arm is returned to the side, it is in **adduction**. An example can be seen in Figure 5-7.

To hold a bowl of soup in the palm of your hand, you must turn your palm upward in **supination**. Turning the palm of the hand downward is called **pronation**. See Figure 5-8 for an example.

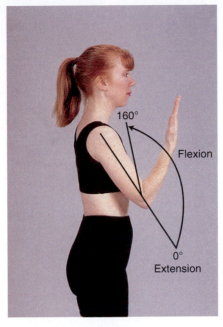

FIGURE 5-6 Flexion and extension.

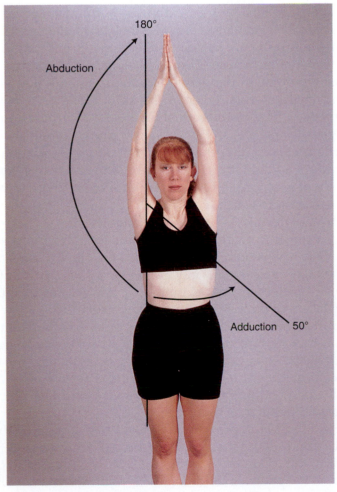

FIGURE 5-7 Adduction and abduction.

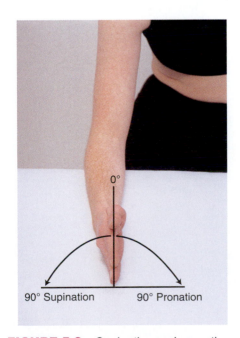

FIGURE 5-8 Supination and pronation.

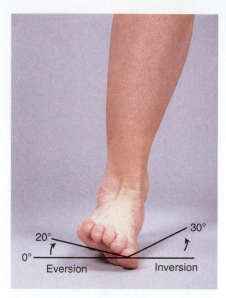

FIGURE 5-9 Eversion and inversion.

Athletes often injure their ankles, and the EMT may be called onto the playing field. If the athlete's foot turned outward, this is called an **eversion** injury. It is more likely that an athlete will twist his ankle inward and sustain an **inversion** injury. Figure 5-9 illustrates these two mechanisms for ankle injury.

The new EMT should practice using these terms in documentation and then have the report reviewed by an experienced EMT. The accurate use of these terms is important. When in doubt as to how to describe an injury, an EMT should use plain English. Other health care professionals will be more impressed with a simple but accurate description than with a "flowery" but vague or even inaccurate description of an injury.

THE INTEGUMENTARY SYSTEM

The skin is made up of many different tissues working together as a system. The skin is called the **integumentary system**, which means "covering."

The skin's outermost layer, the **epidermis**, is actually made up of layers of dead cells. These dead cells are constantly being rubbed, or abraded, off the body. At points where wear is intense, the skin actually develops calluses, or areas of thickened epidermis, to protect the underlying tissues.

Beneath the top skin layer is the **dermis**. Within the dermis are tiny blood vessels called capillaries and nerve endings that can sense heat, cold, pain, and pressure. The ability to feel these sensations is a very important safety mechanism. Feeling heat or pain allows an individual to sense a potentially dangerous situation. Without the nerve endings found in the dermal layer of the skin, these useful warnings would be missed, putting individuals at greater risk for serious injury.

Sweat glands and hair follicles are also found within the dermis. These structures are important in temperature regulation. Sweat glands produce a liquid that can bathe the skin and then evaporate to rid the body of excess heat. In cooler environments, hair serves as an insulator to maintain warmth.

Beneath the dermis is the **subcutaneous tissue** (*sub-* means "beneath," *cutaneous* means "skin"). The subcutaneous tissue connects the skin to the underlying muscular layer. Fat is also stored within this layer, serving not only as an energy reservoir but also as insulation to protect against extremes of temperature. Figure 5-10 shows the layers of the skin and important structures.

The skin has many functions. Perhaps one of its most important functions is that it protects the underlying structures from the external environment. One of the greatest environmental hazards the skin protects us from is disease-causing organisms. Bacteria and viruses do not usually penetrate intact skin. This is a protective mechanism against some types of infection.

Whenever an EMT approaches a patient, one of the first things he may notice about that patient is the appearance of the skin. Careful examination of the skin can provide the EMT with a wealth of information about the patient's condition, such as the quantity of blood circulating. The color of the patient's skin can reveal a lack of oxygen,

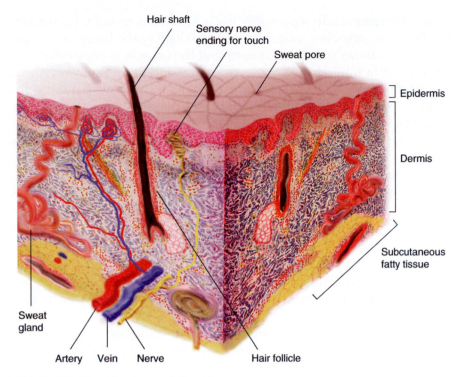

Hair shaft

Sensory nerve ending for touch

Sweat pore

Epidermis

Dermis

Subcutaneous fatty tissue

Sweat gland

Artery   Vein   Nerve

Hair follicle

FIGURE 5-10   Structures of the skin.

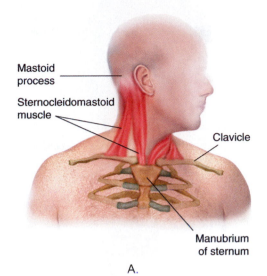

Mastoid process

Sternocleidomastoid muscle

Clavicle

Manubrium of sternum

A.

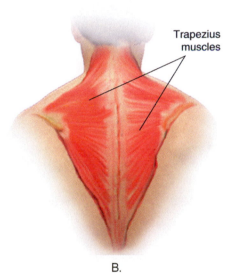

Trapezius muscles

B.

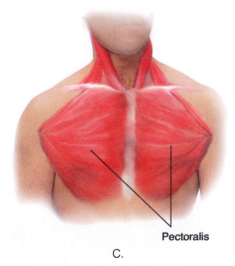

Pectoralis

C.

FIGURE 5-11   Muscles of the thorax. A. Sternocleidomastoid muscle. B. Trapezius muscles. C. Pectoralis muscles.

liver failure, or severe carbon monoxide poisoning. The use of skin color as a diagnostic tool is discussed more in Chapter 10.

THE MUSCULAR SYSTEM

Our ability to walk upright is a function of the unique musculoskeletal makeup of the human body. The ability of muscles to shorten, and in doing so to move the associated bone ends, is what permits movement. There are 206 bones in the human body and more than 650 muscles. An EMT should know a few of the larger muscles and bony structures. Most muscles can be remembered by either what they do or where they are. For example, the temporal muscle is attached at the temple of the forehead and moves the jaw. This muscle helps to chew food.

The **sternocleidomastoid muscle** is named for its points of origin and insertion. This muscle, also called the strap muscle, connects the sternum with the clavicle and the mastoid process and helps to lift the chest wall. Because of this action, it is often referred to as an accessory muscle of breathing as it aids in expansion of the chest wall in times of respiratory distress.

The upper chest wall is blanketed, front and back, by large muscles. The triangular **trapezius muscles** cover the upper back and help to lift the shoulders. The **pectoralis major muscles** cover the anterior chest wall and help to lift the sternum and upper ribs. These important muscles of the thorax are shown in Figure 5-11.

Each shoulder and upper arm is covered and protected by a **deltoid muscle**. The deltoid muscle forms a triangle over the shoulder, with the base covering the shoulder and the apex pointing toward the elbow about two-thirds down the length of the upper arm. This is a site commonly used for intramuscular injections.

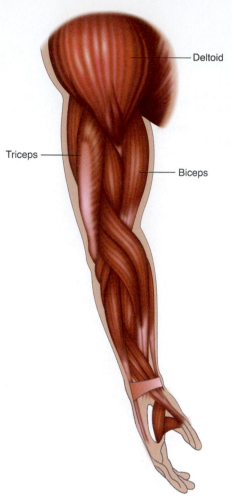

The **biceps muscle** is probably the best-known muscle. The request to "flex your muscles" usually means to display the biceps muscle of the upper arm as the elbow is bent and the muscle is contracted. The antagonist (a muscle that works in opposition to another muscle) to the biceps muscle is the **triceps muscle**, which straightens out the arm at the elbow. A depiction of the muscles of the upper extremity is found in Figure 5-12.

The anterior abdomen is protected by several strong layers of muscles. The **diaphragm** is another important muscle; it anatomically divides the abdominal cavity from the space enclosed within the rib cage, also known as the chest cavity, or the **thoracic cavity**. This muscle is vital in allowing normal breathing and is discussed in more detail later in this chapter. These structures are shown in Figure 5-13.

The legs have a number of muscles that permit a person to stand, walk, and run. The larger muscles of the buttock, called the **gluteus muscles**, are important in allowing proper leg movement. Because of their easy identification, they are also another common site for intramuscular injections.

The **quadriceps muscle** runs down the anterior portion of the upper leg and permits us to extend our leg, such as when kicking a ball. The **gastrocnemius muscle**, or calf muscle, has been called the toe dancer's muscle because it enables a person to stand on his toes. Figure 5-14 shows the muscles of the lower extremity.

THE SKELETAL SYSTEM

The skeletal system constitutes the bony framework of the body. This framework serves two distinct purposes. The skeleton protects vital organs of the body and provides support for erect posture.

FIGURE 5-12 Muscles of the upper arm.

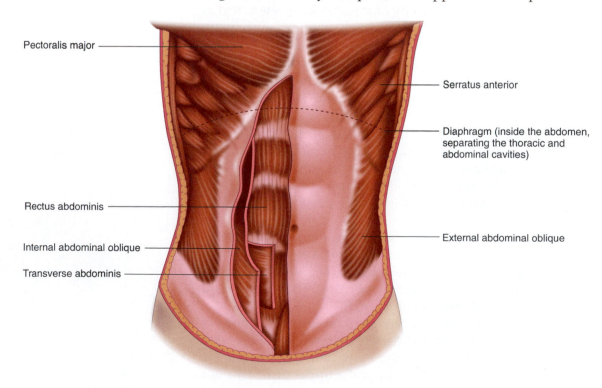

FIGURE 5-13 Muscles of the anterior abdominal wall.

The Axial Skeleton

The **axial skeleton** includes the skull, the spinal column, and the bony ribs that are attached. These form the axis, or core, of the support structure of the body. The primary function of these bones is to protect the underlying brain, spinal cord, and thoracic and abdominal organs. The axial skeleton is illustrated in Figure 5-15.

The Skull

The skull actually consists of multiple facial bones and several bones that make up the cranium itself. Figure 5-16 shows these in detail.

The face contains several large bones that provide support and a form to the jaw, cheeks, and nose. They are also involved in the act of chewing. The lower jawbone, or the **mandible**, is semicircular and contains teeth.

The **maxillae** are actually two bones that fuse at the midline to form the upper jaw. Attached to these bones is the anterior portion of the **hard palate** (the bone that forms the roof of the mouth).

The cheekbones are two bones that give shape and definition to our face. The cheekbones, or **zygomatic bones**, are attached at the temples and arch of the nose. The zygoma forms part of the eye's bony housing, or **orbit**. Parts of the orbital bones are thin and easily broken.

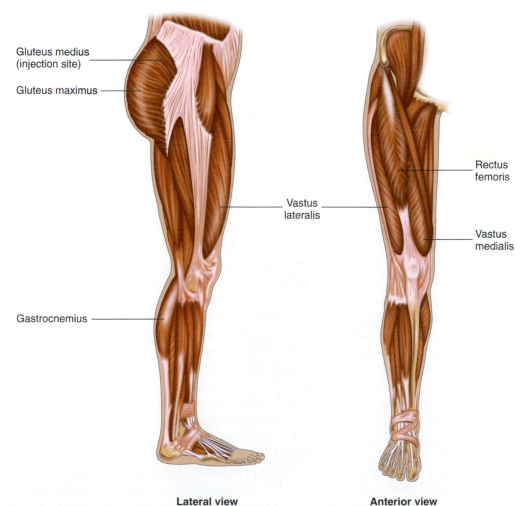

Gluteus medius (injection site)

Gluteus maximus

Rectus femoris

Vastus lateralis

Vastus medialis

Gastrocnemius

Lateral view   **Anterior view**

FIGURE 5-14   Muscles of the lower extremity.

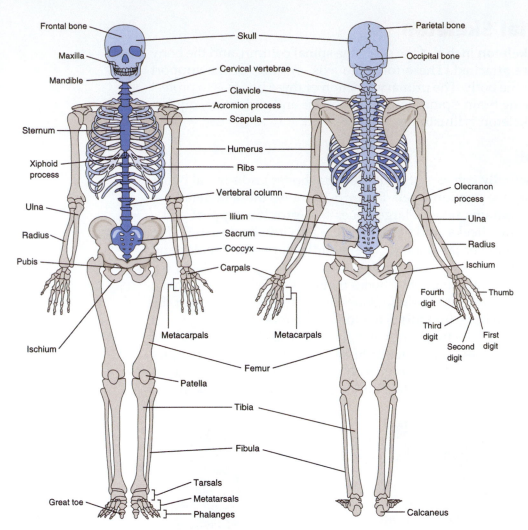

FIGURE 5-15 Axial (highlighted in blue) and the appendicular skeleton.

The **cranium** itself is an oblong egg-shaped collection of bones that is designed to protect the important anatomic structure underlying it, the brain.

The anterior bone that makes up the forehead is called the **frontal bone**, and it is very strong. The **temporal bone**, which makes up the sides of the skull, along the temples, is weaker and more easily fractured with a direct blow. Located in the temporal bone, behind the ears, is the **mastoid sinus**, sometimes called the mastoid process. The term *sinus* means a cavity within a bone.

The posterior bone in the cranium is the **occipital bone**. The spinal cord passes through the occipital bone through a large opening called the **foramen magnum**, which translated means "big hole."

The largest of the bones of the skull is the **parietal bone**, which, by nature of its size and lateral position, protects a large part of the brain.

All the cranial bones are joined at immovable joints called **sutures**. The infant skull is not yet completely fused, and the sutures actually allow the skull to expand as the child's brain grows. Soft, flexible fibrous regions exist where several suture lines meet. These regions, called **fontanels** (Figure 5-17), are easily felt at the front and back of the head as "soft spots." Fontanels normally close and are no longer easily felt by about 18 months of age.

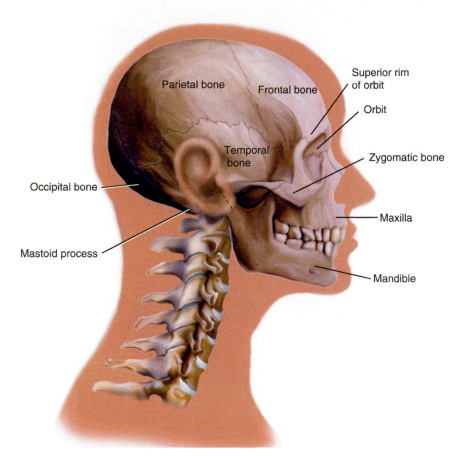

FIGURE 5-16 Bones of the skull and face.

The Spinal Column

The **spinal column** is made up of a series of bones stacked one on top of another in a strong, yet flexible column. This unique design permits the spinal column to act as a series of joints, permitting bending, and to bear the weight of the entire body. The spinal column serves to support the head and provides for attachment of the ribs. Another important function is to protect the spinal cord, which lies within it.

The individual bones are called **vertebrae**. Each vertebra, except for the first two, has a drum-shaped center, called the vertebral body, that bears weight. A fibrous pad called an **intervertebral disk** cushions each vertebra. Posterior to the vertebral bodies are rings of bone that create the **vertebral foramen**, which houses the **spinal cord** (a collection of nerves that runs from the brain through the spinal column and branches to body organs and tissues). Figure 5-18 illustrates the anatomy of the spinal column.

The spinal column has five distinct sections. The first is the cervical spine (or curvature), then the thoracic spine, followed by the lumbar spine, and finally the sacrum and coccyx.

The **cervical spine** (the uppermost section of the spinal column) is of particular importance to EMTs because it is particularly susceptible to injury during any traumatic event. In total, there are seven cervical vertebrae.

The posterior portion of the vertebra is called the **spinous process**. The spinous process of the seventh cervical vertebra can be easily felt, or palpated, at the base of the neck.

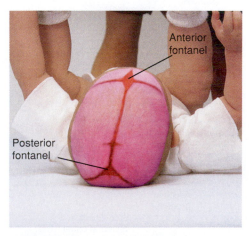

FIGURE 5-17 Fontanels of an infant's skull.

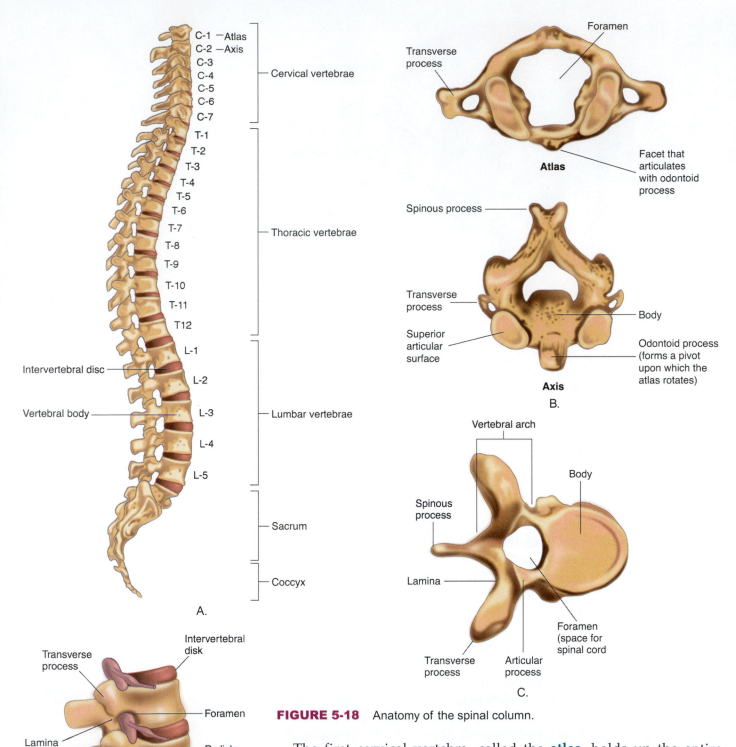

FIGURE 5-18 Anatomy of the spinal column.

The first cervical vertebra, called the **atlas**, holds up the entire weight of the skull, like the mythical giant who is depicted as holding up the weight of the world. The second cervical vertebra is called the **axis**. This vertebra allows the head to turn from side to side, as the axle in a car allows the wheels of the car to go around.

An injury to any area of the cervical spine is potentially lethal if it damages the cervical spinal cord. The cervical portion of the spinal column is supported by muscles and ligaments but is not as well supported as the remainder of the spinal column, thus leaving it open to injury. To visualize the relative fragility of this portion of the spinal column, imagine a 22-pound bowling ball on the end of a broom handle. This would be analogous to the skull and the cervical spine (refer to Figures 5-15 and 5-16).

With a sudden force, such as might occur in a motor vehicle collision, either the muscles of the neck are strained or torn or the bones break. The broken bones may then protrude into the spinal canal and injure the fragile spinal cord, or the injury may produce such instability in the vertebral column that injury to the spinal cord may result.

The next 12 vertebrae are called the **thoracic vertebrae**. There is one spinal vertebra for each rib. These ribs originate at the spine and come together at the front of the chest, forming the **rib cage** (bony structure that surrounds and protects the organs of the chest).

The next portion of the spinal column is the workhorse of the spine. The five **lumbar vertebrae** support the weight of the entire upper body. When an EMT bends and lifts a patient, he can put several hundred pounds of pressure on just a few of the five lumbar vertebrae. This pressure can cause quite a strain and if done improperly can result in serious injury.

The **sacral vertebrae** are actually a portion of the pelvic girdle. The five sacral vertebrae are usually joined or fused together to form a more solid point of contact for pelvic bones.

The last portion of the spinal column is called the tailbone, or the **coccyx**. If this bone were broken, for example after a fall, sitting would likely be very painful. The relationship between the cervical, thoracic, lumbar, sacral, and coccygeal vertebrae can be seen in Figure 5-18.

The Thoracic Cage

The heart and lungs, both vital organs, are protected and surrounded by a bony cage. This cage is called the rib cage and is made up of bony ribs, cartilage, and the sternum. Figure 5-19 shows the thoracic cage.

In the middle of the chest is the breastbone, also called the **sternum**. During CPR classes, all students are taught to identify the sternum and its landmarks. To review, the sternum has a **sternal body** or midportion. This is the section of the sternum upon which external cardiac compressions are performed. Logically then, the heart must be under the body of the sternum.

The top section of the sternum is called the **manubrium**. The manubrium meets the body of the sternum at a bony ridge called the **sternal angle**; it is also called the **angle of Louis** and is an important anatomic landmark on the chest wall.

Located at the uppermost border of the manubrium is the **suprasternal notch** (*supra-* is a prefix meaning "above"). Underneath the suprasternal notch lies the windpipe, or **trachea** (a cartilaginous tube that serves as the passageway for air to get to the lungs).

Returning to the main body of the sternum and running the fingers to the inferior portion, the EMT will palpate the **xiphoid process**. This bony protrusion is occasionally broken during external cardiac compressions if the hands are placed too low on the sternum. Underneath the xiphoid process lies the edge of the liver. Pieces of broken bone can injure the liver if external cardiac compressions are improperly performed. Figure 5-20 shows the anatomy of the rib cage and sternum.

The bulk of the rib cage is made up of ribs. These ribs attach posteriorly to the thoracic vertebrae. The top seven pairs of ribs are attached

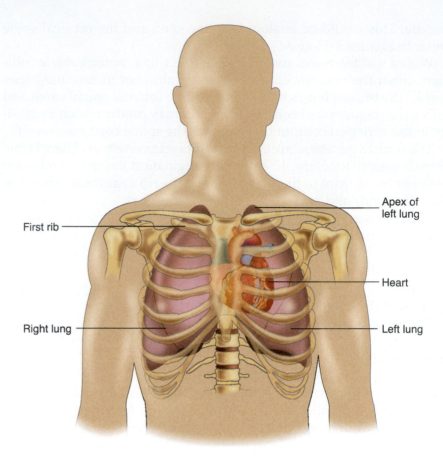

First rib

Right lung

Apex of
left lung

Heart

Left lung

FIGURE 5-19   The thoracic cage. Note how it protects the heart and lungs.

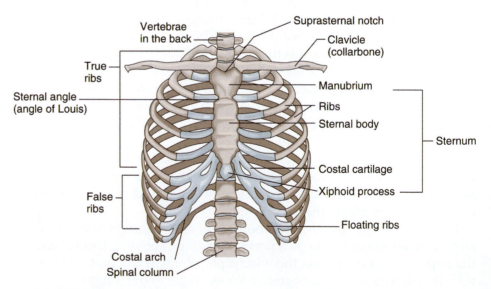

Vertebrae
in the back

True
ribs

Sternal angle
(angle of Louis)

False
ribs

Costal arch

Spinal column

Suprasternal notch

Clavicle
(collarbone)

Manubrium

Ribs

Sternal body

Costal cartilage

Xiphoid process

Floating ribs

Sternum

FIGURE 5-20   Anatomy of the rib cage and sternum. (The sternum and rib cage
are connected by cartilage.)

anteriorly to the sternum by cartilage. These seven pairs of ribs are
called the **true ribs**. The next three pairs of ribs are attached anteriorly
by cartilage to the seventh rib, not directly to the sternum. These are
naturally called the **false ribs**. The false ribs form an umbrella-appearing curvature anteriorly called the **costal arch**. The remaining two ribs
are unattached anteriorly and are therefore called the **floating ribs**.

The true ribs actually protect the vital organs in the thoracic cavity. The false ribs protect other important organs, such as the liver and the spleen, that are parts of the **abdominal cavity** (the space between the chest and the pelvis) but do extend up into the chest. The diaphragm divides these two cavities. See Figure 5-21 for an illustration of this division.

Posteriorly, where the tenth rib and the spine meet is the **costovertebral angle**. Underneath the costovertebral angle lies the kidney, somewhat protected from injury by the overlying ribs. The kidneys lie within the posterior part of the abdomen called the **retroperitoneal cavity**.

The Appendicular Skeleton

The remainders of the bones are a part of the appendages, or limbs, and are used primarily for support and movement. This **appendicular skeleton** is composed of the shoulder girdle, arms, pelvic girdle, and legs. See Figure 5-15.

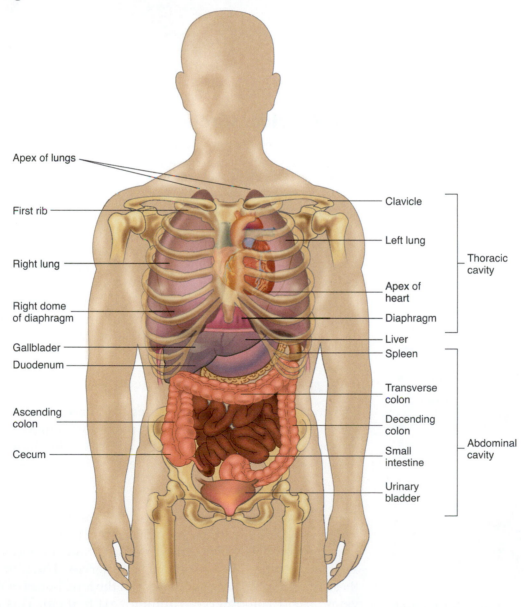

FIGURE 5-21   The abdominal and thoracic cavities are separated by the muscular diaphragm.

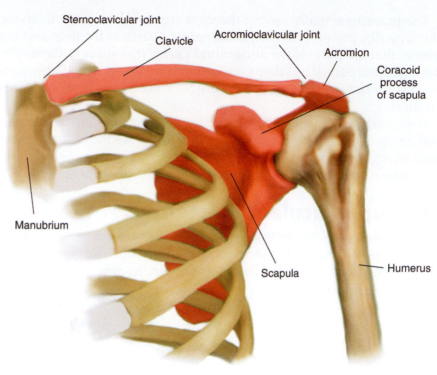

FIGURE 5-22 The shoulder girdle.

The Shoulder Girdle

The shoulder girdle consists of two sets of bones, the clavicles and the scapulas. These bones create an insertion point for the arm to attach to the trunk.

The first bony prominences at the superior, anterior part of the chest that the EMT should identify are the collarbones, or the clavicles. The clavicles protect the thoracic organs from blows from above.

Another pair of bones that lie over the top of the rib cage are located posteriorly and superiorly. These are the shoulder blades, or **scapulas**. The scapulas, imagine the term *blades*, are large flat bones that protect the posterior rib cage. Together, the scapula and the clavicles create the point of insertion for the arms, forming the shoulders. Figure 5-22 shows the scapula and the clavicles and illustrates the interrelation between the two sets of bones.

The Arms

The arms, or the **upper extremities**, and particularly the hands, provide us with the ability to perform uniquely human functions such as grasping and carrying. The arms can be divided into three sections: the upper arm, the forearm, and the hand.

The Upper Arm

The upper arm has only one bone, called the **humerus**. This long bone attaches to the body at the shoulder joint. The forearm attaches to the upper arm at the elbow. Along the shaft of the humerus run veins, an artery, called the brachial artery, and nerves. The humerus protects these important structures. Almost all the long bones of the body have veins, arteries, and nerves running next to them. This association is shown in Figure 5-23.

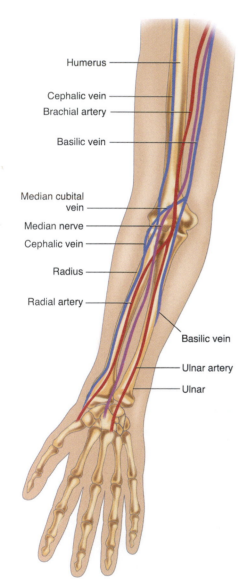

FIGURE 5-23 Note the relationship of veins, arteries, and nerves to the bone.

When a patient strikes an elbow against a hard surface, the nerve along the humerus is pinched between the surface and the bone. Laypeople call this "hitting your funny bone," but the pain created by the impact of the humerus upon the nerve is anything but funny to those who have experienced it.

The Forearm

The forearm has two bones that are attached at the elbow and to the wrist. The bones of the forearm are the **ulna** and the **radius**. These bones are sometimes fractured during falls on an outstretched hand.

The ulna lies on the medial side, closest to the little finger of the hand. This bone provides firm support for the forearm.

The radius attaches to the wrist proximal to the thumb. The radius turns around the ulna whenever the palm of the hand is turned over. When the palmar surface of the hand is facing downward, in pronation, the ulna and radius are crossed. When the hand is turned upward, in supination, the radius bone completes a radius, in a circular motion, and the bones are parallel. The bones of the lower arm are labeled in Figure 5-24.

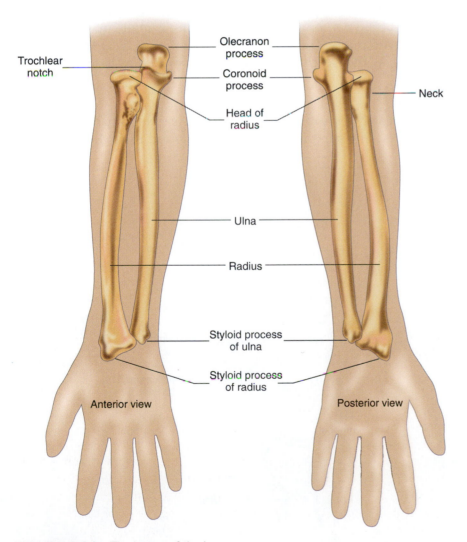

Trochlear notch

Olecranon process

Coronoid process

Head of radius

Neck

Ulna

Radius

Styloid process of ulna

Styloid process of radius

Anterior view

Posterior view

FIGURE 5-24   The bones of the lower arm.

The brachial artery that parallels the humerus divides, or bifurcates, at the elbow, and one artery runs down each of the bones of the forearm. EMTs often take a count of the heartbeat, called a **pulse**, at the point where the radial artery crosses over the radius bone in the wrist. A heartbeat felt at this site is called a radial pulse.

The Hand

Each hand is made up of 27 bones. These bones have been divided into carpals, metacarpals, and phalanges. Together, these small bones enable an individual to perform complex and intricate tasks.

Starting at the wrist, the **carpal bones** form two rows consisting of four bones each. The **metacarpals** form the framework for the palm of the hand. The fingers are formed by bones called **phalanges**. These bones are identified by their position relative to the wrist. The most distal bones are called distal phalanges; the most proximal to the metacarpals are the proximal phalanges. All the fingers except for the thumb have a third phalanx in the middle, called the middle phalynx. The bones of the hand are identified in Figure 5-25.

The Pelvic Girdle

The bony pelvis supports the organs of digestion, elimination, and reproduction. This bony bowl-like structure is made up of the ilium, ischium, and pubis. The spine inserts into the pelvis at the rear; consequently, all the weight of the body is supported by the pelvis.

The Ilium

The most easily recognized part of the pelvis is the "hip bones," or the **iliac bones**. The superior portions are referred to as the iliac wings

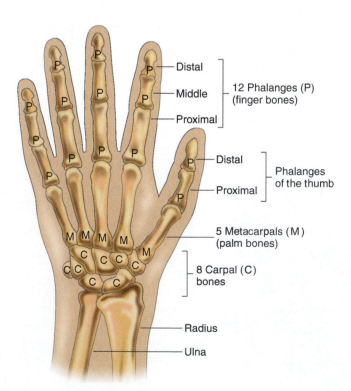

FIGURE 5-25 Bones of the hand.

because of their shape. The iliac crests, at the top of the wings, can be felt on most patients at the point where it is common to put the hands on the hips. The iliac bones create the main shape of the pelvis. The female pelvis is wider than the male pelvis and is well adapted for childbirth.

The Ischium

The portion of the pelvis that supports our weight as we sit is called the **ischium**. A bony prominence of the ischium is used as a point of fixation for splints of the lower legs.

The Pubis

At the very front of the pelvis is the **pubis**, consisting of two bones that complete the pelvic ring anteriorly. The joint formed by the union of the two pubis bones is called the **symphysis pubis**. Directly underneath the symphysis pubis lies the urinary bladder. EMTs may sometimes apply a gentle downward pressure to the symphysis pubis, while assessing for injury, to see if the pelvic ring has been disturbed. The bony pelvis is shown in Figure 5-26.

The Legs

The legs, or **lower extremities**, permit us to stand erect, walk, and run. Performance of all these activities requires a large number of well-coordinated muscles as well as the support of some major bones. Like the arm, the leg can be divided into upper and lower portions.

The Upper Leg

The upper leg has only one bone, like the upper arm, and it is called the **femur**. Found deep within the thigh, the femur is the longest and strongest bone in the body. The femur turns inward at the hip and inserts into its socket in the pelvis, called the **acetabulum**. The area where the femur meets the acetabulum is referred to as the hip. These structures can be seen in Figure 5-27.

The Patella

The **knee** is the joint between the femur and the lower leg. The **patella**, or kneecap, is a bony disc that lies over the anterior aspect of the knee, helping to protect the inner joint. Many people accidentally displace or dislocate their kneecap. However, it takes a great deal of force to dislocate the knee itself. A dislocated knee is a surgical emergency, whereas a dislocated kneecap is not. The patella is labeled in Figure 5-28.

The Lower Leg

Many people have "skinned the shin bone" after falling. The shinbone, or the **tibia**, is the bone along the front of the lower leg, and it is covered anteriorly with only a thin layer of skin. The other bone in the lower leg is the **fibula**, which is found at the lateral aspect of the lower leg.

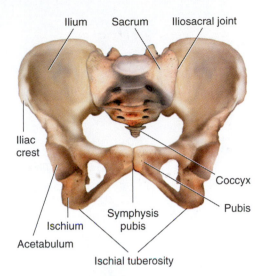

FIGURE 5-26   The pelvic girdle.

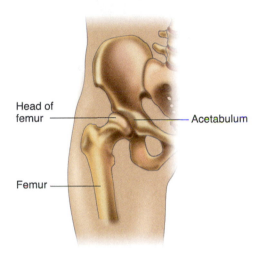

FIGURE 5-27   The ball-shaped head of the femur fits smoothly into the socket-shaped acetabulum to form the hip joint.

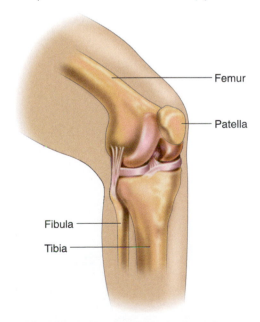

FIGURE 5-28   The knee and patella.

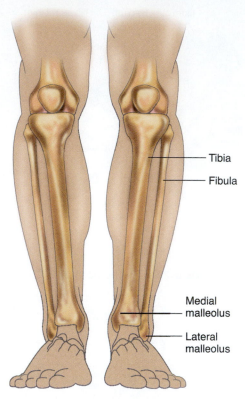

FIGURE 5-29 The lower leg.

On both sides of the ankle are bony prominences of the distal tibia or fibula called the medial and lateral **malleolus**. There is a pulse point posterior to the medial malleolus called the **posterior tibial pulse**. Figure 5-29 illustrates these structures of the lower leg.

The Foot

The saying goes "man is like a monkey, his feet are like his hands." This is true of the bones of the foot with one exception. Instead of being called carpals, the bones are called **tarsals**. The largest bone in the foot is the **calcaneus**, or heel bone. Figure 5-30 shows the bones of the foot in detail.

The Joints

Joints are the points where bones meet bones. Joints permit a degree of movement called the range of motion. Each joint has its own normal range of motion. An injury to a joint may result in a decrease in this range of motion.

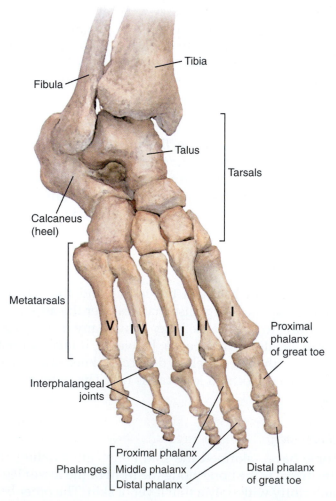

FIGURE 5-30 The foot.

PHYSIOLOGY

The study of the bodily processes of an organism is called physiology. An understanding of how the body works serves as a foundation to understanding how disease affects the body and how drugs help decrease the damage done by disease.

Equilibrium

The body strives to maintain a steady optimal state for growth and development and resists any influence, internal or external, that would upset this balance. This constant state of internal equilibrium is called **homeostasis**.

   The term, first coined in 1932 by Walter Cannon, speaks of the ability of the body to regulate itself internally to maintain those optimal conditions; the "wisdom of the body." Two organ systems are specifically involved in maintaining homeostasis: the endocrine system and the nervous system. The endocrine system is responsible for the more general adjustments in the body's internal organs, whereas the nervous system is responsible for the moment-to-moment fine adjustments.

THE NERVOUS SYSTEM

The **nervous system** controls and coordinates all bodily functions. This complex task involves interactions between three main subdivisions of the nervous system. These subdivisions are the central, peripheral, and autonomic nervous systems. Figure 5-31 illustrates this interaction.

The Central Nervous System

The **central nervous system** is made up of the brain and the spinal cord and is involved in the initiation and transmission of all control-oriented messages throughout the body.

The Brain

The seat of all higher intellect, the human brain is thought to make us different from other creatures. However, in many ways our brains are very similar to those of other mammals. The human brain consists of a brainstem, cerebellum, and cerebrum. These areas of the brain have further subdivisions, each of which has its own unique functions. Figure 5-32 shows these subdivisions.

The Brainstem

The most basic part of the human brain is the brainstem. The **brainstem** acts like a junction box for the complex wiring system of the central nervous system. The upper regions of the brain send all signals to the brainstem to be passed to the spinal cord for distribution to the body. The brainstem consists of the midbrain, pons, and medulla oblongata. All mammals have a brainstem that is involved in the control of life-sustaining functions such as breathing and heartbeat.

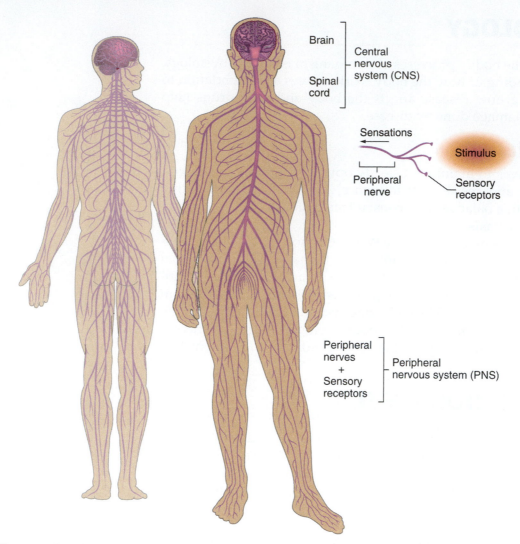

Brain
Spinal cord
Central nervous system (CNS)

Sensations
Peripheral nerve
Stimulus
Sensory receptors

Peripheral nerves + Sensory receptors
Peripheral nervous system (PNS)

FIGURE 5-31   The central, peripheral, and autonomic nervous systems.

The Cerebellum

The word **cerebellum** means little brain. Actually, it can be thought of more as the "athletic brain." The cerebellum controls muscular coordination and complex actions, such as shooting a basketball or driving a car. When a police officer stops a car and tests the driver's sense of balance, as part of a drunken driver assessment, the police officer is testing the person's cerebellar functions.

The Cerebrum

The seat of all higher thinking is the **cerebrum**. The cerebrum is the largest area of the brain and occupies the majority of the cranial vault. The cerebrum is divided into a right and a left hemisphere. The cerebrum can be further divided into different lobes with each having its own specific duties and functions.

The Meninges

We can use the analogy of an egg to describe the organization of the brain. The brain is protected by a hard bony shell. Inside the shell there are membranes, called **meninges**, that surround the brain and

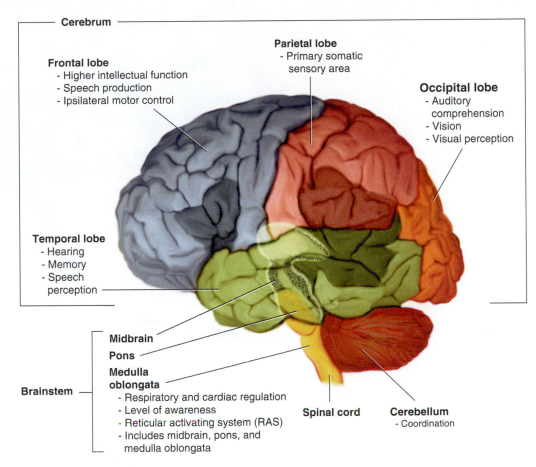

Cerebrum

Parietal lobe
- Primary somatic
  sensory area

Frontal lobe
- Higher intellectual function
- Speech production
- Ipsilateral motor control

Occipital lobe
- Auditory
  comprehension
- Vision
- Visual perception

Temporal lobe
- Hearing
- Memory
- Speech
  perception

Midbrain

Pons

**Medulla
oblongata**
- Respiratory and cardiac regulation
- Level of awareness
- Reticular activating system (RAS)
- Includes midbrain, pons, and
  medulla oblongata

Brainstem

Spinal cord

Cerebellum
- Coordination

FIGURE 5-32   The brain and its subdivisions.

continue along the spinal cord. These meninges pad the brain from impact. The innermost layer is called the **pia mater** and clings to every surface of the brain. The next layer of the meninges is the **arachnoid**. The arachnoid spreads, weblike, over the entire brain. The outermost layer is called the **dura mater**, which literally means "tough mother." Together, the *p*ia mater, the *a*rachnoid, and the *d*ura mater act together to "pad" the brain from injury.

As in an egg, there is a great deal of fluid, called **cerebrospinal fluid (CSF)**, within the skull that further absorbs impact. The CSF also carries nutrients to and removes some wastes from the brain cells.

The combination of the bony skull, the protective meninges, and the shock-absorbing CSF protects the brain itself from impact and injury. These protective layers are seen in Figure 5-33.

The Spinal Cord

The spinal cord originates at the base of the skull and runs down the spinal column. All messages between the body and the brain pass along the spinal cord. The spinal cord can be compared to the trunk-line of a telephone company. Cut the trunk line and all outgoing and incoming calls stop.

The cross section of the spinal cord is about the diameter of a dime in some areas. Moreover, the space between the spinal cord and the surrounding bony spinal canal can be as little as the thickness of a

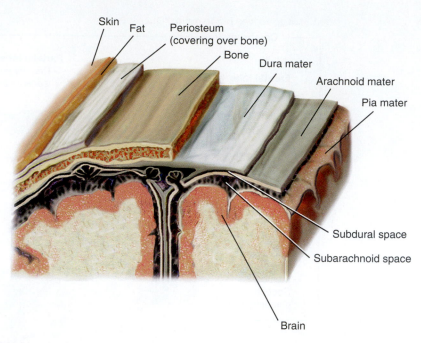

FIGURE 5-33 The meninges are made of the pia mater, the arachnoid, and the dura mater.

pencil's lead. This sometimes precarious positioning can lead to injury to the spinal cord in accidents involving spinal trauma.

The Peripheral Nervous System

The **peripheral nervous system** is made up of nerves that originate in the spinal cord and take messages to the body. Some nerves originate in the body's organs and tissues and transmit information back to the spinal cord, where it is then relayed to the brain. These peripheral nerves are very important and necessary for movement and sensation. Figure 5-34 illustrates the actions of the peripheral nervous system. Part of an EMT's exam will be to test for movement and sensory function. This exam will be testing the interactions between the peripheral and central nervous systems.

The Autonomic Nervous System

The heart muscle, smooth muscles of the body, and certain other structures controlling automatic body functions are under the control of the **autonomic nervous system**. This is a collection of nerves that originate in the brainstem and transmit vital impulses to these organs of the body. Many medicines that doctors prescribe affect the functioning of the autonomic nervous system.

THE ENDOCRINE SYSTEM

The nervous system provides the immediate moment-to-moment control of the body. Helping the nervous system maintain a more constant control of the body is the **endocrine system**.

The endocrine system is probably best known for the hormones that it produces. **Hormones** are chemicals that are produced by certain organs called **glands** and excreted into the bloodstream.

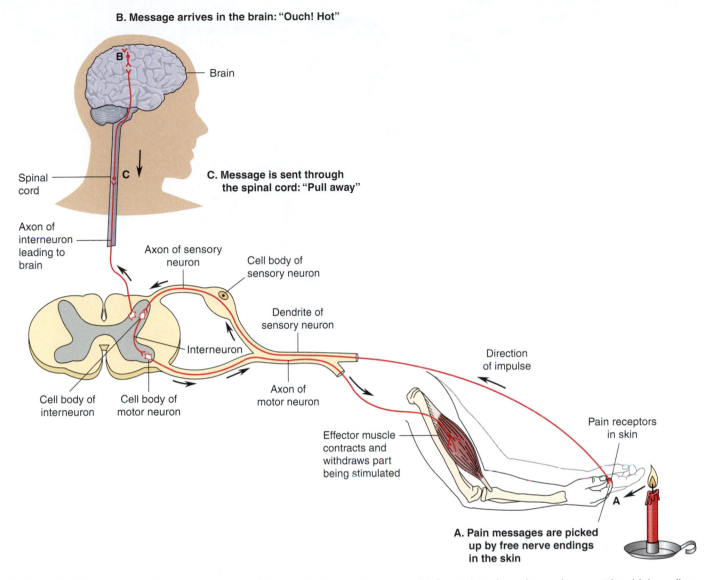

B. Message arrives in the brain: "Ouch! Hot"

Brain

Spinal cord

C. Message is sent through the spinal cord: "Pull away"

Axon of interneuron leading to brain

Axon of sensory neuron

Cell body of sensory neuron

Dendrite of sensory neuron

Interneuron

Direction of impulse

Cell body of interneuron

Cell body of motor neuron

Axon of motor neuron

Effector muscle contracts and withdraws part being stimulated

Pain receptors in skin

A. Pain messages are picked up by free nerve endings in the skin

FIGURE 5-34 The peripheral nerves provide the brain with a rich source of information about the environment in which we live.

Once in the bloodstream, these hormones affect certain **target organs** or cells and change the way that organ or cell is functioning. This sort of chemical message transmission can be affected by prescription medicines. Figure 5-35 depicts many of the glands and target organs of the endocrine system.

An example of an endocrine gland and its hormone that will be relevant to the EMT is the pancreas. The **pancreas** is a rather large gland that is located in the center of the abdomen and under the liver. One of its functions is to produce a hormone called insulin.

Insulin helps the body to use glucose. The pancreas produces more insulin when glucose levels are high, as is typical after a meal. Diabetics cannot produce insulin as needed and are therefore unable to use their glucose, resulting in high blood glucose levels. Diabetics are treated with insulin injections to replace the insulin that their pancreas cannot produce. Insulin replacement is discussed in more detail in Chapter 30.

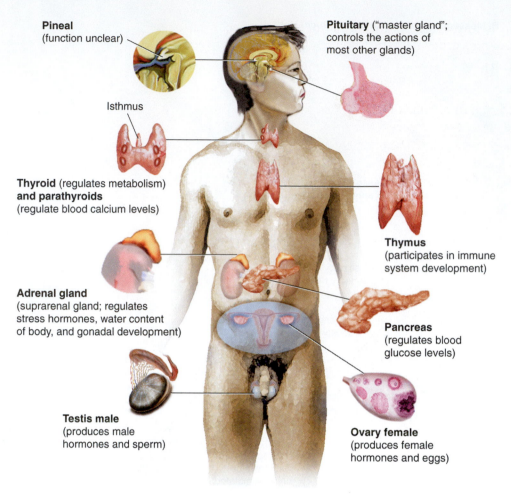

Pineal
(function unclear)

Pituitary ("master gland";
controls the actions of
most other glands)

Isthmus

Thyroid (regulates metabolism)
and parathyroids
(regulate blood calcium levels)

Thymus
(participates in immune
system development)

Adrenal gland
(suprarenal gland; regulates
stress hormones, water content
of body, and gonadal development)

Pancreas
(regulates blood
glucose levels)

Testis male
(produces male
hormones and sperm)

Ovary female
(produces female
hormones and eggs)

FIGURE 5-35 The endocrine system regulates many body functions.

THE CIRCULATORY SYSTEM

Every day the heart pumps gallons of blood around the body one beat at a time. The distribution of blood vessels around the body and back to the heart is called a circuit, and the action of blood flowing in that circuit is called **circulation**.

The purpose of this regular flow of blood is to transport oxygen and other nutrients to all of the organs of the body and to simultaneously remove their metabolic wastes. The **heart** acts as the pump for this amazing system to ensure adequate flow throughout the body. The **blood vessels** are the pipes. Their size and the distribution of blood flowing in them can be altered depending on the area most in need of blood flow. The **blood** is the medium for transport of oxygen and vital nutrients and removal of waste products. It also carries disease-fighting white blood cells, stabilizes body temperature, restricts fluid loss through clotting, and regulates acid levels. The circulatory system is illustrated in Figure 5-36.

The life-sustaining activity of the circulatory system is often taken for granted. However, the circulatory system is so essential to life that any interruption of the function of the heart or damage to the integrity of the blood vessels can have serious and even life-threatening consequences. It is important that EMTs understand the circulatory system and be able to recognize when it is not functioning properly.

The Heart

The heart is a unique muscular organ located slightly left of center in the chest, between the sternum and the spine.

The heart is surrounded by a tough fibrous covering called the pericardium (*peri-* means "around"; *cardium* refers to the heart) that separates it from the lungs on either side of it within the chest cavity.

Cardiac Function

The heart is a remarkable feat of engineering. In fact, two muscular pumps operate independently yet in tandem. The first pump, the right pump, circulates blood through the **pulmonary circuit** so that it may pick up oxygen in the lungs and be rid of carbon dioxide and other wastes. The pulmonary circuit consists of the lungs and the blood vessels within them. This is a very short route and requires very low pressures.

The left side of the heart pumps blood to the entire **systemic circuit** so that oxygen and other nutrients may be brought to the tissues of the body and metabolic wastes may be removed. The systemic circuit involves all the body organs and tissues except the lungs. Therefore, the left side of the heart must pump effectively from the tip of the nose to the tip of the toes. This is a very long pathway and requires the left heart to pump at great pressures to provide adequate flow to all these areas. The pulmonary and systemic circuits are pictured in Figure 5-37.

The pumps of the heart are two-staged pumps. Each pump has a receiving chamber, called the **atrium**, which serves to prime the pump. The primary chamber for each pump, called the **ventricle**, actually performs the work of circulating blood to the lungs and organs and tissues. This relationship is depicted in Figure 5-38.

Direction of Blood Flow

After delivering oxygen to and removing wastes from body tissues, the blood returns via the vena cava to the right atrium, where it is pumped into the right ventricle. One-way valves between the atria and the ventricles ensure continued forward flow. Between the right atrium and the right ventricle is the **tricuspid valve**, so named because of its three-cusp construction.

Once in the right ventricle, the blood is pumped past another valve, the **pulmonary valve** (prevents the backflow of blood), through the **pulmonary artery** (the artery that transfers blood to the pulmonary circuit for oxygenation), and into the pulmonary circulation. In the pulmonary circulation, the blood passes close to tiny air spaces, where it can pick up oxygen and be rid of carbon dioxide and other wastes.

From the pulmonary circulation, the now-oxygenated blood passes through the **pulmonary vein** into the left atrium. From the left atrium, this oxygenated blood passes through the **mitral valve** (also prevents backflow) and into the left ventricle.

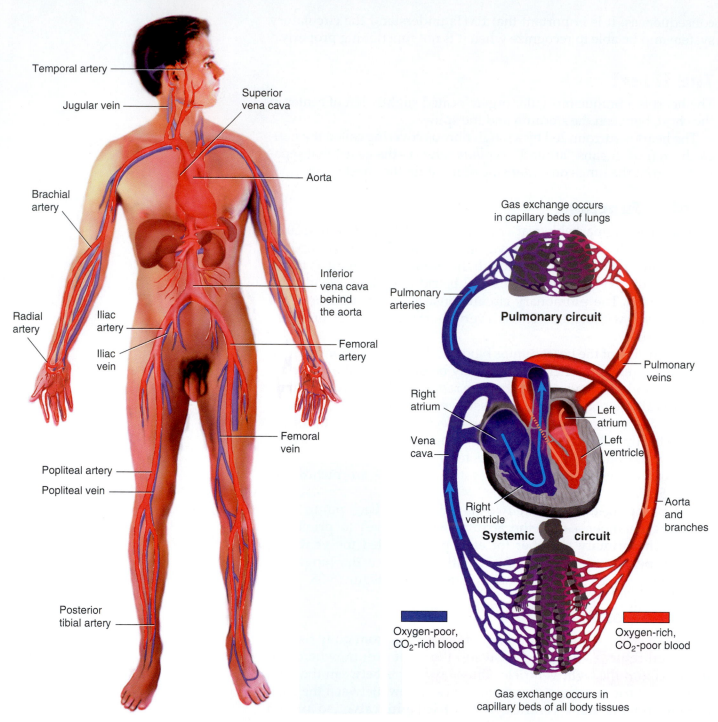

Temporal artery

Jugular vein

Superior vena cava

Aorta

Brachial artery

Inferior vena cava behind the aorta

Radial artery

Iliac artery

Iliac vein

Femoral artery

Femoral vein

Popliteal artery

Popliteal vein

Posterior tibial artery

Gas exchange occurs in capillary beds of lungs

Pulmonary arteries

Pulmonary circuit

Pulmonary veins

Right atrium

Vena cava

Left atrium

Left ventricle

Right ventricle

Systemic circuit

Aorta and branches

Oxygen-poor, CO_2-rich blood

Oxygen-rich, CO_2-poor blood

Gas exchange occurs in capillary beds of all body tissues

FIGURE 5-36   The heart is at the center of the circulatory system.   **FIGURE 5-37**   The pulmonary and systemic circulation.

The left ventricle contracts strongly about 70 times each minute, pumping blood rich in oxygen through the **aortic valve** into a large artery called the aorta and out to the body organs and tissues, where the oxygen and nutrients may be utilized. Once the nutrients have been delivered, the blood returns to the right atrium via a large vein called the vena cava. Now deoxygenated, or without oxygen, the blood is ready to begin another cycle. This continuous cycle is depicted in Figure 5-37.

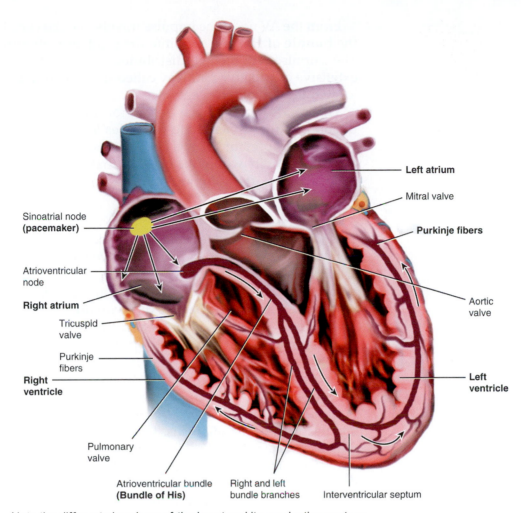

Left atrium

Mitral valve

Purkinje fibers

Sinoatrial node
(pacemaker)

Atrioventricular
node

Aortic
valve

Right atrium

Tricuspid
valve

Purkinje
fibers

**Right
ventricle**

**Left
ventricle**

Pulmonary
valve

Atrioventricular bundle
(Bundle of His)

Right and left
bundle branches

Interventricular septum

FIGURE 5-38   Note the different chambers of the heart and its conduction system.

Electrophysiology

The heart is unique as muscles go, as it is able to generate its own electrical impulses. This feature is referred to as automaticity and is unique to the heart muscle.

Specialized cells within the heart muscle, known as the conduction system, are designed to provide the most efficient means of electrical stimulation of the heart muscle. These unique conduction cells possess several other properties that allow them to do their job efficiently. They not only have the ability to generate their own electrical impulses but also can accept impulses from the cells around them and in turn transmit the message to surrounding cells.

The conduction system within the heart has several distinct cell types (refer to Figure 5-38). The **sinoatrial node**, or **SA node**, is the primary pacemaker of the heart. It generally initiates the electrical impulse that will result in an electrical response from the rest of the heart muscle and lead to a heartbeat.

From the SA node, the electrical impulse will travel down the most efficient pathway through internodal atrial pathways to the **atrioventricular node**, or **AV node**. The AV node slows the electrical impulse momentarily to allow for the mechanical contraction of the heart to catch up to its electrical activity.

From the AV node, the impulse travels into the ventricles by way of the **bundle of His** and then into the right and left **bundle branches**. The impulse will then be distributed through the ventricles via an extensive conductive pathway called the **Purkinje fibers**, which are located throughout the ventricles.

This conduction pathway allows for the efficient and orderly contractions of the atria and the ventricles leading to an effective heartbeat. It is important for the EMT to understand the concept of the electrical activity within the heart so that he may intervene when an abnormality exists, as in cardiac arrest.

The Blood Vessels

The heart is connected to pipelines, called blood vessels, which transmit blood to the organs and the tissues of the body.

A blood vessel is a hollow pipe that carries blood. Blood vessels that carry blood away from the heart are called **arteries**. The blood vessels that carry blood back to the heart are called **veins**.

With one exception, arteries carry oxygenated blood and veins carry deoxygenated blood. The pulmonary artery carries deoxygenated blood away from the right heart and into the lungs, and the pulmonary vein returns to the left heart with oxygenated blood from the lungs.

Capillaries are tiny blood vessels that receive blood from arteries and pass it into adjacent veins. They are so small that **red blood cells**, the oxygen-carrying cells, must pass through them in single file. This may seem like a very ineffective method of circulating blood, but it provides tissues in those capillary beds the opportunity to extract oxygen and excrete carbon dioxide. The relationship of the arteries, veins, and capillaries is exhibited in Figure 5-39.

The Arteries

The largest artery of the body is the **aorta**. The aorta carries all of the blood from the left side of the heart to the body. As the aorta travels downward through the chest, it is referred to as the thoracic aorta. From the point where this large artery passes into the abdomen, it is then called the abdominal aorta. Many smaller arteries branch off the aorta. Figure 5-36 illustrates many of the major arteries of the body.

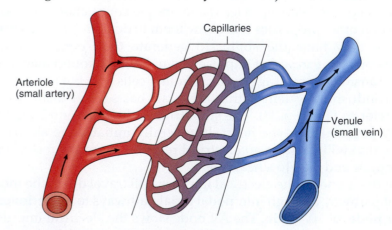

FIGURE 5-39 Arteries deliver oxygenated blood to capillaries and once the oxygen has been extracted, the blood is returned to the venous system.

Each of the terminal arteries is named after a bone that lies close to the artery. Because of the proximity of arteries to bones, a pulse can be felt at each of these points. Perhaps even more important, if a pulse can be felt then, with gentle direct pressure, circulation can be stopped. Therefore, rapid arterial bleeding beyond these **pressure points** could be halted. It is imperative that all EMTs know the exact location of the major pressure points in the body, shown in Figure 5-40.

The Veins

Blood is returned to the heart via blood vessels called veins. Unlike arteries, which start very large and keep subdividing into smaller and smaller arteries, veins start very small and grow bigger and bigger. Some veins are visible, like those on the back of the hand, and are called superficial veins.

Those veins that originate from the internal organs are said to be deep veins. Bleeding from a deep vein can become life-threatening in a very short amount of time. One of the few deep veins that come to the surface is the **jugular vein** in the neck. An injury to the jugular vein is a serious wound.

As mentioned earlier, veins and arteries run together next to bones. As are the partner arteries, most veins are named after the bone that they also parallel. This system makes identifying veins and arteries easier for the EMT.

The largest vein in the body is called the **vena cava**. It has a superior and an inferior portion. The superior vena cava drains the brain, the neck, and the arms; the inferior vena cava drains the majority of the body.

Veins from the legs (iliac veins), the kidneys (renal veins), the liver (hepatic vein), and the intestines (mesenteric veins) all drain into the inferior vena cava. Figure 5-36 shows the main venous structures of the body.

The Blood

The purpose of this elaborate human plumbing system is to transport the blood. Blood has many functions, all of which serve to continue the life of the body.

The human body is a machine. To run such a machine requires fuels such as glucose, or sugar, and oxygen. The use of such fuels by the body is referred to as **metabolism**. There has to be a means to get these fuels to the individual cells in the tissues and the organs of the body. Blood is that means of transportation.

Blood that circulates to all the tissues of the body is perfusing the body. **Perfusion** is a Latin term meaning "to pour through," and that is exactly what blood does in the body.

Beyond the transportation of oxygen-carrying **red blood cells**, the blood also circulates disease-fighting white blood cells.

Finally, the blood has a self-repair mechanism. The complicated coagulation cascade is activated any time there is bleeding, allowing a clot to form and bleeding to stop. Coagulation prevents the loss of blood and helps maintain its steady supply. This entire process of blood clotting is called **hemostasis**, which literally means to stop bleeding.

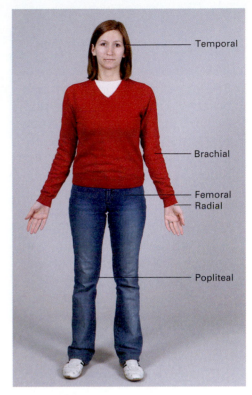

Temporal

Brachial

Femoral
Radial

Popliteal

FIGURE 5-40 The arterial pressure points of the body.

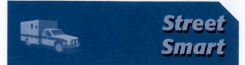

THE LYMPHATIC SYSTEM

Paralleling the circulatory system is another circulatory system of sorts called the **lymphatic system**. The lymphatic system is filled with an almost colorless fluid that is very similar to blood plasma. This fluid, called **lymph**, carries away infectious microorganisms such as bacteria to the **lymph nodes**, solid glandlike bodies such as the tonsils, where white blood cells destroy them. Lymph nodes can be found in the neck, armpits, chest, spleen, abdomen, and pelvis.

The lymphatic system also assists the circulatory system to drain the body's tissues of excess fluids, returns that fluid to the central circulation, and discharges it into the vena cava via the lymphatic duct.

THE RESPIRATORY SYSTEM

An important mission of the circulatory system is to distribute oxygenated blood. Naturally, the next question should be how does the blood get the oxygen to circulate. The answer is through the respiratory system.

The term **ventilation** refers to the actual movement of air into and out of the lungs. The mechanism that produces this air movement is discussed later in this section. The term **respiration** refers to the exchange of gases, such as oxygen and carbon dioxide, at the capillary level. The EMT will be able to improve a patient's ventilation but will often have no direct impact upon the actual respiration at the cellular level.

The respiratory system can be easily divided into the upper airway and the lower airway. Essentially, the lower airway is the start of the "sterile airway." That means that one of the main burdens of the upper airway is to clean the outside air of any contamination, including disease, before it enters the lungs.

The Upper Airway

The largest opening, or orifice, of the body is the mouth. The mouth permits large volumes of air to enter into the airway and eventually into the lungs.

The inside of the mouth is referred to as the **oropharynx**. It is the portion of the airway that is visible to the EMT when the mouth is opened wide, such as when suctioning the airway.

The nose also permits the movement of air into the lungs. The nostrils of the nose have fine hairs, called cilia, that clean the air as it passes over them. The nasal passage, also called the **nasopharynx**, is also coated with a thick sticky liquid material, mucus, that traps and holds dirt, dust, and any other particulate contamination. The nasal passages also are rich in blood vessels that serve to heat the air that passes over them to a warm 98.6 degrees Fahrenheit, or body temperature. Figure 5-41 shows the structures of the upper airway.

The Larynx

The windpipe, or trachea, is a long funnel that channels air into the lungs. It starts at a structure called the **larynx**. The larynx is a cartilaginous boxlike structure that contains the vocal cords; hence, it is

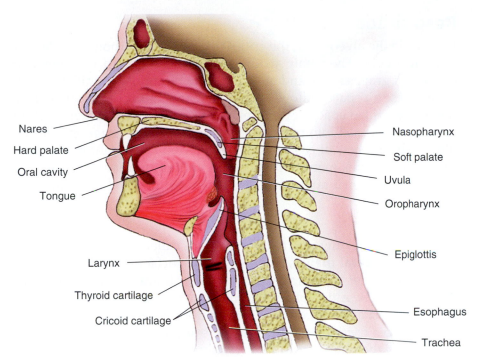

Nares
Hard palate
Oral cavity
Tongue

Nasopharynx
Soft palate
Uvula
Oropharynx

Larynx

Epiglottis

Thyroid cartilage

Cricoid cartilage

Esophagus

Trachea

FIGURE 5-41 The structures of the upper airway.

sometimes called the voice box. The vocal cords vibrate when air passes over them and create sound. In males, the voice box is larger than in females and externally can be identified as the Adam's apple.

Above the larynx is the **epiglottis**. The epiglottis is a cartilaginous structure that protects the trachea from foreign bodies. When the epiglottis fails and a foreign body enters the trachea, it may block the passage of air. The maneuvers to remove a foreign body airway obstruction (FBAO) must be performed so that air may pass again. These techniques are vital for the EMT to know.

The warmed, filtered air continues to pass into the lungs via the trachea. The trachea is a semirigid tube that can be felt anteriorly in the midline of the neck. The trachea and its related structures are illustrated in Figure 5-41.

The Lower Airway

The trachea ends at a division, or bifurcation. This point is called the **carina**. The right and left mainstem **bronchi** start here and continue deep into the lungs. The bronchi are cartilaginous tubes that divide into smaller passages called **bronchioles** and keep dividing into smaller passages until they become very narrow **terminal bronchioles**. Lining the inside of the bronchioles are **goblet cells** and **cilia**. The goblet cells produce a mucous blanket that is designed to entrap particles and microorganisms, such as bacteria, and prevent them from entering the alveoli. This thick mucous blanket is constantly moving upward, propelled by small hairlike projections called *cilia*, into the back of the throat to be coughed up. Toxins in cigarette smoke, for example, can paralyze the cilia and allow the bacteria-laden mucous blanket to stagnate, causing an infection called *bronchitis*. Attached to the terminal bronchioles are the clustered **alveoli**. These structures are shown in Figure 5-42.

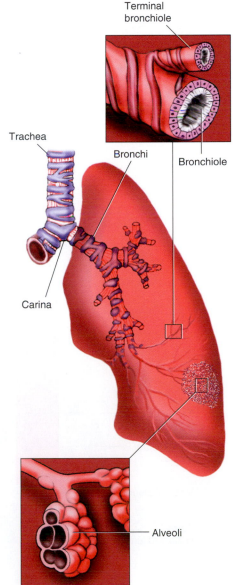

Terminal bronchiole

Trachea

Bronchi

Bronchiole

Carina

Alveoli

FIGURE 5-42 The lower airway structures.

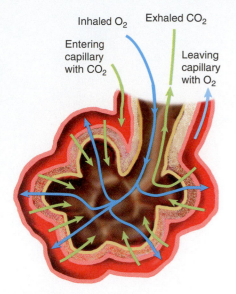

FIGURE 5-43 Exchange of oxygen and carbon dioxide takes place at the alveoli.

Inhaled O₂ Exhaled CO₂

Entering capillary with CO₂

Leaving capillary with O₂

Respiration

It is inside the alveoli that the critical exchange of carbon dioxide and oxygen occurs. The small saclike alveoli are clumped together like clusters of grapes at the end of a vine. Tiny pulmonary capillaries surround these air spaces, allowing deoxygenated blood to pass closely by the oxygen-filled spaces. As the blood passes by these alveoli, carbon dioxide is released into the air space and oxygen is taken up into the blood. This process of gas exchange is referred to as pulmonary respiration. It is in this manner that certain wastes are removed from the blood and oxygen is taken on. This process is illustrated in Figure 5-43.

The Pleurae

Surrounding the lungs are two membranes called pleurae. One membrane, the **visceral pleura**, is found on the surface of the lungs themselves. The other membrane, the **parietal pleura**, lines the inside of the rib cage. These two pleural linings move against each other as the lungs expand and deflate with ventilation. A very small amount of fluid reduces friction by lubricating the space between them. Figure 5-44 shows the pleurae and their relationship to the lungs and chest wall.

The Diaphragm

The diaphragm is a large muscle that lies within the lower part of the chest and is unique in that it is similar to other skeletal muscles in structure but is not completely under voluntary control. It is controlled by the brainstem via nerves from the cervical spinal cord. A

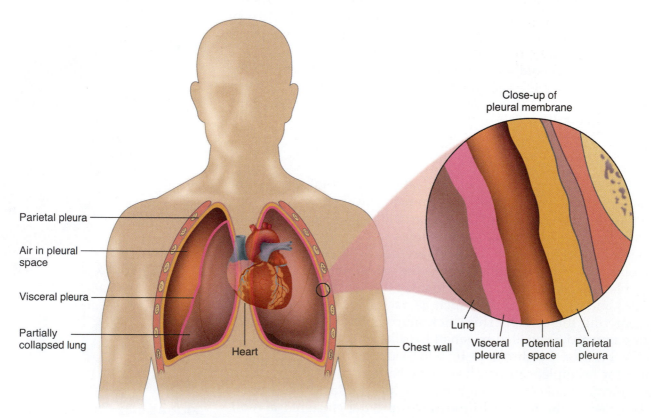

Close-up of pleural membrane

Parietal pleura

Air in pleural space

Visceral pleura

Partially collapsed lung

Heart

Chest wall

Lung

Visceral pleura

Potential space

Parietal pleura

FIGURE 5-44 The pleural membranes allow the lungs to move smoothly within the chest.

complex interaction of signals between the body and the brain signals how often the diaphragm needs to contract. Figure 5-45 illustrates the nervous control of the diaphragm.

Ventilation

When the diaphragm contracts, it is pulled down into the abdomen, creating a negative pressure, or vacuum, within the thoracic cavity. This negative pressure then forces the intake of air through the mouth and nose into the lungs to equalize the pressure. When the diaphragm then relaxes, it is pushed back up into the chest and a positive pressure is created that forces the air out of the lungs. This is how we inhale and exhale. Figure 5-46 illustrates this physiology.

THE DIGESTIVE SYSTEM

Ventilation and respiration account for part of the intake of fuels and removal of wastes, but the remainder of this metabolic process is maintained by organs involved in digestion and elimination. By digesting foods, the body is able to extract the sugars and other nutrients that it needs to survive. The nutritional flow starts at ingestion and ends with elimination of wastes and indigestible substances. This process is illustrated in Figure 5-47.

The Abdominal Cavity

The organs of digestion are contained, for the most part, within the abdominal cavity. The abdominal cavity is bordered inferiorly by the pelvic floor, superiorly by the diaphragm, and anteriorly and laterally by abdominal wall musculature, as shown in Figure 5-48.

Phrenic nerves

Diaphragm

FIGURE 5-45 The diaphragm is controlled by the phrenic nerves.

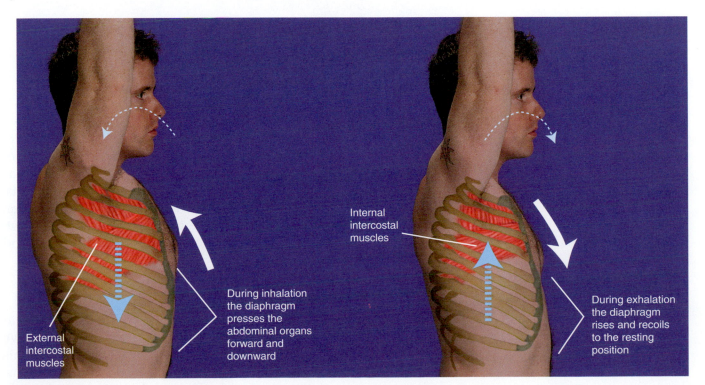

External intercostal muscles

During inhalation the diaphragm presses the abdominal organs forward and downward

Internal intercostal muscles

During exhalation the diaphragm rises and recoils to the resting position

FIGURE 5-46 Inhalation and exhalation.

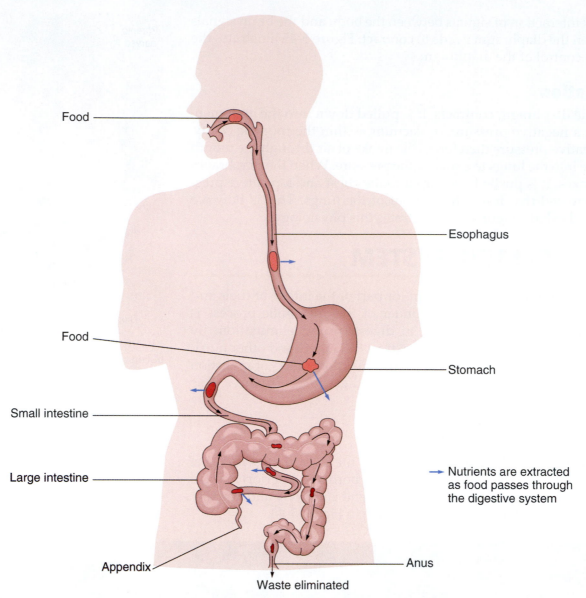

Food

Esophagus

Food

Stomach

Small intestine

Large intestine

→ Nutrients are extracted as food passes through the digestive system

Appendix

Anus

Waste eliminated

FIGURE 5-47 Nutrient flow in the gastrointestinal tract.

The abdominal cavity can be thought of as a large shallow bowl. Unfortunately, the only reliable distinguishing landmark on the anterior abdominal wall is the umbilicus. This point is used as a point of reference for describing areas of injury or pain. With the umbilicus as the center point, the abdomen has been divided into four quadrants. Each quadrant is named either left or right and upper or lower. Although other systems of descriptive topographic anatomy exist, this method is the most commonly used in emergency medicine and is pictured in Figure 5-49.

The Digestive Organs

The first portion of the digestive process occurs in the mouth. It is in the mouth that food is chewed, or masticated, mixed with digestive enzymes found in saliva, and swallowed as a mass, or a bolus. This bolus is then passed down the oropharnyx, past the closed epiglottis, and swallowed into the **esophagus**. The esophagus, approximately

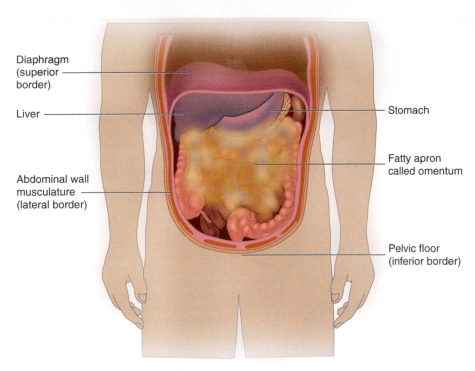

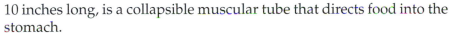

Diaphragm (superior border)

Liver

Abdominal wall musculature (lateral border)

Stomach

Fatty apron called omentum

Pelvic floor (inferior border)

FIGURE 5-48 The abdominal cavity and its contents.

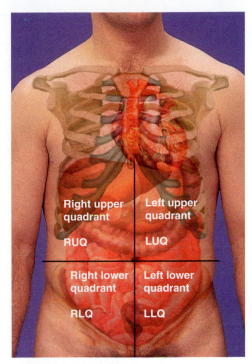

Right upper quadrant

RUQ

Left upper quadrant

LUQ

Right lower quadrant

RLQ

Left lower quadrant

LLQ

FIGURE 5-49 The four quadrants of the abdomen.

10 inches long, is a collapsible muscular tube that directs food into the stomach.

Once past the thoracic cavity and safely into the stomach, the bolus of food is further broken down by stomach acids and digestive enzymes. The stomach then empties its contents into the **small intestine**. About 90% of digestion (the breakdown and absorption of sugars and nutrients) occurs in the small intestine.

The small intestine is the largest digestive organ, taking up the majority of the abdominal cavity. The small intestine can be found in all four quadrants.

Other digestive enzymes excreted from the **gallbladder**, such as bile, aid in the process of digestion. The gallbladder is found in the upper right quadrant under the liver and is an important aid to digestion of fatty foods.

The large intestine encircles the abdominal cavity. At the end of the small intestine, the **large intestine** ascends within the right side of the abdomen then crosses the superior abdomen and descends in the left side. The large intestine terminates at the midline **rectum**. The rectum forms and stores the feces that is eventually expelled out of the **anus**. This material consists of indigestible or unusable food products as well as other metabolic waste products. The pathway of digestion and gastrointestinal elimination can be seen in Figure 5-50.

The Appendix

The **appendix** is a tubular organ attached to the large intestine that has no known function. Generally, most people go through life unaware that they have an appendix until this half-inch-thick pouch becomes inflamed by material trapped within it, a condition called *appendicitis*.

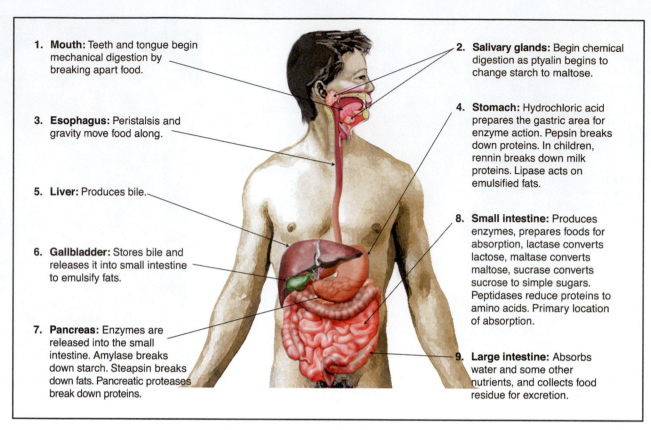

1. **Mouth:** Teeth and tongue begin mechanical digestion by breaking apart food.

3. **Esophagus:** Peristalsis and gravity move food along.

5. **Liver:** Produces bile.

6. **Gallbladder:** Stores bile and releases it into small intestine to emulsify fats.

7. **Pancreas:** Enzymes are released into the small intestine. Amylase breaks down starch. Steapsin breaks down fats. Pancreatic proteases break down proteins.

2. **Salivary glands:** Begin chemical digestion as ptyalin begins to change starch to maltose.

4. **Stomach:** Hydrochloric acid prepares the gastric area for enzyme action. Pepsin breaks down proteins. In children, rennin breaks down milk proteins. Lipase acts on emulsified fats.

8. **Small intestine:** Produces enzymes, prepares foods for absorption, lactase converts lactose, maltase converts maltose, sucrase converts sucrose to simple sugars. Peptidases reduce proteins to amino acids. Primary location of absorption.

9. **Large intestine:** Absorbs water and some other nutrients, and collects food residue for excretion.

FIGURE 5-50 The gastrointestinal system.

Externally, the appendix can be found in the lower right quadrant of the abdominal cavity. More specifically, if a mental (imaginary) triangle starting at the umbilicus (belly button) extending to the crest of the hip then to the pubis bone and then back to the umbilicus is formed, the appendix can be found in the middle of that triangle at a position called *McBurney's point*. Pain and tenderness at McBurney's point is highly suspicious for appendicitis.

The Liver

The **liver** is a solid organ in the right upper quadrant that serves to create the digestive bile stored in the gallbladder and has a number of other functions. All blood from the intestines must first pass through the liver before it can be circulated to the rest of the body. The liver neutralizes, or detoxifies, any poisons (toxins) that are in the bloodstream.

The liver also contributes to the production of factors that allow blood clotting (coagulation). Finally, the liver stores an emergency sugar supply called glycogen that is released whenever a person's blood sugar gets too low.

The Pancreas

The pancreas is located in the center of the abdomen, behind several other structures. It creates some of the most powerful digestive fluids, or enzymes, in the digestive tract. In fact, the pancreas can create up to 2 quarts of these fluids every day! The pancreas is also where the hormone insulin is produced as previously discussed.

The Retroperitoneal Cavity

Clearly, the majority of the vital organs are contained within the cranial cavity, the thoracic cavity, and the abdominal cavity. There is another, often-overlooked, cavity—the retroperitoneal cavity.

The retroperitoneal cavity is located in the posterior of the abdomen. It is separated from the abdominal cavity by a thin lining called the peritoneum. Some of the intra-abdominal structures lie partially in the retroperitoneal cavity. Several structures lie completely within the retroperitoneal cavity: namely, the kidneys, the abdominal aorta, and the inferior vena cava.

The Kidneys

The **kidney** is an organ that is densely packed with blood vessels. The purpose of the paired kidneys is to filter blood and from that filtrate eliminate unnecessary volumes of fluid, salts, and other wastes as urine. These organs are located on either side of the spine in the retroperitoneal cavity, well protected by the overlying lower rib cage.

Each kidney collects this urine in a collecting chamber within its center, called the renal pelvis. From the renal pelvis, the urine flows into pipelike structures called the **ureters**. The ureters are pencil-lead thick and may easily become blocked by solid collections of salts known as kidney stones.

The ureters are safely buried within a bed of muscle and fat within the retroperitoneal cavity. They empty into the **bladder**, which is an expandable container in the pelvis that can hold up to a quart of fluid. The kidneys and their associated structures are pictured in Figure 5-51.

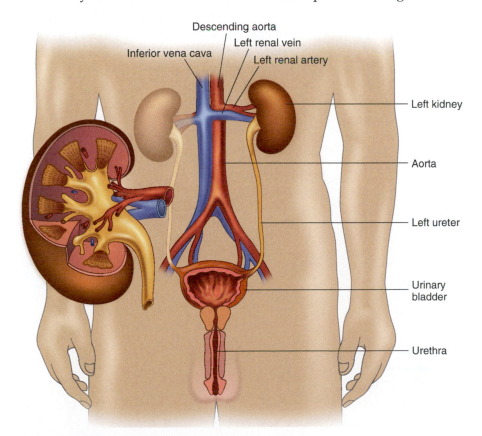

Descending aorta
Left renal vein
Inferior vena cava
Left renal artery

Left kidney

Aorta

Left ureter

Urinary bladder

Urethra

FIGURE 5-51 The structures of the urinary system.

THE REPRODUCTIVE SYSTEM

There are obvious differences between male and female reproductive anatomy. Both sexes have organs of reproduction called glands or **gonads**. In the male, these are the testes, and in the female, the ovaries. All other features of these two systems are distinctly different between male and female.

Male Reproductive Organs

The male reproductive organs are situated outside of the abdominal cavity and consist of the testes and penis.

The Testes

The **testes** are the main sex hormone-producing glands in the male and are suspended outside of the body in a pouch called the **scrotum**. This pair of gonads produces the hormone called testosterone. Testosterone is responsible for the secondary sex characteristics of the male. These include facial hair, deep voice, broad shoulders, and profuse body hair. The testes are also responsible for producing the sperm that will fertilize a female's egg during conception.

The Penis

The **penis** is a conduit for the passage of both urine and semen. Semen is the fluid that contains not only the **sperm** (male reproductive material) from the testes but also fluid from the seminal vesicles and the **prostate gland** that assists in transport of the sperm.

The prostate gland also serves to block urine flow while it assists with the expulsion of semen, called ejaculation. If this gland becomes enlarged, as sometimes occurs in old age, then normal urine flow may become interrupted.

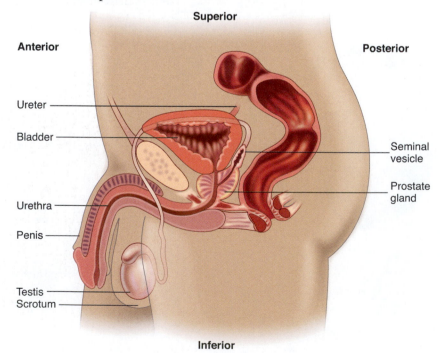

FIGURE 5-52 The male reproductive system.

Chapter 5 Anatomy and Physiology **117**

Because of the relatively unprotected location of the male genitalia, the penis and testes are prone to injury from trauma. Figure 5-52 shows the structures of the male genital system.

Female Reproductive Organs

The female reproductive organs are located in the pelvic cavity. This positioning protects these organs somewhat during nonpregnant states. During pregnancy, however, the enlarged uterus extends out of the pelvis and into the abdominal cavity.

The Ovaries

The primary female gonad is the **ovary**. The ovary produces characteristic female sex hormones, such as estrogen and progesterone. These hormones are responsible for the development of female secondary sex characteristics such as breasts, wide hips, and typical distribution of fat.

The ovaries contain a woman's entire life supply of eggs. On average, every 28 days a mature woman's ovary releases an egg for fertilization. The egg passes through a structure called the **fallopian tube**. It is usually inside the fallopian tube that an egg may unite with a sperm and become fertilized, resulting in pregnancy.

The Uterus

The **uterus** is a muscular pouch that is known to the layperson as the womb. It is inside the uterus that the fertilized egg becomes implanted and where it grows and becomes a fetus. Stages of pregnancy are discussed further in Chapter 36.

If the egg is not fertilized or the implantation is incomplete, then the egg and the uterine lining are swept out of the uterus in a menstrual flow. This flow occurs monthly and is referred as **menstruation**.

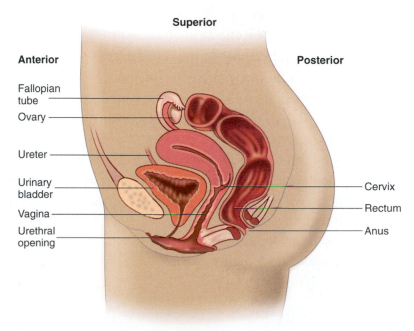

FIGURE 5-53   The female reproductive system.

The Vagina

The **vagina** serves several functions. First, it is the path by which the menstrual flow exits the body. Second, it is the conduit for the acceptance of the male penis during coitus, the act of sexual intercourse.

Finally, the vagina serves as the birth canal. When an infant is ready to be delivered, the head passes down the vaginal canal and out of the vaginal opening. Figure 5-53 shows the structures of the female genitalia.

CONCLUSION

This chapter has described and illustrated much of human anatomy and physiology, as it is relevant to the EMT. There is much more complexity to every aspect of the human body than can be taught in the confines of this course. Although this review has been brief, it is important for the EMT to be familiar with basic anatomy and to know the normal functioning of the human body. It is only with this knowledge that a health care provider can begin to recognize when a physical problem exists and how to go about remedying that problem.

TEST YOUR KNOWLEDGE

1. Describe the standard anatomical position.
2. Draw a picture of the human body in anatomical position and then place the following lines of reference on the body: the midline, the midclavicular line, the four quadrants of the abdomen.
3. A patient has an injury of the inner wrist. Describe the location of that injury using the following anatomic terms: proximal, distal, lateral, superior, inferior, and palmar.
4. List the most important function of the skin.
5. List the names of the bones of the cervical spine.
6. List the bones of the appendicular skeleton.
7. What is the function of the nervous system?
8. What is the name of the hormone responsible for the metabolism of sugar?
9. What are the three types of blood vessels in the body?
10. What are the portions of the upper and lower airway called?
11. Name the organs of the digestive system starting at the mouth and ending at the anus.
12. What is the function of the kidneys?
13. Name the male and female gonads.

INTERNET RESOURCES

Visit the following Web sites for more information of anatomy and physiology. Many of these Web sites have interactive activities that aid in increasing one's understanding of how the body works.

- Inner Learning Online, http://www.innerbody.com
- Instant Anatomy, http://www.instantanatomy.net
- Net Anatomy, http://www.netanatomy.com
- Visible Human Project, http://www.nlm.nih.gov/research/visible/visible_human.html

FURTHER STUDY

Scott, A. S., & Fong, E. (2004). *Body structures and functions* (10th ed.). Clifton Park, NY: Thomson Delmar Learning.

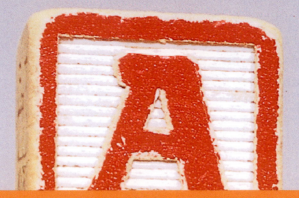

While working in a rural community in western New York, we responded to a call for a man not feeling well. With me was my partner and a paramedic from our service. After going up and down a dirt road trying to find the house, as there were no house numbers, we were finally flagged down by a woman. She appeared calm as she approached us and told us that her husband was inside in a chair. She didn't know what was wrong with him. "He has been like this for about 20 minutes, but maybe it is his sugar. He's a diabetic, you know."

We followed her into the house where a very large man in coveralls with a long beard (similar to ZZ Top) was sitting in a chair in an extremely cluttered room. His head was down and he was supporting himself with a cane (hands folded on top of the cane). My partner and I each reached to check a pulse; I grabbed the wrist, he the carotid. Nothing. We looked at each other, baffled, and switched pulse locations. Again nothing. Oh darn (those weren't the exact words), he's in arrest. My partner maneuvered behind the patient, and I grabbed the patient under his thighs, just above the knees. Our goal was to lay him down in this cluttered home. He was big and heavy, so it took everything that we had to get him out of this chair. I prepared myself, wide stance, knees bent, back straight, ready to heave ho. "1-2-3-LIFT!" With all my might, I lifted as hard as I could, only to find myself falling backward and the patient not moving. I looked down to find that both of the patient's legs have become longer and are now twisted around, one backward. The wife then says, "Oh, I'm sorry, he has prosthetic legs."

The look on my face must have been priceless because whenever I return to that area, almost 10 years later, I'm still known as "legs."

Kyle Bates, MS, NREMT-P
County EMS, Ellsworth, Maine
Mayo Regional Hospital EMS, Dover-Foxcroft, Maine

Fundamentals of Emergency Medical Care

The foundation of an EMT's practice is laid upon several fundamental skills, such as airway management and bleeding control. Often these basic skills are all that is needed to save a patient's life. In every case, these basic skills must be performed before the EMT can use more advanced skills to care for the patient.

All EMTs, from the EMT–Basic to the EMT–Paramedic, must practice these fundamental skills until they become second nature. Only then can an EMT expect to be able to provide competent emergency medical care.

Infection control, airway management, ventilation, and bleeding control are reviewed in this section, as well as taking vital signs and lifting and moving patients. All of these topics include skills that are a part of the emergency medical care an EMT provides to every patient.

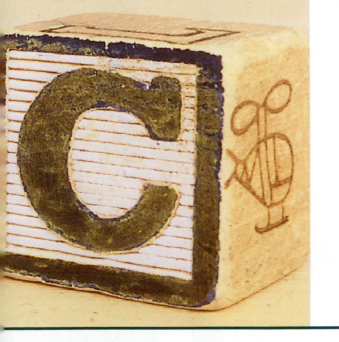

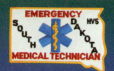

CHAPTER 6

Infection Control

KEY TERMS

antibody

biohazard

body substance isolation

carrier

contagious

decontamination

designated officer

direct contact

immunity

immunization

immunocompromise

indirect contact

infection control

infection control officer

microorganism

mucous membrane

pathogen

personal protective
  equipment (PPE)

portal of entry

prophylaxis

risk management

risk profile

Ryan White Law

safety officer

sharps

sharps container

Standard Precautions

sterilization

transmission

vector

OBJECTIVES

Upon completion of this chapter, the reader should be able to:

1. Explain the importance of infection control.
2. List the elements of OSHA 1910.1030.
3. List five of the more common infectious illnesses an EMT will encounter.
4. Explain the different modes of disease transmission.
5. Explain what is meant by the term *portal of entry*.
6. List possible personal defenses against infectious disease transmission.
7. Define what is meant by the terms *body substance isolation* and *personal protective equipment*.
8. Define the term *Standard Precautions*.
9. Describe the methods of infection control used for typical medical procedures performed by EMTs.
10. List the different levels of disinfection.
11. Explain what an infection control plan is and where it can be found.
12. Explain the importance of documenting a potential infectious disease exposure.
13. Describe how notification laws affect the EMT.
14. Describe what is proper medical follow-up for an infectious disease exposure.

OVERVIEW

When an emergency medical technician (EMT) approaches a sick or an injured patient, there is always a possibility of exposure to disease. Some patients carry infections that may be inadvertently transmitted to health care workers if preventive measures are not taken. Over the past two decades, health care workers have become increasingly knowledgeable about this issue. Today, EMTs are regularly taught about prevention of disease transmission through infection control measures.

Workplace Exposure

"It was when we were transferring the patient over to the hospital stretcher when I got the blood on me," Don explained to the emergency physician, Dr. Bosco.

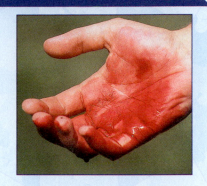

The patient had cut his own wrists in an apparent suicide attempt. The engine company had bandaged the wrists securely before the ambulance arrived and helped the crew secure the combative patient to the gurney. The patient was then transported to the local hospital for a medical evaluation. Sam, Don's partner, rode with the patient while Don drove. Don took off his gloves before he started to drive.

When the ambulance got to the hospital, the crew unloaded the stretcher and took the patient to the triage nurse. She advised them that isolation room 1–A was prepped and ready.

As they rolled the gurney into the room, the patient immediately started to buck and pull at his restraints. It took an orderly, a nurse, and the two EMTs to move him over to the stretcher.

That's when it happened. Don was holding the patient's wrist when the bandage slipped. Blood started spurting all over the place and all over Don's bare arms. They quickly finished restraining the patient, and the nurse reinforced the original bandage to control the bleeding.

Don immediately washed his hands and then went out to the desk to speak with the doctor.

- Why should this EMT be concerned?
- What could he have done to prevent this from happening?
- Was this a significant exposure? Why or why not?

This chapter discusses infectious disease and how EMTs can prevent transmission of disease in the workplace. It is important for an EMT to understand the principles of infection control and prevention measures. The EMT who fails to learn these lessons may be putting her life and the lives of those she cares for in jeopardy.

INFECTION CONTROL

An infection is a disease that is caused by some type of **microorganism** (microscopic life form) that flourishes in the body, sometimes causing illness. Infections can be acquired in many different ways, all requiring the microorganism to contact the person and enter the body in some way. Each microorganism has a particular mode of **transmission**, or moving, from one place to another. If an EMT understands the most common means of transmission of infectious disease, measures can be taken to prevent infection. Attempts to prevent the spread of infectious disease can be referred to as **infection control** measures.

The benefits of simple infection control measures were described by Dr. Semmelweis, an Austrian obstetrician, in 1847. He reported a significant drop in infection rates when health care providers washed their hands before caring for each patient. Before hand washing was common, 18% of young mothers died in the hospital from postchildbirth infections (Figure 6-1). After Dr. Semmelweis insisted that all providers wash their hands between patients, the maternal death rate dropped to less than 1%. This simple infection control measure had dramatic results in preventing the spread of disease in these patients.

Personal Safety

The EMT's personal safety is one of the reasons why infection control is necessary. Emergency medical services (EMS) is a profession with many potential risks. It is important that measures be taken to prevent the EMT from acquiring an infectious disease on the job.

The smart EMT looks for potential dangers in the work environment and takes preventive action. This kind of behavior is called **risk management**. Infection control plays a major role in risk management for all health care professionals.

When an EMT is evaluating the risk of infectious disease in the work environment, the potential for infection in the community served should be considered. Is there a large homeless population that may not have easy access to medical care? Is there a large immigrant population that may not have received the routine "American" immunizations or that is a population known to have a high incidence of a certain infectious disease?

When an EMT considers the potential for disease process within the community, she is creating a **risk profile** (Figure 6-2). An EMT who operates in a community known to have a high incidence of a particular infectious disease or injury risk would regularly take specific precautions to prevent transmission of that disease or to prevent that type of injury. The more that is known about the health of the community, the more specific the EMT can be about infection control. The local or county health departments can be very helpful in determining a community's risk profile.

Although there are local variations in the disease risk profile, the major diseases EMTs are concerned about are seen on a broad basis,

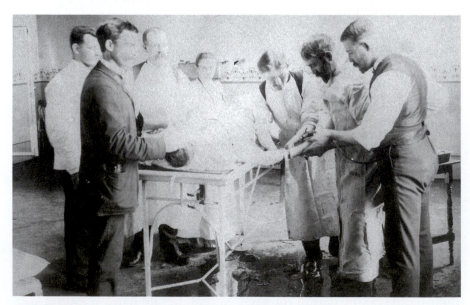

FIGURE 6-1   Doctors were slow to accept infection control principles.

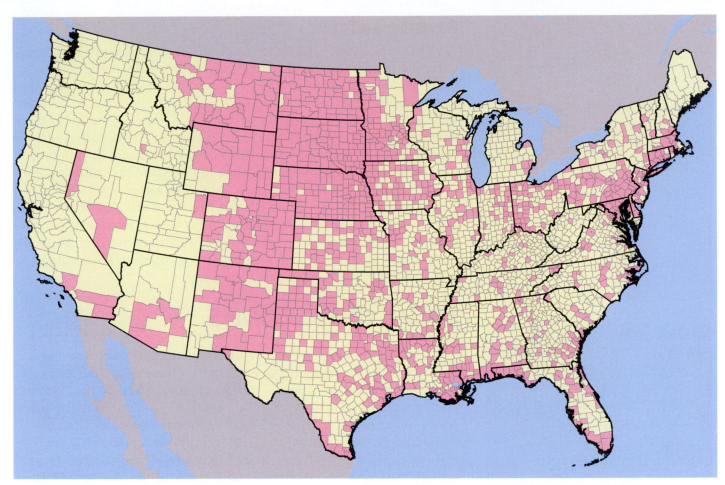

FIGURE 6-2 County health departments are a rich source of information about disease and local outbreaks of disease. This map shows reports of West Nile Virus as collected by the U.S. Geographical Survey and the Centers for Disease Control and Prevention. (Courtesy of the Centers for Disease Control and Prevention, West Nile Virus Map—2003: USA Human Map.)

and general approaches to managing these risks have been adopted by EMS.

Patient Safety

An essential principle of medicine is to "do no harm." The assistance an EMT renders should not cause the patient more health problems. This issue is exemplified in the observations of Dr. Semmelweis. A medical professional, whether a doctor, a nurse, or an EMT, should not bring an infectious disease to the patient.

Infection control is a two-way street. Just as the EMT does not want to get exposed to an infectious disease through interaction with the patient, the patient does not want to be exposed to an infectious disease through interaction with the EMT. Most of the patients an EMT will care for are in a stressful situation. This stress can make the patient's body more susceptible to infection.

Even without the added stress of an emergency, some medications and disease processes can leave a patient with a weakened immune system and little or no resistance to disease. This weakened immune state is called **immunocompromise**. Infections that would not make an average healthy person sick can cause serious illness in the immunocompromised patient.

Family Safety

An EMT who is exposed to an infectious disease at work may inadvertently bring it home. The EMT may not become ill after exposure to the organism, but a significant concern for the EMT is the potential of transmitting an infectious disease to family members. Children, who have immature immune systems; elderly parents, who have declining immune systems; and any ill persons in the household are all at a greater risk of becoming ill when exposed to an infectious disease. To protect these loved ones, the EMT needs to take infection control precautions to avoid becoming a disease carrier.

A carrier of an infectious disease harbors within the body the microorganism that causes an illness yet does not necessarily become ill as a result. Carriers of an infectious disease may not even be aware of their carrier state, yet they can pass the microorganism along to other people, who may become ill as a result.

LEGAL OBLIGATIONS

The Centers for Disease Control and Prevention (CDC) is an organization within the federal government that monitors outbreaks of infections and advises affected groups on how to handle the situation and control the spread of disease. The CDC has issued many advisories regarding common disease outbreaks such as hepatitis B caused by the hepatitis B virus (HBV) and tuberculosis (TB).

To encourage compliance with these advisories, another federal agency, the Occupational Safety and Health Administration (OSHA), produces standards for infection control practice in EMS. One of the first standards and practice rules was the Bloodborne Pathogens Rule (29 CFR 1910.1030) published in 1992. This set of rules had very clear provisions for employers regarding infection control practices. Table 6-1 outlines the rules and regulations of this standard.

Another group that has an interest in the health and welfare of its members is the fire service. The majority of EMS has been and still is provided by EMTs in the fire service. Senior fire service leaders and other fire service experts periodically meet to discuss and agree upon the standards of practice that the fire service should utilize. The National Fire Protection Association (NFPA) Standard 1581 specifically addresses the issue of infection control (Table 6-2).

The Safety Officer

There are such a large number of state and federal rules, standards, and laws that the average EMT could easily become overwhelmed. Most progressive EMS agencies have created a position called the infection control officer or safety officer. The infection control officer is responsible for reviewing publications from agencies such as the CDC, OSHA, and the NFPA for new rules and standards that could affect EMS operations.

The position of infection control or safety officer is so common in fire departments and EMS agencies that there is a National Association of Safety Officers. These officers discuss methods of obtaining and

TABLE 6-1

OSHA Standard 1910.1030, Occupational Exposure to Bloodborne Pathogens

Intent: To eliminate or minimize occupational exposures to bloodborne pathogens.

Applicable to: All employees with potential for occupational exposure to blood or other potentially infectious material.

Requirements:
- Exposure control plan
- Exposure determination
- Methods of compliance
  Universal precautions
  Engineering controls
  Work practice controls
  Personal protective equipment
  Housekeeping/waste disposal
  Hepatitis B vaccination
  Signs and labels on hazardous materials
  Training
- Postexposure follow-up

Source: 29 *Code of Federal Regulations* 1910.1030.

TABLE 6-2

NFPA Standard 1581, Fire Department Infection Control

Intent: To reduce the exposures to infectious diseases by responders in both emergency and nonemergency situations.

Applicable to: Any organization providing rescue, fire suppression, and other emergency service functions.

Requirements: Describes minimum standards for infection control programs:

- Policy
- Training and education
- Infection control liaison person
- Immunization and testing
- Exposures
- Cleaning and disinfecting areas
- Storage rooms
- Infection control garments and equipment
- Personnel handling of sharp objects
- Skin washing
- Disinfectants
- Emergency medical equipment
- Protective clothing
- Disposal of material

distributing important information about infection control to their members.

The infection control or safety officer (the chief operating officer, if there is no formally designated infection or safety control officer), is the person to approach if an EMT has a question regarding infection control (Figure 6-3).

Reporting Exposure

The first question naturally is, what is an occupational exposure? An occupational exposure occurs when an EMT, while in the course of regular and routine duties, comes into contact with a potentially

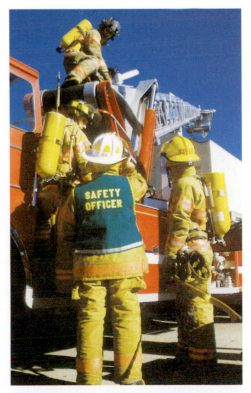

FIGURE 6-3 The key person in charge of infection control in many EMS organizations is the infection control officer or safety officer.

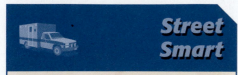

infectious material, such as blood or other body fluids. Contact occurs when the potentially infectious material contacts a mucous membrane, open wound, cut, or laceration or is introduced, by injection, under the skin.

An EMT who believes that she has been exposed to a potentially infectious material must seek out medical treatment and follow-up. The first step is usually to notify the infection control or safety officer. In most cases, the infection control or safety officer will direct the EMT to see a designated physician immediately. In all cases, the EMT should follow departmental procedures.

On the basis of the nature of the exposure, the physician may recommend that the EMT initiate treatment to try to prevent or at least lessen the likelihood of becoming ill as a result of the exposure. This type of treatment is called **prophylaxis**. For prophylaxis to be effective, it must begin as soon after the exposure as possible. Some prophylaxis regimens should be started within 1–2 hours of the exposure. The sooner it is begun, the better the chances of avoiding illness. Therefore, all incidents of potential exposure must be reported immediately.

Notification by Hospitals

If a patient who is transported by EMS to a hospital is found to have an infectious disease that may have posed a danger to EMS providers, the hospital is obligated, under the **Ryan White Law**, to notify the EMS agency's **designated officer**.

The Ryan White Comprehensive AIDS Resource Emergency (CARE) Act mandates that all EMS agencies have procedures in place for notifying "emergency response employees," including EMTs, whenever they have been exposed to a potentially infectious disease. The list of infectious diseases include common infections such as hepatitis B and human immunodeficiency virus (HIV) and some not so common diseases such as the plague.

An EMT may either request that the designated officer of the agency follow up on a patient to see if he has an infectious disease, for example, after a blood splash into the eyes of an EMT, or the hospital's infection control nurse may contact the designated officer to report a potential exposure to an infectious disease to an EMT, for example, an exposure to the airborne pathogen TB.

While it is often necessary to get the patient's permission for testing, in many cases the patient agrees after an adequate explanation is provided regarding the EMT and the requirements that EMTs have to maintain patient confidentiality.

The designated officer of an agency is the person who is responsible for receiving notifications of potential exposures and following up on them as appropriate. This person is also usually the infection control or safety officer, who is the person in the agency most likely to have the necessary background and to be familiar with the policies regarding such exposures.

EMTs are notified of a potentially infectious disease exposure and must follow through with the usual exposure process. Notification is usually made within 24–48 hours.

CAUSES OF DISEASE

The agents of infectious diseases, microorganisms, exist just about everywhere. Microorganisms that can cause infection and disease are classified into three major groups: fungi, bacteria, and viruses.

Although the study of microbiology is vast, an EMT need know only about a few of the more common disease-causing agents. Chickenpox, measles, strep throat, and influenza (Figure 6-4) are diseases that are commonly known to the public. Except under special circumstances, these illnesses are eliminated by the body over a relatively short period of time and pose no long-lasting threat to the EMT.

Patients with other infections, such as HIV and HBV, may pose a threat to the EMT in certain circumstances. EMTs are often in direct contact with a patient's blood or other bodily substances through which these diseases are transmitted. Table 6-3 lists common diseases an EMT may encounter during the course of routine patient care.

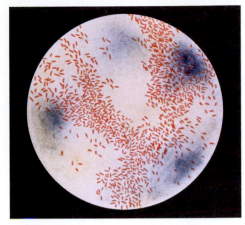

FIGURE 6-4　Most disease-causing agents are too small to be seen with the naked eye, such as *Haemophilus influenzae* as seen in this microscopic image. (Courtesy of the Centers for Disease Control and Prevention Public Health Image Library.)

TABLE 6-3

Common Disease-Causing Organisms and Infectious Illnesses

Organism/Illness	Signs and Symptoms	Mode of Transmission
Adenovirus (the common cold)	Runny nose, cough, sore throat, congestion	Contact with droplets, airborne
Varicella virus (chickenpox and shingles)	Rash (itchy or painful)	Contact with open lesions, airborne
Mycobacterium tuberculosis (tuberculosis)	Cough, sweats, weight loss	Airborne
Hepatitis Type A virus	Fever, nausea, vomiting, yellow skin color	Contaminated food or water
Hepatitis Types B, C, D viruses	Fever, nausea, vomiting, yellow skin color, abdominal pain	Direct contact with blood or other body fluid
Herpes simplex 1 virus (oral herpes)	Painful lesions, usually around mouth	Contact with saliva or wound
Herpes simplex 2 virus (genital herpes)	Painful lesions, usually in genital area	Contact with lesions
Human immunodeficiency virus (cause of AIDS)	Multiple infections such as pneumonia, thrush, herpes	Contact with blood or body fluids
Influenza virus (causes the flu)	Cough, fever, headache, vomiting, diarrhea, general malaise	Airborne
Methicillin-resistant *Staphylococcus aureus* (MRSA)	None (a bacterium that can inhabit a wound or healthy skin)	Contact with contaminated area
Neisseria meningitidis (a bacterium, one cause of meningitis)	Fever, rash, headache, stiff neck	Airborne respiratory secretions

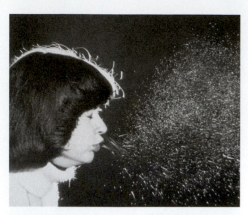

FIGURE 6-5 Airborne particles can travel far and contaminate many inanimate surfaces. (Courtesy of Lester V. Bergman/Corbis.)

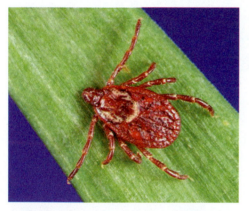

FIGURE 6-6 Disease is spread rapidly with the help of vectors such as the tick. (Courtesy of the Centers for Disease Control and Prevention Public Health Image Library.)

DISEASE TRANSMISSION

Disease transmission occurs between people by either **direct contact** (person to person) or **indirect contact** (via a contaminated object). The specific means of transmission are directly by contact, indirectly via air, another vehicle such as food or water, or a vector.

Contact Transmission

Contact transmission occurs through direct contact with a substance harboring an infectious agent, such as blood or another body substance. Hepatitis B and HIV infection are examples of diseases transmitted through direct contact.

Airborne Transmission

The most common means of disease transmission is via droplets in the air. These particles are carried in the air until they settle onto a surface. Sneezing and coughing are the means by which airborne diseases such as the common cold and influenza are transmitted (Figure 6-5).

Vehicle Transmission

Vehicle transmission is an indirect method of disease transmission in which food or water is a carrier of the disease-causing organism. For example, food poisoning is actually the result of ingestion of food contaminated with a bacterium such as *Salmonella*.

Vector-Borne Transmission

Around the world, a common source of disease is animals or insects. Ticks and mosquitoes transmit diseases such as Lyme disease or malaria. A living creature that is involved in the transmission of disease is called a **vector**. Deer ticks carry the organism that causes Lyme disease and transmit it to humans when they bite. The deer tick is the vector for Lyme disease (Figure 6-6).

PORTAL OF ENTRY

To cause illness in a person, an infectious organism must first enter the body. The means of entry for the organism is called the **portal of entry**. A common portal of entry is through the relatively unprotected mucous membranes in the mouth, nose, and eyes. An infectious agent that comes into contact with the well-vascularized mucous membranes can settle onto the surface and multiply or work its way into the superficial blood vessels and move throughout the body.

Another common, but often preventable, portal of entry for disease is through nonintact skin. The skin normally serves as a fairly impenetrable defense system, but broken skin can allow bacteria and other infectious organisms to enter the body.

Potential for Exposure

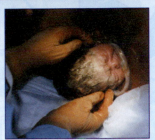

The call was for a "woman in labor." This was the fourth pregnancy for this mother of three, and she was telling the crew that she was "ready." The question that the crew had was, were they ready?

Helping the mother to an overstuffed chair, an EMT confirmed that the baby was "crowning," and they had better prepare to deliver the infant right there.

Following local protocols, one EMT contacted medical control via the telephone, another prepared the birthing kit, as still another donned personal protective equipment. A paramedic had been requested to respond to the scene in the event the delivery became complicated or the infant needed advanced-level care.

Everyone was ready, and the delivery went naturally. It was a girl. The mother and child were transported, without lights or siren, to the birthing center, and the crew went back into service.

Back at the station, as the crew cleaned up, the captain came out and affixed a pink stork emblem to the front quarter panel of the ambulance.

- What body substances could an EMT encounter during childbirth? Are they potentially infectious?
- What protective equipment should be utilized for this type of call?
- What postcall activities must occur?
- How would an EMT report a suspected infectious disease exposure?

SUSCEPTIBILITY TO DISEASE

The body does not necessarily become infected every time it is exposed to a disease. Actual illness caused by exposure to an infectious agent is dependent upon two factors: the strength of the organism, or its virulence, and the strength of the person's immune resistance. To create an illness, the organism must be virulent enough to overcome the resistance of the host.

Often, a virus or bacterium is weakened as a result of contact with air, drying in the environment, or other physical degradation. This weakened infectious particle may not have the strength to cause an infection. Hand cleaners and other cleaning solutions chemically weaken bacteria and viruses and may even kill them. These cleaning agents are often labeled "antibacterial."

Whenever a foreign particle, such as a virus or bacterium, enters the body, that body's defenses are set in motion. The disease-fighting white blood cells engulf the bacterium and subsequently remove it from the system.

This immune defense is very effective against small numbers of microorganisms. However, if the number, or dose, is large, then these defenses may become overwhelmed and illness may result. For example, one cubic centimeter of blood can have as many as 100 million

HBV particles. The larger the number of particles present, the harder the immune system must work to overcome the invasion.

Once an EMT has been exposed to a disease-causing organism of sufficient dose and virulence to overcome the body's resistance, illness results. This process can take days, weeks, or, rarely, years. It is during this time or shortly thereafter that the EMT can transmit the disease to others. The time when the EMT is **contagious** and can transmit the disease is the time when the EMT is a potential danger to family, friends, coworkers, and patients. Certain diseases such as influenza (flu) are highly contagious, and the EMT should take measures to protect herself and others.

One method of protection is isolation. An EMT should not work whenever suffering from a contagious illness. A doctor's advice is helpful when deciding when to return to work after any illness.

DEFENSE AGAINST DISEASE

The skin is a remarkable organ. It not only helps regulate our internal body temperature but also protects the body from the outside environment. The uppermost layer of skin is composed of dead cells. These cells shed regularly, carrying any surface contamination away. The skin represents the first barrier to disease. Unless there is a break in the skin, this barrier is relatively impenetrable to most infectious microorganisms.

The surfaces of the respiratory and gastrointestinal tracts that come into contact with the outside environment are lined with **mucous membranes**. A mucous membrane creates a liquid, called mucus, that can wash bacteria off the surface. However, these mucous membranes are quite porous and well lined with blood vessels. These features allow for an easy portal of entry for an infectious agent.

A healthy body is the best defense against disease. Annual physicals and ongoing health assessments are rapidly becoming standards in the health care industry. Employers, and the health care organizations that they pay insurance premiums to, have learned that it is less expensive to prevent disease than to treat it.

EMTs can also try to augment their immune system with regular immunizations. The body develops certain defense cells within the blood, called **antibodies**, that attack specific types of microorganisms. These antibodies need prior exposure to the microorganism in order to mount the most effective attack.

People are routinely provided exposure to common disease-causing agents (**pathogens**) in an attenuated, or weakened, form in order to allow the body to develop these specific antibodies. This process of exposing or inoculating the body to weakened pathogens is called **immunization**.

Every EMT should receive a broad spectrum of immunizations. Some immunizations are given only once in a lifetime. Others, such as the tetanus vaccine, must be given regularly in order for **immunity** to be maintained (protection from a disease as a result of exposure or immunization).

OSHA has required that every EMT have the opportunity to receive the hepatitis B vaccine. If used as recommended, this vaccine is helpful in preventing hepatitis B infection after an exposure to the virus. Any time a vaccination is made available in this way, the EMT should seriously consider the risks of being exposed to the disease and the benefits and protection of the immunization.

Not all diseases have immunizations available. For example, there is no vaccine to protect against TB or HIV. The EMT is advised to get regular testing for these infections if she is at risk of exposure to them. Early diagnosis can lead to early treatment. Early treatment can have a dramatic impact on the quality of life that an EMT enjoys or can cure certain diseases entirely.

Hand Hygiene

Proper hand hygiene is an important but often overlooked aspect of an EMT's practice. The single action that can best prevent the spread of disease is hand washing.

Many soaps claim to be "antiseptic" or "antibacterial," but the type of soap used is not nearly as important as is the hand washing technique. The single most important action in hand washing is the scrub. The forceful scrubbing and friction on the skin remove the top layer of skin, and the water washes the dead skin away along with the bacteria.

Soap dispensers and faucets should be the kind that can be operated hands free. Alternatively, "paddle" faucets should be available. Paddle faucets are turned off with an elbow to avoid using freshly washed hands to touch the "dirty" faucet.

If neither of these types of plumbing is available, then the faucet is turned off with a clean hand towel, never with the bare hand. Skill 6-1 demonstrates the proper procedure for hand washing.

Hand washing is part of the routine care of every patient. After every patient contact and before the next patient contact, the EMT must wash the hands. In addition, open wounds must be covered because they are a portal of entry for an infection. An EMT should not work if an open wound exists on the hands that cannot be effectively covered or that is draining and soaking through an applied bandage.

The convenience of soap and running water is not always available to the EMT. In those cases, alternatives, such as waterless cleansers, should be available and used. These often portable alcohol-based hand washes help to reduce harmful pathogens such as viruses, bacteria, and fungi on the skin.

The Association for Professionals in Infection Control and Epidemiology (APIC) recommends using alcohol-based hand washes after removing gloves, such as occurs between procedures, and after each patient contact; for example, during a multiple casualty incident. The EMT should completely coat the hands with the alcohol-based hand wash and perform a vigorous 1-minute rub to reduce the majority of pathogens. If the EMT's hands are visibly soiled, then she should use soap and water. Furthermore, the EMT should wash the hands with soap and water after every call regardless of whether waterless cleansers were used or not.

Personal Protective Equipment

The question most often asked by EMTs is, "When do I protect myself?" Seemingly the answer would be, Whenever there is a risk of exposure.

Street Smart

Many EMTs who wash their hands several times a day ignore the drying effect that hand washing has on the hands. Dried hands can crack and become reddened or sore. A crack in the skin is a portal of entry for disease.

There are moisturizing hand lotions available that will help reverse the drying effects of frequent hand washing. The EMT should find an effective brand of hand lotion, preferably unscented, and use it regularly after hand washing.

SKILL 6-1 *Hand Washing*

PURPOSE: To remove any contamination by blood or other bodily fluids from the EMT's hands.

STANDARD PRECAUTIONS:

- ☑ Soap
- ☑ Water
- ☑ Hand brush

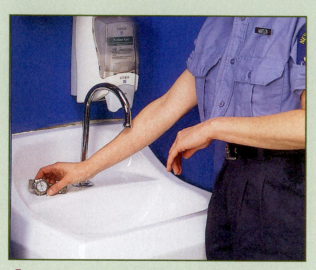

1 The EMT should remove any rings, watch, or other jewelry that could trap contamination.

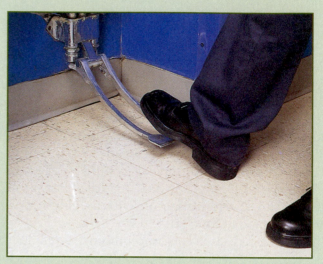

2 A deep basin sink and foot-pedal water faucets are preferable to wash hands. The EMT should adjust the hot and cold water to a comfortable lukewarm temperature.

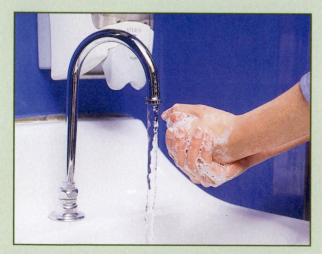

3 The EMT should then wet the hands to the mid-forearm. After applying a liberal amount of soap, the EMT should wash the hands carefully. The areas between the fingers deserve special attention. A hand brush may be used for difficult-to-remove contamination.

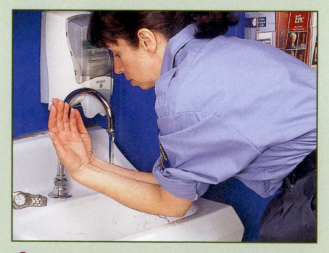

4 The EMT should then thoroughly rinse the hands, allowing the contaminated water to run off the elbow.

(continues)

SKILL 6-1 (continued)

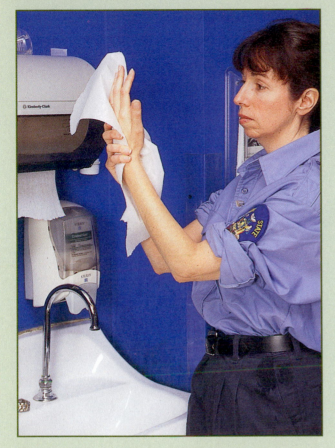 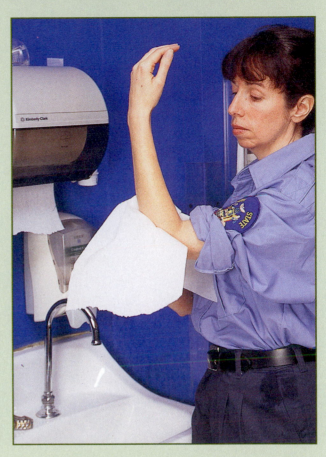

5 The EMT should then turn the water off. Grasping a clean towel, the EMT can turn off the faucet and discard the towel. Using a clean towel, the EMT should dry the hands, starting at the fingers and working toward the elbow.

Firefighters have what could be called a "dress down" philosophy. Firefighters enter into an unknown situation with full turnout gear—coats, gloves, pants, boots, and helmets with face shields—then remove what is not needed.

For EMS, a similar approach would be very expensive. Every time an EMT had a contact with a patient, the EMT would need to wear a complete isolation suit. This approach would be cost prohibitive.

Even more important, this extent of protection is unnecessary for the vast majority of patient encounters. Clearly, the majority of patients are seen and cared for on a daily basis with a minimum of equipment and commotion.

EMS has a "dress up" philosophy when it comes to **personal protective equipment** (PPE; gear used to protect against exposure to disease or injury); when you need it, you put it on. Equipment such as gloves, facemask, goggles, and a gown can be used by the EMT as protection against pathogens when needed (Figure 6-7). Occasionally

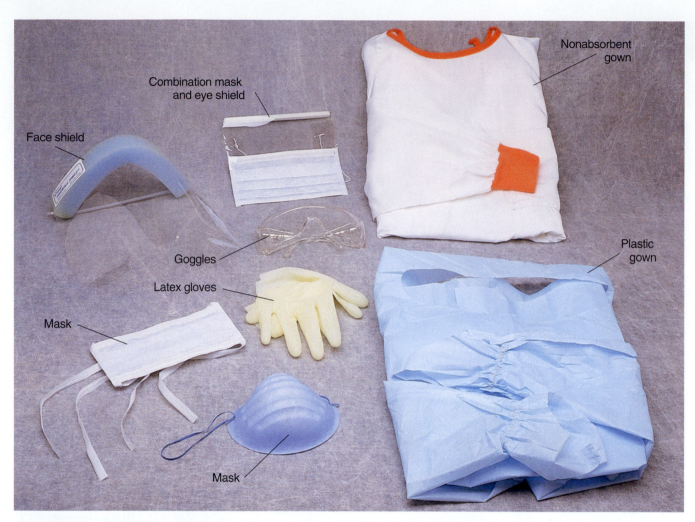

Face shield

Combination mask and eye shield

Nonabsorbent gown

Goggles

Plastic gown

Latex gloves

Mask

Mask

FIGURE 6-7 A variety of personal protective equipment is available for the EMT to use in infection control.

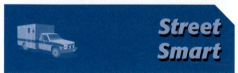

Street Smart

Many health care providers are sensitive to latex. This sensitivity may have already existed before the person became an EMT, or it may have developed over time after repeated exposure to latex. In either case, the EMT is advised to avoid wearing latex-containing gloves and to choose another material instead.

Some gloves are powdered with talc or other powders to make it easier to put the gloves on. Some EMTs are sensitive to the powder in the gloves. Many EMS agencies have stopped using powdered gloves entirely.

there is a delay while "gowning up," but the delay seldom creates a problem for the patient and it protects the EMT.

The first rule of infection control in EMS is to treat all bodily fluids as if they are potentially infectious. Table 6-4 lists potentially infectious body fluids that an EMT should avoid direct contact with. Remember that "an ounce of prevention is worth a pound of cure." Whenever an EMT asks herself whether she needs personal protective equipment, she probably does. This level of protection was formerly called **body substance isolation**, referring to protection against any body substance that could be considered potentially infectious. This term has been replaced with perhaps the more appropriate **Standard Precautions**. This terminology describes the need to assume that all patients have the potential to have some form of infectious disease and the protective measures should be considered standard for every patient encounter.

Barrier Devices

Barrier devices are any articles that create a physical partition between the EMT and the environment. These devices act like a second layer of skin, affording the EMT another layer of protection.

Gloves

Because so much of what an EMT does involves the hands, the barrier devices used most often are gloves. Gloves are a very important reality in every health care provider's daily practice. A glove, when it is used properly, is an excellent barrier to transmission of disease by direct contact. Gloves can be made from several different materials, all of which are effective barriers to disease transmission.

"Surgical" gloves fit very snugly and are preferred by doctors and nurses for certain procedures. These special gloves are sterilized. Sterile gloves have gone through the process of **sterilization**, in which they are treated to remove any microorganisms. In general, sterile gloves are not necessary for EMTs, except under specific situations. The added cost of routinely using sterile gloves is unjustifiable.

Before the start of any duty shift, the EMT should find the appropriate type and size of gloves. Gloves of different sizes must be provided to the EMT. Many times an EMT will put on a pair of gloves at the start of patient care and not remove them until the patient is at the emergency department, perhaps an hour or so later. Comfort is important when gloves are worn for long periods of time.

Nonsterile gloves, the type EMTs commonly use, are designed for one use and one patient only. Gloves should never be washed off and reused.

If the glove becomes torn when caring for the patient, the EMT should stop, wash the hands, and replace the gloves with a new pair of gloves before returning to patient care. If soap and water are not readily available, then waterless hand cleaners or antiseptic towelettes should be used. The EMT responsible for driving the emergency vehicle should deglove and wash the hands before beginning transport. Once at the emergency facility, the EMT should then reglove before handling and transferring the patient.

The importance of hand washing after wearing gloves in all instances cannot be stressed enough. Although gloves provide a substantial amount of protection, they do not provide perfect protection and microscopic tears sometimes occur. These microscopic tears may allow small amounts of blood or other material through, where they may come into contact with the EMT's skin. Any tiny breaks in the skin can then serve as a portal of entry.

Goggles

The eyes represent one of the largest exposed mucous membranes of an EMT. The eyes have many special self-protective capabilities that other mucous membranes do not have. Despite this fact, the eyes remain very vulnerable to splashes with body fluids if the EMT is unprotected.

Keeping the concept of barrier devices in mind, the EMT can protect the eyes by using goggles or protective safety glasses. Eye protection is a large concern in many industries in addition to EMS. Responding to this demand, manufacturers have created dozens of styles and types of protective eyewear. An EMT should shop around for the eyewear that fits the best and then practice wearing it regularly.

Some EMTs wear eyeglasses for reading and other everyday activities. These glasses are satisfactory, provided they also fulfill their

TABLE 6-4

Potentially Infectious Body Fluids

Blood
Amniotic fluid
Vaginal discharge
Semen
Cerebrospinal fluid
Pleural fluid
Synovial fluid
Peritoneal fluid
Pericardial fluid

Fluids with little potential to transmit blood-borne diseases:

- Tears
- Nasal discharge
- Vomitus
- Sputum
- Saliva
- Feces
- Urine

Street Smart

Always change gloves between patients to eliminate cross-contamination between two patients. An EMT should always carry spare gloves for use when assessing multiple patients on a scene such as a motor vehicle collision.

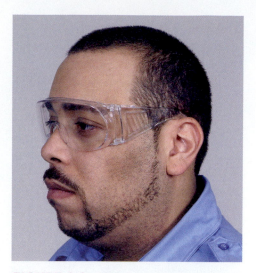

FIGURE 6-8 Without side guards, regular eyeglasses provide incomplete protection against splashes.

primary purpose in EMS, splash protection (Figure 6-8). Without side-splash protection, the EMT with eyeglasses is at risk for an accidental exposure.

Masks

Masks provide protection from blood and other fluids splashing into the open mouth of the EMT. This problem is most common when an EMT is performing a procedure, such as suctioning the airway, that requires the EMT to be close to the patient.

Masks provide another protection as well. A mask will protect the EMT from inhaling airborne infectious particles. These particles are often carried on microscopic water droplets in the air around the patient when the patient coughs or sneezes.

One specific airborne disease, a drug-resistant strain of TB, has become a problem to all health care workers in recent years. This systemic illness is discussed in greater detail later.

The increased incidence of resistant TB makes it necessary that any EMT caring for a patient with a cough must wear a protective mask. A protective mask, such as the N95 mask, should be carried with the EMT so that it is readily available (Figure 6-9). The mask is another barrier device that prevents exposure of the EMT to disease.

Some masks come as a mask/eye protection combination device (Figure 6-10). These "face shields" are often very convenient for the EMT. They both provide mouth, nose, and eye protection and speed the process for application of PPE. EMTs should refer to their agency infection control manual to determine the appropriate type of mask to use for a given situation.

Pocket Mask

An EMT who comes upon a nonbreathing patient must always consider her own protection by using a pocket mask to ventilate the patient (Figure 6-11).

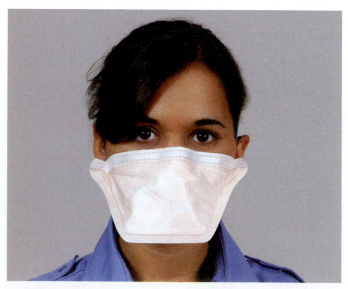

FIGURE 6-9 A mask provides the EMT with protection from airborne diseases.

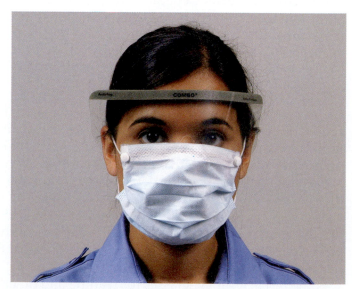

FIGURE 6-10 A mask and eye shield combination is both practical as well as effective.

If a pocket mask is not readily available, the EMT should have a transparent shield device at hand. Both the pocket mask and the shield are barrier devices that allow effective ventilation while preventing direct contact of the rescuer's mouth with the patient's oral secretions.

Gowns

Seldom does an EMT wear a protective gown. Most EMTs depend on their duty uniform to provide the first layer of protection against accidental blood or body fluid splatter. However, there are occasions when another layer would prevent gross contamination. These situations include childbirth and severe arterial bleeding.

Most gowns tie in the back and are impermeable to fluids. Some of these gowns are made of specially coated paper material. The more durable gowns are made of cloth and can be recycled. For the limited use that EMTs make of gowns, most EMS services provide the paper style of gown.

In the few cases in which more head-to-toe protection is needed, an EMT should consider wearing a disposable one-piece jumpsuit. These garments are used frequently in hazardous materials spills and are relatively inexpensive.

In the majority of high-risk cases, the EMT should wear a long paper gown. This will usually provide more-than-adequate protection while still being functional.

Table 6-5 illustrates the use of different personal protective gear as a part of Standard Precautions.

Donning and Removing Protective Apparel

EMTs are told what personal protective apparel to wear, but seldom are they told how to apply these articles or how to take them off. Improper application or careless removal of soiled protective apparel can result in accidental exposures.

Before putting on other personal protective apparel, the EMT should first put on a mask and eye protection. The ties should be tight, and the mask secure so that it will not fall down accidentally. The EMT should then put on a gown if necessary. Assistance tying the back of the gown is often needed. Last, gloves should be applied over the sleeves of the gown.

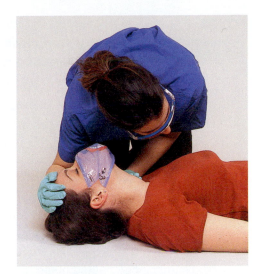

FIGURE 6-11 Barrier devices provide the EMT another margin of safety when performing cardiopulmonary resuscitation (CPR).

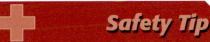
Safety Tip

To date, there has not been a documented case of disease transmission from patient to the EMT providing mouth-to-mouth; however, the EMT should not take the risk and attempt mouth-to-mouth ventilation unless there is absolutely no alternative. Proper preparation promotes good EMS practice. All EMTs should carry a barrier device with them.

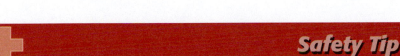
Safety Tip

In the past, a bloodied uniform was seen by some EMTs as a badge of courage. Today, a bloodied uniform is a hazard to the EMT, her partners, her patients, and the public. As soon as a uniform is soiled with blood or bodily fluids, the EMT should immediately change clothing, being careful to wash the exposed area thoroughly, and report any possible infectious fluid exposures. If heavy contamination is thought to be likely, an appropriate protective gown should be worn over the duty uniform.

TABLE 6-5

Standard Precautions for Infection Control

Wash Hands (Plain soap)

Wash after touching **blood, body fluids, secretions, excretions,** and **contaminated items.**

Wash immediately **after gloves are removed** and **between patient contacts.**

Avoid transfer of microorganisms to other patients or environments.

Wear Gloves

Wear when touching **blood, body fluids, secretions, excretions,** and **contaminated items.**

Put on **clean** gloves just **before touching mucous membranes** and **nonintact skin.**

Change gloves between tasks and procedures on the same patient after contact with material that may contain high concentrations of microorganisms. Remove gloves promptly after use, before touching noncontaminated items and environmental surfaces, and before going to another patient, and wash hands immediately to avoid transfer of microorganisms to other patients or environments.

Wear Mask and Eye Protection or Face Shield

Protect mucous membranes of the eyes, nose, and mouth during procedures and patient-care activities that are likely to generate **splashes** or **sprays** of **blood, body fluids, secretions,** or **excretions.**

Wear Gown

Protect skin and prevent soiling of clothing during procedures that are likely to generate **splashes** or **sprays** of **blood, body fluids, secretions,** or **excretions.** Remove a soiled gown as promptly as possible and wash hands to avoid transfer of microorganisms to other patients or environments.

Patient-Care Equipment

Handle used patient-care equipment soiled with **blood, body fluids, secretions,** or **excretions** in a manner that prevents skin and mucous membrane exposures, contamination of clothing, and transfer of microorganisms to other patients or environments. Ensure that reusable equipment is not used for the care of another patient until it has been appropriately cleaned and reprocessed and single-use items are properly discarded.

Linen

Handle, transport, and process used linen soiled with **blood, body fluids, secretions,** or **excretions** in a manner that prevents exposures and contamination of clothing and avoids transfer of microorganisms to other patients or environments.

Use **resuscitation devices** as an alternative to mouth-to-mouth resuscitation.

(Courtesy of BREVIS Corporation.)

To take off the personal protective apparel, the EMT should go in reverse order. First, the EMT would remove her gloves, then the gown, mask, and eye protection. In the case of gross contamination from blood or other fluid, the risk of accidental exposure is too great for an EMT to disrobe alone. The assistance of another EMT should be requested to ensure better safety and to decrease the risk of self-contamination. Specific instructions on application and removal of personal protective equipment are provided in Skills 6-2 and 6-3.

SKILL 6-2 *Donning and Removing Personal Protective Equipment (PPE)*

PURPOSE: To protect the EMT from blood and other bodily fluids. The task to be performed dictates the appropriate barrier devices to be worn.

STANDARD PRECAUTIONS:

   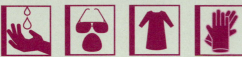

- ☑ Mask
- ☑ Goggles
- ☑ Gown
- ☑ Nonsterile examination gloves (EMTs with latex sensitivity should wear vinyl gloves)

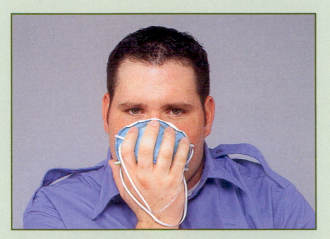

1 The EMT grasps the top ties of the mask and positions the metal strip in the mask over the bridge of the nose.

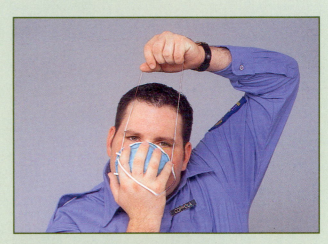

2 Pull the elastic straps over the head.

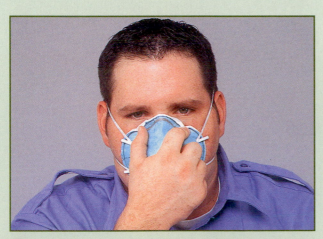

3 Grasp and pinch the metal strip around the bridge of the nose.

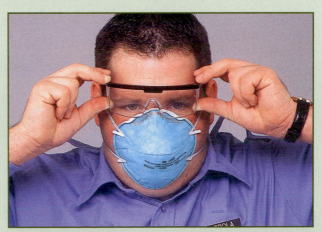

4 Pick up and apply the protective eyewear.

(continues)

SKILL 6-2 (continued)

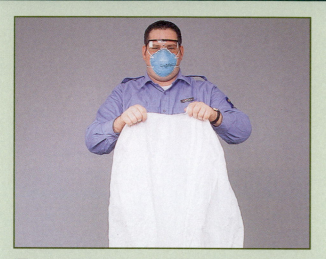

5 The EMT then grasps the gown by the collar and allows it to hang with the inside of the gown toward the EMT.

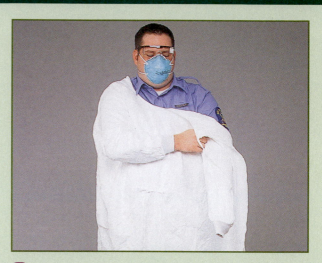

6 Next, the EMT places his arms in the sleeves.

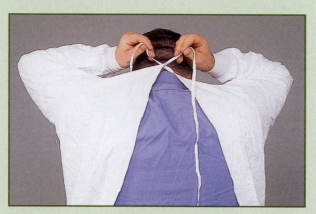

7 Then the EMT ties the gown behind the neck.

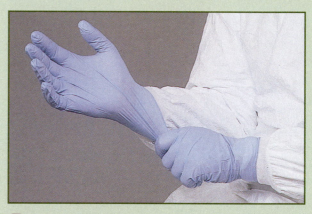

8 Next, the EMT pulls on properly sized examination gloves. Each glove's collar should be over the sleeve of the gown.

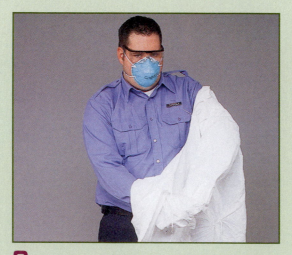

9 To remove the PPE, the EMT would reverse the order and wash the hands afterward.

SKILL 6-3 *Donning and Removing Gloves*

PURPOSE: To protect the EMT from blood and bodily fluids.

STANDARD PRECAUTIONS:

☑ Nonsterile gloves
☑ Hazardous waste container

APPLICATION OF NONSTERILE GLOVES

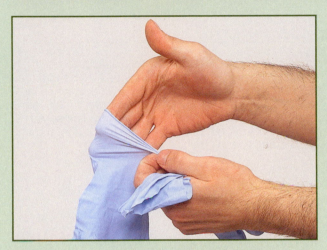

1 Choose an appropriate size and type of glove for the task at hand. Arrange one glove so that the thumb is aligned with the thumb of the hand it is intended to go on.

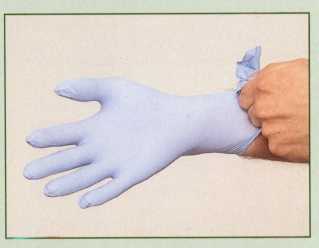

2 Grasp the front of the cuff with one hand, while inserting the other hand into the glove. Be sure to place each finger within the appropriate finger section. Pull at the cuff to ensure that the glove is completely applied to the hand.

REMOVAL OF CONTAMINATED GLOVES

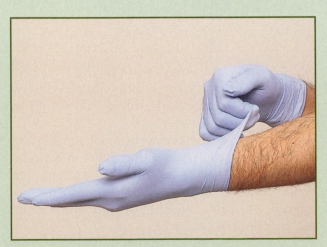

3 Repeat the process for the other hand.

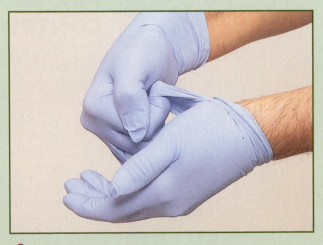

4 Grasp the palm or outside cuff of the left glove with the gloved right hand.

(continues)

SKILL 6-3 *(continued)*

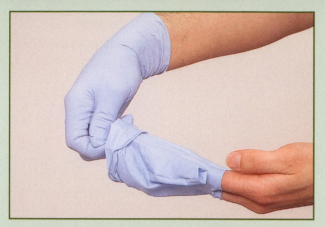

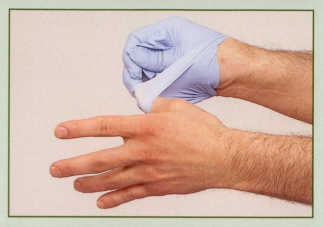

5 Pull the left glove toward the fingertips. The glove should turn inside out as it is removed.

6 Hold the removed glove in the still-gloved right hand. Insert the thumb of the ungloved left hand under the cuff of the right glove, carefully avoiding any contaminated areas. Pull the right glove toward the fingertips, turning it inside out as it is removed. The soiled left glove should remain in the palm of the right glove as it is removed.

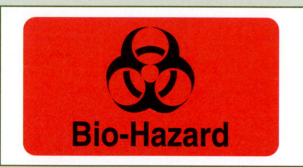

7 Dispose of the gloves in a container clearly marked with the biohazard label and wash hands thoroughly.

PREPARING FOR INFECTION CONTROL

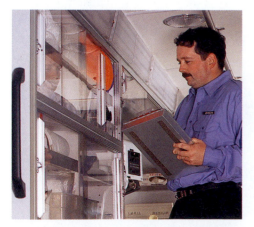

FIGURE 6-12 All emergency response vehicles must have an adequate stock of personal protective equipment for all personnel on board.

Before an emergency call occurs, it is important that the EMT be prepared. Chapter 2 describes much of the preparation involved in training, education, and equipment readiness. An infection control plan is a part of that preparation.

Emergency service agencies will have written plans relating to infection control practices. These plans are found in the infection control manual. The EMT should know the location of the infection control manual. An infection control manual should list typical situations that may be encountered and how the EMT would protect herself from potential disease exposure in each case.

At the start of every shift, or tour of duty, the EMT should be sure that there is an adequate supply of gloves, gowns, and masks as well as prepare the ambulance or emergency response vehicle (Figure 6-12). Floors should routinely be mopped with a cleaning solution that includes a disinfectant such as bleach. The entire interior of the vehicle must be cleaned regularly, according to departmental standards contained within the infection control manual.

House Rules

Many EMTs reside at a station when they are on duty. The rules listed in Table 6-6 represent good health practices in the station house. When followed, these practices will result in a work environment safe from unnecessary contamination.

Responding to a Call

Prearrival instructions from the communications center can offer the EMT an opportunity to prepare PPE. On the basis of the information given, the EMT can decide what PPE to use.

For example, a patient with a cough, fever, and chills would represent several potential hazards to the EMT, including blood-borne and airborne infections. The EMT would minimally need a pair of non-sterile gloves and a mask that also offers eye protection.

On the Scene

Infectious disease precautions taken upon arrival to the scene are usually based on the patient's chief complaint (CC) or on the emergency medical procedures that are required. Complaint-driven PPE assumes that the EMT spoke to the patient and has considered the patient's chief complaint and the PPE that should be used. Table 6-7 lists common patient complaints and the PPE that the EMT should use.

While assessing a patient, an EMT may discover certain signs of disease. For example, a person with a rash and fever may have an infectious disease and should be assumed to be contagious.

Whatever the case, the EMT must have PPE readily available. Eye protection left in the ambulance cannot protect the EMT in the house.

TABLE 6-6

House Rules

1. EMTs may not eat food, apply makeup, or smoke until after hands have been washed thoroughly.

2. No hand washing is allowed in the same sink that food is prepared in.

3. Hands must be washed after:
   - every EMS call
   - whenever toilet is flushed
   - whenever hands are soiled

4. All contaminated clothing must be removed before entering the dayroom.

5. Any potential infectious disease exposures must be reported immediately.

TABLE 6-7

Common Chief Complaints and Personal Protective Equipment

Chief Complaint	Gloves	Mask	Eyewear	Gown
Fever	X	X		
Rash	X	X		
Seizures	X	X		
Coughing	X	X	X	
Bleeding wounds	X (if spurting)	X	X (if spurting)	X (if spurting)
Neck stiffness	X	X		
Vomiting	X	X		

TABLE 6-8

Common EMS Tasks and Personal Protective Equipment

Task	Gloves	Mask	Eyewear	Gown
Taking pulse rate	X			
Measuring blood pressure	X			
Controlling bleeding (minimal visible blood)	X			
Giving an injection	X			
Inserting oropharyngeal/ nasopharyngeal airway	X	X	X	
Suctioning	X	X	X	
Intubation	X	X	X	
Arterial bleeding control	X	X	X	X
Assisting childbirth	X	X	X	X
Disinfecting equipment	X	X	X	X

Procedure-driven PPE implies that the first step of every emergency medical procedure performed by an EMT is to don PPE. For example, whenever suction is used, the EMT should minimally have on gloves, eye protection, and a mask. Table 6-8 lists common emergency medical procedures performed by EMTs and the PPE that must be used.

Needle Disposal

EMTs will often work side by side with paramedics who are using IV needles and other sharp instruments. Some EMTs will assist a paramedic with the administration of certain drugs that require a needle to inject them into the skin. In any case, the needle must be safely discarded.

The single largest risk of occupational exposure to blood-borne diseases is by accidental needle stick. It is important for EMTs to know how to handle any needle, syringe, or sharp blade. These groups of potentially hazardous instruments are commonly referred to as **sharps**.

Once used, all sharps must go directly into an approved **sharps container**. These containers, either bright red or white with a biohazard label on the side, are essentially puncture proof. To be effective, the sharps container must be readily accessible to the EMT. Carrying a sharp any distance for disposal is risky. Small sharps containers are frequently carried to the scene by paramedics so that needles may be immediately and safely disposed of.

A sharp should be dropped into the sharps container, as demonstrated in Figure 6-13. Sharps should never be forced into a container because they may break and cause injury to the EMT. When transfer-

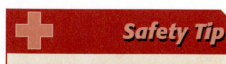

Safety Tip

Although it may be tempting to do so, the EMT should never recap a needle or other sharp instrument. The risk of injury while replacing a cap over a contaminated needle is unnecessary.

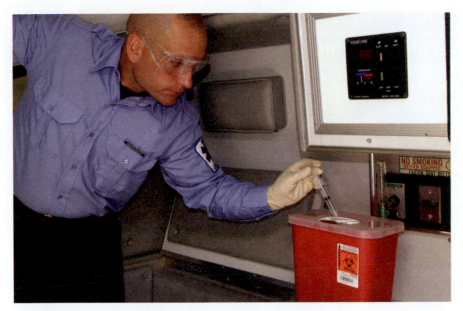

FIGURE 6-13 Sharp objects, such as IV needles, must be properly disposed of immediately.

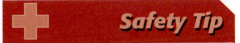

ring a sharp object to a container, the EMT should always point the needle or sharp edge downward.

It is the responsibility of all EMTs, both basic and advanced, to be accountable for all sharps. The scene must be clear of all sharps before it is considered safe. In some EMS systems, the person responsible for the sharps calls out "all sharps clear" to indicate to other team members that the scene is safe.

Disposal of Waste

Bloody bandages and other contaminated waste must be disposed of properly before leaving the scene. These potentially infectious materials are considered a **biohazard**. A biohazard is any material that is potentially contaminated with biological waste. There are strict rules regarding the collection and management of biohazardous waste.

Biohazardous waste must be placed in a red plastic bag that is clearly marked with the biohazard sign, as shown in Figure 6-14. The red-bagged waste must be treated as infectious waste and placed in a proper disposal unit.

Not all waste on a scene is a biohazard. Oxygen masks, clear plastic wrappers, and the like should be put into regular garbage containers. Table 6-9 illustrates potentially infectious items typically used on the scene and where they should be disposed of. Of course any item that is covered with blood or other body fluids should be considered biohazardous waste and disposed of properly.

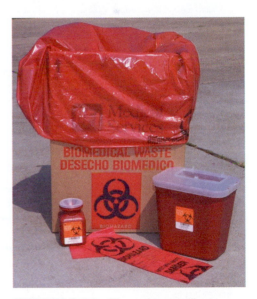

FIGURE 6-14 The red bag indicates that the contents are biohazardous.

After the Call

After the patient has been turned over to another health care professional, the EMT must turn her attention to getting back in service.

The EMT should remove any contaminated clothing and put on a clean change of clothes. Being careful to avoid further contamination, the EMT should place her soiled clothing into the proper bin for soiled laundry.

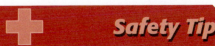

TABLE 6-9

Disposal of Potentially Infectious Materials

Item	Regular Waste (white bag)	Biohazardous Waste (red bag)	Sharps Container (hard plastic box)
Airway equipment	X		
Tissues	X		
Nasal cannula	X		
Oxygen mask	X		
Bag-valve-mask	X		
Plastic wraps	X		
Gloves	X		
Paper gowns	X		
Filled emesis basin		X	
Bloody dressing		X	
Vaginal pads		X	
Absorbent pads		X	
Soiled adult undergarments		X	
IV needles			X
Injection needles			X
Blood-filled glass tubes			X

The EMT should then wash her hands thoroughly, in the same manner as described previously. The importance of washing hands before doing anything else cannot be stressed enough. An EMT should not apply any makeup, smoke any cigarettes, or eat any food until the hands have been washed.

If a sink with running water is not immediately available, then the EMT should use either a waterless, alcohol-based cleansing gel or an antiseptic cloth made just for that purpose.

Documentation

Documentation is a very important part of an EMT's responsibilities. Documentation of infectious disease can be divided into patient reporting and exposure reporting.

When an EMT is reporting a patient's condition on the patient care report, all signs and symptoms considered significant must be listed, even if they do not appear to be related to the chief complaint (Figure 6-15).

Cleaning Up

When the paperwork has been completed, or while it is being done, the emergency equipment must be returned to service. This process includes cleaning equipment, noting defective or damaged equipment, and reporting it or replacing it.

One of the essential tasks before a piece of equipment can be returned to service is removal of obvious contamination, or **decontamination**. Decontamination is the use of either chemical or physical means to remove or neutralize any disease-causing organisms. After completion of the decontamination process, the equipment must not be capable of transmitting disease to another person. There are several levels of decontamination.

The lowest level of decontamination is really just plain old-fashioned housekeeping. If there is no visible blood or body fluids, then the object is simply wiped down with a hospital disinfectant designed for such low-level disinfection.

High-level disinfection requires sterilization. Sterilization, as the name implies, kills all microorganisms on the surface. Sterilization is required for any piece of equipment that might enter into another person's body, such as an IV catheter. Obtaining this level of decontamination often involves special procedures such as hot steam and pressure processing, autoclaving (Figure 6-16), or gas sterilization, with expensive equipment.

Typically, EMTs do not sterilize their equipment. It is more cost-effective to use disposable equipment. Disposable equipment is discarded into appropriate waste receptacles once it has been used.

Occasionally, EMTs who either work with paramedics or who perform special procedures, such as intubation, need to sterilize individual pieces of equipment. In those cases, special chemicals are used. This process can take up to 12 or 24 hours, depending on the chemical sterilant. Strict adherence to cleaning guidelines is required.

Emergency Equipment Cleanup

A majority of the cleanup concerns EMTs have are related to handling equipment contaminated with blood or other body fluids. First, the EMT should don a pair of gloves (heavy-duty kitchen-type gloves are preferred). An impermeable apron or gown may be required if splashing can reasonably be anticipated.

The next step is to remove the gross contamination with plain soap and water. The equipment should be cleaned down to the surface, and no visible blood should remain.

The next step depends on what the piece of equipment is used for. If the equipment would touch only a patient's skin, then only intermediate-level disinfection is necessary. If the equipment would touch a patient's mucous membranes, then high-level disinfection is required.

With intermediate disinfection, the surface is wiped down with an Environmental Protection Agency (EPA) registered germicide. A cleaner that can kill pathogens, as written on the product label, is considered to be a germicide.

Alternatively, many EMTs use a bleach-and-water solution (1:100 mixture). This is a cost-effective and practical method of achieving

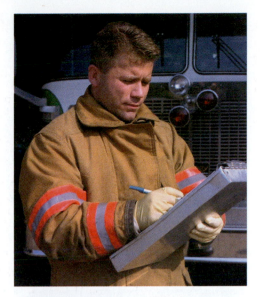

FIGURE 6-15 Documentation of the symptoms that the patient gave provides other health care providers a basis for more treatment.

Street Smart

A word of caution: Documentation of a patient's AIDS/HIV status is controversial. Questions about breaches of a patient's right to confidentiality and right to privacy have been raised. In some states, a court hearing is required before HIV information can be released.

All EMTs are advised to follow the instructions of their local medical control and county or state health departments regarding documentation of AIDS/HIV status. The advice of legal counsel can also be valuable in this circumstance.

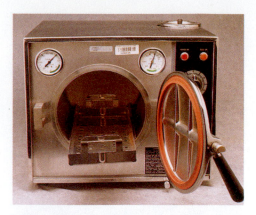

FIGURE 6-16 Sterilization, using an autoclave, is the highest level of disinfection.

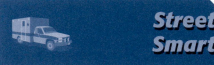

Street Smart

If it is not possible to remove visible blood, vomitus, and so on, such as often occurs when Velcro® is soiled, then the equipment should be discarded.

Safety Tip

Many cleaning solutions are potentially toxic if ingested, inhaled, or contacted for prolonged periods. Read the Material Safety Data Sheet (MSDS) as well as the label and package for safe use instructions for these products.

Street Smart

Avoid wiping down clear plastic surfaces with bleach solution because it can fog the surface.

intermediate-level disinfection. Table 6-10 lists the types of equipment an EMT might use and the level of decontamination that is necessary.

Cleaning Areas

In all emergency departments, there is an area that is usually referred to as the "dirty utility room." This area is marked with a biohazard sign that warns people that inside are dangerous chemicals as well as potentially infectious materials.

The room is usually well designed for its purpose. The area should be both well lighted and well ventilated. All drains from large sinks or hoppers (Figure 6-17), toilets, and floor drains empty into a separate sewer system for proper disposal. There is usually a large nonporous work surface as well as hoses or sprayers that permit equipment from bedpans to backboards to be washed down.

Equipment may be dried, in racks, in the dirty utility room, but it is never stored there. Equipment that is cleaned in these dirty utility rooms is never to be used in the kitchen, bathrooms, or living areas of an EMS station.

Cleaning the Ambulance

After all contaminated equipment and waste have been removed, it is important to clean the vehicle. The rules for cleaning an ambulance are the same as for cleaning the equipment.

If no visible blood or other body fluids are present, then wiping the exposed surfaces with a hospital disinfectant is all that is necessary. Airing out the ambulance for a few minutes is also a good idea.

TABLE 6-10

Decontamination of EMS Equipment			
Item	Low	Intermediate	High
Stretcher		X	
Linen	X	X	
Surfaces	X		
Benches	X		
Stethoscope		X	
Blood pressure cuff		X	
Splints		X	
Cervical collars		X	
Backboards		X	
Intubation equipment			X

If blood or other biohazard is visible, soak up any blood or other body fluids with an absorbent towel, taking care to dispose of it properly. Then scrub the surface with soap and water to further remove grossly visible contamination (Figure 6-18). Next, disinfect the surface with either a bleach solution or a germicidal solution.

Next, air out the vehicle until all exposed surfaces are dried. This step usually takes only 10 or 15 minutes.

It is important that the ambulance be cleaned thoroughly on a regular basis. Many EMS agencies have instituted a mandatory cleaning schedule that includes such tasks as wiping down the underside of the ambulance stretcher and cleaning the walls and ceiling of the ambulance. Small blood splashes, invisible to the naked eye, can harbor such potentially infectious diseases as hepatitis B for weeks.

The last step of every EMS call is restocking the vehicle. Do not forget to replace the personal protective equipment that was used. Glove boxes need to be full. All portable kits need to be complete with eye protection, gloves, masks, and gowns.

CONCLUSION

The importance of infection control to the daily practice of an EMT cannot be overemphasized. Training beyond what is received in an EMT class must occur at the agency level. Training at the agency level must be continual, reemphasizing the potential hazards and infection control precautions that are specific to the local community. Regular immunizations and annual health monitoring are necessary for all health care workers. EMTs must become educated about infection control and integrate that education into their practice.

TEST YOUR KNOWLEDGE

1. What is the importance of infection control?
2. What are five of the more common infectious illnesses that an EMT will encounter?
3. What are the different modes of disease transmission?
4. What is meant by portal of entry?
5. What are all of the items of personal protective equipment an EMT should have available to prevent an accidental exposure to an infectious disease?
6. What is meant by the term *Standard Precautions*?
7. What are the different levels of disinfection?
8. What is an infection control plan, and where can it be found?
9. Why is it important to document a potential infectious disease exposure?
10. How do notification laws affect the EMT?
11. What is proper medical follow-up for an infectious disease exposure?

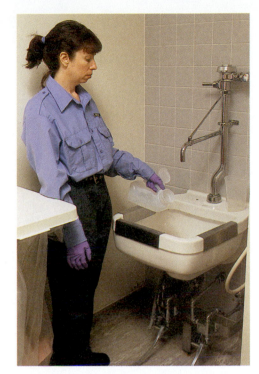

FIGURE 6-17 Liquid waste should be disposed of in a toilet or similar device, such as the hopper shown here, and flushed into the sanitary system.

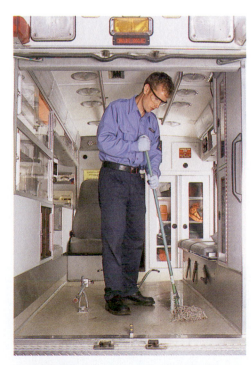

FIGURE 6-18 Regular cleaning of an ambulance is part of the regular routine of every EMT.

INTERNET RESOURCES

Visit the Web sites of the following organizations for information on infection control:

- Occupational Safety and Health Administration (OSHA), http://www.osha.gov
- National Fire Protection Agency (NFPA), http://www.nfpa.org
- Centers for Disease Control and Prevention (CDC), http://www.cdc.gov

FURTHER STUDY

Centers for Disease Control and Prevention. (1997a). Immunization of health-care workers: Recommendations of the Advisory Committee on Immunization Practices (ACIP) and the Hospital Infection Control Practices Advisory Committee (HICPAC). *MMWR Morbidity and Mortality Weekly Report*, 46(RR-18), 1–42.

Centers for Disease Control and Prevention. (1997b). Recommendations for follow-up of health-care workers after occupational exposure to hepatitis C virus. *MMWR Morbidity and Mortality Weekly Report*, 46, 603–606.

Centers for Disease Control and Prevention. (1998). Public Health Service Guidelines for the management of health-care worker exposures to HIV and recommendations for postexposure prophylaxis. *MMWR Morbidity and Mortality Weekly Report*, 47(RR-7), 1–33.

Guide to managing an emergency service infection control program. (2002). Publications Center, United States Fire Administration, 16825 South Seton Avenue, Emmitsburg, MD 21727.

Occupation Safety and Health Administration. (1991, December 6). *Occupational exposure to bloodborne pathogens* (Final Rule No. 29, CFR Part 1910.1030). Washington, DC: U.S. Department of Labor.

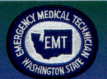

CHAPTER 7

Basic Airway Control

KEY TERMS

airway

apnea

cross-fingered technique

cyanosis

epiglottis

esophagus

French catheter

gag reflex

head-tilt, chin-lift

jaw thrust

larynx

mandible

maxilla

nasal flaring

nasopharyngeal airway (NPA)

occlusion

oropharyngeal airway (OPA)

pharynx

recovery position

saliva

sputum

sublingual

tonsils

trachea

uvula

ventilation

Yankauer

OBJECTIVES

Upon completion of this chapter, the reader should be able to:

1. Name and label on a diagram the major structures of the respiratory system.
2. Describe the steps in performing the head-tilt, chin-lift.
3. Relate mechanism of injury to methods of opening the airway.
4. Describe the steps in performing the jaw thrust.
5. State the importance of having a suction unit ready for immediate use when providing emergency care.
6. Describe the technique of suctioning.
7. Describe how to measure and insert an oropharyngeal (oral) airway.
8. Describe how to measure and insert a nasopharyngeal (nasal) airway.

OVERVIEW

The ability to open and maintain a patent airway in a patient is the single most important lifesaving skill an emergency medical technician (EMT) can learn. Remarkably, the most common airway obstruction is created by the patient's own tongue. The most basic airway maneuvers can relieve that obstruction. EMTs, as the largest group of prehospital medical care providers, must be experts at airway control.

The mantra for the EMT is simple: *Open, assess, suction, and secure.* This simple order of tasks represents what could be the most important actions an EMT can take to save a life.

ANATOMY REVIEW

In discussions of the management of a patient's airway, it is useful to have a clear picture of the relevant anatomy. Starting at the lips, the first structures encountered are the teeth. Teeth are usually fairly stable, primarily because they are embedded in bone. Blunt trauma can dislodge the teeth, making them potential airway obstructions. The teeth also have an excellent blood supply and can bleed profusely when disrupted. The loose teeth and blood can then block the airway, decreasing free airflow.

The teeth are embedded into two jawbones. The lower jawbone, the **mandible**, serves as the floor of the mouth. Attached to the mandible, at the back of the throat, is the tongue. Therefore, if the mandible is moved, the tongue is also moved. The upper jawbone, or **maxilla**, holds the roof of the mouth, or the hard palate. The palate is the border between the floor of the nose and the roof of the mouth.

Most normal breathing occurs through the nose. The nose not only smells aromas in the air it also adds moisture to the airway and raises the temperature of the air to body temperature. The nose consists of two nostrils that are divided by a septum. Taking in a deep breath results in **nasal flaring**, or widening of the nostrils. Persistent nasal flaring is a sign of respiratory distress. The nostrils, acting as air intake ports, open larger to take in larger and larger amounts of air.

The area in the back of the throat, where the oral cavity and the nasal cavity meet, called the **pharynx**, contains several easily identified structures. As seen in Figure 7-1, the most obvious structure is the small piece of flesh that is hanging off the roof of the mouth called the

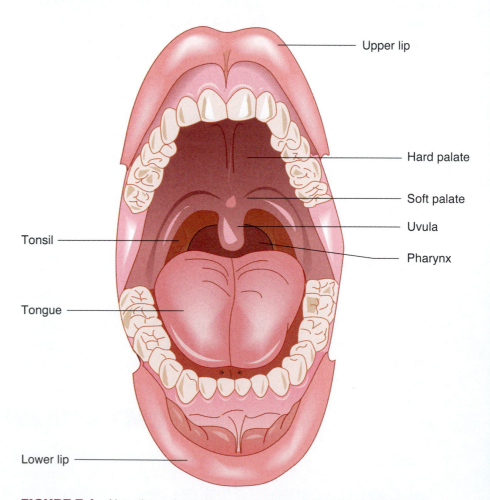

Upper lip

Hard palate

Soft palate

Uvula

Pharynx

Tonsil

Tongue

Lower lip

FIGURE 7-1   Note the various structures in the mouth visible from the front, including the teeth, tonsils, and palate.

uvula. The uvula swings up to help protect the nasal cavity when a swallow occurs. It is also the farthest point that is visible to the EMT without special equipment.

On each side of the back of the throat are two pillars of soft tissue called the **tonsils**. These tissues are very fragile, and vigorous suctioning can result in serious bleeding.

The tongue is probably the most important structure in the mouth. The tongue enables us to taste our food when we eat and helps with our speech. The entire surface of the tongue is covered with a liquid called **saliva**. This saliva is created by salivary glands lining the mouth. Bacteria and other harmful microorganisms are entrapped in saliva to be swallowed and destroyed in the stomach's acid, or "spit" out. This feature of saliva makes the entire interior of the mouth a potential source of infectious body fluids. An EMT working within the mouth (oral cavity) must observe proper Standard Precautions (body substance isolation).

The tongue is vascular, meaning it has many blood vessels. The source of the blood supply for the tongue comes from under the tongue in an area called the **sublingual** area. Because the area is so rich with blood, medications are often deposited under the tongue to be absorbed into the bloodstream.

In the back of the throat, not visible to the EMT, is the base of the tongue. As seen in Figure 7-2, the base of the tongue is at the top of both the windpipe, called the trachea, and the food passage, called the **esophagus**.

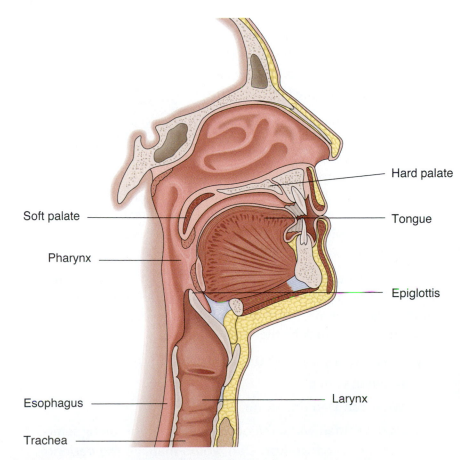

FIGURE 7-2 Note the relationship of the esophagus to the trachea.

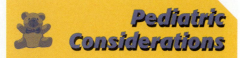

Pediatric Considerations

The epiglottis in a child is relatively larger and less rigid than that of an adult. As a result, swelling and inflammation can result in a complete blockage of the airway. This condition, called *epiglottitis*, is clearly very serious.

Street Smart

When placing a suction catheter into a patient's mouth, an EMT may stimulate a gag reflex. This reflex will often result in retching as the patient tries to expel the catheter from the mouth. Not uncommonly, such a reflex will also lead to vomiting. Vomiting will certainly not assist in airway clearance. The EMT should always take care when suctioning a patient who has an intact gag reflex.

The base of the tongue also abuts a very important structure called the **epiglottis**, which means "above the glottis." The glottis is the opening to the sound-producing portion of the throat, the voice box or **larynx**. More important, it is the uppermost structure of the lower airway.

To prevent the accidental passage of food into the airway during swallowing, the epiglottis blocks off the trachea. If a food particle enters the trachea, the patient will cough vigorously in an attempt to dislodge it from the airway. This coughing also brings up mucus from the airway called **sputum**.

If a piece of food is too large to be swallowed, it will strike the walls of the back of the throat, and the patient will gag. Stimulation of this protective response, called the **gag reflex**, results in the objects being expelled from the mouth, protecting the airway from blockage by the food.

For a more complete review of the structures of the upper airway, please refer to Chapter 5.

He's Not Breathing

The phone rang, and a frantic voice at the other end cried, "Come quick, Brian's not breathing!" Dan, the resident adviser for the dorm, quickly called campus public safety and reported a possible medical emergency in room 951.

Dan had been an EMT back in his hometown of Spring Valley, so he knew that he could help. He grabbed his first aid bag and ran up the nine flights of stairs.

Stopping long enough to catch his breath, Dan looked into the room. He saw Brian, a freshman, lying unconscious on the floor next to the couch. Looking around the room, he quickly concluded that there had been a dorm party. Dozens of empty beer bottles were scattered on the floor, and a couple of half-empty whisky bottles were on the table. Everyone was huddled against the far wall.

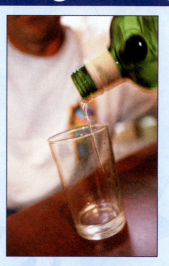

(Courtesy of PhotoDisc.)

Brian had obviously been laid on the floor. His head had been propped up on a pillow, and he was making a loud snoring sound. As Dan approached Brian, donning gloves in the process, he was suddenly struck by the smell of vomit.

- Why is Brian snoring? What are the implications of smelling vomit?

- What can Dan do, alone, to help Brian?

- Assume Brian was semiconscious. Would his being semiconscious change how Dan would manage the patient?

PHYSIOLOGY

The human body needs oxygen to allow the cells of the body to produce energy. Without oxygen, the body dies in a process called *shock*. This process is discussed in detail in Chapter 9.

The lungs supply the body with oxygen. The lungs get oxygen from the air inhaled into the airway. The airway is a passage starting at the mouth and ending in the lungs. This airway is not a simple open conduit. It takes many muscles and nerves to keep the airway open. Whenever a patient cannot maintain this airway as an open passageway, the EMT must assist in its maintenance.

Control of the airway essentially involves the realignment of the structures of the upper airway until they create an open passageway for air movement. This movement of air into and out of the lungs is called *breathing*, or **ventilation**. Ventilation is not possible without a clear airway.

Signs of an Obstructed Airway

Loss of consciousness often results in relaxation of the muscles, including the muscles in the airway. The immediate result is that the soft tissues of the throat, and particularly the tongue, collapse into the airway. Therefore, any unconscious patient is assumed to have a potential airway obstruction.

The collapse of the pharyngeal soft tissues makes the smooth passage of air more difficult. If the obstruction created by these collapsed tissues is not complete and air is able to get through, the patient may make a characteristic snoring sound as the air pushes past the tongue and pharyngeal tissues. The EMT should recognize a snoring sound in the unconscious patient as a partial airway obstruction. The tongue is the single most common cause of airway obstruction in the unconscious patient, as seen in Figure 7-3.

If the collapsed pharyngeal tissue, or any other object, has completely occluded the airway, no air movement will occur; therefore, no noise will be evident. Breathlessness, or **apnea**, is a potential sign of a completely obstructed airway. A blue discoloration to the skin, called **cyanosis**, is an indication that blood is not getting oxygen, possibly because of an airway obstruction. As demonstrated in Figure 7-4,

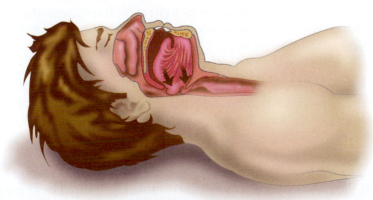

Obstructed airway (tongue against pharynx)

FIGURE 7-3 The tongue commonly creates an airway obstruction in the supine, unconscious patient.

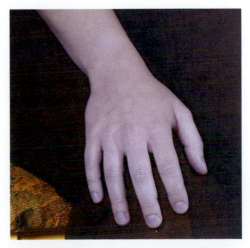

FIGURE 7-4 Look for cyanosis at the fingernail beds.

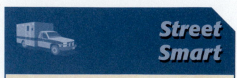

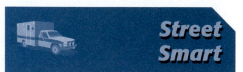

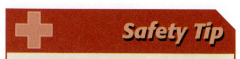

cyanosis is often most visible in the fingernail beds, the inner eyelid, called the *conjunctiva*, and the inside of the lips. No matter the cause, the EMT must quickly recognize the patient with a complete airway obstruction and provide an effective remedy.

PERSONAL PROTECTIVE EQUIPMENT

An EMT protecting the airway is at an increased risk of exposure to blood, sputum, and saliva. All of these body fluids are potential carriers for infectious disease.

EMTs rarely forget to wear gloves but are often careless in regard to eye protection and masks. A cough is a forceful and sometimes violent exhalation of air. A cough can easily expel microorganism-laden sputum as far as 3–4 feet. Some vomiting, called *projectile vomiting*, can go even farther.

When suctioning a patient's airway, or performing any task, determine whether your eyes and mouth are within 3–4 feet of the patient. If they are, those areas are at risk for exposure to sputum, saliva, or vomit. The EMT should always follow Standard Precautions as appropriate for the situation.

OPEN

The first question the EMT should ask when assessing a patient is whether an open (patent) passageway for air exists. Because life depends upon breathing, and breathing depends upon a clear passageway for air movement, the first priority must be to open the air passageway, or **airway**.

The patient with a clear passage for air movement will be able to breathe quietly without any evidence of mechanical obstruction. Air should be noted to move into and out of the patient's mouth and nose without any difficulty.

Recognition of a potential airway blockage, or **occlusion**, is of key importance to the EMT. An EMT who cannot recognize that a problem exists will not know to fix it.

There are several techniques that can be used by the EMT to create a clear air passageway, or airway. The method that is used depends upon the patient's condition. The patient who has a neck injury will need to have special care taken to avoid any movement of the neck during airway management.

Proper Positioning

Often, an unconscious patient is found on the ground or flat on a surface such as a bathroom floor or a bed. If the patient is facedown, or prone, the EMT must decide whether it is necessary to roll the patient over.

The decision to roll the patient onto the back should not be taken lightly. If the patient has a spinal injury, movement must be done with great care to avoid worsening of the injury. This change in position is best done by several EMTs together. The techniques for moving the patient with a possible spine injury are detailed in Chapter 11.

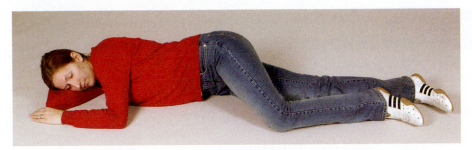

FIGURE 7-5 The recovery position allows natural drainage of airway secretions.

If the EMT is alone and the potentially spine-injured patient is in a prone position, the EMT must consider whether the patient has an open airway in that position. If the EMT finds that the patient's airway is open and is not likely to be occluded in that position, then he is well advised to leave the patient prone until more help arrives.

If the EMT does not suspect a spinal injury, then he may choose to place the patient in a position that allows better airway maintenance. One such position, as seen in Figure 7-5, involves rolling the patient onto the side to allow for easy drainage of oral secretions. This position was formerly called the coma position and is now known as the **recovery position**.

If the patient is prone and does *not* have a patent airway, the EMT is forced to act immediately. Unfortunately, most of the airway techniques an EMT can employ require that the patient be lying on the back, or supine.

If the EMT is alone with an unconscious patient who does not have an adequate airway, he must perform a one-person logroll. The one-person logroll is *not* the preferred method of handling a trauma patient with a potential spinal injury. It should be used only when the risk of death from airway collapse is great.

Once the patient has been placed in a supine position, there are several techniques that the EMT may use to open the airway. The best technique for the situation is decided on the basis of the suspicion, or lack of suspicion, that a spine injury exists.

Head-Tilt, Chin-Lift

The most common airway maneuver used by EMTs is the **head-tilt, chin-lift**. This procedure is reserved for patients for whom trauma, specifically neck injury, has been ruled out. This category would include the patient who is found in bed and a patient who was observed to go unconscious without striking the head when collapsing. The head-tilt, chin-lift is easily done by a single EMT and is detailed in Skill 7-1.

Jaw Thrust

Whenever a possible neck injury is suspected, or when the patient's condition is unknown, spinal precautions must be taken. Spinal precautions involve careful attention to stabilization and immobilization of the head, neck, and back to prevent any further injury to the delicate spinal cord. This concept and techniques of spinal immobilization are discussed in Chapter 22.

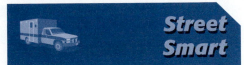

Street Smart

Although, as a general rule, any foreign bodies in the airway of an unconscious patient should be removed, intact dentures should be left in place as long as they do not occlude the airway. These dentures will help serve as a foundation for the mask of the bag-valve-mask to rest upon when the patient is being ventilated.

Pediatric Considerations

Infants who have choked on a foreign body and have a complete airway obstruction (evidenced by the inability to cry or breathe) are too small to undergo the standard Heimlich maneuver. Instead, a technique of alternating back blows and chest thrusts is used to try to forcibly expel the object from the airway.

SKILL 7-1 *Head-Tilt, Chin-Lift*

PURPOSE: To allow the EMT to open the airway of a nontrauma patient.

STANDARD PRECAUTIONS:

☑ Gloves
☑ Goggles
☑ Mask

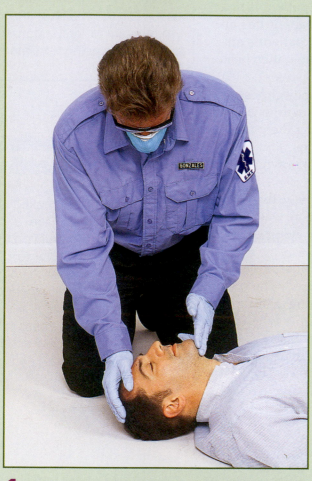

1 After donning the appropriate PPE, the EMT positions himself at the side of the patient's head.

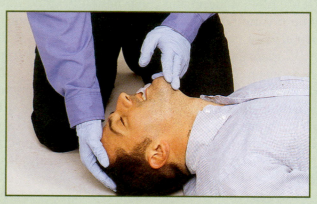

2 The palm of one hand is placed on the patient's forehead, and the fingertips of the other hand on the patient's jaw.

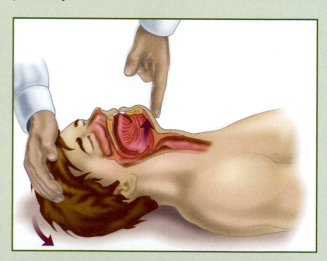

3 The patient's head is tilted back using a firm pressure on the forehead while the jaw is gently lifted up to pull the tongue off the back of the throat. Care should be taken not to push backward on the jaw as doing so will only force the patient's mouth closed.

If the patient with a potential neck injury is in need of airway assistance, the EMT should not hesitate to provide it. There are a few special techniques to use when managing the airway of the trauma patient. The first component to trauma airway maintenance involves stabilization of the head and neck. When neck injury is suspected, it is important to minimize any movement.

The usual techniques of airway management would involve too much movement, so a different maneuver is used. This maneuver, the **jaw thrust** maneuver, involves lifting the mandible. Because the tongue is attached to the mandible, lifting the mandible will serve to lift the tongue off the back of the airway. This technique is detailed in Skill 7-2.

ASSESS

After the airway has been either opened with one of the techniques discussed or determined to be spontaneously open, a moment should be taken for a more detailed examination. Any condition that may affect the patency of the airway should be found and addressed. The EMT should use a light and look into the patient's mouth for any accumulation of secretions or foreign matter that may cause an airway obstruction. Broken teeth or partial bridges and other dental hardware may occlude the unconscious patient's airway and should be removed.

If the airway is obstructed and simple airway maneuvers such as the head-tilt, chin-lift or jaw thrust do not remedy the problem, then the EMT should consider the possibility of a foreign body airway obstruction. A history of choking will often lead the EMT quickly to this conclusion.

If an airway foreign body is suspected and the patient is unable to speak or breathe, indicating complete airway obstruction, the EMT should perform the maneuvers recommended by the American Heart Association and American Red Cross for management of such a condition. Abdominal thrusts are recommended for the conscious patient with a complete airway obstruction, whereas a combination of chest compressions and finger sweeps is used in the unconscious victim of a foreign body airway obstruction.

SUCTION

A conscious person may be able to effectively clear oral secretions, but an unconscious person cannot. Saliva and possibly other foreign matter accumulate in the mouth and throat of the unconscious patient. Therefore, every unconscious patient *must* be suctioned.

Many EMTs have come to depend on mechanical suction to clear airways that are filled with vomitus, blood, or other secretions. Unfortunately, the design of mechanical suction devices often does not match the reality of the patient who is vomiting solid materials. In those cases, two fingers must be used to clear out the solid debris first.

These finger sweeps should be done carefully so as not to push the material farther into the throat. Many EMTs hesitate to place their fingers into the mouth of an unconscious patient, for fear of being accidentally bitten by the patient. An oropharyngeal airway can be placed between the upper and lower molars and held there. The oral airway works very effectively as a bite block to prevent finger injury.

Even if another EMT is using the head-tilt, chin-lift or jaw-thrust method to open the airway, it may be necessary to open the patient's

Street Smart

Take a moment and lie in bed. Now try *not* to swallow. Upon completion of this exercise, the EMT will quickly realize that a person swallows many times in an hour in order to clear the mouth of secretions. However, if you are unconscious, you may not be able to swallow. How long did it take you before you *had* to swallow to remove the accumulation of saliva? Five minutes? Ten minutes? Now consider how long your patient has been lying there, waiting for EMS. Five minutes? Ten minutes? Longer?

SKILL 7-2 *Jaw Thrust Maneuver*

PURPOSE: To allow the EMT to open the airway of a nontrauma patient.

STANDARD PRECAUTIONS:

☑ Gloves
☑ Goggles
☑ Mask

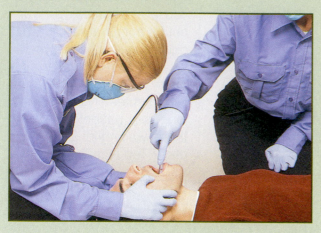

1 After donning appropriate PPE, the EMT should positions herself above the patient's head.

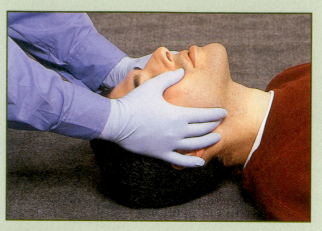

2 The EMT places her middle and index fingers on the angles of the patient's jaw and her thumbs on the cheekbones.

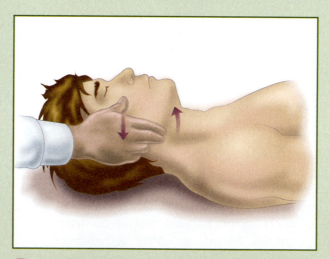

3 The middle and index fingers lift the jaw and the tongue up off the back of the throat while avoiding any movement of the neck.

mouth even further in order to fully visualize the oropharynx or to introduce the suction catheter tip. To accomplish this the EMT should use the **cross-fingered technique**.

The EMT would place his left hand's forefinger against the lower incisors and his thumb against the upper incisors proximal to the midline of the mouth opening. With a scissorslike action, the EMT would gently pry the teeth apart and open the mouth even further (Figure 7-6). It should be emphasized that the cross-fingered technique is not a replacement for either the head-tilt, chin-lift or jaw-thrust airway opening techniques, but it is an adjunct technique that improves visualization and control of the airway.

The Suction Machine

All suction machines have one quality in common: they are designed to vacuum the debris from a patient's mouth. There are many machines on the market. Each claims to have a special feature that makes it better than all the other machines.

The first category of suction machine, sometimes called an "aspirator," is the manual suction. As the name implies, the power for the suction machine comes from the operator, in this case an EMT. Many models on the market claim rapid evacuation of the fluid and vomit. Many of these machines are portable, making them attractive for the EMT. Clearly, the single largest advantage of the manually powered suction machine is the presence of a dependable power supply, the EMT.

The next category of suction machine is the electric suction unit. Some electric suction units run off standard wall current; others are battery dependent. Most can be powered by both. These machines, in many respects, resemble the suction machines in the hospital. For this reason, they are familiar to many providers. One option that can be attractive in certain situations is the ability for electric suction to vary its vacuum power.

Finally, many ambulances are equipped with a suction machine that operates off the power created by either an oxygen device or the ambulance engine. The benefits of this approach include a reliable power source; its main drawback is that a leak anywhere within the system can lessen the suction power.

All suction machines have a collection chamber. Many of these chambers are self-contained, a feature that decreases the likelihood of accidental spillage. Others require cleaning and decontamination.

Most suction devices have a length of tubing that extends from the collection canister to the suction catheter. This tubing is usually clear plastic and, more important, disposable. The tubing allows the machine to be placed a distance away from the patient. Figure 7-7 highlights the features of a suction machine.

Suction Tubing

Suction tubing stretches from the suction machine to the suction catheter and serves as a conduit for the suctioned material to the machine and for the suction to the patient. Prior to using a suction device it is customary to bend and occlude the suction tubing to see if adequate suction is being produced by the suction machine. Typically, suction pressures of at least 300 cm H_2O should be produced within 4 seconds of activation (KKK specification 3.12.4).

The EMT should check all connections between the suction machine and suction tubing to ensure a tight fit if the suction machine fails to produce an adequate vacuum. If the problem persists, then the

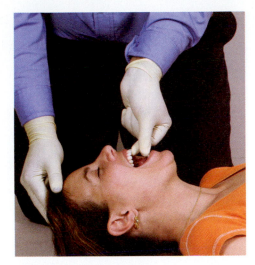

FIGURE 7-6 The cross-fingered technique can be used to further open the mouth in order to suction.

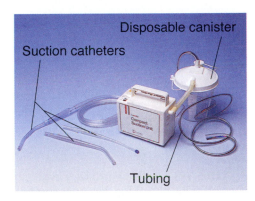

FIGURE 7-7 The suction machine has several disposable parts, including the suction catheter, the tubing, and the canister.

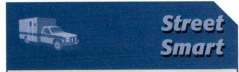

Street Smart

It is important to remember that suction not only removes unwanted secretions but removes needed oxygen as well. Some EMTs make it a practice to hold their breath while performing suctioning. When they feel the need to take a breath, it is a good clue that the patient needs one also.

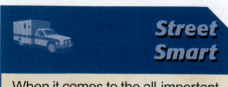

EMT should troubleshoot the suction system and correct any problems prior to using it on a patient.

The Catheter

There are a variety of suction catheters available, each designed with a different purpose in mind. The EMT should decide what he needs a suction catheter for and then select the correct catheter for that use.

The tonsil tip catheter is made of a rigid plastic that makes it easy to use even when wearing a pair of gloves. The tip of the catheter is blunted so that when suction is applied it does not injure soft tissue, such as the tonsils at the back of the throat. The tonsil tip catheter is an excellent choice when used to suction large amounts of saliva or liquid material such as blood.

However, when the EMT needs to suction thick secretions such as blood clots, a **Yankauer** suction catheter with large open tips is more practical. Caution is advised so as not to inadvertently increase the bleeding by injuring soft tissues.

As seen in Figure 7-8, both the tonsil tip and the Yankauer suction tip have a whistle port. If the EMT places his thumb over the whistle port, suction occurs at the distal end of the catheter. Release the thumb and the suction is broken.

Another type of suction catheter used by EMTs is the flexible **French catheter**, sometimes called a "spaghetti" catheter. Most flexible catheters today are disposable clear plastic (Figure 7-9). They are used by EMTs either to suction the external nares of the nose or to suction the opening of a tracheostomy, called a stoma. These long, flexible catheters are also used when suctioning through an endotracheal tube. This procedure is discussed in Appendix A.

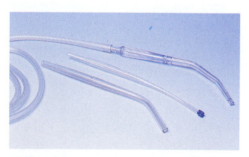

FIGURE 7-8 Note the relatively large opening at the end of the Yankauer suction catheter compared to the opening of the tonsil tip.

Water

Suction setup would not be complete without an available source of water. Often during suctioning the catheter becomes clogged with debris. All it takes to unclog the catheter is a dip in the water and a little vigorous suctioning. Water can save time that would have otherwise been wasted changing clogged catheters.

The Procedure

The EMT must remember that suctioning removes not only fluids but oxygen-laden air as well. Logically, the first step before suctioning is to ensure good oxygenation whenever possible. Occasionally the patient must be suctioned to clear a pathway for the oxygen. Even in those cases, the EMT must keep in mind that the patient may be going without oxygen. Skill 7-3 lists the steps used in suctioning a patient's airway.

If it is necessary to resuction, after properly reoxygenating the patient, then the catheter should be flushed in water and the procedure repeated as many times as necessary until the airway is cleared.

In some serious trauma cases involving massive facial injuries, an EMT may spend his entire time with the patient suctioning the airway clear of blood. This single task may make the difference between life and death for the patient. Without an airway, there is no breathing; without a breath, there is no life.

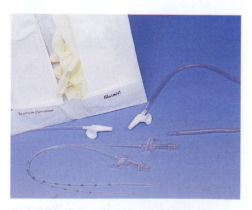

FIGURE 7-9 Flexible catheters are useful when suctioning through an endotracheal tube.

SKILL 7-3 *Suctioning the Airway*

PURPOSE: To clear the airway of secretions that may be preventing air exchange.

STANDARD PRECAUTIONS:

- ☑ Gloves
- ☑ Goggles
- ☑ Mask
- ☑ Suction device (electric or mechanical)
- ☑ Tubing
- ☑ Catheter
- ☑ Water

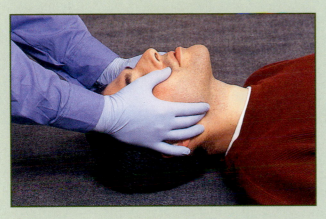

1 One EMT opens and assesses the airway, using the technique appropriate to the patient's situation.

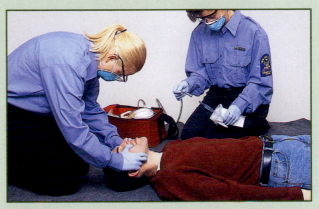

2 Another EMT removes the rigid suction tip from its protective covering, attaches the tip to the tubing, and then the tubing to the intake of the suction machine. Once the equipment is assembled, the EMT tests the machine's suction.

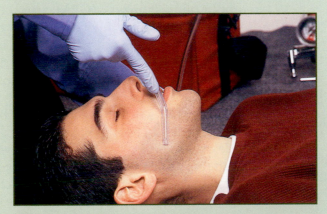

3 One EMT measures the length of the suction tip against the distance from the opening of the mouth to the angle of the jaw.

(continues)

SKILL 7-3 *(continued)*

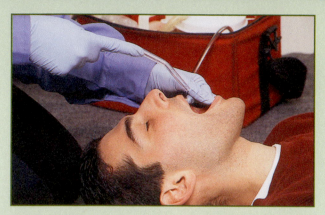

4 The EMT then opens the mouth with the nondominant hand, using a cross-fingered technique. Placing the thumb on the lower teeth and the forefinger on the upper teeth, the EMT holds the teeth apart by a finger-snapping type of motion.

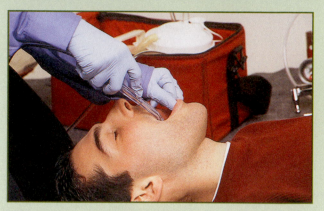

5 The rigid suction tip is then inserted to the depth of the measurement. Suction is applied only as the tip is withdrawn, usually by placing a thumb over a whistle port. Repeat suctioning as often as necessary but never for more than 15 seconds. It is important to oxygenate the patient between suction attempts.

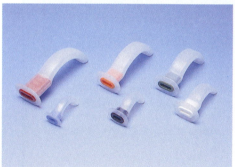

FIGURE 7-10 The correct OPA must be chosen from selection available.

Pediatric Considerations

An alternative method of using the OPA is to use a tongue blade or other tool to hold the tongue while the OPA is inserted following the curvature of the tongue. This method is useful in small children or in the patient who has suffered injury to the palate at the roof of the mouth.

SECURE

An EMT must maintain a constant vigil of the airway. A moment's inattention can lead to airway collapse. The single most important aspect of airway control in the field is the continuous maintenance of the manually controlled airway. The EMT can augment his efforts at airway control with adjunctive devices. However, these are an adjunct to, not a replacement of, good manual airway control.

The Oropharyngeal Airway

An **oropharyngeal airway (OPA)**, also called an oral airway, is a disposable molded plastic device designed to help keep the tongue off the roof of the mouth and from falling into the back of the mouth (Figure 7-10). The OPA also creates an artificial channel for the passage of oxygen into the trachea. It can also act as a bite block, preventing the patient from accidentally biting the tongue or the EMT's finger. What it does *not* do is actually lift the tongue off the back of the throat; only manual control can do that.

There are several types of OPAs; however, all have some sort of flange that rests against the lips and prevents the OPA from accidentally being swallowed. Although some have "channels" to assist the passage of a flexible soft catheter, the use of an OPA for this purpose is *not* encouraged. Occasionally, the catheter, especially if it is not properly lubricated, becomes lodged and the OPA must be removed.

Whenever an OPA is used to assist with airway control, several cautions must be remembered. It is very common for an OPA to stimulate a gag reflex. The EMT must be prepared to immediately remove the OPA if this occurs to prevent vomiting. Suction *must* be ready whenever an OPA is being inserted.

An improperly measured OPA can actually occlude the airway by pushing the tongue into the back of the throat. This problem should be suspected whenever the OPA is seen to advance then retract with every respiration, in a see-saw type motion. An OPA that is too small will simply be swallowed into the mouth and create an airway obstruction.

It is important to remember to completely suction the mouth before inserting an OPA. If the EMT fails to completely suction the airway, any debris can be pushed farther into the airway and even into the trachea.

Using the OPA

The majority of unconscious patients need an OPA to assist with control of the airway. Therefore, every EMT must be skilled at control of the airway and use of the OPA. Skill 7-4 illustrates the insertion of the OPA.

The Nasopharyngeal Airway

The **nasopharyngeal airway (NPA)**, or nasal airway, is used infrequently in the prehospital setting, yet it is easy to use and provides significant benefits over the oral airway. The NPA is a soft, flexible tube that extends from the external nostril, through the nose and into the back of the throat. Figure 7-11 shows various NPAs. Because of its unique position in relation to the structures of the airway, the NPA does not induce a gag reflex as frequently as does an OPA (Figure 7-12).

The rigid nature of the OPA makes it the adjunct of choice in the unconscious patient, in whom definitive airway control is needed. However, in cases in which the patient will not tolerate the OPA because of a gag reflex, the airway adjunct of choice is the more flexible nasal airway.

It is impossible to pass an OPA into the mouth of a patient with clenched teeth, as sometimes occurs during seizures. The nasal airway assists in providing a patent airway in those patients during the event and can be easily removed later when the patient's problem has resolved. Skill 7-5 reviews the procedure for insertion of an NPA.

Once the airway is in place, the entire process taking less than 30 seconds, the patient should be reoxygenated as needed. The NPA still does not substitute for manual control of the airway, and an EMT should maintain either the jaw thrust or the head-tilt, chin-lift maneuver as needed.

CONCLUSION

The maintenance of an open airway is the first priority in all patient contacts by an EMT. Without a patent airway, the patient has little chance of survival. Fortunately, the manipulation of the airway becomes relatively easy for most EMTs after a little practice.

Practice is the key to gaining mastery of this fundamental skill. The simple mantra of open, assess, suction, and secure will serve the EMT well during airway management.

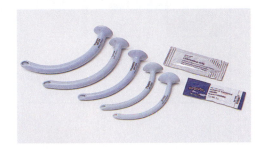

FIGURE 7-11 NPAs, like OPAs, must be properly fitted to the patient.

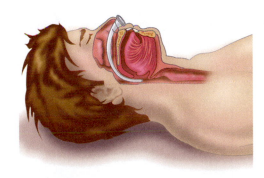

FIGURE 7-12 In this model, the NPA is clearly behind the tongue in a position where it can help to protect the airway, yet it does not often stimulate a gag reflex.

Safety Tip

The soft tissues within the nose are very vascular. Sometimes very slight trauma, such as that involved in placing an NPA, can cause bleeding. Therefore, great care must be exercised to never force an NPA if it does not go in smoothly and easily. The majority of NPA insertions are done without any significant bleeding.

SKILL 7-4 Oropharyngeal Airway Insertion

PURPOSE: To use a mechanical adjunct to assist the EMT who is manually maintaining the airway.

STANDARD PRECAUTIONS:

☑ Gloves
☑ Goggles
☑ Mask
☑ Assortment of oral airways

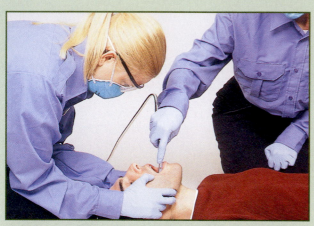

1 First, an EMT must manually open the airway, using the technique appropriate to the patient's condition. The patient's airway should be suctioned as needed.

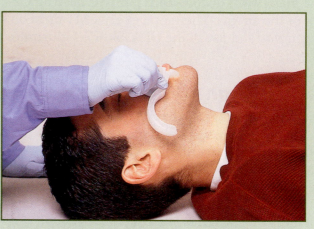

2 The EMT then chooses an oral airway that fits the patient. The length of the oral airway should match the distance from the angle of the jaw to the opening of the mouth.

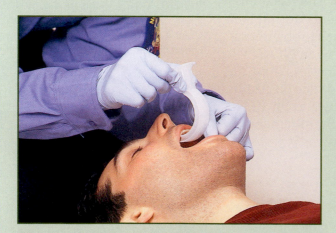

3 Using the cross-fingered technique, the EMT opens the mouth. The EMT begins to insert the airway, curved portion downward, toward the jaw, to about midway.

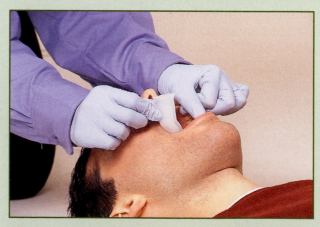

4 The EMT then rotates the oral airway 180 degrees so that the airway naturally follows the curve of the hard palate.

(continues)

SKILL 7-4 *(continued)*

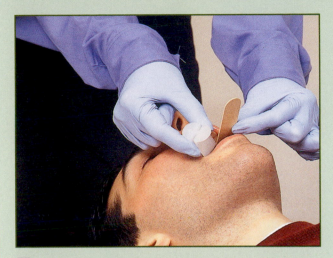

5 Alternatively, the EMT can use a tongue depressor to press the tongue downward and forward. Then an oral airway may be inserted directly into the oral cavity, following the curve of the hard palate.

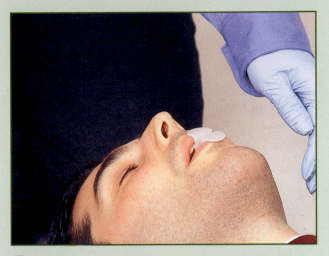

6 The airway is correctly placed when the flange of the airway rests on the patient's teeth.

TEST YOUR KNOWLEDGE

1. List the steps for performing a head-tilt, chin-lift maneuver.
2. When is the jaw thrust preferred over the head-tilt, chin-lift?
3. Describe how a jaw thrust maneuver is performed.
4. What is the most commonly forgotten piece of EMS equipment?
5. What is the danger of suctioning for too long a period of time?
6. How do you measure an oral airway?
7. What are the two techniques for inserting an oral airway?
8. What is the most significant advantage of a nasal airway over an oral airway?
9. How do you measure a nasal airway?

INTERNET RESOURCES

Visit the Web sites of the following organizations for information on how to manage airway obstruction:

- American Heart Association, http://www.americanheart.org
- American Red Cross, http://www.redcross.org

Look up information on foreign body airway obstruction. What other resources are available on this topic?

SKILL 7-5 *Nasopharyngeal Airway Insertion*

PURPOSE: To provide an airway for patients who cannot tolerate an oral airway but also cannot protect their own airway.

STANDARD PRECAUTIONS:

- ☑ Gloves
- ☑ Goggles
- ☑ Mask
- ☑ Assortment of nasal airways
- ☑ Water-soluble lubricant

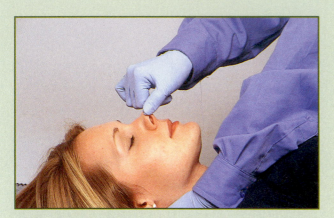

1 The EMT first examines the nostril opening to determine an approximate size of nasal airway that will be needed.

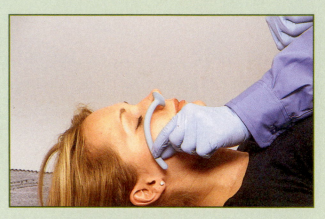

2 The EMT then compares the length of the nasal airway with the distance between the nostril and the tip of the earlobe.

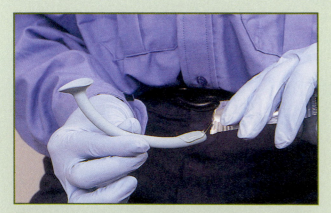

3 The EMT then applies a generous layer of water-soluble lubricant to the length of the nasal airway.

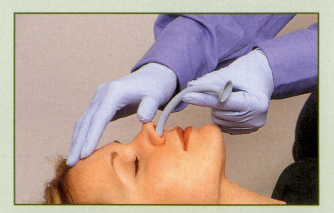

4 The nasal airway is then gently introduced to the nostril. The bevel of the airway should be facing inward toward the nasal septum.

(continues)

SKILL 7-5 (continued)

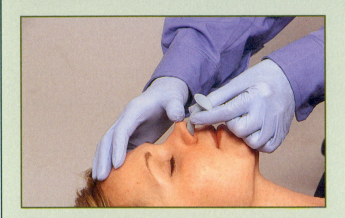

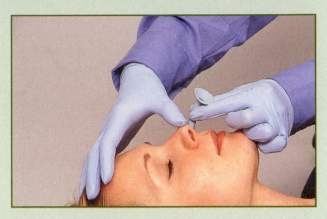

5 A gentle corkscrewing action, back and forth, as the EMT gently pushes straight backward usually allows the nasal airway to be placed.

6 If resistance is met, then the nasal airway should be withdrawn and insertion into the other nostril attempted.

EMS in Action

My partner and I were dispatched priority 1 for a patient complaining of chest pain and difficulty breathing. The call came from a convalescent home for retired nuns, priests, and high-ranking officials in the Catholic church.

Upon arrival, we were met at the door by two frantic nursing assistants. As soon as we entered the doorway, they took off running down a long hallway. It was all we could do to keep up with them, as we were toting a gurney loaded down with all our equipment. We were led into a cafeteria where an elderly female was hunched over in a chair, extremely cyanotic and unresponsive. The staff was screaming, "Help her!" They reported that the patient had been eating her lunch and began to choke. I quickly got into position and performed the Heimlich maneuver, but with no success. My partner and I lowered her to the floor, and I instructed him to begin the unconscious adult choking series while I set up my laryngoscope and Magill forceps. He looked back at me with eyes as big as saucers then quickly took action. The basic life support maneuvers proved unsuccessful, so I inserted the laryngoscope and visualized a completely obstructed airway. I proceeded to remove a significant amount of chewed-up French bread from the patient's airway.

At this time, I noticed a large figure standing over me. It was a large man dressed in a uniform consistent with what a bishop might wear. The gentleman leaned down over me while I was still clearing the airway, anointed the patient's airway, and proceeded to read the last rites. I thought to myself, Give me a chance, I'm not done yet! About this time I removed the remaining pieces of bread and the patient took a deep breath. I immediately ventilated the patient and the patient regained consciousness and was back to normal mental status within a minute or two.

The staff was extremely happy and so were we! At this point, I asked, "Was this the patient having chest pain?" The staff replied, "No, he's down the hall."

Steve Melander, NREMT-P, CCEMT-P
Clinical Coordinator
WestMed Training, San Jose, California

FURTHER STUDY

American Heart Association. (2001). *Basic life support for healthcare providers*. Dallas, TX: Author.

American Red Cross. (1993). *Cardiopulmonary resuscitation for the professional rescuer*. Author. Washington, D.C.

Metcalf, W., & McSwain, N. (2001). *Professional rescuer CPR*. Boston: Jones and Bartlett.

Scott, A., & Fong, E. (2003). *Body structures and functions* (10th ed.). Clifton Park, NY: Thomson Delmar Learning.

CHAPTER 8

Respiratory Support

KEY TERMS

accessory muscles of
respiration
air hunger
artificial ventilation
auscultate
bag-valve-mask (BVM)
contraindication
cricoid pressure
dead space
dentures
dyspnea
flow-restricted oxygen-
powered ventilation
device (FROPVD)
humidification
hypoventilation
hypoxia
indication
nasal cannula (NC)
non-rebreather mask (NRB)
onboard oxygen
palpate
pocket mask
pursed lip breathing
regulator
resuscitated
stoma
tachypnea
tracheostomy
tripod position

OBJECTIVES

Upon completion of this chapter, the reader should be able to:

1. List the signs of adequate breathing.
2. List the signs of inadequate breathing.
3. Define the components of an oxygen delivery system.
4. Identify a non-rebreather facemask and state the oxygen flow requirements needed for its use.
5. Describe the indications for using a nasal cannula versus a non-rebreather facemask.
6. Identify a nasal cannula and state the flow requirements needed for its use.
7. Describe how to artificially ventilate a patient with a pocket mask.
8. Describe the steps in performing the skill of artificially ventilating a patient with a bag-valve-mask while using the jaw thrust.
9. Describe the steps in performing the skill of artificially ventilating a patient with a bag-valve-mask for one and two rescuers.
10. Describe the steps in artificially ventilating a patient with a flow-restricted oxygen-powered ventilation device.

OVERVIEW

Even in ancient times, breathing was associated with life. In 800 BC, Elijah was reported to have given a breath of air to an apparently dead child and the child arose. The ancient Greeks also understood that breathing was the very essence of life. They called it *pneuma*, and they attached great significance to it. It is easy to understand the importance that was placed on this body function. Breathing is a clearly visible sign of life.

Over the centuries, it became known that a patient who had stopped breathing could potentially be revived, or **resuscitated**, with artificial respiration. Early pioneers, such as the Royal Society for the Resuscitation of the Apparently Dead, and, more recently, the American Red Cross taught these techniques to health care providers as well as the lay public.

173

Trouble Breathing

Grandma Smith had been having trouble breathing for the past several days. When asked why she was having trouble breathing, she would quickly dismiss her grandchildren by saying, "It's just old age."

Tonight was different. Grandma had gone to bed at her usual bedtime, which was nine o'clock. Not more than 3 hours had passed when she called out to her grandson Todd.

Todd rushed to the room. Grandma was standing at the open window, her arms bracing herself on the window ledge. "I can't . . . catch . . . my breath," she said.

Todd, not sure what to do, called 9-1-1.

- What are the signs and symptoms of difficulty breathing?
- What abnormal breath sounds would typically be heard in this case?

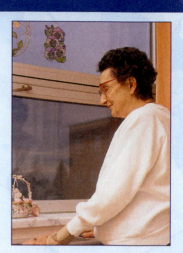

Modern techniques of artificial respiration have become a mainstay of EMS. The administration of these lifesaving techniques has been responsible for many favorable outcomes. The public has come to expect that EMTs are experts in the techniques of respiratory support.

BREATHING

Although the act of breathing seems simple, it is actually a fairly complex activity. The lungs, chest muscles, brain, nerves, heart, and blood must all work together in order to get the right amount of oxygen to the cells of the body.

The oxygen we breathe in comes from the air in our environment. Air consists of 21% oxygen, with the remainder being composed of primarily nitrogen and a little carbon dioxide. In certain oxygen-poor environments, such as in confined spaces or at high altitudes, there may not be sufficient oxygen in the air to sustain life indefinitely. In these environments, workers or rescuers would collapse and die without supplemental oxygen.

Although 21% oxygen in the inspired air is sufficient for most people in most circumstances, there are some illnesses that may lead to a need for increased oxygen intake. Certain conditions impair the body's ability to utilize the inspired oxygen, requiring increased intake in order to maintain necessary levels of oxygen to the body tissues.

Because oxygen is a necessary fuel for all organ systems, insufficient oxygen supply can lead to system failure. **Hypoxia** is a term used to describe insufficient body stores of oxygen. One of the body's responses to hypoxia is to increase the respiratory rate. People with hypoxia will feel as though they need to breathe faster, creating a feeling of shortness of breath.

An increased respiratory rate and feeling of shortness of breath can result in a patient's exerting more effort to breathe than is normally used. The usual effortless manner of breathing can become very labored and require a lot of effort and energy. Severe difficulty with breathing can lead to a failure of the respiratory system as the patient tires of working so hard to breathe. Untreated respiratory failure can lead to death. The emergency medical technician (EMT) must recognize respiratory difficulty before it progresses to respiratory failure and death.

The act of breathing can be divided into two portions, ventilation and respiration. The first part, ventilation, refers to the mechanical act of moving air into and out of the lungs. Respiration refers to the process of allowing inspired oxygen to get into the bloodstream. Chapter 5 discusses the physiology of ventilation and respiration in further detail.

The EMT must be able to assess the efficiency of a patient's ventilation and respiration and should be able to support each of these functions if it becomes necessary to do so.

ASSESSMENT

The initial steps in the assessment of the respiratory system are "look, listen, and feel." Each of these actions will provide the EMT with information that will enable her to make decisions about patient care.

Level of Consciousness

Immediately upon arrival the EMT needs to make a rapid determination if the patient is conscious or not. The determination of consciousness is made easier if the patient is walking around or active. However, even a patient who is seated upright with the eyes open may not be conscious.

To check consciousness on a patient who is not obviously awake the EMT should first call the patient's name at a normal conversational level. If the patient fails to respond, then the EMT should increase the volume of her voice and shout out the patient's name.

If the patient remains unresponsive to loud verbal stimuli, then the EMT should proceed to physical stimuli. Like verbal stimuli, the EMT should escalate her physical stimulus from tapping to a slight pinch of the skin and proceed to painful stimuli. EMTs commonly use a sternal rub to illicit a response from the patient. The patient's response is noted, using the Alert, Verbal, Pain, Unresponsive (AVPU) scale. More about the sternal rub and the AVPU scale is contained in Chapter 13, Initial Assessment.

Because oxygen is needed for efficient brain function, the patient who has severe respiratory difficulty and is not effectively oxygenating his blood may show evidence of brain dysfunction. A common sign of hypoxia is confusion or decreased mental status. The patient who shows evidence of respiratory distress and is confused or combative should be considered to be hypoxic. The patient who is not alert or interactive may have severely depressed oxygen levels and must be treated immediately to avoid further decompensation.

Quick Check

In the unconscious person, the EMT should perform what is known as a *quick check* of the respiratory system. This involves the assessment triad of look, listen, and feel. After opening the airway using the techniques outlined in Chapter 7, the EMT should *look* for the chest to rise and fall. This is an indication that air is moving and the patient is actually breathing. Simultaneously, she should place her face close to the patient's mouth and nose to *listen* and *feel* for air movement, also indicating the presence of breathing (Figure 8-1). While this respiratory assessment is being done, the EMT can also check for the presence of a carotid pulse at the side of the neck. This quick check takes a mere 15 seconds and is key in the initial assessment of the unconscious patient.

Look

The experienced EMT knows that by standing in the doorway and watching the conscious patient for a moment she can learn a great deal about the patient's breathing. The alert, interactive patient who greets the EMT at the door is not quite as distressed as the tired-appearing patient who is slumped in a chair and does not acknowledge the EMT's arrival.

Position

The position the patient has assumed can be revealing. The patient who is working very hard to breathe will often be in an upright position, leaning slightly forward, supporting himself with his hands against his knees. Although it does not seem very comfortable, this position allows the patient to better expand his lungs and draw in more air than if he were leaning back into a chair. This characteristic position is known as the **tripod position** and is usually indicative of significant respiratory distress (Figure 8-2).

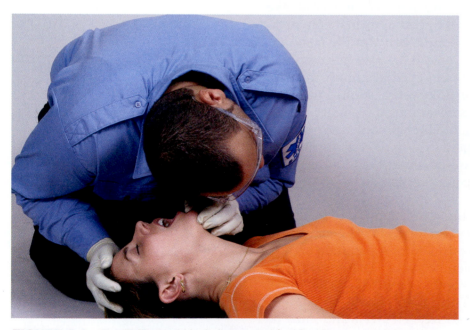

FIGURE 8-1 The EMT should look, listen, and feel for air movement during the initial assessment of the unconscious patient.

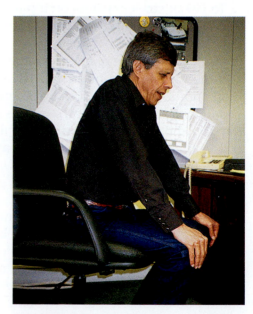

FIGURE 8-2 Patients with significant respiratory distress may sometimes be found in the tripod position.

Color

A close look at the light-skinned patient may reveal that the skin has a bluish tinge. Blood lacking oxygen gives the skin a dusky, bluish color known as cyanosis. The presence of cyanosis tells the EMT that the patient's body is lacking oxygen.

Respiratory Rate

Remembering that effective ventilation is necessary for adequate respiration, as the EMT approaches a patient, she should observe the patient's efforts at breathing. The first obvious quality that would be noted is the rate of breathing, or respiratory rate.

The normal rate of breathing for an adult is between 12 and 20 breaths per minute. Children normally breathe at 15–30 times per minute and infants at 20–40 times per minute. To count the respiratory rate exactly, the EMT must watch the patient's breathing carefully for 1 minute and count how many breaths are taken. This procedure is detailed in Chapter 10. Although an accurate count of respirations is very important, initially all the EMT is concerned with is whether the patient's breathing is too fast, too slow, or about normal.

Because rapid breathing, or **tachypnea**, is often associated with shallow breaths, each breath may not be providing enough air to get deep into the lungs where it is needed. The space in the airway above the lungs, including the trachea and larger bronchi, does not have the ability to participate in gas exchange. The air that enters this so-called **dead space** is therefore not utilized in oxygenation. With very shallow, rapid breathing, much of the inhaled air may stay in the dead space and not be useful in oxygenation.

On the other extreme, a patient who is breathing too slowly is not moving enough air into and out of the lungs. The air inside the lungs becomes stagnant in between breaths. This condition leads to hypoxia and possibly cyanosis. The patient, who is breathing too slowly, regardless of the cause, is experiencing **hypoventilation**. In both cases it may be necessary for the EMT to assist the patient's breathing to allow more effective oxygenation. Patterns of respiration are shown in Figure 8-3.

Effort

The next thing that should be noted by the EMT is the effort that the patient seems to be expending to breathe. Remembering that normal breathing requires no conscious effort, the EMT should consider any exertion seen with breathing to be abnormal.

Starting at the top of the airway, watch the patient breathe. Is he breathing through the nose or the mouth? In normal breathing, most patients breathe through the nose. When the patient is trying to inhale

1. Eupnea (normal)

2. Tachypnea (too fast)

3. Bradypnea (too slow)

4. Apnea (no breathing)

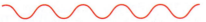

FIGURE 8-3 Patterns of respiration.

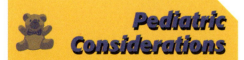

Pediatric Considerations

Nasal flaring is very evident in infants and small children when they experience respiratory difficulty. The EMT should look carefully for this sign in every infant and child assessed.

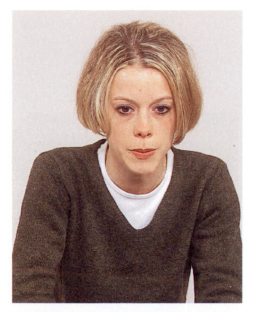

FIGURE 8-4 Breathing through pursed lips is a sign of respiratory distress.

Pediatric Considerations

Abdominal breathing is an indication of respiratory distress that is commonly seen in children. In a supine position, the small child using abdominal muscles to assist respiration may appear to have a see-saw motion of the chest and abdomen evident with each respiration. This paradoxical abdominal motion is an indication of significant respiratory distress in a child and should not be missed.

more air, the nares of the nose can widen to allow increased air entry. This nasal flaring permits more air into the nose and is a sign of extra respiratory effort.

A patient's breathing through an open mouth is an indication of **air hunger**. The patient has such a need for air that his body is bypassing the normal safeguards (air filtration and warming) provided by the nose in order to get the volumes of air that it needs. Mouth breathing is usually seen only in patients with respiratory difficulty or in patients with severe nasal congestion.

Pursed lip breathing, as demonstrated in Figure 8-4, is an effort to maintain pressures in the airways during exhalation by keeping the lips half closed and breathing out forcefully against them. This pressure during exhalation is necessary in patients with some chronic lung diseases whose airways can easily collapse. Maintaining a constant airway pressure in this manner keeps airways from collapsing and makes inhalation easier. Although this manner of breathing is characteristic for patients who have chronic lung disease, it can be seen in many patients in respiratory distress.

Normally the primary muscle of respiration is the diaphragm. When the diaphragm alone is unable to provide the ventilation that the body needs, additional muscles are used. Muscles of the neck, chest, and abdomen can act as such **accessory muscles of respiration**.

In the adult, the muscles of the neck and shoulders are useful in lifting the upper ribs and expanding the chest cavity. The muscles of the neck, sometimes called the strap muscles, are easily visible when being used to assist respiration. The muscles between the ribs, called the intercostal muscles, also help to expand the chest cavity so that air can be drawn in. The large muscles of the abdomen can also contract, decreasing the volume of the abdominal contents and therefore allowing a greater space for the lungs to expand. Use of the abdominal muscles to assist respiration is evident when the abdomen is seen to expand with exhalation instead of inhalation as normally occurs.

When their efforts are combined, the accessory muscles of respiration can greatly assist the patient's breathing, although their use expends a significant amount of energy. The patient using accessory muscles of respiration will quickly tire and progress to respiratory failure.

To properly assess a patient for evidence of accessory muscle use, the EMT may have to remove some of the patient's clothing. Neck muscle use is often evident with clothing on, as seen in Figure 8-5. Intercostal muscle use may be difficult to see, even with clothing removed, owing to increased external musculature and body fat in many adults.

Pulse Oximetry

Pulse oximeters are machines that measure the percentage of red blood cells that are saturated with oxygen. The pulse oximeter depends on oxygen-rich blood having a characteristic bright red color and oxygen-poor blood a bluer color. A pulse oximeter is used by many EMTs as an additional tool in the assessment of a patient with respiratory distress (Figure 8-7). The use of the pulse oximeter is detailed in Chapter 11.

Well-oxygenated blood has an average oxygen saturation of 96%–100%. Many systems require that oxygen be administered when-

Pediatric Considerations

Intercostal muscle use is common in small children with respiratory difficulty. This important physical finding is evidenced by retraction of the skin between the ribs with each breath. Such intercostal retractions obviously are seen only if the shirt is lifted up or removed for the assessment (Figure 8-6).

With increasing distress, a child will often have retraction of the skin above the sternum and even of the sternum itself as every muscle in the child's chest tries to assist with breathing. The finding of sternal retractions is an ominous sign in the child with respiratory distress.

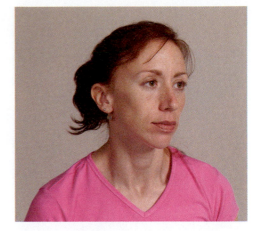

FIGURE 8-5 The strap muscles in the neck are useful in assisting in respirations in times of distress.

ever the oxygen saturation falls below 95%. The patient is significantly hypoxic when the oxygen saturation falls below 92%. It is important to remember that there are several factors that may impair the accuracy of the pulse oximeter. If the EMT's assessment suggests that the patient is hypoxic, then he should be treated as such, regardless of the reading on the oximeter.

Listen

After the EMT has properly identified herself and asks the question "What is the problem," it is important to listen carefully not only to what is said but also to how it is said. Patients will complain of "trouble breathing," or of being "short of breath," or of not being able to "catch my breath." Each of these phrases indicates a subjective feeling of respiratory distress. The chief complaint should be documented, preferably in the patient's own words. A term referring to the feeling or the appearance of respiratory distress is **dyspnea**.

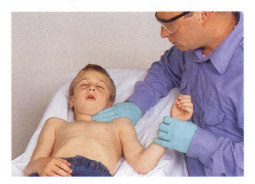

FIGURE 8-6 Intercostal retractions is a valuable physical finding that is only seen when the patient's shirt is removed.

Speech

The EMT should note how easily the patient is able to speak. If he is able to speak in full sentences without stopping at every word or two to catch his breath, severe distress is likely not present. However, if the patient answers in short and broken sentences or is able to give only monosyllabic answers, such as "yes," "no," or "OK," severe respiratory distress is present.

This conservation of words is the patient's effort to save breath for living and not speaking. The patient should never be pressed to answer questions more fully in this circumstance. Such pressure leads only to frustration and anger on the part of the patient and generally a worsening of the patient's condition.

Obvious Noise

As the EMT approaches the patient, she should note any noises associated with breathing. Normal respirations occur without much noticeable noise. Any noise heard should be noted and considered to be a sign of a respiratory problem. As discussed in Chapter 7, a snoring sound indicates an upper airway obstruction, often created by the

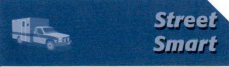

Street Smart

Although modesty is important to maintain, the EMT must perform an adequate assessment of the patient's work of breathing. Lifting the back of the patient's shirt will often provide a good look at the muscle use while still maintaining modesty of the patient in a public place.

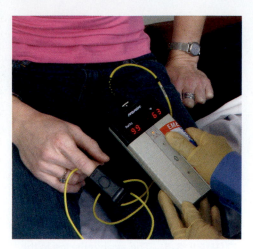

FIGURE 8-7 A pulse oximeter can be a valuable tool in assessing a patient but must never replace the EMT's own judgment.

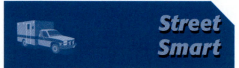

Always treat the patient and not the machine. If the patient says he is short of breath and needs oxygen, give him oxygen despite what the reading on the pulse oximeter says. The pulse oximeter is an assessment tool for an EMT. The pulse oximeter should never replace good judgment in patient care.

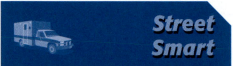

A useful way to quantify a patient's respiratory difficulty is to count the words he is able to speak between breaths. The patient who is initially able to speak five words at a time and progresses to only two words at a time is clearly getting worse, whereas the patient who is able to speak only one word at a time but later is able to speak five words at a time is obviously improving.

patient's own tongue. Other characteristic respiratory noises are discussed in Chapters 16 and 27.

Breath Sounds

Finally, the EMT should quickly listen to, or **auscultate**, the patient's lungs. Normal air entry and exit from the chest creates a characteristic sound pattern. This pattern consists of the sound of smooth airflow throughout the chest. Any obstruction to that airflow will create abnormal sounds. The specific sounds that are associated with different respiratory diseases are discussed in Chapter 27.

Auscultation of the lungs should reveal several important pieces of information. Air movement should be evident in both lungs by normal breath sounds heard over both sides of the chest. The absence of breath sounds over an area in which they are expected to be heard indicates lack of air movement in that area. Diminished breath sounds may indicate poor airflow or lung abnormality.

The easiest areas in which to auscultate breath sounds are anteriorly just under each clavicle and laterally, at the nipple line. The EMT in Figure 8-8 is demonstrating auscultation of the lungs. When using a stethoscope to auscultate breath sounds, the EMT should place the earpieces forward into the ears, following the natural path of the ear canal. The flat diaphragm at the end of the stethoscope is pressed firmly against the patient's skin, and sounds underneath it will be transmitted through the tubing to the examiner's ears. Use of the stethoscope is addressed in more detail in Chapter 10.

Feel

To conclude the assessment of the respiratory system, the EMT should take a moment to quickly feel, or **palpate**, the chest wall for tenderness, deformity, and equality of movement. This step is useful whenever assessing, in particular, a trauma patient who is short of breath. With the hands under the armpits, the EMT applies a small amount of pressure to the entire rib cage in order to discover any major sources of pain, as is demonstrated in Figure 8-9. The chest assessment of the trauma patient is described in more detail in Chapter 14.

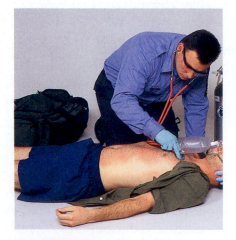
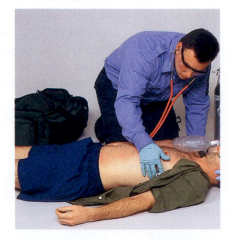

FIGURE 8-8 Auscultation of lung sounds can reveal important physical findings.

OXYGEN THERAPY

Although oxygen is found in the air around us, it is considered a medication and is used in the treatment of many medical conditions. Oxygen is the most common medication administered by the EMT. Therefore, EMTs need to be intimately familiar with its indications, contraindications, and methods of administration.

Indications

The primary reason, or **indication**, to administer oxygen is to reverse hypoxia. Because an EMT does not routinely directly measure oxygen levels, he must rely upon other indicators of hypoxia. Physical signs of hypoxia are restlessness, anxiety, confusion, tachypnea or hypoventilation, and tachycardia (rapid heart rate) or bradycardia (slow heart rate). In addition, the presence of cyanosis indicates hypoxia, but the absence of cyanosis does not indicate the opposite.

Although many EMTs do use a pulse oximeter to measure oxygen saturations, as pointed out in the previous section, this is not a perfect test, and the EMT should always rely on her clinical judgment when it comes to oxygen use. When in doubt, erring on the side of administration is always safe.

In practice, the decision to administer oxygen is based on the patient's chief complaint. If the patient complains of feeling short of breath or of having trouble breathing, even if the physical examination does not immediately reveal any reason why the patient should feel that way, he should be given oxygen. Throughout the remainder of this text, the use of oxygen will be discussed as it is related to each medical condition presented. Table 8-1 lists some indications for oxygen administration.

Contraindications

A **contraindication** is a reason not to use a medication. Although there is no absolute reason not to administer oxygen if there is an indication for it, there are several situations in which it should be used with caution.

Oxygen toxicity, a problem of prolonged oxygen use, is a contraindication to high-concentration oxygen. This most often occurs in premature newborn infants and will rarely affect the EMT.

In the past, EMTs were taught to administer oxygen cautiously to patients with emphysema or chronic obstructive pulmonary disease (COPD). This caution was based on a belief that a small percentage of patients with COPD will actually lose the drive to breathe if given high-flow oxygen. This outcome has been found to occur very rarely, and *the EMT should never withhold oxygen from a patient who needs it*. The danger of allowing hypoxia to progress is much greater than the small risk of causing respiratory depression in such a patient.

On the other hand, careless administration of oxygen to patients when there is no indication can also have potential complications. It is inconsistent with the standard of care for an EMT to administer 100% oxygen to a patient when the patient's sole complaint is ankle pain after twisting his foot. Therefore, the EMT should always know why

Street Smart

The patient with respiratory distress who is quiet is trying to conserve energy. This is a reliable sign of distress. Keep questions brief and to the point, and ask questions that can be answered with a yes or a no.

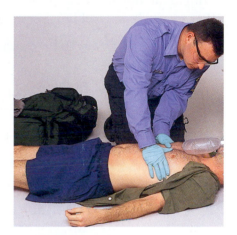

FIGURE 8-9 Palpation can reveal problems with chest wall expansion and ventilation.

TABLE 8-1

Indications for Oxygen Administration

Respiratory distress or failure

Cardiopulmonary arrest

Chest pain

Headache

Dizziness

Weakness

Abdominal pain

Hypoperfusion

Altered mental status

A Tumble Downstairs

Thud. Everyone in the family heard it. Even the baby was startled. Ahmed was the first to go investigate.

The sound came from the kitchen. Stepping into the center of the kitchen, Ahmed saw the open door to the basement. Then the faint voice, "I'm down here!"

The voice that he heard was his Uncle Hameed. Uncle Hameed, who frequently had bouts of confusion, had apparently opened the wrong door. He had fallen down a dozen stairs to the landing in the basement.

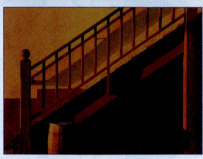

(Courtesy of PhotoDisc.)

Ahmed ran down the stairs, while the family stood in the doorway. Kneeling next to his uncle, he noticed that his uncle was holding his ribs with one arm and straining to breathe.

Ahmed called upstairs to his mother, "Call the ambulance, I think Uncle Hameed is hurt, maybe some broken ribs."

Using the *Buddycare* he had been taught in the army, Ahmed helped his uncle lie down and told him not to move until the ambulance arrived.

Ahmed noticed that his uncle's breathing was getting much worse.

- What is the primary respiratory problem in this case?
- What can be done to assist the patient?
- What can one EMT do? Two EMTs?

she is giving oxygen and under what medical authority she is doing so. Medical protocols will often guide oxygen administration.

Oxygen Humidification

Oxygen blowing into the nose or mouth can dry the mucous membranes. For the short period of time involved during most transports, less than 1 hour, this is not a major problem.

However, in the case of a long-distance transport, this drying action can cause significant discomfort and injury to the delicate airway tissues. Instillation of moisture, or **humidification**, of the inspired oxygen can help to prevent such injury.

A humidification system, can provide sterile, cool moisturization of the oxygen administered. For this mist to actually move through the tubing, the tubing must be of larger diameter than the standard oxygen tubing.

An effective means of administering humidification to a patient is to use a standard small volume nebulizer. Instead of placing medication in the bowl the EMT would instill about 3–5 ml of sterile water, often available in a self-contained package, called *pearl of saline*. The oxygen regulator flow should then be placed at 8 liters per minute.

Alternatively, the oxygen reservoir can be removed from the partial non-rebreather mask and nebulizer attached to the bottom of the mask. The oxygen regulator flow should remain the same.

Under no circumstance should an EMT deprive a patient of needed oxygen, and the EMT should follow local medical protocols. However, these two methods of administering humidification with oxygen are useful and should be considered if the patient has croup, asthma, or inhalation burns.

OXYGEN DELIVERY SYSTEMS

EMS providers use two types of oxygen delivery systems, fixed and portable. The fixed systems are found on board the ambulance and operate very much like the wall oxygen in the hospital. The portable systems are easily movable and are designed to be brought to the patient's bedside.

Although different in size, both systems operate off a tank of compressed gas. Oxygen on the ambulance, **onboard oxygen**, may have 3,000 liters of oxygen, whereas the small handheld portable tank may have only 350 liters. Table 8-2 displays the liter volumes of each size of oxygen tank commonly used by the EMT.

Oxygen tanks hold oxygen under pressure, which is measured in pounds per square inch (psi). By observing the pressure gauge on an oxygen tank, the EMT can determine how much oxygen is in the tank, or "bottle," as it is sometimes called. A tank of any size can generally be filled to about 2,000 psi. Many EMTs have the portable tanks refilled before they fall below 200 psi.

At the start of every tour of duty the EMT should fill the portable oxygen tanks to capacity. This ensures that the EMT will have the oxygen when it is needed. In some cases, such as a long-distance transport or a woodland rescue, it may be necessary to calculate the time the oxygen tank will last. To calculate the time, the EMT would measure the pressure in the tank (seen on the regulator gauge), subtract 200 psi (the safe minimum residual), and multiply that number by the tank factor, seen in Table 8-2. Taking the result, the EMT would then divide that number by the flow rate on the regulator and the subsequent result is the estimated time that the tank will last. Some emergency medical services (EMS) calculate these values and place them on the inside of the oxygen tank compartment for quick reference.

Street Smart

A blue-ridged plastic tubing is usually used for administering humidified oxygen. Standard oxygen tubing placed on a humidifier does not provide any appreciable amount of moisture in the oxygen to benefit the patient.

$$\frac{[\text{Pressure in tank} - 200\ (\text{safe residual})] \times \text{tank factor}}{\text{flow rate}} = \text{tank duration}$$

TABLE 8-2

		Oxygen Tank Capacity				
Use	Size	Capacity (liters)	Factor	6 lpm	8 lpm	10 lpm
Portable	D	300–350	0.16	50 min	35 min	30 min
Portable	E	600	0.28	1 $^3/_4$ hr	1 hr 10 min	1 hr
Onboard	M	3.450	1.37	9 $^1/_2$ hr	7 hr	5 $^3/_4$ hr

Note: lpm = liters per minute; hr = hours; min = minutes

Street Smart

A new system of oxygen delivery is available using liquid oxygen, or LOX. These systems require that the EMT become familiar with the manufacturer's recommendations before operation. These systems have the advantage of supplying the same amount of oxygen as a standard large tank in about one-third the space.

Safety Tip

The weakest part of every oxygen tank is at the point where the stem is inserted into the top of the tank. If a tank is dropped or falls on its side, the stem can fracture at the neck and the tank could explode.

Therefore, all unsecured oxygen cylinders should be carefully laid down flat. Large oxygen cylinders need to be firmly secured to the wall. It is preferable to secure every oxygen tank to decrease the risk of injury.

Street Smart

One of the worst feelings an EMT can have is to open an oxygen duffel and find that the oxygen wrench is missing. If there is no means of opening the tank, the oxygen inside is useless to the EMT. The supply officer should consider purchasing oxygen tanks with a built-in toggle or having a wrench attached to a chain that is secured to the tank.

Example:

$$\frac{(3{,}000 \text{ liters} - 200 \text{ liters}) \times 1.37 \text{ (M)}}{15 \text{ lpm}} = 256 \text{ minutes or approximately } 4\,{}^{1}\!/_{2} \text{ hours}$$

Anatomy of an Oxygen Delivery System

Each oxygen delivery system has a cylinder that holds oxygen under pressure. If not properly sealed and cared for, this cylinder could leak or rupture. All oxygen tanks therefore undergo regular hydrostatic testing to ensure that they are safe. If the tank is deemed safe, then it is stamped with a time date and symbol indicating the length of time that the tank is considered safe under normal circumstances. Because EMS often operates under abnormal circumstances, oxygen tanks should probably be hydrostatically tested every 5 years.

An oxygen tank is usually turned on or off with either an oxygen wrench or a toggle. If a wrench is used, it is placed on the valve like a key and turned in a counterclockwise direction until all the way on. Many EMTs make a practice of turning an oxygen tank all the way on then turning the valve back one-half turn to ensure that everybody knows that the tank is on.

Oxygen flows out of an oxygen tank through a **regulator**, sometimes called a flowmeter. Safeguards have been put into place to prevent oxygen regulators from accidentally being placed on tanks containing other gases. For one, all oxygen tanks are either painted green or have a green head on the cylinder. In addition, the stems of the tanks are milled with an array of pinholes that will accept only the pins of an oxygen regulator. The National Standard Pin Index System prevents crossover of one type of regulator with another type of tank. Figure 8-10 shows the relationship of an oxygen regulator and the oxygen tank.

Once the regulator has been mated with the proper tank, they are tightened together, usually by way of a T-piece on the yoke of the regulator. Even after the regulator has been tightened to the tank's stem, there is often a leak. All regulators require a washer to prevent these leaks. The washer is often made of plastic, though some are metal with a rubber insert.

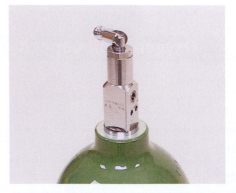
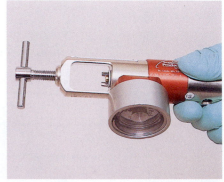

FIGURE 8-10 The pins of the regulator must exactly match the holes in the tank's stem.

The regulator is the active portion of the system. It regulates the amount of oxygen that will flow, usually in liters per minute (lpm). Most modern regulators have a built-in pressure gauge, which tells the EMT the amount of oxygen in the tank as well as provides a method of controlling the flow rate.

Some regulators control flow using a variable-opening dial; others use a flow gauge that allows the EMT to "dial in" the flow rate. All regulators should be able to reliably produce flow rates from 2 lpm to 15 lpm.

Wall oxygen regulators work on the same principle as those on portable tanks. The Bourbon system uses the pressure of a column of oxygen against a small ball in a chamber to measure the flow rate while using a constant flow selector valve. Some wall regulators are screwed onto a fitting; others use a quick-release spring mechanism. Figure 8-11 shows a type of wall regulator. Oxygen tank assembly is described in Skill 8-1.

Street Smart

Broken, dried, or even missing washers are the most common reasons oxygen tanks will leak. Although these washers are relatively inexpensive, they are one of the most important pieces of the assembly. Without a washer, the oxygen delivery system does not work. Therefore, experienced EMTs always have a couple of extra oxygen washers close at hand.

Safety Tip

Never allow combustible materials such as oil or grease to touch the oxygen cylinder, regulator, or valves. Under pressure, oxygen and oil will ignite and possibly even explode. Furthermore, caution is advised when using tape around an oxygen tank as many of the adhesive tapes have a petroleum base.

Safety Tip

When a patient is delivered to a hospital and then transferred to a hospital gurney, usually the oxygen supply is transferred from the ambulance tank to the hospital's wall system. Care should be used when transferring the oxygen over. Many hospitals also have pressurized air piped into the emergency room. The only difference between an air regulator and an oxygen regulator may be the color of the connection at the wall. Oxygen is always identified by green. Air may be denoted by yellow.

A mistake in identifying the correct gas for administration could have serious consequences for the patient.

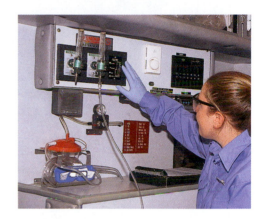

FIGURE 8-11 Regulators in the ambulance are very similar to the regulators used on the wall in the emergency department.

Safety Tip

Never smoke near oxygen tanks.

Never allow petroleum products near tank or fittings.

Never store oxygen in extreme temperatures.

Never use a modified regulator from another gas cylinder.

Never leave an oxygen tank on unattended.

Never leave an oxygen tank standing upright.

SKILL 8-1 *Oxygen Tank Assembly*

PURPOSE: To permit the EMT to use an oxygen regulator-tank assembly to administer oxygen.

STANDARD PRECAUTIONS:

☑ Oxygen tank
☑ Regulator

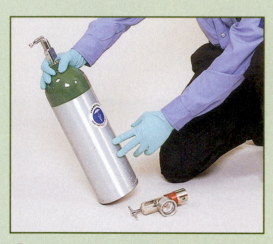

1 The EMT starts by confirming that the tank is an oxygen tank. By convention, all oxygen tanks are standardized with green paint.

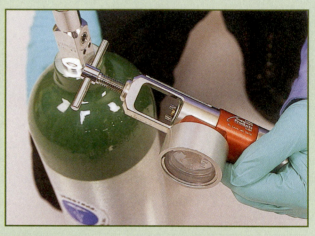

2 Then the EMT compares the oxygen regulator's pins with the contacts on the oxygen bottle's stem. Again, by convention, oxygen regulators have a specific pin configuration that fits only oxygen bottles.

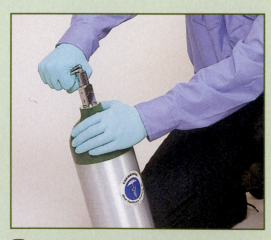

3 Using an oxygen wrench, the EMT mates the key to the latch and quickly opens and closes the oxygen tank. This procedure, called "cracking the tank," blows out any dirt and dust in the outlet.

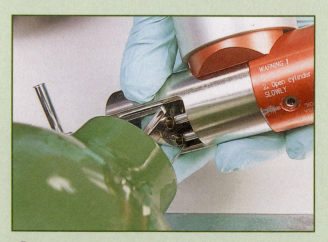

4 Then the EMT mates the regulator to the oxygen tank, being sure to tightly seal the regulator. Often, a plastic washer is needed for an airtight fit.

(continues)

SKILL 8-1 *(continued)*

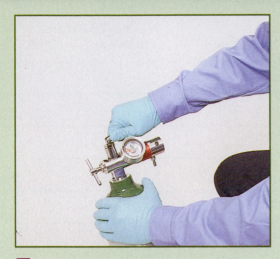 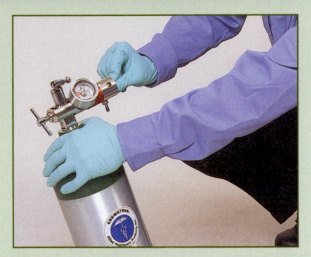

5 The oxygen tank may now be safely opened, and the pressure within the tank noted.

6 To adjust the liter flow rate, the EMT turns the knob in a counterclockwise motion until the correct liter flow appears.

OXYGEN DELIVERY DEVICES

There are a large number of oxygen delivery devices available on the market. Fortunately, the EMT needs to be familiar with only two devices, the partial **non-rebreather mask (NRB)** and the **nasal cannula (NC)**.

There are other oxygen delivery devices that the EMT should be familiar with, in case she should come across them in the field. These devices include the simple facemask and the Venturi mask. The simple facemask is used when modest amounts of oxygen are desired or the patient needs more oxygen than nasal prongs (cannula) can provide. The percentage of oxygen delivered by a simple facemask is a function of the patient's respiratory rate. Alternatively, the Venturi mask is a special mask that is engineered to deliver a specific percentage of oxygen regardless of the patient's respiratory rate. The Venturi

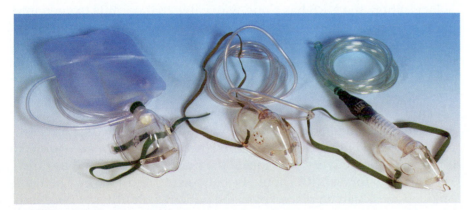

FIGURE 8-12 Partial non-rebreather mask, simple facemask, and Venturi mask (left to right).

TABLE 8-3

Oxygen Percentage from Flow Rate at Normal Respiratory Rate (16–20 bpm)

Liter Flow	Nasal Prongs (Cannula)	Simple Facemask	Venturi Mask	Partial Non-Rebreather Mask
1	24%			
2	28%			
3	32%			
4	36%		28%	
5	40%			
6	44%	40%		60%
8		60%	35%	80%
10				90%
12			60%	>95%

Safety Tip

The oxygen reservoir of an NRB should never be allowed to collapse more than halfway. Collapsing will cause the patient to receive a lower concentration of oxygen than is desired. If the reservoir does collapse significantly with patient inspiration, it can easily be remedied by increasing the oxygen flow rate that is being provided to the device.

mask is used for some patients with lung disease, like emphysema, who can tolerate neither too much nor too little oxygen. Examples of these devices can be seen in Figure 8-12. Table 8-3 lists the oxygen percentages for various flow rates and devices.

The Partial Non-Rebreather Mask

The most commonly used oxygen delivery device in the prehospital situation is the partial non-rebreather mask, or NRB. This oxygen delivery device can provide high concentrations of oxygen when the liter flow is greater than 10 lpm. In fact, if the NRB is fit well to the patient's face, oxygen concentration can approach 80%–100%.

The NRB has a clear plastic mask that is designed to fit snugly over the patient's mouth and nose while a clear plastic bag serves as a reservoir for supplemental oxygen.

In addition, the NRB has a one-way valve that permits oxygen into the mask but does not allow the expired air into the reservoir to be breathed again. Oxygen supply tubing provides oxygen directly to the device. Finally, the mask has two exhaust ports to permit the escape of expired air. This design allows delivery of high-concentration oxygen while preventing rebreathing of exhaled air.

Before applying an NRB to a patient, the EMT must attach the tubing to the oxygen tank, turn on the tank, and allow the oxygen reservoir bag to fill. Filling can be accomplished by placing a clean gloved finger over the delivery port inside the mask until the bag has filled. The liter flow for an NRB should be between 10 and 15 lpm. Then, the prefilled mask can be placed over the patient's mouth and nose. It is important to secure the nosepiece of the mask to the bridge of the patient's nose snugly and to secure the head strap around the patient's head to provide the closest fit of the mask and prevent accidental dislodgment of the device.

It is important to remember that, although an NRB is capable of delivering high concentrations of oxygen, the gas is not delivered to the patient's lungs unless he is breathing effectively. *Without adequate ventilation, the oxygen will not be delivered. The patient who is being given oxygen via an NRB must be continually monitored to ensure that the respiratory status is not changing and another oxygen delivery device is not needed.* Application of an NRB is described in Skill 8-2.

Tracheostomy Mask

A variation of an oxygen facemask is the tracheostomy mask. As the name implies, the "trach mask" fits over tracheostomy opening, called a stoma, and provides oxygen (Figure 8-13). Some trach masks even come with an opening at the front that will permit a flexible French catheter to be used for suctioning.

SKILL 8-2 *Application of a Non-Rebreather Mask*

PURPOSE: To permit the EMT to use a non-rebreather oxygen mask to deliver oxygen to a patient.

STANDARD PRECAUTIONS:

☑ Oxygen tank and regulator
☑ Non-rebreather mask
☑ Gloves

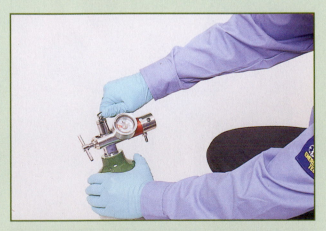

1 First, the EMT must ensure that the oxygen tank and regulator are correctly assembled. The oxygen tank should have sufficient pressure to provide continuous flow.

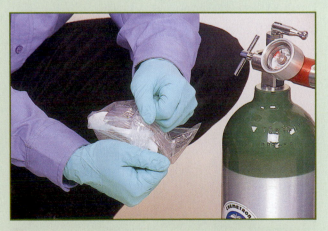

2 Then the EMT should choose the correct oxygen administration device. A non-rebreather mask is used when high concentrations of oxygen are desired.

(continues)

SKILL 8-2 *(continued)*

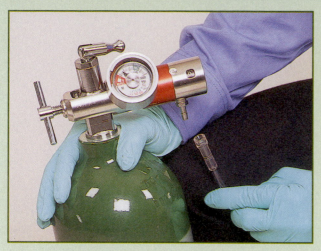

3 To use the non-rebreather mask, the EMT must attach the oxygen tubing to the regulator and turn on the regulator. As a rule, 10 to 15 liters per minute is sufficient. The regulator should never be turned below 6 liters per minute.

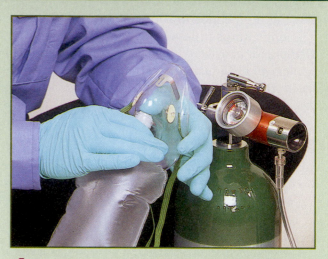

4 The EMT then places his thumb over the valve between the bag and the mask, permitting the bag to fill completely.

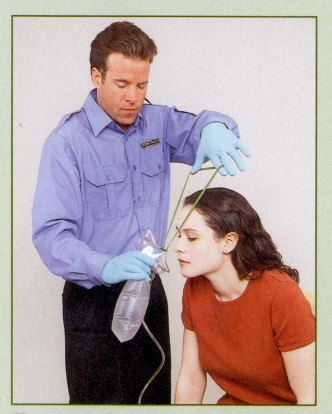

5 Grasping the mask in one hand and the elastic band in the other, the EMT seats the mask firmly on the bridge of the nose and drapes the elastic band around the head. The EMT should pinch the metal strip around the nose.

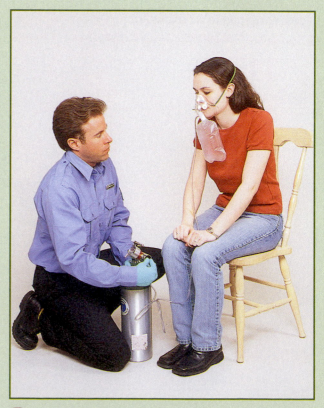

6 The EMT then adjusts the liter flow to ensure that the oxygen bag is always filled to about one-half.

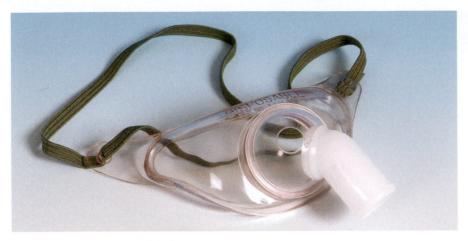

FIGURE 8-13 The tracheostomy mask is designed to provide high-concentration oxygen to patients with a tracheostomy.

The Nasal Cannula

The NC is a flexible plastic device that is composed of two small prongs attached to a length of tubing. The prongs are designed to fit somewhat comfortably into a patient's nose, while the tubing is attached to an oxygen source at relatively low flows. Flow rates for the nasal cannula vary from 1 to 6 lpm. Table 8-4 indicates the oxygen concentration delivered by the NC and NRB at different flow rates.

Because there are not many situations in which the EMT would decide to use low-flow oxygen over high flow, use of an NC by the EMT is generally restricted to patients who are already on low-flow oxygen at home or who absolutely cannot tolerate the NRB. Application of an NC is described in Skill 8-3.

TABLE 8-4

Oxygen Concentrations and Flow Rates

Device and Flow Rate	Concentration of Oxygen Delivered (in ideal circumstances)
Nasal cannula, 1 lpm	24%
Nasal cannula, 2 lpm	28%
Nasal cannula, 3 lpm	32%
Nasal cannula, 4 lpm	36%
Nasal cannula, 5 lpm	40%
Nasal cannula, 6 lpm	44%
Non-rebreather mask	80%–100%

Safety Tip

Some patients have a latex sensitivity or allergy. Before applying an oxygen device, the EMT should make sure that (1) the patient is not latex sensitive and (2) if he is, that the device being used is latex free. Many manufacturers of oxygen delivery devices have removed any latex from their products for this reason.

Street Smart

The "Rule of Sixes" is useful to remember for oxygen delivery devices. This rule states, Never put on any type of *mask* at less than 6 liters per minute and never increase the liter flow on a *nasal cannula* to greater than 6 liters per minute. This precaution prevents both hypoventilation and unnecessary nasal trauma from inappropriate liter flow rates.

Safety Tip

While a patient is receiving supplemental oxygen, the tubing should never be covered from view. Care should be taken to avoid strapping the tubing under blankets or other items to prevent inadvertent kinking. Such kinking of the tubing may decrease the oxygen flow that the patient receives.

SKILL 8-3 *Application of a Nasal Cannula*

PURPOSE: To permit the EMT to use a nasal cannula to deliver oxygen to a patient.

STANDARD PRECAUTIONS:

☑ Oxygen tank and regulator
☑ Nasal cannula
☑ Gloves

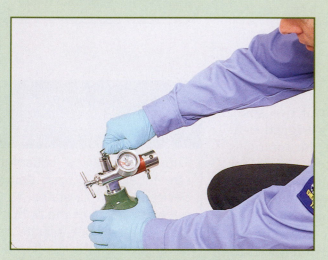

1 First, the EMT must ensure that the oxygen tank and oxygen regulator are correctly assembled. The oxygen tank should show sufficient pressure to provide continuous flow.

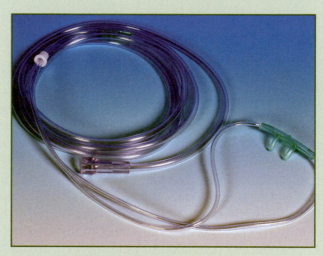

2 Then the EMT chooses the correct oxygen administration device. A nasal cannula is used when the patient cannot tolerate the non-rebreather mask or when low concentrations of oxygen are required.

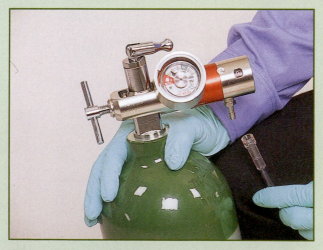

3 To use the nasal cannula, the EMT must attach the oxygen tubing to the regulator and turn on the regulator. As a rule, 4 to 6 liters per minute is sufficient. The regulator should never be turned below 6 liters per minute.

(continues)

SKILL 8-3 (continued)

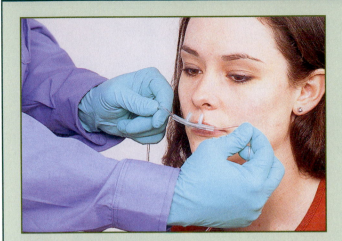

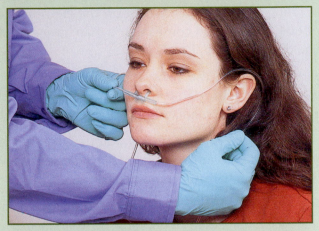

4 The nasal prongs are gently introduced into the nostrils so that they appear to be lying on the floor of the nostril.

5 The tubing is draped over the ears and the tubing cinched loosely under the chin with the ring. The nasal cannula should not be draped over the head like a necklace; the danger of injury from strangulation is too great. The EMT then adjusts the liter flow to ensure that the patient is receiving an adequate liter flow.

ARTIFICIAL VENTILATION

If air is not being brought into the lungs through adequate ventilation, then the blood will not become oxygenated. Therefore, the EMT must pay particular attention to the patient's ventilation. Fortunately, this is relatively easy to do and requires only keen observational skills.

If the patient is not breathing at all, a condition called apnea, then it is quite obvious that air is not getting into the lungs and no oxygenation is occurring. In this situation, the treatment is simply to provide ventilation for the patient. Providing ventilation to a patient is referred to as **artificial ventilation**, or *rescue breathing*. This can be accomplished by a variety of methods.

Use of a Barrier Device

To protect herself from unnecessary exposure to potentially infectious body fluids, the EMT should use a barrier device when performing artificial ventilation. There are many types of these devices on the market. One such device is shown in Figure 8-14. Each barrier device should have an impervious plastic shield that is accompanied by a ventilation port of some kind.

The Pocket Mask

When an EMT arrives at the side of a patient who is not breathing and additional help is not immediately available, she should begin artificial ventilation using a **pocket mask**. A pocket mask is a clear plastic dome-shaped tool that is used as a barrier device for artificial ventilation and also allows supplemental oxygen administration. The side

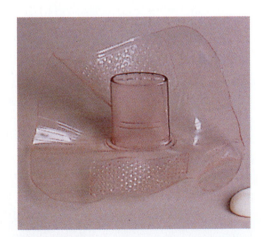

FIGURE 8-14 Many commercially made face shields can be used as a barrier device during the performance of mouth-to-mouth ventilation.

✳ *Respiratory Compromise*

After riding six floors, Tamesha got off the elevator and proceeded to apartment 604. The call had come in as "a man having trouble breathing." The name on the door said "Fish, Ron."

"Hello, Mr. Fish? It's the ambulance," Tamesha called out, while knocking on the door. After getting an invitation to come in, Tamesha stepped into the doorway. She was immediately aware of the acrid smell of cigarette smoke.

Mr. Fish was in the kitchen, sitting bolt upright on a chair at the table, wearing only a T–shirt and briefs. In front of him was an ashtray overflowing with cigarette butts and a half–full cup of coffee.

As Tamesha introduced herself, she noted the oxygen cannula he was wearing. Mr. Fish was a frail elderly man. Now he was hunched over, hands on his knees. His breathing was rapid and shallow. He was blowing out air through pursed lips.

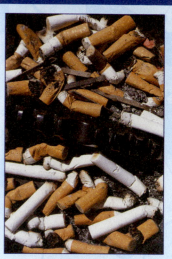

(Courtesy of PhotoDisc.)

While assessing his airway, Tamesha noted that his lips were a pale blue, as were his fingernail beds. She quickly listened to his lungs.

He was moving good air, but the lung sounds were muffled. Tamesha even quickly checked her stethoscope to see that it was adjusted properly.

Mr. Fish's chest was barrel–shaped and did not expand very much with each breath. Tamesha also noticed that the skin between his ribs was retracting every time he took a breath.

Tamesha quickly applied the pulse oximeter, remembering that a high reading may be misleading because of carbon monoxide.

Suddenly, Mr. Fish appeared to be having more trouble breathing. He reached out and grabbed Tamesha by the shirt sleeve. All he could say was "I . . . can't . . . breathe!"

- What indications (signs and symptoms) of respiratory compromise is this patient displaying?
- What treatments are indicated in this case? Is one treatment more desirable than another?
- If these initial treatments are unsuccessful, what actions can the EMT be reasonably expected to take?

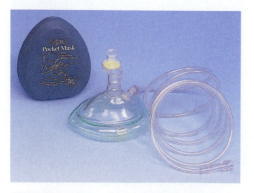

FIGURE 8-15 Supplemental oxygen has been attached to this pocket mask with oxygen tubing.

facing the patient usually has a soft air-filled cushion that helps the EMT maintain a tight fit of the mask to the patient's face.

The other side of the mask has a ventilation port. It is designed for the EMT to put her lips around the ventilation port and blow into the mask to deliver ventilation. This port often has a filter device that allows air to go into the patient's mouth and nose but blocks air and other material from coming out of the mask and entering the EMT's mouth.

Many masks also come with an oxygen inlet (Figure 8-15). When oxygen tubing, running from an oxygen source, is attached to the inlet, the percentage of oxygen delivered to the patient increases from the 16% that is in a typical exhaled breath to about 40% through the use of supplemental oxygen. Whenever possible, a pocket mask should have oxygen attached. The proper use of a pocket mask is described in Skill 8-4.

SKILL 8-4 *Use of a Pocket Mask*

PURPOSE: To permit the EMT to ventilate the apneic patient while using a barrier device for personal protection.

STANDARD PRECAUTIONS:

- ☑ Pocket mask with oxygen inlet
- ☑ One-way valve
- ☑ Oxygen tubing
- ☑ Oxygen tank
- ☑ Oxygen regulator
- ☑ Gloves
- ☑ Goggles

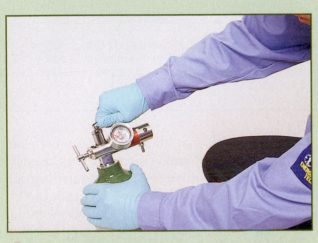

1 First, the EMT must ensure that the oxygen tank and oxygen regulator are correctly assembled. The oxygen tank should have sufficient pressure to provide continuous oxygen flow.

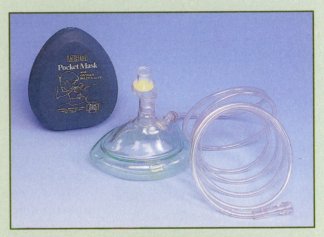

2 Then the EMT chooses the correct oxygen administration device. A pocket mask with an oxygen outlet is preferred when one EMT must ventilate an apneic patient alone.

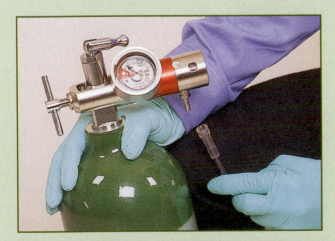

3 To use the pocket mask, the EMT must attach the oxygen tubing from the pocket mask to the regulator and turn on the regulator. As a rule, 10 to 15 liters per minute is sufficient.

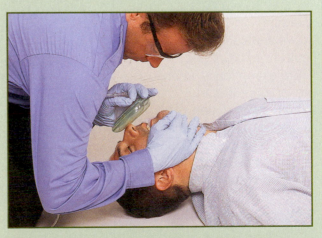

4 The EMT then places the apex of the mask over the bridge of the nose and lays the mask over the patient's nose and mouth. An oropharyngeal airway (OPA) should already be in place.

(continues)

SKILL 8-4 (continued)

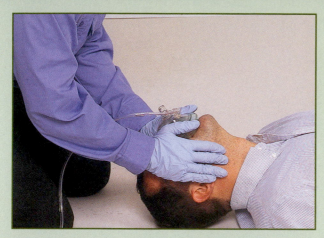

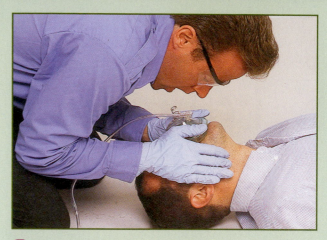

5 The EMT then uses a two-handed grasp around the chimney of the mask while grasping the jaw with the remaining fingers.

6 Tilting the head backward and pulling the jaw upward, the EMT blows into the mask for about 1 1/2 to 2 seconds. The EMT should repeat ventilation every 5 seconds.

Street Smart

Many elderly people have false teeth, called **dentures**. When an EMT is ventilating a patient, these dentures should be left in to serve as a base for the mask to seal upon. Without such a base, the mask seal is quite challenging to maintain and effective ventilation may be very difficult.

The exception is when loose or broken dentures may create a potential obstruction. In this case, they should be removed as soon as the problem is identified. Care should be taken not to lose dentures because they are frequently quite expensive to replace.

The pocket mask is the device that allows for the most effective patient ventilation by the single EMT and is therefore to be used by the EMT who must quickly provide ventilation to a nonbreathing person.

Initial ventilations by the single EMT are generally provided without supplemental oxygen to avoid any delay in beginning ventilation. The 16% oxygen that the EMT can deliver with straight mouth-to-mask ventilation is sufficient for the first minute. When help arrives, supplemental oxygen can be added, or a different device may be used to provide ventilation.

The Bag-Valve-Mask

Despite the speed with which it can be set up and its effectiveness in the hands of the single EMT, mouth-to-mask ventilation has several drawbacks. This method of artificial ventilation can become very tiring to the EMT after a relatively short time. Furthermore, the percentage of oxygen provided through a pocket mask, even with supplemental oxygen, is low when compared with the percentage provided by other devices. Therefore, alternative ventilation methods may be more desirable if additional assistance is available.

The **bag-valve-mask (BVM)** is a device that is used to ventilate the nonbreathing patient. The importance of this task is clearly obvious. What may not be as obvious is the practice that is necessary to become proficient with the device. The EMT should become well acquainted with all aspects of the BVM and become competent in its use in the classroom before using it in the field. For this reason the anatomy of a BVM is reviewed in depth (Figure 8-16).

Anatomy of a Bag-Valve-Mask

The BVM device originated from the anesthesia bags used in the operating room. The most outstanding feature of a BVM is the self-inflating bag. Originally the bag was made of soft collapsible rubber that filled with a gas, such as oxygen, from a source or tank. This soft texture allowed the operator to have a "feel" of the resistance that was present when ventilating the patient.

Resistance is the firm feel to the bag when it is squeezed to deliver a breath. Resistance to ventilation is the result of chest wall and lung stiffness. A certain amount of stiffness is normal; however, it should not be so great that it is difficult to deliver a breath in normal circumstances.

The BVM still has the characteristics of the early soft rubber anesthesia bags. Modern bags are self-inflating. This means that once the bag is emptied by delivery of a breath to the patient, it will automatically refill with air for the next breath to be delivered.

All bags come with a port for supplemental oxygen. Oxygen tubing is run from either the wall source or a portable oxygen tank to the bag. At the typical rate of oxygen flow, the bag with supplemental oxygen can deliver from 40% to 60% oxygen. This oxygen inlet port is usually found at the back of the bag.

Many bags have an attached oxygen reservoir to improve the percentage of oxygen delivered. This reservoir provides a large source of oxygen, which is immediately available, when the bag self-inflates. An oxygen reservoir can allow the EMT to deliver 100% oxygen to the patient. Some reservoirs are corrugated tubes that attach to the rear of the bag. Other reservoirs are collapsible bags that fill with oxygen.

Between the bag and the reservoir most BVMs have a safety valve. This safety valve permits the bag to reinflate with room air whenever the reservoir is collapsed partially or completely. This feature allows continuous supply of airflow to the bag for delivery to the patient.

The delivery valve is perhaps the most important part of the BVM. Among its several purposes, it first provides a unidirectional flow of gas (oxygen-enriched air) to the patient. The valve is designed to fit all types of ventilating masks and endotracheal tubes that are used to provide direct tracheal ventilation.

When an EMT squeezes the bag, the oxygen-enriched air is forced out the delivery valve and toward the patient. The one-way valve prevents any of the gas from returning into the bag and diluting the mixture.

This one-way valve also blocks any bloody secretions or vomit from entering into the bag. Therefore, the bag and the oxygen reservoir always remain clean on the inside.

Another unique feature of this valve is that it allows for the air that is exhaled by the patient after each breath to exit the valve through a port. This feature prevents exhaled air from entering the bag and diluting the oxygen-rich air that is stored there for the next ventilation.

The facemask of a BVM is very similar to the pocket mask. In fact, a pocket mask can be used as a facemask during an emergency. The facemask, like the pocket mask, is a clear plastic dome-shaped mask with a soft air-filled cushion. It is applied to the face in the same manner as a pocket mask. The mask seal for a facemask is also important, as was the face seal of a pocket mask.

Early facemasks, used in the administration of surgical anesthesia, were made completely of black rubber. Rubber was used to reduce the chance of an accidental spark, as many early anesthetic agents were

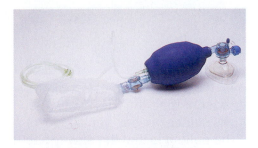

FIGURE 8-16 The bag-valve-mask device is a useful prehospital tool.

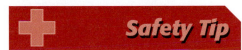

Safety Tip

The EMT should realize that if a BVM is not attached to an oxygen source, the bag will refill with room air. Room air is certainly not as beneficial to the patient as 100% oxygen, which should be delivered via the BVM. The EMT should always ensure that the oxygen source has been turned on and is working properly. Frequently checking the tank capacity is recommended so that when the tank runs low on oxygen, the EMT has a few minutes to find another tank and make the switch.

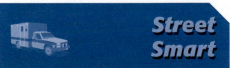

Street Smart

The collapsible reservoir bags have both advantages and disadvantages. On the positive side, these reservoirs visibly expand when filled with oxygen. This expansion is unmistakable evidence that the oxygen source is running. On the negative side, these collapsible reservoirs are usually made of plastic and therefore are easily torn during use, rendering the reservoir useless. Remember to try to keep the reservoir half filled with oxygen at all times.

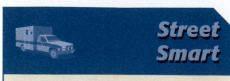

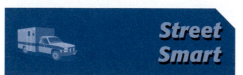

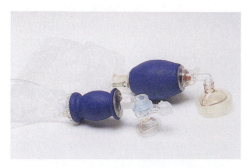

FIGURE 8-17 There are multiple sizes of bag-valve-mask device available for the EMT to choose from based upon the size of the patient.

highly flammable. Some of the better facemasks on the market still have the black rubber cushion. However, it is important that any facemask used have a clear dome so that the patient's airway can be monitored for blood or vomit.

Facemasks, like faces, come in different sizes. The mask should be fitted to the patient. The correctly fitting facemask should extend from the bridge of the nose to the cleft in the chin while covering both the nose and mouth completely. The experienced EMT has several sizes of facemasks on hand when preparing to ventilate a patient.

Ventilation Technique

It is important for the EMT to become proficient in the technique of ventilation. Because the patient's life depends on adequate ventilation and the skill requires practice to perform properly, the EMT should be sure that she is adequately practiced in this skill.

Air Volume

Because all patients are different sizes, not every patient's lungs need the same amount of air delivered when performing artificial ventilation. Care should be taken to deliver a breath to the patient that is sufficient to result in chest rise, but not beyond that. Overaggressive ventilations can result in distention and even rupture of the lung. Furthermore, excess air with overaggressive ventilation can overflow into the esophagus and stomach. This overflow will result in stomach distention and vomiting. Vomiting in the nonbreathing patient is a serious airway problem and should be avoided at all costs. Alternatively, insufficient delivery of a breath can lead to inadequate ventilation and hypoxia.

The EMT should be familiar with the appropriate rates with which to ventilate adult, pediatric, and infant patients who require manual ventilation. Providing ventilations at a rate lower than what is needed can lead to inadequate oxygen levels and buildup of carbon dioxide in the patient's bloodstream. Conversely, overly rapid ventilations can result in an excessive drop in carbon dioxide levels in the bloodstream. Inappropriately high or low carbon dioxide levels can lead to significant complications of many conditions and should be avoided. There are rare conditions in which providing ventilations at a rate more rapid than usual might be appropriate. This is called hyperventilation and is addressed later in this text. Age-appropriate rates of ventilation are noted in Table 8-5.

Two-Person Ventilation

The most effective method of ventilating a nonbreathing patient is to have two EMTs working as a team. The first EMT should be the *airway* person. The airway person is responsible for maintaining an open airway with either the jaw thrust or the head-tilt, chin-lift method while maintaining a good mask seal. The airway person also watches the airway for blood and vomit or other potentially obstructing materials.

If the airway does become obstructed, then the airway person must be prepared to immediately suction. A suction machine should be readily available. Needless to say, the EMT at the airway needs to wear gloves, goggles, and a mask to protect herself from potentially infectious bodily fluids.

The second EMT becomes the *breathing* person. The breathing person focuses his attention on properly ventilating the patient by squeezing the bag, with eyes focused on the chest rise while simultaneously looking for abdominal distention.

Obviously, in the cardiac arrest situation, there would be an additional person performing compressions. This *circulation* person would work with the breathing person to effectively intersperse ventilations with compressions. Figure 8-18 demonstrates how three EMTs can effectively perform CPR without interfering with one another. Skill 8-5 describes ventilation with a BVM.

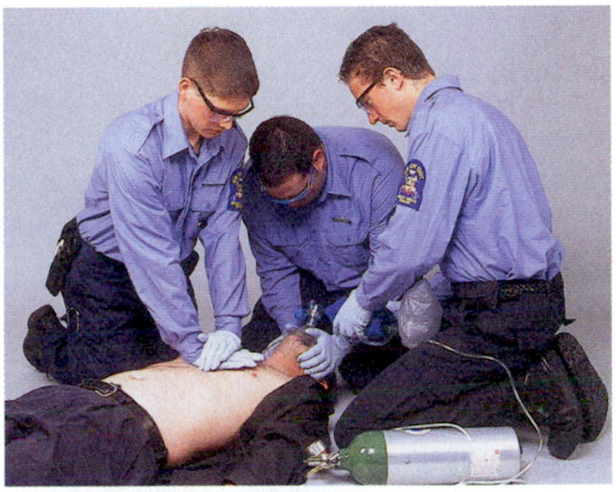

FIGURE 8-18 This team of EMTs are performing effective CPR.

Cricoid Pressure

Whenever possible, and provided that a free hand is available, gentle **cricoid pressure** should be applied to the trachea. The cricoid is a cartilaginous ring that supports and helps hold open the trachea. The cricoid ring is found just below the Adam's apple, or larynx. The EMT uses her forefinger and thumb to press the cricoid ring gently posteriorly. This action compresses the esophagus, not allowing air to easily enter. Cricoid pressure is being applied to the patient in Figure 8-19.

TABLE 8-5		
Age Appropriate Rates for Manual Ventilation		
Age	**Normal Rate**	**Hyperventilation**
Adult	10	20
Children	20	30
Infants	25	35

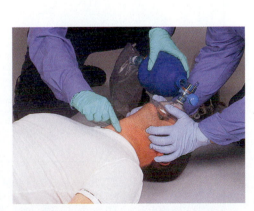

FIGURE 8-19 Notice that the EMT ventilating the patient is using a free hand to apply some gentle cricoid pressure to the patient.

SKILL 8-5 *Ventilation with a Bag-Valve-Mask*

PURPOSE: To permit two EMTs to provide positive-presure ventilation to the apneic patient.

STANDARD PRECAUTIONS:

  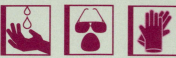

☑ Bag-valve-mask (BVM) assembly
☑ Oxygen tubing
☑ Oxygen regulator
☑ Oxygen tank
☑ Gloves
☑ Goggles
☑ Mask

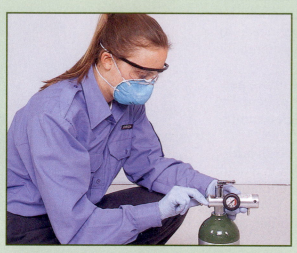

1 First, the EMT must ensure that the oxygen tank and oxygen regulator are correctly assembled. The oxygen tank should have sufficient pressure to provide continuous oxygen flow.

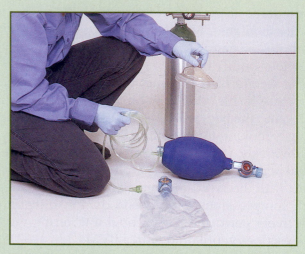

2 Then the EMT chooses the correct oxygen administration device. A BVM assembly is used when an apneic patient needs to be ventilated by two EMTs.

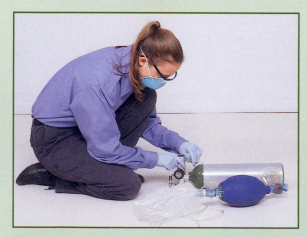

3 To use the BVM, the EMT must first attach the oxygen tubing to the regulator and turn on the regulator. As a rule, 10 to 15 liters per minute are sufficient.

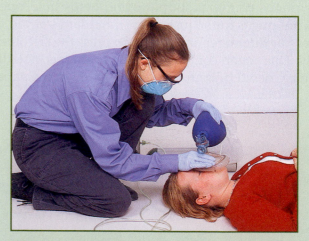

4 Next, the EMT chooses a properly fitting face-mask. The facemask should fit securely over the bridge of the nose and extend to the cleft of the chin.

(continues)

SKILL 8-5 (continued)

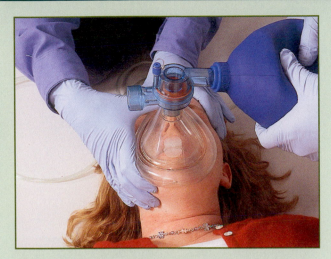

5 Ensuring that the airway is patent and an OPA (oropharyngeal airway) is in place, the EMT places the mask over the apneic patient's face.

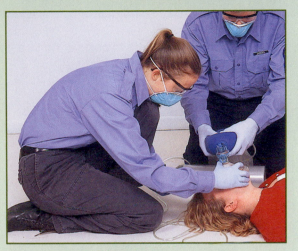

6 One EMT holds the mask in place using the two-handed "OK" grasp while another EMT compresses the bag with two hands. The patient should be ventilated every 5 seconds.

Oxygen-Powered Ventilation Device

Early EMTs frequently used an oxygen-powered device called the demand valve. The demand valve worked simply; the patient could either inspire air and trigger the oxygen valve to come on, hence the name "on demand," or the EMT could press a trigger and automatically provide oxygen to the patient. The problem occurred when the trigger was pressed for too long and the stomach became grossly distended. Whenever the demand valve was used during a cardiac arrest, the patient would invariably vomit, then aspirate, thereby making a bad situation worse.

With technical improvements to the design of the demand valve, the modern **flow-restricted oxygen-powered ventilation device (FROPVD)** has returned to favored status among many EMTs. Because of the ease of being able to hold a tight mask seal while effectively ventilating the patient, the EMT can single-handedly ventilate the patient with 100% oxygen. Caution is advised, however, because it is still easy to overinflate the patient's stomach with this device.

Another downside to the oxygen-powered ventilation device is that the EMT cannot feel the resistance created by the patient's lungs. Increasing resistance is a clue that something has changed in the patient's lungs. This can be a valuable clue that is not available when using this device. Skill 8-6 demonstrates the use of the FROPVD.

Single-Person BVM Ventilation

The EMT who is ventilating a patient alone is doing the work of two EMTs. Frequently, because of poor technique and fatigue, the value of one-person ventilation is debatable.

For these reasons the EMT should consider first ventilating with a pocket mask, then with an FROPVD; if neither is available, then start

SKILL 8-6 *Ventilation with a Flow-Restricted Oxygen-Powered Ventilation Device*

PURPOSE: To ventilate a hypoxic or nonbreathing patient.

STANDARD PRECAUTIONS:

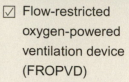

- ☑ Flow-restricted oxygen-powered ventilation device (FROPVD)
- ☑ Oxygen regulator
- ☑ Oxygen tank
- ☑ Gloves
- ☑ Goggles

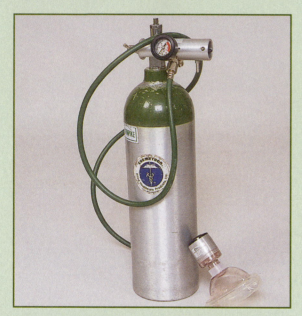

1 First, the EMT must ensure that the oxygen tank and oxygen regulator, with the FROPVD, are correctly assembled. The oxygen tank should show sufficient pressure to provide continuous oxygen flow. Then the EMT chooses the correct oxygen administration device. An FROPVD is used when an apneic patient needs to be ventilated by a single EMT.

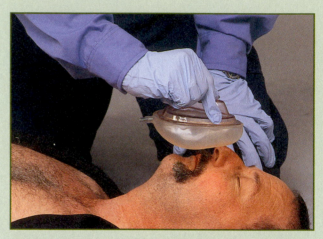

2 Next, the EMT should choose a properly fitting facemask. The facemask should fit securely over the bridge of the nose and extend to the cleft of the chin.

(continues)

with a BVM alone. Single EMT use of a BVM should be considered as a last resort and only then as a temporary measure until the arrival of additional EMTs.

Because only one hand is available to compress the bag and the other is busy trying to maintain an open airway, insufficient volumes of oxygen are often generated. The efficiency of the BVM can be improved by pressing the bag against the face of the patient. This technique not only increases the volume delivered but also helps maintain the mask seal (Figure 8-20).

Ventilation of the Breathing Patient

Many patients with extreme difficulty breathing can be assisted with a BVM. Although ventilating a breathing patient may seem confusing, remember that these patients often are breathing ineffectively and to delay assistance is only inviting disaster.

SKILL 8-6 *(continued)*

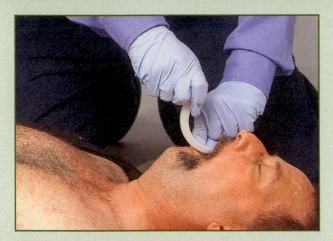

3 Ensuring that the airway is patent and that an OPA (oropharyngeal airway) is in place, the EMT places the mask over the apneic patient's face.

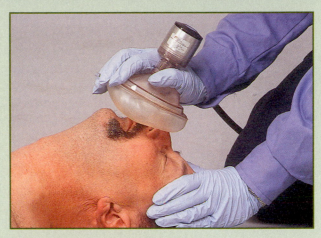

4 The patient's head should then be tilted backward.

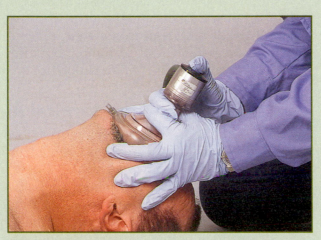

5 The EMT holds the mask in place, using the two-handed "OK" grasp while compressing the trigger of the FROPVD for about 2 seconds or until the lungs rise. The patient should be ventilated every 5 seconds.

To review, the patient who may be a candidate for assisted ventilation is usually fatigued to the point of exhaustion or is breathing so rapidly that air does not have time to get into the lungs. In both cases, the patient will become hypoxic (evidenced by blue skin color), tired, and confused. Eventually the patient who is in respiratory failure will cease breathing altogether. By assisting ventilations, the EMT can avoid periods of hypoxia associated with respiratory failure and respiratory arrest.

The patient with severe respiratory difficulty is usually sitting upright and should be allowed to remain so as long as he can support himself. The procedure about to be attempted should be described to the patient in terms that he can understand. For example, "Mr. Jones, I am going to help you breathe using this mask. You will notice that

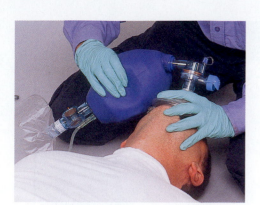

FIGURE 8-20 When forced, an EMT might have to use a BVM alone. Use the side of the patient's face to compress the bag more completely and help maintain the facemask seal.

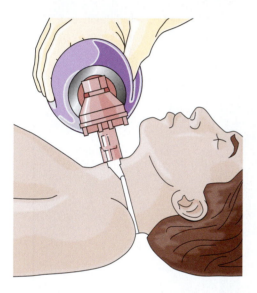

FIGURE 8-21 The BVM will attach to all standard tracheostomy tubes. Less volume is needed to ventilate the patient, so caution is advised.

your lungs will feel a little fuller and you should start to feel better. Let me know if you want me to stop."

Next, gently place the BVM over the patient's mouth and let him draw in some oxygen from the bag. Remember that oxygen from a BVM with a reservoir is almost 100%, the percentage that should be administered to any patient in distress. The patient will be able to draw in enough air as long as he is breathing; the BVM acts like a demand valve in these cases.

Carefully watching the patient's respiration, gently collapse the bag as the patient ends an inspiration, thereby filling the lungs. If a little pressure is applied to the bag with the fingertips, the EMT can feel when the patient inspires and should then gently squeeze the bag. These two techniques—gently squeezing the bag while feeling for inspiration and watching the chest rise—should enable the EMT to perfectly time each assisted ventilation.

Eventually a regular, often slower, rate will be established. Do not be surprised if the patient stops breathing entirely and allows you to ventilate him. These patients are exhausted, and the respite from the work of breathing provides them with a much-needed break. Continue to reassure the patient while constantly monitoring the level of consciousness and the airway.

Many EMTs are somewhat uncomfortable with assisting a conscious patient with breathing, but after a few experiences, the EMT will realize the incredible difference he has made for these patients.

Ventilation of the Surgical Airway

Some patients who have either a long-standing history of lung disease or cancers of the throat undergo a surgical procedure that bypasses the natural airway and creates a new airway. This surgical airway usually consists of an opening to the trachea that is made in the front of the neck. This can allow for easier breathing in the patient who has severe lung disease or diseases of the upper airway.

Although there are several types of surgical airways that are created for different reasons, the most common surgical airway the EMT will encounter is the **tracheostomy**. A tracheostomy is a hole that is surgically created in the front of the neck that allows air to enter the trachea directly without passing through the mouth and nose. Normally, a rigid plastic tube is left in that hole to protect it from collapse or obstruction. This tube is called a tracheostomy tube. The tracheostomy tube looks just like a very small endotracheal tube. The single feature that should be of interest to EMTs is the fact that the

Street Smart

Routine airway maneuvers, such as the jaw thrust or the head-tilt, chin-lift, are *not* necessary when ventilating the tracheostomy tube or the stoma. The neck should be maintained in a neutral position, keeping the trachea in a straight line. A folded towel placed under the neck will help to maintain a neutral position while also providing a platform for the EMT to ventilate.

external connection of the tracheostomy tube will fit onto the bag-valve-mask device connector if ventilation becomes necessary. Figure 8-21 shows how the EMT can easily ventilate these patients.

Ventilation of a patient with a tracheostomy tube is very simple. First, connect the BVM to the 8 mm adapter on the tracheostomy tube and then begin to ventilate, paying special attention to the amount of air being ventilated. Because the mouth, nose, and upper airway are not being filled by this air, less air is needed to ventilate the tracheostomy patient.

Another type of surgical airway involves rerouting the trachea to open at the front of the neck. This type of airway is often used for patients with severe cancers of the upper airway. Initially this opening will be maintained by a tracheostomy tube also, but as time goes on the opening "matures" and will remain open, or patent, without the tracheostomy tube. This opening, called a **stoma**, is now the patient's airway (Figure 8-22).

Ventilating a stoma at first may seem frightening. The EMT should size the stoma's opening for a properly fitting mask, usually an infant-sized or small child-sized mask. This mask may be placed over the stoma, and ventilation may proceed as usual.

Because of the lack of adequate humidification normally provided by the nose and mouth, many surgical airway patients develop thick mucus collections around their tracheostomy. These secretions can even obstruct the airway and are called mucous plugs. If such an obstruction prevents the patient from ventilating effectively, the EMT should use a flexible French catheter to suction the tracheostomy. The catheter should be inserted only as far as the EMT can see into the opening. The tracheostomy patient in Figure 8-23 is being suctioned with a flexible catheter. If suctioning is unsuccessful in clearing the airway, then standard obstructed airway procedures should be instituted and the airway reassessed.

CONCLUSION

Oxygen administration is one of the most commonly used tools of the EMT. Oxygen administration performed properly can have truly lifesaving results. Careful assessment of the patient and thoughtful decision making regarding oxygen administration and artificial ventilation are tasks that the EMT should become very comfortable with.

TEST YOUR KNOWLEDGE

1. What are some signs of shortness of breath?
2. What is hypoxia? What are the signs of hypoxia?
3. What is cyanosis? Where can cyanosis be found?
4. Starting at the tank, list all the parts of an oxygen delivery system.
5. What is the minimal acceptable flow rate for a non-rebreather mask? What is the maximal acceptable flow rate for a nasal cannula?

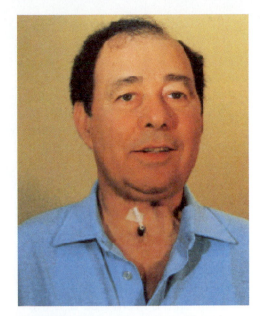

FIGURE 8-22   The patient with a stoma breathes through a surgically created opening in the anterior neck.

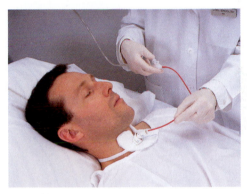

FIGURE 8-23   Tracheostomy tubes often become clogged with mucus and can be suctioned gently, using a French catheter.

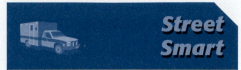

Street Smart

Advances in biomedical technology have reduced the size of bedside ventilators that are seen in a hospital's intensive care unit to ventilators that can be placed on a bedside stand in the home or even on the shelf of an ambulance. Although these machines offer many advantages for long-term ventilation, if the patient goes into respiratory or cardiopulmonary arrest, the ventilation should be removed and the patient manually ventilated with a BVM.

6. When would a nasal cannula be preferred over a non-rebreather mask?

7. What is the preferred method of ventilation when a rescuer is alone? What is the optimal number of rescuers needed to perform cardiopulmonary resuscitation (CPR)?

8. What is the first step in the process of ventilating the breathing patient with a bag-valve-mask?

9. What is the single greatest danger when using a flow-restricted oxygen-powered ventilation device?

INTERNET RESOURCES

- Search the Web for information on respiratory support. What additional information can you find that is pertinent to working in the EMS field on calls of this nature?

- Is there any additional research being done in the field of EMS on how to improve the care provided on calls of this nature?

FURTHER STUDY

Menegazzi, J. J., & Winslow, H. J (1994). In-vitro comparison of bag-valve-mask and the manually triggered oxygen-powered breathing device. *Academic Emergency Medicine*, 1(1), 29–33.

Terndrup, T. E., & Warner, D. A. (1992). Infant ventilation and oxygenation by basic life support providers: Comparison of methods. *Prehospital Disaster Medicine*, 7(1), 35–40.

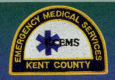

CHAPTER 9

Shock: A State of Hypoperfusion

KEY TERMS

anaphylactic shock

anaphylaxis

capillary refill time

cardiac output

cardiogenic shock

compensated shock

decompensated shock

evisceration

hemorrhagic shock

hypoperfusion

hypovolemia

hypovolemic shock

irreversible shock

military anti-shock trousers (MAST)

neurogenic shock

orthostatic vital signs

perfusion

pneumatic anti-shock garment (PASG)

postural hypotension

septic shock

shock

stroke volume

tilt test

urticaria

OBJECTIVES

Upon completion of this chapter, the reader should be able to:

1. Define *perfusion* and identify the significance of hypoperfusion.
2. Identify five specific etiologies of shock.
3. List the signs and symptoms of compensated shock.
4. Explain the importance of capillary refill in children.
5. Define *decompensated shock*.
6. Describe the appropriate initial evaluation of the patient in shock.
7. List appropriate steps in management of the patient with signs and symptoms of shock.
8. List the indications and contraindications for the use of MAST/PASG.
9. Describe the application of MAST/PASG.

OVERVIEW

Cells in the human body require oxygen to function properly. When cells are without oxygen for a period of time, they will not be able to function properly and eventually will die. When many cells in a particular organ die, the organ will fail. When several organs in the human body fail, the patient may die. Oxygen is carried throughout the body in the bloodstream. **Perfusion** is the term describing the distribution of blood, nutrients, and oxygen throughout the body. **Hypoperfusion** refers to inadequate blood flow and oxygenation of body tissues and organs.

Extended periods of hypoperfusion will lead to cell death and organ failure. The state that the body is in when parts of it are hypoperfused is called **shock**.

There are many causes of shock, although the end result is similar. It is crucial that the Emergency Medical Technician–Basic (EMT-B) recognize the early signs of hypoperfusion and be prepared to provide treatment that may help to halt the progression of shock. It is also helpful to recognize and differentiate between the different etiologies of shock, as there are some specific treatments that may be required for each.

This chapter reviews the physiology leading to shock and the body's means of compensating for it. Recognition of compensated shock is stressed as well as the management priorities of the EMT-B.

PERFUSION

Perfusion is the delivery of oxygenated red blood cells to tissues and organs. All tissues and organs in the human body require constant perfusion to function at their best.

The amount of blood that the heart pumps to the body in 1 minute is called the **cardiac output**. The cardiac output depends on the volume of blood pumped out with each beat, called the **stroke volume**, and the rate at which the heart beats.

The formula for determining cardiac output is CO = SV × HR (CO, cardiac output; SV, stroke volume; HR, heart rate). This formula illustrates how the cardiac output can be increased by increasing the heart rate, the stroke volume, or both.

Because the cells, tissues, and organs of the body are dependent upon an adequate cardiac output to survive, the body can usually regulate stroke volume and heart rate as needed. There are times, however, when such regulation is not possible or not effective in maintaining the cardiac output. In these cases, the inadequate cardiac output translates into hypoperfusion of body tissues.

HYPOPERFUSION

Hypoperfusion means inadequate perfusion. Hypoperfused tissue is no longer being given enough oxygen and will stop working optimally. The body has some defenses against this type of problem. Some organs are better equipped to survive temporary decreases in perfusion than others.

The organ in the body most sensitive to decreases in blood and oxygen supply is the brain. After just a few seconds of no blood flow, the brain will cease to function optimally, resulting in loss of consciousness or other signs of neurologic compromise. After just 4 minutes of hypoperfusion, brain cells are irreversibly damaged.

In contrast, skeletal muscle can survive several hours without adequate perfusion and suffer no permanent consequences. However, this ability to withstand hypoperfusion does not translate into optimal functioning. When muscles are without adequate oxygen and other nutrients, they do not function optimally. Pain and inability to move the muscle group are common findings in patients with inadequate perfusion to a muscle group.

Causes of Hypoperfusion

If we think about the makeup of the circulatory system, several things that can lead to poor perfusion in the human body can be identified. The three basic components of the circulatory system that can affect

Industrial Accident

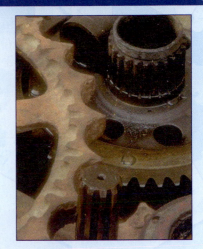

Jon was just completing his equipment check when his pager went off. "Medical emergency, building 12, man caught in machine, EMS has been notified, time 13:44."

Jon had just completed his first emergency medical technician (EMT) course. The EMT course had been a part of his job training as plant security officer at the Greenwood Industrial Park. He was eager to show everybody what he had learned, so he grabbed his kit, jumped into the company pickup, and sped off.

Upon arrival, Jon was met by the plant supervisor, Paul, who led him to the patient. Jon found a young man seated on the floor next to a machine in which his arm seemed to be entangled. His coworkers were in the process of dismantling the machine in order to free his arm.

There was significant tissue damage to the man's upper arm. Then Jon noticed the rather large pool of blood on the floor next to the machine. Looking around, Jon also noted additional blood inside the machine.

The man cried out in pain as a piece of machinery shifted. Then he looked up to Jon and yelled, "My arm's caught!"

- Is this patient at risk of developing any life–threatening conditions?
- What signs and symptoms would this patient predictably develop?
- What treatment and transportation decisions are indicated?

perfusion are the fluid, the container, and the pump. This simple description of cardiovascular anatomy and physiology is useful when identifying the causes of shock.

Basic differentiation of the causes of shock is necessary to the EMT-B because certain interventions are indicated only in particular conditions. These interventions are discussed in more detail later in the chapter. The EMT should attempt to identify the cause, although the initial treatment and transport priorities are similar for all types of shock.

The Fluid

The fluid of the cardiovascular system is blood. As discussed in Chapter 5, the blood is made up of several components. The red blood cells carry oxygen; the white blood cells fight infection; the platelets help blood to clot; and the plasma carries all of these cellular components as well as other important clotting factors, immunologic components, and other substances.

If there is not enough fluid (blood) to fill the container (the blood vessels), hypoperfusion will occur. Hypoperfusion may occur also if the blood does not contain enough oxygen-carrying red blood cells. Hypovolemic and hemorrhagic shock are examples of shock resulting from a fluid problem.

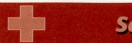
Safety Tip

Personal protective equipment, such as gloves, should always be worn when assessing a patient for bleeding. Gowns and eye protection may also be necessary.

Hypovolemic Shock

When body fluids are lost and not adequately replenished, we say that the total body fluid volume is low. A term used to describe this condition of low fluid volume is **hypovolemia**.

A state of hypoperfusion that results from hypovolemia is referred to as **hypovolemic shock**. There are several causes of low fluid volume. Perhaps the most easily recognized cause is the actual loss of blood, as was the situation described in the case study on page 209.

When shock results from an actual loss of blood, it can be called specifically **hemorrhagic shock**. Other means of losing total body volume are by other fluid losses such as excessive vomiting, diarrhea, sweating, or urinating.

Treatment will be geared toward halting the fluid loss, helping the body to compensate, and replacing lost fluids. These are discussed in more detail later in this chapter.

The Container

Blood vessels have the ability to significantly alter their diameter by contraction or relaxation of smooth muscles within their walls. This ability to alter the flow of blood to a particular area by changing the size of the vessels supplying it is useful in many circumstances.

For example, if an injury is sustained to the radial artery in the wrist, the artery proximal to that can constrict to decrease the blood flow to that injured section of blood vessel, thereby limiting the amount of blood lost. Figure 9-1 illustrates this concept.

The body can cause generalized constriction of blood vessels in order to decrease the total capacity of the entire vascular system if needed. There are many uses for this complex management of vessel size by the body.

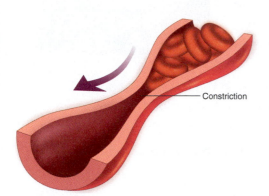
Constriction

FIGURE 9-1 Localized arterial constriction can limit blood flow to a particular area if needed.

Pneumonia

Mrs. Gray was diagnosed with "pneumonia" after she was seen for a persistent cough. Her doctor prescribed a 10-day course of antibiotics and strict bed rest.

On the third day after her diagnosis was made, Mrs. Gray became increasingly lethargic. Her granddaughter, who was concerned about her change in condition, called the doctor's office.

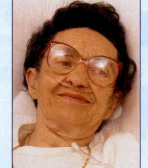

She told the nurse that her grandmother was periodically running high fevers and was not eating well. She also related that her grandmother's pulse, at her wrist, was rapid and weak.

This morning, she told the nurse, her grandmother was very difficult to arouse and then would not even take a sip of water. The nurse advised her to call an ambulance.

When the ambulance arrived, the granddaughter met the EMTs at the door. She told them, "My grandmother has pneumonia."

- Why is this patient exhibiting the signs and symptoms of shock?
- What are other possible causes of hypoperfusion, and what is the pathophysiology involved?

This ability to change the size of individual blood vessels and therefore the total capacity of the system can also be harmful in some circumstances, such as anaphylactic, septic, or neurogenic shock.

Anaphylactic Shock

Anaphylaxis is a condition brought on by exposure to something that the patient is extremely allergic to. Once exposed, the body reacts by releasing several substances into the bloodstream that cause a number of things to happen.

Most commonly, blood vessels that are close to the skin will dilate (become wider) in small areas, resulting in a pink or red color to areas of skin as the red blood comes closer to the surface.

In addition, release of certain chemical factors from white blood cells causes leaking of plasma from these blood vessels. This leakage results in swelling, or edema, in the area involved. The area of edema may be localized to patches of skin, as seen in hives (also called *urticaria*), or it may be more extensive. Further discussion regarding types of allergic reactions is found in Chapter 35. Extensive edema from a severe allergic reaction may cause narrowing of the airway and must be recognized rapidly or airway compromise will occur. Figure 9-2 depicts a patient with hives and Figure 9-3 depicts a patient with severe edema.

Similarly, if the dilation of the blood vessels is not strictly localized, as seen in hives, the capacity of the vascular system can be increased. Unfortunately, the volume of blood in the system is not increased proportionately, and, as a result, the pressure in the system will be lower.

A simple way to think about this concept is to imagine a set of pipes that represent the blood vessels. If there is a certain amount of liquid in the pipe system, and the pipes are replaced by pipes with a much wider diameter without increasing the amount of the liquid, there will be less volume within the pipes. This concept is illustrated in Figure 9-4.

In terms of an anaphylactic reaction, widening of the vessel diameters translates into a dropping blood pressure, unless compensatory measures are effective.

The patient with **anaphylactic shock** will have urticaria (hives), airway swelling (evidenced by wheezing or stridor), and hypotension (low blood pressure) as a result of a severe allergic reaction. There is usually a history of a suspicious exposure, such as a bee sting.

The definitive treatment is to stop the reaction and reverse the harmful effects. Epinephrine is a medication that can halt many of the bad effects of a severe allergic reaction, but additional medications are needed to halt the progression of the anaphylactic shock.

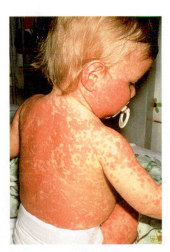

FIGURE 9-2 This patient has an allergic reaction as evidenced by generalized hives. (Courtesy of Robert A. Silverman, MD, Clinical Associate Professor, Department of Pediatrics, Georgetown University, Georgetown, MD.)

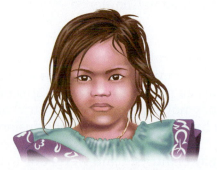 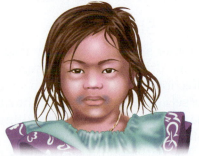

FIGURE 9-3 An anaphylactic reaction can range from simple hives to severe, life-threatening airway edema and shock.

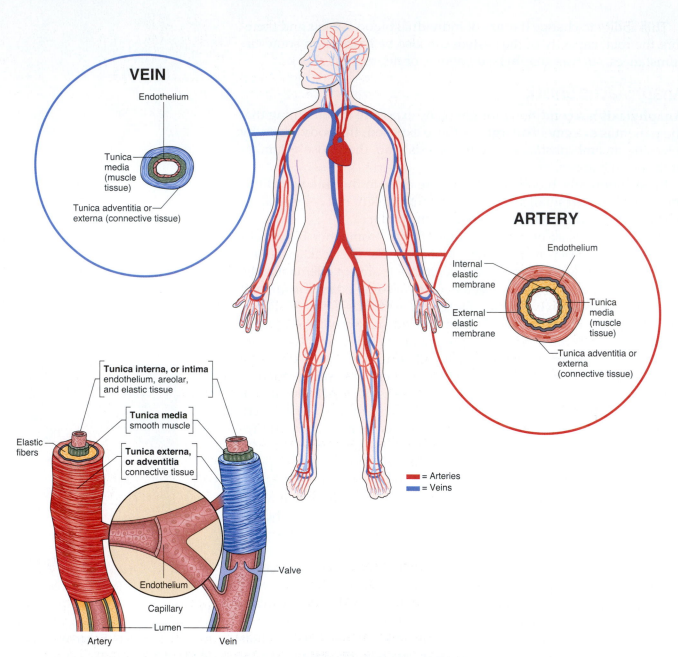

FIGURE 9-4   Generalized dilation of the blood vessels will cause a decrease in blood pressure as the container becomes too big for the amount of fluid in it.

Epinephrine is often prescribed to people who have severe allergic reactions resulting in anaphylactic shock. The use of this medication by the EMT-B in anaphylaxis is discussed in Chapter 35.

Septic Shock

Another situation that may lead to generalized blood vessel dilation with a drop in blood pressure and diminished perfusion is a severe infection. Certain types of bacteria can produce toxins that affect the vessels in such a way that they may not appropriately constrict and may become leaky. The resulting hypotension and hypoperfusion is referred to as **septic shock**.

The patient with septic shock may be flushed and warm due to the generally dilated blood vessels and the proximity of the blood to the skin. More often, however, as the condition progresses and volume losses and other chemical factors associated with the infection become more significant, the presentation varies from this description.

The patient with septic shock may have a history that suggests some sort of infection. Definitive treatment lies in the hospital, where a clear diagnosis can be made and antibiotic treatment can be started.

Neurogenic Shock

One final cause for an inappropriate increase in total vessel capacity is the loss of control of the smooth muscles in the vessel walls. This may occur as a result of a spinal cord injury because the nerves that control the constriction of the vessels come from the spinal cord.

If the nerve connections from the spinal cord to the vessels are interrupted, the vessels no longer have the ability to constrict when appropriate. All of the vessels supplied by the injured nerves will dilate.

This dilation results in a flushed appearance caused by the proximity of the blood to the skin surface as blood is allowed to pool freely in the capillary beds. Despite the appearance of adequate perfusion to the skin, other organ systems may not be receiving adequate perfusion owing to low system pressures.

Hypoperfusion resulting from spinal cord injury and disruption of the nerve control to the blood vessels is called **neurogenic shock**. This condition has also been termed "spinal shock."

The Pump

The final main cause of hypoperfusion is related to inadequate pumping action provided by the heart. If the pump does not have enough power to generate adequate forward flow, the amount of blood pumped (stroke volume) will be smaller, and the smaller volume will result in a lower cardiac output.

Cardiogenic Shock

If the heart muscle is damaged, as during a heart attack, it does not pump at its full capacity. After a heart attack, if sufficient muscle damage was sustained, the inefficient pumping action of the heart can lead to inadequate perfusion and shock.

Shock that results from inadequate cardiac pumping action is called **cardiogenic shock**. This condition is treated by attempting to improve oxygenation and perfusion while addressing the underlying cardiac problem. The patient suffering from cardiogenic shock benefits from timely care and transport to a hospital.

PHYSIOLOGIC RESPONSE TO SHOCK

The human body is quite smart. When faced with hypoperfusion, the body takes compensatory actions to attempt to prevent organ failure and death. These actions can often sustain the body until the source of the shock can be addressed by medical providers.

Compensated Shock

When the body recognizes hypoperfusion, it responds in several ways. Some responses are immediately evident to the examining EMT.

Recall that cardiac output is dependent upon both the stroke volume and the heart rate. If perfusion is decreased for any reason, increasing either the volume of blood pumped with each stroke or the heart rate will serve to increase the available blood supply to the body.

Improving the oxygenation of the blood by increased respiratory rate is also a compensatory mechanism. An additional mechanism used in compensation for hypoperfusion is to adjust the blood flow to only the areas that absolutely need it at that time. This adjustment is made by constricting arteriolar circulation at particular places.

The body will preferentially sacrifice the perfusion of particular organs to maintain the blood supply to others. This concept is illustrated in Figure 9-5. The patient who exhibits these signs of compensation for hypoperfusion is said to be in **compensated shock**.

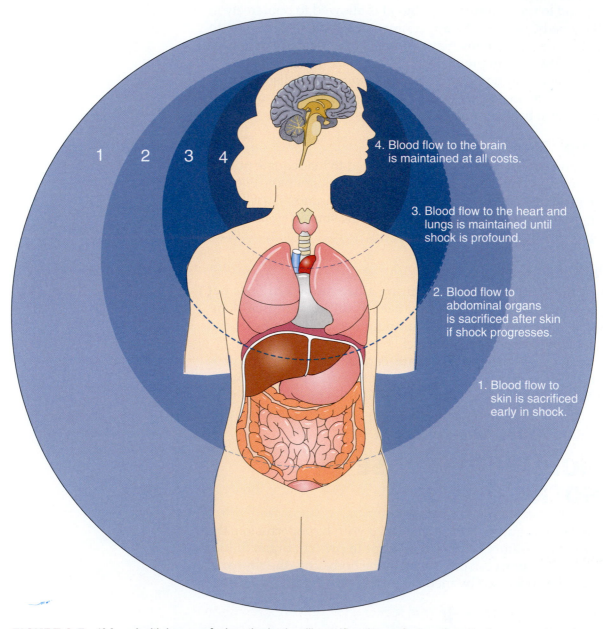

1   2   3   4

4. Blood flow to the brain is maintained at all costs.

3. Blood flow to the heart and lungs is maintained until shock is profound.

2. Blood flow to abdominal organs is sacrificed after skin if shock progresses.

1. Blood flow to skin is sacrificed early in shock.

FIGURE 9-5 If faced with hypoperfusion, the body will sacrifice the perfusion of particular organs to maintain the blood supply to others.

Pecking Order

We can think about the order in which the body will preferentially sacrifice perfusion as a sort of pecking order. The tissues that most easily survive without adequate oxygenation for the longest period of time, and that are the most expendable (the least vital to maintain life), are the first to be cut off.

The skin, soft tissues (e.g., muscles), and bones can function for several hours without oxygen, using anaerobic metabolism. After several hours, damage to tissue becomes evident. When blood supply to the skin is reduced, the light-skinned patient will be pale and cool to the touch, as the warm, red blood is drawn farther from the skin's surface. The more peripheral pulses (pedal and radial) will become weaker as further vascular constriction occurs.

If the hypoperfused state persists, the blood supply to the abdominal organs is then decreased so that the remaining blood can be sent to the more vital organs. This change may be evidenced by a feeling of nausea as the stomach loses blood supply. The kidneys also will cease to function optimally, and urine output will greatly diminish (evident if the patient has an indwelling catheter, sometimes seen in nursing-home or hospitalized patients). The abdominal organs can tolerate less than 1 hour of decreased blood supply before showing evidence of permanent tissue damage.

If hypoperfusion persists and further shunting of blood supply is needed, some decrease in brain perfusion will occur. This is evidenced by confusion and agitation because the brain does not function well under conditions of poor perfusion. Brain tissue does not tolerate more than 4 minutes of complete lack of blood supply before suffering permanent damage.

In addition to the brain, the organs in the body least tolerant of hypoperfusion are the heart and lungs. The body will attempt in every way to maintain adequate blood and oxygen supply to these organs. If the heart and lungs suffer hypoperfusion, they malfunction in a matter of minutes. When they do, blood pressure falls and decompensation is evident.

Signs and Symptoms

Knowing how the body compensates for hypoperfusion, the EMT can recognize the extent of a patient's illness by a careful examination. Except in certain cases, such as neurogenic shock, the patient in compensated shock will be pale, cool, and clammy and will have weakening peripheral pulses. Heart rate will be elevated, as will respiratory rate.

The patient in compensated shock may complain of nausea or may even vomit. An altered mental status in the shock patient is an ominous sign because it indicates poor brain perfusion.

Table 9-1 lists the signs and symptoms of compensated shock with the reason for their presence.

Decompensated Shock

Once systolic blood pressure drops to less than 90 mm Hg, the condition is termed **decompensated shock**. This low blood pressure (hypotension) can be thought of as the point at which the body is no

Street Smart

Although the vital signs described here are seen in most patients with compensated shock, there are notable exceptions. The patient with neurogenic shock has an interruption in the nerve relays between the spinal cord and the brain. This can result in an inability to generate the classic tachycardia that the EMT may expect to see in shock. With this "relative bradycardia" in the presence of other indicators of shock, the EMT should suspect a spinal cord injury and neurogenic shock.

Geriatric Considerations

Many older people take multiple medications for different chronic medical problems. Some medications can impede a patient's ability to increase the heart rate, even when an increase is needed, as in shock. Most of these medications are those that are prescribed for control of high blood pressure and other cardiovascular problems.

In addition, the body's ability to compensate for shock may become less effective as it ages. Classic vital signs and physical findings that the EMT can use as warning signs of a serious illness may not be present early on.

Knowing the effects of aging, the EMT must continue to assess for other signs of shock in the elderly patient because the vital signs may not be particularly revealing.

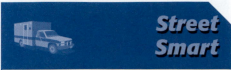

Street Smart

Pale skin color may be difficult to appreciate in a dark-skinned person. The EMT should look at the patient's nail beds or the mucous membranes of the mouth or the eyes. These areas may be pale, indicating possible shock.

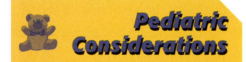

Pediatric Considerations

One physical finding that is particularly useful in children is the perfusion of the skin. This can be measured by using **capillary refill time**. This measurement refers to the time it takes to observe capillary filling (evidenced by return to normal color) at the skin after blanching (loss of color in an area of skin pressed with a finger).

As perfusion decreases to the skin, capillary refill time will become prolonged. Normal capillary refill time is less than 2 seconds. The longer the time necessary for complete refill to occur, the poorer the perfusion to the area.

This sign is a reliable measure of the overall perfusion status in children. For multiple reasons, capillary refill measurement may not always be accurate in adults. The actual technique used to measure capillary refill time is reviewed in Chapter 10.

TABLE 9-1

Signs and Symptoms of Compensated Shock

Sign or Symptom	Reason
Tachycardia	To maintain cardiac output
Tachypnea	To increase oxygenation
Cool, pale skin	Due to shunting of blood to core of body, away from skin
Nausea	Due to shunting of blood to core of body, away from stomach and other abdominal organs
Thirst	Due to the body's recognition of need for more fluid
Confusion, agitation	Due to poor perfusion of brain

longer able to compensate for the event. When hypotension is noted, the patient is considered to be in decompensated shock and must be aggressively treated if survival is going to be possible.

Decompensated shock will lead to multiple organ failure and death of the patient unless the source of the problem is quickly corrected and the hypoperfused state reversed.

Irreversible Shock

If multiple body organs are without oxygen for enough time to cause permanent damage, the patient is unlikely to have a good outcome. Once a patient has been in decompensated shock for a period of time and multiple organs have failed, the patient is said to be in **irreversible shock** and will almost certainly not survive.

ASSESSMENT

In assessing a patient, the EMT must be careful to look for the signs of compensated shock. If you don't look for it, you won't find it! It is necessary to begin to treat the patient in shock *before* she decompensates and becomes hypotensive.

The "Look Test"

Before examining any patient, the EMT must ensure his own safety. The safety of the environment must be assessed, and proper personal protective equipment must be used.

As the EMT approaches the patient, he should form a quick general impression. On the first look, does the patient appear to be very sick or not? This impression is often based on experience and is referred to as the "look test." The EMT will base his immediate priorities in patient care and scene management on this initial impression of the patient.

Mental Status

The patient's ability to communicate and interact with the rescuers is a good indication of brain perfusion. The initial assessment of the patient's level of consciousness is an important piece of information. It is useful to reassess the patient's mental status throughout the incident as a measure of brain functioning.

ABCs

The ABCs of assessment are airway, breathing, and circulation. To have adequate oxygenation of the blood, the patient must have an open airway and be ventilating effectively. It is for this reason that airway and breathing management is the primary priority for medical providers at any level.

Once assured that the airway is patent and ventilations are adequate, the EMT should turn his attention to the circulation. He should look for signs of hypoperfusion, such as cool and clammy skin, tachycardia, tachypnea, and weak peripheral pulses. The details of this initial assessment are reviewed in Chapter 13.

Vital Signs

The EMT should obtain an initial heart rate, respiratory rate, blood pressure, and pulse oximetry as well as note the skin temperature, condition, and color. It is important to be complete in this assessment and to continue to reassess the patient for any change during the course of treatment and transport. These procedures are detailed in Chapter 10.

Orthostatic Vital Signs

If a patient's blood volume is low and she stands up suddenly, blood will pool in the legs and the blood pressure will fall. The result is that the brain is temporarily deprived of oxygen. The patient may complain of feeling dizzy or may even pass out. This change in blood pressure associated with a change in position, or posture, is called **postural hypotension**.

The EMT can test for postural hypotension by checking the patient's vital signs in the supine position, having the patient stand up, and rechecking the vital signs in the standing position. Dizziness, a rise in heart rate of more than 20 beats per minute, and a fall in blood pressure of more than 20 mm Hg is referred to as a positive **tilt test**. This may be indicative of volume loss. This process of measuring the vital signs in two different positions is called taking **orthostatic vital signs**. Skill 9-1 describes this process.

When taking orthostatic vital signs, the EMT should be prepared for the patient to become dizzy or even lose consciousness. If this should happen, lay the patient on the stretcher and assume that the tilt test is positive.

Orthostatic vital signs are useful for determining borderline shock patients. This procedure is not used on any patient with suspected spinal injury or whose initial vital signs indicate shock.

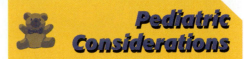

Pediatric Considerations

Children compensate very well for hypoperfusion. They tend to not show external signs of shock until it is very advanced. Once a child becomes hypotensive, the situation is very serious and usually rapidly progresses to an irreversible state. It is imperative that the EMT recognize the signs of compensated shock in the pediatric patient and take appropriate action to prevent decompensation.

SKILL 9-1 *Taking Orthostatic Vital Signs*

PURPOSE: To obtain a baseline set of vital signs lying and standing for assessment and comparison.

STANDARD PRECAUTIONS:

☑ Stethoscope
☑ Blood pressure cuff
☑ Watch with second hand
☑ Gloves

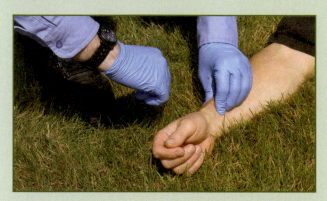

1 Obtain a full set of vital signs from the lying patient.

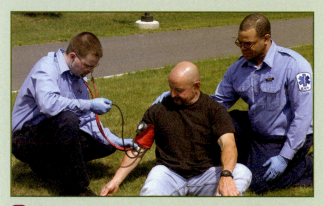 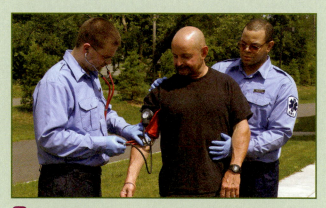

2 Assist the patient to a sitting position with an assistant behind the patient for support. Reassess vital signs.

3 Assist the patient to a standing position with an assistant behind the patient for support. Reassess vital signs.

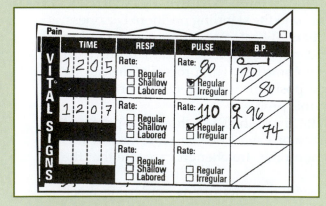

	TIME	RESP	PULSE	B.P.
VITAL SIGNS	1205	Rate: ☐ Regular ☐ Shallow ☐ Labored	Rate: 80 ☑ Regular ☐ Irregular	120 / 80
	1207	Rate: ☐ Regular ☐ Shallow ☐ Labored	Rate: 110 ☑ Regular ☐ Irregular	96 / 74
		Rate: ☐ Regular ☐ Shallow ☐ Labored	Rate: ☐ Regular ☐ Irregular	

Pain

4 Compare vital signs lying, sitting, and standing.

MANAGEMENT OF HYPOPERFUSION

The treatment of shock is geared toward restoring adequate oxygenation, ventilation, and circulation. Specific interventions such as epinephrine may be useful in selected situations such as anaphylactic shock. However, the majority of patients with signs of hypoperfusion have conditions that are not definitively treated by BLS (basic life support) techniques. The EMT must maximize the perfusion while rapidly transporting the patient to a hospital, where definitive treatment may be available.

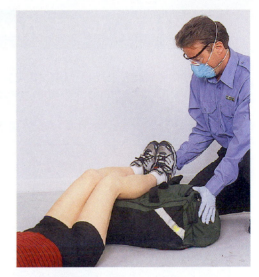

FIGURE 9-6 Elevation of the lower half of the body serves to allow increased blood flow to the torso and vital organs.

Oxygen

After securing the airway and assisting with ventilations as needed, the EMT should apply supplemental oxygen. The patient in shock is suffering from a lack of sufficient oxygen delivery to the tissues. Regardless of the etiology, increasing the oxygen content of the blood is useful to the tissues.

If you think about it, if the amount of oxygen in the blood is increased, then there is more of a chance that some of that oxygen will get to the affected tissues and organs. It is always appropriate to administer 100% oxygen to the patient in any stage of shock.

Control Bleeding

If the patient is suffering from hemorrhagic shock, the EMT should locate the source of the bleeding and, if external, should control it in whatever way possible. Controlling bleeding will hopefully halt any further progression of the shock state. Techniques used in bleeding control are dealt with in Chapters 13 and 24.

Modified Trendelenburg

The EMT has two ways to support the blood pressure of the patient in shock. The first and easiest means of blood pressure support in the shock patient is to elevate the patient's legs. The effects of gravity in this position serve to increase the blood volume in the thorax and abdomen, while decreasing that in the lower extremities.

This positioning is called the modified Trendelenburg position and can be easily accomplished by placing blankets or an equipment bag under the patient's legs while keeping the patient's torso supine. Review Chapter 9 for proper positioning of patients.

The patient with suspected fractures of lower extremities or back injury cannot be placed in this position for fear of displacing any possible fractures. This concept is demonstrated in Figure 9-6.

MAST/PASG

The **pneumatic anti-shock garment (PASG)**, also called **military anti-shock trousers (MAST)**, is a device that also may serve to support blood pressure in certain circumstances. A balloonlike set of pants is applied to the patient's lower body and then inflated. Skill 9-2 describes the process. MAST/PASG improves the blood supply to the

SKILL 9-2 *Application of MAST/PASG*

PURPOSE: To use MAST/PASG to improve perfusion to vital organs in a patient suffering from decompensated shock due to abdominal or pelvic bleeding.

STANDARD PRECAUTIONS:

☑ MAST/PASG with foot pump attachment
☑ Stethoscope
☑ Blood pressure cuff
☑ Patient Care Report and pen
☑ Gloves

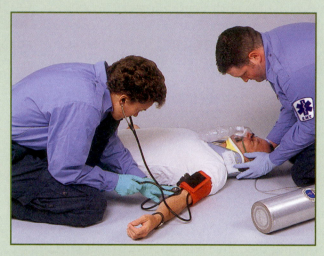

1 Perform initial assessments and vital signs. Identify indications for MAST/PASG application: injured patient with severe hypotension (systolic blood pressure less than 50 mm Hg) or hypotension (systolic blood pressure less than 90 mm Hg) with associated pelvic instability and with other signs of shock (more than two of the following: altered mental status, persistent tachycardia, cool and clammy skin, diaphoresis [profuse perspiration], thirst, or nausea).

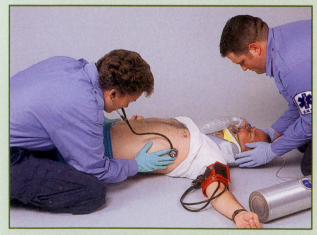

2 Ensure lack of absolute contraindications (pulmonary edema, penetrating chest injury) and relative contraindications (pregnancy, impaled object, evisceration).

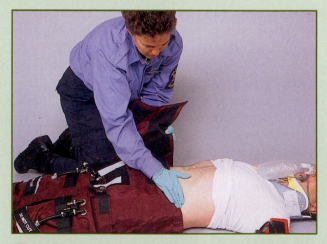

3 Pull MAST/PASG up to the level of the lower ribs and secure Velcro fasteners. Adjust length of legs as needed.

(continues)

SKILL 9-2 *(continued)*

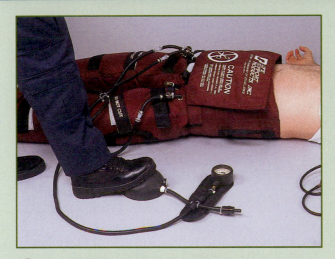

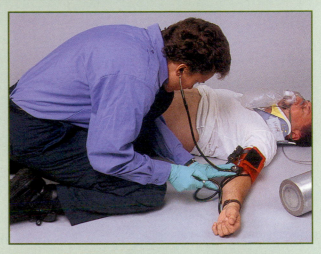

4 Attach air hoses and set to open position. Use foot pump to inflate trousers until gauge reaches 106 mm Hg or pop-off valve releases. All valves should be opened and in-line.

5 Set air pump hoses to closed position. Reassess patient's ABCs and vital signs.

upper body and vital organs. The device is separated into three individual sections (abdomen, right leg, left leg) that may be inflated individually or in order to support blood pressure.

Indications

According to the medical literature, MAST/PASG has been shown to be useful for patients who have severe hypotension (systolic blood pressure less than 50 mm Hg) or who are hypotensive (systolic blood pressure less than 90 mm Hg) because of severe pelvic injuries. In these patients, the pressure exerted by the inflated pants may serve to limit bleeding within the pelvis while improving the blood supply to the upper body and the vital organs.

Contraindications

MAST/PASG can create complications. It creates an increased pressure within the thorax and may potentially worsen thoracic injuries, if present.

Use of MAST/PASG is not advised, or is absolutely contraindicated, when the patient has a penetrating thoracic injury or has pulmonary edema. The increased thoracic pressure may worsen these conditions.

Relative Contraindications

Relative contraindications to the use of MAST/PASG include pregnancy, penetrating object, and evisceration. The abdominal section of MAST/PASG is not inflated on an obviously pregnant woman to avoid fetal injury.

Street Smart

If MAST/PASG is used in patients with lower extremity fractures, there is an increased rate of complications with the fractures due to the increased pressures. For this reason, MAST/PASG use is discouraged in this situation.

Sometimes, a patient with multiple lower extremity fractures is markedly hypotensive and would benefit from the use of MAST/PASG. In that case, the EMT would treat the more life-threatening problem first—that is, the hypotension.

Street Smart

Because the application of MAST/PASG does take a minute or two and may be difficult once a patient is already immobilized and secured, it is useful to anticipate the need for MAST/PASG and to apply the device with the initial patient preparation. MAST/PASG is then in place and ready for inflation if the need arises. It never hurts to be prepared and to think ahead!

The abdominal section should also not be inflated if there is a penetrating injury to the abdomen in which bowel is showing through. The medical term for this condition is **evisceration**.

The EMT should never remove a penetrating foreign body from a patient's body, and so will not be able to apply MAST/PASG over a body part that has a penetrating foreign body in it.

MAST/PASG Application

When considering application of MAST/PASG, the EMT must perform an initial assessment (including listening to lung sounds) and obtain an initial set of vital signs. If there are indications for use of MAST/PASG and there are no contraindications, the patient must then be fully exposed. A brief exam of the abdomen and lower extremities before covering them with MAST/PASG is useful because once the trousers have been applied, these areas will be covered and inaccessible to the examiner.

There are several techniques commonly used when applying the trousers; any one may be utilized. The goal is to apply the device quickly with minimal movement of the patient.

Figures 9-7 and 9-8 demonstrate two methods of MAST/PASG application for the supine patient. The first is the *trouser method*. As in

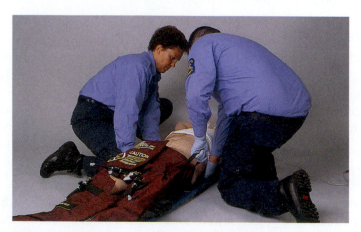

FIGURE 9-7 The *trouser method* for MAST/PASG application.

putting on a pair of pants, one leg is put on, then the other. Finally, the entire garment is pulled up to the bottom of the lower ribs.

Alternatively, the garment may be situated on a backboard and the patient placed on top of MAST/PASG during immobilization. This method, the *wrapper method*, is useful when legs may have fractures or the pelvis is unstable.

Regardless of the method of application, the trousers should be snugly fit to the patient using the Velcro attachments. Once the trousers have been fully applied, the air pump should be attached and the hoses opened for filling.

The EMT then must use the foot pump to inflate MAST/PASG. Inflation takes several minutes and may be done in the ambulance during transport. The MAST/PASG device is completely inflated when a pressure gauge attached to the device reads 106 mm Hg or the pop-off valve releases.

Once inflation is complete, the hoses should be turned so that air cannot escape. The patient must then be reassessed for the ABCs and vital signs. As should any procedure, MAST/PASG application should be practiced until the provider is comfortable with the process.

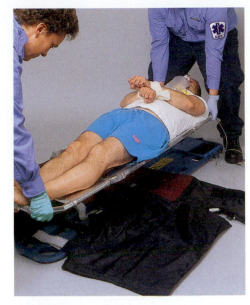

FIGURE 9-8 The *wrapper method* for MAST/PASG application.

MAST/PASG Removal

MAST/PASG should never be deflated by the EMT or in the field. There is a specific procedure followed in deflation that involves adequate intravenous access and fluids to maintain blood pressure.

Physicians in emergency departments should be familiar with the procedure involving slow deflation of the device with frequent blood pressure monitoring, not allowing the blood pressure to fall more than 5 mm Hg at a time. This is often a gradual process and should not be attempted outside of the hospital unless specifically directed by a physician.

Reduce Heat Loss

An injured patient suffering from shock who is allowed to lose body heat is likely to suffer complications. For this reason, the EMT must make every effort to prevent excessive heat loss during the evaluation and treatment of the critically ill or injured patient.

Heat loss may be avoided by preventing prolonged exposure of the patient. Once an assessment has been accomplished, the patient should be covered with blankets (Figure 9-9). Care should be taken to remove the patient from cold, wet surfaces and to remove wet clothing from the patient.

Transport

After assessing a hypoperfused patient and beginning appropriate BLS treatment, the EMT must decide what mode of transportation is most appropriate. The decision-making process that goes into determining whether a patient should be transported by ground ambulance or by helicopter is discussed in a later chapter.

During transport, it is imperative that the EMT reassess the patient at frequent intervals. The patient with signs of hypoperfusion should be constantly observed, with vital signs monitored at least every

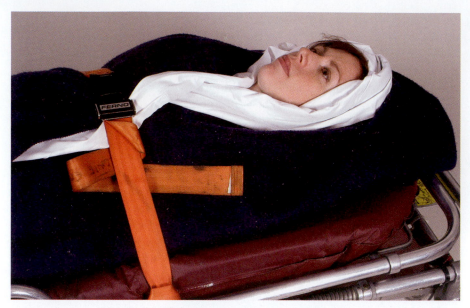

FIGURE 9-9   It is important to keep the injured patient warm.

5 minutes. Changes in mental status or vital signs should be recorded carefully and reported to the destination facility.

ALS Intercept

Some patients will need therapies that are beyond the scope of practice for the EMT. Some of these therapies, such as medication administration and IV therapy, can be initiated by properly trained advanced life support (ALS) personnel.

The hypoperfused patient requires ALS modalities. If the EMT is practicing in a system that has access to ALS personnel, he must decide whether to request assistance at the scene or to go directly to a hospital for such treatment. The need for ALS interventions is addressed throughout this text as each condition is discussed.

Destination Issues

It is important for the EMT to be aware of the general capabilities of the surrounding medical facilities in order to decide which hospital the patient should be transported to. In general, the patient in shock should go to the closest hospital. However, trauma patients often are diverted to a specialized trauma center. Local protocols often govern these issues.

CONCLUSION

Shock is a state of hypoperfusion in which the body tissues are not receiving an adequate supply of oxygenated blood. The patient in shock will show classic signs and symptoms that, if unrecognized and untreated, will lead to death.

The EMT should be knowledgeable about the different etiologies of shock and must be able to recognize and identify signs of compensated and decompensated shock.

Regardless of the cause of the hypoperfused state, the initial treatment consists of maintenance of an adequate airway and ventilations, with oxygen administration and circulatory support if necessary. Recognition of hypoperfusion by the EMT is critical in the management of the ill or injured patient.

TEST YOUR KNOWLEDGE

1. Define *shock* in your own words.
2. Identify five specific causes of shock.
3. List the signs and symptoms of compensated shock.
4. What is the "pecking order" of shock?
5. Define *decompensated shock*.
6. Describe the appropriate initial evaluation of the patient in shock.
7. List appropriate steps in management of the patient with signs and symptoms of shock.
8. Describe the indications for MAST/PASG use.
9. List the absolute and relative contraindications for MAST/PASG use.

INTERNET RESOURCES

- Search for research being done in EMS and the medical field related to emergency treatments of shock and hypoperfusion. What did you find? Share the results with your colleagues.
- Search for information on each of the types of shock discussed in this chapter (hypovolemic, hemorrhagic, anaphylactic, septic, neurogenic, and cardiogenic). Create review cards for each of the types of shock; include signs and symptoms, assessment, and management guidelines. Use these cards for review and study.

FURTHER STUDY

Cayten, C. G., Berendt, B. M., Byrne, D. W., et al. (1993). A study of pneumatic anti-shock garments in severely hypotensive trauma patients. *Journal of Trauma, 34,* 728–35.

Domeier, R. M., et al. (1997). Use of the pneumatic anti-shock garment (PASG). National Association of EMS Physicians. *Prehospital Emergency Care, 1*(1), 32–35.

Emergency Cardiac Care Committee and Subcommittee, American Heart Association. (1992). Guidelines for cardiopulmonary resuscitation and emergency cardiac care. I: Introduction. *Journal of the American Medical Association, 268,* 2171–83.

Mattox, K. L., Bickell, W., Pepe, P. E., et al. (1989). Prospective MAST study in 911 patients. *Journal of Trauma, 29,* 1104–12.

O'Connor, R. E., & Domeier, R. M. (1997). An evaluation of the pneumatic anti-shock garment (PASG) in various clinical settings. *Prehospital Emergency Care, 1*(1), 36–44.

CHAPTER 10

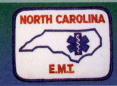

Baseline Vital Signs and SAMPLE History

KEY TERMS

accessory muscle use
anisocoria
antecubital fossa
baseline vital signs
capillary refill time
diastolic
exhalation
grunting
gurgling
inspiration
jaundice
pallor
PERRL
pulse oximeter
pupil
SAMPLE
sign
snoring
sphygmomanometer
stridor
symptom
systolic
wheezing

OBJECTIVES

Upon completion of this chapter, the reader should be able to:

1. Identify the vital signs.
2. Describe how to assess the quality and quantity of respiration.
3. Recognize a normal respiratory rate and quality.
4. Describe how to assess the quality and quantity of the pulse.
5. Recognize a normal pulse rate and quality.
6. Describe the methods to assess blood pressure.
7. Define *systolic pressure*.
8. Define *diastolic pressure*.
9. Describe the methods to assess the pupils.
10. Identify normal and abnormal pupil size, shape, and reaction.
11. Describe the methods to assess the skin color, temperature, and condition.
12. Describe how to assess capillary refill in infants and children.
13. Identify normal and abnormal skin colors, temperatures, and conditions.
14. Identify normal and abnormal capillary refill in infants and children.
15. Discuss the use of pulse oximetry.
16. Describe how to measure oxygen saturation using a pulse oximeter.
17. Identify the components of the SAMPLE history.
18. Differentiate between a sign and a symptom.
19. State the importance of accurately reporting and recording the baseline vital signs.

OVERVIEW

During the course of training, the emergency medical technician (EMT) will learn many skills. Those used most frequently will be obtaining vital signs and a basic history.

The vital signs such as respiratory rate, heart rate, blood pressure, skin temperature, and pulse oximetry will provide a great deal of information about the patient's physical condition and present state of health. Examination of the pupil's response to light can also provide valuable information. Monitoring these vital signs over time will also allow the EMT to identify acute changes in the patient's status.

In addition to obtaining vital signs, every patient encounter must involve some questions regarding basic medical history. The acronym SAMPLE (explained later in this chapter) is helpful to remind the EMT of the most important historical questions that should be asked of every patient.

Because every patient interaction will involve measuring and interpreting vital signs as well as taking a SAMPLE history, the EMT must be competent in these skills.

BASELINE VITAL SIGNS

After the initial assessment and management of the airway, breathing, and circulation, the EMT will take the time to quantify actual vital signs. The first measurement of vital signs is sometimes referred to as **baseline vital signs**.

These numbers serve as a baseline against which subsequent readings, or values, are compared. It is important to obtain an accurate baseline set of vital signs at the onset of care so that any changes can be recognized early and acted upon quickly.

Time should be spent during EMT training practicing measuring vital signs. This section discusses each of the vital signs in detail, review normal and abnormal values, and describe how to measure each of them appropriately.

Respiration

Many parts of an EMT's assessment of a patient will be done by observing the patient. The assessment of breathing is one of these. While the EMT approaches the patient and begins the initial assessment, several aspects of breathing should be noted.

Quantity

First, how quickly does the patient seem to be breathing? Does the patient's breathing seem very fast or particularly slow? To determine the appropriateness of the respiratory rate, the EMT must be familiar with normal respiratory rates. Table 10-1 shows normal respiratory rates for people of different ages.

To determine the exact respiratory rate, the EMT must observe the patient's breathing and count the number of breaths taken in 1 minute. Each breath consists of an **inspiration** (breathing in) and an **exhalation** (breathing out). This breathing rate is then reported as the number of breaths per minute.

Often, it is easier and more convenient to shorten the time necessary to obtain such a respiratory rate. It is acceptable to count the number of breaths taken for 30 seconds then multiply by 2 to equal the number of breaths taken in 1 minute. The EMT should avoid shortening the measurement time any more than this to avoid inaccuracy.

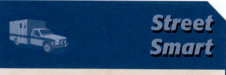

Street Smart

The EMT should practice measuring vital signs on classmates, coworkers, and family members to gain experience in the performance of these important skills.

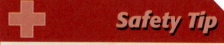

Safety Tip

The EMT must remember to don any needed personal protective equipment before any patient contact. For many situations, gloves alone will be sufficient to protect the EMT against possible exposure to body fluids. If further protection, such as masks or goggles, is necessary, these too should be donned before patient contact.

TABLE 10-1

Normal Respiratory Rates, by Age

Age	Normal Respiratory Rate (breaths/minute)
Adult	12–20
Adolescent (11–14 yr)	12–20
School-aged child (6–10 yr)	15–30
Preschool-aged child (1–5 yr)	20–30
Infant (1 mo–1 yr)	20–40
Newborn (0–1 mo)	30–50

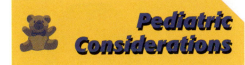

Pediatric Considerations

Nasal flaring is very commonly seen in infants and small children who are having respiratory difficulty. An EMT seeing nasal flaring in a child should be concerned. Respiratory failure is often the cause of death for infants and children, and nasal flaring is one of the first signs of respiratory difficulty. Figure 10-1 illustrates such a finding.

If the patient's breathing is irregular, then the EMT should count the respirations for a full minute to avoid reporting an erroneous respiratory rate.

Quality

In addition to counting the respiratory rate, the EMT should note the quality of the respiration. She should observe for depth, regularity, and any unusual noise or effort.

Normal breathing quality is of a moderate depth (chest rise is visible), regular (approximately one breath every 3–5 seconds for an adult), and quiet. Any unusual effort or noise, indicating that the patient may be struggling for breath, should be noted.

Labored Breathing

The EMT can describe a patient's breathing as being labored if there is any noticeable unusual effort or noise during the respiratory cycle. Patients who are having difficulty breathing for any reason may appear uncomfortable and may show classic signs of increased respiratory effort or difficulty.

The increased use of additional muscles to breathe is a sign of increased respiratory difficulty. The muscles of the chest and neck are thought of as accessory muscles of respiration and normally work together with the diaphragm to create smooth inspiration and exhalation.

When breathing becomes more difficult, these muscles work harder. Increased use of chest and neck muscles is sometimes referred to as **accessory muscle use**. Increased effort is also evidenced by nasal flaring as the patient tries to get as much air in as possible during inspiration. Nasal flaring is the wide opening of the nostrils with each breath.

The patient who is having difficulty breathing may also have abnormal noises during breathing. When air flows through a narrowed upper airway, such as in a common pediatric illness called croup or with any upper airway obstruction, a harsh sound can be heard on inspiration. This sound is called **stridor**.

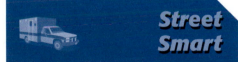

Street Smart

It is important that the EMT avoid telling the patient that she is counting the respiratory rate. The patient may become self-conscious about his breathing and alter his breathing pattern if he is aware that the EMT is counting his respiration.

It is often useful to count the respiratory rate while holding the patient's wrist on the patient's abdomen, acting as if the pulse is being counted. This method provides a distraction to the patient and allows the EMT to count a more accurate respiratory rate.

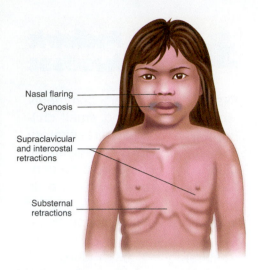

Nasal flaring

Cyanosis

Supraclavicular
and intercostal
retractions

Substernal
retractions

FIGURE 10-1 Child with respiratory distress using accessory muscles.

TABLE 10-2

Normal Pulse Rates, by Age	
Age	**Pulse Rate (beats per minute)**
Adult	60–100
Adolescent (11–14 yr)	60–105
School-aged child (6–10 yr)	70–110
Preschool-aged child (1–5 yr)	80–120
Infant (1 mo–1 yr)	90–140
Newborn (0–1 mo)	120–160

Another sound created by an upper airway obstruction, often because the tongue falls back in the throat of an unconscious patient and partially occludes it, is **snoring**. The patient who is snoring could potentially occlude his airway and therefore needs a manual airway maneuver, such as the jaw thrust, to open his airway to relieve the partial obstruction created by the tongue.

A **gurgling** sound may be heard if liquid material is in the upper airway. This sound should immediately trigger the EMT to think, "I must suction the patient's airway." If the airway is not suctioned, then the patient risks aspirating, or swallowing, the liquid into his lungs. Aspiration is a leading cause of pneumonia.

Immediately after suctioning an airway, the EMT should consider whether the patient would benefit from an oral airway, to help keep the airway open, as well.

Wheezing is a high-pitched sound that is more typical of lower airway obstruction, as seen with foreign body obstruction deeper in the chest or with the lung disease asthma. It is most commonly heard on expiration but may also be heard during inspiration. The EMT should listen for wheezing at the top of the patient's lungs, near the clavicles, or collarbones, as well as at the base of the lungs, below the scapulas, or shoulder blades, in order to describe the extent of the wheezing throughout the entire lung.

A **grunting** sound can also be heard in patients who are working very hard to breathe. This sound is indicative of extreme effort being exerted and should not be ignored. Frequently, small children and infants will continuously grunt when they are having trouble breathing. Grunting is an important physical finding that must be reported immediately.

It is standard practice to also mention any changes from a normal respiratory pattern when describing respirations during a report of vital signs. The combination of the respiratory rate, the quality of breathing, including additional breath sounds, and any patterns of breathing provides an excellent description of the patient's respiratory status. Chapter 8 provides descriptions of abnormal breathing patterns. Measurement of respiration is described in Skill 10-1.

Pulse

The pulse is also an important vital sign to measure in every patient. The rate, strength, and regularity of a patient's pulse can give the EMT information about the severity of the patient's illness or injury. Following these values over time allows the EMT to also note any change in the patient's condition or health.

A pulse can be measured at any point where an artery comes close to the skin, allowing the examiner to feel the pressure of the blood as it is pumped through the artery. The most common sites for a pulse check, in an adult, are over the radial, femoral, and carotid arteries. In infants, the brachial pulse is substituted for the others because it is usually easier to find. Figure 10-2 illustrates where these pulse points are found.

Quantity

As with respiration, to recognize the appropriateness of a particular heart rate, the EMT must be familiar with normal heart rates. Table 10-2 lists normal heart rate ranges for different age groups.

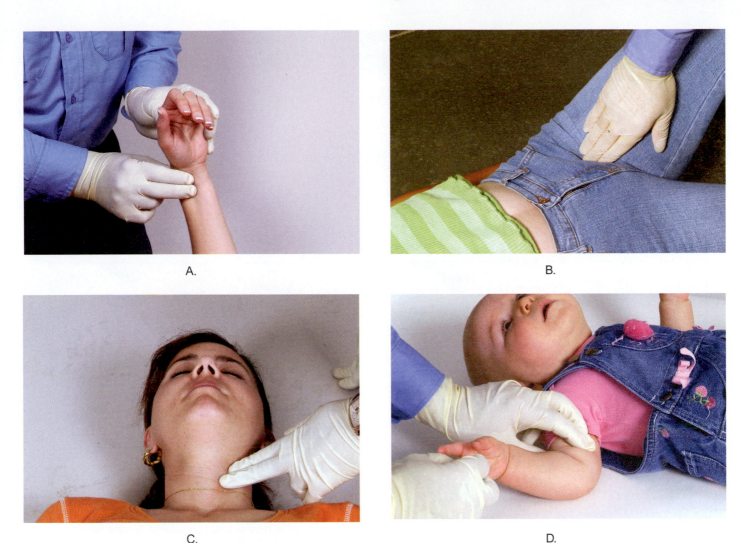

FIGURE 10-2   Pulse points: A. Radial. B. Femoral. C. Carotid. D. Brachial.

To measure the patient's pulse rate, the EMT must choose a pulse site. The most common site initially used in adults is the radial pulse at the wrist. This pulse can be found by placing the pads of two fingers on the wrist, just below the base of the thumb. Figure 10-2A demonstrates this position. Once the pulse is felt, the EMT should count the number of pulse beats felt in 30 seconds, then multiply this number by 2 to calculate the beats per minute. (See Skill 10-2.)

Quality

In addition to counting the pulse rate, the EMT should note the strength and regularity of the pulse beat. Common terms used to describe the strength of a pulse are *strong*, or *bounding*, and *weak*, or *thready*. A pulse can also be described as *regular* if the beats seem to be spaced evenly. If the beats seem to occur in no regular pattern, the pulse is described as *irregular*.

Blood Pressure

The next measurement that is important for the EMT to accurately obtain in every patient is the blood pressure. This is measured using a

SKILL 10-1 *Measurement of Respiration*

PURPOSE: To obtain a baseline respiration number for assessment and comparison.

STANDARD PRECAUTIONS:

- ☑ Watch/clock with second hand
- ☑ Patient Care Report and pen
- ☑ Gloves

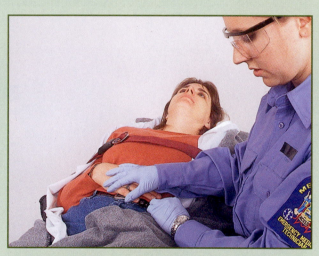

1 The EMT places her hand on top of the patient's hand, then places the patient's hand on top of the abdomen. Observe patient's chest or abdomen for rise and fall with respiration, noting any irregular patterns, noise, or effort. Note whether the respiration is shallow or labored.

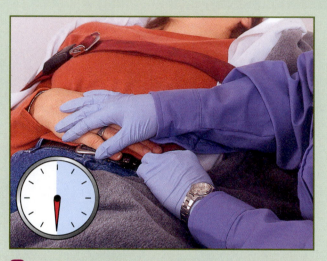

2 Count the number of complete breaths taken (one inhalation plus one exhalation counts as one breath) over a 30-second period.

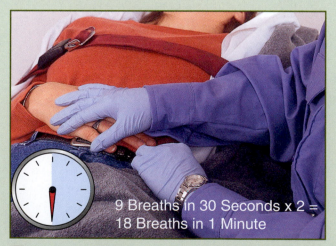

9 Breaths in 30 Seconds x 2 = 18 Breaths in 1 Minute

3 Multiply this number by 2 to obtain breaths per minute.

(continues)

SKILL 10-1 (continued)

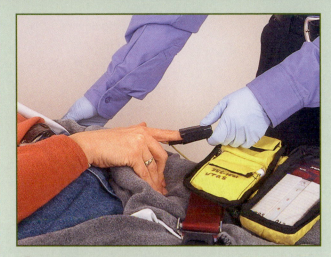

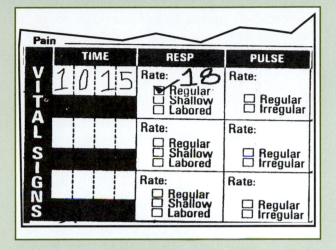

4 The EMT should consider taking a pulse oximetry reading at this time.

5 Record the respiratory rate and quality.

special tool called a **sphygmomanometer**, or blood pressure cuff, and a stethoscope.

Blood pressure is reported in two numbers. The first, or top, number is called the **systolic** pressure. *Systole* means contraction. This number refers to the pressure in the arteries during the contraction phase of the heart. This is the highest pressure created when the heart pumps blood out of the ventricles and into the circulation.

The lower number in the blood pressure is the **diastolic** pressure. *Diastole* means relaxation. The diastolic pressure refers to the pressure in the artery during the relaxation phase, immediately after a pulse. The diastolic pressure may be thought of as the resistance that the heart must pump against with each contraction. Table 10-3 shows normal blood pressure values.

The blood pressure is measured by inflating a special measurement cuff, a sphygmomanometer, around the patient's arm and measuring the pressure at both the contraction (systole) and relaxation (diastole) phases. There are two common methods of measuring the pressure: auscultation and palpation. Auscultation means listening, and palpation means feeling. Auscultation provides more accurate and more complete information than palpation and is generally preferred in most circumstances.

Cuff Application

Before measuring a patient's blood pressure, the EMT should select the proper size cuff. A properly fit blood pressure cuff should cover two-thirds of the upper arm, elbow to shoulder.

The Velcro attachments should securely close the cuff around the arm. Blood pressure cuffs come in several sizes. If an improper size is used, the numbers obtained will be inaccurate and misleading.

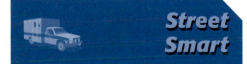

Street Smart

For the patient with an irregular pulse, a more accurate heart rate will be obtained if the pulse is counted for 1 full minute. An irregular pulse can be an indication of a potentially lethal cardiac abnormality. It is important that an EMT report if a pulse is regular or irregular and consider whether advanced life support is needed. In some cases, the patient will tell the EMT that he normally has an irregular pulse. The EMT should always remember to ask the patient whether he normally has an irregular pulse that "skips beats."

In addition, any patient who is very cold may have a slow pulse. The cold patient's pulse should be checked for 1 full minute.

SKILL 10-2 *Measurement of Radial Pulse*

PURPOSE: To obtain a baseline pulse rate for assessment and comparison.

STANDARD PRECAUTIONS:

- ☑ Watch/clock with second hand
- ☑ Patient Care Report and pen
- ☑ Gloves

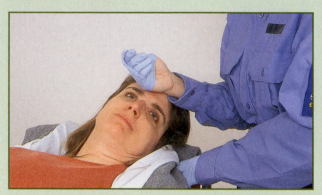

1 First, the EMT notes the condition of the skin as warm or cool, and moist or dry.

2 Next, the EMT finds the radial pulse. The radial pulse is on the anterior surface of the distal forearm, proximal to the thumb. The EMT notes the quality and regularity of the pulse as weak or strong, regular or irregular.

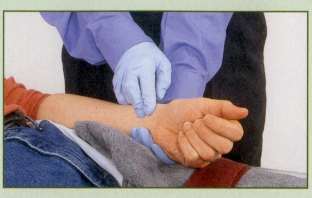

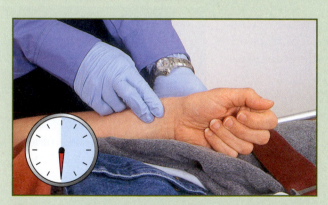

3 The EMT then counts the number of pulse beats felt over a 30-second period. (If the pulse is irregular, then the EMT counts for 1 minute.)

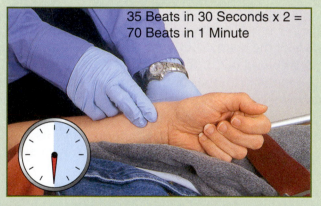

35 Beats in 30 Seconds x 2 = 70 Beats in 1 Minute

4 Multiply this number by 2 to obtain beats per minute.

	TIME	RESP	PULSE	B.P.	LEVEL OF CONSCIOUSNESS	GCS	R	PUPILS	L	SKIN
V I T A L S I G N S	1015	Rate: ☐ Regular ☐ Shallow ☐ Labored	Rate: 70 ☑ Regular ☐ Irregular		☐ Alert ☐ Voice ☐ Pain ☐ Unresp.		☐	Normal Dilated Constricted Sluggish No-Reaction	☐	☐ Unremarkable ☐ Cool ☐ Pale ☒ Warm ☐ Cyanotic ☐ Moist ☐ Flushed ☒ Dry ☐ Jaundiced
		Rate: ☐ Regular ☐ Shallow ☐ Labored	Rate: ☐ Regular ☐ Irregular		☐ Alert ☐ Voice ☐ Pain ☐ Unresp.		☐	Normal Dilated Constricted Sluggish No-Reaction	☐	☐ Unremarkable ☐ Cool ☐ Pale ☐ Warm ☐ Cyanotic ☐ Moist ☐ Flushed ☐ Dry ☐ Jaundiced
		Rate: ☐ Regular ☐ Shallow ☐ Labored	Rate: ☐ Regular ☐ Irregular		☐ Alert ☐ Voice ☐ Pain ☐ Unresp.		☐	Normal Dilated Constricted Sluggish No-Reaction	☐	☐ Unremarkable ☐ Cool ☐ Pale ☐ Warm ☐ Cyanotic ☐ Moist ☐ Flushed ☐ Dry ☐ Jaundiced

5 Record the quality and regularity of the pulse rate and the condition of the skin.

Once the proper size cuff is chosen, it should be applied to the patient's bare upper arm. If clothing is present, either remove it or roll the sleeve up to expose the upper arm. Be careful not to allow the rolled sleeve to form a constricting band around the upper arm, potentially making the blood pressure inaccurate by inhibiting blood flow to the arm.

Measurement by Auscultation

The most complete method of blood pressure measurement is by auscultation. To measure blood pressure by auscultation, the EMT should apply the cuff, then find the brachial pulse. This pulse is usually found toward the medial part of the **antecubital fossa**, the space opposite the elbow on the front of the arm.

The blood pressure cuff is inflated until the brachial pulse is no longer felt, then inflated 20 mm Hg higher. A stethoscope is placed on the area of the brachial pulse, then the pressure in the cuff is released slowly.

The EMT should listen for the sound of the pulse returning. When the return of pulse is first heard, the number on the dial should be read. This is the systolic blood pressure.

As the EMT continues to listen while releasing the pressure in the cuff, the audible pulse will disappear. When it does, the EMT notes the number on the dial at the last beat. This number is the diastolic pressure. The blood pressure is then reported as systolic pressure over diastolic pressure. Skill 10-3 illustrates this procedure.

Measurement by Palpation

In some circumstances, an EMT may not be able to hear the blood pressure because of interference from other noises. Examples of noisy interference include vibrations from a helicopter during flight and noisy machinery in an industrial setting. In these cases, the blood pressure may be estimated by the palpation method, illustrated in Skill 10-4. This is merely an estimation, and blood pressures by palpation are often lower than those obtained by auscultation. Any blood pressure obtained by palpation should be confirmed with a standard auscultated blood pressure as soon as possible.

Blood pressures by palpation are accomplished by palpating the return of the radial pulse during deflation of the cuff and noting that number on the blood pressure gauge as the systolic pressure. Because a stethoscope is not used, the loss of the pulse cannot be heard, and the diastolic pressure is therefore not available. This blood pressure is reported as the systolic number over palpation. For example "one-twenty by palpation" or "120/P."

Skin

As discussed in Chapter 9, the skin can tell us a lot about the patient's circulatory status. For this reason, it is crucial that the EMT pay attention to skin condition when measuring vital signs. Together with the heart rate and blood pressure, skin condition can clue the EMT in to potentially serious circulatory problems.

TABLE 10-3

Normal Blood Pressures

Age	Systolic (mm Hg)	Diastolic (mm Hg)
Adults	90–150	60–90
Children	Approx. 80 + [2 × age (in years) for children over 1 yr]	Approx. 2/3 systolic

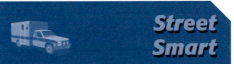

Pediatric Considerations

Although blood pressure cuffs can be purchased in sizes appropriate for tiny infants, the general assessment of the infant and small child is much more valuable than obtaining a blood pressure reading. Blood pressures are often not obtained for children under the age of 3.

Street Smart

New technology has brought with it automatic blood pressure cuffs, sometimes called a *non-invasive blood pressure monitor* (NIBP), and some EMS systems are becoming increasingly dependent on this tool. Every time an NIBP is used, a manual blood pressure should be taken first to compare with the NIBP reading to ensure that cuff placement is correct and the readings are dependable.

SKILL 10-3 *Measurement of Blood Pressure by Auscultation*

PURPOSE: To obtain a baseline blood pressure for assessment and comparison.

STANDARD PRECAUTIONS:

☑ Stethoscope
☑ Properly sized blood pressure cuff
☑ Gloves

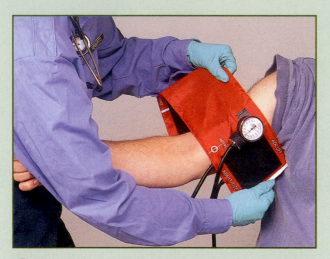

1 The EMT places the blood pressure cuff around the patient's upper arm snugly. The cuff should cover more than half but less than two-thirds of the length of the upper arm.

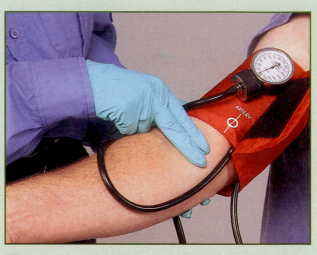

2 The EMT then finds the brachial pulse. The brachial pulse is usually found on the medial side of the elbow.

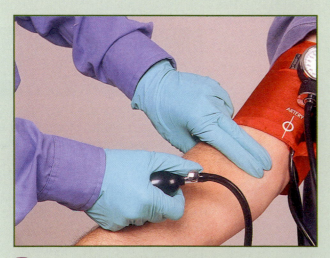

3 Next, the EMT closes the valve on the cuff and inflates the cuff until the brachial pulse is no longer felt, then continues inflating for 20 mm Hg higher.

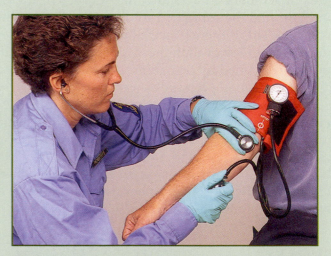

4 Then the EMT places the head of the stethoscope on the brachial pulse and the ear tips in the ears.

(continues)

SKILL 10-3 *(continued)*

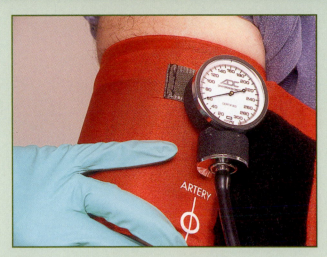

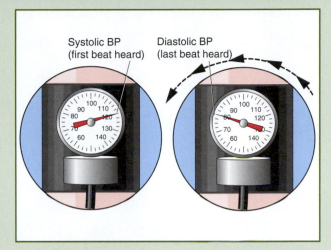

Systolic BP (first beat heard)   Diastolic BP (last beat heard)

5 Slowly deflate the blood pressure cuff, at about 10 mm Hg a second, using the relief valve next to the bulb.

6 Note the systolic and the diastolic pressures.

SKILL 10-4 *Measurement of Blood Pressure by Palpation*

PURPOSE: To obtain a baseline blood pressure for assessment and comparison.

STANDARD PRECAUTIONS:

☑ Properly sized blood pressure cuff
☑ Gloves

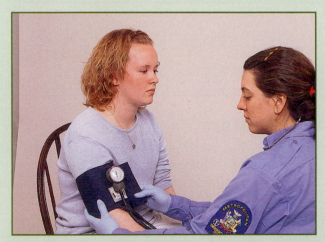

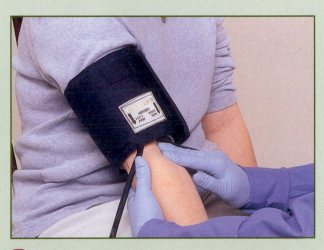

1 The EMT places the blood pressure cuff around the patient's upper arm snugly. The cuff should cover more than half but less than two-thirds of the length of the upper arm.

2 The EMT then finds the brachial pulse. The brachial pulse is usually found on the medial side of the elbow.

(continues)

SKILL 10-4 (continued)

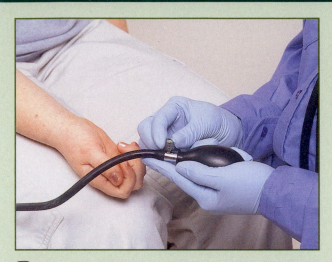

3 Next, the EMT closes the valve on the cuff and inflates the cuff until the brachial pulse is no longer felt, then continues inflating for 20 mm Hg higher.

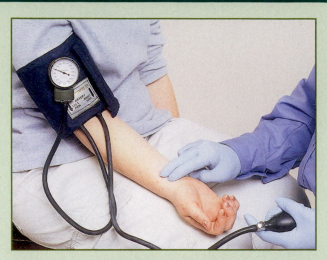

4 Then the EMT places her fingertips over the radial pulse and slowly deflates the blood pressure cuff until the pulse returns.

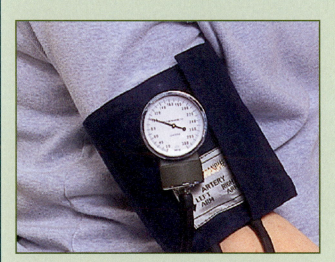

5 The EMT notes the pressure on the valve at the time that she felt the return of the radial pulse.

RESP	PULSE	B.P.
Rate: ☐ Regular ☐ Shallow ☐ Labored	Rate: ☐ Regular ☐ Irregular	120 P
Rate: ☐ Regular ☐ Shallow ☐ Labored	Rate: ☐ Regular ☐ Irregular	
Rate:	Rate:	

6 The EMT records the reading on the Patient Care Report.

Temperature and Moisture

The healthy person normally has warm, dry skin. It is important to actually measure the temperature with your hand on a central part of the patient's body. Measuring temperature peripherally, at the hands for example, may be misleading if the room temperature is at an extreme of hot or cold.

To measure temperature, partially remove a glove and place the bare skin from the back of the hand against the patient's bare skin on either the forehead or the abdomen.

The skin temperature should be described as hot, warm, cool, or cold. A patient who had a fever greater than 101 degrees Fahrenheit would be called *hot to the touch.*

Moisture on the surface of the skin may represent normal sweating if the patient is in a hot environment. Moist or sweaty skin may also represent a nervous system reaction to a stressful situation. *Cool and clammy* skin is different from hot and sweaty skin and usually indicates that the patient has a circulatory problem.

Color

The patient's color should be determined by assessing the nail beds, oral mucosa, or conjunctiva (the pink underside of the eyelid). Color is usually a direct measurement of the adequacy of blood supply to that area. Normally, these areas will have a healthy pink color from good blood flow, or perfusion.

If blood supply is decreased, as in hypoperfusion, the light-skinned patient's skin will become pale. The patient's skin is sometimes described as looking pallid or having a **pallor** (a deficiency of color). A dark-skinned patient will show a lighter complexion as well. This change has been described as looking dusky or gray. Figure 10-3 shows an example of pallor.

If a state of poor oxygenation exists, a bluish discoloration, or cyanosis, may be present. Peripheral cyanosis, a bluish hue to the fingertips, may also represent poor circulation. Central cyanosis, a bluish hue to the lips or inner eyelids, is a sign of hypoxia, or lack of oxygen in the blood.

Other skin colors may give the EMT clues about underlying disease states. A flushed red appearance to the skin may indicate a sunburn, heat exposure, or serious carbon monoxide poisoning. A yellow appearance, called **jaundice**, may indicate liver disease. Figures 10-4 and 10-5 show examples of these skin colors.

Capillary Refill in Children

For children, the EMT has an additional tool that may be useful in assessing the adequacy of circulation and perfusion. Recall that early in a state of hypoperfusion, or shock, the body preferentially shunts blood away from the skin to compensate for poor circulation, and the skin is therefore not supplied with blood. This important bodily response allows continued perfusion of important central body organs when the blood supply is limited. We can see evidence of this selective shunting of blood away from the skin by assessing the time it takes for the blood to return to the skin when the skin is compressed. This measurement is called **capillary refill time**.

The capillaries of a healthy child have a constant supply of oxygenated blood. If the blood were pushed out of a capillary bed, by external pressure on the area, the area would become pale as blood was forced out of the skin's capillaries.

The normal response of the skin is to rapidly refill those capillaries with blood, and the skin becomes pink again. This capillary refill normally occurs in less than 2 seconds. The EMT can test capillary refill by compressing and releasing the fingertip of the child's first finger.

If more than 2 seconds elapse before the capillary bed refills and the area becomes pink, the child's skin can be said to be hypoperfused and the child may be in shock.

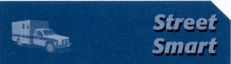

In the past the presence of a radial or carotid pulse was assumed to mean that the patient had a certain blood pressure. Current research has rejected that notion. It is more accurate to assume that the patient with a strong radial pulse has an adequate blood pressure, while a patient without a radial pulse may have a low blood pressure. No further assumptions about the blood pressure can be made without measurement by the EMT.

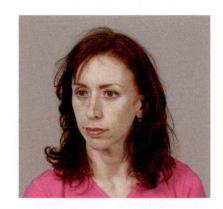

FIGURE 10-3 Note the pallor, a sign of shock.

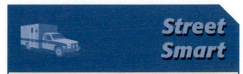

Street Smart

If unsure whether the patient has a pallor, ask a family member or other person who knows the patient whether this is the patient's normal color. Also, look around the room for a picture of the patient to see his normal skin color.

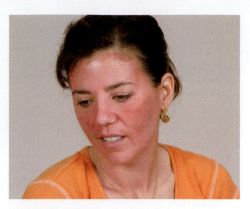

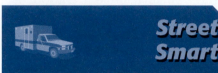

FIGURE 10-4 A flush can occur from embarrassment or disease.

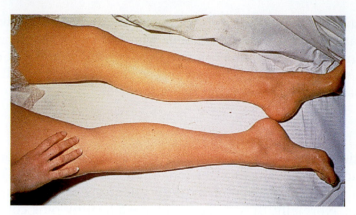

FIGURE 10-5 Jaundiced skin can be caused by liver disease.

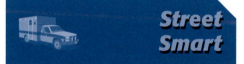

Street Smart

A child's peripheral capillary refill will be delayed in cold weather. To obtain an accurate measure of capillary refill in a cool environment, check a central area, such as the forehead, by pressing on it with a finger.

Street Smart

Normally, when you are measuring capillary refill, the blood flow (i.e., color) should return in the time it takes to say "capillary refill."

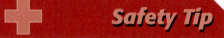

Safety Tip

Jaundice is best seen in the whites of the eyes or the inner eyelids. Although there are many causes of jaundice, hepatitis-induced liver disease is one. When treating a jaundiced patient, use extra caution when handling potentially infectious body fluids.

Although adult capillary refill testing was taught in the past, this test may not be as accurate an indication of hypoperfusion in adults as previously thought. A number of confounding factors—for example, certain medications, old age, and smoking history—make this test less accurate in adults. For these reasons, the results of capillary refill testing in adults are questionable.

Pupils

It has been said that the eyes are the windows to the soul. For the EMT, the eyes are the windows to the brain and how well it is functioning. An essential part of every neurologic exam includes checking the pupil's response to light.

The **pupil** is the black part in the center of the eye. It is usually round and changes size in reaction to changing light conditions. The EMT should check this response during each measurement of the vital signs and note any changes. A change in pupillary reaction may mean the patient's neurologic status, or brain function, is improving or deteriorating.

When checking pupil response, the EMT should shield the patient's eyes from the room light, or turn down the lights and then use a hand-held penlight to assess size, shape, and reaction.

Size and Shape

Pupil diameter can be described using exact millimeters, ranging from 2 mm to 8 mm. Some providers may prefer to use less precise terms, such as *dilated,* meaning large, or *constricted,* meaning small. Figure 10-6B shows dilated pupils, and Figure 10-6A shows contricted pupils.

Table 10-4 lists some terms used to describe pupils. The pupil of the eye is normally round. The two pupils are usually the same size. They tend to react together when one is exposed to light. This is called a consensual response.

If the pupils are not of equal size, this condition is termed **anisocoria**. Figure 10-6C shows a patient with anisocoria. Some people naturally have this condition, but it can be a sign of serious eye or brain injury.

Reactivity

When the eye is exposed to light, the normal response of the pupil is to constrict rather briskly. When the light is removed, the pupil should dilate just as quickly. If this response occurs, the pupil is considered normal and reactive. If no response to light is seen, the pupil is considered nonreactive. If the pupil responds slowly, the pupil is described as being sluggish.

When an EMT shines a light into a patient's eyes, she should observe the size, shape, and reactivity of the pupil. Often the normal response is described with an acronym: **PERRL**. This stands for *p*upils *e*qual, *r*ound, and *r*eactive to *l*ight.

Some neurologic or brain injuries and injuries directly to the eye will alter this normal reaction. It is important that the EMT note the pupil response with each set of vital signs in order to recognize any changes from the initial baseline exam.

Pulse Oximetry

There are times when it is useful to quantify the effectiveness of a patient's breathing. The EMT can count the breaths per minute and describe the quality of the breathing effort. These observations tell a great deal about the effectiveness of the patient's respirations.

An additional tool that can be useful to determine how effectively a patient is breathing is the **pulse oximeter**. The pulse oximeter is a noninvasive machine that indirectly measures the amount of oxygenated blood in a patient's circulatory system. (See Skill 10-5).

This device uses an infrared light to estimate the percent of blood that appears to be oxygenated in the capillaries at a fingertip. The pulse oximeter relies on the difference in appearance of blood cells that are bound to oxygen and those that are not to make this determination. The normal percent of blood that is saturated by oxygen is 96%–100%.

If the respirations are effective, the blood will be well oxygenated and the pulse oximetry reading will be normal. Less than 96% indicates that the blood is poorly oxygenated and that there may be problems with breathing or circulation. Below 90% is considered to be a serious problem in oxygenation.

These numbers are described as percent saturated. So if the device read "97," this reading would be described as "97 percent saturated" and would be considered within the normal oxygen saturation range.

The pulse oximeter should not be used to determine whether a patient needs oxygen. The EMT should base oxygen administration upon the patient complaint and her own assessment of the patient's condition. If the EMT decides that the patient needs oxygen, on the basis of the patient's presenting problem and physical exam, it should be given. Measuring the pulse oximetry when the need for oxygen has already been determined only delays oxygen administration and is inappropriate.

The pulse oximeter can be used to judge the effectiveness of the EMT's treatment. If 100% oxygen has been applied and the pulse oximeter reading is dropping, the EMT should rapidly reassess the patient's status and need for further interventions, such as bag-valve-mask ventilation or even cardiopulmonary resuscitation (CPR).

For the machine to accurately determine the percent of saturated blood, it must "see" an adequate sample of capillary blood. For various reasons, an adequate sample is not always available. For example,

TABLE 10-4	
Descriptive Terms for Pupils	
Pinpoint	Tiny pupils, usually smaller than 2 mm diameter
Constricted	Small, usually 2–3 mm
Midposition	Medium-sized, usually 4–5 mm
Dilated	Large, usually 6–8 mm
Blown	Huge, usually greater than 8 mm

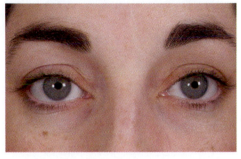

A.

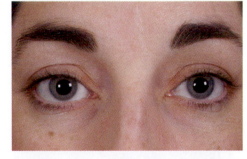

B.

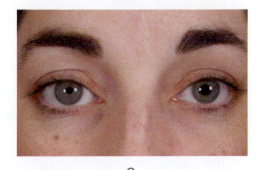

C.

FIGURE 10-6 A. Constricted pupils. B. Dilated pupils. C. Unequal pupils (anisocoria).

SKILL 10-5 *Pulse Oximetry*

PURPOSE: To obtain a baseline oxygen saturation for assessment and comparison.

STANDARD PRECAUTIONS:

☑ Pulse oximeter with indicator light
☑ Nail polish remover
☑ Gloves

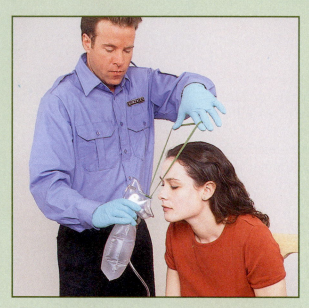

1 Assess the patient. Never withhold oxygen to obtain an oxygen saturation if the patient is hypoxic.

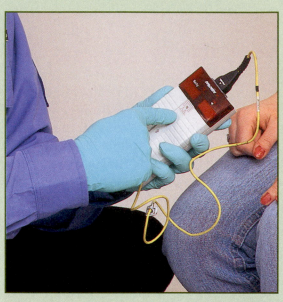

2 Turn on the pulse oximeter and check for self-test results.

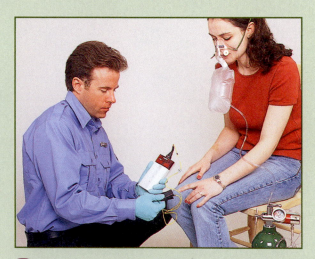

3 Place the probe on the patient's finger (if nail polish is present, remove the polish first).

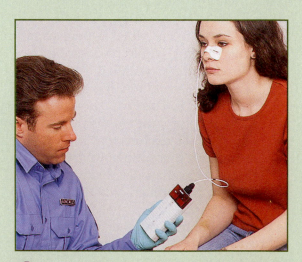

4 If distal circulation is diminished, place a disposable probe over the bridge of the nose.

(continues)

SKILL 10-5 *(continued)*

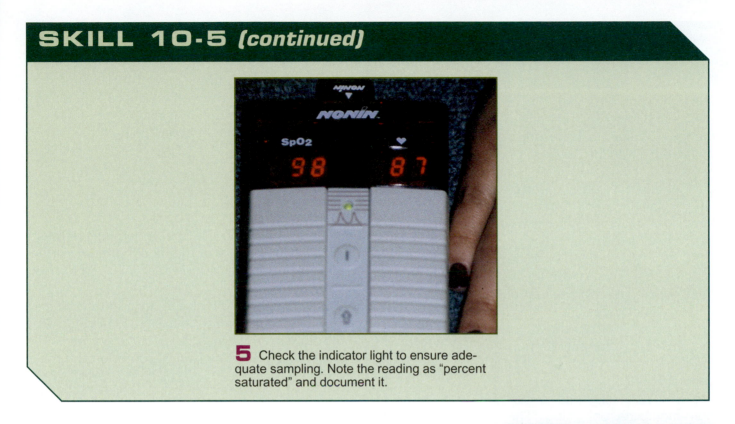

5 Check the indicator light to ensure adequate sampling. Note the reading as "percent saturated" and document it.

if the patient has heavy nail polish, the device may not be able to sense accurately through the polish. The nail polish must be removed, usually with acetone or nail polish remover, in order to get an accurate reading.

If the patient does not have adequate blood flow to the finger that the device is placed on, an adequate sample will not be seen. For example, while a blood pressure is being taken, the pulse oximeter reading may become low temporarily.

Many devices have an indicator light, or a lighted meter, to tell the EMT that an adequate sample has been "seen" and that the number given is accurate. It is recommended that the EMT use a pulse oximeter that indicates when the reading is adequate. A lighted bar meter or a green or yellow light indicator visually confirms that the sample is adequate and reliable.

Street Smart

Bright overhead lights can interfere with a pulse oximeter. If an EMT is having difficulty obtaining a pulse oximeter reading in a bright environment, she should try putting a washcloth over the finger probe to block out some of the environmental light.

REASSESSMENT OF VITAL SIGNS

An EMT will often care for a patient over an extended period of time. During that time it is important that the EMT be aware of any change in the patient's condition. Changes can be determined only if the EMT repeatedly reassesses the patient.

It is imperative that the EMT repeat the assessment of vital signs frequently during care for any emergency patient. If the patient's initial vital signs were within normal range, and the patient seems stable, the vital signs should be repeated every 10–15 minutes to assess for changes.

If the patient is unstable or had abnormal vital signs at the first check, the EMT should repeat the vital signs at least every 5 minutes.

Street Smart

It is important to remember that the pulse oximeter is merely a machine that is to be used in conjunction with the EMT's clinical judgment. If an EMT suspects that a patient is in need of oxygen for any reason, regardless of the pulse oximeter reading, she should provide it.

Oxygen should never be withheld from a patient who needs it because of a normal pulse oximetry reading. There are certain situations in which the pulse oximetry may be normal, but the patient is in need of supplemental oxygen.

One such example is carbon monoxide poisoning. The carbon monoxide binds to the hemoglobin, causing the pulse oximeter to "see" completely saturated hemoglobin (100% saturation). This device cannot distinguish between oxygen and other molecules attached to the hemoglobin and will read a normal saturation despite a lack of oxygen.

If a medication is administered to the patient, the EMT should repeat the vital signs within 5 minutes after the administration of any medication, including oxygen.

All measurements of vital signs should be carefully documented, with the time that they were obtained noted on the record. Noting changes in any vital sign and passing that information on to the hospital providers are crucial and will help them understand the changes in the patient's condition.

HISTORY TAKING

History taking often occurs while other EMTs are obtaining vital signs or immediately afterward. The history of the illness often describes the reason for the patient's present health crisis as well as what treatments may have worked in the past.

It is vitally important that the EMT obtain an accurate history. Obtaining an accurate history is often easier said than done. The patient's anxiety, cultural considerations, interference from family and bystanders, and even the patient's physical condition can make gathering a history difficult.

Patient Rapport

There are several steps the EMT can take to make the patient feel calmer about the stressful situation. The EMT should always remember that every time she is called to care for a patient, regardless of the nature of the problem, it is stressful for that patient.

What may seem like an everyday occurrence to the EMT is likely a once-in-a-lifetime occurrence for the patient. The patient will appreciate the EMT's effort in understanding the patient's stress and taking a few steps to put him at ease and will feel more comfortable during his evaluation and transportation to the hospital.

Proper Introduction of the Crew

The first thing an EMT should do upon encountering a patient is to introduce herself and describe her training and her purpose for being there—for example: "Hi, my name is Jessica Brown. I'm an EMT with Greenville Rescue Squad, and my crew and I have come to help you." It may put the patient at ease to know the names of his caregivers and the level of their training.

Proper Etiquette

After the EMT has introduced herself, she should ascertain the patient's name. It is appropriate and respectful to address adults by their last name—for example, "It is nice to meet you, Mrs. Jones. How can we help you today?" At no time should the EMT address a patient as "sweetie" or "honey." Such terms are considered too familiar in most cases and are generally considered disrespectful.

The EMT should refer to the patient by his first name only if the EMT is about the same age as the patient or if the patient gives the EMT permission.

EMS in Action

People don't call 9-1-1 until the situation is out of their control. It matters not whether the emergency is real or perceived. For some victims, perception is reality. One factor that shapes their perception is past experiences.

I remember a squad run involving an eight-year-old girl who had her foot caught in the chain of her bicycle. Other then a few scratches, she was not injured. However, her mother was screaming, "Don't cut off her leg! Please don't amputate her leg!"

No amount of talking could reassure the mother that we would disentangle her daughter from the bike without using such drastic measures. Within three minutes, we had her leg free, but the mother was still crying uncontrollably.

Later a neighbor informed us that her father just lost his leg to diabetes, so the thought of amputation, real or perceived, weighed heavily on the mother's mind.

Arlene Zang, EMT-P, FF
Public Safety Coordinator, Great Oaks Institute
of Technology and Career Development
Cincinnati, Ohio

Cultural Considerations

Hand gestures have different meanings to different people. Whereas in New England the gesture for "okay"—a circle made with the thumb and index finger—is an accepted positive hand signal, in Brazil and Turkey it is considered an insult.

When a language barrier prevents communication, EMTs often resort to hand gestures and signals. Misunderstood gestures can increase confusion rather than improve communication. The EMT must be conscious of the meanings that her gestures are relaying.

Cultural Considerations

The EMT should be aware of different cultural practices in interpersonal interactions. Some eastern Indian and Mexican cultures may not approve of direct eye contact. Some Arab Americans do not approve of physical contact by EMTs of the opposite gender.

Other cultures, for example Anglo-Americans, may consider someone who looks directly into their eyes trustworthy, and a comforting hand may be invaluable in relieving stress for these patients.

The EMT should become familiar with the practices of cultural and ethnic groups found in her jurisdiction. By understanding cultural diversity, and modifying her practice accordingly, the EMT is demonstrating sensitivity and professional conduct.

In some groups, for example Asian Americans, it is disrespectful to refer to the patient by his or her first name at any time. The EMT should be aware of and be sensitive to these ethnic differences.

Children, however, will usually feel more comfortable when an adult refers to them by their first name. But remember to call their parents by their last name.

Comforting Touch

During the course of caring for a patient, it is comforting to the patient if the EMT remains calm and reassuring in her attitude and in her actions. If it seems appropriate, a hand placed on the patient's forearm or hand may be very reassuring to the patient.

Again, in certain cultures, touching is restricted to only immediate family. For example, Arab Americans may not want a male EMT to "lay his hand on" a female patient except to obtain vital signs or perform procedures.

In other cultures, physical contact is almost an expectation, and if the EMT does not reassure the patient with the touch of a hand, then the EMT might be labeled as cold and unsympathetic.

Often, a mere statement of understanding and reassurance is extremely helpful to the patient. The EMT must be careful not to make promises that cannot be kept and not to lie to the patient in an attempt to comfort him. For example, it is inappropriate for an EMT to tell an obviously sick patient that "everything will be fine." The EMT has no

TABLE 10-5

SAMPLE History

S = Signs and symptoms

A = Allergies

M = Medications

P = Past medical history

L = Last oral intake

E = Events leading up to the illness or incident

TABLE 10-6

Signs and Symptoms

Sign	Symptom
Ankle swelling	Ankle pain
Labored breathing	Shortness of breath
Abdominal tenderness	Abdominal pain
Unsteadiness	Dizziness
Rapid pulse rate	Palpitations

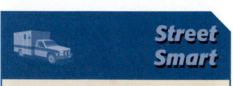

Street Smart

When you are documenting medications, spelling counts. Many medications have very similar-sounding names but very different actions. It is important that the EMT *accurately* write the name of the medication down as well as the dose and frequency of medication administration.

---

way of knowing what the outcome will be and cannot make that promise. Rather, the EMT should make a statement such as, "We are going to take care of you" or "We will be at the hospital soon." Both are truthful and comforting statements.

SAMPLE HISTORY

During the course of caring for any patient, there is certain basic information that the EMT must ascertain. This basic information should be obtained as soon as possible, after all life threats have been properly addressed.

To remember what questions must be asked of every patient, the EMT can use the acronym **SAMPLE**. Table 10-5 defines this term briefly.

Signs and Symptoms

One of the first things the EMT may ask a patient is "What is the difficulty today?" or "What problem can we help you with?" The patient's response to these questions will provide the EMT with useful information.

When the patient tells you about his complaint, he is reporting his symptoms. A **symptom** is the patient's perception of his illness or injury. For example, if a patient reported that he fell and now his ankle hurts, then ankle pain is the patient's symptom. A symptom is a subjective complaint that is not necessarily visible to the EMT but something the patient tells her.

A big bruise and a lot of swelling on the same ankle would be referred to as a sign. A **sign** is an objective condition that is observable by the EMT.

An example of the difference between a sign and a symptom is related to pain and tenderness. Pain is a subjective complaint made by a patient. Tenderness is discomfort initiated by palpation during an exam and demonstrated by the patient's facial grimace or outcry. Pain is a symptom, and tenderness is a sign.

During the initial history taking, the EMT should encourage the patient to discuss any symptoms and signs relative to the complaint. Table 10-6 lists some signs and symptoms.

Allergies

A crucial piece of information for the EMT to gather is whether the patient has any allergies to medications. Even though the EMT may not be administering any medications to the patient, the hospital staff may. It is very important that the EMT pass along any known allergies to hospital staff so that they may avoid mistakenly administering those medications.

Medications

When the EMT is asking a patient what medications he takes, it is often helpful to gather them (if available) and bring them to the hospital. Having the medications enables the hospital staff to know the exact dosage of the medicines and how often they are being taken.

Some systems discourage EMTs from bringing the patient's medications to the hospital. In those cases, the EMT should make an effort to write down the names of the medicines the patient takes, what the doses of the medication are, and how often the patient takes the medication. This information can be found on the prescription label on the medicine.

In addition to the current medication list, the EMT should ask the patient whether the doctor has ordered any changes in his medications recently. Sometimes the medication change creates the problem that the patient is experiencing.

The EMT should also ask whether the patient has been taking his medications as ordered. In other words, is he *compliant* with the instructions that he was given about his prescribed medication. This information should be carefully documented and passed on to the hospital staff as well.

Past Medical/Surgical History

The EMT should ask the patient about any past medical problems, including any previous surgeries, that the patient may have that could be contributing to the problem today. It is often helpful for the EMT to review several general categories of health problems to remind the patient of certain conditions.

Table 10-7 lists some of the more common diseases that the EMT should ask about. It is often helpful for the EMT to ask who the patient's doctor is and then ask why he sees the doctor. For example, if the patient says he sees Dr. Putnam and Dr. Putnam is a well-known

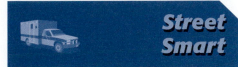

Street Smart

Many patients will take over-the-counter (OTC) medications for relief of symptoms before they call EMS. Do not forget to ask about OTC medications. Many OTC medications have very strong actions that may have contributed to the patient's current problem.

TABLE 10-7

Past Medical History	
Lay Term	**Medical Term**
Stroke	Cerebrovascular accident (CVA)
Seizures	Epilepsy
Heart attack	Myocardial infarction
High blood pressure	Hypertension
Asthma	Asthma
Emphysema, bronchitis	Chronic obstructive pulmonary disease
Sugar sickness	Diabetes
Cancer	Cancer

and respected cardiologist, then the EMT would naturally ask the patient whether he is seeing Dr. Putnam for heart problems.

Last Oral Intake

It is useful to report to the hospital the last time the seriously ill or injured patient had anything to eat or drink. The hospital staff must know when the last oral intake was.

If the patient requires surgery, any food in the stomach can cause the patient to vomit. Vomiting when the patient is unconscious, while under sedation or anesthesia, can create a serious problem such as aspiration pneumonia. The time of the last meal is an important pre-operative consideration. Without an accurate time of last meal, the surgery could be delayed.

Events Leading Up to Incident/Illness

In addition to the signs and symptoms related to the current illness or injury, the EMT should question the patient as to how the incident occurred or what led up to it. The event leading up to the injury or illness is often the cause of the injury or the trigger for the illness. For example, exercise can induce shortness of breath from an asthma attack or chest pain from angina. Specific questions relative to different medical conditions are discussed in later chapters.

If the patient was driving his motorcycle without a helmet and then crashed his motorcycle, then the event preceding his injury was driving a motorcycle without a helmet and the result is a head injury. Driving the motorcycle would be reported as the mechanism of injury, and falling without a helmet would be the event preceding the injury.

CONCLUSION

The EMT is responsible for gathering certain baseline information on every patient she encounters. This information minimally consists of repeated vital sign measurements and a basic history of the patient's medical condition.

The EMT must be well practiced at assessing respiration, pulse, blood pressure, pupils, skin condition, and pulse oximetry. Familiarity with normal values for each of these parameters is important if the EMT is expected to identify abnormal vital signs.

Ongoing assessment of these values is also important. Ongoing assessment is useful in recognition of any changes, positive or negative, in the patient's condition.

Finally, the EMT must be able to obtain a minimal history, using the mnemonic SAMPLE, before she can fully understand the patient's condition.

TEST YOUR KNOWLEDGE

1. Identify the vital signs.
2. Describe how to assess the quality and quantity of respiration.
3. List the normal respiratory rate and quality for adults and children of different ages.
4. Describe how to assess the quality and quantity of the pulse.
5. List the normal pulse rate and quality for adults and children of different ages.
6. Describe the methods to assess blood pressure.
7. Define *systolic pressure*.
8. Define *diastolic pressure*.
9. Describe the methods to assess the pupils.
10. Describe normal and abnormal pupil size, shape, and reaction.
11. Describe the methods to assess skin color, temperature, and condition.
12. Describe how to assess capillary refill in infants and children.
13. Identify normal and abnormal skin colors, temperatures, and conditions.
14. Identify normal and abnormal capillary refill in infants and children.
15. Discuss the utility of pulse oximetry.
16. Describe how to measure oxygen saturation using a pulse oximeter.
17. Identify the components of the SAMPLE history.
18. Differentiate between a sign and a symptom.
19. State the importance of accurately reporting and recording the baseline vital signs.

INTERNET RESOURCES

- Do a search on each of the vital signs discussed in the chapter. What types of resources are available?

- Search for resources for breath sounds. One site to check out is http://www.rale.ca. Listen to a variety of breath sounds that may be available so that when you hear these sounds in the field you can become more adept at identifying them.

- Can you find any research being done on the use of vital signs in the field? Share your findings with your colleagues.

FURTHER STUDY

DeLaune, S., & Ladner, P. (2002). *Fundamentals of nursing: Standards & practice* (2nd ed.). Clifton Park, NY: Thomson Delmar Learning.

Estes, M. E. Z. (2002). *Health assessment and physical examination* (2nd ed.). Clifton Park, NY: Thomson Delmar Learning.

Lindh, W., Tamparo, C., Pooler, M., & Cerrato, J. (2002). *Comprehensive medical assisting* (2nd ed.). Clifton Park, NY: Thomson Delmar Learning.

CHAPTER 11

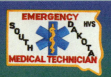

Lifting and Moving Patients

KEY TERMS

arm drag
basket stretcher
bedroll
blanket drag
body mechanics
carry transfer
caterpillar pass
chair carry
clothing drag
cradle carry
cravat
diamond stretcher carry
direct carry
direct lift
draw sheet
draw sheet transfer
emergency drag
emergency move
end-to-end stretcher carry
extremity lift
firefighter's carry
firefighter's drag
flexible stretcher
four corners carry
litter
orthopedic stretcher

(continues)

OBJECTIVES

Upon completion of this chapter, the reader should be able to:

1. Discuss proper back care.
2. Define body mechanics as it pertains to tasks of an EMT.
3. Discuss the guidelines and safety precautions that need to be followed when lifting a patient.
4. State the guidelines for reaching and their application.
5. Describe the guidelines and safety precautions for carrying patients and equipment.
6. State the guidelines for pushing and pulling.
7. Discuss the general considerations of moving patients.
8. State several situations that may require the use of an emergency move.
9. Describe and demonstrate four emergency drags.
10. Describe and demonstrate six emergency carries.
11. Describe and demonstrate two lifts used for routine transportation.
12. Describe the utilization of the following patient-carrying devices:
    a. Orthopedic, or scoop, stretcher
    b. Stairchair
    c. Basket stretcher
    d. Flexible stretcher
    e. Portable stretcher (litter)
    f. Wheeled stretcher
13. Describe correct and safe carrying procedures on stairs.
14. Describe correct and safe carrying procedures for stretchers.
15. Describe proper patient packaging.
16. Describe correct and safe transferring procedures.

OVERVIEW

Packaging, lifting, and carrying of patients are necessary on every emergency medical services (EMS) call. Whether the term is *scoop and run* or *load and go*, the mission has remained the same for EMS: the safe transportation of the patient to definitive medical care.

Although the procedure may seem routine, there are many decisions an emergency medical technician (EMT) makes regarding lifting and carrying that can have a dramatic impact on the patient and the EMT. By choosing the wrong lifting technique, an EMT can get hurt. If an EMT uses a carrying device improperly, the patient can be dropped and further injuries may result.

As more EMTs complain of work-related back injuries, EMS leaders are becoming increasingly attentive to the manner in which EMTs lift and carry. Back braces, reengineered carrying devices, and back care programs are becoming commonplace. The key to a long career in EMS hinges on proper lifting and carrying of patients and equipment.

BACK INJURIES

The scenario is all too common; an EMT lifts someone or something, thinking that the task can be done easily, and disaster strikes. A back injury may occur that could take the EMT out of work, perhaps permanently. Every EMT needs to know how to prevent back injuries.

Anatomy Review

Back injuries are actually injuries of the spine or the muscles adjacent to the spine, or both. The spine carries the weight of the upper body and anything carried by the person. This weight is primarily borne by the lumbar section of the spinal column. The lumbar spine is the victim of about 85% of all back injuries.

The spine is not rigid as are some other bony structures in the body. The spinal column is a series of bone segments, called vertebrae, that are stacked one on top of the other. This arrangement gives the spine an ability to bend and flex as well as to hold great weight.

Although the flexible nature of the spinal column allows the person to bend and move easily, these movements require a great deal of balance and muscle coordination. The spine is supported by a large number of muscles and ligaments to help with support and balance.

Between each two vertebrae is a soft disc that acts as a shock absorber. These discs help the spine absorb shocks and vibrations. They occasionally deteriorate, are crushed, or move and slip out of place. In any case, the result can be severe back pain.

The lower back, and the lumbar spine in particular, can be injured by strains or sprains of the muscles, by destruction or movement of intervertebral discs, or by fractures to the lumbar vertebrae themselves. These injuries are often the result of careless lifting and carrying.

Back Care

EMTs regularly lift and carry patients and equipment. Therefore, it is important that an EMT keep his back strong and healthy.

The key to a strong back is regular exercise. Exercise strengthens the back muscles and prepares them for the hard work ahead. Regular back exercises along with practice in proper lifting techniques and use of certain assistive devices are part of a program of back care. Good back care is essential for long-term survival of the EMT in EMS.

Companies around the world have experienced the benefits of back care programs. Some companies encourage participation or provide for employee exercise programs to strengthen their backs. Others encourage the practice of tai chi or weight training. Exercise has benefits for employer and employee alike. Figure 11-1 shows a number of lower back exercises that will help improve the back strength of the EMT.

An EMT's back must also be flexible and able to withstand the demands of bending and twisting that are required of it. The most common source of back injury is twisting while lifting an object. To prevent these injuries, every EMT should take a few minutes, at the start of every tour of duty to warm up the lower back. These exercises seldom take more than 10 minutes to perform and can help prevent a lower back injury.

Back Exercises

There are many simple back exercises that can help the EMT maintain flexibility and strength as well as reduce the incidence of injury. However, an EMT should never exercise an injured back nor exercise the back to the point of pain. The old adage "no pain, no gain," is simply not true. Exercising during injury only leads to more injury.

The following back exercises are simple, easy to do, and can be done while on the job, for example, first thing in the morning before the vehicle equipment check. To begin the first exercise the EMT should stand and grasp his hands above the head with palms facing upward. Now, the EMT should try to stretch his arm upward as far as possible. It is important to breathe normally during this exercise and not to arch the lower back. Once in position, the EMT should hold the position for a 10- or 15-second count. This exercise, called the tall stretch, helps to exercise the upper back.

For the next upper back exercise, the EMT, while in a standing position with knees slightly bent and hips directly over the feet, should reach out with outstretched hands that are shoulder width apart. With the hands placed on a countertop, the EMT would then bend down at the hips until he feels a gentle stretch and hold that position for a count of 10 or 15. This exercise can be repeated three times.

The next exercise stretches the lower back and is called the standing lower back stretch. Again the EMT assumes a standing position with hips directly over the feet and places his hands on his hips at the back, as if to support the lower back. The EMT would then gently arch the back backward, against the palms of the hands, and then hold that position for a count of 10 or 15. This exercise can also be repeated several times.

The last exercise, illustrated in Figure 11-1, requires that the EMT lie on a firm surface. Called the Tuck stretch, the EMT lays his head flat on the ground and pulls his knees toward the chest while pushing the lower back against the ground. Once in position the EMT should hold

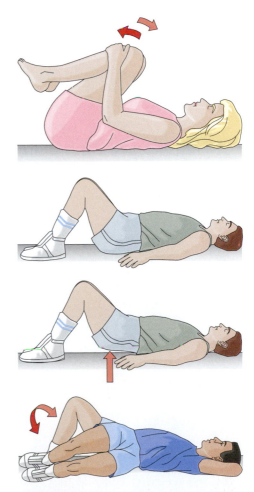

FIGURE 11-1 Back exercises reduce the chance that an EMT will suffer a back injury.

the position for a count of 10 or 15 then relax. A variation of this exercise includes placing the feet flat on the ground and lifting just the lower back or rolling the hips back and forth in a gentle rocking motion.

Know Your Limitations

The EMT should take a moment whenever he is about to lift a patient and ask himself two very important questions: (1) Is there enough help to lift this patient? (2) Is the right equipment being used?

The answers to these questions will affect the patient, the EMT, and the EMS. Failure to answer the questions correctly can mean further injury for the patient, injury and disability for the EMT, and unnecessary expenses for the EMS agency.

Is There Enough Help?

The functional job description for an EMT states that the EMT must be able to lift and carry 125 pounds. Essentially, when two EMS providers respond to a call, they should be able to safely lift and carry the average patient without difficulty.

Additional assistance should be requested for any patient who weighs more than 250 pounds. It may be possible for EMTs to lift a heavy patient, but it is not necessarily wise to do so.

The EMT should factor in the weight of the stretcher as well as any equipment that is being carried. These items can quickly add another 50 pounds.

Patients over 300 pounds present a special challenge to the EMT. Careful planning and additional resources are often needed to ensure that the EMT can safely move the patient without danger to himself or his crew.

What Is the "Right Stuff"?

There are many methods of carrying a patient, as well as adjunctive equipment to assist the EMT in the carry. Careful consideration of the problem at hand and the method that will be used to perform the carry improves the chance that the EMT will perform a safe carry.

Like an Olympic athlete, the well-trained EMT mentally visualizes the carry. Then he considers what equipment he could use to improve his performance. For example, it is much easier to drag a patient on a blanket than it is to carry one draped over the shoulder.

Safety First

Orthopedic back supports are designed to support the lower back and prevent injuries. Whenever a heavy patient is carried, a back support should be worn.

Unfortunately, back supports are frequently misused and can be harmful if not used correctly. A supporting brace should not be worn at all times. Most braces are intended to be worn loosely around the waist then tightened up with a belt, or some other means, when needed. If the brace is worn tightly for long periods, the brace may actually weaken the back muscles.

Back support braces come in different sizes. A properly fitted brace will perform as it was designed, as a back support. Some back support braces have foam padding built into the belt to provide warmth as well as support.

Proper footwear is also important. Closed-toe shoes are required for the EMT. An EMT's boots are more than just footwear. Boots serve as the foundation for lifting and carrying as well as protection for toes and feet.

The soles of the boots should be nonskid, preferably with a traction lug sole. A midcalf boot provides additional support to the ankles. This added support is important when the EMT is carrying a patient across uneven terrain (Figure 11-2).

BODY MECHANICS

Body mechanics is the proper or most efficient way to perform physical activities that are safe, are energy conserving, and help prevent the physical strains that may cause injury. The primary goal of understanding proper body mechanics is to learn how to lift and carry without injury to the spine. Awareness of common mistakes and principles of body mechanics can help the EMT achieve this goal. Table 11-1 lists the principles of good body mechanics.

Reaching

Whether the EMT is reaching for a piece of equipment or reaching to grasp a wrist for a pulse, there are several fundamental rules for reaching.

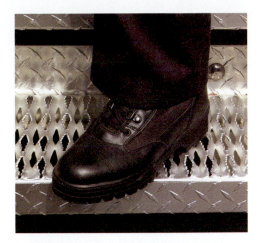

FIGURE 11-2 Proper footwear is an important part of maintaining the health and physical fitness of the EMT.

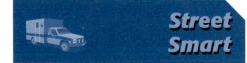

Street Smart

After having a stretcher roll over his toes a couple of times, the experienced EMT buys boots that have a reinforced toe, maybe even a steel toe. Typically, toes are not broken, but the pain and discomfort that can be avoided make the extra money spent on safety boots worth every penny.

TABLE 11-1

Principles of Good Body Mechanics

1. Keep feet apart about shoulder width.
2. Keep chin up and back straight when lifting.
3. Bend at the knees and not at the back.
4. Keep objects close to your body.
5. Do not twist your body when lifting or carrying.
6. Exhale when lifting.
7. Lift with the legs and not with the back.
8. Push or pull instead of lifting.
9. Never reach more than 18 inches away from the body.
10. Avoid fast, jerking motions when lifting.

First, the EMT should never lean backward to grab a piece of equipment. An EMT should not twist his back to reach a piece of equipment either. Twisting and arching the back backward can lead to injury.

Instead, the EMT should pivot on his heels and face the object that he is reaching for. While facing the object, and keeping the back straight, the EMT can reach to grasp the object.

The EMT should never reach more than 18 inches away from the body to grasp an object. That's about the length of the arm from elbow to hand. In addition, the elbows should not leave the side of the body. Equipment that is not readily accessible in this manner should be rearranged.

If the object is heavy, more than 10 pounds, the EMT should bend at the knees, while keeping the back straight, and lift the object to him. Again, the elbows should be close to the body but never farther out than the knees.

Lifting

When lifting an object off the ground, the EMT should carry the load as close to the body as possible. A straight back, with good vertical spinal alignment, will place the weight of the load on the pelvis and strong leg muscles while taking the weight off the lower back.

The Power Lift

Whenever a person or heavy object is lifted, the EMT should use a **power lift**. This technique, sometimes called the **squat lift**, utilizes the stronger muscles of the legs instead of the weaker muscles of the lower back. The power lift is useful when lifting baskets or stretchers or even when moving heavy furniture out of the way.

An EMT first stands within 6 inches of the object to be lifted. The closer the body's center of gravity is to the object, the more powerful the lift. Notice how an Olympic power lifter will place his feet under the bar before lifting. As the lift is accomplished, the bar moves parallel to and next to the center of mass. The EMT should use the image of an Olympic power lifter when he is performing this lift.

The EMT's feet are the foundation of the lift. One slip of a foot spells disaster for both the EMT and the patient. Good footwear, discussed previously, is imperative. A comfortable stance, with the feet evenly placed, is important. Finally, the EMT's feet should be flat on the ground, with the soles of the boots making firm contact with the surface.

The Power Grip

When preparing to perform a power lift, the EMT squats to reach the item to be lifted, such as a backboard. The EMT should obtain a firm grasp, usually palms up. The palms-up grasp, sometimes called the **power grip**, utilizes the most powerful muscles of the arm. The amount that can be lifted is limited only by the strength of the grip.

The EMT's arm should be *locked out*, meaning that the elbows are straight and the arm is one long rigid structure. This maneuver ensures that the EMT is using his back and legs to lift rather than his weaker arm muscles.

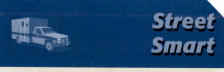

On signal, usually from the EMT at the head, two EMTs should slowly lift together. The lift should never be jerky or so fast as to jolt the patient. The lift is complete when, and only when, the EMT is in an upright position and the weight is being suspended directly in front of him.

Skill 11-1 shows an EMT lifting a backboard. Notice that the back is straight. He has knelt down to the load. He has not bent down. He carefully secures his hand grasp on the litter grips. His arms are straight, and his elbows are locked out. He then crouches to a squatting position. The load is very close to the center of his body, the center of his mass.

SKILL 11-1 *Proper Lifting Techniques*

PURPOSE: To allow the EMT to lift objects without causing back injury.
STANDARD PRECAUTIONS:

- ☑ Appropriate personal protective equipment
- ☑ Appropriate back support
- ☑ Proper footwear
- ☑ Adequate numbers of trained assistants

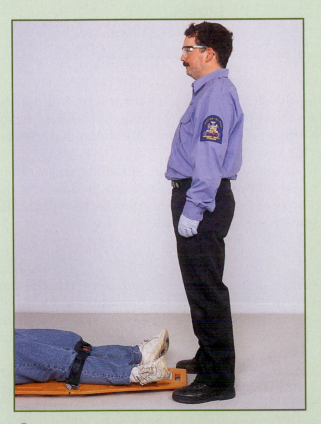

1 The EMT positions his feet about shoulder length apart, facing forward.

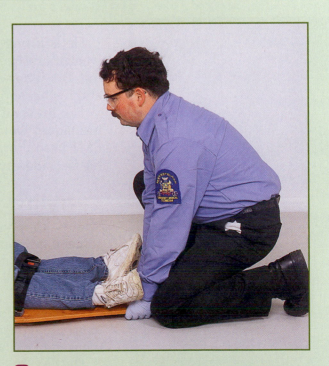

2 The EMT then lowers his body by bending at the knees, one knee down, keeping the back straight.

(continues)

SKILL 11-1 *(continued)*

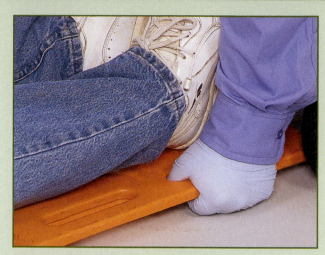

3 The EMT grasps the object with both hands, palms upward (power grip), then lifts evenly and smoothly.

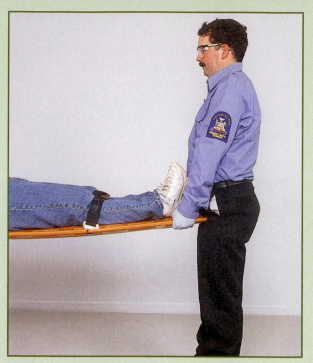

4 With arms locked out straight, the EMT stands fully upright.

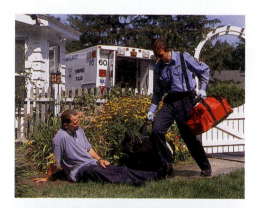

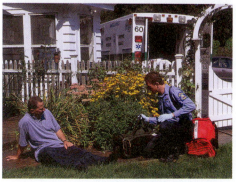

FIGURE 11-3 With knees bent and back straight, heavy objects can be carried safely.

He is lifting using the strong muscles of his thighs and not the weaker muscles of his lower back. As he is lifting, he is slowly exhaling. Exhaling while lifting helps him tighten his abdominal muscles and further support his lower back.

The lift should occur in one fluid motion, smoothly and without hesitation. Note that the elbows are never beyond the knees. If the EMT has to turn, to transfer the patient, for example, he will shuffle his feet sideways rather than twist his back.

Carrying

Radios, jump kits, suction units, backboards, and oxygen bottles are some of the equipment an EMT carries every day. Improved technology has translated to more equipment for an EMT to carry to a scene. Sometimes, the EMT feels more like a pack mule than a health care provider.

Whenever possible, a bag or case should be carried by a shoulder strap slung over the shoulder. This method of carrying tends to keep the weight of the object close to the body.

The EMT in Figure 11-3 is carrying two jump kits. Note that his back is straight and that he has a balanced load—that is, one kit in each arm. Notice that when he arrives at the patient's side, he is bending his knees and slipping the bag straps off his shoulders, to release the load, while using the handles to gently place the bags on the ground.

Fire Rescue

The smoke was choking and the pace was maddeningly slow as fire-fighter-EMT Santulli crawled along on all fours. He had been detailed to the rescue company today to cover a sick call-out. The first alarm this morning was a fire in an abandoned house.

"The house fire was probably the work of arsonists," he thought as he did the room-by-room search.

Suddenly, he felt something move. Yes, something or someone had grabbed his leg. He yelled out, "Someone's in here!"

Turning, he saw an elderly man. He appeared to be coughing in fits and then collapsed to the ground. Santulli thought, "Maybe he was trying to crawl out and got lost. It's easy to understand how someone could get lost in all this thick black smoke."

Firefighter-EMT Deso joined him at the patient's side. Yelling at the top of his lungs, through his mask, he told Santulli that the ambulance was at the backdoor "standing by."

- What about this situation makes it urgent that the firefighter-EMT move the patient?
- Are there any risks with moving the patient?
- Is the move justified in light of those risks?
- What method could the firefighter use to move the patient if he is ambulatory? If the patient is injured but conscious?
- How could the EMT move the unconscious patient to a safe area? What can the EMT do if there is another EMT available?

Pushing and Pulling

Whenever possible, an EMT should try to push an object rather than pull it. Trying to pull patients out of cars and other confined spaces has resulted in back injuries for many EMTs.

By following a few simple rules when pushing and pulling objects, listed in Table 11-2, the EMT can avoid back injuries and enjoy a long career in EMS.

PLANNING A MOVE

The EMT should always have a plan for how he wants to move a patient. Even in an emergency, there are several methods of quickly moving a patient. The advantage to having a plan is that the patient can be moved quickly, without further injury, while the safety of the EMT is not compromised.

First, survey the scene and determine the priorities. The means to move someone at a house call is different from the means to remove someone from a motor vehicle collision (MVC). The scene often dictates the best means of carry.

What is the patient's priority? Is it a life-or-death emergency? If the patient is high priority, then time is of the essence and only a few

TABLE 11-2

Pushing and Pulling Guidelines

1. Avoid pulling objects. Push objects whenever possible.

2. Whenever an EMT is moving an object, either by pushing or by pulling, the EMT should attempt to keep his back straight.

3. Push while standing and walking only if the object is at waist height.

4. If the object is below the waist, either kneel or use a rope, or similar device, to extend the arm's reach.

5. The EMT should try to keep his elbows bent and close to his sides while pushing.

Safety Tip

Most EMS agencies do not permit the assistance of civilians with a carry as a matter of policy. An EMT who is injured during a carry will be afforded medical care under workers' compensation and disability, but civilians who help and get hurt are left to their own resources. A back injury can be a lifelong affliction, so to ask a family member, or any civilian, to help may be exposing the person to unnecessary injury, long-term medical care, and perhaps no chance of recovering related costs.

carries are useful. If the patient is low priority, then more time can be taken to safely move the patient.

What are the resources at hand? The EMT carefully assesses the amount of "muscle" that will be needed. Calling for help from the middle of the staircase is a little too late.

Communicate the plan of carry to everyone involved. Sometimes a more experienced EMT may have an alternative approach that saves time or energy. Once the decision has been made, it is important that everyone stick to the plan. Typically, the person at the head of the patient makes the calls for when to lift, turn, and move.

The heaviest end of a stretcher is the top half, where the torso lies. Typically, when a heavy person is being carried, the strongest EMT takes the head. When the patient is being brought down a flight of stairs, the situation is reversed, and the strongest person should be at the feet.

Whenever a carry is being planned, the most important point for the EMT to remember is to know his personal limits. Stopping a carry to rest the back or relax the fingers can prevent fatigue from replacing common sense. Every EMT wants to get the job done. However, no EMT wants to get hurt or to cause further injury to the patient while getting the job done.

Obese Patients

Overweight or obese patients provide the EMT a unique transportation challenge. Most standard EMS carrying devices are not designed to carry the additional weight of these patients. For example, a typical backboard may only be rated for 300 pounds maximum. Loading a heavier patient onto these backboards risks having the backboard break and the potential of dropping the patient. Every EMS system should make arrangement, also known as preplan that includes both manpower and equipment, to be able to provide care, including transportation, to these patients.

Emergency Moves

In some situations, the patient needs to be moved immediately. The risk of serious injury, or even death, outweighs the risk of harm that might occur from moving the patient in a hasty extrication.

In those emergencies, the EMT should first consider whether he is prepared and capable of entering the scene and removing the patient. The first priority of every EMT is personal safety.

In the case in which the EMT can reasonably enter the scene safely and rapidly remove the patient, he should attempt to do so. Table 11-3 lists the four principal reasons that a patient should be removed quickly using an **emergency move** technique.

Emergency Drags

When the situation is critical and time is of the essence, the EMT cannot afford to wait for additional support. He must act quickly and efficiently. In these cases, he should perform an **emergency drag**. When an EMT, using a minimum of supplies, grabs a patient and hauls her to safety, he is performing an emergency drag.

The Clothing Drag

The easiest emergency drag to perform is the **clothing drag**. As shown in Skill 11-2, the shirt collar or a handful of clothing is grabbed from behind the neck. Using two hands, the EMT walks backward while dragging the patient along with him. The patient's head remains cradled between the rescuer's forearms.

TABLE 11-3
Reasons for an Emergency Move
1. Presence of fire or immediate danger of fire
2. Explosions or immediate danger of explosions

3. Inability to protect the patient from life-threatening hazards
  a. Potential for structural collapse
  b. Gathering hostile crowd
  c. Gunfire in the vicinity

4. Access to another more seriously injured patient is blocked by the patient

Safety Tip

Although car fires do occur, the number of fires that occur in MVCs is extremely small, as little as 1%. Patients in MVCs should be properly assessed before a decision is made to remove them.

The danger of creating permanent paralysis from aggravating a cervical spine injury is greater than the theoretical danger of the patient's becoming burned in an automobile fire that does not exist. A rule of thumb is that the patient should remain in the car unless smoke is clearly visible. Consult the fire officer on scene for guidance in such matters.

Street Smart

Patients frequently collapse in cardiac arrest while in the bathroom. Although it is possible to attempt a resuscitation in the bathroom, it is frequently more reasonable to move the patient to an adjoining hall before starting cardiopulmonary resuscitation (CPR).

The additional room provided helps to ensure that everybody has space to work without interfering with or injuring someone else.

SKILL 11-2 *The Clothing Drag*

PURPOSE: To permit the EMT to drag the patient to safety using the patient's clothing.

STANDARD PRECAUTIONS:

☑ Appropriate personal protective equipment

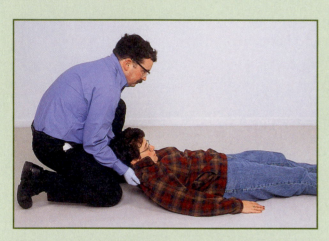

1 The EMT grasps the patient's clothing at the collar, while cradling the patient's head on his forearms.

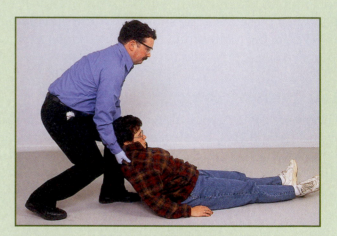

2 Crouching down, with back straight, the EMT walks backward.

The Arm Drag

If a good handhold on the clothing cannot be obtained, then the EMT can try an **arm drag**. The EMT, as seen in Skill 11-3, grasps the wrists of the patient, pulls her arms to her chest, and drags her by the arms. The arm drag can be very effective provided the patient can hold her head up. If the patient is unconscious, do not use the arm drag. The head of an unconscious patient may fall forward, blocking the patient's airway, or fall backward, injuring the head and neck.

First, the EMT must partially prop the patient up to a semireclined position, holding the patient upright against his knee. The EMT then slips each of his arms under the patient's shoulders. Grasping the patient's right wrist with the left hand and the patient's left wrist with the right hand, and crossing them over the patient's chest, the EMT has a tight grasp of the patient.

The EMT then squats and then stands erect, walking backward to safety.

The Blanket Drag

If the patient is large or the EMT is having trouble dragging the patient, a blanket can be an invaluable tool. The EMT can logroll the patient onto a blanket, sheet, or drape, then drag the patient to safety.

SKILL 11-3 *The Arm Drag*

PURPOSE: To permit the EMT to drag the patient to safety using the extremities.

STANDARD PRECAUTIONS:

☑ Appropriate personal protective equipment

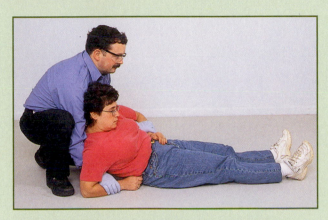

1 Kneeling down, the EMT slides his arms under the patient's arms and grasps the wrists across the chest.

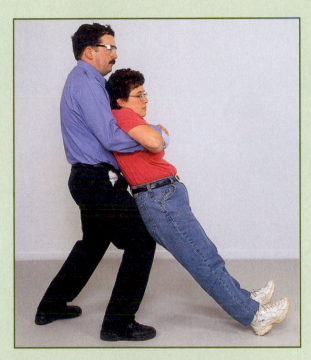

 Standing up, the EMT walks backward.

The EMT should quickly straighten the patient's legs, place his forearm along the patient's spine while cradling the patient's head in the palm of the hand. Using the other arm, the EMT should reach under the patient's arm and grasp the patient by the shirt or chest, then carefully roll the patient over onto his back, trying to move the patient as a unit.

Once the patient is supine, the EMT rolls up the edges of the blanket to form a horseshoe-shaped collar. The patient's head, now partially supported by the blanket, is protected from striking the floor. The patient can now be dragged, using a **blanket drag**, across the floor quickly.

A distinct advantage of the blanket drag is that when other help arrives, there are many readily available handholds to help with the drag, and with enough hands the body can even be lifted and carried. Skill 11-4 demonstrates the blanket drag.

> **Safety Tip**
>
> The one-person logroll is *not* the preferred method of handling a trauma patient with a potential spinal injury. It should be used only when the patient is in danger of serious injury, or even death, if not moved quickly.

SKILL 11-4 *The Blanket Drag*

PURPOSE: To permit the EMT to drag the patient to safety using a blanket.

STANDARD PRECAUTIONS:

☑ Appropriate personal protective equipment

☑ Blanket, tarp, drape, or similar covering

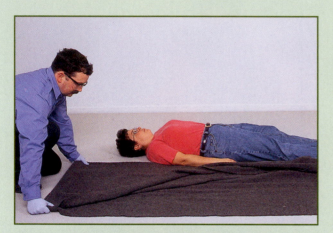

1 Place the blanket along the long axis of the body, leaving about a foot of material at the head.

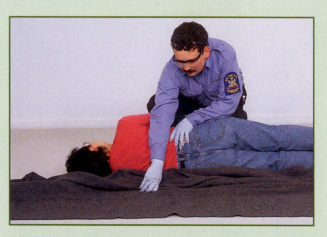

2 Logroll the patient onto the blanket, pulling the blanket underneath the patient.

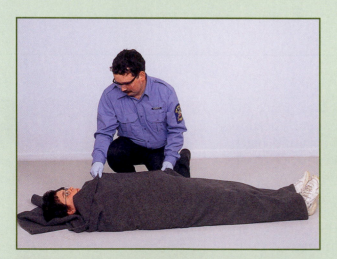

3 Wrap the patient with the blanket, protecting the patient.

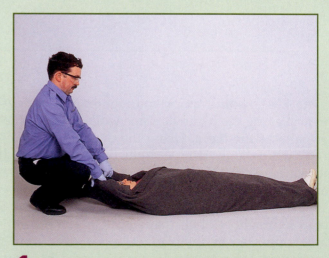

4 Roll up the excess material at the head and grasp the roll.

The Firefighter's Drag

All of the preceding drags require that the EMT drag the patient backward. These drags are effective when the patient has to be moved only a few yards. However, these drags are physically exhausting for a single EMT to perform. The **firefighter's drag** uses a simple cotton triangular bandage, called a **cravat**, to make the work of moving the patient much easier.

The EMT uses the cravat to secure the patient's wrists together. A hitch over each wrist and then a knot will securely tie the wrists together.

With the hands securely fastened together, the wrists are draped over the neck and shoulders of the EMT while the EMT is on hands and knees. The patient is then dragged under the EMT. The EMT can still look forward and see where he is going, as shown in Skill 11-5. The patient is also protected from any falling debris by the body of the EMT.

SKILL 11-5 *The Firefighter's Drag*

PURPOSE: To permit the EMT to drag the patient to safety while still looking forward.

STANDARD PRECAUTIONS:

☑ Appropriate personal protective equipment
☑ Triangular bandage

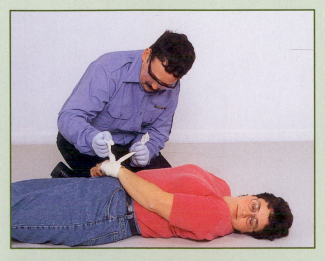

1 Using the triangular bandage, folded into a cravat, the EMT secures the patient's wrists together.

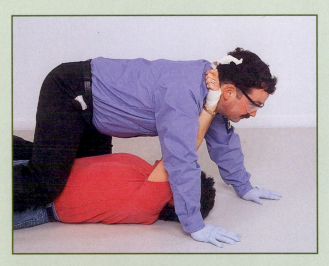

2 While on all fours, the EMT drapes the tied hands over his shoulders and drags the patient underneath him.

Street Smart

Securing a patient's wrists together whenever the patient is being moved is so common that many EMTs keep a cravat in the pocket of their turnout coat. Practice tying someone's wrists together until it becomes second nature.

Emergency Carries

If the EMT has the strength or the patient is small enough, it may be easier to just pick up the patient and carry her. Such a carry, although more difficult to perform than a drag, will result in the patient's being moved farther from the danger more quickly.

The Rescuer Assist

If the patient is able to walk and an EMT is available, then he can assist the patient. While assisting the patient, with the **rescuer assist**, the rescuer is acting like a crutch.

The distinct advantage of a rescuer assist is that if the patient suddenly becomes weak, the EMT can drag the upright person to safety. This rescue move is used by soldiers to assist exhausted or "walking wounded" comrades. Skill 11-6 demonstrates the techniques used.

SKILL 11-6 *The Rescuer Assist*

PURPOSE: To permit the EMT to assist the walking, but injured, patient to safety.

STANDARD PRECAUTIONS:

☑ Appropriate personal protective equipment

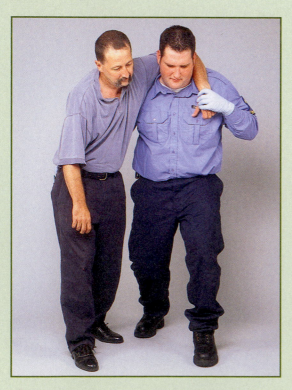

1 The EMT crouches to the patient's level and swings one arm over the EMT's shoulders.

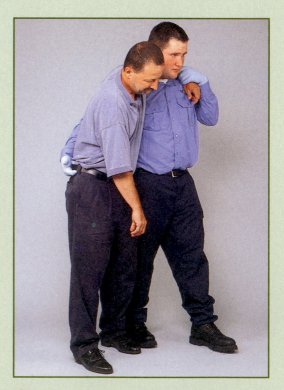

2 With one hand grasping the patient's beltline, and another grasping the patient's wrist, the EMT stands and assists the patient with walking.

Note that, if necessary, the EMT can let go of the wrist and waist and the patient can drop flat on the ground. Also, if another rescuer suddenly becomes available, he can take the patient's other side and assist the first rescuer.

The Pack Strap Carry

If during an assist a walking patient becomes weak or even loses consciousness, the EMT can quickly change from a walking assist to a **pack strap carry**. The EMT simply lets go of the arm under the patient's shoulder, steps in front of the patient, reaches back, and grabs the now hanging arm by the wrist. Once the EMT has a firm grasp of the wrist, the EMT pulls both arms forward while he is bending over. When the pack strap carry is done correctly, as shown in Skill 11-7, the patient's weight should be on the EMT's back and the

---

SKILL 11-7 *The Pack Strap Carry*

PURPOSE: To permit the EMT to carry an injured person on his back to safety.
STANDARD PRECAUTIONS:

☑ Appropriate personal protective equipment

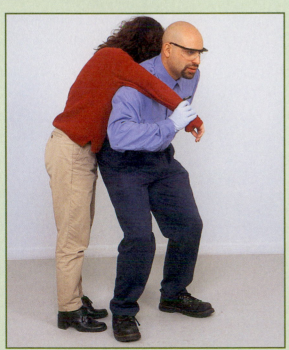

1 Crouching in front of the seated patient, the EMT grasps the patient's wrists and then pivots on his heels, draping the patient's arms over his shoulders in the process.

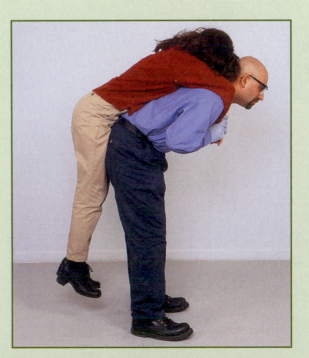

2 The EMT then stands, hoisting the patient onto his shoulders and off her feet. (This carry is also useful if the patient who is being assisted suddenly tires and needs to be carried. The EMT would simply release the belt and step in front of the patient, grasping the free hand and placing it over his shoulders.)

patient's feet should be off the ground. This technique is very hard on the EMT's back and should be done only in an emergency when no other means of transport are feasible.

The Cradle Carry

If the patient is a small adult or a child, often the EMT can pick the patient up in his arms. Skill 11-8 demonstrates this **cradle carry** technique. This technique permits the EMT to quickly move the patient to safe ground. It also places a great deal of stress upon the EMT's back. Only small adults or a child should be picked up and carried in this manner.

The Firefighter's Carry

If the patient is unconscious and needs to be moved quickly from the scene, the **firefighter's carry** remains one of the most effective carries. Unfortunately, although it is effective, it is also difficult to master and takes a great deal of practice to perform correctly. Skill 11-9 demonstrates the series of maneuvers that must be performed to properly execute the firefighter's carry.

The patient must start supine in front of the EMT. The patient's knees must be flexed. Flexing the patient's knees is accomplished by pushing the patient's feet backward toward the body utilizing the

SKILL 11-8 *The Cradle Carry*

PURPOSE: To permit the EMT to carry a non-ambulatory or unconscious patient to safety.
STANDARD PRECAUTIONS:

☑ Appropriate personal protective equipment

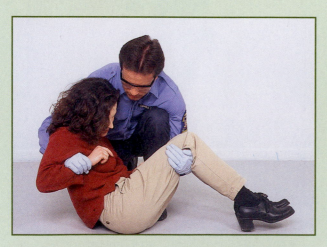

1 The EMT first kneels next to the supine patient, placing one hand under the shoulders and the other hand under the knees.

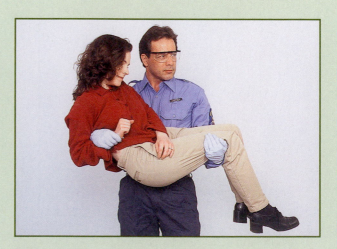

2 The EMT then stands, keeping the patient's body close to his.

SKILL 11-9 *The Firefighter's Carry*

PURPOSE: To permit the EMT to carry an unconscious patient quickly to safety.

STANDARD PRECAUTIONS:

☑ Appropriate personal protective equipment

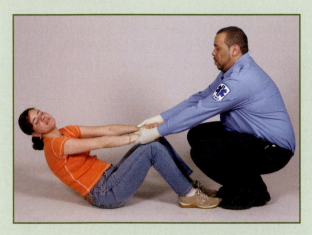

1 The EMT starts by standing toe to toe with the supine patient. Crouching down, he grabs the patient's wrists and proceeds to roll the patient to a seated position.

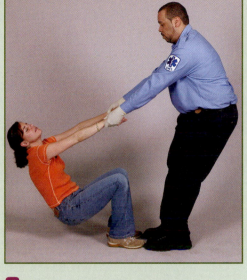

2 Without stopping, the EMT then pulls the patient as nearly erect as possible.

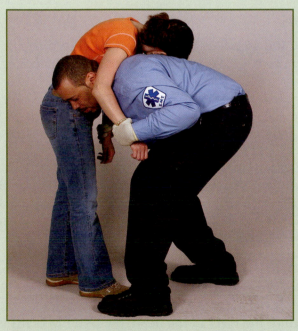

3 Quickly crouching again, the EMT places his shoulder into the patient's abdomen, while simultaneously standing.

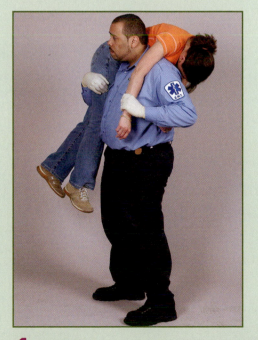

4 The EMT then puts one arm through the patient's legs and grasps the patient's hand with his free hand. (Another EMT may help hoist the patient up onto the shoulders of the EMT. The second EMT waits until the patient is up and over the first EMT's shoulders, then, grasping the patient's knee, helps hoist the patient.)

EMT's feet. Locking the patient's feet down by stepping on the toes with the tip of the EMT's boots, the EMT reaches forward and grasps the two wrists of the patient.

The next step is very important and must be done in a fluid motion. A moment's hesitation and the EMT could drop the patient. The patient is quickly moved to a near-standing position by being pulled upward to her feet. At the same time, the EMT ducks under the patient and then drops a shoulder down under the patient.

When the patient is squared over the EMT, the EMT stands up. Putting his arm between the patient's legs and coming around the front of the knee, the EMT grasps the arm that is dangling in front. Locking his hand and arm around the patient's wrist and leg effectively fixes the patient onto the EMT's shoulders. The EMT now has one hand free to open doors or carry bags. The bulk of the patient's weight is over the EMT's shoulders and is easier to carry.

The Seat Carry

If the patient is able to assist with his own rescue and there are two EMTs available, then the **seat carry** is useful. With the seat carry, the two EMTs form a seat by grasping wrists, as demonstrated in Skill 11-10. With arms locked out at the elbows, the two EMTs drop to opposite knees and the patient sits.

The patient can now place her arms around the shoulders of the two EMTs for balance. Standing upright, the two EMTs are able to walk while carrying the patient.

Note that the patient must remain capable of assisting with the carry. This carry is very useful if the patient has a leg or foot injury and is unable to walk.

The Chair Carry

Carrying a person by the wrists or clothing can be very difficult at times. When there are two EMTs, and time permits, transferring a patient to a carrying device, such as a backboard or a stairchair (a specially designed chair for carrying patients down stairs), can be very helpful. If no such devices are available and the patient needs to be moved quickly, any standard kitchen chair can be used for a **chair carry**.

The patient should be supine. Lift the patient's legs. Lay the chair down and slide it in under the patient's buttocks. While grasping the patient's waistband, advance the chair until the patient appears to be sitting in the chair, flat on his back. Now lift the chair to the normal seated position, as shown in Skill 11-11.

If the patient is unable to assist the EMT with sitting in the chair, a cravat secured to the chair can be wrapped around the chest. One EMT turns and, facing forward, grasps the legs of the chair. The other EMT grabs the back of the chair.

Together, on the call of the EMT at the head, the two EMTs lift the chair and proceed to walk out of the room. Skill 11-11 demonstrates how two EMTs perform the chair carry.

Although this carry is very useful for the debilitated patient, it should not be used with unconscious patients.

SKILL 11-10 *The Seat Carry*

PURPOSE: To permit two EMTs to assist an injured, but conscious, patient to safety.

STANDARD PRECAUTIONS:

☑ Appropriate personal protective equipment

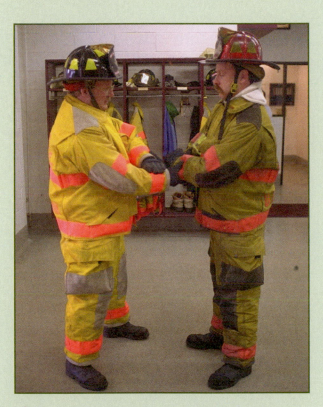

1 The two EMTs clasp arms. Each EMT grasps the other EMT at the elbow as shown here.

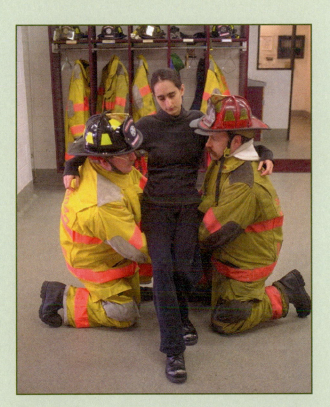

2 With one pair of arms high, the patient sits back into the seat that has been created. The EMTs then stand together, at the same time.

Street Smart

Before using a kitchen chair, check to see whether the chair legs can hold the patient's weight. Chairs are not designed to be used in this fashion, and only sturdy chairs should be selected. If in doubt, the EMT should choose another means of moving the patient.

SKILL 11-11 *The Chair Carry*

PURPOSE: To permit two EMTs to safely move a conscious patient, using a chair as a carrying device.

STANDARD PRECAUTIONS:

☑ Appropriate personal protective equipment

☑ Hardback chair

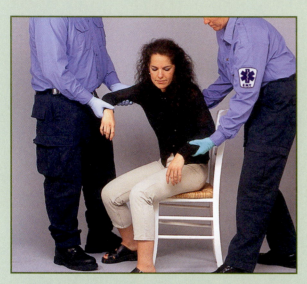

1 The patient is assisted to sitting in the chair.

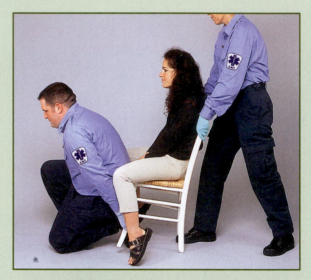

2 One EMT kneels in front of the chair, facing forward and between the patient's legs. He reaches back and grasps the legs of the chair.

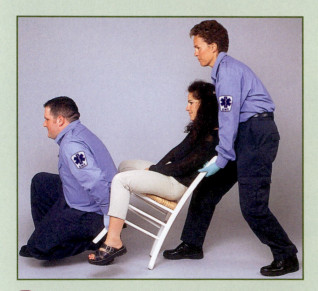

3 The second EMT, at the back of the chair, grasps the uprights of the chair and leans the chair backward.

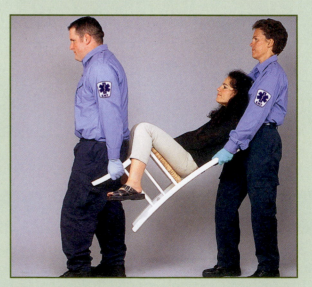

4 Simultaneously, the two EMTs lift the patient up and proceed to walk forward together.

Nonurgent Moves

Most of the time, patients are not urgent. When an EMT takes the time to carefully prepare for the carry, it is a low-priority move. The patient's safety and comfort, as well as the safety of the entire prehospital team, are the EMT's primary concerns. There are a number of devices and methods to safely move a patient from the scene, to an ambulance cot, to the hospital gurney.

Command and Coordination

One misstep can turn a simple lift and carry into a disaster. Without coordination of all team members, a fall may occur that could injure the patient, the crew, or the EMT. A few simple rules, agreed to ahead of time, can prevent tragedy from striking.

Almost by convention, the EMT at the head of the patient or to the patient's left side is in charge. That EMT decides when to lift, when to turn, or when to stop.

It is expected that the team's leader will exercise his command by giving specific orders, for example, "Turn on three—one, two, three."

To be understood, orders must be loud and clear. There is no room for confusion or misunderstanding. The EMT should state the objective clearly and ensure that all members of the team, even if it is just one more EMT, understand.

✴ *A Fall at Home*

The scene is a house call for a medical emergency. An elderly patient, who has fallen, called EMS. Paramedics from the fire department are already on scene.

As A. J. steps out of the ambulance, he looks up at the three-story house. Located in an older section of the city, the house is in the old Victorian style, including narrow halls and even narrower stairs.

Once A. J. reaches the top of the stairs, he is greeted by the fire lieutenant. Lt. Groat explains that the patient had slipped on a throw rug, fallen, and appears to have broken her hip. The patient's vital signs are stable. A routine transfer is needed to a local hospital for further evaluation and possible surgical repair of the hip.

The only problem is that she fell in the bathroom between the toilet and the bathtub. There is plenty of help available. She is not urgent at this time, so the EMT discusses the method of removal with the paramedic.

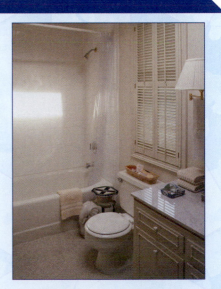

(Courtesy of PhotoDisc.)

- What methods could the EMT use to move the patient in this case?
- Suppose the patient had fallen in the dining room. Would that location change the method used?
- What method would be used if the patient's problem were shortness of breath instead of a probable hip injury?

By agreeing to these simple rules of lifting and moving, the EMTs can ensure that the patient's transport will be uneventful and the EMTs can decrease their risk of back injury.

The Extremity Lift

The **extremity lift** is perhaps one of the most commonly used lifts in EMS. It is used to transfer a patient from a bed to a stretcher or from the floor to a stretcher. It *cannot* be used to transfer a trauma patient to or from a stretcher because the extremity lift does not protect the spine.

The first EMT comes from behind the patient and slips his hands under the patient's arms. The first EMT then grasps the opposite wrist of the patient from his own. It is helpful if the second EMT grasps the patient's wrists and brings them to within reach of the first EMT.

The second EMT then slips his hands under the patient's knees. If the patient were to be carried any distance, then the second EMT would kneel between the patient's knees, grasp each knee with his hands, and, while facing forward, stand up, while lifting the patient and then walking. Skill 11-12 demonstrates this useful technique.

SKILL 11-12 *The Extremity Lift*

PURPOSE: To permit two EMTs to lift a patient onto a carrying device.

STANDARD PRECAUTIONS:

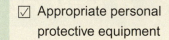
☑ Appropriate personal protective equipment

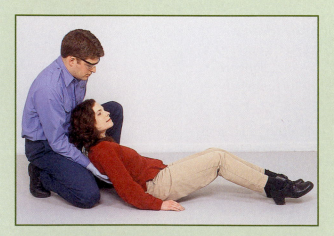

1 The first EMT kneels behind the patient and helps the patient up to a sitting position. The patient can be rested against the EMT's knee for a moment.

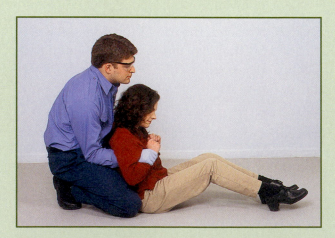

2 The EMT then reaches under the patient's arms and grasps the patient's wrists, pulling them against the patient's chest tightly.

(continues)

SKILL 11-12 *(continued)*

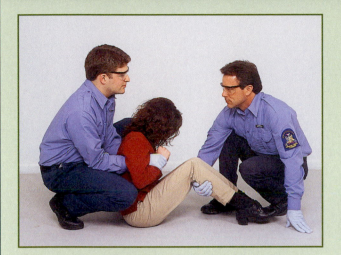

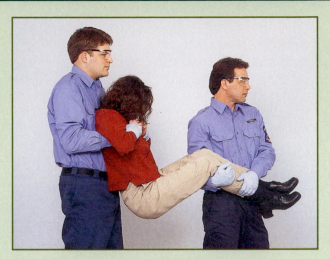

3 The second EMT then crouches. Reaching down on each side, the EMT grasps under the patient's knees. (In some cases, it may be more convenient to crouch beside the patient's knees and hook arms under the patient's knees.)

4 Simultaneously, the two EMTs stand with the patient and walk forward together.

The Direct Lift

When the patient needs to be moved from the floor to a bed or to a stretcher, and only one side of the patient is accessible, the EMTs can try a **direct lift**. It takes disciplined teamwork to perform a direct ground lift correctly. The direct ground lift does not protect the spine during movement and is *not* used for trauma patients.

The two or, preferably, three EMTs line up next to the patient. All three kneel with one knee down and one knee up. The EMT at the patient's head cradles the patient's head and neck with his hand. The same EMT slides his arm under the patient's shoulders.

The second EMT slides one hand under the lumbar section of the patient's back, in the hollow of the back, and the other hand under the patient's buttocks. The third EMT slides one hand in the hollow under the back of the knees and the other hand under the patient's ankles.

On command, all three EMTs lift the patient, as a unit, to their knees. The patient should be resting comfortably, with arms crossed upon the chest, in the arms of the three EMTs. Skill 11-13 demonstrates the position in which the patient should be resting.

If the patient needs to be moved only a foot or so, to an awaiting stretcher, for example, then all three EMTs, on command, lean forward while dropping the raised knee to the ground.

If the patient needs to be moved a greater distance, across a room for example, then all three EMTs, on command, roll the patient toward their chests. This technique keeps the patient's weight centered over the EMT's center of gravity and helps prevent back injuries.

The three EMTs then stand and walk, in unison, lock-step fashion, to the stretcher or bed.

SKILL 11-13 *The Direct Lift*

PURPOSE: To permit two or more EMTs to lift and carry a patient to a carrying device.

STANDARD PRECAUTIONS:

☑ Appropriate personal protective equipment

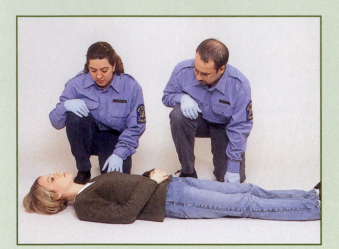

1 All of the EMTs stand on one side of the supine patient, then kneel, on the same knee, beside the patient.

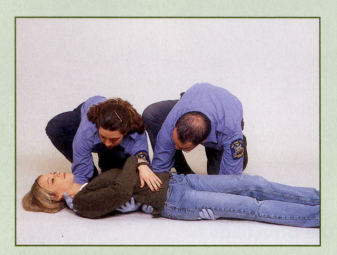

2 The first EMT places one arm under the patient's head and neck and the other arm under the shoulders. The second EMT places his arms under the patient's lower back and buttocks.

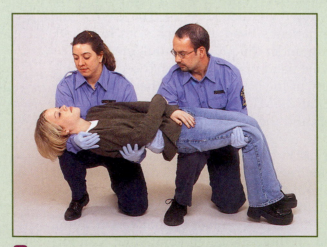

3 Simultaneously, the two EMTs hoist the patient to their knees. If the patient is being transferred to a stretcher on the other side of the patient, they need only drop the one knee to move forward and over the stretcher. If the patient is to be carried any distance, the EMTs should roll the patient against their chests and then walk forward together.

The Scoop Stretcher

The **orthopedic stretcher** was designed to fit into tight spaces, where both sides of the patient could be reached. The orthopedic stretcher is meant to be broken into two halves, utilizing the releases at both ends. Each half of this split stretcher is then slipped under the patient. When the patient is firmly on the orthopedic stretcher, the orthopedic stretcher is reconstructed. In effect, the patient is scooped up by the two halves of the orthopedic stretcher. This is why the orthopedic stretcher became labeled as the **scoop stretcher**.

Although the operation of the scoop stretcher, demonstrated in Skill 11-14, appears easy, the EMT must be cautious. Often the patient's clothing, floor coverings, and even the patient himself, are pinched by the scoop stretcher.

The scoop stretcher has a void in the middle and therefore does *not* support the spine directly. For this reason, the scoop stretcher is used as a temporary transfer device while a patient is moved to a backboard for routine spinal immobilization.

SKILL 11-14 *The Scoop Stretcher*

PURPOSE: To permit two EMTs to carry a patient on an orthopedic, or scoop, stretcher to another carrying device.

STANDARD PRECAUTIONS:

☑ Appropriate personal protective equipment
☑ Orthopedic stretcher

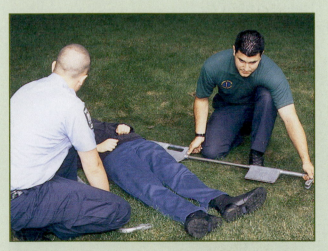

1 The scoop stretcher must be split into its two halves, and the two halves adjusted to the patient's length.

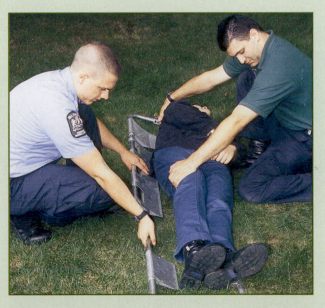

2 The patient is then logrolled to one side, and the scoop stretcher half placed along the patient's axis. This process is repeated with the other side, and the two ends are secured.

**Street
Smart**

Current models of stairchairs offer the advantages of rollers or slides that decrease the lifting and carrying required by the EMT. Whenever they are available the EMT should consider taking advantage of these labor-saving devices, which also help to reduce the danger of back injury.

**Street
Smart**

It is the wise EMT who buckles the patient's arms inside the straps of the stairchair or other device. Securing the arms prevents the patient from reaching out and grabbing a rail suddenly.

It is the wise EMT who tells the patient to keep his hands inside the blankets and explains to the patient why. A few moments reassuring the patient may prevent a disastrous fall due to the patient's suddenly flailing and grabbing, throwing the EMTs off balance.

Scoop stretchers are designed to be narrow and are made of rigid tubular aluminum, which adds strength to the frame. Some design features make the scoop stretcher ideal for transfers out of cramped quarters, confined spaces, or narrow hallways. For example, if a sailor became ill and had to be carried out through narrow ship corridors, the scoop stretcher would be very useful.

Stairchairs

Occasionally a patient will not tolerate lying flat on a litter, scoop stretcher, or Reeves stretcher. Most such patients have some difficulty breathing while lying flat. The solution is simple. Use the chair carry that was described earlier.

Manufacturers of patient-carrying devices have taken the simple chair carry to its logical conclusion. By adding seat belts for the patient and handles for the EMT, they created the **stairchair**.

The stairchair is frequently used in the city or anywhere there are narrow hallways and flights of stairs. It requires two EMTs to move the patient.

Some stairchairs are lightweight and compact, requiring the EMT to carry the patient. Others are designed with rub bars and wheels. The rub bars permit the stairchair to be slid from step to step down a flight of stairs. The wheels permit the stairchair to be used like a wheelchair, rolling the patient down hallways, and to the ambulance.

The Stair Carry

Stair carries, using a stairchair or other carrying device, can be very dangerous. The EMT must concentrate on both balancing and carrying his load as well as stepping from step to step without the benefit of seeing where he is stepping.

Note the EMT in Figure 11-4 at the bottom of the stairs. Her hand is on the small of the back of the EMT at the feet, providing a little reas-

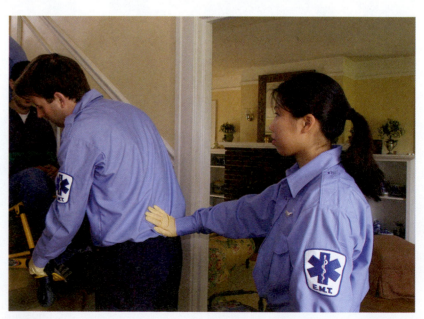

FIGURE 11-4 A hand in the small of the back reminds the EMT that there is help if needed.

EMS in Action

One of the biggest obstacles EMS providers deal with is moving patients. Houses are not built with consideration to cots making corners, long boards turning, or stairs wide enough for people to carry someone down them. I have taken windows out to get coded patients to the ambulance, dragged them on blankets, carried them on folding chairs, and just about any other method of moving that you can come up with.

I recall one call for an elderly female who had a hip and knee transplant. She had gone to the basement to get something, twisted, and dislocated the replacement hip. When we arrived, she was sitting on a chair that she used to bend over to reach low in the cupboard. The prosthetic hip was tenting against the skin on her hip and she was in excruciating pain. The considerations were several:

- How to immobilize her hip with as minimal movement as possible?
- How to get her up the narrow and turning stairs, which would not allow anyone to be beside her?
- How to set her up for transport to the hospital?

We carry a folding stair chair in the rig, so we set this up so that it would go down the stairs and make the corners. To immobilize her hip, we placed pillows between her knees and legs and secured them with triangular bandages. We placed the stair chair beside the chair we found her in and carefully moved her to it. Once on the stair chair, we strapped her to it very tightly, with her hips and legs especially secure. By adding a rope to the chair to pull with, we moved her up the stairs to the yard.

Our next concern was moving her to the cot. This would take an additional move to her hip, which was extremely touchy and fragile. We decided to leave her on the chair, place it on a long board, raise the head of the cot a few inches, and secure the chair to the cot. This way we eliminated one painful and possibly dangerous move. It worked, and she was able to be treated without surgery. The doctor informed her that as weird as it was transporting her in that manner, it may have saved her from another surgery and replacement.

Treatment is not the only complicated decision made by EMS providers. Every call may be one like this, in which you have to step back and figure out what might work.

Tom Chartier, EMT-I
EMS Instructor
Western Iowa Tech Community College, Sioux City, Iowa
Woodbury Central High School, Moville, Iowa

surance as well as some immediate support should the EMT walking backward stumble and fall. It is important that the EMT does not grab the belt. With the hand on the belt, the hand can become trapped; if someone stumbles, then everyone falls.

With each step, the EMT guiding the crew should be calling out the steps until the EMT carrying the patient reaches bottom—for example, "Step, another step, three steps left."

Often the EMT carrying the patient has a difficult time seeing the steps and feels for them with his foot first, then places it flat when he is sure it is on a firm surface. A little reassurance by the guide EMT can be very comforting and ensures patient safety.

The patient should always be carried down the stairs feet first for a number of reasons. One of the most important reasons is to keep the patient from feeling as if he is falling.

Whenever an EMT is carrying a patient down stairs, it is important that he keep his back straight and bend at the hips and knees. The stairchair or stretcher needs to be carried as close to the body as is practical.

Off-Road Stretchers

Walking across uneven terrain and rough ground while carrying a patient is a formula for disaster. A misjudged step or a turn of an ankle and both crew and patient take a fall. The use of special off-road stretchers decreases the hazard that uneven surfaces pose to the EMT and the patient.

The Basket Stretcher

The original **basket stretcher** was made of chicken wire stretched over a rigid steel metal frame. It was designed to carry a patient in the basket, hanging from a cable, between ships during World War II. Basket stretchers were made available to fire rescue after the war by Civil Defense and have seen active use ever since.

Modern basket stretchers, such as the **Stokes basket**, are made of fiberglass-plastic composites that will withstand rugged use. The earlier wire baskets were difficult to use in wilderness situations because they tended to get caught on tree branches and did not protect the patient. The full fiberglass shell of a Stokes basket avoids this problem.

A Hunting Accident

The day was perfect for hunting. The leaves were down, the sky was clear, the sun was warm, and the wind was calm. Everything was perfect, or so Tom thought as he climbed into the old tree stand for a look around. He knew he wasn't supposed to climb up anything he hadn't set up himself, but he just wanted a quick look.

Now, here he was lying on the ground, at the foot of the tree, with an arrow impaled in his thigh. Thank goodness for cellular phones.

One quick call and a lengthy description of where he was and help was on the way. He estimated that he was about 4 miles north of Beaver Dam Road.

He started to wonder, "How are they going to get me out of here?"

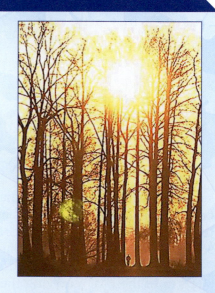

- What method would be used to carry this hunter out of the woods?
- What method would be used if the trail were narrow?
- What would the team do if a fallen tree obstructed their pathway?

Furthermore, a Stokes basket can be pulled across snow and ice much as a sled would be. However, in defense of the wire basket, the Stokes and other similar shell baskets are heavier to carry. For this reason, many rope rescue experts still prefer the lighter wire baskets.

The Flexible Stretcher

A modern cousin of the basket stretcher is the **flexible stretcher**. An example of a flexible stretcher is a SKED. These plastic stretchers are lightweight and can be rolled up. In use, the flexible stretcher wraps around the patient, like a cocoon, and becomes rigid. Because of its small size, it is useful in confined-space rescues and cave rescues.

Moreover, because it is lightweight, it has seen extensive service in wilderness and rope rescues. The U.S. military uses the SKED flexible stretcher in many of its tactical rescue operations.

All baskets have multiple handholds for convenience. Some manufacturers have even attached a tubular metal rail around the top of the basket. This permits a limitless number of handholds. In all cases, these handholds serve as both a grab point for rescuers and a point of fixation for straps or webbing.

For protection, the patient in a basket stretcher must be securely strapped in. While the patient is being carried over rough terrain, he might be tipped over accidentally and may even be dropped. The patient can be securely anchored to the basket using a length of webbing, looped like a shoestring, between handholds.

Another device commonly used in transporting a patient out of a house is the **Reeves stretcher**. This flexible stretcher was designed by a Philadelphia police officer, named Reeves, and a tent maker, named Smith.

The problem they had was carrying patients out of the two- and three-story walk-ups in the city. Using a little imagination, they created a flexible stretcher that worked something like the corsets commonly worn at the time.

The Reeves stretcher has long thin slats that run lengthwise down the stretcher. These slats are sewn into a canvas litter. The result is that the Reeves can be rolled up and carried under the arm. Yet, when a patient is placed on top of the Reeves the slats create a rigid surface to carry the patient.

Handholds for carrying are provided at each corner of the Reeves as well as on the sides. The patient is usually rolled to one side, the Reeves is slid under the patient, then the patient is rolled to the other side, and the Reeves is pulled through. Three straps, sewn into the stretcher, secure the patient.

 Street Smart

A common problem with carrying a patient on a Reeves flexible stretcher is that the patient's feet rub against the pant legs of the EMT. To prevent this problem, the EMT places the patient on the Reeves flexible stretcher with about a foot of material left below the feet. When the patient is lifted, the extra material folds over the feet and protects the EMT's pants.

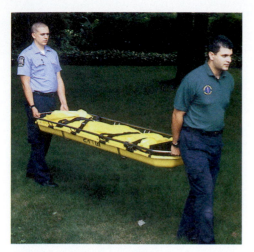

FIGURE 11-5 The end-to-end stretcher carry can be used to carry patients long distances.

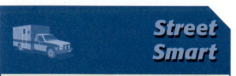

Street Smart

Experienced EMTs know that it is safer to lift and stand with the patient while someone else rolls the ambulance stretcher under the backboard than it is to try to walk with the patient to the ambulance stretcher.

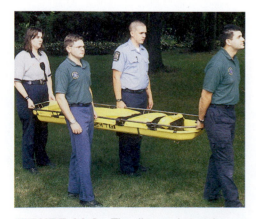

FIGURE 11-6 The diamond stretcher carry is used to transport patients over uneven terrain.

Off-Road Carries

There are a number of methods of carrying a stretcher off-road. Some are more suited to short hauls, while others are more suited to long wilderness carries.

Each carry is also dependent on the number of providers available. Whereas four people can carry a stretcher, it may be preferable to let two carry the stretcher if the hallway, or trail, is narrow.

Rescuer fatigue, the patient's weight, and the distance to be covered must all be factored into the decision of which carry is to be used.

The End-to-End Carry

Since early history, wounded soldiers have been removed from the battlefield to an aid station or field hospital by fellow soldiers, paramedics, or corpsmen using a portable stretcher called a **litter**.

The U.S. Army litters were typically made of sturdy canvas and two rigid poles. Some of these portable litters even had legs that could be used to convert the litter to a temporary bed when needed. A quick emergency litter can be rigged up using two pike poles and a woolen blanket.

Usually only two EMTs are available to carry the patient. In those cases, each EMT grabs the end of the litter and lifts: an **end-to-end stretcher carry** (Figure 11-5). If any amount of distance needs to be covered, the two EMTs need to be facing the same direction. Careful observation of army medics evacuating a wounded soldier will reveal that no one is walking backward. Both carriers face forward because the danger of tripping is greater when walking backward.

However, if the ground is level and the patient is being moved only a few feet, then the two EMTs can face one another during the carry. If the carry is more than 20 feet, then both EMTs should be facing forward.

The Diamond Stretcher Carry

If the trip is more than a dozen or so feet and the ground is uneven, then it is not safe for two people to carry a patient. It is important that all sides of the litter, basket, or backboard be supported.

As described earlier, the first two EMTs each take an end of the carrying device, facing each other. The next two EMTs take a position at each side of the carrying device. All EMTs are now in a position for a **diamond stretcher carry** (Figure 11-6).

On the signal of the EMT at the head, the four EMTs lift together. All of the EMTs should be using a power grip and be performing a power lift. The lift should be steady and even.

Once all EMTs are fully erect and comfortable with their stance, the EMT at the patient's feet will turn around and face forward, in the direction of travel. Notice that the EMT at the head of the patient is facing the patient. He is monitoring the patient's condition—mental status, airway, and so on—while carrying the patient.

Now the team is ready to move, again on the signal of the EMT at the head. Once the team has arrived at the destination, the procedure is reversed. The patient has now been moved safely and effectively.

The Four Corners Carry

Very similar to the diamond carry is the **four corners carry** (Figure 11-7). The four corners carry is useful when carrying a basket or similar device over a great distance: for example, for several miles out of the backcountry. As many as six or even eight EMTs can be involved in this carry. Therefore, it is a very useful carry for extremely heavy patients or when patients and equipment are heavy.

Each EMT grabs either the corner of the basket or somewhere in the middle, and they all face one another. It is preferable to pair EMTs across from each other according to height and strength. This arrangement works to even the load when it is carried and to create a balance.

On the signal of an EMT at the head, everyone squats, and then they all lift together. After the team has adjusted their stance and is ready, the team turns, together, in the same direction. This means that only one hand is in contact with the basket. It is important to remember to lift with the legs and not with the back.

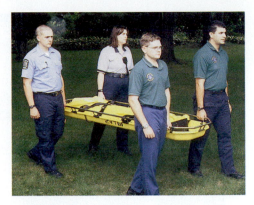

FIGURE 11-7   The four corners carry is used to transport a patients over long distances and rough terrain.

The Use of Slings

It is tiring to carry a patient on a litter or in a basket with one hand. The body has a tendency to twist to one side, and the muscles of the back have to compensate in order to keep the back straight. Loops of webbing called **slings** are used to help even the load.

The sling, as demonstrated in Skill 11-15, is looped in a half-hitch through the handhold or rail. It is then slung over the shoulder to the opposite hand. After the load is lifted, the EMT grasps the sling, or **stringer**, and pulls down. Pulling down on the stringer uses the shoulders as a fulcrum and helps to balance the load.

Passing over Obstacles

In the course of moving a patient, many obstacles may get in the way. A common obstacle is the guardrail along the roadside. The EMT must be careful not to drop the patient while overcoming the obstacle.

The best way to overcome an obstacle is to pass the patient over the obstacle to waiting EMTs on the other side. This maneuver is called the **caterpillar pass**.

Stopping in front of the obstacle, the EMTs turn and face each other, firmly grasping the backboard or basket with two hands. Two or more EMTs line up on the other side. The backboard or basket is now handed over, hand over hand, to the EMTs on the other side.

The key is to have all EMTs standing still. No feet should be moving. If the obstacle is a low embankment, in which case establishing a rope system would be time consuming or unnecessary, then a human chain is created up the embankment. Skill 11-16 shows a group of EMTs working together to carry a patient up the embankment.

When the EMTs become fatigued, they use the caterpillar pass to hand off the patient to other EMTs. Two EMTs, who may have been ahead clearing the path, stop at the front of the basket. The team turns and grabs the basket with two hands.

The two fresh EMTs replace the two EMTs at the head. The two EMTs at the head slide down to the middle, and the two EMTs in the middle

SKILL 11-15 *Use of a Stringer*

PURPOSE: To aid the EMT who is carrying a stretcher a distance.

STANDARD PRECAUTIONS:

☑ Appropriate personal protective equipment
☑ Loop of webbing, approximately 6 feet long
☑ Stretcher

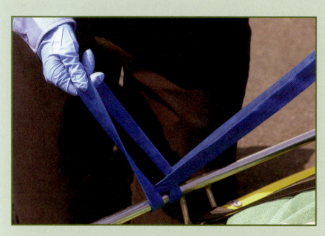

1 The EMT places the webbing under the bar, or under the handhold, and loops it back through itself, in effect creating a half-hitch.

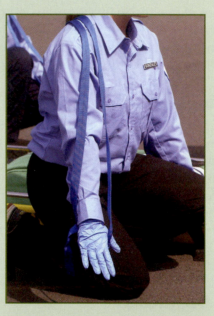

2 The EMT then kneels next to the stretcher and slips the loop of webbing over his shoulder, being sure that the webbing knot is not on the shoulder.

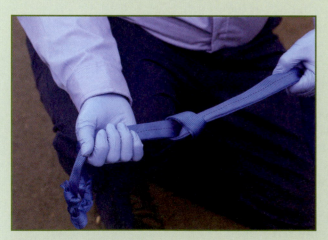

3 Then the EMT slips his opposite hand inside the loop. It may be necessary to shorten the length of the loop by tying a knot in the webbing.

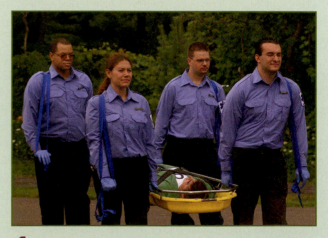

4 Once standing, the EMT adjusts the loop over his shoulders. One hand should be carrying the stretcher, and the other hand should be exerting downward force on the loop, in effect balancing the load.

SKILL 11-16 *The Caterpillar Pass*

PURPOSE: To permit the EMT to move the patient on a stretcher or litter over an obstacle.

STANDARD PRECAUTIONS:

☑ Appropriate personal protective equipment
☑ Stretcher or litter

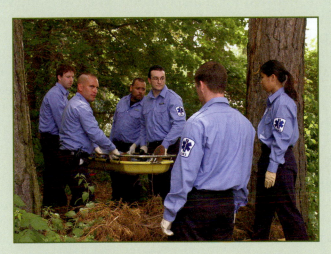

1 Coming to the obstacle, all EMTs stop and turn toward each other.

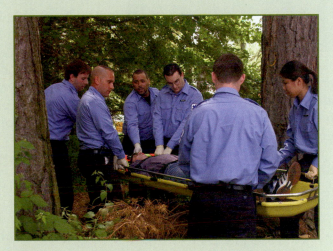

2 Two EMTs go around or over the obstacle and take a position across from the litter. The front of the litter is then handed to them across the object.

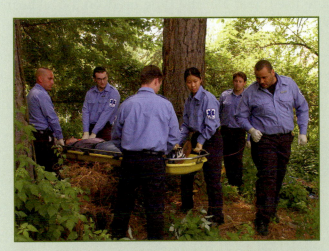

3 As the litter is passed forward, the two EMTs in the rear move forward to take position beyond the obstacle.

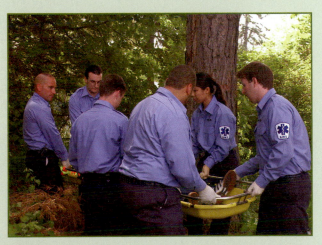

4 All EMTs remain standing with feet firmly planted as the litter is passed. Once the litter is beyond and clear of the obstacle, all EMTs turn and face forward. The EMTs may then move forward together as a unit.

replace the two EMTs at the end. The last two EMTs are now relieved of duty and typically take a position in front of the team as scouts.

PACKAGING THE PATIENT

Trundle, gurney, stretcher, and cot—these are all names for the portable rolling bed in an ambulance. Yet, the ambulance cot is more than just a conveyance. It is part of the plan of treatment. Older litters provide only one position, flat. Modern ambulance cots may be adjusted to different positions according to the patient's needs.

Ambulance cots usually have linens that provide comfort and warmth to the patient. These **bedrolls** are wrapped around the patient when she is prepared for transportation. The EMTs in Skill 11-17 are demonstrating one method of making a bedroll, as well as how to wrap the patient in the bedroll.

A large percentage of body heat is lost from the head and neck. To conserve this heat, and to make the patient more comfortable, the EMT should wrap the head with the bedroll's collar. Loss of body heat can lead to a condition called hypothermia. Hypothermia is an especially serious problem for trauma patients.

Positioning

If the patient's feet are up, more blood goes to the brain; if the head is up, the patient breathes more easily. The EMT must make a conscious decision every time he places a patient on a stretcher as to which position is best for the patient. That decision must be medically motivated.

Strapping

To prevent the patient from being thrown from the ambulance cot during sudden stops, the EMT must secure her to the cot. Usually seat belt–style straps are used, just like the type used on a backboard. Figure 11-8 shows a patient properly secured to the ambulance cot.

The first strap secures the upper torso. If it is cold outside, the patient's arms are bundled inside the blankets and both arms and chest are strapped in. Otherwise, most patients prefer to have their arms outside the strap. Leaving the strap under the arms and over the chest allows the EMT to take blood pressures and pulses more easily.

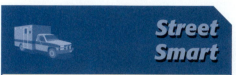

Street Smart

There is nothing worse than being strapped down, flat on your back, and then being forced to endure rain falling on your face.

Experienced EMTs keep a bath towel under the head of the cot, between the mattress and the frame, or wrapped in the bedroll. During inclement weather, the EMT will place the towel loosely over the patient's face.

Courtesy requires that the EMT advise the patient of his intentions before covering the patient's face.

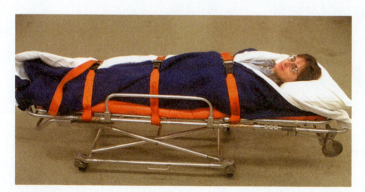

FIGURE 11-8 The patient must be safely secured to the stretcher before transportation can begin.

SKILL 11-17 *The Bedroll*

PURPOSE: To allow the EMT to provide warmth and comfort to the patient.

STANDARD PRECAUTIONS:

☑ Appropriate personal protective equipment

☑ Stretcher, blanket, sheet, pillow, pillowcase

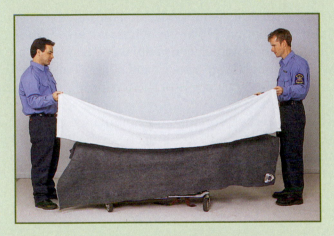

1 The first EMT centers the blanket on the stretcher and then places the sheet on top of that.

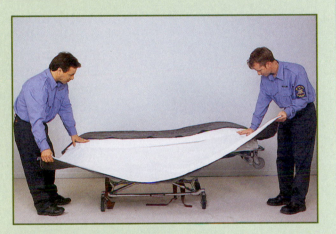

2 The first and second EMT grasp one half of the linen and fold it in half, creating a collar. Then they do the same with the other side. To open the bedroll, the EMTs simply grasp the collar and unfold the edges.

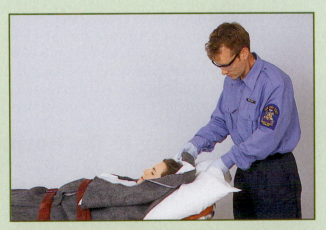

3 With the patient lying supine, the EMTs can fold the upper edge over the patient's head, then secure the edge with the lower edge. The pillow should then be placed behind the head, outside the linen.

The middle strap is usually adjusted over the pelvis, as a seat belt would be. It is important to place the middle strap over the bony pelvis. If the seat belt is riding higher on the abdomen and the ambulance is struck from behind, the patient may experience internal damage to his abdominal organs because of the whiplash effect.

The last strap is across the legs, usually at or about the knees. Often equipment, such as an oxygen tank, is secured with this strap as well. It should be emphasized that whenever a hard object is placed against soft tissue and then securely strapped in place, there is a potential that the object will hurt the patient. A pad, such as a small pillow, should be placed over the patient's knees to prevent this discomfort.

Transferring to the Ambulance

Ambulance cots come with wheels for a reason. Ambulance cots are usually rolled to their destination. However, whenever an ambulance stretcher is in the high position, which is usually waist height for most EMTs, it can tip over. Although large wheels and a large base provide some stabilization, the ambulance cot is prone to tipping, especially when going around corners.

For this reason, many rescue squads and ambulance companies have policies that state that "loaded" cots must be in the low position every time the patient is moved. In every case in which the ground is rough or uneven, an EMT should be on each side of the cot to protect the patient from a fall.

Loading the Ambulance

How an EMT loads an ambulance cot depends on the ambulance manufacturer's recommendations. Nevertheless, the principles of lifting remain the same. The EMT must have his feet firmly planted and his back straight, lifting with the legs and not the back, using a power grip and lifting as a team member.

The hardware placed on the floor of the ambulance is designed to hold the ambulance cot in place in case of a collision (Figure 11-9). These pieces of hardware are subject to some of the most grueling conditions of any equipment on board an ambulance. Consider the fact that the ambulance cot is the single most used piece of equipment aboard any ambulance. For this reason alone, ambulance cots need to be inspected daily and given preventive maintenance regularly.

Transferring to the Hospital Bed

Arriving at the hospital, the crew would unload the ambulance cot, following good back care practices, and proceed to roll the patient into the hospital. Some patients, when lying flat and moving backward, complain of feeling nauseated. As a matter of practice, most EMTs roll the cot feet first. As noted earlier, many EMTs leave the cot in the low position, decreasing the likelihood that the cot will tip over.

The first person the crew is likely to encounter is the triage nurse. He will assign a room and maybe even the nurse who will be taking the report. Occasionally, the patient is transferred from the ambulance cot to a hospital wheelchair. The extremity lift is very effective in those

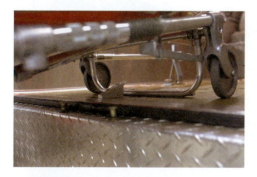

FIGURE 11-9 Ensure that the ambulance cot has firmly engaged the locking hardware.

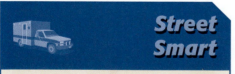

Street Smart

Whenever the patient is on the stretcher, one EMT should have at least one hand on the stretcher at all times. Wheeled devices always have a tendency to roll. If a wheel should strike a pothole, for example, the stretcher could inadvertently tip over, potentially further injuring the patient in the process.

cases. Be sure the wheels on the wheelchair are locked before moving the patient over.

Once the patient's room has been found, the EMTs will prepare to transfer the patient over to the hospital gurney. Be sure the wheels of the hospital gurney are in the locked position. Leave the hospital gurney flat. It is easier to transfer a patient to a flat surface than it is to an incline. Once the patient is on the hospital gurney, the head can be elevated as needed.

There are a number of transfer devices that can be used to move a patient from the ambulance cot to the hospital gurney. By far the most common device used to transfer patients is the backboard.

Get the two stretchers as close to each other as possible. Be sure to lower any side rails that would interfere with the transfer. Next, release the ambulance cot straps but *not* the backboard straps. Check the backboard straps, and make sure they are secure. Often, straps are loosened during transport to access arms for blood pressures and the like.

One EMT takes a position on each end of the backboard and they move the patient over as a unit, on the signal of the EMT at the head. If the patient is heavy, consider either having two EMTs on each end or lifting the patient and having a third EMT switch the two stretchers.

The Carry Transfer

Occasionally a cubicle, at a doctor's office or a clinic, is too narrow to accept the crew, the ambulance cot, and the gurney. In those cases, the ambulance cot is placed against an adjunct wall and the crew performs a direct carry, or a **carry transfer**, from the ambulance cot to the gurney. Skill 11-18 shows the position of the two stretchers.

The EMT should take the time to plan this move. Standing in the middle of the room holding a patient in midair and then realizing that the stretcher is positioned incorrectly can be embarrassing.

The Draw Sheet Transfer

For many decades, nurses have used **draw sheets** to transfer patients from one bed to another or from hospital bed to gurney. A draw sheet is either a regular sheet folded over in half or a sturdy linen of equal length. The advantage was that a patient could be pulled across from bed to bed with ease.

Many EMTs utilize the **draw sheet transfer** technique for transferring patients from the ambulance cot to the hospital gurney. With the two stretchers next to each other, and with side rails down, each EMT grabs a side of the cot's linen. If the patient is heavy, the EMT may have to climb onto the hospital gurney; remember to lock those wheels.

Each EMT grabs a handful of sheet and rolls it into a stiff collar. Taking a moment, each EMT pulls against the other. This pulling performs two functions. First, it checks the integrity of the sheet; if it is going to tear, it will do so now. Second, it ensures that all the slack has been taken out from under the patient. Skill 11-19 shows how the patient is transferred in an almost hammocklike affair.

SKILL 11-18 *The Carry Transfer*

PURPOSE: To permit the EMT to move the patient from one stretcher to another stretcher.
STANDARD PRECAUTIONS:

☑ Appropriate personal protective equipment

☑ Two stretchers, gurneys

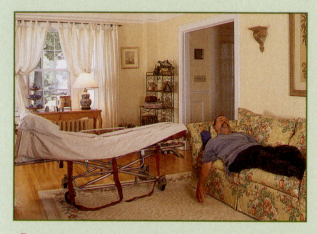

1 The first stretcher is placed with the patient's head at the foot of the other stretcher at a 90-degree angle.

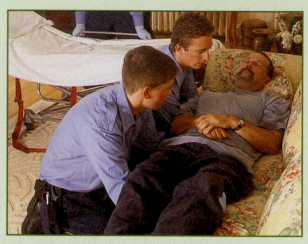

2 The two EMTs stand on the side of the patient, and the first EMT places one arm under the patient's head and neck and the other arm under the shoulders. The second EMT places his arms under the patient's lower back and buttocks.

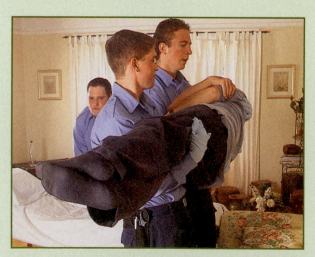

3 Simultaneously, the two EMTs hoist the patient to their chest. Shuffling sideways, the two EMTs move the patient to the awaiting stretcher.

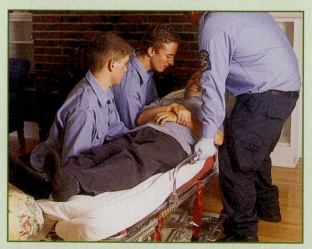

4 The patient is then gently laid onto the awaiting stretcher. The EMT should be sure that all stretcher straps are attached before moving the patient.

SKILL 11-19 *The Draw Sheet Transfer*

PURPOSE: To allow a patient to be moved from stretcher to hospital gurney.

STANDARD PRECAUTIONS:

☑ Appropriate personal protective equipment

☑ Two stretchers, draw sheet or bed linen

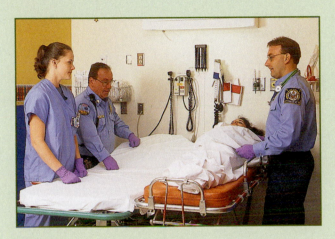

1 The two stretchers are placed side by side. The EMT should be sure that the stretcher brakes are engaged before moving the patient. Any side rails present will have to be lowered.

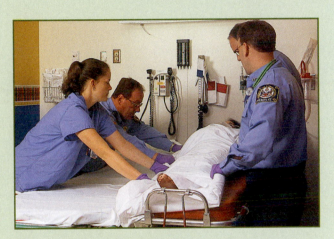

2 Two EMTs are on the one open side of both stretchers. Rolling the edge of the draw sheet or bed linen into a collar, the EMTs grab a firm purchase. (It is a good practice to have the two teams of EMTs pull vigorously against each other to test the strength of the sheet.)

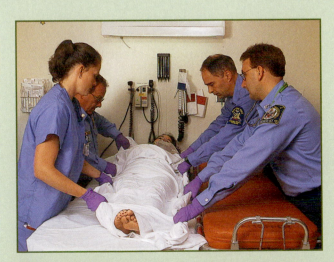

3 Simultaneously, the four EMTs slide the patient from one stretcher to the other in one fluid motion.

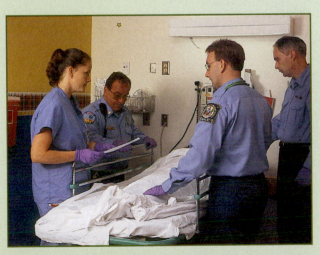

4 Once the patient is on the new stretcher, the side rails should be replaced.

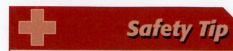

EMTs are cautioned that it is very easy to overextend the back in these cases, with resultant injury. If in doubt, consider alternatives such as the transfer board.

The Use of a Transfer Board

In response to the alarming rise in back injuries, many hospitals have purchased **transfer boards**. Transfer boards, also called slide boards, act as a smooth surface on which to slide the patient from one stretcher to another. Some newer-model hospital gurneys have a transfer board built into the frame.

The transfer board simply reduces the friction, and therefore the work, between the patient and the stretcher. With the hospital gurney slightly lower than the ambulance cot, the patient is pulled across using the draw sheet technique.

CONCLUSION

Without exception, every EMS call involves several lifts, carries, or transfers. That means that every EMS call could also end with a back injury or worse. Unfortunately, transfers are so commonplace that the EMT forgets to practice good back care principles and injuries occur.

Exercise, use of braces, and proper lifting and carrying help prevent back injuries. Most important, every EMT should know his limits. An EMT should never be afraid to ask for lifting assistance.

Every back injury means pain and suffering for the EMT as well as another provider potentially lost to EMS.

TEST YOUR KNOWLEDGE

1. What is proper back care?
2. What are the proper body mechanics that an EMT should observe?
3. What safety precautions should an EMT observe before lifting?
4. What are the guidelines for reaching?
5. What are the guidelines for lifting?
6. What are the guidelines for carrying?
7. What are the guidelines for pushing and pulling?
8. What concerns must be addressed before moving a patient?
9. Why would an emergency move be necessary?
10. What are the four emergency drags?
11. What are the six emergency carries?
12. How does an EMT lift a patient from the ground to the stretcher?
13. How are the following patient-carrying devices used?
    a. orthopedic, or scoop, stretcher
    b. stairchair
    c. basket stretcher

    d. flexible stretcher

    e. portable stretcher (litter)

    f. wheeled stretcher

14. What precautions must be taken when carrying a patient down a flight of stairs?

15. What methods are available to carry a litter or stretcher?

16. How is a patient packaged for transport?

17. What are the safe transferring techniques EMTs use at the hospital?

INTERNET RESOURCES

- Search the Web for additional exercises you can do for your back such as those you can find at http://www.thermacare.com and http://www.exrx.net.

- Search for additional resources on proper techniques for lifting such as those at http://www.stronghealth.com (search for "tips for proper lifting").

- Search for the various lifts and equipment discussed in this chapter and take notes on additional information you are able to find. Share your findings with your colleagues.

FURTHER STUDY

Hegner, B. R., & Caldwell, E. (2004). *Nursing assistant: A nursing process approach* (9th ed.). Clifton Park, NY: Thomson Delmar Learning.

U.S. Fire Administration and Federal Emergency Management Agency. (1994). *EMS safety: Techniques and applications* (Publication No. FA-144). Emmitsburg, MD: USFA Publications.

EMS *in Action*

You can, in fact, drive from a scene with all the ambulance doors open. They *will* close if you are driving fast enough.

My partner and I, along with a rookie observer, responded one midnight to a "liver pain" call. My partner and the rookie knocked on the door, with no response. I had returned to the truck to talk to dispatch about making a call-back to the house when the front door opened. I saw my partner running back to the ambulance, shouting in a whisper. Since my partner was a seasoned, methodical EMS provider who almost never ran, I thought we had a code or other critical situation. I started grabbing equipment to take to the house.

When my partner got close enough for me to hear him, I realized he was whisper-shouting, "He's got a gun. He's got a gun!" I was between the ambulance and the front door, so I dove into the truck, landing between the front seats and on top of two PASG hard cases. The rookie was at the driver's door, running in place and getting nowhere.

A seasoned provider and driver *can* pick up a 200-pound rookie, throw her across the driver's seat and on top of a 150-pound crew chief. Two women *will* recline, though not terribly comfortably, in the space between the front seats of a van ambulance with two PASG cases! And the doors *will* close when you drive off quickly enough, regardless of the rookie saying, "But the doors are open!"

Points to be taken:

- Get enough information from your dispatcher.
- Do not get yourself into a situation like this (and only *you* can prevent that from happening).
- Always park your unit so it is positioned for a quick, forward exit.
- Know safe and appropriate approach techniques.
- *Always* know your cover and concealment options.
- Know what a "kill zone" is and be aware of where you are in it.
- *Always, always* listen to any "hinky" feeling that you may get on any call or from any patient. It's almost always right!

EMS safety is not an option, nor should it ever be an afterthought. It is more essential to you than the ABCs! It should be proactive, practiced, and policy.

The rookie went on to become a good paramedic. My partner that night was my husband, and if something should have gone wrong, we would have left our three-year-old daughter an orphan. Remember, and be safe.

Allisynne Dunlap, EMT-P
Program Director II
West Virginia EMS Technical Support Network
Elkview, West Virginia

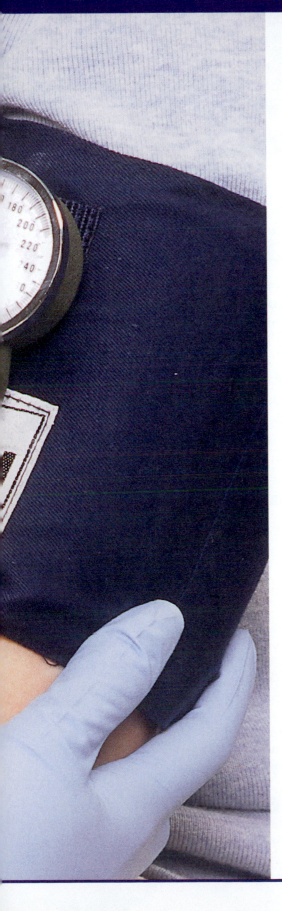

Patient Assessment— General Principles

Before an EMT can apply the new skills she has acquired, she must learn how to assess the patient and determine what help is needed.

In some cases, the EMT must quickly make an assessment, decide what needs to be done, and then prioritize care so that the patient may receive the maximum benefit from on-scene care without needless delay to definitive treatment.

In every case, the EMT must be vigilant, constantly assessing and reassessing, looking for those changes that may signal a deterioration in the patient's condition and intervening before the patient suffers further harm, or even death.

This section begins with an explanation of the initial assessment and takes the EMT through the entire patient contact, ending with the ongoing assessment.

CHAPTER 12

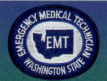

Scene Size-Up

KEY TERMS

crumple zone

dangerous instrument

deadly weapon

environmental assessment

global assessment

high index of suspicion

initial report

loaded bumper

Occupational Safety and
Health Administration
(OSHA)

perimeter

risk factors

safety corridor

size-up

staging

step blocks

triage

OBJECTIVES

Upon completion of this chapter, the reader should be able to:

1. List important safety regulations that pertain to EMS.
2. Describe a "standard approach" to an EMS call.
3. List the scene information that may be obtained from the pre-arrival instructions.
4. Discuss the importance of staging as a protective behavior.
5. Describe what is meant by the term *scene size-up.*
6. List risk factors at residential EMS calls.
7. List the elements of a global survey.
8. List risk factors at the scene of a motor vehicle collision.
9. Describe how the EMT can manage on-scene risks.
10. Describe how to protect the public's safety.
11. Describe what to look for during a damage survey.
12. Demonstrate the minimum actions to stabilize an automobile.

OVERVIEW

Many emergency medical technicians (EMTs) will admit that the excitement of the red lights and sirens, and the possibility of danger, attracted them to the field. However, no one really joined emergency medical services (EMS) expecting to get hurt. Unfortunately, injuries—preventable injuries—do occur.

Chapter 4 stresses the importance of personal well-being and a healthy lifestyle in reducing the chances of injury or illness. Those strategies to prevent injuries are important. This chapter stresses the protective behaviors an EMT should practice while on scene. Please read this chapter carefully. The life you save may be your own!

HISTORY OF SAFETY IN EMS

EMTs have always faced hazards while providing patient care. Extremes of weather, hazardous road conditions, and infectious diseases are just a few of the more common hazards EMTs routinely face.

However, until recently, not much attention was given to responder safety and injury prevention. In 1973, the federal report *America Burning* drew attention to the growing problem of on-the-job injury in the fire and emergency services. Since that report, the fire service, the country's largest EMS provider, has made injury prevention and responder safety a top priority.

National focus groups, such as the National Fire Protection Association (NFPA), started to publish recommendations and standards for safe emergency operations. Yet many of these recommendations and standards were not actively pursued by many fire and EMS agencies.

The complacency of fire and emergency services toward safety standards, particularly related to infectious disease, all changed on March 6, 1992, when the federal **Occupational Safety and Health Administration (OSHA)** issued the blood-borne pathogens rule, OSHA 1910.1030 (29 CFR 1910.1030). The blood-borne pathogens rule simply says that EMS agencies are responsible for the safety of their employee-members. It further states that the government can enforce that responsibility.

With that single regulation, the federal government assumed a prominent role in EMS safety. The intent of the rule was to eliminate or reduce the incidence of EMS workers' exposure to blood-borne pathogens. The effect of the rule was to shake up the emergency services community and awaken them to the serious safety concerns that exist. Table 12-1 reviews a number of important regulations and standards that have had a dramatic impact on emergency services nationwide.

In response to this challenge, EMS and the fire service have institutionalized safety practices, have distributed standard operating guidelines, and are starting to employ safety officers.

Street Smart

Although the National Fire Protection Association (NFPA) only establishes standards and has no ability or authority to enforce them, these standards are frequently adopted, in part or in whole, by OSHA. Therefore, many EMTs monitor the changes in the NFPA standards closely for the opportunity to see what OSHA may require in the future.

TABLE 12-1

Rules, Regulations, and Standards That Affect EMS

1. Occupational Safety and Health Administration (OSHA) Regulations
   1910.10.146, *Confined Spaces*
   - Outlines training and precautions, including a permit, required to enter confined spaces
   1910.134, *Respiratory Protection*
   - Provides guidelines for use of respiratory masks, fit testing, and physical performance requirements
   1910.120, *Hazardous Waste Operations and Emergency Response*
   - Also known as HAZWOPER, established requirements for hazardous materials awareness for all emergency responders
   1910.1030, *Occupational Exposure to Bloodborne Pathogens*
   - Requires emergency responders be protected from blood-borne pathogens; includes training mandates as well as exposure procedures

(continues)

TABLE 12-1 (continued)

Rules, Regulations, and Standards That Affect EMS

2. National Fire Protection Association (NFPA) Standards

   NFPA 473, *Competencies for EMS Personnel Responding to Hazardous Materials Incidents*
   - Established standards for emergency responders to hazardous materials incidents

   NFPA 1500, *Fire Department Occupational Safety and Health Program*
   - Established standards and guidelines for fire service health programs

   NFPA 1521, *Fire Department Safety Officer*
   - Established standards for the safety officer, outlining duties and responsibilities

   NFPA 1561, *Fire Department Incident Management System*
   - Established standards for a common approach to public safety incidents for the fire service

   NFPA 1581, *Fire Department Infection Control*
   - Established standards for infection control programs and departmental guidelines

   NFPA 1582, *Fire Department Medical Requirements for Fire Fighters*
   - Established standards for physical requirements, including immunizations, for firefighters

   NFPA 1999, *Protective Clothing for Emergency Medical Operations*
   - Established standards for protective clothing, including protection against infectious materials

3. Centers for Disease Control and Prevention (CDC)
   - Provides guidelines for prevention of transmission of human immunodeficiency virus

4. Ryan White Comprehensive AIDS Resource Emergency Act of 1990
   - Requires the creation of a designated officer as well as disease-reporting requirements

5. Environmental Protection Agency (EPA)

   40 CFR 311, *Hazardous Materials Response*
   - Established requirements for responders to hazardous materials incidents

These safety officers are charged with upholding applicable federal and state law as well as departmental regulations. This duty includes training EMTs and firefighters about safe practices. On the scene of a major incident, the safety officer performs as a member of the incident management's command staff.

Today's modern EMS agency cannot afford to ignore the risks associated with being an EMT. Whenever possible, the EMT must be afforded protection against foreseeable injury or illness. The EMT

Accident on the Interstate

"Ambulance 24, motor vehicle collision on Interstate 66 at mile post marker 124, unknown injuries, time out 16:20." After throwing out their lukewarm coffee, Joe and Kenny fasten their seat belts and turn on the emergency lights.

As is typical, the situation is an unknown collision. The 9-1-1 caller probably was on a cell phone and cannot be reached again. Looking ahead, they can see that traffic is backed up for about half a mile. Joe carefully turns the ambulance onto the shoulder of the roadway and slowly proceeds toward the scene.

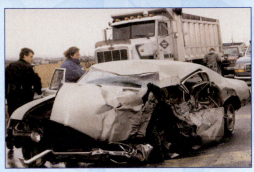

(Courtesy of David J. Reimer Sr.)

- What are the risk factors on the scene of a motor vehicle collision?
- If this had been a house call, would the risk factors be different?
- How does an EMT routinely approach every scene?
- How do you prepare for the hazards involved in a motor vehicle collision?
- What type of additional resources would be needed to handle those hazards?

must also be trained to identify scene hazards, mitigate those hazards, and implement scene safety in general.

Times have changed, and a reckless disregard for one's personal safety is no longer acceptable. Whenever an EMT is responding to an EMS call, the first question the EMT must answer is, "Is the scene safe?"

STANDARD APPROACH

When EMTs approach a scene, they are all thinking the same thought: "Is the scene safe?" The only thing that may be different is the circumstances on scene. Only when the EMT has assessed the scene for hazards and has controlled those hazards can an EMT make a decision to care for the patient.

Careful attention to this process of scene approach, assessment, and hazard control helps to ensure the safety of the EMT. Eventually the EMT will automatically integrate the process of approach, assessment, and control into practice. This level of behavior is usually seen in the most experienced EMTs.

Dispatch Information

The EMT should use every resource available to assess the scene for hazards. The first source of good information about scene hazards is the information from the communications center.

The dispatch information may describe the mechanism of injury or the nature of illness. The nature of the call, be it medical or trauma, illness or injury, will have to be confirmed on arrival, but the EMT can assume, with some confidence, that the dispatch information is accurate.

Street Smart

A senior EMT will often sense that something is "just not right." She will take in all the information on the scene, compare it with her own experience, and come to a subconscious conclusion that danger is present. This so-called *intuition* is often the result of right-brain thinking, and all of this information processing is often accomplished in a matter of seconds. Whenever a senior EMT has a "sixth sense" that the scene is not safe, listen!

Listening carefully to the dispatch of other emergency services can also provide the EMT with additional information regarding on-scene hazards. For example, when a fire engine is dispatched to a motor vehicle collision (MVC), the EMT might conclude that there may be a fire hazard present. Or, if a police unit is dispatched for a fight in progress, the EMT might conclude that there is violence on scene and weapons may be present.

When a heavy rescue has been requested by the first arriving law enforcement units, the EMT might conclude that patients might be entrapped. If multiple emergency services are responding to the same accident, then perhaps there are several cars, and multiple patients, involved.

All this information is filtered by the EMT as she tries to make a mental picture of the scene and the hazards that might exist.

Prearrival Instructions

The dispatch information provided by the emergency medical dispatcher, or communications specialist (COMSPEC), contains an abundance of clues regarding the character of the scene. By paying careful attention to the details of the initial dispatch report and prearrival instructions, the EMT can get an early idea, or a *heads up*, on what she is going to encounter.

Table 12-2 lists some of the information that the communications specialist may have available. Today's modern telecommunications centers are electronically linked to a marvelous array of computers and information sources. Weather information, minute-to-minute road conditions, global positioning coordinates, as well as a "history"

TABLE 12-2

Dispatcher Information

1. Nature of emergency—medical versus trauma

2. Patient's level of consciousness

3. Patient's breathing

4. Presence of life-threatening physical conditions—for example, loss of consciousness, chest pain, shortness of breath, abdominal pain

5. Violence on scene—police en route or on scene

6. Fire or smoke condition reported

7. Special equipment needed—heavy rescue extrication

8. Special rescue—for example, confined space, hazardous materials

9. Traffic conditions—fastest route and traffic delays

10. Other responding emergency vehicles

of prior calls at the same location are often available. All the EMT has to do is ask for the information in many cases.

Personal Protective Equipment

Next, the EMT begins to protect herself by donning personal protective equipment (PPE). The type of PPE needed is determined by the nature of the call. Medical calls may require gloves, goggles, and a mask. A trauma call may require the EMT to wear a complete set of turnout gear, including a helmet with an eye shield, a rescue coat, heavy-duty gloves, and a pair of boots.

The dispatch information will provide a clue to the nature of the call and therefore the PPE that will be needed. Please review Chapter 6 for more information on a symptom-based approach to personal protective equipment for medical calls.

Staging

After careful consideration of the dispatch information, the EMT prepares herself physically, perhaps by donning gloves, and mentally, by imagining what she will see when she arrives.

It is important that the EMT does not hastily enter the scene. It is better to proceed slowly into a scene, making assessments for hazards, than to pull into a dangerous situation and try to make a hasty retreat.

Some situations call for the EMT to place the emergency vehicle a safe distance from the scene and observe the scene first (Figure 12-1). Stopping the emergency vehicle a safe distance from the scene is called **staging**.

Staging serves two purposes. First, it may keep the EMT out of harm's way. The best defense against explosions, gunfire, hazardous materials exposure, and the like is distance.

Second, it gives the EMT time to assess the scene from the relative safety of the vehicle. Staging should be a part of the routine response to many hazardous calls.

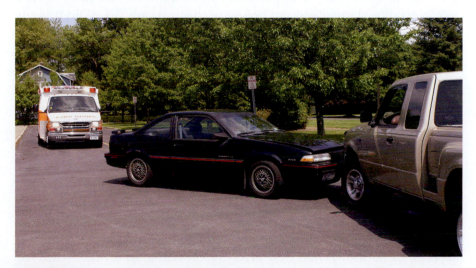

FIGURE 12-1 Parking the ambulance away from the scene provides safety for the EMT and the crew while allowing for an assessment of hazards and needed resources.

Scene Size-Up

The EMT would next perform a scene **size-up**, a term borrowed from the fire service. A size-up is the process of observing a scene and making judgments about the equipment, resources, and personnel that will be needed to stabilize the scene.

The scene size-up, in many ways, started with the prearrival instructions, when the EMT started to visualize the scene in her mind. The size-up continues when EMS first arrives on scene.

The on-scene size-up consists of several parts that are normally done in sequence. Circumstances may require the EMT to be flexible, to perform certain elements of the scene size-up as the opportunity becomes available.

First, the EMT is concerned with the entire scene and what hazards may be present. The EMT is "taking in the big picture," or performing what is called an **environmental assessment**.

Having identified the hazards, the EMT then proceeds to either mitigate the hazards or move the patient to safety, if moving the patient is possible without endangering the EMT.

The EMT then determines the exact nature of the illness or inspects the mechanism of injury. And, finally, the EMT calls for whatever resources are needed to help stabilize the scene.

To get those needed resources, the EMT usually calls in an **initial report**. The initial report establishes that EMS is on scene and in the process of controlling the scene. It also typically describes the scene. Finally, any additional resources needed are often requested at the end of the initial report.

Why Do a Scene Size-Up?

It is natural for an EMT to become engrossed in the excitement of an emergency scene. Rolled-over cars, burned patients, and gunshot wounds can distract the EMT from seeing potentially life-threatening hazards that are ever present on scene.

Yet, these scenes could contain some serious hazards to the EMT. The standardized size-up approach ensures that the EMT does not fail to identify the danger present before rendering care. To avoid this situation, and to improve the chances of survival, the EMT should take a careful *stop, look, and listen* approach.

Stop the ambulance several hundred feet from the scene and visually scan the scene. The EMT should observe for hazards, such as downed power lines.

An EMT can use a pair of binoculars to extend sight and improve vision of the scene (Figure 12-2). Binoculars can be an invaluable tool and should be readily available in the front compartment of every emergency vehicle.

The EMT should also consider rolling a window down and listening. The sounds of breaking glass and gunfire are clearly signs of danger ahead.

Perhaps more alarming than gunshots or shouting is the complete absence of sound. When first arriving on scene, to a house call, for example, the EMT would expect to see a light on the porch or someone at the door waving them down.

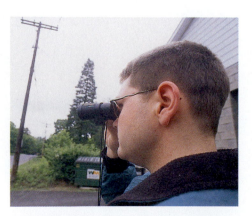

FIGURE 12-2 Binoculars can extend an EMT's field of vision, helping him identify hazards earlier.

If the house is dark and the scene is quiet, there are two possibilities. One, the EMT has simply responded to the wrong address. Or, two, the EMT could be walking into an ambush. The EMT should first call to confirm the address, then consider requesting law enforcement to the scene.

Global Assessment

Once the EMT has performed an environmental assessment for hazards; has taken actions to reduce or eliminate those hazards; and has performed a complete scene size-up, including considering the mechanism of injury or nature of the illness and determining the number of patients, she should stop and make a **global assessment**.

With a global assessment, the EMT takes in all the information she has gathered, considers it, and then makes her initial action plan.

This process of assessing and deciding is turned into action as the EMT gives the initial report and proceeds either to care for the first patient or to establish EMS command.

HAZARD IDENTIFICATION

The EMT must identify hazards on a call. Safety is everyone's job. An example can help illustrate the point.

Take the case of a single patient with a gunshot wound. If law enforcement officers are on hand, creating a perimeter with a safe zone, and the scene is quiet, the EMT might decide to do lifesaving treatments on scene such as airway control.

If a hostile crowd has gathered at the perimeter, the EMT may decide to quickly transport the patient to the relative safety of the ambulance, or to "scoop and run" with the patient, rather than risk an exposure to violence on the street. There have been cases in which EMTs were trying to save a gunshot wound victim, only to have a gang member reach over the EMT's shoulder and shoot the patient again!

These two illustrations represent the same situation, the same mechanism of injury, but different on-scene hazards. The patient's condition was not different. It was the hazards that created a unique environment.

Risk Factors

A risk, by definition, is an exposure to a hazard that could lead to injury. EMS is a risky business, and injuries do occur, but many hazards are predictable and therefore many risks are preventable.

Certain risks are so common, so predictable, that they are almost routine. For example, broken glass would be a typical hazard found on the scene of many motor vehicle collisions, and every EMT knows to wear heavy-duty gloves.

These predictable risks, those seen commonly at certain scenes, can be grouped together and called **risk factors**. Table 12-3 lists risk factors common to certain typical EMS calls.

TABLE 12-3
Risk Factors

Motor vehicle collisions
1. Oncoming traffic
2. Passing traffic
3. Spilled fuels—rear
4. Spilled antifreeze—front
5. Wires down
6. Utility pole suspended
7. Smoke from vehicle
8. Fire visible
9. Surface—slope or uneven
10. Broken glass
11. Loaded bumpers

House calls
1. Animals
2. Damaged stairs
3. Loose rugs
4. Poor lighting

High Index of Suspicion

A **high index of suspicion** describes a way of thinking. This term, borrowed from medicine, precisely describes the viewpoint an EMT should always take whenever she is approaching a scene. When a medical provider is given a fact, she may suspect, or have a high index of suspicion, that other complications that are corollaries to the initial fact may be present.

For example, an EMT may have a high index of suspicion that a patient with chest pain may also have shortness of breath. If the EMT is told that the call is a motor vehicle collision, she should have a high index of suspicion that broken glass, spilled fuel, and a traffic jam may be present on arrival.

The EMT should carefully consider what hazards could be present, then focus her senses, using her eyes and ears, and decide whether the hazard is present. The EMT who approaches a scene unaware or, worse, uncaring, risks bodily harm for herself and for her crew. If the EMT is not looking for hazards, she will not see them. The mental connection between what is seen and the danger that it presents is key to rescuer survival.

Information Overload

Too much information about scene conditions and hazards can lead the EMT to feel frustrated from *information overload*. Information overload can lead to inaction or, worse, inappropriate action. How is an EMT expected to sift through the incredible amount of information that is present on scene?

First, learning how to size up a scene, while at the side of an experienced EMT, can be invaluable. An EMT should be coached. A mentor should tell the EMT what she sees and the danger it represents so that the EMT can see what she is seeing.

If a more experienced EMT is not available, then the EMT should maintain a high index of suspicion and use *Sutton's law*. Willie Sutton was a bank robber. When he was asked why he robbed banks, he replied, "Because that's where the money is." Applied to EMS that means that one should look for specific hazards where they are most likely to be.

Flammable liquids flow and are likely to be under a vehicle or in a low depression. Similarly, smoke rises and would more likely be seen in the sky. An EMT uses her intelligence and a high index of suspicion to ascertain hazards.

Hazards at a House Call

Residential or house calls are the most common calls that an EMT responds to. In many cases, the patient or the patient's family has a pet in the house. Pets can range from the common house cat to the exotic boa constrictor. Many of these animals, under the right conditions, can pose a danger to the EMT.

Possibly the most common animal an EMT will encounter on scene is the dog. Dogs, both large and small, can be a very formidable obstacle, especially when the animal thinks that it is protecting its fallen master (Figure 12-3). In most cases, it is a good idea to insist that the dog be shut in another room before attending the patient.

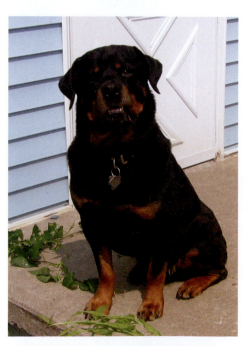

FIGURE 12-3 Dogs represent a real and common hazard to EMTs.

The EMT should never approach an unfamiliar dog without first asking the owner for permission to touch it. After the owner gives permission the EMT should extend the back of her hand to the dog and allow it to come forward and sniff the hand. The EMT should not move forward into the dog's territory; she should wait for the dog to approach her.

The EMT should be cautious around a mother dog with pups or a dog that is feeding; it is at these times that the dog is more aggressive. If the dog should run toward the EMT, the EMT should remain motionless, with hands at her side, and avoid eye contact with the dog. The EMT should never run or scream because the dog's natural instincts will be to pursue her. If the dog knocks the EMT off her feet then she should roll into a ball and keep quiet; the dog will quickly lose interest and disengage from the attack. Above all, the EMT should never look directly into the dog's eyes because the dog may see this as threatening.

Another constant threat to the EMT's safety is poor lighting. Poorly lit hallways and entranceways obscure trip hazards. The EMT risks slipping and falling on loose floorboards or throw rugs. An experienced EMT uses a flashlight to illuminate the doorway or hallway.

Physical hazards to the EMT can often be identified and dealt with accordingly. It is the unseen, or unsuspected, hazard that can be the most dangerous. Family members who initially welcomed the EMT and ushered the EMT into the house can suddenly change their attitude and pose a formidable risk to the EMT. Experienced EMTs always keep an eye on the family.

As a matter of practice, an EMT will always try to keep the pathway to the nearest door clear, permitting a quick exit if needed. Many EMTs work in pairs for safety. One EMT will focus her attention on the patient while the other EMT is observing the scene, and family members, for any sign of danger. This practice, commonly referred to as "watching your partner's back," is an example of a safe practice.

When an EMT enters a room, she should perform a visual sweep of the room for any deadly weapons or potentially dangerous instruments. A **deadly weapon** is any device that, by its nature, is intended to produce death. Knives, rifles, and shotguns are examples of deadly weapons. EMTs usually do not have any difficulty identifying a deadly weapon. However, EMTs frequently fail to identify **dangerous instruments**. Dangerous instruments are things capable of producing death or serious bodily injury when used in certain circumstances. For example, a pair of sewing scissors can be used as a dangerous instrument. Another example of a dangerous instrument is a broken whiskey bottle.

Stairs also represent a serious hazard to the EMT. Loose boards and broken handrails can cause an EMT to lose her equilibrium and fall. Many EMTs lean against the inside wall when carrying a patient down the stairs rather than trust the handrail.

Hazards at a Motor Vehicle Collision

The scene of a motor vehicle collision can be one of the most dangerous places an EMT has to work. Flammable liquids, slippery antifreeze, sharp glass, and jagged metal edges are some of the more common hazards an EMT will encounter.

When a truck is involved in a motor vehicle collision, look at the truck carefully. Are fumes visible? If fumes are visible, are the fumes white, like steam, or tinged with color? Do the fumes stream skyward, or do they hug the ground?

Are there any diamond-shaped hazardous materials placards on the side of the truck? What is the name of the carrier? Gasoline company trucks usually transport gasoline.

These are all signs of a potential hazardous materials spill. More information on hazardous materials identification, and the EMT's response to hazardous materials, is provided in Chapter 44, Public Safety Incident Management.

Downed Power Lines

When a vehicle strikes a utility pole, it can bring electrically charged wires down. The EMT should look for downed power lines on the scene of any motor vehicle collision (Figure 12-4). Smoldering grass fires, so-called hot spots, or clearly visible sparks flying are indications of a downed power line.

Occasionally, downed lines are telephone lines or television cables. However, the EMT should never assume that a downed telephone line or television cable is harmless. These lines can be draped across charged power lines and become energized. The EMT must treat *all* downed lines as potentially dangerous.

It is important for an EMT to also look up for downed power lines. Disrupted power lines can be found either sagging dangerously low, but not touching the ground, or one end can be dangling over the EMT's head. If the EMT's head should come into contact with the line then her body will complete the circuit and she could be electrocuted.

Also, the EMT should never assume that a downed power line that is safe now will remain safe. Power is routinely interrupted by squirrels and other animals. When these interruptions occur, the power company reroutes electricity through other paths in the power grid in order to bypass the short in the line and restore electricity to the affected customers.

A downed power line is not safe until the power company physically removes or otherwise isolates the power line. Until the power company arrives, *all* downed lines are assumed to be energized, and therefore dangerous, until proved otherwise.

New housing developments routinely bury unsightly power lines underground to obscure them from view. The only sign that a power line may be buried is the aboveground splice box or a transformer. These splice boxes and transformers are often hidden in the shrubbery. When a car comes crashing across someone's lawn, and through the shrubs, the car can come to rest on one of these boxes and become energized. It is important to look both under the car and over the top of the car for power lines.

If downed power lines are visible on scene, do *not* approach the scene. Park the ambulance at least *one* full span of wires away from the pole with the downed wires. Use the public address (PA) system in the ambulance to warn the occupants of the motor vehicle to stay in the car. They are safer inside the car.

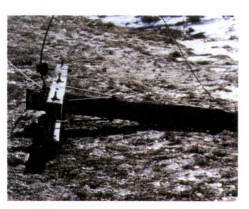

FIGURE 12-4   Downed power lines pose a serious threat to the EMT.

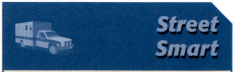

Street Smart

A car may strike a telephone pole so hard that it shears the pole from its foundation. The only thing holding the pole upright is the power lines. Unsuspecting EMTs may be hurt if the wires snap and the pole drops. All broken poles should be treated with the same respect as a downed power line.

Street Smart

Downed power lines create a "field" of energy around the point where they contact the ground. When the unsuspecting EMT approaches the scene, she will feel a kind of tingling sensation in her legs. The tingling sensation indicates that the EMT has entered an electric field.

Once an EMT realizes that she has entered the energy field of a downed power line, the *worst* thing she can do is turn and run. Lifting one leg and then placing it down creates a pathway, or a circuit, for the electricity to travel.

Instead, the EMT should stand completely still until the power is turned off. If standing still is not practical, then the EMT has two choices. The EMT can either "shuffle" off the scene, keeping her feet and knees in contact at all times, or the EMT can "hop" off the scene, again with both feet together. Shuffling and hopping prevent a circuit from being created and injury from occurring.

Also, warn curious onlookers to stay away from the vehicles, again using the PA system. After warning the vehicle occupants and onlookers, call for the power company or fire department, or both, according to the service's standard operating guidelines.

RISK MANAGEMENT

Whenever a hazard has been identified, the EMT must act to protect herself, the public, and the patient, in that order, from bodily harm and risk of injury. The process of identifying hazards and ensuring protection is called risk management.

The fact that a patient has gotten himself into a dangerous situation does not automatically mean the EMT must endanger herself to rescue the person. The EMT's *first duty is to herself*. The courts have upheld the idea that an EMT can refuse to enter an inherently dangerous situation. An EMT, however, cannot simply refuse to act. The EMT must act to try to mitigate the danger and make it safe to provide care. However, until that danger has been reduced to an acceptable risk, or eliminated, the EMT should not enter the scene (Figure 12-5).

Risk Management at a Motor Vehicle Collision

The single largest danger to the EMT at the scene of a motor vehicle collision is not on scene when she arrives! The danger is traffic. Every year, passing motorists strike and kill law enforcement officers, firefighters, and EMTs while they are performing their duty.

Careless drivers, called rubberneckers, focus on the carnage of twisted metal and bleeding patients and fail to notice the people working around the scene trying to rescue those patients. The use of

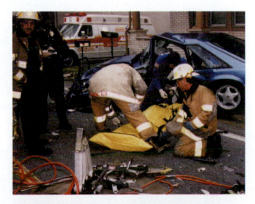

FIGURE 12-5 Risk management is a team effort requiring the cooperation of many public safety agencies. (Courtesy of David J. Reimer Sr.)

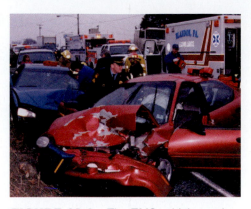

FIGURE 12-6 The EMS vehicle can be used as a physical barrier, creating a safety corridor in front of it. (Courtesy of David J. Reimer Sr.)

effective warning devices and proper vehicle placement can reduce the chance of an EMT's being struck by passing motorists.

Vehicle Placement

When the EMT is in the first arriving emergency services unit, it becomes the EMT's responsibility to protect herself, her crew, and the patients in the motor vehicle collision. There are several tactics an EMT can use to improve the odds of survival.

Consider how law enforcement officers position their patrol vehicles purposefully when they make a vehicle stop, using the vehicle as a physical barrier. What the law enforcement officer has created, in effect, is a **safety corridor** between his patrol car and the stopped vehicle. Figure 12-6 demonstrates the effect of positioning the emergency vehicle at the roadside of a scene to create a safe zone from within which the EMT can work more safely.

The next decision an EMT must make is how close to park the vehicle to the scene. How close the emergency vehicle should be placed to the scene depends on several factors. First, the types of vehicles on the road affect the decision. Second, the average speed of the traffic on the road affects the decision. Third, the type and weight of the emergency vehicle must be factored in.

In situation one, demonstrated in Figure 12-7, the roadway is an interstate, and the vehicles range from personal cars to tractor-trailers. Remember that the emergency vehicle is serving as a barricade. The object of a barricade is to either stop or slow another vehicle from coming down on the EMTs or at least to allow them enough time to escape when the vehicle strikes the ambulance.

How far back an ambulance should be positioned on a busy interstate, where vehicles are driving by at 60 to 70 miles per hour (mph), is dependent on how far a tractor-trailer can push an ambulance. The EMT should consider placing the ambulance at least 30 yards, or about three roadside markers, from the scene.

Contrast the scene above to a motor vehicle collision within a small village. Local traffic is light, and the posted speed limit is 30 mph. This

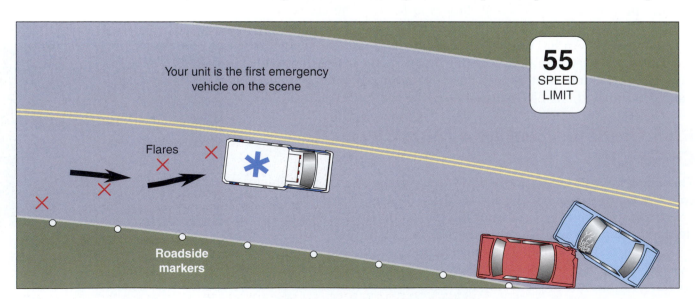

FIGURE 12-7 The EMS vehicle should be at least three roadside markers away from the scene on a controlled-access highway.

scene presents a different picture than the previous scenario. The degree of danger may be less, but danger still exists. In all cases, the *minimum* safe distance to position an emergency response vehicle is about 50 feet.

Warning Lights

The emergency warning lights are a valuable tool for safety. Arguments flourish among EMTs about the best array of emergency lights. Some prefer beacons because they strike overhead power lines and reflect back to oncoming drivers. Others prefer strobe lights that emit a powerful glow visible for miles.

The colors of the emergency lights are important as well. Some states have adopted blue lights for all emergency vehicles; others have adopted red lights. Some studies have indicated that blue lights are more visible after dark than red lights. However, the most visible color at night is yellow light. Recently, the federal ambulance specifications have required the presence of one rearward-facing yellow light on all ambulances. Yellow light has been generally accepted as a "warning light" by the public.

There is one point of agreement among emergency responders. Emergency lights are an important part of scene safety. The EMT should turn them on and leave them on whenever an emergency vehicle is on scene.

The best situation for an EMT is one in which other responders have already shut down the closest lane when she arrives on scene (Figure 12-8). From a safety standpoint, the safest place for an ambulance is ahead of the collision site. The EMT would pull the emergency vehicle ahead of the others and leave the corner, or secondary lights, flashing. Too many flashing lights on scene can blind drivers or distract them from driving.

Typically, traffic is backed up behind the collision site. If the ambulance is in front of the scene, then it is not blocked by traffic and has a clear exit to the hospital. Whenever possible, the EMT should position the ambulance facing the direction of travel to the appropriate hospital.

If the patient is seriously injured, rapid transportation to a trauma center may be needed. Precious time can be lost trying to a make a three-point turn on a narrow roadway.

Road Flares

Flares are commonly used by EMTs as a traffic warning device. Portable and highly visible both day and night, flares can also be very dangerous. By following a few simple rules, the EMT can safely use flares.

First, the EMT should put on PPE before lighting a flare. A lit flare is actually burning metal. When lit, flares tend to sputter and throw sparks in every direction. These sparks can cause serious burns to the unprotected EMT.

Firefighter-grade gloves and protective eyewear are the minimum PPE. It is preferable that the EMT wear a turnout coat, or similar flame-resistant coat, if available, to prevent sparks from falling on the EMT's forearm. Flying sparks can fly into the eyes of the EMT as well

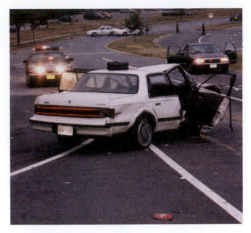

FIGURE 12-8 Police officers will often secure the scene of a motor vehicle collision before EMS arrives. (Courtesy of Craig Smith.)

Street Smart

Often drivers approaching the scene of a collision come from around a curve on the road or from the top of a hill and therefore cannot see the flashing hazard lights of the emergency vehicles. In those cases, the EMT should use safety devices, such as flares or cones, to enhance scene visibility.

and lead to permanent blindness. Eye protection, safety glasses or a helmet shield, must be worn by an EMT who is lighting a road flare.

To light the flare, the EMT removes the striker from the head of the flare. Firmly grasping the shaft of the flare about 6 inches from the head with one hand, the EMT lights the flare by placing the *striker* on the head, or igniter, of the flare and firmly striking the flare, with the striker, *away* from the body. Sometimes it takes several hits before ignition occurs. Always follow the manufacturer's instructions to light flares properly.

Once the flare is ignited, either stand the flare up with wire legs or use the spike to stick it into the ground. Use caution whenever spiking a flare, as falling embers can severely burn the EMT. Skill 12-1 describes the procedure for lighting a road flare.

The position and pattern of flare distribution will determine the effectiveness of the flare as a warning device. The farthest flare should be placed so that the oncoming driver can see the flare, react, and bring the vehicle to a stop, if needed, before entering the scene.

To estimate where the first flare should be placed, take the posted speed limit, convert it to feet, and then multiply by 4. If the posted speed is over 50 mph, add 100 feet to the total. This figure is the number of feet away from the scene that the first flare should be dropped. Table 12-4 lists the suggested distance from the first flare to the scene according to the posted speed.

The distribution of the flares is also very important. On a straight road, the EMT would calculate the distance needed to the first flare, as shown in Table 12-4, and then place the first flare there.

If the crash scene is on a curve, then the EMT must add the radius of the curve to the total distance calculated. Finding the radius sounds difficult, but it really is not that hard. The EMT simply calculates the distance from the bottom of the curve to the top of the curve and then adds that to the distance given in Table 12-4.

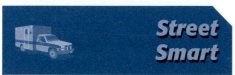

Street Smart

The EMT should be careful what surface the flare is placed on. Telephone poles can ignite from the heat of a flare. Dried underbrush will act like kindling and start a grass fire. Fumes, from spilled fuels, for example, are frequently heavier than air and, when carried to the flare, can ignite. Spilled gasoline has been known to run downhill to a lit flare, ignite, and follow the stream back to the automobile.

An EMT always surveys her surroundings before placing a flare on the ground to ensure the safety of everyone on scene.

TABLE 12-4

Flare Distances		
Speed Limit (mph)	Conversion to Feet	Distance of First Flare (feet)
30	30	120
40	40	160
45	45	180
50	50	200
55	55 (+100)	320
60	60 (+100)	340
65	65 (+100)	360

SKILL 12-1 *Lighting a Road Flare*

PURPOSE: To protect the EMT from injury while lighting a road flare.

STANDARD PRECAUTIONS:

- ☑ Road flare
- ☑ Helmet with eye shield
- ☑ Gloves
- ☑ Turnout coat

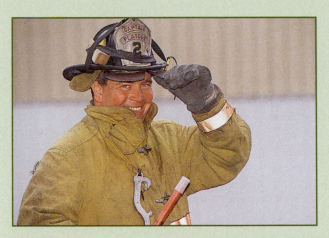

1 The EMT first puts on eye protection and gloves, minimally. It is preferable for the EMT to wear a turnout coat as well.

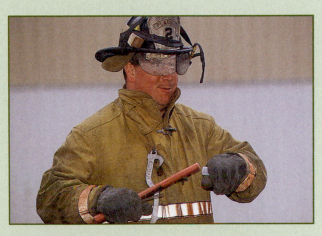

2 The EMT holds the flare 6 inches below the head and then removes the striker from the end of the flare.

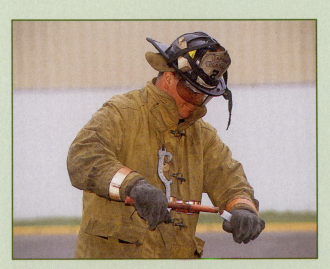

3 The EMT then briskly strikes the striker against the flare's igniter while aiming it away from his body.

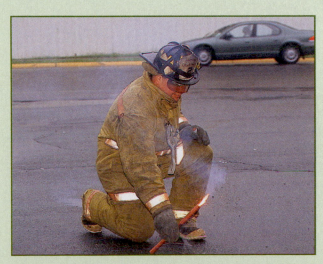

4 The EMT then keeps the lit flare away from his body and places it on the ground.

The same theory is applied for collisions that have occurred in a hollow or even a ravine off road. The EMT would add the distance from the bottom of the hill to the top of the hill to the distance given in Table 12-4.

If the crash is a head-on collision in the middle of the roadway, then flares must be placed both in front of and behind the site, effectively isolating the scene. If the road is a two-lane road, it is often safer to close the road and reroute traffic around the scene.

The EMT, having determined where to place the flares and how many she will need, should walk to the farthest point *first*. The EMT should always face traffic when walking and walk on the shoulder of the road.

Starting at the farthest point, the EMT would proceed to "drop flares" every 50 feet or so, as the situation dictates. While walking along the shoulder of the road, the EMT should *never* turn her back to the oncoming traffic.

Figure 12-9 demonstrates the proper distribution, as well as the order of flare placement, for crash scenes on straight roads, curves, and hollows. Note that flares should never be placed closer than 100 feet from any spilled fuels.

Despite the proper use of flares, the danger of fire and explosion still exists. For this reason, many EMS agencies are using electric, or battery-operated, hazard lights instead of flares. These hazard lights are an excellent alternative to flares. EMS agencies that have EMTs who may have little or no experience using flares should consider using electric hazard lights instead of flares.

During daylight hours, traffic cones provide an excellent alternative to flares as well. Used by highway construction crews for years, these cones provide a highly visible and generally recognized hazard warning device.

Highway traffic cones also make a loud noise when they are struck, alerting the driver to the hazard ahead. Finally, traffic cones are reusable and therefore are a cost-effective traffic warning device.

Public Safety

When an EMT is setting up flares, she is establishing a **perimeter** for motor vehicle traffic. This is one aspect of public safety. The EMT must also be concerned about pedestrian traffic. Motor vehicle collisions tend to draw the attention of people, especially children.

High-speed limited-access highways usually have wire fences along the roadside to prevent pedestrians from wandering onto the highway. Local roads and secondary roads usually do not have fences. The EMT on scene should make some effort to protect pedestrians. Ensuring pedestrian safety usually involves enlisting the aid of law enforcement officers or fire police.

Damage Survey

Starting at the driver's side, the EMT starts a clockwise walk around the car. If the driver or passengers are conscious, the EMT should call out to them to stay seated and not to move. When the walk is completed, the EMT should be at the driver's-side door.

The EMT would start by looking at the front bumpers to see if there are **loaded bumpers**. A bumper becomes loaded when the shock

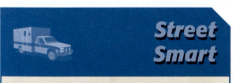

Street Smart

Many EMS agencies have reduced their use of flares in favor of traffic cones. Drivers who are mesmerized by the flashing lights have been known to drive toward the scene instead of diverting away from the lane, thus unknowingly driving over the flares. On the other hand, whenever a vehicle drives over a traffic cone there is a tremendous amount of noise that tends to awaken the driver in time for evasive driving maneuvers.

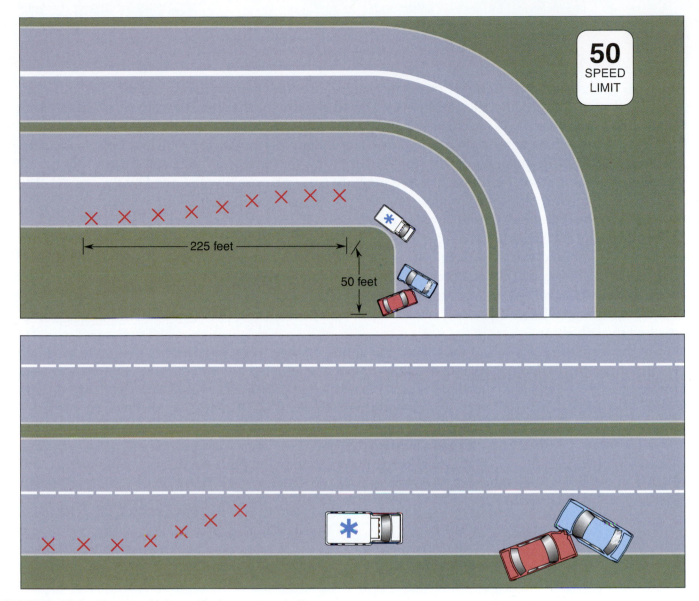

FIGURE 12-9 Proper vehicle positioning ensures better response.

absorbers behind the bumper are compressed but not allowed to release. The energy is stored in the bumper, and the now-loaded bumper can suddenly release, injuring nearby rescuers. An EMT should always keep several feet between herself and a loaded bumper.

The EMT should look for damage to the bumper as well. Current bumpers are designed to absorb a low-speed impact, preventing damage to the car. If the bumper and the fender behind the bumper are severely damaged, then the EMT can assume that the car was moving faster than 10 mph.

The fenders of modern cars are also designed to absorb energy by deforming in **crumple zones**. Any car with a crumpled fender can be assumed to have been in a moderate-speed collision.

A crack at the base of the windshield indicates that a great deal of force traveled through the engine compartment and into the passenger compartment. The front windshield is designed to withstand a great deal of force without cracking. The EMT should carefully examine the windshield.

EMS in Action

Rescue 47 rolled out with Engine 47 on a balmy summer evening, just after dusk for a "car vs. pole." Arriving first on the rescue truck, my partner and I slowly approached the vehicle. It was a black Chevy Blazer on its side. It had hit the guy wire of a power pole so hard that the wire lacerated through the chrome bumper right at the turn signal, snapping the car to an instant halt. Noting the size and height of the pole, we knew from our training that it was a 7,200-volt transmission line. The pole also had a street light attached and the light was out, possibly damaged by the impact. The wires were intact but were drooping low over the residential intersection. There was little traffic and the engine arrived and began to secure the area for us.

We cautiously walked around the car to check for hazards. No fluids on the ground, and the driver was kind enough to crash with the gas filler pipe on the upward side. We then checked to see if any wires were in contact with the vehicle. As we were looking through the broken windshield, a girl about 18 years old walked up to us from across the street.

"I was driving," she said proudly. "Last month, they sent me to the hospital on BayFlite when I wrecked my other car."

I put my hand on the hood of the Blazer and shook my head. She gave us permission to evaluate her, although she had no complaints. While my partner evaluated her and began the refusal process, I looked up at the pole and suddenly noticed that the guy wire was covered on top by a fiberglass sheath. The sheath-enclosed wire was pulled down by the weight of the car and was contacting a smaller 120-volt wire for the street light. I could have, should have, and would have been dead but for that insulator. Not all guy wires have them.

Scene safety is paramount. I have taught it for years myself, yet I missed that one smaller wire and nearly lost my life.

Patrick Shepler, BS, NREMT-P
EMS Development and Marketing Coordinator
Continuing Medical Education
St. Petersburg College, St. Petersburg, Florida

While looking at the windshield, the EMT should look for a small fracture in the glass, called a star. A star indicates that something struck the windshield at one specific point. The object could have been the top of the patient's head. A starred windshield could be equated to head and neck injuries for a passenger. The EMT should always examine the windshield for a star.

As the EMT circles the car, assessing damage, she should open all unlocked car doors. Leaving the door slightly ajar permits rapid entry into the vehicle during the extrication process.

If the mechanism of injury is a lateral-impact motor vehicle collision, the EMT should be focusing on the amount of intrusion into the passenger compartment. If it is greater than 12 inches, then the EMT should have a high index of suspicion that the occupants may have serious injuries.

Looking into the passenger compartment, the EMT should see if the car has air bags and whether they are deployed. Some modern cars have both passenger-side and lateral-side air bags as well as the driver-side air bags. Be careful around undeployed air bags. On rare occasions, these air bags will spontaneously inflate, injuring EMTs in the process. Although air bags are ordinarily very safe, some EMS agencies choose to disarm or even remove air bags to prevent further injury.

The fact that an air bag has deployed does *not* mean that the patient was protected. Air bags are most effective against frontal impacts. The forces that result from a lateral or rotational impact may throw the driver out of the path of the air bag.

The EMT should always lift up and look under the air bag to see whether the patient's body struck the steering wheel hard enough to bend it.

When an air bag does deploy, it literally slaps the patient in the face. This violent action can leave a mild superficial burn, and the patient may complain of a burning sensation. This burning sensation is generally short-lived. If the patient is wearing glasses the glasses may fragment and cause lacerations as well. The patient's face should be examined for injuries following an air bag deployment.

Once an air bag has been deployed, it cannot be reused. Therefore, if the car is struck from behind after striking another car in front, the air bag will not protect the driver. These so-called double taps occur most often on congested city streets or in limited-visibility conditions such as fog or rain. Drivers in cars with a double tap should be assessed for both frontal and rear impact injuries. Table 12-5 summarizes what an EMT should assess on a vehicle involved in a motor vehicle collision.

Number of Patients

On the scene of a motor vehicle accident, there is frequently more than one patient. When more than one patient is present, the EMT must decide who will get treatment first and who will wait for additional responders. In short, the patients must be sorted according to the severity of their injuries.

This decision-making process requires a special approach called **triage**. Triage should take only a few minutes and can potentially save more lives than an approach that assesses one patient at a time. Triage is discussed in more detail in Chapter 44, Public Safety Incident Management.

Triage is a part of the total incident management system (IMS). The IMS is an effective means of caring for multiple patients. The IMS is discussed in fuller detail in Chapter 44.

The entire IMS depends on the first-arriving EMT or emergency services worker to establish that there are multiple patients. It is important for the EMT to determine the number of patients during the scene size-up and to call for additional resources during the initial report. Calling for additional personnel and equipment immediately to care for the additional patients prevents unnecessary delays in transportation or care.

If the EMT fails to perform her duty and instead runs up to the first patient that she comes to and starts to render care, other patients, who otherwise might have survived, will die needlessly.

First Contact

As the EMT approaches the first patient, she should confirm whether the seat belt was worn. Occasionally, the seat belt is still on the patient.

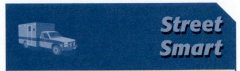

Street Smart

Air bags are covered in starch, which helps the air bag deploy more evenly. After the air bag does deploy, a cloud of smoke may be visible. Some occupants may think that the car is on fire. The explosive charge to inflate the air bag is contained and self-limiting. Danger of fire from an air bag is almost nonexistent.

TABLE 12-5

Assessment of Vehicle Damage

Damage to Vehicle	Point of Patient Impact
Star on windshield	Forehead
Rearview mirror broken	Forehead
Air bag deployed	Face or torso
Locked seat belt	Torso
Steering wheel bent	Torso
Broken headrest	Head
Broken dashboard	Knees
Broken or bent pedals	Feet or legs
Seat broken off pedestal	Body
Side-door intrusion	Body, same side

Frequently, it is not. A quick tug on the free end of the seat belt will reveal if the seat belt locked up during the accident.

If the seat belt is not locked up, pull the seat belt out to its full length. A seat belt is really just a flat rope. And, like most ropes, when the seat belt is stretched beyond its maximum strength, threads will break and it will fray before it fails. When a passenger's weight is thrown against the seat belt during a collision, the seat belt will stretch and may become frayed. The EMT should carefully examine the seat belt for signs of fraying.

Vehicle Stabilization

All motor vehicles involved in a collision should initially be assumed to be unstable. Even cars that are on all four tires have been known to roll or shift. *Any* vehicle that is *not* on all four wheels *must* be stabilized with wood blocks or cribbing, or both, before any EMT enters the vehicle to perform patient care.

An EMT should never enter a vehicle that is not stable. Instead, the EMT must immediately take action to either stabilize the vehicle, with cribbing, or to call for resources, such as heavy rescue.

Fortunately, most motor vehicles can be made safe with a few simple actions. These actions, taken by the first EMT on scene, can remarkably improve EMT safety as well as decrease the chance of further patient injury. Every EMT should make these actions a routine part of her initial entry into a car involved in a collision.

First, the EMT should take the car with automatic transmission out of drive. This step seems obvious, but most drivers do not stop and think to take their car out of gear after a collision. Whenever a car's automatic transmission is still engaged, the car can move and the EMT is at risk of personal injury.

Next, the EMT should turn the car's engine off. A car that is still running is energized and capable of moving. In the northern climes, EMTs are sometimes reluctant to turn a car off. The heat from the car helps prevent hypothermia. However, a misplaced elbow or knee, while moving the patient, can shift the car into drive. It is always safer for the EMT to turn the car off.

Before turning off the car, be sure that if the car has power windows or door locks that they are left open. Also, check the seat to see whether it is electric. The EMT may want to move the seat backward, for easier patient extrication, before turning off the car and after manually stabilizing the patient's head.

The EMT should immediately engage the parking brake. Severe damage to the car's engine may disrupt the hydraulic lines to the power brakes, allowing the car to roll. Applying the mechanical parking brake greatly enhances the margin of safety for the EMT.

Finally, the EMT should block the wheels. Some EMS agencies, as a matter of practice, automatically place a wedge, or chock, behind two wheels on opposite sides of the car. Using a chock prevents the vehicle from rolling even if both braking systems have failed.

If the car is still unstable, it may be necessary for properly trained personnel to isolate the wheels from the frame of the car by using special cribbing called **step blocks**. Step blocks are designed to be placed under the frame of the vehicle to lift it off its wheels.

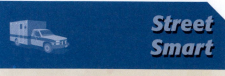

Street Smart

In some EMS agencies, it is standard practice to throw the vehicle's keys on the driver's-side floor. Then, when the tow truck needs to move the car, the tow operator knows where to find the keys.

When cribbing is needed to stabilize a car, the EMT should consider requesting a heavy rescue unit or fire service assistance. Skill 12-2 describes vehicle stabilization.

SKILL 12-2 *Vehicle Stabilization*

PURPOSE: To protect the EMT from hazards created as the result of a motor vehicle collision.

STANDARD PRECAUTIONS:

☑ Flashlight
☑ Turnout coat
☑ Helmet

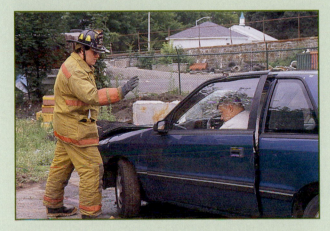

1 The first EMT circles the car starting from the driver's side. The EMT advises the patient to sit still for a minute. The EMT is checking for vehicle damage.

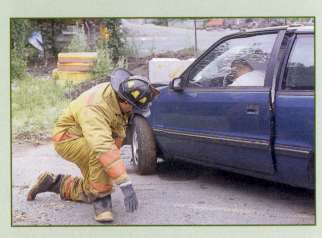

2 The second EMT circles the car from the opposite side. The EMT is checking for hazards above and beneath the car.

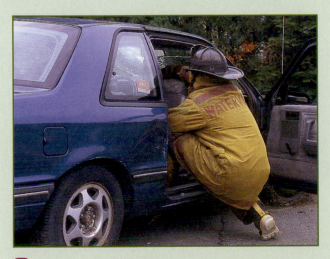

3 After the second EMT calls "all clear," the first EMT enters the passenger side and stabilizes the patient's head.

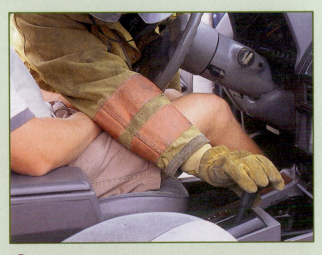

4 The second EMT then reaches in and checks to see that the car is in park.

(continues)

SKILL 12-2 *(continued)*

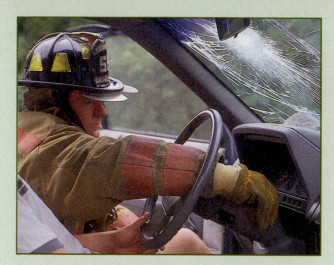

5 After checking for electric locks, windows, and seats, the EMT confirms that the car is turned off.

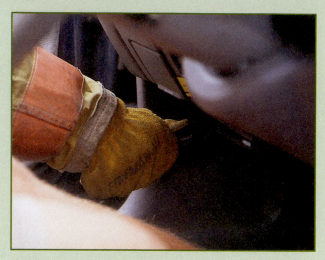

6 Finally, the EMT confirms that the car's emergency brake is engaged.

CONCLUSION

All EMTs approach a scene in a similar manner and ask themselves the same questions. Am I safe? Is the scene safe? What is the nature of the call? How many patients do I have? What other resources do I need?

The answers are frequently different, but the questions remain the same. The EMT should practice reciting these questions whenever she approaches a scene. The EMT should practice running these questions through her mind until the questions become second nature.

The most important person on any EMS call is the EMT. There is nothing more disturbing to any EMT than to learn that another EMT failed to follow a few simple guidelines, ignored hazards, and lost her life needlessly. By completing the scene size-up correctly, the EMT can prevent this type of tragedy from occurring.

TEST YOUR KNOWLEDGE

1. Name several regulatory agencies that have established safety rules for EMS.

2. What is meant by the standard approach to an EMS call? Please describe it.

3. What information can be obtained from the prearrival instructions?

4. What is the importance of staging to an EMT's safety?

5. What risk factors exist on the scene of a medical emergency? Of a trauma emergency?

6. What resources should be called to manage these risks?

7. Whose safety is first? The patient's? The public's? The crew's? The EMT's?

8. How would an EMT protect the public from becoming injured?

9. What are the minimal actions an EMT should take to stabilize a motor vehicle?

10. What are the elements of the global survey?

INTERNET RESOURCES

- Review safety standards as outlined by the National Fire Protection Association, http://www.nfpa.org, and the Occupational Safety and Health Administration, http://www.osha.gov.

- Search for information on some of the hazards you read about in this chapter. What additional information can you find about dealing with these hazards? What other hazards can you think of that were not addressed in the chapter? Keep review cards of the various hazards and techniques for safely managing the hazards for self-study and review.

FURTHER STUDY

Dernocoeur, K. B. (1996). *Streetsense: Communication, safety, and control* (3rd ed.). St. Louis, MO: Mosby.

Elling, B., & Elling, K. (2002). *Principles of patient assessment in EMS.* Clifton Park, NY: Thomson Delmar Learning.

Krebs, D. (2002). *When violence erupts: A survival guide for emergency responders.* Boston: Jones and Bartlett.

Leisner, K. (1989). Managing the pre-violent patient. *Emergency Medical Services, 18*(7), 18–20, 23, 26, 28–29.

Rice, M. M., & Moore, G. (1991). Management of the violent patient: Therapeutic and legal considerations. *Emergency Medical Clinics of North America, 9*(1), 13–30.

Richards, E. (1995). *Knife and gun club: Scenes from an emergency room.* St. Louis, MO: Mosby.

CHAPTER 13

Initial Assessment

KEY TERMS

ABCs

alert

AVPU

crepitus

flail chest segment

general impression

initial assessment

paradoxical motion

responsive to painful stimuli

responsive to voice

sternal rub

sucking chest wound

unresponsive

OBJECTIVES

Upon completion of this chapter, the reader should be able to:

1. Summarize the reasons for forming a general impression of the patient.
2. Discuss methods of assessing mental status.
3. Differentiate between assessing the mental status in the adult, child, and infant patient.
4. Discuss methods of assessing the airway in the adult, child, and infant patient.
5. Describe methods used for determining whether a patient is breathing.
6. State the care that should be provided to the adult, child, and infant patient with adequate breathing.
7. State the care that should be provided to the adult, child, and infant patient without adequate breathing.
8. Differentiate between a patient with adequate breathing and one with inadequate breathing.
9. Distinguish between methods of assessing breathing in the adult, child, and infant patient.
10. Compare the methods of providing airway care to the adult, child, and infant patient.
11. Differentiate between obtaining a pulse in an adult, child, and infant patient.
12. Discuss the need for assessing the patient for external bleeding.
13. Describe normal and abnormal findings when assessing skin color, temperature, and condition.
14. Describe normal and abnormal findings when assessing capillary refill in the infant and child patient.
15. Explain the reason for prioritizing a patient for care and transport.

OVERVIEW

Every patient an emergency medical technician (EMT) encounters will be different in some way from all the others. Many may have similar complaints, but each patient must be evaluated thoroughly by the

EMT. This chapter covers the recommended method of initially assessing patients.

It is important for the EMT to attempt to perform this assessment the same way every time. Of course, it will vary slightly depending upon patient situations, but the order of the assessment and the priorities must always remain the same. If assessments are done systematically, the EMT will be less likely to leave something out or to forget to assess something.

Chapters 14 through 17 discuss further assessment techniques for both medical and trauma patients.

THE INITIAL ASSESSMENT

The priorities when assessing a patient must be to find and treat any life-threatening problems first. The assessment that is done first to find such life threats is called the **initial assessment**. It is a quick, yet systematic, assessment of the most important functions of the human body: the airway, breathing, and circulatory status.

The purpose of the initial assessment is to allow the EMT to rapidly find and treat any immediate life-threatening problems, such as an occluded airway. During the initial assessment, life-threatening problems are fixed as they are found. In contrast, less urgent problems will be managed at the completion of the appropriate assessments.

Because every patient has the potential to have a life-threatening problem, every patient the EMT encounters will get an initial assessment upon first encounter. We will discuss how the initial assessments differ according to the patients' status.

✳ *Chest Pain*

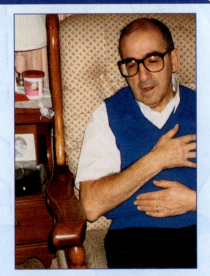

After a scene size-up proves not to show any danger to his crew, Will enters the patient's living room and observes a man seated in a chair. The patient is an older man, in his 70s, who looks quite pale and sweaty.

He is leaning back in the chair, with both hands rubbing his chest, complaining of a "heavy" sort of chest pain and slight difficulty in breathing.

- What is your general impression of this patient?
- Does he seem to be acutely ill?
- Are any immediate treatments indicated?

Steps of the Initial Assessment

You will recall from Chapter 12 that the first thing an EMT should do as he approaches a scene is to perform a scene size-up and ensure that it is safe to approach the patient. The EMT should also be using the appropriate personal protective equipment that is expected for the situation. Once the scene has been deemed safe, the next step is to approach the patient and begin the initial assessment.

The abbreviation used to remember the essential parts of the initial assessment is ABC: airway, breathing, and circulation. The **ABCs** are commonly referred to in emergency care as the top priorities in care. There are two tasks the EMT may accomplish while approaching the patient to assess the ABCs; these are to note the patient's general appearance and her mental status.

General Appearance

An EMT must learn to use his powers of observation. While approaching a patient, the EMT should be looking around the scene to find any clues that may help in determining what the problem could be due to. The EMT should then concentrate his attention on the patient.

A **general impression** of the status of the patient can be formed in the first 15 seconds of observation. The more experience the EMT has, the more confident he may be in this initial impression. The EMT should ask several questions at this time.

- Does the patient appear to be awake?
- Does the patient appear to be very ill or very uncomfortable?
- Does the problem seem to be related to a medical illness or to a traumatic injury?

The first general impression is formed as the EMT walks across the room toward the patient and will determine how quickly and how urgently he must direct his crew to act.

The general impression is often referred to as the "look test." That is, when you first look at the patient, does she look sick? The man in the case study looks quite ill, so the EMT might say he has "failed the look test." This impression should stimulate the EMT and his crew into moving more quickly to assess and manage this patient.

Mental Status

As the EMT approaches the patient, the general state of consciousness should be easily noted. Does the patient seem to be awake? There is a standardized way to evaluate and report the patient's general mental status, or state of consciousness.

The abbreviation **AVPU** is often used in reporting level of consciousness. *A* stands for **A**lert; *V* stands for responsive to **V**oice, *P* stands for responsive to **P**ain; and *U* stands for **U**nresponsive.

Alert

As the EMT approaches, if the patient's eyes are open and she seems aware of the crew approaching, she is referred to as **alert**. This can be further qualified as the EMT speaks with the patient by reporting whether she is oriented or not. Three common questions to test orientation are related to person, place, and time. Table 13-1 lists examples of questions the EMT might ask to determine orientation.

If the patient correctly answers each of these questions, the patient is determined to be alert and oriented to person, place, and time. Sometimes this status is abbreviated as "A/OX3," or "alert and oriented times three," referring to person, place, and time.

If the patient is unable to answer any of these questions, the patient is said to be disoriented. If the patient knows her name but not the place or time, the patient is said to be oriented to person but not to place or time. It is useful to specify which question the patient is oriented to and which she is disoriented to so that health care providers who care for the patient later on can compare their exam with the EMT's and know whether anything has changed.

Responsive to Voice

If the patient does not seem to be awake as the EMT approaches, the EMT should attempt to arouse the patient first by speaking. "Are you all right?" is a good way to start. If the patient opens her eyes when spoken to but closes her eyes again when not spoken to, she is considered to be **responsive to voice**.

If a normal tone of voice does not arouse the patient, then a louder tone may be used. If this arouses the patient, we say that she is responsive to loud verbal stimuli. The difference between the "alert" and the "responsive to voice" categories is that the alert patient does not require verbal stimuli to keep her awake and interactive. When not being spoken to, the *V* patient will close her eyes and withdraw from interaction.

Responsive to Pain

If the patient does not respond to loud verbal stimuli, the next most appropriate action would be to attempt to awaken her with physical stimuli. A firm tap on the shoulder is a good way to start. If this awakens the patient, the terminology used is "responds to physical stimuli." If this does not awaken the patient, a more noxious physical stimulus must be used.

A common maneuver used by EMS providers in this situation is the **sternal rub** (Figure 13-1). The knuckles of the EMT's hand are rubbed against the patient's sternum firmly in an attempt to arouse the patient. If this stimulus arouses the patient, we say that she is **responsive to painful stimuli**. The EMT should describe what the patient did in response to this stimulus.

Unresponsive

If no response is elicited by verbal or painful stimuli, the patient is truly **unresponsive**. The unresponsive patient is very ill and requires rapid interventions.

Airway

Once the general impression has been formed and the level of consciousness determined, the EMT must address the state of the patient's airway. If the patient is awake and alert, the airway is most

TABLE 13-1

Questions to Determine Orientation

Person:	What is your name?
Place:	Where are you right now?
Time:	Can you tell me the time of day? What day is it today?

Pediatric Considerations

When assessing infants and small children, who don't speak or are not old enough to know where they are or what the day is, we cannot use the same criteria as for adults. If a child is awake, the EMT should observe how the child interacts with the parents or caregiver.

If the child is awake and clinging to the caregiver, looking around at things going on in the immediate environment, and acting in a manner appropriate for a child of that age, we refer to that child as being awake and *appropriate*, rather than oriented.

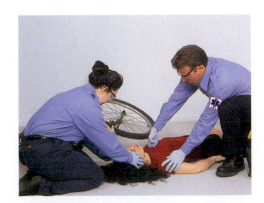

FIGURE 13-1 Use a sternal rub to check for a patient's response to a painful stimulus.

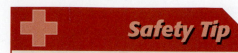

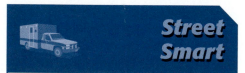

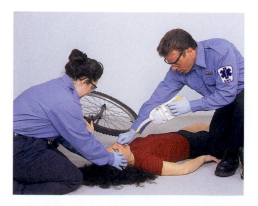

FIGURE 13-2 *Open, assess, suction,* and *secure* the airway.

likely being maintained without difficulty. The EMT can confirm this assumption by observing the patient's effort to breathe and speak. If the patient is speaking and seems to be moving air in and out without difficulty, then the airway is considered open, or patent.

If the patient is awake but cannot speak, or has the appearance of struggling to breathe air in, the EMT must further assess the airway. Drooling is also a sign that the patient is having difficulty with the airway. Normally, a person can swallow his or her own saliva. In the case of an airway obstruction, the saliva may not be able to get by the obstruction to be swallowed. This means that air may not be able to get by either.

If the patient is not awake, then the EMT must be immediately concerned about the status of the airway. The less responsive the patient becomes, the more likely it is that the airway will not be maintained on its own and remain clear of saliva and debris.

The EMT should use a methodical method of assessing and managing a patient's airway. The order in which actions are taken is "open, assess, suction, secure" (Figure 13-2). Such airway assessment and management techniques are discussed in detail in Chapter 7 and should be reviewed.

Once the EMT has assessed and appropriately secured the airway, he can move on to the next step in the assessment.

Breathing

After ensuring that the patient has a patent airway, the EMT turns his attention to the patient's breathing.

The first question the EMT must answer is whether the patient is breathing at all. To determine the presence of breathing, the EMT should bend down over the patient and look, listen, and feel for air movement. Look for chest rise, listen for air coming from the mouth and nose, and feel for the air against your cheek.

If the patient is not breathing, then the appropriate actions must be taken to establish effective ventilations as described in Chapter 8.

If the patient is breathing upon this initial assessment, then the EMT should assess the adequacy of the breathing by determining a respiratory rate. If the patient's respiratory rate is between 10 and 28 and appears to be adequate in volume, then supplemental oxygen should be administered by means of a non-rebreather mask.

If the patient is breathing, but the breathing is too fast or too slow, is of inadequate depth, or requires marked effort, then the EMT should assist the patient's ventilations using a bag-valve-mask with 100% oxygen.

All patients who are not completely awake and oriented should be given high-concentration supplemental oxygen via non-rebreather mask.

Patients who are awake and oriented may also require oxygen, depending on the presenting medical condition. Complaints such as chest or abdominal pain, difficulty breathing, or any signs or symptoms of shock are indications for high-flow oxygen by non-rebreather mask. The use of oxygen in the management of specific complaints will be addressed throughout the book.

After assessing the presence and the adequacy of breathing, the EMT must assess for potential problems with breathing. This assessment involves a careful examination of the patient's chest for any injuries that may cause problems with adequate respirations. Again, the EMT should *look, listen, and feel*.

Look

First, the patient's chest should be exposed sufficiently to inspect for any obvious wounds or uneven breathing. Open chest wounds, such as stabs or gunshot wounds, create problems with effective breathing because they allow air into the chest via the wound, and air in the chest can impede adequate lung expansion. These types of open chest wounds are called **sucking chest wounds**. Normal negative intrathoracic pressure pulls air into the chest through the wound and can make bubbling or sucking sounds. The appropriate immediate action for the EMT to take is to cover the open wound with an occlusive dressing that does not allow air to pass through. Management of such chest injuries is described in more detail in Chapter 23.

Other types of injuries that may impair adequate ventilations are broken ribs. An indication that a patient may have broken ribs is poor chest expansion associated with chest pain after trauma. Because ribs are painful when broken, deep breaths may not be possible. A patient will *self-splint* that area to protect it.

If more than three ribs are broken in two or more places, these form a free-floating segment of ribs and are called a **flail chest segment**. This flail chest moves in the opposite direction to the rest of the chest wall. This type of movement is called **paradoxical motion** and can be quite painful and cause damage to the lung underneath it.

The EMT should immediately recognize this type of injury and take action to stabilize it to avoid further movement and lung injury. Further discussion and management techniques for a flail chest segment are discussed in Chapter 23.

Listen

After a rapid inspection of the chest wall, the EMT should use a stethoscope to evaluate the effectiveness of air movement by listening to the chest wall. The best place to listen is just below the clavicles and at their midpoint. This location will allow the EMT to hear the air movement into the lung on that side. Listening to both sides will allow the EMT to assess for equality of the breath sounds.

Figure 13-3 shows the proper position to auscultate, or listen to, lung sounds during the initial assessment. The clear sounds of air moving in and out should be heard. If air movement is diminished when compared with the other side, or if it is not heard at all, the patient may have a serious injury. The EMT should take steps to rapidly transport the patient to the most appropriate hospital. If an advanced life support (ALS) intercept is available, it should also be arranged. It is important for the EMT to note any abnormal sounds when listening to the lung sounds. These abnormal lung sounds may fall into several categories, which are described in Table 13-2.

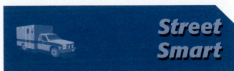

Street Smart

Patients with a sucking chest wound or a flail chest are very seriously injured and must be quickly managed and transported to an appropriate facility. They will often require ventilatory support, so the EMT should pay close attention to their breathing. If the patient starts to breathe too shallowly, then the EMT will need to assist the patient's breathing with a bag-valve-mask.

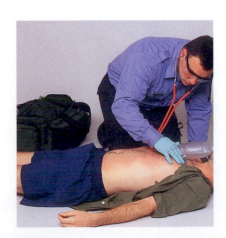

FIGURE 13-3 *Look, listen,* and *feel* for breathing.

TABLE 13-2

Abnormal Lung Sounds	
Sound	**Potential Diagnosis**
Absent	Complete airway obstruction
Diminished (volume of sound)	Collapsed lung (pneumothorax)
Wheezing (whistling sound)	Air moving through narrowed lower airways (asthma or partial airway obstruction)
Crackles (or rales)	Fluid in smaller airways (heart failure)
Rhonchi (rumbling sound)	Fluid in larger airways (bronchitis)

Feel

Finally, the EMT should quickly feel for any deformity or instability within the chest by using both hands to press on both sides of the chest wall and the sternum. Any point of tenderness on the chest wall suggests a rib fracture. If a rib fracture is ignored, it can eventually puncture a lung.

Evidence of subcutaneous air, or **crepitus**, should be noted. Crepitus is the sensation of air under the skin that feels like Rice Krispies popping under the fingertips. This indicates a potentially serious chest injury.

Only after completing the assessment of the breathing, and managing any life threats in that step, can the EMT move on to circulation in the initial assessment.

Circulation

Once the airway and breathing have been assessed and managed appropriately, the EMT must then direct his attention to the C step of the initial assessment. This involves assessment and support of the circulatory system.

Assess for a Pulse

The first step in assessing the circulatory status is to check for a pulse. It is useful to check the radial pulse first. If a radial pulse is present, the EMT can assume that the patient has enough blood pressure to supply blood to that peripheral site. In addition to noting whether the pulse is present, the EMT should note its strength, rate, and regularity.

If a radial pulse is not present in either wrist, the EMT should move directly to the carotid pulse. If the carotid pulse is present but the radial pulse was not, the EMT should assume that the blood pressure is quite low. If a carotid pulse is not present after a 5- to 10-second pulse check, the EMT should begin external chest compressions.

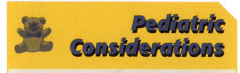

Pediatric Considerations

In children younger than 1 year of age, the radial pulse is often quite difficult to palpate, so the brachial site is used for pulse checks.

Assess for Bleeding

After assessing for the presence of a pulse, the EMT should quickly assess the patient for evidence of a problem that may compromise the circulatory system. Massive bleeding may cause a patient to go into shock and die. The EMT must assess the patient for evidence of life-threatening hemorrhage.

External hemorrhage can be easily found by swiping gloved hands under each part of the patient's body and checking the hands to see whether any blood was recovered from that area. Any areas of active bleeding should be immediately assessed more carefully.

If the amount of bleeding seems small and not life threatening, the EMT should leave that wound to be addressed at a later point in the assessment. If the amount of bleeding seems large and is potentially life-threatening, the EMT should immediately control the bleeding. The first step in controlling bleeding is to apply direct pressure to the wound, usually with a gloved hand. This pressure should be initiated immediately when extensive bleeding is found.

After assessing for gross external hemorrhage, the EMT should assess the patient for hidden, or occult, bleeding. This type of bleeding can be determined by assessing the patient for signs of hypoperfusion.

At this point, the EMT has already assessed mental status, respiratory rate, and heart rate. The next part of the assessment should involve checking the skin temperature, condition, and color.

The details of how to check skin temperature and condition can be reviewed in Chapter 10. Pale, cool, and clammy skin along with rapid breathing and a rapid pulse are signs of shock and should be rapidly found during the initial assessment.

Circulatory Support

If circulatory status is in need of support, it should be immediately provided. CPR should be done immediately as needed. Severe bleeding should be controlled. If patients exhibit any signs of hypoperfusion, they can be placed in the Trendelenburg position to improve circulation to the torso. If indications are present for use of MAST/PASG (military anti-shock trousers/pneumatic anti-shock garment; MAST/PASG local protocols will vary), then they should be applied immediately.

Only after completing the assessment of the circulatory status and addressing any life threats in those steps can the EMT move on in the assessment process.

DETERMINE PRIORITY

Once the initial assessment has been completed, the EMT must make a decision about the priority of the patient. On the basis of the findings in the initial assessment, does the patient have any life-threatening problems that require immediate, rapid transport to the hospital? Do the EMTs need to arrange for an ALS intercept or aeromedical transport?

Certain conditions are considered to be life-threatening emergencies or potentially life-threatening emergencies. At the end of the

Street Smart

A profoundly cold, or hypothermic, patient can have a very slow heart rate. Therefore, the hypothermic patient's pulse should be taken for a full minute. If the patient remains pulseless after 1 minute, CPR should be initiated.

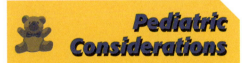

Pediatric Considerations

Remember that for children and infants, capillary refill should be measured as an indicator of peripheral blood flow. Capillary refill time of greater than 2 seconds is indicative of poor circulation and perfusion and is suggestive of shock.

initial assessment, the EMT must determine whether he thinks any of these conditions exist. Table 13-3 lists findings on the initial assessment that should be considered potentially life-threatening. Patients with these findings should be identified as high-priority patients in need of rapid transport and ALS assistance.

High Priority

If a patient is identified as a high-priority patient, the patient must be appropriately packaged and loaded into the ambulance for transport to the closest appropriate hospital. Sometimes the phrase "load and go" is used to describe the actions needed when a high-priority patient has been identified. Most patients in this category will require an ALS intercept if one is available. Local protocols will dictate which hospital to take the patient to and when ALS should be called.

Low Priority

If a patient is identified as a low-priority patient and does not have any immediate life-threatening problems, then the EMT must continue in the assessment of the patient. The remaining assessment will depend upon the type of problem, medical or trauma. Although scene time is not extended beyond that necessary to complete the relevant assessment, a phrase that is sometimes used to describe the disposition of the low-priority patient is "stay and play," indicating that immediate rapid transport is not necessary.

In the remainder of the assessment, the EMT will focus in on the patient's presenting problem or complaint and will assess the particular

TABLE 13-3

Life-Threatening Physical Assessment Findings

Poor general impression

Unresponsive

Decreased level of responsiveness

Responsive but not following commands

Difficulty breathing

Shock (evidence of hypoperfusion)

Complicated childbirth

Chest pain

Uncontrolled bleeding

Severe pain anywhere

areas that are involved. Further history will be elicited on the basis of the type of presenting problem. Chapters 14 through 17 describe these assessment techniques. Figure 13-4 shows the order of assessment, and Skill 13-1 describes the procedure for an initial assessment.

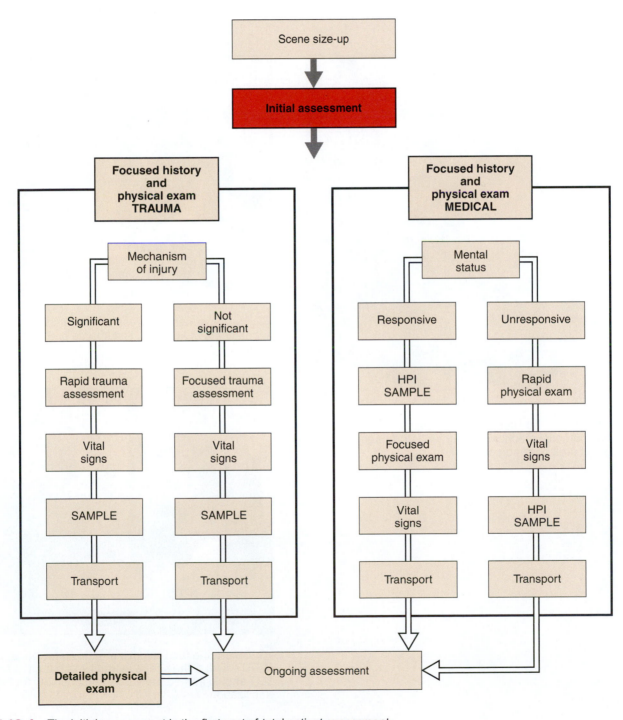

FIGURE 13-4 The initial assessment is the first part of total patient assessment.

SKILL 13-1 *The Initial Assessment*

PURPOSE: To obtain a baseline examination for assessment and comparison as well as to detect and treat life-threatening injuries.

STANDARD PRECAUTIONS:

☑ Personal protective equipment

☑ Stethoscope

☑ Scissors

☑ Airway management equipment

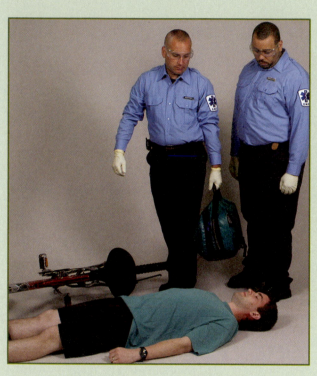

1 Survey the scene for safety hazards as well as any potential mechanism of injury. Don needed personal protective equipment.

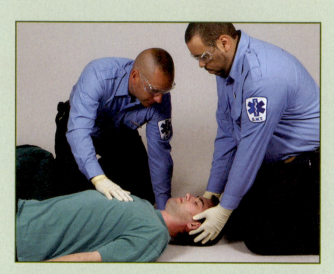

2 Form a general impression of the scene upon approaching the patient. Is it trauma or medical in nature?

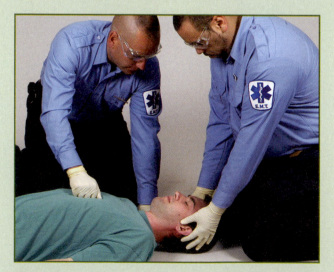

3 Determine the patient's mental status on an AVPU scale. If the scene is trauma in nature, a second EMT should immediately take responsibility for head stabilization.

(continues)

SKILL 13-1 *(continued)*

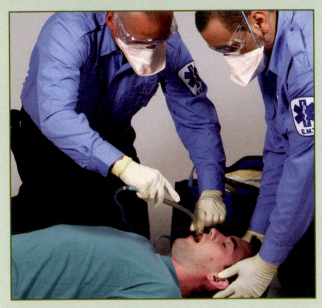

4 Assess and manage the airway as needed.

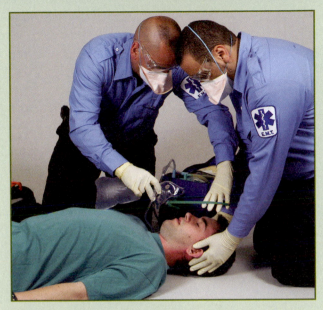

5 Assess and manage breathing.

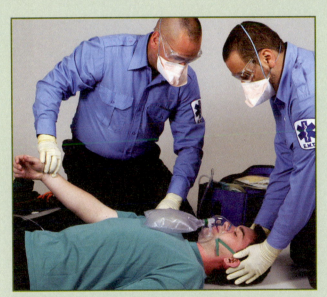

6 Assess and manage circulation. If the patient is a high-priority patient, he should be transported immediately.

CONCLUSION

The initial assessment is completed by the EMT on every patient in order to expediently find and address life-threatening problems.

A general impression will help guide the EMT to prioritize the care in this initial assessment. The patient's mental status is assessed so that any changes may be noted during later assessments.

Airway, breathing, and circulation are quickly assessed, with any life-threatening problems addressed as soon they are found. At the completion of the initial assessment, the EMT has enough information to assign a priority to the patient and to guide further assessments and care.

TEST YOUR KNOWLEDGE

1. Why should an EMT form a general impression of the patient?
2. What are the levels of consciousness?
3. How does an EMT determine the patient's level of consciousness?
4. How is the patient's airway assessed?
5. What can be done if the airway is not patent?
6. How is the patient's breathing assessed?
7. What can be done if the breathing is inadequate?
8. How is the circulation assessed?
9. What can be done to support the circulation?
10. What is the difference between a high-priority patient and a low-priority patient?

INTERNET RESOURCES

Search the Web using these key words:
- Initial assessment
- AVPU
- Airway
- Breathing
- Circulation

Share interesting Web sites and facts that you find with your colleagues.

FURTHER STUDY

Dalton, A. L., Limmer, D., Mistovich, J. J., & Werman H. A. (1999). *Advanced medical life support*. Upper Saddle River, NJ: Brady/Prentice Hall.

Elling, B., & Elling, K. (2002). *Principles of patient assessment in EMS*. Clifton Park, NY: Thomson Delmar Learning.

CHAPTER 14

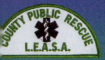

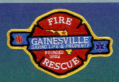

Focused History and Physical Examination of the Trauma Patient

KEY TERMS

abrasion

burn

contusion

DCAP-BTLS

deformity

focused trauma assessment

guarding

jugular venous distension (JVD)

laceration

puncture

rapid trauma assessment

swelling

tender

OBJECTIVES

Upon completion of this chapter, the reader should be able to:

1. State the main objectives for a rapid trauma assessment.
2. Give examples of patients who should, and should not, have a rapid trauma assessment.
3. Describe the importance of the patient-physician relationship to the practice of EMS and its impact on the performance of a focused history and physical examination.
4. Discuss the reasons an EMT should consider mechanism of injury.
5. List those mechanisms of injury that would cause an EMT to have a high index of suspicion that significant injuries exist.
6. Describe the advantages that an advanced life support provider can bring to the injured patient.
7. List the steps in the assessment of a trauma patient with a significant mechanism of injury.
8. Describe each of the components of DCAP-BTLS.
9. Describe the rapid trauma assessment by body regions.
10. Describe the importance of obtaining a baseline set of vital signs and a SAMPLE history.

OVERVIEW

The objective of the initial assessment is to discover and treat life-threatening injuries. Immediate transportation quickly follows in the case in which the patient is seriously ill or injured. However, if the initial assessment is completed and no immediate life threat is discovered, the emergency medical technician (EMT) should continue the assessment while giving special attention to injuries that might have arisen owing to the mechanism of injury. The focused history and physical examination of the trauma patient will allow the EMT to find injuries that may not have been apparent during the initial assessment or that were not immediately life threatening and to discover any minor injuries that need field stabilization before transportation.

This chapter reviews the focused history and physical assessments of minor trauma patients and major trauma patients. These two cases represent the extremes of trauma injury, one minor and one major. What both cases emphasize is the approach an EMT would use to assess these types of patients.

High-Speed Rollover

"Ambulance one, high-speed crash, possible rollover on Cornish Hill."

"Ambulance one en route."

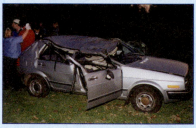

Upon arrival, the ambulance pulls ahead of the crash scene. A teenager can be seen lying on the side of the road, covered with a blanket. Sue, the EMT in charge, prepares to care for the patient, while Carrie carefully goes down the hill to check out the car in the ravine.

(Courtesy of David J. Reimer Sr.)

Walking completely around the car, Carrie observes the driver's-side front fender damage. Then she notices that, although the car is now on four wheels, the roof is caved in.

Carrie then peers into the driver's-side window. The windshield is broken, and a deflated air bag is hanging from the steering wheel. She lifts the air bag off the steering wheel and observes that the steering wheel is bent. Continuing, she tugs on the seat belt and notes that it unrolls easily.

Returning to the ambulance, Carrie finds that Sue has completed her initial assessment. The patient's only complaint is sore wrists.

- Does this patient need a rapid trauma assessment?
- What observations should make an EMT have a high index of suspicion that there may be serious hidden injury?
- How does the possibility of hidden injury affect the patient's priority?

DETERMINATION OF TRAUMA

In most cases, the EMT decides that the patient's injuries are traumatic because of an apparent mechanism of injury. For example, when a patient in a motor vehicle collision (MVC) complains of forearm pain and has an obvious swollen deformity of the forearm, then the assumption is that the patient suffered a broken arm as a result of the MVC.

Sometimes the mechanism of injury is *not* apparent. Take the case of the unconscious woman who is found by the sheriff's patrol on the side of a road on a hot summer day. Was she hit by a car or did she pass out from the heat? If an EMT is in doubt as to whether the patient is ill from a medical condition or injured as a result of trauma, it is safest to assume that the condition is related to trauma and to take the appropriate precautions. These precautions will avoid aggravation of injuries that may not be immediately obvious.

Following the initial scene size-up, which include a consideration of the mechanism of injury and the initial assessment for life-threatening injuries, the EMT should make a determination if the patient is high priority or low priority. This decision is important to determining the next step.

If the patient is high priority then efforts should be made to immediately package and transport the patient before proceeding with the physical examination and history. In some cases, with sufficient personnel, the EMT may continue with physical examination while the patient is being prepared for transport.

Alternatively, if the patient is low priority then the EMT may elect to continue her physical examination of the patient on scene. This decision tree is represented in Figure 13-4.

FOCUSED HISTORY AND PHYSICAL ASSESSMENT

The physical assessment of the trauma patient is geared toward finding the patient's injuries. Because early identification of injuries will guide the management of the trauma patient, the physical assessment is performed before the medical history.

The mechanism of the accident often allows prediction of the type and severity of injury. The more significant the mechanism, the more serious the injuries may be. Whenever a major mechanism of injury is encountered, the EMT should perform a complete head-to-toe **rapid trauma assessment**. By performing an organized examination of the patient from head to toe, the EMT can quickly discover hidden or suspected injuries.

However, most trauma involves an isolated minor injury. It is unnecessary for an EMT to perform a complete head-to-toe assessment on a patient with an isolated minor injury. For example, a patient who cut his finger with a knife while slicing bread has an injury that is obviously isolated to the finger. The chances of hidden injury as a result of this mechanism are fairly low. A rapid head-to-toe trauma assessment is unnecessary and would be an unnecessary intrusion into the patient's privacy. In cases in which there is minor isolated trauma, the EMT should perform a **focused trauma assessment** based on the patient's specific injury.

After the focused trauma assessment is complete, the EMT should obtain a baseline set of vital signs as well as a SAMPLE history, as described in Chapter 10. In some cases, the injury is treated at the same time as, or immediately after, the vital signs are taken.

General Principles of Physical Examination

When an EMT touches a patient she is assessing, she is performing a medical examination of that patient. She will use these assessment findings to make decisions about the care needed by that patient. The patient consents to the touching because it is a medical examination. The EMT is exercising a relationship similar to the physician-patient relationship when the physician is performing a medical examination.

The relationship between the EMT and the patient is based on trust and respect. It is an EMT's duty to gain the patient's trust and maintain respect for the patient. For this reason, every EMT should exercise the following principles whenever performing a physical examination:

1. Be polite. After an initial introduction, giving her name and title, the EMT should refer to the patient by title, Mr. or Ms. Jones. Using the patient's first name is appropriate only if the patient is of similar age or younger; otherwise, using the patient's first name may be construed as impolite. Consider asking the patient how he would prefer to be addressed. A patient should never be called "honey" or "bud" or other such terms.

2. Offer explanations. A patient has a right to know what an EMT is going to do. It is common courtesy for an EMT to explain to the patient how and why she intends to assess the patient for further injuries.

3. Maintain the patient's privacy. If a patient is awake or is in a public place, the EMT should endeavor to unclothe the patient only when necessary and only those portions of the body that need assessment. Once the assessment is complete, the patient should be covered.

4. Make eye contact. Eye contact, in most cases, demonstrates a caring attitude on the part of the EMT. Always make an effort to reestablish eye contact after assessing each portion of the body.

5. Be honest. A medical emergency is, by definition, a crisis for the patient. The patient is fearful about pain or suffering. An EMT should use honesty to help comfort the patient and alleviate the anxiety the patient is experiencing. As far as is practical, an EMT should always speak honestly about matters that the EMT knows—for example, that the oxygen should help make the patient feel better.

6. Focus the patient's attention. In times of crisis, patients have a tendency to focus on one person, to see one individual as the healer. It is important for the EMT to provide that focus. Although several EMTs may be treating a patient, only one should be performing the assessment and giving verbal instructions to the crew.

Reconsider the Mechanism of Injury

Obvious injuries are usually discovered and treated during the initial assessment. In many trauma cases, it is not what can be seen that will kill the patient; it is what *cannot* be seen. Therefore, an EMT needs to reconsider the mechanism of injury and ask herself, "In the worst case scenario, what injuries could this patient have?"

A serious mechanism of injury will create a high index of suspicion that a serious hidden injury may exist. The American College of Surgeons Committee on Trauma has developed a list of mechanisms that can produce serious injury. A summary of this list can be found in Table 14-1. The amount of force that is involved in each of these types of incidents is often associated with serious injury, even without obvious initial physical findings.

The mechanism of injury for a trauma patient can be thought of as the history of the present illness (HPI), which is often obtained for the medical patient; this is discussed in more detail in Chapter 16. The EMT should gather as many details as she can regarding the mechanism of injury.

Whenever an EMT discovers a serious mechanism of injury, a rapid trauma assessment should be completed. Any of the events listed in Table 14-1 fit the category of a serious mechanism of injury; however, this list is not all inclusive by any means. Experience with trauma often teaches EMTs that a seemingly minor mechanism can have a major impact, especially in certain patient populations. Elderly patients and patients with chronic illness are often highly susceptible to serious injury, even with a minor mechanism. Such patient factors must be considered when determining the risk of injury from a particular mechanism.

Certain other high-risk patients may also benefit from a rapid trauma assessment. An example is the patient who was not wearing a seat belt at the time of a crash who may have bounced around within the vehicle. Or a bent steering wheel may be an indication that the patient's chest was injured on impact. These patients may appear stable initially, but they can have internal injuries that can cause deterioration. These patients should have a rapid trauma assessment to help in early identification of serious injury.

TABLE 14-1

Serious Trauma by Mechanism

1. Falls of 20 feet or more

2. Crash speed 20 mph or greater

3. Twenty inches of front-end impact damage

4. Twelve inches of side-impact damage from same side

5. Twenty inches of side-impact damage from opposite side

6. Death of another occupant in automobile

7. Ejection from a motor vehicle

8. Rollover MVC with unrestrained patient

9. Pedestrian struck by a vehicle at 20 mph or greater

Street Smart

Seriously injured patients can have very painful and gruesome injuries. These injuries, called *distracting* injuries, can divert the attention of the EMT away from less painful, but more life-threatening, injuries.

Experienced EMTs know that the patient who is yelling the loudest is usually hurt the least. Avoid becoming distracted by gruesome injuries or by loudly yelling patients. Instead, stick to the discipline and assess each patient methodically. Assessing the patient methodically increases the likelihood that truly life-threatening injuries will be discovered.

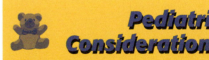

Pediatric Considerations

Because children are smaller than adults, they are susceptible to serious injury as a result of lesser mechanisms in some circumstances. For example, a fall of greater than 10 feet should be considered a serious mechanism of injury for a small child. Bicycle collisions with motor vehicles also contribute to pediatric trauma and should be regarded as a potentially serious mechanism.

Unconsciousness after trauma implies serious injury that has altered perfusion to the brain. After completion of the initial assessment and management of immediately life-threatening problems, all unconscious trauma patients should have a rapid trauma assessment. This rapid trauma assessment should be performed while en route to the closest appropriate hospital. If transportation is not immediately available, this assessment can be done on scene.

Any patient with more than one obvious injury, the multiple-trauma patient, should have a rapid trauma assessment to identify other potential injuries. Multiple injuries may put the patient at high risk of developing shock, and the EMT should keep this possibility in mind when assessing multiple-trauma patients.

Basic Assumptions

When caring for injured patients in the prehospital environment, the EMT is forced to make several assumptions. Because the diagnostic capabilities of the EMT in the field are somewhat limited, injuries often are assumed to be present if there is suspicion based on the mechanism of the injury. This assumption may result in overtreatment of many patients but will avoid the disaster of undertreatment with a bad outcome.

This assumption of injury is crucial in the situation of spinal injury. A patient who has sustained any significant force applied to the body has the potential to have an injury to the somewhat vulnerable cervical spine. As will be discussed in detail in Chapter 22, any movement of the patient's head or neck in the presence of certain types of spinal injuries can result in worsening of the injury. Spinal cord injuries carry with them a very high rate of morbidity and mortality.

It is best to assume that the patient who has sustained a significant mechanism of injury has a spinal injury and to treat that patient presumptively by stabilizing the head and neck to avoid any movement and potential of worsening a less than obvious injury. A good rule of thumb is that all trauma patients have spinal injuries until proved otherwise. All trauma care begins with manual stabilization of the head.

This concept of presumed injury based on mechanism applies to any injuries suspected in the field. If an EMT suspects the possibility of an injury, she should assume it is present and treat for it. This practice will make it less likely that the EMT will miss an injury that may cause harm to come to the patient.

ALS Backup

Serious trauma can have serious consequences. A life may depend on the EMT's ability to maintain an airway. In such cases, the assistance of more highly trained EMTs could be lifesaving. If advanced life support (ALS) personnel (i.e., EMT–Intermediates or paramedics) are not on scene, then an ALS unit should be called to the scene or should be asked to intercept the ambulance while it is en route to the closest appropriate hospital (Figure 14-1).

ALS backup is called when the EMT arrives on scene and is a part of the scene size-up. This decision to call for ALS is largely based on the EMT's assessment of the mechanism of injury. However, some patients who have experienced what appears to be a minor mecha-

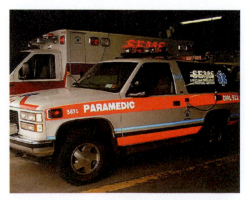

FIGURE 14-1 Consider advanced life support backup for a seriously injured patient. (Courtesy of Deborah Funk, MD, Albany Medical Center, Albany, NY.)

nism of injury may be seriously hurt. These patients may have vital signs that are unstable or significant presenting injury following physical examination or a confounding medical condition that is revealed during the patient's history. These three factors—unstable vital signs, significant physical injuries, or a significant past medical history—are reasons to call for ALS backup at this point in the patient's care (Table 14-2).

THE RAPID TRAUMA ASSESSMENT

Any trauma patient who has been exposed to a significant mechanism of injury should undergo an initial assessment followed by a rapid trauma assessment. As discussed previously, this rapid head-to-toe assessment is geared toward identifying injuries that may not be initially obvious, yet may be quite serious. The rapid trauma assessment, as the name suggests, is rapid. It should take an EMT about 1–2 minutes to complete a rapid trauma assessment. Taking longer than 2 minutes is wasteful and unnecessary and could compromise the patient by further worsening his condition if he is seriously injured.

While the EMT is performing the rapid trauma assessment, she must also be continually monitoring the patient's condition. Is the patient still awake? Is the patient maintaining his airway? Is the patient breathing adequately? If at any point the patient's condition changes, then the EMT must immediately stop the rapid trauma assessment and resolve the life-threatening problem.

During the rapid trauma assessment, the EMT is looking for indications of obvious or hidden trauma. Although accuracy is important, time should not be wasted on details that are not significant at this point. The rapid trauma assessment is short and to the point. A more detailed physical exam of areas of injury will be performed at a later time.

Physical Signs of Injury

The signs an EMT looks for that may indicate serious underlying injuries are abbreviated by the initials **DCAP-BTLS**. Table 14-3 lists the initials and their meanings. The EMT should memorize this abbreviation and use it every time she does a rapid trauma assessment.

Deformity

Any irregularity outside of the normal body shape should be considered a **deformity** and possibly the result of trauma. For example, a deformity is often the first indication of a broken or fractured bone under the skin. The forearm of the patient in Figure 14-2 is deformed.

Contusion

A bruise is a layperson's term for a **contusion**. Bruises are the result of blood pooling under the skin. Therefore, any contusion should be considered a sign of potentially serious bleeding under the skin. Contusions usually take around 15–20 minutes to form and therefore may not be immediately apparent to the EMT. The presence of a contusion, as seen in Figure 14-3, may indicate that the trauma occurred

TABLE 14-2

When to Call for ALS Backup

Unstable Vital Signs
- Glasgow coma scale <14
- Respiratory rate <10 or >29
- Systolic blood pressure <90
- Revised trauma score <11

Significant Injury
- Open or depressed skull fracture
- Flail chest
- Pelvic fractures
- Paralysis
- Two or more proximal long bone fractures
- Amputation proximal to the wrist and ankle
- Penetrating wounds of the head, chest, abdomen, or pelvis and of the extremity proximal to the knee or elbow
- Major burns
- Trauma with burns

Significant Past Medical History
- Age <5 or >55
- Cardiac disease
- Respiratory disease
- Diabetes
- Pregnancy
- Immunosuppressed
  - AIDS patient
  - Leukemia patient
  - Cancer patient undergoing chemotherapy
- Bleeding disorders
  - Hemophilia
- Anticoagulant medication
  - Heparin
  - Coumadin

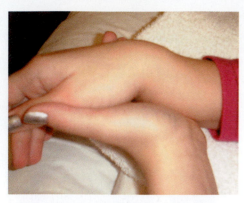

FIGURE 14-2 A fractured bone can result in a painful, swollen, deformed extremity. (Courtesy of Deborah Funk, MD, Albany Medical Center, Albany, NY.)

TABLE 14-3

DCAP-BTLS		
Term	**Meaning**	**Lay Term**
Deformity	Distorted, unnatural	Looks funny
Contusion	Injury where the skin is not broken	Bruise
Abrasion	Scraping away the top layer of skin	Skinned knee
Puncture	A wound that pierces the skin	Knife wound
Burns	Tissue injury due to heat or chemicals	Burn
Tenderness	Pain when pressure is applied	Tender, sore
Laceration	Torn skin	Cut
Swelling	Abnormal enlargement	Swollen

some time ago. The exact location and size of any contusion should be noted in the report.

Abrasion

Abrasions occur whenever the skin is scraped and underlying tissue is exposed. A skinned knee from a fall off a bike is an example of an abrasion. An abrasion in and of itself is not serious, but it delineates the area where a force was applied, as in a fall. Most of the bleeding, as seen in Figure 14-4, is self-controlled.

Puncture

A **puncture** wound is an injury caused by an object's penetrating the skin and soft tissues. Puncture wounds can be quite deep despite a relatively small skin wound. Any penetrating wound to the head, neck, chest, abdomen, or pelvis should be considered serious. The

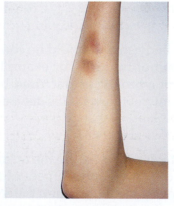

FIGURE 14-3 A large bruise, or contusion, can represent serious bleeding.

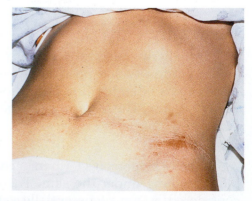

FIGURE 14-4 Abrasions indicate that force was applied to the body. (Courtesy of Deborah Funk, MD, Albany Medical Center, Albany, NY.)

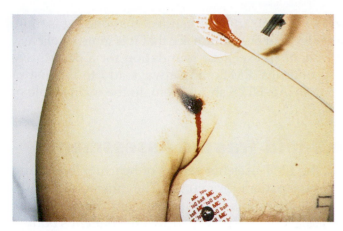
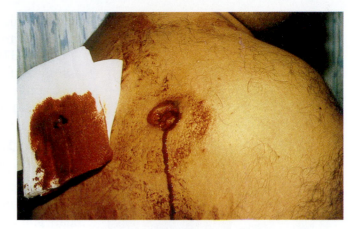

FIGURE 14-5 Puncture wounds can result in serious underlying injury. (Courtesy of Deborah Funk, MD, Albany Medical Center, Albany, NY.)

EMT cannot know how deep the puncture could have gone or what organs may have been damaged along the way. The gunshot wound in Figure 14-5 may have damaged organs that are 6 inches, or farther, away from the entrance wound. All wounds need to be reported to the hospital staff immediately so that further assessment of underlying organs may be immediately initiated.

Burn

Burns are created whenever a significant source of heat damages the outer layers of the skin. Although a superficial burn, such as sunburn, may not be serious, other deeper burns are considered more serious. Any burn involving the hands, face, feet, or genitals, such as the burn seen in Figure 14-6, is considered a serious burn regardless of the depth of the burned skin.

Tenderness

While assessing the patient, the EMT should be gently pressing her fingertips against the skin. Any area that is sensitive or even painful to the touch is said to be **tender**. Such areas, or points, of tenderness usually indicate tissue damage under the skin. Signs of tenderness include a facial grimace or guarding of the injured area (Figure 14-7). The patient may even push the EMT's hand away from his body. If the area is tender, the patient will usually complain of *pain*, a symptom.

Laceration

Any deep cuts in the skin, called **lacerations**, should be noted and reported. Lacerations often need to be *sutured*, or sewn, closed. More important, lacerations can indicate where a significant external force was applied to the body. The deep laceration seen on the patient's leg in Figure 14-8 may have damaged nerves and tendons as well as muscle.

Swelling

The EMT should note any **swelling** under the skin. This last sign can be difficult to assess. The best method of determining whether something is swollen is to compare the suspect area with the other side of the body,

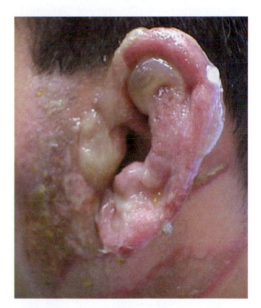

FIGURE 14-6 Burns can range from minor in severity to life threatening. (Courtesy of Deborah Funk, MD, Albany Medical Center, Albany, NY.)

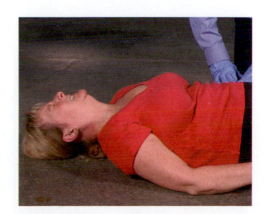

FIGURE 14-7 Facial expressions often reveal areas of tenderness.

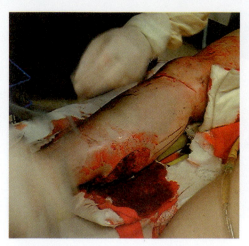

FIGURE 14-8 Lacerations can result in injury to underlying nerve, vessel, and muscle structures. (Courtesy of Deborah Funk, MD, Albany Medical Center, Albany, NY.)

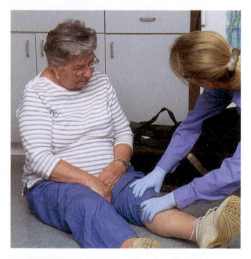

FIGURE 14-9 Swelling is often felt and not seen.

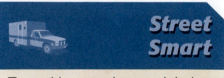

Street Smart

To avoid worsening any injuries, as well as to maintain the patient's trust, most EMTs assess obviously injured areas only after they have looked for less obvious injuries.

as shown in Figure 14-9. Often, an EMT can feel that one leg is more swollen than the other leg, but she cannot see that it is more swollen.

DCAP-BTLS represents an excellent foundation for a descriptive assessment of injury findings. EMTs may always add to this list of descriptive terms, but DCAP-BTLS should remain the main staple of any assessment.

Steps of the Rapid Trauma Assessment

Starting at the head, the EMT uses her senses of hearing, touch, and sight to rapidly assess the patient for injuries. The mnemonic DCAP-BTLS reminds her of all the points of the assessment. Starting at the head, she will methodically work her way down the patient's body.

Head and Neck

Injuries to the head and neck are often very serious. Bleeding can cause problems with the airway. Blows to the head can injure delicate brain tissue, causing the patient to lose consciousness. Neck injuries can lead to permanent paralysis. Therefore, a moment should be taken to carefully assess the head and neck. The abbreviation DCAP-BTLS should be recalled as the EMT looks for signs of injury to the head and neck.

Starting at the top of the head, the EMT should run her fingers through the patient's hair, somewhat like kneading bread dough. She should first run her fingers a short distance, feeling for any deformities, then pull her fingers out, looking for any blood on the fingertips of the gloves.

Attention should then be given to the bony structures that surround and support the airway. Grasping the angle of the jaw, the EMT would run her fingers over the length of the jawbone, ending by pressing gently on the teeth. Next, she would check inside the mouth and nose for any signs of bleeding or foreign objects.

Turning her attention to the neck, the EMT starts by assessing the anterior neck for DCAP-BTLS. Is the trachea damaged? Is the trachea midline? Is there any swelling that could threaten the airway?

An important sign to assess for is **jugular venous distension (JVD)**. Veins on the side of the neck, running from the angle of the jaw to the shoulders, are normally visible but not bulging. Bulging jugular veins in the neck can be a sign of fluid overload in the medical patient or serious internal chest injuries in the trauma patient. Significant JVD, as seen in Figure 14-10, should be reported.

Sliding her hands downward to the posterior neck, the EMT should palpate for point tenderness along the midline, starting at the base of the skull and ending at the shoulders. Any pain or tenderness should be reported. All seriously injured patients are assumed to have spinal injury until proved otherwise. Therefore, if a rigid cervical immobilization device (CID) has not already been applied, then one should be applied now.

Chest

The chest cavity contains the heart and the lungs. Injuries to the chest are potentially life threatening. An EMT's skill in quickly, but accurately, assessing the chest wall for signs of chest injury can mean the difference between life and death.

"You can't treat what you don't see." This statement could not be truer when it comes to chest injuries. It is important for the EMT to balance the patient's right to privacy against the patient's need for effective medical attention. The two can be accomplished simultaneously. Unbutton or pull down the shirt, one section at a time. Perform all aspects of the assessment at one time, then cover that section of the patient back up. If serious injury, for example, a gunshot wound, is discovered, then the need for immediate lifesaving treatment should supersede any concerns about privacy.

The EMT should begin her assessment of the chest by looking carefully at the entire chest wall. What is the quality of breathing? Does the patient appear to be straining or working hard at breathing? Problems with breathing should be addressed immediately.

Then the EMT should proceed to assess each section of the chest—upper, lower, and sides—for DCAP-BTLS. Starting at the top of the anterior chest wall, the EMT should first *look and listen,* then *feel,* that section.

Look, or inspect, for signs of chest injury: DCAP-BTLS. Are there abrasions, from seat belts, or punctures, from gunshot wounds? A quick visual inspection of the chest wall usually reveals any injuries. Paradoxical motion from a flail chest or air escaping from a sucking chest wound should be noted now if they were not picked up in the initial assessment. These findings are discussed in Chapter 13.

Using a stethoscope, the EMT should listen to, or auscultate, the lungs. Place the stethoscope against the bare skin; clothing can muffle the breath sounds. The head of the stethoscope rubbing against clothing can also create false impressions of the lung sounds. A more thorough assessment of lung sounds is done in the rapid trauma assessment than was done in the initial assessment.

At this time, the EMT should listen minimally in four places. The most useful areas to hear breath sounds are in the apices at the midclavicular lines and at the bases, in the midaxillary lines, high in the axillae. The EMT should determine whether breath sounds are present in each of these places, and, if they are present, whether they sound equal from one side to another.

Next, the EMT should feel, or palpate, the entire chest wall, looking for any injuries. In addition to the usual DCAP-BTLS, when assessing the chest, the EMT should note the presence of crepitus. Crepitus is a crunching sensation felt during palpation of an injury. Crepitus can be caused by air accumulation under the skin from a lung injury, creating the sensation of Rice Krispies when palpated, or by broken bone ends rubbing together. These physical findings indicate serious chest injury and should be reported to the hospital staff immediately upon arrival.

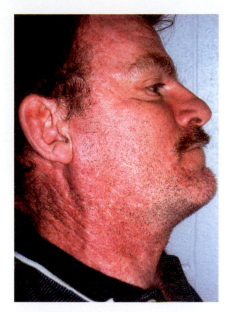

FIGURE 14-10 Jugular venous distension in the trauma patient can indicate serious internal chest injuries.

Abdomen

The abdominal cavity is home to a large number of solid and hollow organs. These organs all lie within a large bowl-like cavity formed by the pelvis and the diaphragm. This abdominal bowl can hold a great deal of blood without demonstrating significant outward signs. The rapid trauma assessment will not only discover some of the more subtle signs of intra-abdominal injury but also perhaps more important, can establish a baseline abdominal exam for comparison later.

The abdomen lacks any distinct landmarks. For this reason, the belly button, or umbilicus, serves as the midpoint of the abdomen, and the abdomen is divided into four quadrants. Each quadrant is labeled left or right, upper or lower, as the case may be. Review Chapter 5 for a discussion of abdominal anatomy.

The EMT should assess the abdomen using the "look first, then feel" concept that was described in the chest assessment section. The abdomen should be exposed for assessment, and the EMT should first look for DCAP-BTLS.

Although seat belts are very helpful in reducing injuries sustained in MVCs, they can cause some injury also. A seat belt applies pressure across the abdomen and torso; this pressure can be significant in the event of a high-speed crash. The pressure from the seat belt can cause contusions and abrasions to the abdominal wall, which can be seen by the EMT during her assessment, and may result in internal abdominal organ injury. These internal injuries are most often seen when the seat belt is worn incorrectly and are invariably not as severe as the injuries sustained by unbelted occupants of a vehicle involved in a high-speed crash.

After a complete visual inspection, the EMT should gently palpate each quadrant. The abdomen should be soft and nondistended. Any distension should be noted as well as any attempt by the patient to *guard* the abdomen. **Guarding**, a tightening of the abdominal muscles, is a protective reflex when abdominal injury exists and is evidenced by a localized firm feeling upon palpation of the abdomen. A patient's grimace or loud protest may indicate that an area is very painful. The exact location of any tenderness should be carefully noted and reported.

The pelvis is a strong ring of bone that protects many important organs and large blood vessels. Damage to these organs and vessels can lead to a substantial amount of blood loss. It takes a great deal of force to break this bony ring. However, if the pelvis is fractured, then it is likely that the underlying structures are also damaged.

To assess the bony pelvis, the EMT should gently press downward, then inward on the pelvic wings. A fractured pelvis is painful, and the conscious patient will likely make this discomfort known. If bony fractures are present when this compression is done, the EMT may feel crepitus as bone ends grate against one another. If tenderness or crepitus is elicited during the exam, that maneuver should not be repeated.

Finally, the EMT should press downward on the pubic bone to assess for fractures of the anterior pelvis. Some EMTs find it more acceptable to take the patient's hand, provided it is not injured, and place it over the pubis. Then the EMT lays her hand on top of the patient's hand and gently presses down. Again, patient modesty or EMT inhibition should not prevent the patient from receiving a complete medical assessment.

Extremities

Although a broken bone itself is usually not life threatening, the bleeding that can come with a broken bone can be significant. Therefore, one of the objectives of an extremity check is to determine whether there is severe bleeding within the tissues.

Street Smart

Always end the abdominal assessment by palpating the most painful quadrant last. Palpation of a painful quadrant may make the patient reluctant to allow further examination of the rest of the abdomen.

As usual, the EMT should assess each extremity using DCAP-BTLS. Any deformity noted may be an indication of a broken bone. Contusions and abrasions indicate where a force has been applied. The EMT should carefully assess for deformity and tenderness in those areas particularly. Often the only sign of bleeding into the soft tissues, for example, the thigh, is swelling. Again, this swelling may not be readily apparent to the naked eye, but careful comparison of one leg with the other will reveal the swelling occurring inside.

Any lacerations that are accompanied by deformity may indicate that an open fracture of the bone has occurred. An open fracture carries with it serious risk of bleeding and infection and will be discussed further in Chapter 25.

Major arteries, veins, and nerves run parallel to the large bones of the body. Therefore, if a large bone breaks, there is a great likelihood that the sharp broken ends will puncture these vessels or damage the nerves. The result is severe bleeding or loss of function. To assess whether a blood vessel has been damaged, the EMT should check for peripheral pulses.

The most accessible peripheral pulse in the arm is the radial pulse at the wrist. The radial pulse can be found on the palmar surface of the wrist proximal to the thumb. The most accessible peripheral pulse in the leg is the pedal pulse. The pedal pulse can be found along the midline of the top of the foot, about halfway between the ankle and the great toe.

Whenever an EMT is checking for the pulse in an extremity that has been injured, she should also check for nerve function. Nerves have both fibers that create movement—motor nerves—and fibers that create feeling—sensory nerves. Therefore, a check of motion and sensation is part of the assessment.

A complete assessment of peripheral pulses and motor and sensory nerve functions (PMS; pulses, movement, and sensation) should be completed on all four extremities. Typically, an EMT will report "PMS×4 intact." Any loss of these functions should be reported.

Back and Buttocks

When the patient is being logrolled onto a backboard, a moment should be taken to assess the back and buttocks. The EMT should quickly perform a check for DCAP-BTLS. After a visual inspection for signs of injury, a hand should be run down the length of the spine from the top of the shoulders to the top of the buttocks. Any wounds or tenderness should be noted and reported.

Careful control of the spine, using a rigid cervical immobilization device as well as continuous manual in-line stabilization, is required. It takes a minimum of three providers to properly logroll the patient to assess the back and buttocks. The concepts involved in spinal immobilization are discussed further in Chapter 22.

Baseline Vital Signs and SAMPLE History

A baseline set of vital signs is a part of every physical assessment. Some EMTs will *clear* an arm so that another EMT can start vital signs while the rapid trauma assessment is being performed.

A SAMPLE history is then performed. An abbreviated history of the present illness is often obtained on scene. Once the rapid assessment is complete, the EMT must take the time to obtain as complete a SAMPLE history as possible. Frequently, this history is taken while en route to the hospital.

Skill 14-1 describes the procedure for a rapid trauma assessment.

SKILL 14-1 *Rapid Trauma Assessment*

PURPOSE: To assess the major trauma patient for injuries that are not life threatening.

STANDARD PRECAUTIONS:

☑ Appropriate personal protective equipment
☑ Stethoscope
☑ Blood pressure cuff
☑ Scissors
☑ Cervical collars

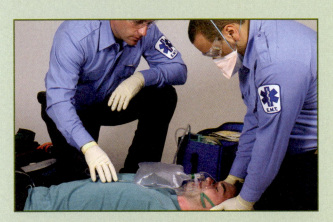

1 After completing an appropriate scene size-up and initial assessment, the EMT performs a rapid trauma assessment on the trauma patient with a significant mechanism of injury. Manual head stabilization should be maintained for the duration of the rapid trauma assessment.

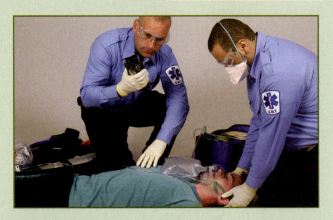

2 Before beginning the rapid trauma assessment, the EMT considers a request for ALS backup and reconsiders his decision for transport priority. Most seriously injured trauma patients are en route to the hospital while the rapid trauma assessment is being done.

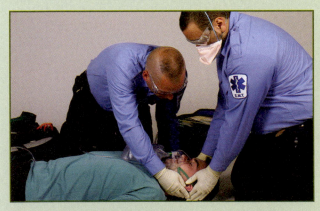

3 The EMT next assesses the head by careful inspection and palpation for any signs of injury. Deformities, contusions, abrasions, punctures or penetrations, burns, tenderness, lacerations, or swelling should be noted. Moving in a methodical fashion, the EMT then inspects and palpates the neck.

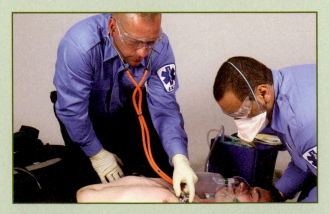

4 The EMT next looks, listens, and feels the chest to assess for the presence of any signs of injury. Breath sounds should be carefully assessed at the apices and the bases. Presence and equality of air movement should be noted.

(continues)

SKILL 14-1 (continued)

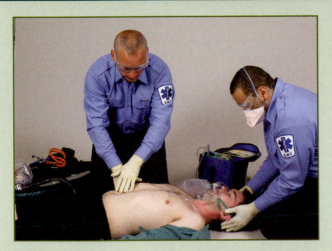

5 The abdominal assessment includes looking and feeling for any signs of injury. The pelvis is visually inspected, then gently compressed downward and inward in order to find any signs of injury.

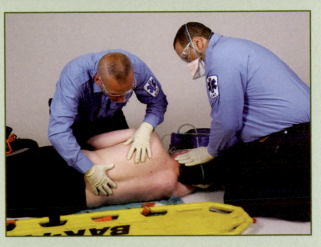

6 After rolling the patient to the side, using a logroll technique and maintaining spinal immobilization, the EMT inspects and palpates the back and buttocks to find any signs of injury.

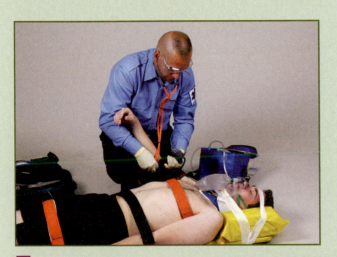

7 After the rapid trauma assessment has been completed, a complete baseline set of vital signs must be taken.

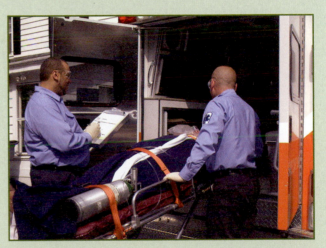

8 A SAMPLE history is then elicited. Bystanders may provide information if the patient is unconscious. Transport should have been initiated by this point.

THE FOCUSED TRAUMA ASSESSMENT

Not every trauma call is a life or death emergency. In fact, most are not. That is not meant to imply that these patients do not need prompt medical attention but simply that the nature of the injury permits the EMT to assess and stabilize the injury on scene. This assessment and stabilization before transport prevents further injury from occurring.

If the injury is obviously isolated and the mechanism does not suggest further injury potential, it is unnecessary to perform a head-

✳ *Ankle Injury*

The radio crackled. "Officer Sherman, go to the lower level food court escalator for a woman who may have fallen." The mall had trained its security officers as EMTs about 6 months ago. This was Officer Sherman's first call as an EMT.

When Officer Sherman arrived, he did a quick scene size-up. There was one patient sitting on the floor at the foot of the escalator. Officer Sherman quickly donned a pair of gloves and reached under the rail to turn the escalator off.

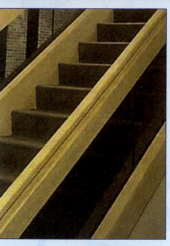

(Courtesy of PhotoDisc.)

A woman in her 20s was sitting cross-legged on the floor. Officer Sherman directed another officer to perform manual stabilization of her neck while he asked the woman what had happened. As she was answering, Officer Sherman did a quick initial assessment. He noted that she was awake and alert, her airway was patent, and she was breathing a little fast but not too fast. He further noted that she had no obvious bleeding and her pulse was a little rapid.

"Where do you hurt, ma'am?" Officer Sherman asked. She replied that she had been distracted for "just a minute" and had tripped at the bottom of the stairs when getting off; now her right ankle is hurt.

- What potential does this mechanism of injury have?
- What sort of assessment does the woman need?
- What priority does this type of injury create?

to-toe rapid trauma assessment. If the mechanism of injury is minor or the injury is isolated, it is more appropriate to focus on the injured part.

A physical assessment that is limited to the area of injury is called a focused trauma assessment. Except for the fact that it is limited to one body part or region, it is otherwise performed in the same manner as the rapid trauma assessment.

After an appropriate scene size-up and initial assessment reveal that the patient has no significant mechanism or obvious signs of serious injury, the EMT should begin a focused trauma assessment based on the patient's specific injury. Focusing on the affected area, the EMT should assess for DCAP-BTLS.

Naturally, treatments will follow in accordance with the type and severity of the injury. Figure 14-11 presents a flowchart for assessment. It is a safe practice to assume the worst injury and hope for the best.

Every patient, regardless of the severity of the injuries, needs a baseline set of vital signs and a SAMPLE history. Appropriate preparation for transport should be accomplished, and the patient should be brought to the most appropriate hospital for further evaluation of the injury. Skill 14-2 demonstrates the focused trauma assessment.

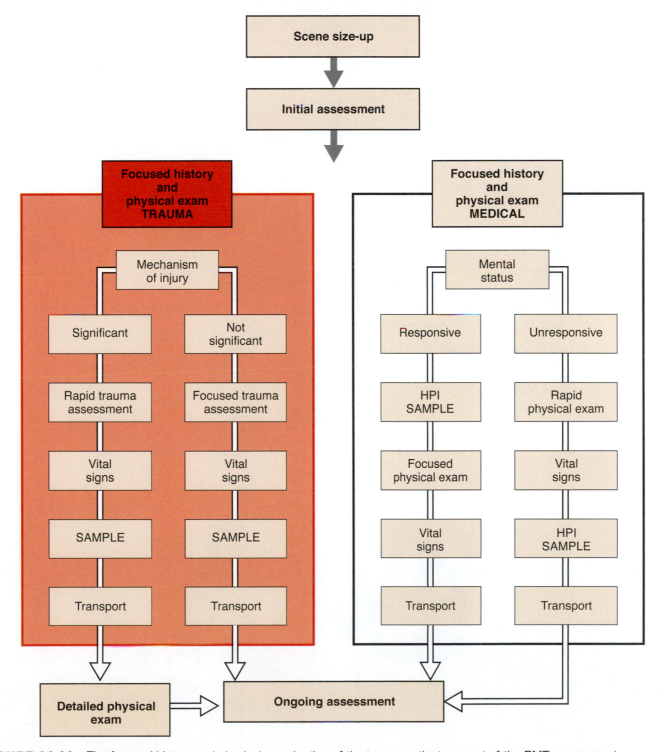

FIGURE 14-11   The focused history and physical examination of the trauma patient are part of the EMT assessment.

SKILL 14-2 *Focused Trauma Assessment*

PURPOSE: To obtain a baseline physical examination for assessment and comparison of the minor trauma patient.

STANDARD PRECAUTIONS:

☑ Stethoscope
☑ Blood pressure cuff
☑ Assortment of cervical collars

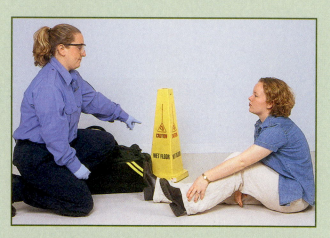

1 The EMT considers the mechanism of injury. Depending on the mechanism of injury, the EMT decides whether to perform a rapid trauma assessment or a focused physical examination.

2 The EMT next determines the chief complaint.

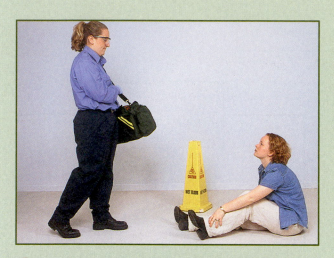

3 The EMT performs a focused examination specific to the injury.

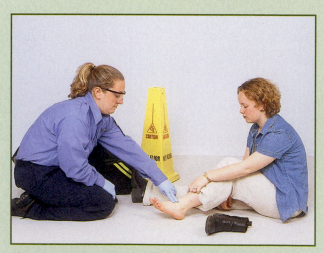

(continues)

SKILL 14-2 *(continued)*

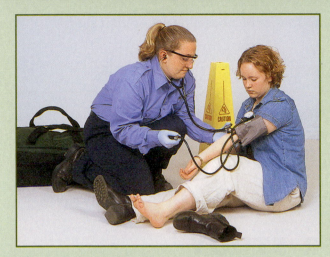

4 The EMT then obtains baseline vital signs.

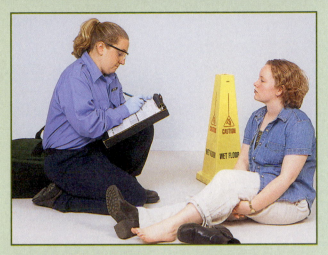

5 The EMT completes the assessment with a SAMPLE history.

CONCLUSION

The decision whether to perform a rapid trauma assessment on a patient or a focused physical examination is a function of the severity of the injury as well as the mechanism of injury. Whenever an EMT is in doubt about which type to perform, then the EMT should perform a rapid trauma assessment.

The usefulness of a rapid trauma assessment is in discovering potentially life-threatening injuries. To find an injury, one has to suspect an injury might exist in the first place. Consideration of the mechanism of injury can help the EMT obtain a high index of suspicion that a serious underlying injury may exist.

Most injuries are minor and a focused physical examination is sufficient to determine the right course of treatment. However, keep an open mind and always suspect that other injuries may have occurred.

TEST YOUR KNOWLEDGE

1. What is the main objective of the rapid trauma assessment?
2. Give several examples of trauma patients who would receive a rapid trauma assessment.
3. Why must EMTs maintain the dignity of their patients during a physical examination?
4. Give examples of mechanisms of injury that have a high potential for serious bodily harm.
5. List each step in the assessment of a seriously injured trauma patient, starting at the scene size-up.
6. What does each of the initials in DCAP-BTLS mean?

7. In addition to DCAP-BTLS, list one extra assessment finding for each of the following body regions: head, neck, chest, abdomen, pelvis, extremities, and back.

8. What is the importance of a baseline set of vital signs?

INTERNET RESOURCES

Search the Web using these key words:

* Trauma assessment
* Mechanism of injury
* DCAP-BTLS

Share any interesting Web sites and facts with your colleagues.

FURTHER STUDY

Elling, B., & Elling, K. (2002). *Principles of patient assessment in EMS*. Clifton Park, NY: Thomson Delmar Learning.

Prehospital Trauma Life Support Committee of National Association of Emergency Medical Technicians and American College of Surgeons/Committee on Trauma. (1999). *Basic and advanced prehospital trauma life support* (4th ed.). Philadelphia: Mosby.

CHAPTER 15

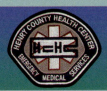
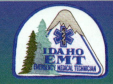
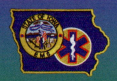

Detailed Physical Examination

KEY TERMS

Battle's sign
cerebrospinal fluid (CSF)
hyphema
raccoon's eyes

OBJECTIVES

Upon completion of this chapter, the reader should be able to:

1. List the patients who require a detailed physical examination.
2. Describe the primary objective of the detailed physical examination.
3. Describe how the detailed physical examination is similar to and different from the rapid trauma assessment.
4. List the points of examination for the following areas of the body: head, neck, chest, abdomen, pelvis, extremities, and back.

OVERVIEW

The detailed physical examination is a patient-specific, injury-specific examination. It is patient specific because it is typically used for patients who are unconscious or who have a decreased level of consciousness. It is injury specific because it is performed on all patients who have endured a significant mechanism of injury or who have sustained significant injuries. This chapter reviews the detailed physical examination in depth.

DETAILED PHYSICAL EXAMINATION

The primary objective of the detailed physical examination is to discover all signs of injury that may not have been uncovered during the rapid trauma assessment. Because it is a more extensive assessment that takes time to complete, a detailed physical examination should not be performed on scene, except if transport to the hospital is not yet available.

The goal of an emergency medical technician (EMT) in completing a detailed physical exam is to uncover those signs of injury that could be treated while en route to the hospital. The fact that the detailed physical examination must be conducted during transport substantially limits the length of time available to complete it. Nevertheless, it may take an EMT 10 minutes to properly complete a detailed physical examination.

A detailed physical examination is always performed *after* the initial assessment and rapid trauma assessment have been completed. The rapid trauma assessment creates a baseline physical examination for the EMT. The detailed physical examination measures the effectiveness of prehospital treatments that were initiated early on in the assessment. In addition, further attention is paid to details of the physical exam that were not addressed in the more rapid previous assessments.

Changes in a patient's condition, especially deterioration, may require the EMT to rethink decisions. Should the patient's priority be upgraded? Would the patient benefit from the assistance of an advanced life support (ALS) unit? Is the destination hospital still appropriate, or should the patient be diverted to a specialized trauma

Silo Accident

The high-angle rescue team had successfully lowered the patient from the pinnacle of the silo to the ground using a basket. The patient, a 16-year-old male, had climbed the conveyer to fix a jam when it suddenly lurched forward, throwing the youth some 20 feet to the grain pile below.

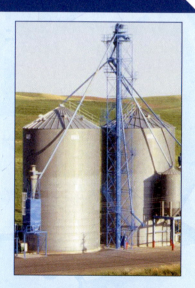

The initial assessment was unremarkable, and the rapid trauma assessment uncovered only some minor contusions on his arms and legs. Because of the height of the fall and the length of time that it took to rescue him, the EMTs decided to transport him to the regional trauma center. The youth was quickly assessed and packaged for immediate transportation to the hospital.

- On the basis of the mechanism of injury, what injuries should be suspected?
- What, if any, further signs of injury would the detailed physical examination uncover?
- On the basis of the limited information provided, what conditions could develop en route that would necessitate either an ALS intercept or a change in the patient's transportation priority?

center? These decisions are based on changes in the patient's condition that are often noted during the detailed physical exam.

The detailed physical exam is a methodical head-to-toe physical examination. All patients who may have further injury that was not uncovered by the initial assessment and rapid trauma assessment should be given a detailed physical examination. This category includes any trauma patient who had a significant mechanism of injury or who shows signs of serious or multiple injuries. The detailed physical exam should be performed during transport to the hospital only if enough personnel are present and time permits. Ongoing treatment of life-threatening conditions may preclude the completion of this examination.

The detailed physical examination need *not* be done on trauma patients with an isolated injury. Performing a detailed patient assessment on these patients would be too intrusive and therefore inappropriate.

Steps in the Detailed Physical Examination

The detailed physical examination is very much like the rapid trauma assessment. The mnemonic DCAP-BTLS is used to describe the signs of injury that should be sought. However, there are more special elements to the detailed physical examination that will be discussed as each body section is addressed.

Head

Beginning at the head, the EMT should carefully palpate the entire skull (see Skill 15-1). Starting at the rear of the skull, in the occipital area, the EMT should look and feel for DCAP-BTLS (see Table 14-3 for a definition of this term). Even small external injuries may indicate the possibility of serious internal head injury and should be carefully noted.

Carefully remove any glass shards that might cause injury. Use a penlight to improve your vision. If a spot of blood is found, take a piece of gauze and blot the area gently. Is there a small laceration that is causing the bleeding? This detailed exam of the head can reveal signs of injury that may be important in the care of the patient.

Street Smart

The patient may question the necessity of another physical examination. It is important to explain to the patient that the first physical examination was very brief and that you are going to now perform a complete physical examination.

The added privacy of the ambulance should be pointed out to the patient. A professional attitude, coupled with the seclusion of the ambulance compartment, is usually enough to convince the patient to agree to a detailed physical examination.

SKILL 15-1 *Detailed Physical Examination*

PURPOSE: To obtain a more thorough physical examination of injuries to a trauma patient; usually performed en route to the hospital.

STANDARD PRECAUTIONS:

☑ Penlight
☑ Stethoscope
☑ Blood pressure cuff
☑ Scissors

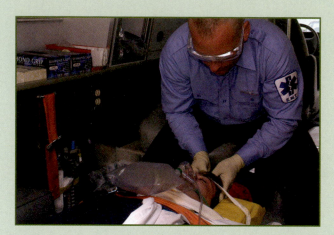

1 The EMT starts at the top of the head and assesses the scalp and the face for DCAP-BTLS.

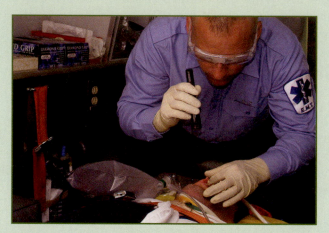

2 Next, he assesses the ears, nose, and throat, noting any bleeding or drainage of fluids as well as jugular venous distension or displacement of the trachea.

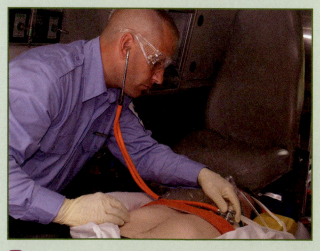

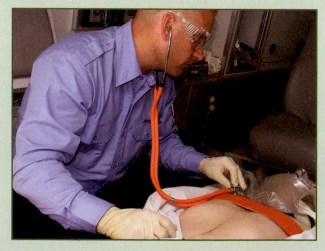

3 Then the EMT proceeds to looking, listening, and feeling the chest wall for injury, including crepitus and paradoxical motion.

(continues)

SKILL 15-1 *(continued)*

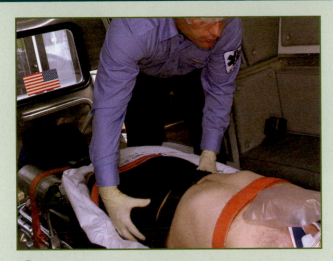

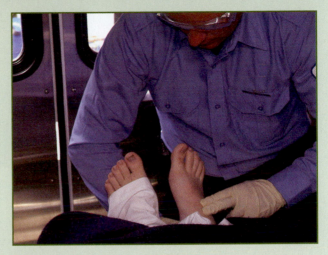

4 Turning next to the abdomen and the pelvis, the EMT assesses for DCAP-BTLS. Assessment of the pelvis should include gentle pressure inward on the hips to check for hip fracture.

5 Then the extremities are assessed for pulses, movement, and sensation as well as DCAP-BTLS.

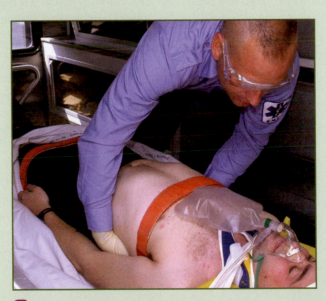

6 After checking as much of the posterior as possible, the EMT obtains another set of vital signs.

Ears

Next, the EMT should examine the ears, looking for DCAP-BTLS. In addition, the EMT should quickly look into the ears for the presence of any drainage. Clear fluid from the ear may be **cerebrospinal fluid (CSF)** (Figure 15-1). This is the nutrient-rich fluid that bathes and protects the brain and spinal cord. Because this clear fluid comes from inside the skull, the presence of CSF in the ears indicates a skull fracture. *Never* attempt to stop the flow of CSF because doing so can result

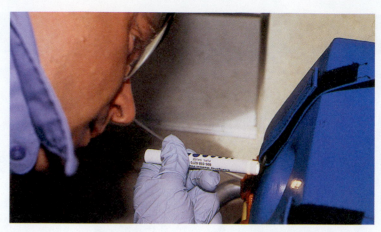

FIGURE 15-1 Clear fluid from the ear could be cerebrospinal fluid (CSF).

in increased pressure inside the skull. The EMT can use clean gauze to absorb the fluid that is leaking. Chapter 21 discusses skull fractures in more detail.

Certain types of skull fractures can create characteristic physical findings. The EMT should carefully look for these findings and report them to hospital staff if found. Bruising behind the ears, called **Battle's sign**, can indicate a fracture to the base of the skull. This condition will be discussed further in Chapter 21.

Eyes

Moving toward the front of the skull and the face, the EMT should take time to thoroughly examine the patient's eyes. Although trauma to the eyes may not be life threatening, it can have a lifelong impact on the patient. It is useful to compare one eye with the other to look for differences while looking for DCAP-BTLS.

In addition to the usual signs of injury that the EMT is looking for, there are several findings that may be specifically sought out in the eye examination. Discoloration such as bruising around the eye should be noted. Bruising around the eyes is sometimes called **raccoon's eyes** and may be indicative of a fracture to the base of the skull.

During the eye examination, the pupils should be carefully assessed for size, shape, and reaction to light. Any inequality, irregular shape, or lack of constriction to light may indicate serious eye or brain injury and should be carefully noted. Chapter 10 discusses the examination of the pupils in detail.

Any foreign material, such as dirt or glass, should be brushed away from the eyes if possible. If this material does not easily brush away, the EMT should leave it alone and allow the hospital staff to remove any objects that are stuck in the eye.

Injuries to the eye can result in bleeding both outside and inside the eye. Accumulation of blood inside the eye can sometimes be seen as a haziness in the front of the eye. This haziness may settle out into a layer of blood that is visible in the front of the eye. The term for blood that has accumulated inside the eye is **hyphema** (Figure 15-2).

Occasionally, an EMT will observe a pupil that is irregularly shaped. This irregularity is often the result of surgery to remove

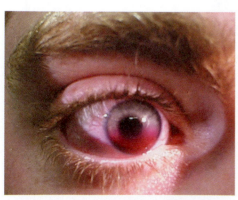

FIGURE 15-2 Blood in the front of the eye is called a hyphema. (Courtesy of Kevin Reilly, MD, Albany Medical Center, Albany, NY.)

abnormal growths in the front of the eye, called cataracts. The irregularly shaped pupil resulting from surgery may not react well to light.

If the pupils of the eye are equal in size, round, and react to bright light by constricting bilaterally, then EMTs will document PERRL. PERRL means the *pupils* are *equal*, *round*, and *reactive* to *light*.

Face

Moving away from the eyes, the EMT should next carefully assess the rest of the face. Careful inspection and palpation of each of the bony prominences in the face will reveal any evidence of DCAP-BTLS.

Nose

The EMT should turn his attention to the nose next. Inspection and palpation for DCAP-BTLS should reveal any injuries. Injuries to the nose may not in and of themselves be life threatening, but they may have implications for the EMT. A painful, swollen, and deformed nose may be broken. Excessive bleeding may result if a nasopharyngeal airway is inserted into a broken nose.

To assess for any bleeding or drainage, the EMT can use a penlight to look into the nares. Blood running down the back of the throat may nauseate the patient and cause vomiting. Any clear fluid running from the nose should be reported immediately. It may only be mucus, but it can also be CSF. Any CSF draining from the nose indicates that a serious head injury may have occurred.

Mouth

The mouth is the beginning of the airway. Injury to the mouth can create a potential airway problem. Careful inspection for signs of injury to the inside or outside of the mouth should be performed. Assessment for DCAP-BTLS will reveal such injuries.

In addition, the EMT should examine the inside of the mouth carefully because anything that is in the mouth could block the airway. The stability of the teeth should be assessed by gently pressing on them with a gloved finger. Broken pieces of teeth and any other foreign object should be immediately removed from the mouth to prevent aspiration. Any secretions or bleeding should be immediately suctioned.

If a bleeding source can be identified, direct pressure on the site may help to slow the bleeding, decreasing the potential for an airway problem. Lacerations to the cheek can be controlled by direct pressure applied to both the inside and the outside of the mouth.

Is the tongue swollen, or are the surrounding tissues reddened or otherwise discolored? Swelling, from burns for example, in the mouth can mean swelling in the lower airway as well. Continued swelling can lead to a complete airway obstruction. A hoarse voice after airway injury is one sign of lower airway swelling and should be considered a true emergency.

What about dentures or other oral hardware? If a piece of a dental appliance is loose in the mouth, then it should be removed and stored safely in a cup. If the dentures are intact, then leave them in place. The

Street Smart

What if the eye does not react and the patient has not experienced any head trauma? Ask the patient if she has a glass eye; they are more common than one might expect.

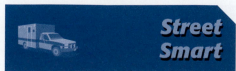

dentures serve as a platform for a mask seal if the patient needs to be ventilated.

Neck

Moving down to the neck, the EMT should gently palpate the anterior soft tissues. When injured, these tissues can quickly swell and threaten the airway. Careful inspection for DCAP-BTLS should reveal evidence of injury.

When assessing the anterior neck, the EMT should identify the position of the trachea. It is normally easily palpated anteriorly at the base of the neck right in the midline. A displaced trachea is a sign of increased pressure in the chest.

Chest

In the detailed physical examination, the chest should be thoroughly examined and the presence or absence of signs found in the rapid trauma assessment should be reaffirmed.

Using the *look, listen, and feel* methodology, the EMT should examine the entire chest wall, front and back. DCAP-BTLS should be sought during this assessment. Check the armpits and under the breasts for wounds, as small punctures can easily hide in these places.

Take a moment to watch the patient breathe. Is the breathing comfortable and effective? Is the patient *catching* her breath when the EMT asks her to breathe deeply? This could be a sign of a broken rib because deep inspiration will cause pain. Shallow breathing can also mean that there are rib fractures.

Using a stethoscope, the EMT should reassess the same four areas on the anterior chest as were assessed in the rapid trauma assessment (see Skill 15-1). It is important to keep the "scope on the skin" to avoid extraneous sound.

The EMT should also listen to the posterior lung fields if possible. Sliding the stethoscope between the patient and the backboard, the EMT should attempt to listen at the apices by placing the head of the stethoscope at the top of the shoulder blades. The EMT can slide the

Safety Tip

Rigid cervical immobilization devices are often placed on the patient quickly, sometimes before a complete neck assessment has been performed. Most cervical immobilization devices have holes in the front or sides, or both, to allow for examination after placement. If these spaces do not allow the necessary examination and the EMT must open the collar anteriorly, he must be sure to maintain adequate cervical spine immobilization during this assessment. A second EMT manually holding cervical spine stabilization is appropriate in this case.

If it is not absolutely necessary to the care of the patient, the cervical collar should not be removed once it has been applied. Keeping it in place avoids any unnecessary movement of a potentially unstable neck injury.

stethoscope in laterally behind the patient to better assess the base of the lung. In the supine patient, assessing lung sounds posteriorly can reveal sounds that may not have been noted during the initial exam.

A patient can fracture a rib without creating a deformity; this is called a nondisplaced rib fracture. These fractures can be discovered only by running your fingers over the bones until the patient complains of tenderness in one particular area.

Starting at the sternum, the EMT should place his forearm flat against the sternum and press firmly but gently downward. In this way, fractures of the sternum, or the rib attachments to the sternum, can be detected. Gentle palpation of the ribs anteriorly from top to bottom should reveal areas of tenderness or deformity, as well as any crepitus.

If an area of tenderness or bony crepitus is found, the EMT should take care not to cause further pain or injury by repeated palpation of the area. Finding no tenderness, the EMT should gently, but firmly, compress the rib cage (Figure 15-3). Any crepitus or paradoxical motion of a section of rib cage should be noted.

Starting at the top of the sternum, the EMT should run his fingers along the clavicles, feeling for deformity as well as tenderness. Once both hands are on the shoulders, the EMT should gently squeeze the shoulders together to see whether the shoulder girdle is intact.

Abdomen

Before starting the examination of the abdomen and pelvis, explain to the patient what is about to happen. The look, listen, and feel philosophy works well for an abdominal assessment. *Look* for any injuries as evidenced by DCAP-BTLS. Identify landmarks, such as the umbilicus and the margins of the ribs. Assess for any distension, which may indicate bleeding internally.

Note the presence of urinary incontinence. Injuries to the spine can cause the patient to lose control of her bladder. Local trauma to the bladder, for example, a penetrating knife wound, can cause incontinence also. Finally, certain medical conditions, such as seizures, can lead to incontinence.

Always document the presence of urine on clothing. Frequently, clothing is cut away from the patient and discarded. After that, it may be impossible to know whether the patient was incontinent on scene unless the EMT documents it.

Listen to what the patient tells you. Where is the pain? Does one area of the abdomen hurt more than another? Next, *feel* the anterior abdomen gently (Figure 15-4). Does the abdomen feel firm or soft when palpated? A firm, tender abdomen indicates the natural muscular guarding of an injury. Such guarding is suspicious for abdominal bleeding.

If the patient either has complained of abdominal pain in one area or has shown signs of tenderness and guarding on previous physical exams, then it is unnecessary to reassess those areas. Little more can be gained from the information, and the unnecessary creation of pain is cruel.

The final step of the detailed physical examination of the abdomen involves compression and flexion of the pelvis. Gently compress

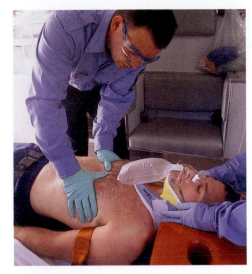
FIGURE 15-3 Gentle chest compression will reveal rib fractures.

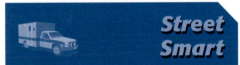
Street Smart

Seat belts often leave a red mark on the abdomen. Look for the "seat belt sign." Some patients, often obese or pregnant patients, wear their seat belt over the waistline instead of over the hips as it is designed to be worn. The result is that in a sudden stop or deceleration, the unprotected hollow organs of the abdomen can be crushed. Stop and think what organs are under that abrasion.

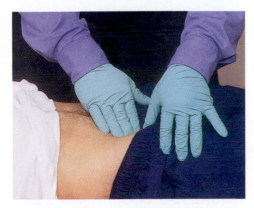
FIGURE 15-4 Careful examination of the abdomen will reveal tenderness.

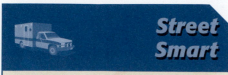

downward on the iliac wings, watching the patient's face for signs of discomfort. Pressing inward on the hips will help to discover a hip fracture. Finally, gently press downward on the pubis to stress the bony pelvic ring (Figure 15-5). Tenderness during any part of this exam indicates possible fracture. If bony pelvic pain is present, a very gentle palpation of the area should be performed to assess the area of tenderness. Compression and flexion is not indicated for the patient in whom a pelvic injury is already suspected.

Extremities

The detailed physical examination for the limbs is very similar to the rapid trauma assessment for the limbs described in Chapter 14. However, in this phase of the assessment, more attention is paid to injuries that are not life or limb threatening, such as superficial wounds.

Starting with a visual inspection, the EMT should look for any evidence of injury in the presence of DCAP-BTLS. Then, each limb should be carefully and firmly palpated along the length of each bone.

Each limb should be examined separately. Take time to discover any localized tenderness that might indicate an injury of the bone underneath. A nondisplaced bone fracture will be straight, and the bone may even support some weight. Treat any bone pain as if it were a fracture, until an x-ray proves otherwise. Management of bony injuries is described in Chapter 25.

During the assessment of the extremities, it is often helpful to compare one extremity with the other. Most extremities are quite symmetric in appearance. Look for differences in size and coloration.

Every examination of the extremities ends with a reassessment for pulses, movement, and sensation (PMS). Each peripheral pulse should be checked (pedal and radial pulses) and compared from side to side. An absent pulse on one side indicates injury to that extremity. The patient's ability to move an extremity should be tested. To assess for movement in the hands, ask the patient to grasp your index finger and squeeze. You should be assessing the *equality* of the grasp as well as the strength.

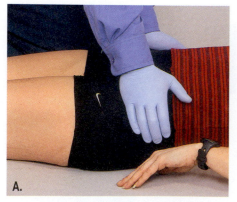 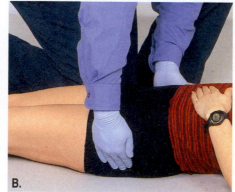 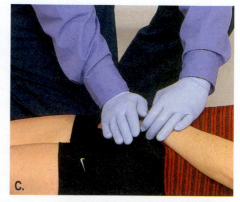

FIGURE 15-5 A. Gentle pressure downward on the iliac wings may reveal fractures and sites of patient discomfort in the pelvic area. B. Gentle pressure inward on the hips may reveal a hip fracture. C. Gentle downward pressure on the pubis will reveal pelvic fractures.

To assess for movement in the feet, ask the patient to flex and extend her feet, as shown in Figure 15-6. Ask the patient to "point your toes to your nose and then press on the gas." This instruction encourages the patient to fully extend and flex both feet. No further movement should be requested in the multiple-injured patient to avoid aggravating any existing injuries. Last, the sensation in each extremity is checked by gentle squeezing of a toe or a finger.

Back and Buttocks

The patient's back and buttocks can hide many wounds, for example, lacerations or exit wounds. While maintaining continuous manual stabilization of the head, preferably with a cervical collar in place, the EMT should carefully examine the back and buttocks for injury. Any deformity, contusion, abrasion, punctures, burns, tenderness, lacerations, or swelling should be carefully examined and noted in the patient's report.

Common examples of back injuries include stab wounds in the upper back from an overhead knife and abrasions caused by the road surface after the patient has been ejected from a vehicle. A common example of a buttocks wound would be a partial avulsion of the buttocks following a motorcycle collision.

Vital Signs Revisited

Every prehospital medical examination should be followed up with a full set of vital signs. This set of vital signs should then be compared with the baseline set obtained after the rapid trauma assessment to establish a trend. Any changes should be noted. A rising heart rate could be a sign of shock. An increasing respiratory rate may indicate worsening chest injuries. Any significant changes in vital signs should be reported to the hospital staff.

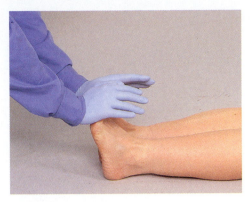

FIGURE 15-6 Flexion and extension of the toes can test the strength of the lower extremities.

Street Smart

Most EMTs obtain a full set of vital signs as often as is indicated. However, many EMTs will follow or *track* a pulse rate or respiratory rate continuously. During a major trauma call, new EMTs may be assigned to get a radial pulse every minute and report them aloud to the crew.

A report might go like this. "Radial pulse 100, strong and regular. Radial pulse 120 and weaker. I can't find the radial pulse anymore." That is an excellent description of consequences of blood loss and hypoperfusion.

CONCLUSION

The detailed physical examination (Figure 15-7) is a comprehensive head-to-toe examination of the patient, looking more specifically for injuries that need to be addressed.

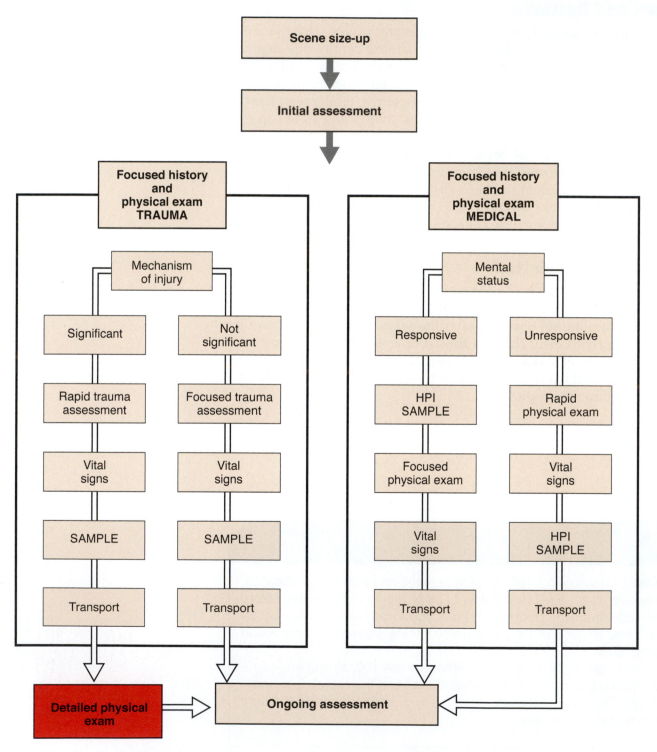

FIGURE 15-7 The detailed physical examination is part of the EMT's assessment of the trauma patient.

TEST YOUR KNOWLEDGE

1. Which patients should always receive a detailed physical examination?

2. What is the primary objective of the detailed physical examination?

3. How is the detailed physical examination similar to and different from the rapid trauma assessment?

4. List the additional points of examination beyond DCAP-BTLS for the following body areas: head, neck, chest, abdomen, pelvis, extremities, back.

INTERNET RESOURCES

Search the Web using these key words:

- Battle's sign
- Raccoon's eyes
- Hyphema

List the interesting Web sites and facts you discover. Share them with your colleagues.

FURTHER STUDY

Elling, B., & Elling, K. (2002). *Principles of patient assessment in EMS.* Clifton Park, NY: Thomson Delmar Learning.

McSwain, N., et al. (1999). *Basic and advanced prehospital trauma life support* (4th ed.). Philadelphia: Mosby.

CHAPTER 16

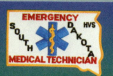

Focused History and Physical Examination of the Medical Patient

KEY TERMS

chief complaint

focused physical examination

MedicAlert® emblems

ongoing assessment

OPQRST

rapid physical examination

vial of life

OBJECTIVES

Upon completion of this chapter, the reader should be able to:

1. Describe the different priorities when assessing a medical versus a trauma patient.

2. List the steps followed when assessing a responsive medical patient.

3. Identify the importance of eliciting any past medical history from the medical patient.

4. List the steps followed when assessing an unresponsive medical patient.

5. Identify the importance of eliciting information regarding the present illness and any past medical history from the family of an unresponsive medical patient.

6. Differentiate between the assessment that is performed for a patient who is unresponsive or has an altered mental status and other medical patients requiring assessment.

OVERVIEW

The initial assessment is performed to discover and quickly manage life-threatening problems in all patients. Once this has been completed, the emergency medical technician (EMT) moves on to the next phase of the assessment, which will vary somewhat depending upon whether the patient is traumatically injured or medically ill.

The assessment of the trauma patient is discussed in Chapters 14 and 15. The management of the medical patient is somewhat different. This chapter examines the focused history and physical examination of the medical patient.

ASSESSMENT OF THE MEDICAL PATIENT

The priorities of a patient suffering from a medical illness are somewhat different from those of the patient suffering from trauma. These priorities differ depending on whether the medical patient is awake and responsive or unresponsive.

History

It is very important to identify and examine the mechanism of injury for the trauma patient. The medical patient does not have a mechanism of injury. The medical patient has an illness that progressed in some way to result in a call for emergency care and transport.

The EMT can elicit the specifics of this progression by obtaining a history. The history provides the information needed to prioritize the care of the medical patient.

Sometimes the history is easily obtained from the patient. Other times, the history might be obtained from family members or bystanders if the patient is unable to provide the details himself.

Regardless of how it is obtained, the history for the medical patient is the equivalent of the mechanism of injury for the trauma patient.

Physical Examination

In the assessment of the medical patient, the EMT will use the history to guide the physical examination. The physical examination findings will often confirm the suspicions the EMT formed on the basis of the history. For example, a patient who gives the history of extensive vomiting and diarrhea for several days will likely be severely dehydrated and may even be in hypovolemic shock. Physical examination may reveal evidence of dehydration and shock.

Street Smart

The EMT should pay careful attention to the surroundings on a scene and make use of the things she sees. Some people have a very useful container of information in their home called a **vial of life**.

Usually there is a sticker or indication near the front door that there is a vial of life in the home. The vial is usually kept in the refrigerator. This vial is a small plastic tube with a piece of paper inside that contains the patient's name, address, and essential medical information.

Allergies, medicines, medical problems, and contact names are also included in this vial. This is a very important clue not to be missed if present on a scene. Figure 16-1 shows a typical identifying sign in a home with a vial of life.

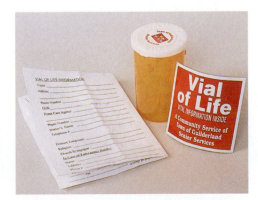

FIGURE 16-1 The patient's vital information is in the vial of life.

Palpitations and Dizziness

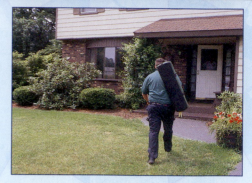

Crystal and Jeremy responded to a call for a woman having chest pain. Upon their arrival, they were greeted by a young girl who directed them into the living room, where they found the girl's mother seated in a chair, with one hand clutched to her chest. She was holding herself upright and was awake but did seem to be quite uncomfortable.

Jeremy approached the woman and introduced himself and his partner as EMTs with the local ambulance service. He asked the woman what the problem was. She responded easily and told him that she was feeling palpitations and chest pain and felt too dizzy to stand up. The woman's respirations did not appear to be labored and seemed of a normal rate. Jeremy felt her radial pulse and noted it to be quite rapid and weak.

- What is the general impression of this patient? Is this trauma or medical?
- What treatments are indicated immediately?
- What are the priorities for further management?

THE RESPONSIVE MEDICAL PATIENT

The responsive medical patient is probably one of the most common types of patient an EMT will encounter. This patient has a medical illness and is usually able to communicate the details of it to the EMT.

The initial assessment of the alert patient is very easily done. Once the initial assessment has been completed and the priorities for transport have been addressed, the EMT should then gather historical information from the patient. This historical information will guide further assessment and treatment.

History of the Present Illness

When obtaining a history, the EMT must be clear and organized in her questioning in order to quickly get the information she is looking for. Many patients will attempt to give long-winded accounts of their entire medical history. This may be a nice way to pass the time during transport to the hospital, but it should be allowed only after the needed information has been obtained and the assessment has been completed.

Chief Complaint

The first and most important part of the history of the present illness is the **chief complaint**. The chief complaint is the main reason why the patient called for help. This can be determined by asking the patient what made him call or what is bothering him.

Sometimes a patient will have multiple complaints. Each of these must eventually be addressed, but the EMT should ask the patient to distinguish what seems to be the primary complaint; what is bothering him the most.

Cultural Considerations

EMTs may encounter patients who do not speak English well or at all. In these circumstances, the EMT may be forced to use family members as interpreters. This practice is acceptable if the EMT remembers a few caveats. One, be cautious about having younger family members give direction and information to older family members. Instead, wait until the patient is in the emergency department.

Two, personal questions, such as those that probe into sexuality, may make all concerned parties very uncomfortable. Again, wait until the patient is in the emergency department, where these questions can be asked more privately.

Street Smart

It is important to ask open-ended questions when trying to obtain historical information. Giving the patient choices such as Yes or No, or Sharp or Dull may limit what he will tell you. It is wise to ask the questions in an open manner to allow the patient to find his own answer. If the patient is obviously struggling for an answer, provide a complete list of optional answers.

OPQRST

Once the chief complaint has been determined, the EMT should ask some other specific questions regarding that chief complaint in order to better define the problem and determine the needed treatment.

An acronym that can be used to remember the questions that should be asked to further define a chief complaint and the history of the present illness is **OPQRST**. Table 16-1 defines each of these letters.

TABLE 16-1

OPQRST			
Letter	**Meaning**	**Determines**	**Example of Question**
O	Onset	When the symptoms began	When did these symptoms begin?
P	Provocation	Provoking factors	What were you doing when the symptoms started? Does anything seem to make it worse?
Q	Quality	Quality of the symptoms (sharp, dull, heavy, etc.)	How would you describe these symptoms?
R	Radiation	Radiation of discomfort from primary location	Does the discomfort go anywhere else?
	Region	Part of the body affected by the symptoms	What part of your body does the symptoms affect right now?
	Relief	Relieving factors	Is there anything that seems to make the symptoms better?
S	Severity	Severity of the symptoms	On a scale of 1 to 10, 1 being very mild and 10 being the worst thing you could ever imagine, where are your symptoms right now? Give a number.
T	Time	Length of time symptoms present	How long do you think these symptoms have been going on?

SAMPLE History

In addition to the specific questions asked regarding the chief complaint, the EMT must also obtain the usual SAMPLE history of the medical patient. This history was examined in detail in Chapter 10.

In review, the SAMPLE history covers important elements of the patient's medical history that may help further define the current problem. **S**igns and symptoms will be covered by the OPQRST quite well. **A**llergies to medications must be determined for every patient and must be carefully documented and passed on to the hospital staff. Current **m**edications should be written down and ideally should be gathered up and put into a bag to be brought with the patient to the hospital for review by the hospital staff. **P**ast medical history, especially anything similar to the current event, should be determined. For certain conditions (such as chest pain, difficulty breathing, and allergic reactions), local protocols may allow an EMT to help a patient use previously prescribed medications. These will be discussed in detail in later chapters. The time of **l**ast oral intake should be determined. The **e**vents leading up to the event will likely have been elicited during the OPQRST questioning.

Focused Physical Examination

After obtaining a thorough history via OPQRST and SAMPLE, the EMT will focus the physical exam on the body area that seems affected by the current problem. This assessment is called the **focused physical examination**.

The history is used to guide the physical exam of the responsive medical patient. Table 16-2 lists common chief complaints with body areas that should be examined.

Further details regarding each chief complaint and the specific exam findings will be dealt with in later chapters. As she does for the trauma patient, the EMT will be looking at the particular body area for DCAP-BTLS, as discussed in Chapter 14.

TABLE 16-2

Chief Complaint with Body Area Focus

Chief Complaint	Body Area
Headache, weakness, sensory problems, fainting	Head
Neck pain	Neck
Chest pain, shortness of breath	Chest
Abdominal pain, nausea or vomiting	Abdomen
Back pain	Back
Arm or leg complaint	Extremities

Baseline Vital Signs

At this point in the assessment of the medical patient, the EMT has addressed any life threats, has obtained a complete history, and has assessed the relevant body parts. Now it is appropriate to obtain a full set of vital signs as a baseline before any further treatment or transport decisions.

As covered in Chapter 10, the signs to be measured are respiration, pulse, blood pressure, skin temperature and condition, pupils, pulse oximetry, and capillary refill in children. Once obtained, these vital signs should be carefully documented and integrated into the plan for further treatment of the responsive medical patient.

Any abnormal vital signs should prompt the EMT to consider the patient a high priority and initiate immediate transport. Further treatment decisions can be made while en route to a hospital.

Treatment and Transport

Treatment for life threats is provided during the initial assessment. Oxygen will have been applied during the "B" step (breathing) if it was deemed appropriate. During the course of the focused history and physical, the EMT will find additional information about the patient's condition. The baseline vital signs provide even more information about the patient's condition.

Some patients are designated a high priority on the basis of findings in the initial assessment. These patients are transported immediately. Further treatment and assessment can be administered during the transport.

For patients not considered a high priority, the EMT may complete the focused history and physical with baseline vital signs on the scene before transport. In general, this complete assessment should take no longer than 10 minutes.

On-Line Medical Control

There are certain medical conditions that will be discussed in further detail later in this text that may require the EMT to assist a patient in using previously prescribed medications. Often, contact with a medical control physician will be necessary in order to obtain permission to administer these medications. The process of talking to a physician at the time of the call is referred to as on-line medical control. Local treatment protocols will dictate when this is to be done and how to accomplish it.

Consider ALS

If the EMT feels the patient would benefit from treatment that is beyond her scope of practice, she may choose to arrange to meet up with an advanced life support (ALS) provider. Local protocols often govern when ALS would be indicated.

Ongoing Assessment

During transport, it is crucial that the EMT continue to assess the patient and any interventions that have been provided. Details of this ongoing assessment will be discussed in Chapter 17. Skill 16-1 describes the focused medical assessment of the responsive patient. Figure 16-2 outlines the steps in the assessment of the responsive medical patient.

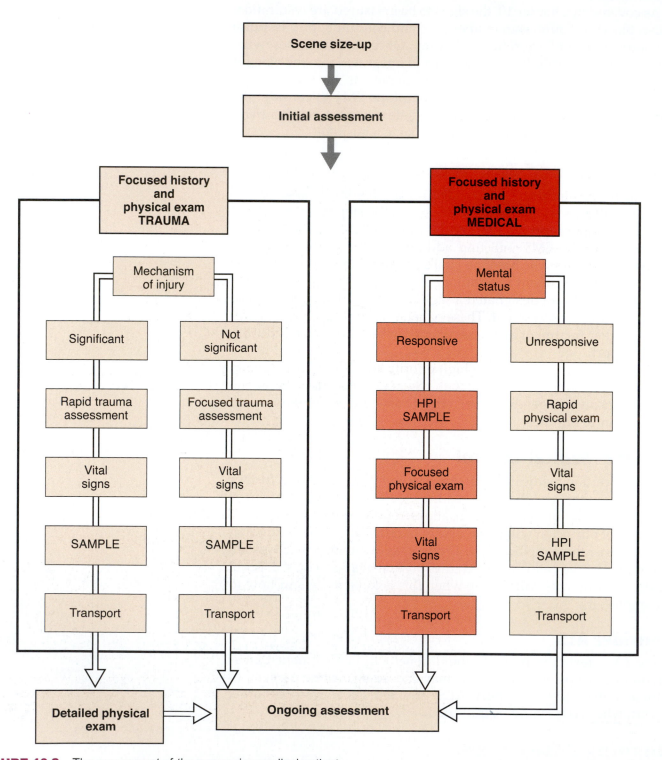

FIGURE 16-2 The assessment of the responsive medical patient.

SKILL 16-1 *Focused Medical Assessment—Responsive Medical Patient*

PURPOSE: To obtain a baseline examination of the responsive medical patient.

STANDARD PRECAUTIONS:

- ☑ Penlight
- ☑ Stethoscope
- ☑ Blood pressure cuff
- ☑ Scissors

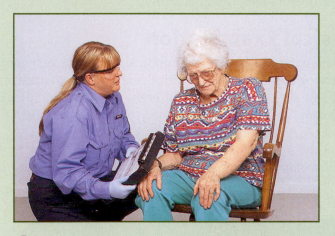

1 The EMT proceeds with obtaining a chief complaint and a history of the present illness, using the OPQRST format when appropriate.

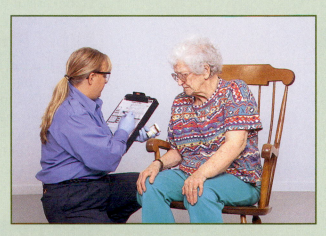

2 After obtaining the history of the present illness, the EMT takes the patient's SAMPLE history.

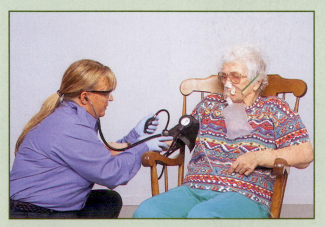

3 On the basis of the patient's chief complaint, the EMT performs a focused physical examination of the affected area. After the physical examination, the EMT obtains a baseline set of vital signs.

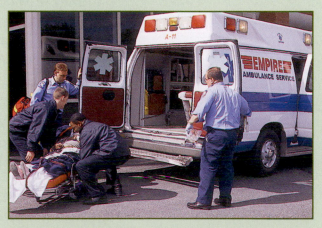

4 It may be necessary for the EMT to assist the patient with medications or transport the patient to the hospital. An ongoing assessment should be continued en route to the hospital.

THE UNRESPONSIVE MEDICAL PATIENT

The unresponsive medical patient requires the EMT to shift her mind-set slightly. Whereas the responsive medical patient provided a history to guide further assessment and management, the unresponsive patient, or the patient with an altered mental status, cannot give this history.

The EMT must perform a rapid physical exam to search for sources of the unresponsiveness, then measure vital signs, and if possible obtain a history from the family or bystanders before leaving the scene. Notice that the history is taken after the physical exam is done in the case of the unresponsive medical patient.

Rapid Physical Examination

The **rapid physical examination** for the medical patient is very similar to the head-to-toe rapid physical exam described for the trauma patient. The findings may be somewhat different, but the principles of performing the exam in a systematic manner, looking for abnormalities in the form of DCAP-BTLS, are the same.

Remember that the medical patient who is unresponsive may have fallen, and therefore spinal injury is a possibility. The EMT should be

Unresponsive Male

Ann Marie and Pedro arrived on scene and approached their patient. The call was for an unresponsive male in his 60s. Ann Marie began to perform an initial assessment while Pedro asked the family what had happened.

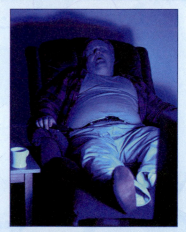

(Courtesy of PhotoDisc.)

Apparently, while watching television, the patient had suddenly complained of a severe headache and then passed out. The family has not been able to wake him. Ann Marie found the man unresponsive, with snoring respirations, requiring her to manually open his airway. He had a strong but slow radial pulse and had no evidence of external hemorrhage.

- What is your general impression of this patient?
- What treatments are immediately indicated?
- What is the priority of this patient?
- What further assessment should be done?

sure to maintain cervical spine immobilization when spinal injury cannot be ruled out.

Head and Neck

The patient's head should be assessed for any abnormalities. Any deformities or bruises may lead the EMT to suspect traumatic head injury as a source for the unresponsiveness.

During the assessment of the head, it is important for the EMT to evaluate the eyes, ears, nose, and mouth. Pupils are an essential part of the head exam. Their shape, size, and reactivity should be noted. Any drainage from the ears or nose should also be noted. Any problems in the mouth would have already been addressed in the airway step of the initial assessment, but this area should be reassessed now.

The neck should be examined next. Any evidence of injury should certainly be noted, as should any scars or venous distension. Increased jugular venous distension may indicate an increased pressure in the circulatory system.

Chest

The chest should be exposed and examined for abnormalities. Any injury should be noted. The EMT should assess for evidence of accessory muscle use. This increased use of the chest muscles and neck muscles to aid in breathing was introduced in Chapter 8. Auscultation of the patient's lungs should be accomplished, and any abnormal sounds noted.

Abdomen and Pelvis

The abdomen should be exposed, and the EMT should observe for any abnormalities. After a careful visual assessment, the examiner should carefully palpate the four quadrants of the abdomen (with the umbilicus as the center point). The EMT should feel for any firmness, masses, or apparent tenderness.

To assess for tenderness, the EMT must observe the facial expression of the patient while palpating the abdomen. A pained expression, or grimace, would suggest that the patient is feeling discomfort.

The pelvis should be assessed by compression of the iliac wings, hips, and pubis as was done for the trauma patient. The EMT should also note any obvious vaginal bleeding or incontinence of urine or stool.

Extremities

The extremities should be assessed for any abnormalities, as was done for the trauma patient. The EMT should pay careful attention to the location of any edema found. Patients who have excess fluid retention may have edema of their feet and ankles. The more excess fluid there is, the higher up the leg the edema might extend.

The presence of peripheral pulses should be noted as well as the patient's ability to move and feel each of the extremities. The pulse, movement, and sensation check can be remembered as PMS.

While examining the extremities, the EMT should look for **Medic-Alert®️ emblems** as an indication of the patient's past medical history.

Street Smart

By wearing the MedicAlert emblem, the patient has consented to the release of the information to emergency responders. The MedicAlert member's emblem typically has three engravings. Members' stored medical profiles have an average of 8 additional items. These can include DNR status, conditions, allergies, medications and dosages, implanted devices, insurance information, and physician and family contacts. It also may contain scanned documents such as ECGs, living wills, and advance directives. Figure 16-3 shows an example of the MedicAlert patient directive.

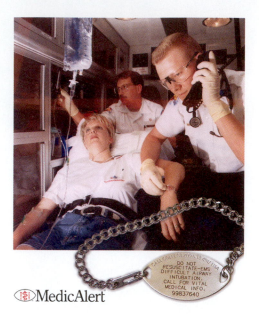

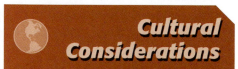

FIGURE 16-3 Always check for a MedicAlert® emblem. (Courtesy of the MedicAlert Foundation, Turlock, CA.)

This emblem represents a patient directive that allows EMS to access the patient's stored medical information by calling the MedicAlert Foundation 24-Hour Emergency Response Center (1-800-625-3780).

Back and Buttocks

The EMT must not forget to assess the patient's back. As the patient is lifted or rolled onto a transport device, the EMT should take a moment to assess the back for any abnormalities. Listening to the lungs from the back may also be useful and should be done if the EMT is able.

Vital Signs

After completing the rapid physical assessment on the unresponsive medical patient, the EMT should obtain a complete set of vital signs, including respirations, pulse, blood pressure, pupils, skin temperature and condition, pulse oximetry, and capillary refill in children. This set of vital signs should be carefully recorded and referred to as a baseline.

The vital signs, along with the physical exam, will help the EMT determine the priority of the patient and the need for further treatment.

History

Once the initial assessment, rapid physical examination, and vital signs are done, the EMT should quickly question the family or bystanders about the patient's history. Any information provided about the history of the present illness, past medical history, allergies, or medications could be very important, and the EMT should take a few moments to gather this information before leaving the scene.

Explanations should be provided to the family as to what treatment the EMT has provided and the plans for transport. It is important to advise the family of the destination so that they can come and be with their family member and possibly provide hospital staff further information. It is sometimes useful to bring a family member along, buckled up in the front seat of the ambulance, so that this relative can stay with the loved one and be present at the hospital immediately upon the patient's arrival.

Treatment and Transport

Any treatments of life-threatening problems would have been provided during the initial assessment. Any additional treatments indicated by the findings in the remainder of the physical examination should be addressed at its completion.

If the patient was considered high priority at the completion of the initial assessment, transport would have likely been initiated already. If transport had not yet been initiated by the completion of the physical exam, then it should be addressed at that point.

Medical Control/ALS

If the EMT feels that the patient requires treatment that she as a basic-level provider cannot provide, then she should arrange for an ALS provider to evaluate the patient. Some systems provide ALS-level care to every patient; others will arrange it only when the EMT deems it necessary.

If local protocols dictate contacting medical control for a particular condition, then the EMT should do so when appropriate. Contacting medical control is always appropriate if the EMT has a question about whether to provide a specific treatment for a patient.

Ongoing Assessment

As must any other patient, the unresponsive medical patient must be repeatedly assessed during transport to find any changes. The details of the ongoing assessment are discussed in Chapter 17.

Contact should be established with the destination hospital to warn the staff of the nature of the patient's injury or illness and to allow them to prepare for the patient's arrival. Finally, it is always appropriate to explain all procedures and actions to the patient and the family if present. These issues will be dealt with in more detail in later chapters.

Skill 16-2 describes the rapid physical examination of the unresponsive medical patient. Figure 16-4 outlines the steps in the assessment of the unresponsive medical patient.

SKILL 16-2 *Rapid Physical Examination— Unresponsive Medical Patient*

PURPOSE: To obtain a baseline examination of the unresponsive medical patient.

STANDARD PRECAUTIONS:

☑ Penlight
☑ Stethoscope
☑ Blood pressure cuff
☑ Scissors

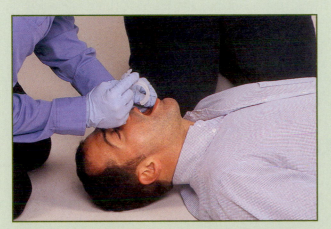

1 The EMT quickly performs an initial assessment.

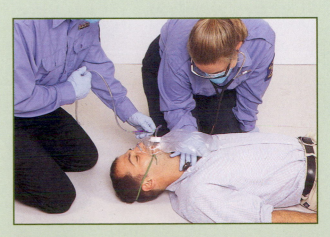

2 The EMT then proceeds to a rapid physical examination of the patient.

(continues)

SKILL 16-2 *(continued)*

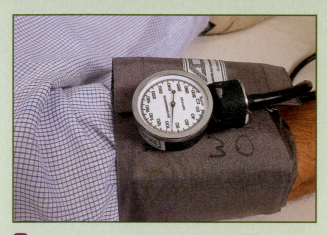

3 As soon as is practical, a baseline set of vital signs should be obtained as well.

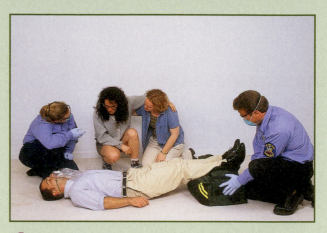

4 Bystanders or family members should be questioned about the patient's illness and past medical history.

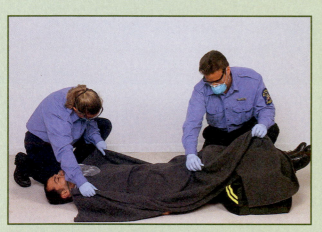

5 The patient is transported as soon as possible.

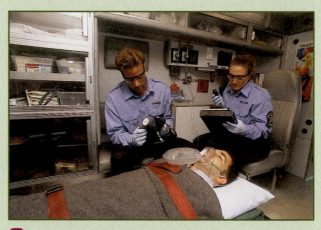

6 En route to the hospital, the EMT contacts medical control and should consider meeting with ALS.

CONCLUSION

The EMT must be proficient in performing a patient assessment for any type of patient. The medical patient is managed somewhat differently, depending upon whether he is responsive or unresponsive.

The important difference between the medical and trauma patient is that the "mechanism of injury" for the medical patient lies within the history. It is for this reason that the EMT must also be proficient at obtaining a history from a patient or family members.

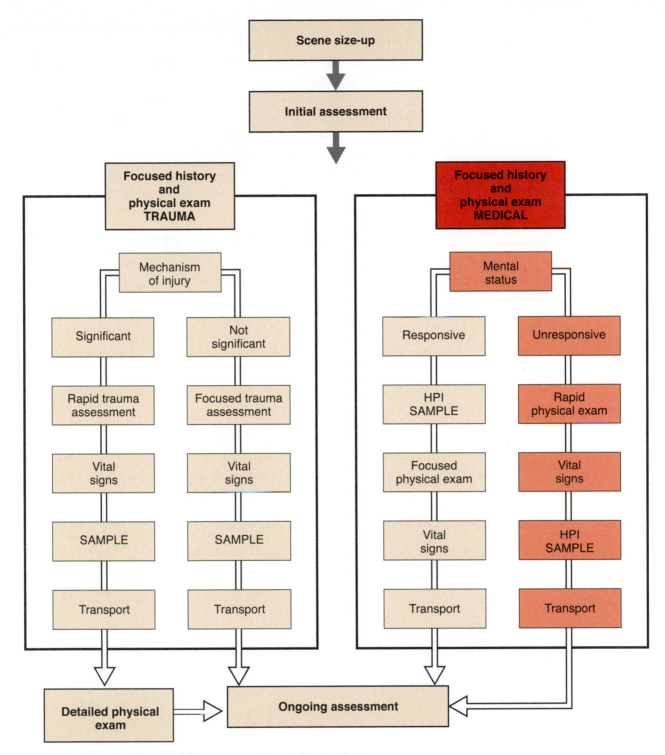

FIGURE 16-4   The assessment of the unresponsive medical patient.

TEST YOUR KNOWLEDGE

1. Describe the different priorities when assessing a medical versus a trauma patient.
2. List the steps followed when assessing a responsive medical patient.

3. Identify the importance of eliciting any past medical history from the medical patient.

4. List the steps followed when assessing an unresponsive medical patient.

5. Identify the importance of eliciting information regarding the present illness and any past medical history from the family of an unresponsive medical patient.

6. Differentiate between the assessment that is performed for a patient who is unresponsive or has an altered mental status and other medical patients requiring assessment.

INTERNET RESOURCES

Search the Web using these key words:

- MedicAlert
- Vial of life
- OPQRST
- SAMPLE

Share any interesting facts and Web sites with your colleagues.

FURTHER STUDY

Elling, B., & Elling, K. (2002). *Principles of patient assessment in EMS.* Clifton Park, NY: Thomson Delmar Learning.

CHAPTER 17

The Ongoing Assessment

KEY TERMS

trend

OBJECTIVES

Upon completion of this chapter, the reader should be able to:

1. List the purpose of performing an ongoing assessment.
2. Describe the ongoing assessment in detail.
3. Give several examples of changes to be monitored.
4. Define the term *trend*.
5. List the frequency of reassessment for different types of patients.

OVERVIEW

In the days of the hearse ambulance, the attendants would sit in a small seat next to the door. During transport to the hospital, there was not enough room to do much with the patient. Simple airway management was difficult, and effective cardiopulmonary resuscitation (CPR) was almost impossible.

Today, prehospital care has evolved to a point where we have enough room and enough training to be able to continue to provide care to patients in the back of the ambulance during transport to the hospital. Sometimes this transport time can be lengthy. No matter how long it is, the emergency medical technician (EMT) is responsible for observing and caring for that patient until arrival at the hospital, where care will be turned over to hospital staff.

Patients who require ambulance transport are at risk for having an unstable, or changing, medical condition. It is therefore critical that the EMT continue to observe the patient and assess for any changes during transport. In this chapter, the importance of continuous reassessment are discussed and emphasized.

ONGOING ASSESSMENT

Once the patient has been thoroughly assessed, vital signs have been measured, and a transport decision has been made, the next step is to begin ongoing assessment.

The purpose of the ongoing assessment is to identify any significant changes in the patient's condition that need immediate attention. Using the ongoing assessment, the EMT evaluates the effectiveness of medical care by comparing baseline vital signs and assessment findings with repeat assessments that are done periodically during transport. The ongoing assessment is conducted after the focused history and physical examination of the trauma or medical patient.

Components of the Ongoing Assessment

The ongoing assessment consists of repeating the initial assessment, taking vital signs, and checking any areas that were previously of concern. Any interventions that were provided, such as oxygen, a splint, or bleeding control, should be reassessed to see whether the patient is improving as a result of implementation. Any changes should be addressed and documented.

The Initial Assessment Repeated

The first step of the ongoing assessment is to repeat the initial assessment. The patient's condition will dictate whether this step will take more than a moment. An EMT should take the time to carefully reassess the primary elements of an initial assessment for a seriously injured patient.

Mental Status

During the ongoing assessment, the EMT reassesses the patient's mental status. AVPU (*a*lert, *v*oice, *p*ain, *u*nresponsive) is the method that will be used to do this reassessment, just as it was in the initial assessment. Mental status changes may occur very gradually but may have devastating consequences if not recognized and quickly acted upon by the EMT.

Airway

The patient's airway is critical. The EMT must maintain a constant vigil over the airway, making sure that it remains open and clear (Figure 17-1).

If the patient is unconscious, the airway is being manually maintained by the EMT. If the EMT is tiring, he should switch roles with his partner.

Breathing

Oxygen is probably one of the most commonly administered treatments in emergency medical services (EMS). Once the oxygen has been given to a patient, its effectiveness must be evaluated. Did the oxygen relieve the patient's pain or make her feel better? If not, why not? A common problem is that the oxygen tubing becomes kinked under linen or the patient. Always leave oxygen tubing in plain view on top of the linen.

Oxygen in a tank is limited. Failure to notice an empty oxygen tank could force the patient to breathe room air, or worse, rebreathe her own exhaled air. Oxygen tanks, both onboard and portable, need to be

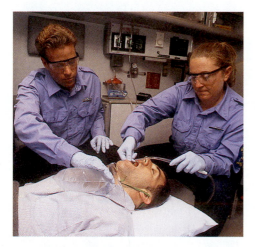

FIGURE 17-1 Some treatments must be repeated while en route.

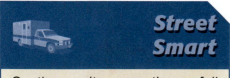

Street Smart

Suction units sometimes fail because batteries run low or suction connections become loose or dislodged. Probably the most common reason suction fails is that the opening of the catheter becomes clogged. Extra suction catheters and water should be available.

checked frequently. Some EMTs check the tank whenever they take a set of vital signs.

Although a patient may have been breathing adequately while on scene, the patient's condition may worsen and cause respiratory decompensation. Oxygen via a non-rebreather mask may not be enough. The EMT may have to ventilate the patient if she is no longer able to breathe effectively on her own.

The pulse oximeter aids the EMT in his assessment of the patient's breathing. Constant readings confirm the EMT's assessment findings (Figure 17-2). It is important to remember that the pulse oximeter reading is a supplement to, not a replacement for, a good assessment of the patient's respiratory effort. Many EMTs place the pulse oximeter on the patient in the ambulance, if they have not already done so.

Circulation

On the scene, vigorous external bleeding would have been controlled. Less obvious, slowly bleeding wounds also need attention.

During the ongoing assessment, the EMT should turn his attention to ensuring that all bleeding has been addressed and remains controlled. That includes reassessing any external bleeding that was discovered and initially managed on the scene.

An EMT can assess and control external bleeding, but he cannot control internal bleeding directly. A high index of suspicion based on the mechanism of injury would make an EMT suspect that the patient may be bleeding internally.

Constant reassessment of indicators of perfusion, such as distal pulses and skin temperature and color, gives an EMT a clue about the presence of internal bleeding.

Reevaluate Patient Priority

Occasionally, patients deteriorate while en route to the hospital. Rarely does a high-priority patient recover sufficiently to be considered low priority. The EMT should always be prepared to upgrade the patient's priority on the basis of the most current assessment findings.

If the hospital has been notified of an impending arrival and the patient's condition changes, the EMT should reestablish contact. Early notification of patient changes permits the emergency department to properly prepare.

If a patient is deteriorating, an advanced life support (ALS) intercept should be arranged if it is possible. Often, a patient who suddenly becomes unmanageable for an EMT can be successfully stabilized by a paramedic (Figure 17-3).

Destination

If the patient's condition changes, a change in destination facility may be necessary. These decisions should be based upon knowledge of local resources and regional transportation protocols.

Reassess Vital Signs

The first set of vital signs the EMT takes establishes a baseline. This baseline requires another set of vital signs in order to establish

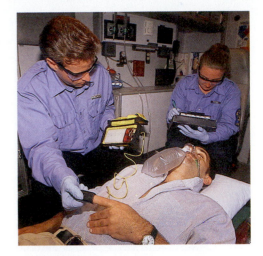
FIGURE 17-2 The pulse oximeter provides continuous reassessment of oxygenation.

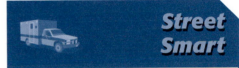
Street Smart

During cold weather, the body shunts blood away from the skin and into the body's core. When the injured patient is moved from a cold environment to the warmth of the ambulance, the process reverses.

The result is that wounds that were relatively bloodless out in the cold may suddenly begin to bleed profusely in the back of the ambulance.

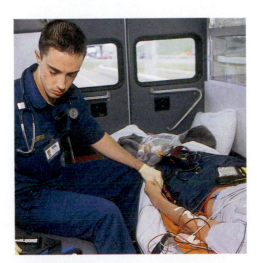
FIGURE 17-3 Patients do deteriorate, and advanced life support can help.

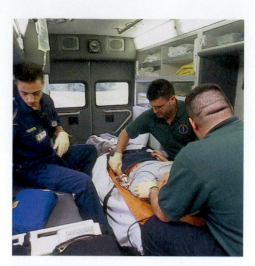

FIGURE 17-4 A repeated history improves reliability.

whether there has been any change. Every patient, regardless of circumstances, should have at least two sets of vital signs obtained and recorded.

Repeat History

People, in general, do not think clearly when they are under stress. When the patient was giving a historical account of her illness on scene, distractions may have confused her. In the relative calm of the back of an ambulance, and away from the distractions, the patient may give a more accurate account of her injury or illness (Figure 17-4).

Reaffirming a patient's history improves the reliability of that history. A reliable history gives the EMT confidence that the treatments he is administering are correct. Perhaps more important, new historical findings, like new physical findings, give the EMT an opportunity to adjust treatments and patient priorities.

Repeat Physical Examination— Focused or Detailed

Physical findings, such as bruising and swelling, take time to develop. Bruises across the abdomen from a seat belt may not appear for 20–30 minutes.

The EMT should reassess the patient using DCAP-BTLS (see Table 14-3 for a definition of this term). Comparisons should be made between on-scene assessment findings and the new assessment.

It is best if the EMT who did the scene assessment also does the ongoing assessment. It is impossible to determine whether a leg is more swollen if there was no baseline to compare it against. Only the first EMT would have that information.

Check ABCs and Interventions

After completing the reassessment, the EMT should check all treatments in progress and adjust them as needed. "Is it working?" is the central question on the EMT's mind.

Previously applied dressings should be examined to ensure proper placement and adequate bleeding control. Splints that were applied for suspected broken bones should be assessed and readjusted as needed for patient comfort. As you will learn in Chapter 25, when splints are applied it is important to assess the distal pulse, motor function, and sensation frequently. It is during the ongoing assessments that this process may be repeated.

If the EMT assisted the patient in taking previously prescribed medications as allowed by local protocols, the effects of these medications should also be reassessed. For example, if an inhaler was used for the asthma patient with difficulty breathing, the EMT should carefully reassess the breathing and determine the effectiveness of the medication.

Note Changes

All changes in the patient's condition from the time on the scene and while en route, must be noted. Observant EMTs may notice that these changes represent a pattern. For example, pale, cool, and clammy skin, with steadily dropping blood pressures and increasing pulse rates, is indicative of progressing shock.

Ongoing assessments will reveal these patterns, or **trends**. A patient's trend, either positive or negative, should be reported and recorded.

How Often?

The frequency with which these repeated assessments are performed is determined by the priority of the patient. If the patient is considered to be a high-priority patient, it is appropriate to continually monitor the ABCs and recheck vital signs every 5 minutes.

Patients who are not considered high priority should be reassessed every 10–15 minutes during transport to find any changes in condition.

Table 17-1 provides a list of suggested patient classifications based on patient problem. Remember that if a patient deteriorates, the priority may change from a low priority to a high priority and the issues involved in the transport as well as the frequency of repeated assessments would need to be readdressed.

It is important that the EMT use these frequent reassessments to note any trending, or changes over time, in the patient's condition. The EMT should carefully document any changes in condition or any trends noted during the transport. Passing this information along to hospital staff upon arrival will also help them to better care for the patient.

Skill 17-1 describes the ongoing assessment. Figure 17-5 outlines the steps of the ongoing assessment.

TABLE 17-1

Patient Classification Guidelines

High priority:	Cardiac or respiratory arrest
	Ventilations require assistance
	Severe upper airway difficulties
	Serious chest trauma
	Decompensated shock
	Decreasing level of consciousness
	Uncontrollable external hemorrhage
	Penetrating injury to head, neck, chest, abdomen, pelvis
Intermediate priority:	Early signs of compensated shock
	Kinematics or injuries suggest hidden injury
	Major isolated injury
Low priority:	Minor isolated injuries
	Uncomplicated extremity injury

SKILL 17-1 *Ongoing Assessment*

PURPOSE: To continue to monitor the patient for assessment and comparison with baseline examinations.

STANDARD PRECAUTIONS:

- ☑ Penlight
- ☑ Stethoscope
- ☑ Blood pressure cuff

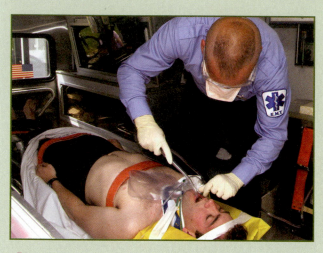

1 While en route to the hospital, the EMT repeats the initial assessment, reassessing the patient's mental status using the AVPU scale and monitoring the airway.

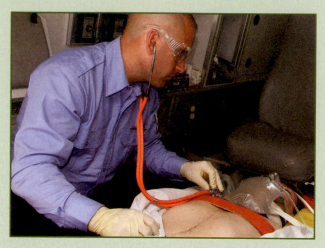

2 The patient's breathing must be reassessed for rate and quality, and lung sounds must be monitored.

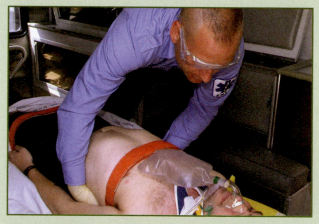

3 The EMT then reassesses the patient's circulatory status, including skin temperature, and notes any additional bleeding.

(continues)

SKILL 17-1 (continued)

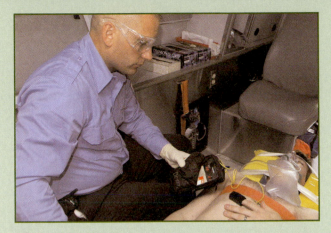

4 After mentally reviewing the patient's priorities, the EMT reassesses the vital signs and repeats a physical examination as needed.

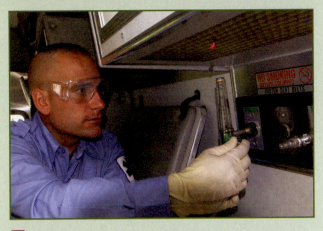

5 The EMT rechecks the interventions, such as oxygen tank pressures.

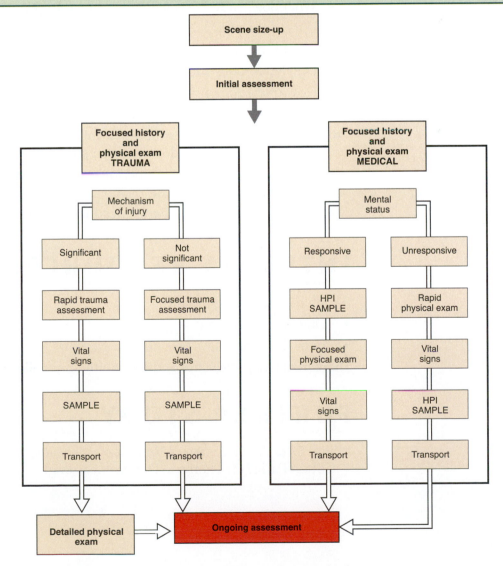

FIGURE 17-5 The ongoing assessment is part of every EMT's patient examination.

CONCLUSION

Once an EMT has assessed a patient, he must continue to reassess in regular intervals in order to notice any trends or changes over time. These repeated assessments should continue during the entire time that the EMT is caring for the patient.

This ongoing assessment is of key importance in caring for emergency patients, who may have changes in condition over time and need different treatment because of these changes. It is the responsibility of the EMT to recognize these changes and take appropriate action.

TEST YOUR KNOWLEDGE

1. What is the purpose of the ongoing assessment?
2. What about the patient's mental status should the EMT reassess?
3. What does an EMT reevaluate in the airway?
4. What does an EMT reevaluate in breathing?
5. What does an EMT reevaluate in circulation?
6. What is meant by the term *trend*?
7. How often does a low-priority patient need reevaluation?
8. How often does a high-priority patient need reevaluation?
9. When would an EMT call for an ALS intercept?
10. What is the minimum number of initial assessments an EMT should complete and document on any patient?
11. What is the minimum number of sets of vital signs an EMT will obtain on any patient?
12. When would an EMT change destination hospitals?

INTERNET RESOURCES

Search the Web using these key words:
- Ongoing assessment
- Vital signs trends

Share interesting Web sites and facts with your colleagues.

FURTHER STUDY

Elling, B., & Elling, K. (2002). *Principles of patient assessment in EMS.* Clifton Park, NY: Thomson Delmar Learning.

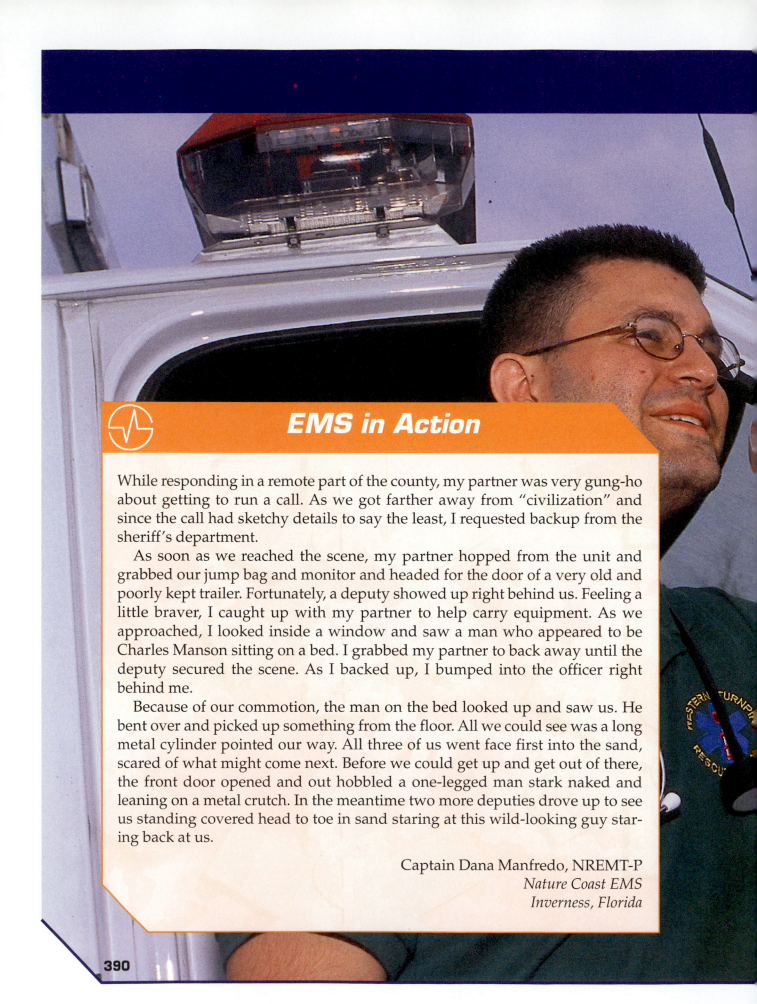

EMS in Action

While responding in a remote part of the county, my partner was very gung-ho about getting to run a call. As we got farther away from "civilization" and since the call had sketchy details to say the least, I requested backup from the sheriff's department.

As soon as we reached the scene, my partner hopped from the unit and grabbed our jump bag and monitor and headed for the door of a very old and poorly kept trailer. Fortunately, a deputy showed up right behind us. Feeling a little braver, I caught up with my partner to help carry equipment. As we approached, I looked inside a window and saw a man who appeared to be Charles Manson sitting on a bed. I grabbed my partner to back away until the deputy secured the scene. As I backed up, I bumped into the officer right behind me.

Because of our commotion, the man on the bed looked up and saw us. He bent over and picked up something from the floor. All we could see was a long metal cylinder pointed our way. All three of us went face first into the sand, scared of what might come next. Before we could get up and get out of there, the front door opened and out hobbled a one-legged man stark naked and leaning on a metal crutch. In the meantime two more deputies drove up to see us standing covered head to toe in sand staring at this wild-looking guy staring back at us.

Captain Dana Manfredo, NREMT-P
Nature Coast EMS
Inverness, Florida

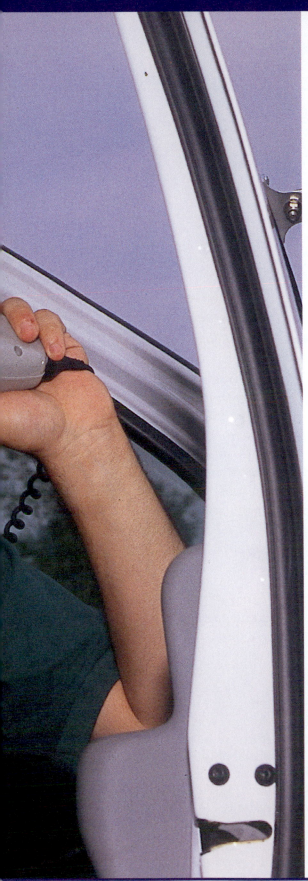

EMS Communications

The sixth and final arm of the Star of Life symbolizes the patient's transfer to definitive care. The transfer to definitive care begins when the EMT communicates the patient's condition to the hospital via a radio. The transfer of care continues when the EMT gives a verbal report at the bedside and ends when the EMT documents the patient's care in a written report. Communication, either spoken or written, is an important aspect of patient care. This section explains the three Rs of EMS: radio, report, record.

Radio

OBJECTIVES

Upon completion of this chapter, the reader should be able to:

1. Discuss the role of the communications specialist.
2. Diagram a typical radio system.
3. Describe the role of the Federal Communications Commission.
4. Describe how modern technology has advanced communications.
5. Describe basic radio procedure when initiating and terminating a radio call.
6. List the elements of an alert report.
7. List the elements of a medical consultation report.
8. List the correct radio procedures used throughout the course of an emergency call.

OVERVIEW

Before the advent of modern radio and paging systems, rescue squads were often summoned by a telephone operator who called a designated telephone, often called the "hot line," to alert the squad of a call for emergency medical services (EMS). The rescue squad member who received the notification would then call the next crew member. Precious minutes were lost trying to round up the crew.

After World War II, radios made their way into civilian emergency services, in large part owing to efforts of the Civil Defense. The result was a more rapid dispatch and arrival of lifesaving aid units.

In the past, the public thought of emergency medical technicians (EMTs) as *ambulance drivers*. Similarly, EMTs used to think of the professional **communications specialist (COMSPEC)** as the *dispatcher*. Modern telecommunications has evolved into a complex field of work involving not only radios but also computers, digital technology, and even satellite linkups.

Car off the Road

In the middle of the night, in a desolate spot, a car slides off the wet pavement and into a tree. The driver is unconscious. The horn blares while steam rises from the hood. Driving home, a local volunteer comes upon the scene.

- What various means of telecommunications could this EMT take advantage of to alert the EMS system?
- What are the advantages of each telecommunications system?
- What is meant by "standard radio procedure"?

(Courtesy of PhotoDisc.)

Although their knowledge need not be as extensive as that of a communications specialist, all EMTs need a basic understanding of communications systems and how to operate them.

COMMUNICATIONS SYSTEMS

Modern communications systems are made up of many pieces of equipment and as many equipment operators. The public accesses emergency services through a central point, usually by dialing 9-1-1 on a telephone. The information is recorded by a communications specialist, who then dispatches the closest emergency crews to the scene to render aid and assistance. Finally, the patient is transported to the hospital and the hospital is alerted to the patient's condition and urgency. Each phase of this emergency call is recorded in some manner at a central point. All of the notifications that are necessary throughout this process are done via the emergency services communications system.

Effective communication between the public, the emergency services personnel, and the hospital staff is necessary to rapidly access, treat, and transport the patient to definitive care. For some medical conditions, every second counts. Modern communications systems facilitate the rapid treatment and transport of a critically ill or injured patient to the hospital.

Communications Specialist

The communications specialist, previously referred to as the dispatcher, is a person who has been trained to facilitate communications between the public, the emergency service personnel, and the hospital staff. These professionals help to coordinate all aspects of emergency care through the use of radios, computers, and telephones. Table 18-1

TABLE 18-1

Roles of Communications Specialists

Role	System Support
Telephone interrogation	9-1-1 telephone systems
Triage	Emergency medical dispatch
Radio dispatch	Computer-aided dispatch
Logistics coordination	System status management
Resource networking	Public safety critical incident management
Prearrival instructions	Emergency medical dispatch

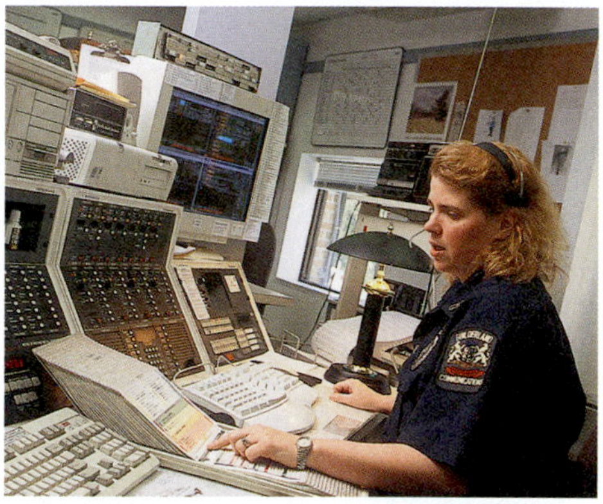

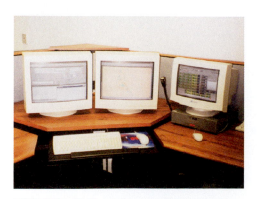

FIGURE 18-1 Predetermined protocols, such as those outlined on these dispatch cards, facilitate safe dispatch of emergency units to a medical emergency.

lists some of the roles of communications specialists and the pieces of the communications system that facilitate their job.

Through guided interrogation of the caller, the communications specialists will determine the number and types of units needed for any given emergency. By utilizing predetermined protocols and a knowledge of the location and capabilities of each unit within the region, the communications specialist can dispatch the closest appropriate units with the safest priority for the situation (Figure 18-1).

Radio dispatch of emergency units is often done through the use of a CAD, or computer-aided dispatch system. This computerized program, together with a status management system, helps the communications specialist to track each of the units that are in service. Such organization also helps maintain efficiency and allows effective networking of resources when needed.

One of the other very important jobs of the communications specialist is to provide prearrival instructions. Under the best of conditions, EMS may take several minutes to arrive on the scene. Simple first-aid instructions given to a bystander or family member can mean the difference between life and death.

Radio Systems

The core of most modern emergency service communications systems is the **two-way radio**. The two-way radio is a wireless electronic device that permits the transmission of messages to distant radio receivers as well as receipt of signals from those distant radios.

The original radio transmitters were large, cumbersome **base stations** that used large amounts of electricity to transmit a signal. Modern base station radios have evolved into powerful compact base units capable of fitting under a desk (Figure 18-2). The base station radio is a large, powerful radio that is located at a stationary site such as a dispatch center.

Radio signals are created in the base station and transmitted from a radio tower via an antenna. The antenna of a receiving radio unit converts the signal back into sound and the message is heard.

FIGURE 18-2 A fixed radio communications point is called a base station.

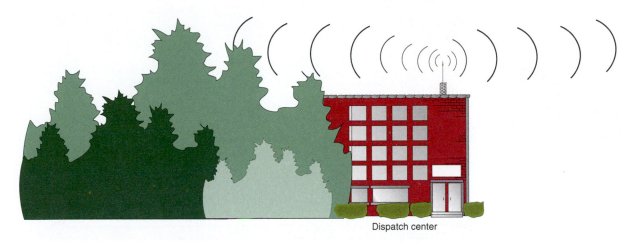

Dispatch center

FIGURE 18-3 Foliage and buildings can dampen the radio wave coming from an antenna.

Radio signals travel in concentric arcs emanating straight out from the source. Therefore, the distance a radio signal can travel is influenced by many factors. Dense foliage or large buildings can either block or absorb some of the radio signal, thereby decreasing the distance the signal will travel (Figure 18-3).

The most important barrier to a long-distance radio signal is the curvature of the earth. More powerful radios, their strength measured in watts, are often used to overcome the impact of the earth's curvature, allowing farther transmission of a radio signal. Tall radio towers place the antenna high above the ground, allowing farther transmission of signal. Therefore, many radio towers are located on the top of a mountain or tall building.

An airplane flying at 38,000 feet can use a very low-powered radio and still transmit over hundreds of miles. Why? Because the airplane acts like a 38,000-foot-tall antenna!

Mobile Radios

A radio that is mounted inside a vehicle is referred to as a **mobile radio**. Most mobile radios transmit at a lower power than base stations, typically 20–50 watts. Therefore, the typical transmission range will be less than that of the more powerful radios. Over average terrain, a mobile radio may transmit 10–15 miles.

The advent of the mobile radio allowed emergency service units to be dispatched from the streets. This advancement in radio technology permitted communications between a central dispatch point, or a **communications center**, and mobile EMS units.

Most EMS units have a mobile radio mounted inside the vehicle, in the trunk or a compartment, while the **radio head** is mounted in the driver's compartment. The radio head includes the microphone and volume and channel controls (Figure 18-4). This allows the driver or passenger to choose radio channels, control volume, and transmit messages.

In cases in which there is a great deal of interference from buildings or a long distance between the mobile radio and the base station, a **repeater** is used. A repeater is a radio receiver/transmitter that picks up the signal from a mobile radio transmitter and increases, or boosts, the signal to the base station receiver (Figure 18-5).

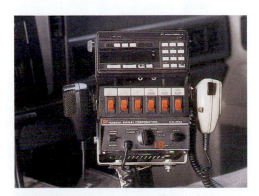

FIGURE 18-4 Modern EMS command/control is accomplished via the mobile radio.

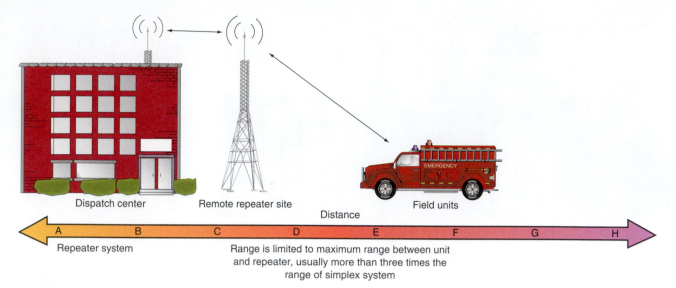

FIGURE 18-5 Repeaters are used to transmit messages over distances.

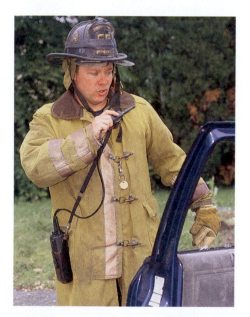

FIGURE 18-6 Portable radios provide added safety and quick access to resources.

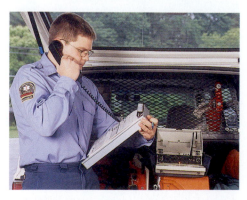

FIGURE 18-7 The push-to-talk feature is a feature of a simplex radio.

Portable Radios

The **portable radio** revolutionized emergency services at every level. This handheld radio allows an EMT at the patient's side to request additional resources, consult with a physician, or slow (downgrade) responding units (Figure 18-6). More important, if an EMT discovers a dangerous situation, she can warn others. This advantage cannot be overemphasized.

These portable radios are small and transmit with less power than a larger radio. The power output of 1–5 watts limits their range somewhat.

Radio Array

The first portable radios, dubbed walkie-talkies, permitted one-way communication. The portable radio could either receive or transmit but could not do both at the same time. These **simplex** radios are largely still in use today.

To use a simplex radio, the EMT would pick up either the entire radio or just the handset. The handset looks like a telephone handset (Figure 18-7). The handset has a button in the cradle. By pushing the button and speaking into the microphone, the EMT could transmit a message.

The problem with a simplex radio was that the receiver had to wait until the transmitter was finished before she could speak. To solve that problem, electronic engineers created **duplex** radios. Duplex radios allow the EMT to both speak and listen at the same time, like a telephone.

In the early days of EMS, paramedics used an electrocardiogram (ECG) machine to obtain an electrocardiographic tracing and then transmit that to a hospital base station for a physician to interpret. This process was called **telemetry**. Telemetry made it necessary for radios to be able to transmit and receive spoken messages as well as complex data.

These multiple-channel radios, called **multiplex** radios, fell out of use as paramedics learned to interpret the ECG on their own.

Radio Frequencies

Radio waves, a part of the electromagnetic spectrum, are used to transmit messages. Each radio wave has a length and a height. Early radios were primarily amplitude modulation (AM) radios. Modern radios are frequency modulation (FM) radios. These FM radios alter or modulate the speed, or frequency, of the radio waves. These frequencies are measured in megahertz (MHz).

There are as many radio frequencies in the radio spectrum as there are colors in a rainbow, which is a spectrum of light. These ranges of radio frequencies are divided into **VHF**, for very high frequency, and **UHF**, or ultrahigh frequency.

Communication by radio has become increasingly popular with the government, businesses, and even the public. The result has been that often many users are sharing radio frequencies. Although considerate use of a radio frequency, or channel, should allow for multiple users, problems can arise.

Channel crowding has become such a problem that some services use **channel guards**. Channel guards, sometimes called private lines (PLs), prevent extraneous interference by blocking radio transmissions from outside the base station.

The Federal Communications Commission

In an effort to prevent problems and maintain some control of the radio airwaves, Congress established the **Federal Communications Commission (FCC)**. The FCC is charged with allocating radio frequencies, licensing base stations, issuing **call signs**, and monitoring radio operations. A call sign is a group of letters or numbers, or both, that is assigned to a particular group using a frequency.

In 1974, the FCC set a specific group, or band, of radio frequencies aside for use by EMS providers. From 460 MHz to 470 MHz is restricted to EMS providers only. These 10 frequencies, called **Med channels**, are frequently used by paramedics and EMTs to speak to base hospital physicians.

In a given region, certain frequencies are dedicated to a particular purpose. For example, in many communities Med channel 4 is the standard **hailing frequency**. This frequency is used to call the base hospital. After contact is made, the EMT is advised to go to another channel for the report.

In 1993, the FCC set the 220 MHz band aside for EMS. Despite these two restricted-access bands, EMS still does not have enough channels (frequencies) to operate without occasionally experiencing channel crowding.

Radio Channels

Once an emergency call is received, it is transmitted to the appropriate EMS units. The *dispatch frequency* is reserved for communications between EMS units in the field and the communications center.

During a multiple-casualty incident, or when several EMS calls are occurring simultaneously, frivolous radio *chatter* may prevent much-needed resources from being dispatched. In cases in which communications between EMS units and other emergency services must occur

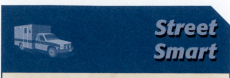

Street Smart

Although radio technology has made great advances, occasionally a radio system will fail. Lightning strikes, battery failure, and computer lockups are some of the problems that can cripple a radio communications system. Consequently, there should always be a backup plan. Many EMS systems use cellular telephones as a backup system. This prevents problems when communications fail and ensures the safety of the public.

on scene, all on-scene units should select a **tactical channel**. A tactical channel is a channel that is kept free for nondispatch-related radio traffic. The use of such a channel permits efficient scene coordination without interfering with system management.

Many communities have a predesignated tactical frequency, such as 155.715, that all EMS units switch to when they arrive on scene. This kind of *preplanning* decreases scene confusion and keeps essential radio channels open for emergency radio traffic.

Hospital communications is usually done on another frequency entirely. This frequency, like one of the Med channels discussed earlier, permits privacy and no interruptions. Because of the nature of these communications, many Med channels are recorded.

Computers and Radios

Most of the time, a radio frequency is not in use. Therefore, multiple users could hypothetically share a frequency. Nevertheless, there are times when radio messages will clash, or be *stepped on*, unwittingly by another user. Certain messages should take priority over others. For example, the message from a police officer calling for help should take precedence over a message from water department truck calling back into service.

A computer can sort through the incoming messages and allow priority messages to be transmitted on any available frequency while diverting or delaying lower-priority messages to an available channel. The use of computers to assist radios allows for truncated frequencies, so-called **trunked lines**. The newer 800 MHz radios, along with computers, are frequently used by municipalities for these trunked lines.

Telephones

Telephones are a vital link between the public and emergency services. Although 9-1-1 access to emergency services is not universal, most communities are moving toward that goal.

Telephones also serve as a link between the EMT and the communications center and the EMT and the hospital. To ensure that the EMT can reach either the communications center or the base hospital, EMS agencies install separate dedicated telephone lines (Figure 18-8). These limited-access phone lines are often used by emergency physicians to give EMTs medical orders. For this reason, these lines are often recorded.

Cellular Phones

Cellular telephones are actually low-powered duplex radios that communicate with a series of interconnected radio repeaters. This series of repeaters creates a grid, and, within the grid, there are cells that permit the EMT an ability to roam around inside the grid and still transmit.

Although commercial cellular services usually charge for the service, most provide 9-1-1 calls for no charge. This is a valuable public service.

When a patient calls 9-1-1 on a telephone, in many cases the exact location of the telephone is displayed in the communications center. Cell phones, on the other hand, are mobile and therefore the commu-

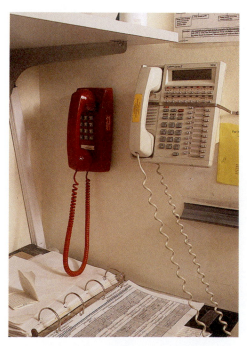

FIGURE 18-8 Dedicated hot lines assure EMTs unimpeded access to the physician.

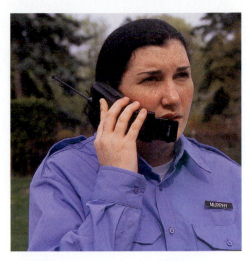

FIGURE 18-9 It is sometimes difficult to pinpoint the location of a cellular call.

nications center does not know the location of the phone. That means that the caller has to describe her location exactly (Figure 18-9). Technology is being developed to allow tracking of the location of a cellular phone for emergency purposes.

Digital Technology

Digital technology converts messages into digitally coded signals, then transmits them at a very high rate of speed. The receiver reconstructs the signal into a readable form. This technology can be used for written, verbal, or electronic data. The fax and an ECG transmitted over a telephone line are examples of the use of digital technology (Figure 18-10).

Satellite Phones

Utilizing a series of low-earth-orbiting satellites, communication is now possible in areas where cellular service may be poor or nonexistent. These satellite phones transmit their digital signal to a satellite, called an uplink, and the satellite retransmits the signal down to a waiting receiver, called a downlink. The use of satellite phones permits radio communications in areas where traditional communication is limited by rough terrain, for example, mountainous terrain, or over great distances, such as ships that are out to sea.

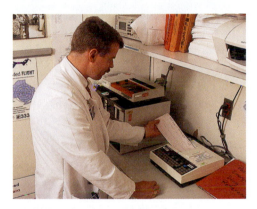

FIGURE 18-10 Digital technology offers new opportunities for EMS.

BASIC RADIO OPERATION

There are many types of radio design. Always take a moment, preferably before the radio is needed, to examine the radio. Where is the power switch? Where is the volume control? Adjust the volume to a comfortable level. Test the radio briefly.

When it comes to using a radio, it is important that the EMT be brief and concise. Careful consideration of the message before transmitting prevents the EMT from rambling in a disjointed fashion. The message should be thought out, then delivered.

Before pressing the transmit button, wait for several seconds to be sure that no other radio traffic is present. If the air is clear, then proceed to transmit. Hold the microphone, or mic, about 2 inches from

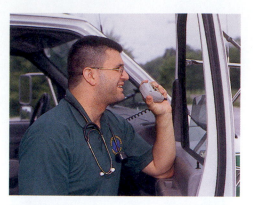

FIGURE 18-11 Press to talk, wait 2 seconds, and speak slowly and clearly.

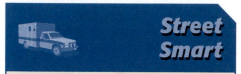

Street Smart

Some EMS calls occur in a noisy environment, as when heavy rescue machinery is in use or diesel engines are running. In those cases, a special *noise-canceling mic* can be helpful. This device has two microphones. One picks up the EMT's voice while the other picks up the sounds in the environment. The EMT's message is transmitted, and the environmental interference is canceled out.

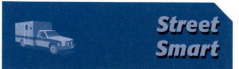

Street Smart

Never say anything over the radio that you would not say in front of your supervisor. The public listens closely to all emergency service channels. Words spoken with anger or sarcasm are heard over radio scanners. A professional EMT always maintains a pleasant disposition while using the radio.

the mouth. Speak clearly and slowly in a normal conversational tone (Figure 18-11). If the EMT must raise her voice to hear herself speak, then she should consider rolling up the window or moving to another location to transmit.

Radio Procedures

When an EMT is attempting to call another party, she should take a "you first then me" approach. First identify the other unit or person you wish to call. Then identify yourself by unit identifier—for example, "EMS command, this is Engine 11, requesting instructions."

When speaking to other units, use plain English. In the past, when radios were not as dependable, transmissions were made shorter by using special codes. These codes varied from community to community. Because of the confusion sometimes created and the availability of higher-quality radios, radio transmissions should be made in plain English.

Careful thought beforehand will prevent the EMT from uttering meaningless phrases such as "be advised," "10-4," and the like. These phrases add nothing to the message, waste valuable air time, and generally are seen as the sign of a novice radio operator.

Profanity should not be tolerated on the radio under any circumstance. The FCC monitors transmissions and will investigate complaints of profanity. The FCC is empowered to suspend or cancel a radio operator's license for use of profanity over the air.

It is not necessary to say "please" or "thank you" over the air. These amenities are implicit in a professional radio transmission. Instead, conserve valuable air time.

If a long transmission is necessary, stop every 30 seconds to permit other EMTs an opportunity to interrupt the transmission. This practice ensures that air time is available in case of emergency. It also encourages EMTs to be brief and to the point.

Standard Nomenclature

If the EMT needs to pause the conversation, and wishes the other party to stay near the radio, the EMT should ask the other party to **stand by**. This request means that the EMT will return to the radio shortly.

Whenever an EMT is answering a question over the radio, she should use the term *affirmative* or *negative*. Short answers such as yes and no are frequently not heard or are misunderstood.

When the EMT is done with a statement, she should say the word *over*, which tells the other party that it is now her turn to speak.

When the EMT is completely done with her radio transmission, she should *clear the air*, typically by stating her identifier and saying the word *clear*—for example, "This is Ambulance 2-4 clearing Med channel 1." Other users who are listening now know that the frequency is available for their use.

When giving a number over the radio, always say each number individually. For example, the number 15 may sound like 50. Saying "one-five" leaves little room for doubt.

Alert Report

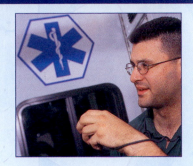

"One, two, three, four, five, bag, one ..." All hands are occupied trying to revive this patient, a 45-year-old male who is in cardiac arrest. Jack is trying to help where he can, not really sure what to do because this is his first cardiac arrest experience. The crew chief looks up and says, "Jack, use the radio to call this one into the hospital."

- What are the fundamental elements of a radio report?
- Does the hospital need to know the complete history and physical findings?
- What specific information does the hospital need to know?

HOSPITAL COMMUNICATION

There are two common reasons for an EMT to use a radio to call the emergency department. The first reason is to confer regarding the patient's condition and obtain any directions or orders that the physician may have regarding patient care. This kind of radio report is understandably longer and more detailed than many other radio transmissions. This type of communication may be referred to as a consultation.

The other reason to make a radio call is simply to alert the emergency department of your impending arrival. This is the most common type of report. Medical orders are not being requested, nor are they expected. This report should be concise. Typically, this report can be given in less than 30 seconds. A nurse usually takes this report and then advises the attending physician, the triage nurse, the charge nurse, and other personnel of the situation. In this case, many important emergency team members may need to be prepared for the patient.

Alert Report

The elements of a complete report are listed in Table 18-2. Some elements are not needed in the brief initial notification report but may be required if the EMT is looking for medical consultation. These are indicated in Table 18-2. First, contact with the emergency department has to be made. Follow your local protocols regarding how to initiate radio contact with the emergency department.

Once contact has been confirmed, the EMT should start by repeating the EMS unit identifier—for example, "Bay State ED, this is

Street Smart

It may be helpful for the EMT to have a radio call form completed that contains those elements listed in Table 18-2. Using this form as a tool, the EMT would then have the information readily available to give in a concise radio report.

TABLE 18-2

Elements of a Radio Report

Item of Information	Alert Report	Consultation Report
Unit ID	X	X
Level of provider		X
Patient's age and sex	X	X
Chief complaint	X	X
Brief history of present illness		X
Relevant past illnesses		X
Mental status	X	X
Vital signs	X	X
Pertinent findings on physical exam		X
Treatments in progress	X	X
Patient's response to care provided		X
Estimated time of arrival	X	X

Ambulance one." Then launch into the report. These first few words should be thought of as a standard introduction. It sets up both the speaker and the listener for the report to follow.

It is traditional among medical professionals to identify the age and sex of the patient at the beginning of the report—for example, "We have a 45-year-old male."

Some EMS systems add the patient's estimated weight. Other systems include the name of the patient's personal physician. If the age is unknown, then an estimate is usually given—for example, "We have an approximately 45-year-old male, a patient of Dr. Putnam."

The patient's chief complaint lends a great deal of insight into the patient's problems. A patient's chief complaint should be stated in the patient's own words, and in a single sentence.

The patient's mental status is key to overall condition. Regardless of the cause, an unconscious patient is seriously ill and considered urgent. Typical descriptions of a patient's mental status include "awake and alert," "conscious but confused," or "unconscious." Use the AVPU (*a*lert, *v*oice, *p*ain, *u*nresponsive) scale when choosing a description.

Proceed to the most recent set of vital signs. Minimally, this should include the patient's respiratory rate, pulse rate, and blood pressure. Major treatments that have been provided should also be relayed.

Consultation Report

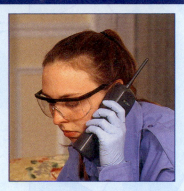

Classic signs of a heart attack. Substernal chest pain radiating into the left arm. The patient took his nitroglycerin tablet without relief. He called EMS. Now he is asking the EMT whether he should take another tablet. His blood pressure is border-line low. The EMT decides to call the base hospital for more directions, using a cellular telephone.

- When is it appropriate to request to speak to medical control?
- What essential elements should be included in this report?
- How does an EMT "accept" a medical control order?

Finally, and perhaps most important, the estimated time of arrival should be given. Simply stated, "Our ETA is 5 minutes," allows the emergency department to adjust to the incoming workload. Patients may be either transferred or discharged to prepare a room for the patient.

Medical Consultation Report

Most of an EMT's instructions for medical care are written in a set of orders called *protocols*. Protocols offer a standardized approach to caring for a typical patient. Some patients are not typical. In those cases, a consultation with an emergency physician is appropriate. The EMT is asking for on-line medical control.

Several goals can be accomplished by calling for medical control. First, the doctor is alerted to the impending arrival of a complex patient. Second, the doctor will have advanced knowledge of the patient's condition and can more adequately prepare. Third, the doctor can give patient-specific medical orders that may ease the patient's complaint or improve his condition.

It is important that the EMT give a complete and accurate report to the doctor. The EMT is the hands and eyes of the doctor in the field. For the EMT to be effective, she needs to give the doctor the best information possible.

Table 18-2 details all the elements of a medical consultation report. Note that there are many similar elements in the short *alert* report and the full *medical consultation* report. It is good practice to have a novice EMT practice several short alert reports before trying to give her first medical consultation report.

All radio reports commence with the standard introduction—that is, hailing the hospital and providing the EMS unit identification. The EMT then proceeds with the patient's demographics: age, sex, and private physician.

Street Smart

Some EMTs have a fear of the radio mic. The thought of speaking to a physician or a nurse is intimidating to them. The best way to get over this fear is through frequent practice.

Start by giving another EMT report, after the call. First, write the report down on a sheet of paper. Then read the report aloud like a movie script. Start by giving short alert reports, then work up to a medical control report.

The report of the patient's mental status and chief complaint are the same as in the alert report, but more information is provided to the physician in the remainder of the medical consultation report.

The EMT should expand on the history of the present illness, following the SAMPLE format (see Table 10-5 for a definition of this term). It is important that the physician hear the patient's entire pertinent past medical history as well as prescription medications being taken.

After describing the pertinent physical findings from the detailed physical examination, using the DCAP-BTLS format (see Table 14-3 for a definition of this term), the EMT should give both the first and the last set of vital signs.

Any treatments the EMT has instituted should be reported as well as the patient's response to those treatments: for example, "The patient was placed on high-flow oxygen and says it gave him some relief from his chest pain." End every report with the expected time of arrival (ETA). Then ask the physician whether she has any more questions. If the patient has a request of the physician, this is the time to ask the physician.

Accepting a Medical Order

When a medical control doctor gives an order, it is important for the EMT to understand the order clearly. Several procedures decrease the likelihood of errors.

First, the EMT should use **echo technique**. In echo technique, the physician gives the order, then the EMT repeats the order back and asks whether her read-back is correct. The physician then confirms the read-back. Notice that there are a minimum of three communications before an EMT accepts the order.

In some systems, another EMT has to hear the order as well. Some radios have a speaker option that facilitates this process. In other cases, the EMT hands the radio or telephone to another EMT.

In any case, if you are unsure of the order, for whatever reason, *do not accept the order*. Question the order if necessary. Repeat the report, or portions of it, if it appears that the physician did not understand the situation. As a last resort, *do nothing*. It is better to do nothing than to cause harm to the patient.

OTHER RADIO COMMUNICATIONS

During the course of daily operation, EMTs will have many opportunities to utilize the radio in order to keep the communications center apprised of their status. The dispatcher should always be made aware of the location of each in-service unit so that he can most efficiently dispatch units to calls.

During the course of an emergency call, the EMT should continue to apprise the dispatch center of the status of the call. Table 18-3 lists the common times the EMT would update the dispatch center. The needs of each emergency system are different, and the EMT should follow local protocols regarding notifications.

TABLE 18-3

Notification Points During an Emergency Call

Event	Example of Transmission
Call received	"Dispatcher, Ambulance one received the information."
En route to scene	"Ambulance one is en route to 123 Main Street."
Arriving on scene	"Ambulance one is arriving at 123 Main Street."
Request additional resources when needed	"Dispatcher, please send an ALS unit to 123 Main Street."
En route to hospital	"Ambulance one is en route to Memorial Hospital."
Hospital communications	As in Table 18-2
Arrival at hospital	"Ambulance one has arrived at Memorial Hospital."
Return to service	"Ambulance one is back in service, returning to quarters."
Arrival at quarters	"Ambulance one is back in quarters."

CONCLUSION

Radio use is an everyday part of the EMT's responsibility. It is important to understand the basic concepts behind radio operation and when to use each form of communication device. Part of the job of every EMT is to be familiar with proper radio terminology and etiquette. The key elements of communication during an emergency call, including hospital notification, should be practiced by the new EMT.

TEST YOUR KNOWLEDGE

1. What are the roles of modern communications specialists?
2. What are the components of a typical radio system?
3. What is the role of the Federal Communications Commission?
4. How has modern technology advanced communications?
5. What are the basic radio procedures for initiating and terminating a radio call?
6. What are the elements of an alert report?
7. What are the elements of a medical consultation report?
8. When is radio communication generally necessary during an emergency call?

INTERNET RESOURCES

Visit the following organizations' Web sites for more information on communications systems:

- National Communications Systems, http://www.ncs.gov
- Federal Communications Commission, http://www.fcc.gov

Search the Web for additional information using these key words:

- EMS radio communications or EMS radio reports
- Mobile radio
- Portable radio
- Alert report
- Medical consultation report

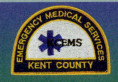

Report

OBJECTIVES

Upon completion of this chapter, the reader should be able to:

1. Describe the importance of a verbal report.
2. Describe the three "rights" of effective interpersonal communication.
3. Describe the barriers to effective interpersonal communication.
4. Describe some techniques EMTs use to overcome these barriers.

OVERVIEW

Typically, a health care provider will transfer patient care to another health care provider and give a **verbal report**. The verbal report narrates the patient's condition for the new provider. The acceptance of the report represents the willingness of the other party to accept the patient. The failure of an emergency medical technician (EMT) to give a report about a patient to the next health care provider could be construed as abandonment.

Beyond the medical-legal justification, giving a patient report offers two health care professionals an opportunity to focus on one patient and exchange observations, records, and physical findings regarding that patient.

Restrictions on radio time, conditions on scene, and the presence of family members near the radio all may prevent the EMT from fully relating the patient's condition to the emergency physician. The verbal report is the opportunity an EMT has to tell the whole story.

THE VERBAL REPORT

The verbal report is an expanded radio report an EMT will give to another health care provider who is taking over, or joining the care of that patient. Using the same information that was provided in the

Transfer of Care

The patient was a middle-aged African American male with a history of hypertension. His wife called 9-1-1 when he started to complain of chest pain.

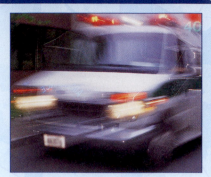

The patient appeared to be having a heart attack. Drew wasn't sure. The wife kept interrupting, and the room started to get noisy. Feeling a little uncomfortable, he directed his partner to package the patient immediately. The patient insisted on going to Center Hospital, all the way across town and out of the district.

At the hospital, still unsure of the entire history, Drew rolled the patient into what could be called chaos. He had obtained a room assignment over the radio, and just wanted to give a report.

The patient was starting to look grayer and was now grossly diaphoretic (perspiring). Drew grabbed the first orderly who went by. The orderly shook him off and told him he was busy.

Drew was starting to feel a little panic himself. He knew the patient was sick and nobody seemed to want to listen. He grabbed the next nurse who went by him.

- What communication barriers has this EMT encountered?
- What are the essential elements of a bedside report?
- Is it necessary for an EMT to provide a bedside report? What are the possible consequences if he does not?

radio report, the EMT describes any changes in the patient's condition and provides a set of the most current vital signs.

The verbal report may be the single most important activity performed by an EMT for a patient, especially for the patient who is unable to speak for herself. The key to effective communication is to tell the right person, at the right place, at the right time about the patient.

The Right Person

Tell the right person the patient's story. This may seem like common sense, but many EMTs have wasted a great deal of time telling the wrong person the patient information. The EMT has to reflect on the nature of the message before deciding who should hear it.

A verbal report is often given to a nurse at the bedside (Figure 19-1). Giving the report to the nurse is appropriate because the nurse will be coordinating the patient's care while she is in the hospital.

There are times when the patient's condition needs to be reported directly to the doctor. Whenever the patient's condition warrants immediate attention to prevent loss of life, then a doctor needs to be notified.

The Right Place

Consideration should be given to where the report is given. Often, family members and friends are standing outside in the hall. These

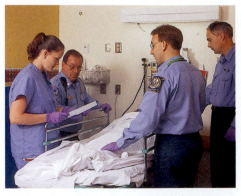

FIGURE 19-1 Most patient reports are received by a registered nurse at the bedside.

well-meaning people are listening for some hopeful news about the patient's condition.

Because they are not the intended audience and may not be knowledgeable about medical terminology, these people may misinterpret what they hear. In addition, the EMT must always remember that every patient has a right to **confidentiality**. The EMT must ensure that private medical information be provided only to those health care providers who will be caring for the patient. The EMT should take measures to ensure that nonprivileged personnel are not able to overhear the report. Failure on the part of the EMT to notice that others are listening may be embarrassing or, worse, a breach of the patient's rights (Figure 19-2).

Most health care providers would prefer to get the patient's history directly from the patient, provided the patient is awake and alert. In those cases, the EMT should provide the health care provider pertinent information about the patient that the patient would not know. For example, vital signs should be reported. Another example is the mechanism of injury and the significance of impact.

Common courtesy dictates that whenever a question can be answered by the patient, then the patient should answer the question. Giving a report while talking over the patient and ignoring the patient is discourteous. Always encourage the patient to enter the conversation at the appropriate time.

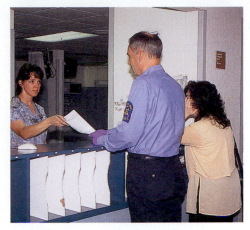

FIGURE 19-2 Caution should be exercised about what is said about the patient. The patient's condition should not be discussed with bystanders.

The Right Time

Every patient is important. However, the patient with a painful, swollen deformity on the hallway stretcher will have to wait while the busy emergency physician treats the patient in cardiac arrest in the trauma room.

The EMT should consider the patient's urgency before insisting on being heard by the emergency department personnel. This simple courtesy improves relationships and ultimately speeds patient care.

INTERPERSONAL COMMUNICATION

Interpersonal communication is part speech and, in larger part, body language. Eye contact, gestures, and posture all communicate a message. Poor eye contact, for example, may indicate that the EMT lacks interest in the patient. This is not the message an EMT wants to convey to another health care professional.

Whenever an EMT gives a verbal report, the EMT should stand straight, look the other person in the eye, and give a clear report of the patient's condition. Facial expressions, tone of voice, and a quick response to questions asked leave the physician or nurse with the impression that the EMT is a caring professional.

Communication Barriers

"I know that's what you heard, but that's not what I said." This statement could be made by many EMTs. Some health care providers may rush to judgment, because of personal bias, emotions, or beliefs, after listening to an EMT's report. A problem arises when they do not understand the patient's problems.

To prevent premature evaluation of a patient's problems, an EMT should try to give a complete report. If giving a complete report is not possible, then the EMT should focus the report on the most important aspects of the patient's condition.

If the message is not getting across to the other individual, the EMT should try a technique that communications specialists use called **repetitive persistence**. While remaining calm and in control, the EMT simply repeats the message until he is sure the message has been understood.

Communication is a two-way street. EMTs can also fail to understand the questions that are asked of them. Simply stop, look, and listen. Stop whatever it is you are doing. Look at the person who is speaking to you. Listen to the person, giving him your undivided attention.

CONCLUSION

The purpose of a patient report is to communicate urgent patient information to someone who can do something. Therefore, careful attention to the right person, place, and time will increase the impact of an EMT's patient report.

The EMT should take the time to stop, look, and listen to the person who is asking questions. You may be the only person who can answer these questions. The answers are important. Failures of communication are costly in terms of money, time, and lives.

TEST YOUR KNOWLEDGE

1. Describe the importance of a verbal report.
2. Describe the three "rights" of effective communication.
3. Describe the barriers to effective communication.
4. Describe some techniques EMTs use to overcome these barriers.

INTERNET RESOURCES

Search the Web using these key words:
- EMS report
- Verbal report

Share interesting facts and Web sites with your colleagues.

CHAPTER 20

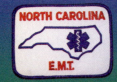

Record

KEY TERMS

affidavit

CHEATED

mandated reporter

minimum data set

objective

patient care report (PCR)

patient refusal form

sentinel PCR

special incident report

subjective

triage tag

OBJECTIVES

Upon completion of this chapter, the reader should be able to:

1. Describe the importance of an EMT's documentation.
2. List the standard elements of every EMT patient care report (PCR).
3. Describe how the PCR fits into the patient's medical record.
4. List four functions of the PCR.
5. Describe a minimum data set.
6. Differentiate open and closed charting methods.
7. List the elements of the acronym SOAP.
8. List the elements of the acronym CHEATED.
9. Describe the importance of standardized abbreviations.
10. List the principles of good documentation.
11. Describe how to correct an error in the record.
12. Describe how to make an addition to the record.
13. List several reasons to write a special incident report.
14. Describe the special documentation an EMT uses at a multiple-casualty incident.
15. Describe what critical elements must be included in every patient refusal.
16. List those people who would make a good witness on a patient refusal form.

OVERVIEW

"The job isn't over until the paperwork is done." State and federal regulations, insurance carriers, and the courts all demand complete and accurate documentation. Complete and accurate documentation of medical care is a fundamental function of every health care professional, including the emergency medical technician (EMT).

411

An EMT, as a part of the medical team, is held to the same documentation standards as any other health care provider. The **patient care report (PCR)** must include the history of the patient's illness, the findings of the physical examination, the treatments rendered, and any difficulties or complications that were encountered in the course of patient care.

An EMT must document patient care as carefully as a physician must. This chapter details the elements and characteristics of a professional EMT report.

THE RECORD

Over decades, each health care profession, from medicine to nursing to physical therapy and so on, developed a method of documentation specific to its specialty. Because of the wide variety of reporting styles, it was often difficult to follow the patient's condition from one record to another.

In the 1970s, Dr. Lawrence Weed of the University of Vermont created a system called problem-oriented medical record-keeping (POMR) as a universal standard of documentation for all health care professionals. POMR quickly gained acceptance in the medical community.

Writing a Report

Mrs. Rocky lived in the third-floor apartment above the barbershop. Every few days she would call EMS for one complaint or another. Today she called because her back hurt; her "sciatica" was acting up, and she had a terrible headache.

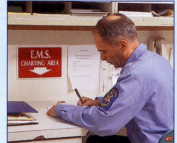

Her past medical history included a heart attack back in 1998, congestive heart failure, a "touch" of emphysema, and a 30-year history of smoking two packs of cigarettes a day.

The EMT completed a focused history and physical exam based upon her complaints. Her physical examination revealed she had jugular venous distension, audible wheezes, and abdominal tenderness, and her legs were swollen from the ankles to the knees.

After turning Mrs. Rocky over to the emergency department nurse, the EMT sat down to write the patient care report.

- What essential elements should be included in the patient care report?
- What format could be used to organize the information?
- What are some important documentation standards?

A problem or diagnosis list is used as an index, and all patient care records are entered under a problem that the patient experiences. This method of record keeping, POMR, is ideal for emergency medical services (EMS).

The patient's chief complaint (CC) is the basis for all care rendered by the EMT. Using the CC, the doctor can link the PCR to a tentative diagnosis in the emergency department. Then the EMT's PCR is attached to a diagnostic group or problem list within the medical record for all health care providers to review.

Functions of the Record

The prehospital PCR is an important part of a complete medical record. It is a record of the patient's condition and the treatment that took place before the patient's arrival at the emergency department.

The PCR can speak for the patient when the patient cannot speak for himself, as when the patient is unconscious, long after the EMT has left the hospital. The PCR can also describe the scene the patient was found in. The EMT is the eye of the physician in the field. The EMT may be the only health care professional who saw the mechanism of injury and can describe it.

Quality Improvement

The PCR is more than just a part of the patient record. The PCR is also used for administrative purposes. For example, some EMS agencies use the PCR as part of their continuous quality improvement (CQI) process.

Other EMTs, in a process called peer review, take all the PCRs on a subject, such as motor vehicle collisions, and review the PCRs for accuracy and compliance with medical protocols (Figure 20-1). If a problem is consistently identified in the PCRs, then a special educational session is created to address the problem.

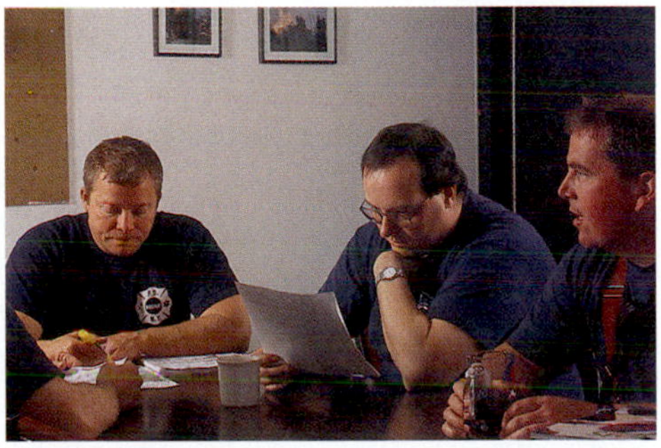

Certain special PCRs may be singled out for call review. These PCRs present an unusual circumstance that deserves special consideration. These designated PCRs, called **sentinel PCRs**, are reviewed by the medical director or a risk management group (Figure 20-2).

FIGURE 20-1   PCRs are used for quality improvement purposes.

Research

Scientific research is relatively new in EMS. Using the experience of other EMTs, as documented on the PCR, researchers strive to improve the practice of EMTs by identifying what works and what does not. Research has helped identify treatments that were not effective in the field and are therefore no longer used. Similarly, collection of data from the PCR can lead to support of a particular practice or suggest ways to improve the care that is given. Research is a part of every profession's development.

Administrative Purposes

The PCR fulfills many administrative purposes that are not directly tied to the patient's care. For example, in order to bill a patient for the services rendered, the business office will minimally need the patient's name, address, date of birth, and Social Security number.

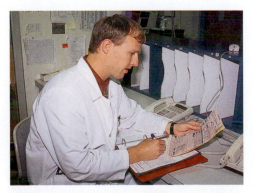

FIGURE 20-2   An emergency physician should review sentinel PCRs.

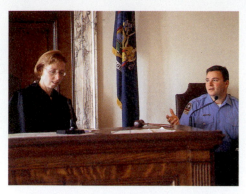

FIGURE 20-3 The PCR is the EMT's written record of care.

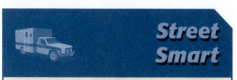

Accurate documentation of time is important on the PCR. Often, the time on the EMT's watch doesn't exactly match that on the dispatcher's desk. Every effort should be made to synchronize timepieces or, at least, work consistently from one clock so that documentation of time on a PCR is accurate.

The PCR also contains information for other reports. Some EMS agencies routinely track figures such as response times. This information is usually found on a PCR.

Legal Document

The PCR is also a legal document. As such, it is used in a court of law to show the events surrounding an illness or injury. When called to court to testify, EMTs are often questioned very closely about the details of an injury or illness as well as about the care they provided (Figure 20-3). A legal case may not reach the courts for months or even years. The EMT must depend on the written record, the PCR, to refresh her memory regarding the circumstances surrounding the call. Therefore, it is in an EMT's best interest to document carefully the entire patient encounter.

Minimum Data Sets

The amount of information an EMT could record on a PCR is almost endless. Recording all the possible information is often wasteful in terms of time and utility. Every PCR requires a minimum amount of information to prevent EMTs from sacrificing accuracy for brevity. These specific bits of information are called the **minimum data set**. For administrative purposes, it is important to have the patient's name, date of birth, address, and other such demographic information. These bits of information represent the administrative data set.

For medical documentation, the patient's chief complaint, vital signs, and a SAMPLE history (see Table 10-5 for a definition of this term) might be considered the minimum data set.

In an effort to standardize prehospital documentation, both state and federal governments have established certain minimum data sets for EMS agencies. Standardization enables EMS administrators to create uniform reports of EMS activity across a state or across the country.

Format for Documentation

Somehow the patient information has to get onto the PCR. How that information is recorded is partly a function of the form. PCR forms can be generally categorized as either open format or closed format.

A closed-format PCR uses either checklists or bubble blanks for patient information (Figure 20-4). This format is useful for recording a large quantity of the same or similar information, such as run numbers and times.

Closed PCRs can also be read directly by a computer, using optical character recognition (OCR) technology. This enables EMS administrators to obtain large amounts of data quickly and accurately.

A disadvantage of the closed format is that little space is provided for any distinctive information regarding the patient. The alternative form developed, utilizing an open format, provides plenty of space for a narrative account of the patient's care.

Looking like a blank sheet of paper, the open PCR gives the EMT space to write her observations in longhand. The open form provides the EMT the opportunity to individualize the patient record. However, it does not provide the EMT the structure in which to organize her

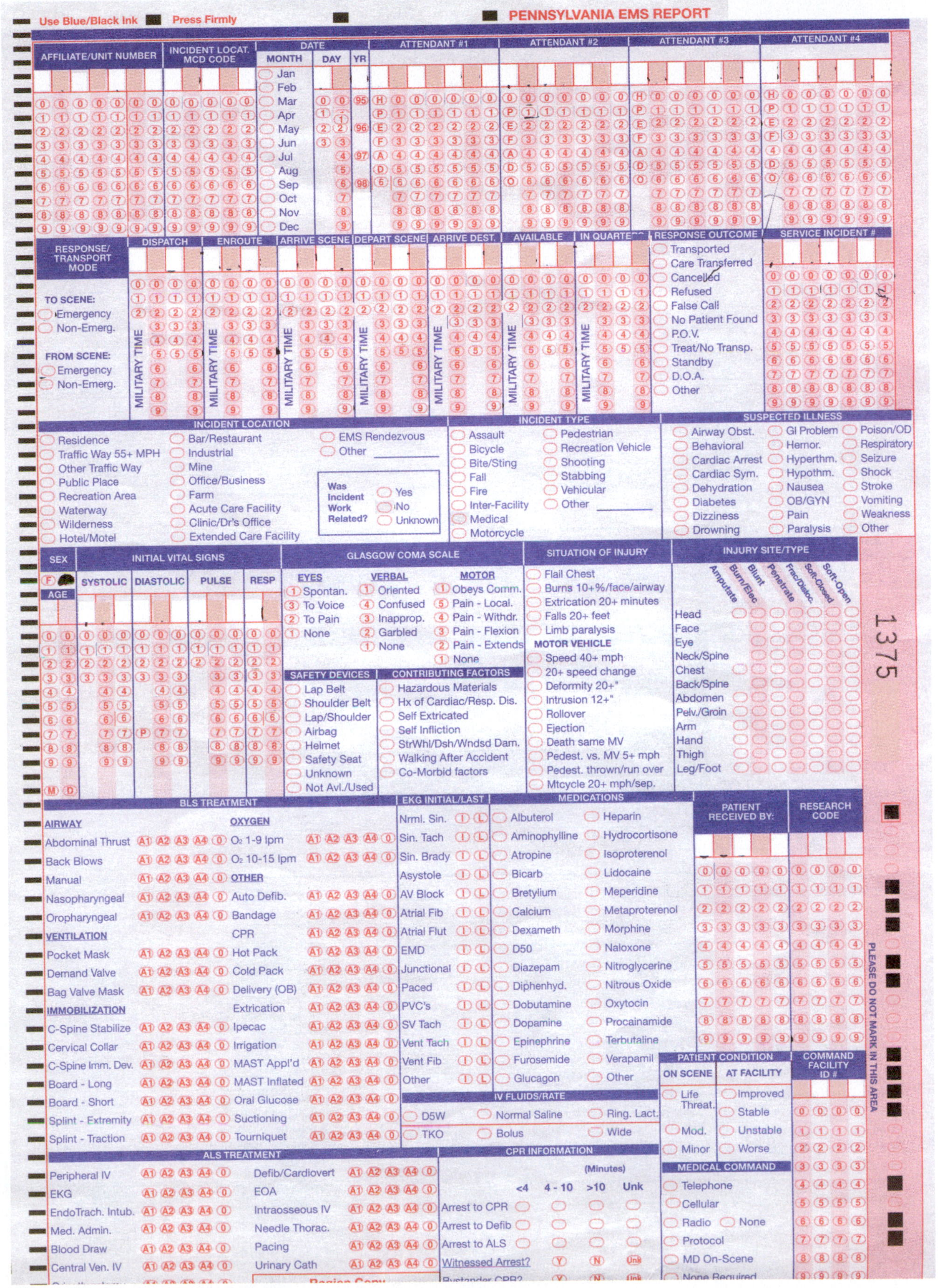

FIGURE 20-4 An example of a closed-format patient care report (PCR).

thoughts. The following section describes several commonly accepted arrangements that an EMT can use to organize her narrative.

Clearly, each format, open and closed, has advantages, but each also is insufficient for effective documentation. For this reason, most PCRs are a hybrid of the two formats, taking the best from each and leaving the worst behind, trying to find that happy medium (Figure 20-5).

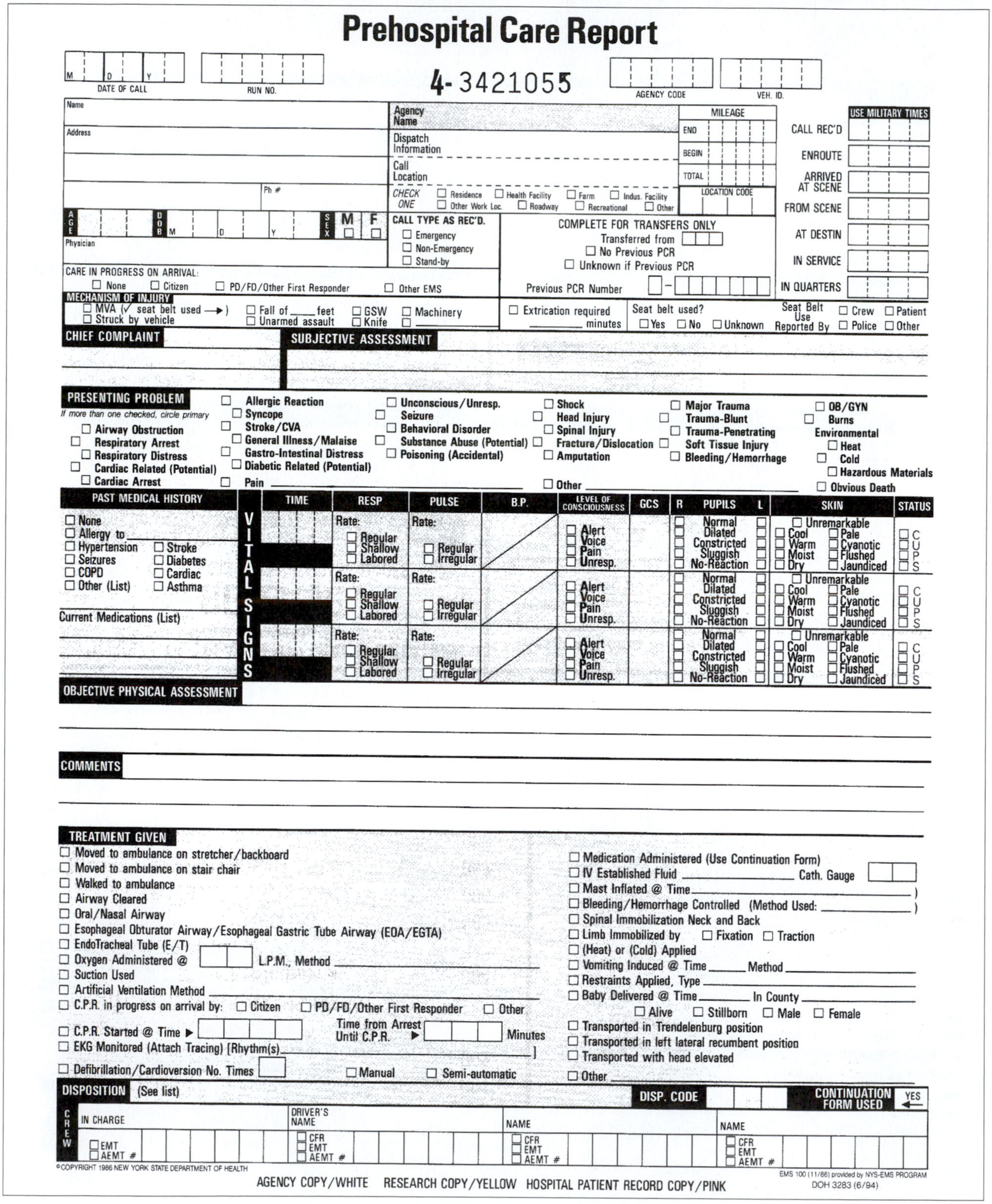

Prehospital Care Report

M D Y DATE OF CALL | RUN NO. | 4-3421055 | AGENCY CODE | VEH. ID.

Name | Address | Ph # | AGE | DOB M D Y | SEX M F | Physician

Agency Name | Dispatch Information | Call Location | CHECK ONE: ☐ Residence ☐ Health Facility ☐ Farm ☐ Indus. Facility ☐ Other Work Loc. ☐ Roadway ☐ Recreational ☐ Other

MILEAGE: END, BEGIN, TOTAL | LOCATION CODE

USE MILITARY TIMES: CALL REC'D, ENROUTE, ARRIVED AT SCENE, FROM SCENE, AT DESTIN, IN SERVICE, IN QUARTERS

CALL TYPE AS REC'D.: ☐ Emergency ☐ Non-Emergency ☐ Stand-by

COMPLETE FOR TRANSFERS ONLY: Transferred from ☐ No Previous PCR ☐ Unknown if Previous PCR; Previous PCR Number

CARE IN PROGRESS ON ARRIVAL: ☐ None ☐ Citizen ☐ PD/FD/Other First Responder ☐ Other EMS

MECHANISM OF INJURY: ☐ MVA (✓ seat belt used →) ☐ Struck by vehicle ☐ Fall of ___ feet ☐ Unarmed assault ☐ GSW ☐ Knife ☐ Machinery ☐ ___ | ☐ Extrication required ___ minutes | Seat belt used? ☐ Yes ☐ No ☐ Unknown | Seat Belt Use Reported By ☐ Crew ☐ Patient ☐ Police ☐ Other

CHIEF COMPLAINT | SUBJECTIVE ASSESSMENT

PRESENTING PROBLEM (If more than one checked, circle primary): ☐ Airway Obstruction ☐ Respiratory Arrest ☐ Respiratory Distress ☐ Cardiac Related (Potential) ☐ Cardiac Arrest ☐ Allergic Reaction ☐ Syncope ☐ Stroke/CVA ☐ General Illness/Malaise ☐ Gastro-Intestinal Distress ☐ Diabetic Related (Potential) ☐ Pain ___ ☐ Unconscious/Unresp. ☐ Seizure ☐ Behavioral Disorder ☐ Substance Abuse (Potential) ☐ Poisoning (Accidental) ☐ Shock ☐ Head Injury ☐ Spinal Injury ☐ Fracture/Dislocation ☐ Amputation ☐ Other ___ ☐ Major Trauma ☐ Trauma-Blunt ☐ Trauma-Penetrating ☐ Soft Tissue Injury ☐ Bleeding/Hemorrhage ☐ OB/GYN ☐ Burns Environmental ☐ Heat ☐ Cold ☐ Hazardous Materials ☐ Obvious Death

PAST MEDICAL HISTORY: ☐ None ☐ Allergy to ___ ☐ Hypertension ☐ Seizures ☐ COPD ☐ Other (List) ☐ Stroke ☐ Diabetes ☐ Cardiac ☐ Asthma; Current Medications (List)

VITAL SIGNS: TIME	RESP	PULSE	B.P.	LEVEL OF CONSCIOUSNESS	GCS	R PUPILS L	SKIN	STATUS
	Rate: ☐ Regular ☐ Shallow ☐ Labored	Rate: ☐ Regular ☐ Irregular		☐ Alert ☐ Voice ☐ Pain ☐ Unresp.		Normal Dilated Constricted Sluggish No-Reaction	☐ Unremarkable ☐ Cool ☐ Warm ☐ Moist ☐ Dry ☐ Pale ☐ Cyanotic ☐ Flushed ☐ Jaundiced	☐ C ☐ U ☐ P ☐ S
	Rate: ☐ Regular ☐ Shallow ☐ Labored	Rate: ☐ Regular ☐ Irregular		☐ Alert ☐ Voice ☐ Pain ☐ Unresp.		Normal Dilated Constricted Sluggish No-Reaction	☐ Unremarkable ☐ Cool ☐ Warm ☐ Moist ☐ Dry ☐ Pale ☐ Cyanotic ☐ Flushed ☐ Jaundiced	☐ C ☐ U ☐ P ☐ S
	Rate: ☐ Regular ☐ Shallow ☐ Labored	Rate: ☐ Regular ☐ Irregular		☐ Alert ☐ Voice ☐ Pain ☐ Unresp.		Normal Dilated Constricted Sluggish No-Reaction	☐ Unremarkable ☐ Cool ☐ Warm ☐ Moist ☐ Dry ☐ Pale ☐ Cyanotic ☐ Flushed ☐ Jaundiced	☐ C ☐ U ☐ P ☐ S

OBJECTIVE PHYSICAL ASSESSMENT

COMMENTS

TREATMENT GIVEN: ☐ Moved to ambulance on stretcher/backboard ☐ Moved to ambulance on stair chair ☐ Walked to ambulance ☐ Airway Cleared ☐ Oral/Nasal Airway ☐ Esophageal Obturator Airway/Esophageal Gastric Tube Airway (EOA/EGTA) ☐ EndoTracheal Tube (E/T) ☐ Oxygen Administered @ ___ L.P.M., Method ___ ☐ Suction Used ☐ Artificial Ventilation Method ___ ☐ C.P.R. in progress on arrival by: ☐ Citizen ☐ PD/FD/Other First Responder ☐ Other ☐ C.P.R. Started @ Time ▶ Time from Arrest Until C.P.R. ▶ Minutes ☐ EKG Monitored (Attach Tracing) [Rhythm(s) ___] ☐ Defibrillation/Cardioversion No. Times ☐ Manual ☐ Semi-automatic

☐ Medication Administered (Use Continuation Form) ☐ IV Established Fluid ___ Cath. Gauge ☐ Mast Inflated @ Time ___ ☐ Bleeding/Hemorrhage Controlled (Method Used: ___) ☐ Spinal Immobilization Neck and Back ☐ Limb Immobilized by ☐ Fixation ☐ Traction ☐ (Heat) or (Cold) Applied ☐ Vomiting Induced @ Time ___ Method ___ ☐ Restraints Applied, Type ___ ☐ Baby Delivered @ Time ___ In County ___ ☐ Alive ☐ Stillborn ☐ Male ☐ Female ☐ Transported in Trendelenburg position ☐ Transported in left lateral recumbent position ☐ Transported with head elevated ☐ Other

DISPOSITION (See list) | DISP. CODE | CONTINUATION FORM USED YES

CREW: IN CHARGE ☐ EMT ☐ AEMT # | DRIVER'S NAME ☐ CFR ☐ EMT ☐ AEMT # | NAME ☐ CFR ☐ EMT ☐ AEMT # | NAME ☐ CFR ☐ EMT ☐ AEMT #

©COPYRIGHT 1986 NEW YORK STATE DEPARTMENT OF HEALTH

AGENCY COPY/WHITE RESEARCH COPY/YELLOW HOSPITAL PATIENT RECORD COPY/PINK

EMS 100 (11/86) provided by NYS-EMS PROGRAM DOH 3283 (6/94)

FIGURE 20-5 An example of a hybrid form PCR. (Reprinted with permission of the New York State Department of Health.)

SOAP Charting

All of the essential elements of an EMT's PCR can be summed up in the acronym SOAP. *S*ubjective, *o*bjective, *a*ssessment, and *p*lan are the components of the SOAP format.

Subjective

The *S* in SOAP stands for **subjective** information. Subjective information is the information that the patient or a family member or bystander tells the EMT (Figure 20-6). It is information that the patient senses or feels. If the patient is describing how he feels, then the information is called a *symptom* and is considered subjective information.

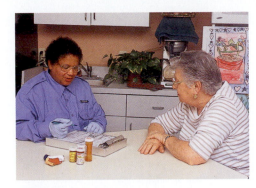

FIGURE 20-6 The patient's history of present illness is subjective.

Objective

Objective information, the *O* in SOAP, is knowledge that the EMT obtains through her own senses. For example, the EMT would feel the patient's pulse. The rate of that pulse is called a *sign* and is considered objective information (Figure 20-7). Heart rates, respiratory rates, and blood pressure are called the vital signs.

Assessment

Using both subjective and objective information, the EMT derives an assessment, the *A* in SOAP, of the patient's problem. For example, for a patient whose subjective chief complaint is "I can't breathe" and whose respiratory rate is 30 times a minute, an EMT would make the assessment that the patient is short of breath.

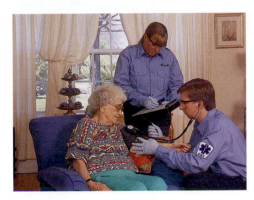

FIGURE 20-7 The EMT's physical examination is objective.

Plan

The EMT would apply oxygen to the patient who is assessed as being short of breath. This is part of the plan (the *P* in SOAP) of treatment for the patient.

Many EMS systems find the SOAP method of charting satisfactory. Others have felt that additional elements of the record, particular to EMS needs, should be included in the charting method for EMTs.

SOAPIE (subjective, objective, assessment, plan, intervention, evaluation), CHART (chief complaint, history, assessment, Rx-treatment, transport), and CHEATED (chief complaint, history, examination, assessment, treatment, evaluation, disposition) represent three examples of expanded charting methods. All of these methods, and many others, still include the fundamental elements contained within SOAP as their basis. It is suggested that the EMT find a method of charting that is complete and that she is comfortable with. Using the same method of charting every time is the best way to develop complete documentation.

CHEATED Charting Method

One of the more EMS-specific charting methods utilizes the acronym **CHEATED**. Table 20-1 lists the components of this charting method. Starting with the initial contact with the patient, the CHEATED method continues with documenting care to the emergency department.

TABLE 20-1

CHEATED

C = Chief complaint

H = History

E = Examination

A = Assessment

T = Treatment

E = Evaluation

D = Disposition

Chief Complaint

The *C* in CHEATED refers to the patient's chief complaint. As far as is practical, the patient's chief complaint should be written in the patient's own words. If the patient is unconscious, then the statement of a family member or bystander should be used.

History

The *H* in CHEATED refers to history. The first history is the history of the present illness (HPI). Some EMTs refer to this as the nature of the illness (NOI). In the case of trauma, the mechanism of injury (MOI) is described.

The patient's past medical history (PMH) also needs to be included. The use of the acronym SAMPLE ensures that the EMT will get the minimum history needed.

Examination

The *E* in CHEATED refers to the examination of the patient—the physical examination. Starting with the initial assessment, the EMT would continue by documenting the detailed or focused physical examination, as the case may be.

Assessment

Then the EMT is asked to make an assessment (the *A* in CHEATED) of the patient's situation. This assessment is the basis for the patient's treatment. The assessment is one of the titles under the EMT's protocols.

Treatment

The EMT would then proceed to document the treatment (the *T* in CHEATED) given to the patient. Typically at this point the patient is either en route to the hospital or being packaged for transportation. Part of the continuum of care an EMT provides is frequent reassessment of the patient.

Evaluation

Both patient improvement and deterioration are noted in the evaluation (the *E* in CHEATED) portion of the patient care report. The patient's response to prehospital treatments helps guide the physician's decision regarding which hospital treatments to proceed with.

Disposition

Patient care is transferred to another health care professional upon arrival at the emergency department. The disposition of the patient (the *D* in CHEATED) is a matter of both medical and legal concern. Patients may be transferred only to another health care provider capable of continuing patient care.

The patient's condition as well as treatments in progress should also be documented. If family members are present, their presence should also be noted. Any personal property of the patient that is given to emergency department staff, for example, canes and dentures, should be documented.

PRINCIPLES OF DOCUMENTATION

Documenting care may seem complicated, but remembering a few general principles can make the EMT's job easier. To begin, the PCR is no place for personal opinions or bias. Record all observations objectively. It is important to document what the patient says, but document only those statements that help bring the patient's condition to light for the physician.

Document all the care that was provided. In legal circles there is a saying, "If it wasn't written, it didn't happen." A failure to document care gives an opportunity for a lawyer to convince a jury that proper care may not have been given or was given poorly.

Submit all PCRs in a timely fashion. Most EMTs complete their PCRs in the emergency department, at the point of transference of care. In those rare cases in which a PCR is not completed before the EMT leaves the emergency department, a copy should be faxed, via a secure line, as soon as possible (Figure 20-8). Always follow a faxed copy of a PCR with a hard copy for the medical record.

Documentation Standards

When it comes to shortening paperwork by using abbreviations, EMTs are some of the most imaginative people alive. However, it must be remembered that the primary purpose of documentation is to communicate the patient's condition to other health care providers, so they must be able to read and understand the patient's record.

Standardized Abbreviations and Symbols

For example, the abbreviation Dx may mean discharge to an EMT but could mean diagnosis to a doctor or even defendant to a lawyer. It is important for the EMT to use accurate abbreviations if she is to use them at all.

To decrease documentation time many medical professionals use abbreviations. Unfortunately, while abbreviations decrease documentation time they occasionally increase confusion. To decrease confusion many hospitals and EMS agencies have adopted standardized abbreviations and symbols. These commonly accepted abbreviations ensure that the message is understood.

Street Smart

Modern electronics has made it easier for EMTs to document care accurately as well as quickly. Instead of using one standardized form for all circumstances, the EMT can choose from multiple standard computerized templates, each designed for a typical situation.

This template, combined with a standard minimum data set, helps ensure accurate documentation. Then, when the EMT arrives at either the emergency department or the station, she can download or transfer the information to another computer.

This use of electronic documentation speeds the transmission and retrieval of patient information while eliminating waste. Other advances in electronics will improve both the speed and the accuracy of EMT documentation.

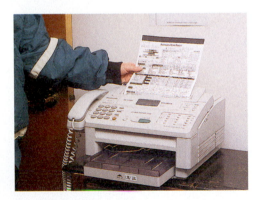

FIGURE 20-8 Always promptly submit or fax a PCR to the emergency department.

Street Smart

To return ambulances to service more quickly, some EMS agencies have obtained the services of a transcription service. Often this service is the same as the one used by the emergency physicians. Transcription services transcribe the EMT's verbal dictation into a typewritten record. This is one way to ensure that the PCR is legible.

The EMT transmits the report via cell phone to a central transcript service, which in turn types and then transmits the PCR to the emergency department, often within 20 or 30 minutes.

The use of some common abbreviations is still unacceptable. For example, medication errors have resulted from mistaking $MgSO_4$ (magnesium sulfate) for morphine sulfate. For this reason it is more appropriate to spell out the words rather than use abbreviations. Whenever an EMT uses an abbreviation or symbol she should refer to the list of accepted standardized abbreviations used in her region or service district. When in doubt about an abbreviation the EMT should spell the word out.

Errors and Corrections

In the course of documenting patient care, errors will occur. Sometimes they are spelling errors or errors in order. Regardless, the EMT should make one single cross-out over the error and then initial the cross-out.

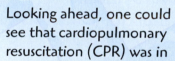

Low Battery

"Man down, CPR in progress." The feet hit the floor before the tones had finished. Down South Pearl to Main and up two blocks. Total response time was 4 minutes.

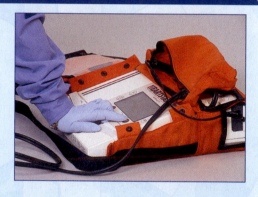

Looking ahead, one could see that cardiopulmonary resuscitation (CPR) was in progress. A middle-aged male was lying on the ground, obviously unconscious. After apnea and pulselessness had been confirmed, the automated external defibrillator (AED) pads were applied and the "analyze" pressed.

The AED warning light came on reading "low battery." Miguel's heart sank. He was sure he had checked the AED at the start of the tour of duty. Miguel quickly replaced the battery with a fresh spare found in the side pocket and proceeded with the defibrillation.

Glancing up quickly, Miguel saw several family members looking down with puzzled expressions on their faces. He proceeded with the shocks and CPR and loaded the patient for the trip to the hospital.

- Should the low battery be reported? To whom?
- Should it be reported on the PCR?
- What information should be included in a report?
- Is this information "discoverable" in a court of law?

Use of white correction fluid or vigorous blackout only creates a question in the mind of the reader, including attorneys, as to what was originally written. Leave no room for guessing on the part of others. A clean, simple cross-out shows that there is nothing to hide (Figure 20-9).

After the PCR is completely written, always initial the last sentence. This indicates that this was the last point of documentation. It is assumed that the date on the PCR is the date the PCR was written. However, some EMS agencies require the EMT to write her initials, date, and time at the end of the document as well (Figure 20-10).

Sometimes after a PCR has been completed, the EMT wishes to add to the record. The EMT can reopen the documentation either by adding to the existing record and then adding initials, time, and date to the last entry or, preferably, by adding to the record another sheet that reflects the new date and time (Figure 20-11).

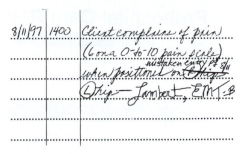

FIGURE 20-9 Cross out errors with one single line, then initial.

Legibility

Illegible documentation helps no one. It is important for the EMT to write clearly. Use block printing if necessary to make the PCR readable.

Most EMS agencies still prefer that PCRs be written in black ink. In the past, old records would be placed on microfilm for storage. Blue ink does not show up well on microfilm. However, today PCRs are photocopied for many reasons. Again, blue ink does not show up on a photocopy as clearly as black ink.

SPECIAL INCIDENT REPORTS

Equipment failure and personal injuries to the crew occasionally occur, but do these incidents belong on the PCR? No, these extraordinary situations should be documented in a **special incident report**. A special incident report is a form that has been designated for

Current Medications (List)	S I G N S				Labored	Irregular	/	Unresp.		No-Reaction		Dry	Jaundiced		S
				Rate:	Rate:		Alert		Normal		Cool	Unremarkable			C
				Regular			Voice		Dilated		Warm	Pale			U
				Shallow	Regular		Pain		Constricted		Moist	Cyanotic			P
				Labored	Irregular	/	Unresp.		Sluggish		Dry	Flushed			S
									No-Reaction			Jaundiced			

OBJECTIVE PHYSICAL ASSESSMENT 40 year old male, awake, alert and oriented to person, place and time. Patient sustained isolated injury to outstretched hand during fall, approximately one inch laceration found on right palm, bleeding controlled spontaneously, no other injury noted. Wound dressed with dry sterile dressing.

COMMENTS Patient refuses transportation to the hospital at this time. Patient advised to seek further medical attention. Patient further advised that failure to seek medical attention could result in infection in his hand, loss of movement in his fingers, and possibly even loss of limb. Patient verbalizes that he understands the warning and still refuses transportation. Patient advised that he may call EMS again, if he changes mind,

TREATMENT GIVEN the wound starts to bleed, or for other symptoms related to the fall. Patient signed refusal on reverse, witnessed by security officer Barnes.
-RB, 8/28/00, 11:30 AM

- ☐ Moved to ambulance on stretcher/backboard
- ☐ Moved to ambulance on stair chair
- ☐ Walked to ambulance
- ☐ Airway Cleared
- ☐ Oral/Nasal Airway

- ☐ Medication Administered (Use Continuation Form)
- ☐ IV Established Fluid _____ Cath. Gauge
- ☐ Mast Inflated @ Time _____
- ☐ Bleeding/Hemorrhage Controlled (Method Used: _____)
- ☐ Spinal Immobilization Neck and Back

FIGURE 20-10 Complete the PCR with your initials, time, and date.

Prehospital Care Report

Page____ of ____

CONTINUATION FORM

USE BALL POINT PEN ONLY

PRESS DOWN FIRMLY: PRINT NEATLY

DATE M D Y	AGENCY NAME	Enter PCR ID# Top Center of PCR	—

PATIENTS NAME	RECEIVING HOSPITAL	RECEIVING HOSP ID	MEDICAL CONTROL ID	Pt's Approx Weight in kgs

TIME	RESP	BREATH SOUNDS	PULSE	EKG	B.P.	G.C.S.	MEDICATIONS	DOSE	ROUTE
	RATE: ☐ REGULAR ☐ SHALLOW ☐ LABORED	R ☐ NORMAL ☐ L; ☐ DECREASED ☐; ☐ ABSENT ☐; ☐ RALES ☐; ☐ RONCHI ☐; ☐ WHEEZES ☐	RATE: ☐ REGULAR ☐ IRREGULAR	☐ DEFIB @ ____ J	/	EO V M Tot	☐ Adenosine ☐ Diazepam ☐ Lidocaine ☐ Albuterol ☐ Epinephrine ☐ Morphine ☐ Atropine ☐ Furosemide ☐ Nitroglyc. ☐ Dextrose ☐ Other________		
	RATE: ☐ REGULAR ☐ SHALLOW ☐ LABORED	R ☐ NORMAL ☐ L; ☐ DECREASED ☐; ☐ ABSENT ☐; ☐ RALES ☐; ☐ RONCHI ☐; ☐ WHEEZES ☐	RATE: ☐ REGULAR ☐ IRREGULAR	☐ DEFIB @ ____ J	/	EO V M Tot	☐ Adenosine ☐ Diazepam ☐ Lidocaine ☐ Albuterol ☐ Epinephrine ☐ Morphine ☐ Atropine ☐ Furosemide ☐ Nitroglyc. ☐ Dextrose ☐ Other________		
	RATE: ☐ REGULAR ☐ SHALLOW ☐ LABORED	R ☐ NORMAL ☐ L; ☐ DECREASED ☐; ☐ ABSENT ☐; ☐ RALES ☐; ☐ RONCHI ☐; ☐ WHEEZES ☐	RATE: ☐ REGULAR ☐ IRREGULAR	☐ DEFIB @ ____ J	/	EO V M Tot	☐ Adenosine ☐ Diazepam ☐ Lidocaine ☐ Albuterol ☐ Epinephrine ☐ Morphine ☐ Atropine ☐ Furosemide ☐ Nitroglyc. ☐ Dextrose ☐ Other________		

NARRATIVE:

MEDICAL CONTROL RECORD	MEDICAL CONTROL FACILITY	ON-LINE MED CTRL PHYSICIAN: PRINT NAME	MD ID#	SIGNATURE (OPTIONAL)

Controlled Substance Destroyed	DRUG	QTY	DATE	DRUG DESTROYED WITNESS: PRINT NAME	SIGNATURE	LICENSE #

INDIVIDUAL ADMINISTERING MEDICATION and/or IN CHARGE - PLEASE PRINT -	SIGNATURE	EMT/AEMT CERT NUMBER

DOH-3411 (2/96)

COPYRIGHT 1995 NEW YORK STATE DEPARTMENT OF HEALTH

EMS 100A

AGENCY COPY

FIGURE 20-11 A continuation sheet can be added at a later date. (Reprinted with permission of the New York State Department of Health.)

documentation of specific incidents such as crew injuries or equipment problems (Figure 20-12).

Most EMS agencies have guidelines for when a critical or special incident report should be generated. Some general guidelines are listed here. The EMT should be aware of the reporting guidelines in her agency.

INCIDENT REPORT

CASE NUMBER	DUTY STATION	FDS NUMBER

ADDRESS

CITY	STATE	ZIP CODE

DATE OF REPORT	DATE OF INCIDENT

TYPE OF INCIDENT
Initial ☐   Follow-up ☐
YES   NO
1. Employee Injury ☐ ☐
2. Patient Injury ☐ ☐
3. Visitor Injury ☐ ☐
4. Medical Device Injury ☐ ☐
5. Property Damage ☐ ☐
6. Hazardous Condition ☐ ☐

SEVERITY
☐ 1. Fatal
☐ 2. Hospitalized
☐ 3. Ambulatory
☐ 4. No Treatment

LOST TIME (days) _____

DISABILITY
☐ 1. Temporary
☐ 2. Partial Permanent
☐ 3. Full Permanent
☐ 4. None

SERIOUS INCIDENT TYPE
(Check one)
☐ 1. Fatal
☐ 2. More than 3 injured
☐ 3. Property damaged $25,000.
☐ 4. Aircraft
☐ 5. Radiation Release
☐ 6. Biological Release

EXAMINED BY PRIMARY CARE PROVIDER ☐ YES ☐ NO	MEDICAL EXPENSE INCURRED: ☐ YES ☐ NO	ESTIMATED COST: $ _____

INVESTIGATION CONDUCTED BY:	PHONE NUMBER ( )

INDIVIDUAL INVOLVED

NAME	TORT POSSIBLE ☐ YES ☐ NO

SOCIAL SECURITY NUMBER	DATE OF BIRTH	SEX ☐ MALE ☐ FEMALE

ADDRESS

CITY	STATE	ZIP CODE

PHONE NUMBER ( )	TIME OF INCIDENT

EMPLOYEE

JOB TITLE	OWCP FORM FILED ☐ YES ☐ NO

PERSONNEL STATUS - CO, GS, WG, TRIBAL, VOLUNTEER, OTHER	GRADE LEVEL / STEP

NUMBER OF DEPENDENTS (Spouse and Children under 18)	SUPERVISOR'S NAME

WORK PHONE NUMBER ( )	SHIFT ONE, TWO, OR THREE ☐ 1 ☐ 2 ☐ 3	TIME ON DUTY BEFORE INCIDENT

PATIENT

DATE OF ADMISSION	DEPARTMENT	DEPARTMENT PHONE NUMBER ( )	CHART NUMBER

DIAGNOSIS ON ADMISSION	MEDICAL DEVICE RELATED ☐ YES ☐ NO

CONDITION BEFORE INCIDENT

MEDICATIONS ADMINISTERED ☐ YES ☐ NO	TYPE OF MEDICATION

COMMENTS

VISITOR

PURPOSE OF VISIT

FIGURE 20-12   A special incident report. (continues)

INCIDENT REPORT

PROPERTY

OWNER

PRIVATE PROPERTY
☐ YES ☐ NO

ADDRESS

CITY

STATE

ZIP CODE

PROPERTY MANAGEMENT NOTIFIED
☐ YES ☐ NO

DATE

NATURE AND EXTENT OF DAMAGE

ESTIMATED REPAIR / REPLACEMENT
$ _____

GOVERNMENT VEHICLE INVOLVED
☐ YES ☐ NO

REGISTRATION / TAG NUMBER

NARRATIVE

Give a factual description of incident, location, and other important specifics (i.e. body part(s), other individual involved, etc.)

FACILITY NAME: _____   DEPARTMENT: _____

DESCRIPTION:

DIAGRAM OF INCIDENT

CODING SECTION

INCIDENT LOCATION CODE:

DESCRIPTION:

OSHA TYPE CODE:

IHS TYPE CODE:

OHSA SOURCE CODE:

ICD NATURE CODE:

OCCUPATION CODE:
___ ___ ___ ___ ___ ___ ___

ICD EXTERNAL CAUSE CODE:

OWCP AGENCY CODE:

SIGNATURE AND TITLE OF REPORTING EMPLOYEE

DATE

PHONE
( )

SIGNATURE AND TITLE OF REVIEWING OFFICIAL

DATE

PHONE
( )

SIGNATURE AND TITLE OF CODING OFFICIAL

DATE

PHONE
( )

The information collected on this form is to be utilized in compliance with the Privacy Act of 1974.

FIGURE 20-12   (continued)

Injury to the EMT

If an EMT is injured while on duty, then that injury needs to be reported immediately to her supervisor. In these cases, the special incident report is very important. The special incident report may serve as the basis for a claim under the workers' compensation system or disability insurance.

Infectious Disease Exposure

Whenever an EMT may have had a potential infectious disease exposure, a special incident report should be completed and returned to the designated infection control officer. The federal Occupational Safety and Health Administration (OSHA) has established very strict guidelines regarding the reporting and management of potential infectious disease exposure. Always follow local protocols for reporting potential infectious disease exposure.

Equipment Failure

Any time equipment fails to operate properly while on an EMS call, the failure should be reported. One reason is to ensure that the piece of equipment is removed from service until it has been properly repaired. Faulty equipment presents a hazard to other patients and EMTs.

All reports of equipment failure should be directed to the attention of a supervisor. In some instances, these reports will be entered as evidence in a court trial. The supervisor should review the report for accuracy.

In the eyes of a jury, it is more acceptable to have had a piece of equipment fail and be repaired than to have had the failure be known but ignored. Table 20-2 lists several common conditions or problems that should be reported to an EMT's supervisor or chief officer.

TABLE 20-2

Problems That Should Be Reported

Confrontations on the scene with the family or public

Confrontations with police or firefighters

Confrontations with hospital personnel

Perceived malpractice by another EMT

Equipment failure

Infectious disease or other hazardous exposure

Lost patient property, such as dentures or glasses

Collision involving an emergency response vehicle

Crime Scene

"Unit 15, man shot, police on scene, proceed to the corner of Moyers and Onondaga and stand by." Proceeding with no lights or siren to the staging area, Mark, the EMT, is approached by Officer Stevens, who advises him that the scene is safe and he may proceed in to care for the patient.

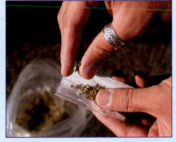
(Courtesy of PhotoDisc.)

Mark introduces himself to the patient, Marvin, and starts to treat the patient, who is lying on the couch. Rolling Marvin over, Mark uncovers a bag of what appears to be marijuana. Officer Stevens, who is standing nearby, reaches over and picks up the bag.

After the call is over and the patient has been properly turned over to the emergency department, Officer Stevens calls and asks Mark to report to the police substation to make a statement.

- Is a statement required?
- Does this incident need to be reported to Mark's supervisor?
- Does Mark's agency need additional paperwork?

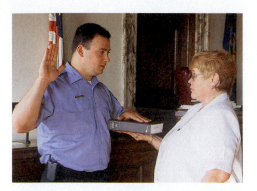

FIGURE 20-13   EMTs may be asked to testify in court about criminal activity.

THE EMT AS A GOOD CITIZEN

An EMT is a good citizen as well as a patient care provider. There are times when an EMT comes across what appears to be criminal activity. In all cases, patient care is the EMT's first responsibility. When the call is completed, then the EMT may have other responsibilities.

In some states, EMTs are required to report suspected child abuse. It is important that an EMT comply with the law in those cases because failure to report them may result in civil or criminal liability.

In all states, it is within the scope of an EMT's practice to report suspected child abuse to a licensed physician or a registered nurse. As **mandated reporters**, physicians and nurses must then investigate the complaint further. In some instances, the involvement of the physician or nurse may relieve the EMT of further responsibility.

Elder abuse has become an increasingly common occurrence. As in child abuse, an EMT's responsibility to report suspected elder abuse is a function of state and local laws.

Every EMS agency should have a procedure in writing to deal with these all-too-common events. In all cases, the advice of a competent lawyer should be sought.

An EMT may be called upon to offer her written testimony, called an **affidavit**, regarding what she saw or heard when on an EMS call. Or she may be called upon to testify in court (Figure 20-13). Frequently, this request is made days, weeks, or even months after the call has occurred.

Multicar Pileup

On a foggy Tuesday morning, the police report that 27 cars and two trucks are involved in a chain reaction motor vehicle collision.

The 9-1-1 communications center dispatches 10 ambulances from three townships to respond to the accident. About 30 minutes later, most of the patients have either been transported or are being staged in a field hospital. EMTs are now directed to report to the field hospital to take vital signs and perform reassessments.

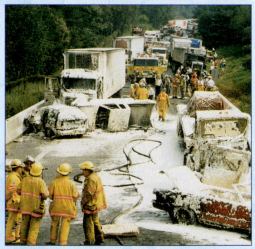

(Courtesy of Baltimore County Fire and Rescue.)

- Is a PCR needed for each patient?
- What minimum information would be required?
- Does this information become part of the patient record?

It is a good practice to write a special incident report for these types of calls. In the future, the EMT may refer to the special incident report for clarification of forgotten details regarding the call.

MULTIPLE-CASUALTY INCIDENT

When there are several patients, from half a dozen to as many as a hundred or more, it is impractical to complete a PCR for each patient. Writing a PCR for each of these patients would slow patient care. In these cases, special documentation records called **triage tags** are used.

These triage tags, shown in Figure 20-14, provide enough space to write a patient's name and address, vital signs, and a few other pertinent facts. The number on each tag is used to track the patient. Other logs and records used by EMS command personnel will also track these patients using that identification number. More details regarding the triage tag systems as well as other logs are provided in Chapter 44.

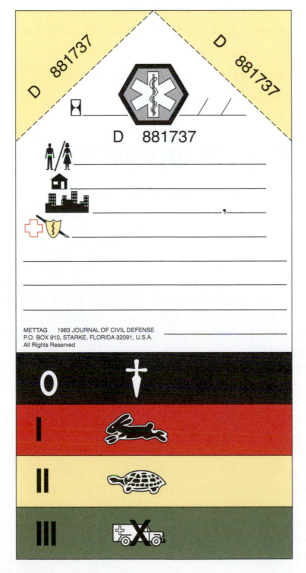

Green (bottom strip):
   Symbol: Ambulance–crossed out
   Meaning: No hospital treatment needed; first aid only
Yellow (second strip from bottom):
   Symbol: Turtle
   Meaning: Nonurgent; hospital care
Red (third strip from bottom):
   Symbol: Rabbit
   Meaning: Urgent; hospital care
Black (fourth strip from bottom):
   Symbol: Cross/dagger
   Meaning: Dead or unsalvageable; no CPR

FIGURE 20-14 Triage tags are used to document care of multiple patients. (Courtesy of American Civil Defense Association.)

Patient Refusal

"Ambulance one-five, Rescue ten, and Engine five-one, respond to the front of Albertson's for a man down, possible diabetic reaction. Time out is 15:33."

Arriving on scene, EMT Shelley sees several people huddled around a twentyish-looking male. He is drinking orange juice.

As Shelley approaches, he says, "Oh no, I'm not going to no hospital. I'm fine. My sugar is giving me a little trouble, that's all."

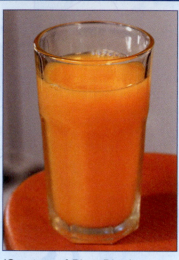

(Courtesy of PhotoDisc.)

- How is a patient refusal documented?
- What critical elements must be contained in the medical warning?
- Should anybody be notified before the patient is allowed to sign himself off?

PATIENT REFUSAL DOCUMENTATION

A patient's refusal to accept either care or transportation runs counter to an EMT's expectation of the patient. When an EMT is called to a scene, she expects the patient to be cooperative and accept the care offered. In cases in which the patient does refuse care or transportation, the EMT needs to carefully examine the patient's reason.

The details of who can reasonably refuse care and the legal ramifications surrounding such a refusal are detailed in Chapter 3. The EMT must document her decision making in this situation very carefully.

When all efforts at swaying the patient have failed, most EMS systems have a **patient refusal form** for the patient to sign (Figure 20-15). Several antecedent conditions are required before a patient refusal can be said to be valid. These are listed in Table 20-3 and must be documented carefully on the refusal form.

Because of the high litigation potential associated with refusals, many EMS systems require that an EMS supervisor be consulted before the patient refuses. In other systems, medical control has decided that contact must be made with an emergency department physician to discuss the case before the patient is permitted to refuse.

In every case, a witness should attest that the patient refused care without threat or duress. This witness should be able to testify that the patient was given a medical warning and that the patient understood this warning. Other EMTs may not be considered good witnesses.

TABLE 20-3

Conditions for Patient Refusal of Care

Patient is older than 18 or is an emancipated minor.

Patient is not obviously intoxicated by alcohol or drugs.

Patient understands potential medical condition and consequences of refusal of care.

Patient is provided with other reasonable options and is given instructions to seek further medical care.

Rensselaer County Emergency Medical Services

REFUSAL OF MEDICAL CARE, TREATMENT, AND/OR TRANSPORTATION

PCR NUMBER:_____ **DATE:**_____ **TIME:**_____

PATIENT: I understand that competent persons maintain the right to refuse medical care, treatment and/or transportation.

I,_____, hereby acknowledge that I have been advised by members of

the _____[AGENCY], that they recommend that I receive medical care, treatment

and/or transportation to a hospital emergency department for further evaluation by a physician.

I further understand that I may refuse medical care, treatment and/or transportation, but do so at my own risk.
I do not have any known physical or mental condition that would prohibit me from making an informed, competent, and intelligent decision to refuse the medical care, treatment and/or transportation that has been offered and recommended.
THE RISK ASSOCIATED WITH REFUSAL MAY INCLUDE POSSIBLE LOSS OF LIMB OR LIFE

I HAVE ALSO BEEN ADVISED THAT IF I DEVELOP ANY MEDICAL COMPLAINTS OR SYMPTOMS, I SHOULD IMMEDIATELY CONTACT AN AMBULANCE, HOSPITAL EMERGENCY DEPARTMENT, OR MY PHYSICIAN.

I hereby release _____[AGENCY], its officers, agents, personnel, and employees from any and all claims, causes of action or injuries, of whatsoever kind or nature, arising out of or in connection with my refusal of medical care, treatment and/or transportation.

Patient's Signature:_____   Date:_____

Patient's Name (print):_____   Patient's Age:_____ Patient refused signature:_____

FOR MINORS OR PERSONS WHO HAVE GUARDIANS: I am the patient's legal guardian. My relationship to the patient is _____.

I am hereby acting on behalf of the patient, _____[PATIENT'S NAME]. I have

read the above information and refuse medical care, treatment and/or transportation on behalf of the patient.

Guardian's Signature:_____   Date:_____

Guardian's Name (print):_____ Guardian's Full Address:_____

_____

WITNESS: I, _____, witnessed members of the _____

_____[AGENCY] recommend to the patient medical care, treatment, and/or transportation to a hospital emergency department for further evaluation and attention. I further witnessed the above-named patient (or patient's guardian) decline such medical care, treatment, and/or transportation.

Witness Signature:_____   Date:_____

Witness Name (print):_____ Witness' Full Address:_____

Occupation:_____   _____

EMS PROVIDER: I, _____[EMS PROVIDER], have offered and recommended to

_____[PATIENT'S NAME OR GUARDIAN'S NAME], emergency medical care and treatment, including transportation to a hospital. The patient (or patient's guardian) has refused my recommendation for medical care, treatment, and/or transportation. I have fully explained the reasons for medical care, treatment, and/or transportation to the patient (or patient's guardian). I have also explained this form to the patient (or patient's guardian) and have requested that he/she personally read it. The patient (or patient's guardian) has expressed to me an understanding of the information contained herein and did not have any questions regarding the content of this form. The patient (or patient's guardian) did not appear to me to be suffering from any illness or injury nor any condition that would affect his/her ability to refuse medical care, treatment, and/or transportation. The patient (or patient's guardian) is alert and oriented to person, place, time, and situation.

EMS Provider Signature:_____   Date:_____

Provider Certification Level / NYS ID Number: _____   Police Agency Present: NO_____YES_____

Police Officer's Name:_____ Police Agency Name:_____

FIGURE 20-15   Many EMS agencies use a separate patient refusal form. (Reprinted with permission of Rensselaer County Emergency Medical Services.)

Choose family members or noninvolved parties, such as police officers or bystanders, whenever possible.

Standardizing the documentation of a refusal of medical assistance (RMA) is important. Some agencies use a standardized form specifically designed for this type of call. If this is not available, the EMT should practice using standard statements that cover the required points. Following is an example: "This 27-yr-old patient is alert and oriented × 3 and refuses to allow further medical care or transport. He verbalizes an understanding of the potential consequences of his refusal to include loss of life or limb. He and his wife signed the RMA form. The patient has been encouraged to seek further medical attention and to call back if he changes his mind."

A written statement such as this at the end of an open-style PCR addresses the necessary questions and requirements for RMA. If a supervisor or physician was contacted regarding the situation, that contact should also be documented.

CONCLUSION

The PCR remains the EMT's primary record of care. Although the PCR may be used for administrative and legal purposes, its primary purpose is as a medical record. The EMT must be mindful that other health care professionals will want to read and understand what happened to the patient in the field. An EMT should focus on a clear and accurate representation of the patient's history and physical as well as initial treatments.

TEST YOUR KNOWLEDGE

1. Why is it important for an EMT to document care?
2. What essential elements should be included in every PCR?
3. Where does the PCR fit into the patient's medical record?
4. Name four primary functions of the PCR.
5. What is a minimum data set? Give an example.
6. What do the letters in SOAP mean?
7. What do the letters in CHEATED mean?
8. What problems are created by using nonstandardized abbreviations?
9. What are several principles of good documentation?
10. How is an error corrected on a PCR?
11. How is an addition added to the PCR?
12. Why is a special incident report written?
13. Why are PCRs not used for multiple-casualty incidents?
14. What are the critical elements of a patient refusal form?
15. Give an example of who would make a good witness of a patient's refusal.

INTERNET RESOURCES

Search the Web using these following key words:

- Patient care report
- EMS legal documents
- EMS minimum data set
- SOAP charting
- Special incident reports

Share interesting Web sites and facts with your colleagues.

FURTHER STUDY

Burstein, J. L., Hollander, J. E., Delagi, R., Gold, M., Henry, M. C., & Alicandro, J. M. (1998). Refusal of out-of-hospital medical care: Effect of medical-control physician assertiveness on transport rate. *Academic Emergency Medicine, 5*(1), 4–8.

Joyce, S. M., Dutkowski, K. L., & Hynes, T. (1997). Efficacy of an EMS quality improvement program in improving documentation and performance. *Prehospital Emergency Care, 1*(3), 140–144.

Ornato, J. P., Doctor, M. L., Harbour, L. F., Peberdy, M. A., Overton, J., Racht, E.M., et al. (1998). Synchronization of timepieces to the atomic clock in an urban emergency medical services system. *Annals of Emergency Medicine, 31*(4), 483–487.

Weaver, J., Brinsfield, K. H., & Dalphond, D. (2000). Prehospital refusal-of-transport policies: Adequate legal protection? *Prehospital Emergency Care, 4*(1), 53–56.

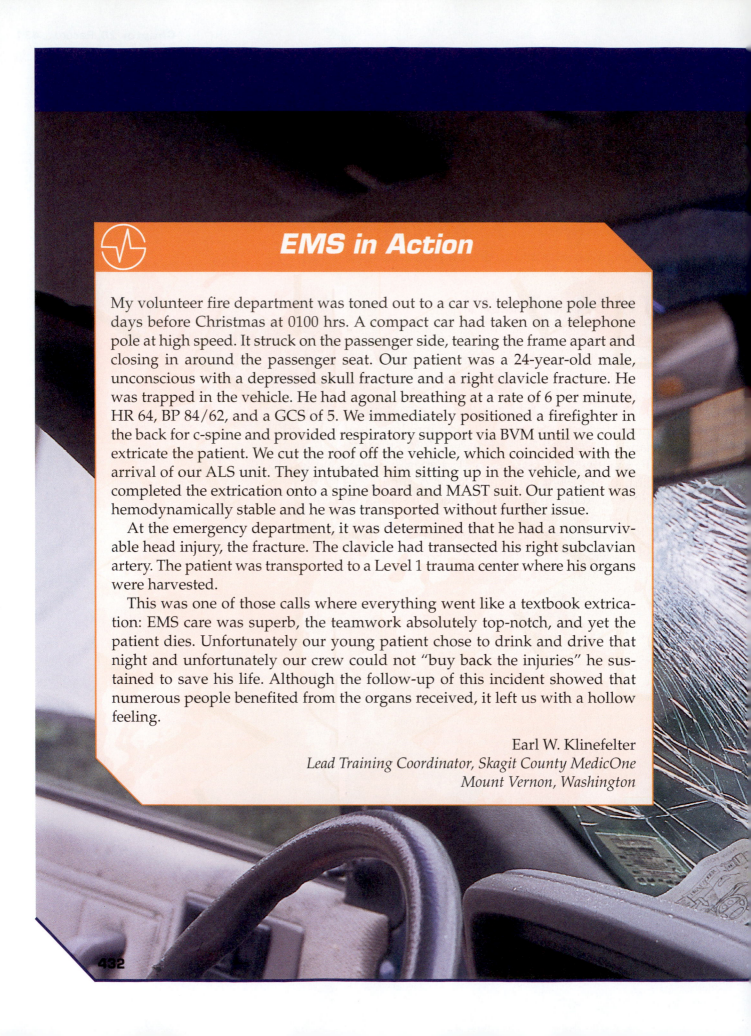

EMS in Action

My volunteer fire department was toned out to a car vs. telephone pole three days before Christmas at 0100 hrs. A compact car had taken on a telephone pole at high speed. It struck on the passenger side, tearing the frame apart and closing in around the passenger seat. Our patient was a 24-year-old male, unconscious with a depressed skull fracture and a right clavicle fracture. He was trapped in the vehicle. He had agonal breathing at a rate of 6 per minute, HR 64, BP 84/62, and a GCS of 5. We immediately positioned a firefighter in the back for c-spine and provided respiratory support via BVM until we could extricate the patient. We cut the roof off the vehicle, which coincided with the arrival of our ALS unit. They intubated him sitting up in the vehicle, and we completed the extrication onto a spine board and MAST suit. Our patient was hemodynamically stable and he was transported without further issue.

At the emergency department, it was determined that he had a nonsurvivable head injury, the fracture. The clavicle had transected his right subclavian artery. The patient was transported to a Level 1 trauma center where his organs were harvested.

This was one of those calls where everything went like a textbook extrication: EMS care was superb, the teamwork absolutely top-notch, and yet the patient dies. Unfortunately our young patient chose to drink and drive that night and unfortunately our crew could not "buy back the injuries" he sustained to save his life. Although the follow-up of this incident showed that numerous people benefited from the organs received, it left us with a hollow feeling.

Earl W. Klinefelter
Lead Training Coordinator, Skagit County MedicOne
Mount Vernon, Washington

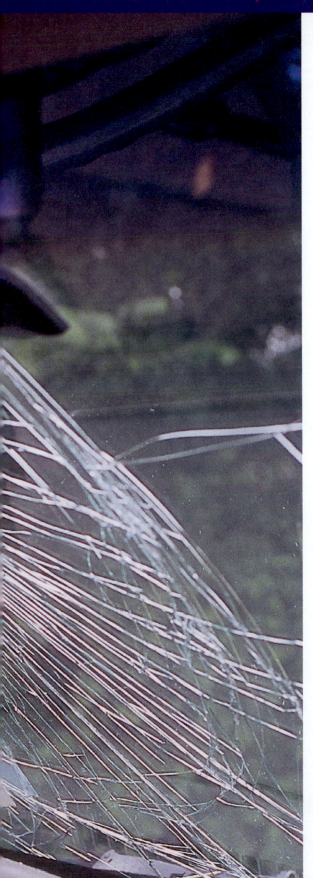

Trauma Care

EMS started in trauma care, and even today, despite the incredible growth of EMS and trauma systems, trauma remains the number one killer of young people.

The EMT must learn how to quickly recognize serious trauma by identifying the mechanism of injury, by assessing the patient for injury secondary to that mechanism, and by instituting immediate lifesaving measures on scene.

Perhaps the greatest challenge to the EMT is to be able to accomplish all these tasks in a minimum of time and initiate rapid transportation to a trauma center. In many cases, the survival of the patient is dependent on the EMT's ability to get the patient to the trauma surgeon quickly.

This section reviews the fundamentals of trauma care and the role of the EMT in the trauma care system.

CHAPTER 21

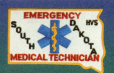

Head Injuries

KEY TERMS

basilar skull fracture

CSF otorrhea

CSF rhinorrhea

Cushing's reflex

Cushing's triad

epidural hematoma

Glasgow Coma Scale (GCS)

hematoma

intracranial pressure (ICP)

mastoid process

post-traumatic seizure

subdural hematoma

OBJECTIVES

Upon completion of this chapter, the reader should be able to:

1. Discuss the relevance of head injuries to trauma deaths.
2. Describe the anatomy of the scalp, skull, and brain.
3. Identify injuries that are commonly associated with head injuries.
4. Discuss the physical findings associated with a scalp injury, a skull injury, and a brain injury.
5. Describe the management priorities of the patient with a scalp injury, a skull injury, and a brain injury.
6. Describe the Glasgow Coma Scale.
7. Discuss the consequences of increased intracranial pressure.
8. Identify the physical findings associated with increased intracranial pressure.
9. Describe the appropriate treatment modalities used by the EMT that can help to decrease intracranial pressure.

OVERVIEW

Approximately half of the trauma-related deaths in the United States are due to head injuries. The mortality rate after a severe head injury is approximately 35%. More than half of those who do survive are left with serious disability as a result of injury to the brain.

Recognition of the signs and symptoms of a serious head injury is a necessary skill for an emergency medical technician (EMT). Appropriate prehospital treatment of these patients is necessary in order to minimize further injury to the brain. It is crucial that the EMT be familiar with the concepts of managing the patient with a head injury.

ANATOMY REVIEW

To understand the presentation of head injuries and the concepts behind their management, the EMT must first have an understanding of the anatomy of the head and surrounding structures. Chapter 5

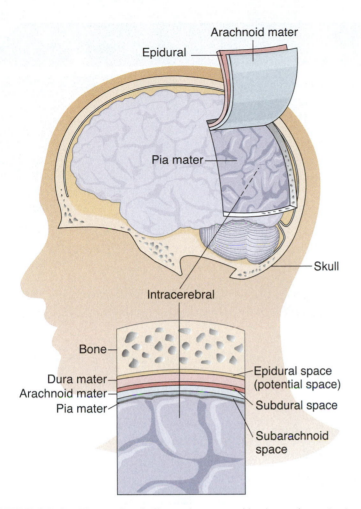

FIGURE 21-1　The scalp, skull, meninges, and brain are important anatomic structures with which the EMT must be familiar.

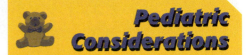

Pediatric Considerations

Children have fusion points in their skulls that do not close until around age 2. These soft spots, or fontanels, leave the underlying brain vulnerable to injury.

When examining a child, the EMT can note the presence of these soft spots on the top and back of the skull. The EMT should note the shape of the scalp over the fontanel.

A bulging fontanel can mean elevated pressures within the skull, whereas a sunken fontanel can mean dehydration. Examination of the fontanels can be a useful tool in the pediatric physical exam.

should be reviewed at this time, with special attention paid to discussions of scalp, skull, meninges, and brain. Figure 21-1 illustrates this anatomy for review.

TYPES OF INJURIES

Trauma to the head can result in many different types of injuries. Some types of head injuries may be instantly fatal; others are not at all life threatening. It is not crucial for the EMT to identify the exact injury that exists, although understanding the mechanisms for these injuries will help in the assessment and management of the head-injured patient.

Scalp

Because of the large number of blood vessels present in the scalp, any injury will result in bleeding. If the injury is from a blunt object, such as a baseball bat, there may be no tear in the skin. If sufficient force was applied, vessels may break and cause bleeding under the skin. This resulting collection of blood underneath the skin is known as a **hematoma**. A scalp hematoma can become very large if not treated quickly. Figure 21-2 shows a patient with a scalp hematoma.

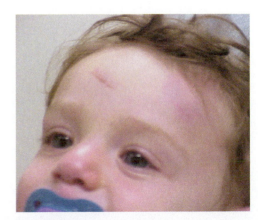

FIGURE 21-2　A collection of blood between the skull and the scalp is called a scalp hematoma. (Courtesy of Deborah Funk, MD, Albany Medical Center, Albany, NY.)

Bar Fight

"The scene is safe," declared Sergeant McNally over the command frequency. "Have EMS enter. We have a man with a head injury." The call had originally been dispatched as a "fight in progress," and EMS had been ordered to stage around the block.

With all emergency lights shut down, the ambulance approached the scene, and the EMTs saw the perpetrator sitting in the backseat of a police cruiser. They entered through the front door.

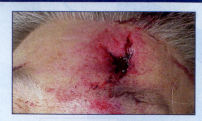

(Courtesy of Ron Straum, MD, Albany Medical Center, Albany, NY.)

Immediately to the right of the door were a broken beer bottle and lots of blood, and immediately to the left stood the source of the blood, a twentyish male with a mean-looking cut over his left eye. His hair may have been blond before, but it was red with blood now.

EMT Johnson immediately took spine stabilization, with gloves on, while EMT Murawski started his assessment. In the meantime, the patient began to complain loudly about the splitting headache he had and loudly declared, "I want something for my pain."

The patient was unsure whether he had been knocked out, and he was also unsure whether the attacker had used any weapons, like a club or a bottle, or just his fists.

- What are the assessment priorities for this patient?
- What is the significance of the patient's symptoms?
- What are the treatment priorities for the patient?
- What signs or symptoms will the patient display if he decompensates?

If the mechanism of injury involved a sharp edge or sufficient force from a blunt object to break the skin, then the bleeding will be outward. Scalp lacerations often bleed extensively. It is not uncommon for blood loss from an isolated scalp wound to result in hypovolemic shock if the patient is not appropriately treated.

Skull

Significant blunt or penetrating trauma to the skull can result in a break in this bony protective covering. Such a break will leave the brain exposed to injury.

There are many specific types of skull injuries, or fractures. Differentiating among them is unimportant to the EMT, with two exceptions. Recognition of these types of skull fractures may affect the care provided by the EMT.

Basilar Skull Fracture

Blunt trauma to the skull may result in a fracture in any area. When a fracture is at the base of the skull, the area posterior to the face, there may be characteristic physical findings. This type of fracture is called a **basilar skull fracture** and will have implications for emergency care of the patient. Figure 21-3 illustrates this fracture.

Bleeding associated with this type of fracture will spread from the fracture site and settle into a few characteristic places. Bruising behind

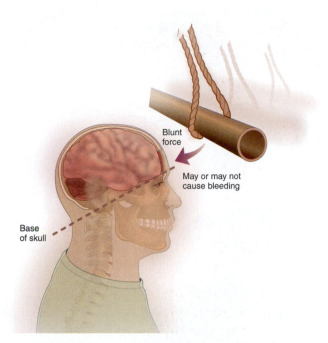

FIGURE 21-3 A basilar skull fracture may have implications for airway management techniques because it is so close to airway structures.

the ears over the bony prominence called the **mastoid process** is known as Battle's sign and can develop within a few hours of a basilar skull fracture. Another characteristic physical finding with this type of injury is bruising around both eyes, commonly called raccoon's eyes (Figure 21-4). Although characteristic for basilar skull fracture, these useful physical findings often will not be present until several hours after the injury.

Injury to the base of the skull may disrupt delicate structures within the ear. If it does, cerebrospinal fluid (CSF) may leak out through the fracture into the ear. The EMT will see a clear or blood-tinged liquid draining from the patient's ear. This condition is called **CSF otorrhea**.

Similarly, if the fracture is at the base of the skull close to the posterior of the nose, CSF may be seen leaking from the nose. This condition, called **CSF rhinorrhea**, is identified as a clear or thin bloody liquid coming from an otherwise uninjured nose.

The EMT should never attempt to halt the flow of any fluid that may be CSF coming from the ear or nose. A sterile dressing may be used to collect the fluids as they leak out.

Open Skull Fracture

An open skull fracture is an obvious opening in the skull, sometimes exposing underlying brain. If an open skull fracture exists, the EMT should take care not to touch the underlying brain tissue. The opening should be carefully covered with a dry sterile dressing. Care should be taken not to apply pressure onto the brain itself while attempting to control bleeding from the scalp.

Although open skull injuries are frightening to view, they are not necessarily correlated with a poor prognosis. The amount of underlying brain injury is the determinant of the final outcome. Figure 21-5 shows an illustration of an open skull fracture.

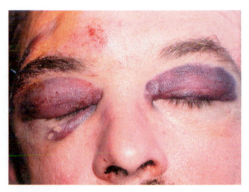

FIGURE 21-4 Raccoon's eyes. (Courtesy of Wayne Triner, DO, Albany Medical Center, Albany, NY.)

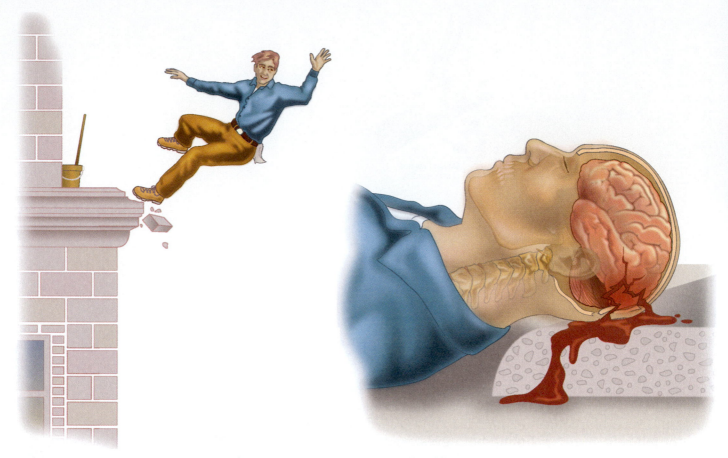

FIGURE 21-5   Open skull fractures leave the brain susceptible to direct injury. Injuries such as this may also contribute to spinal injury.

Penetrating Injury

If an open skull fracture is associated with a penetrating injury, such as a knife or gunshot wound, it should be understood that underlying damage is variable. The extent of intracranial damage is often difficult to determine by looking at the outside of the skull.

Seemingly minor exterior wounds from a gunshot may result in severe intracranial injury. On the other hand, extensive scalp wounds associated with a penetrating injury may not result in serious brain injury.

The EMT should stabilize any remaining foreign body and treat the patient according to the guidelines that will be outlined later in this chapter.

Brain

The most significant component of a head injury is the injury the brain sustains. An EMT will have no way to tell what type of brain injury exists; however, there are several classic presentations of different types of injuries. It is helpful for the EMT to recognize these injury patterns.

Open

Open skull injuries will usually result in direct trauma to the brain, as there no longer is a protective covering. The EMT should take care to protect the exposed brain from further injury.

Closed

Closed head injuries are less impressive to see, but they are much more common and often much more severe. Remember, the skull is rigid, and any swelling or bleeding within its bony confines has no room to expand. The result is pressure upon the adjacent brain tissue. Brain tissue does not respond well to compression.

Compression of blood vessels supplying a section of brain with blood will result in hypoperfusion of the tissue. Brain tissue can survive only a few minutes without oxygenated blood before it is irreversibly damaged.

The EMT must recognize early signs of closed head injury so the patient is treated aggressively in an attempt to prevent irreversible brain damage.

Subdural Hematoma

One of the more common causes of severe brain injury is a collection of blood between the brain and the dura mater. This type of blood collection is known as a **subdural hematoma**.

A subdural hematoma is caused by tearing of multiple small veins that run between the brain's surface and the dura mater. This is often the result of blunt head trauma. Figure 21-6 illustrates this type of injury.

A subdural hematoma can expand, compressing the adjacent brain tissue significantly. When important brain structures are compressed, the brain will malfunction and eventually cause the death of the patient. It is the responsibility of the EMT to recognize the early signs of this brain compression and to treat the patient aggressively to attempt to reduce the likelihood of complications.

Unfortunately, despite aggressive treatment, subdural hematomas often cause severe brain injury and death.

Epidural Hematoma

Another commonly seen intracranial hematoma is the **epidural hematoma**. This collection of blood is found outside the dura mater, just under the skull. The epidural hematoma is most often the result of a skull fracture with an arterial injury. The blood collection in this case is arterial in nature and typically accumulates very quickly. Figure 21-7 illustrates this type of injury.

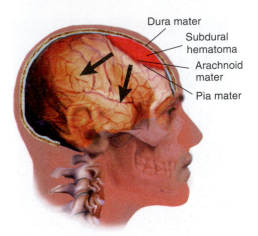

FIGURE 21-6 A subdural hematoma is usually the result of the tearing of small veins under the dura mater.

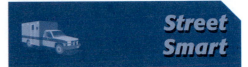

Street Smart

Because a subdural hematoma is the result of venous bleeding, it can sometimes take time to develop. Depending on the size and number of veins that have torn, it may be hours to days before the expanding hematoma causes significant symptoms. The EMT should take a careful history and inquire about any possible head injury over the previous several days and weeks.

Geriatric Considerations

Over the years, the brain of an older adult will shrink, or *atrophy*, leaving extra space between the dura mater and the brain itself. Because the extra space allows these tiny veins to stretch, they can more easily tear. Elderly people are therefore at increased risk of developing a subdural hematoma, even after seemingly minor head trauma.

Chronic alcoholics may suffer premature brain atrophy and are at similar risk, even at a young age.

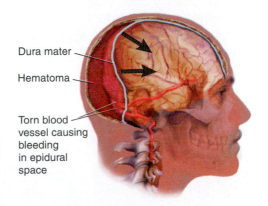

FIGURE 21-7 An epidural hematoma is often associated with a skull fracture and an arterial injury.

TABLE 21-1

Physical Findings Associated with a Rise in Intracranial Pressure

Decrease in mental status

Persistent vomiting

Glasgow Coma Score <8

Unequal pupils

Seizure activity

Hypertension

Bradycardia

Altered respiratory pattern

Street Smart

Definitive treatment for a patient with increased intracranial pressure due to an expanding hematoma often involves surgical decompression. In this situation, seconds count. Every moment the brain is under increased pressure more brain cells are being destroyed.

The EMT must recognize the problem, effectively treat the patient, and provide expedient transport to the most appropriate hospital.

Street Smart

It is important for the EMT to realize that although trauma to the head is a common cause of brain injury, it is also possible to suffer intracranial bleeding without trauma. There are many different non-trauma-related brain injuries. Because the end result within the brain may be similar, the patient presentation may also be similar to that of the head-injured patient. An example of a nontraumatic source of intracranial hemorrhage is a hemorrhagic stroke. This condition is discussed in Chapter 31.

Management priorities of the patient with nontrauma-related brain injury are the same as learned in this chapter. The only exception is, of course, there is no need for cervical spinal immobilization unless trauma to the cervical spine cannot be ruled out.

Despite the accompanying skull fracture and arterial nature of the bleeding, an epidural hematoma alone does not often result in extensive underlying brain injury. Rapid identification of a significant head injury and appropriate treatment by the EMT can contribute to a good outcome.

Intracranial Pressure

Because the skull is a rigid container that does not expand, any increase in volume within it will result in an increase in pressure. The pressure inside the skull is called **intracranial pressure (ICP)**. Elevated pressure within the skull results in compression of brain tissue and subsequent neurologic damage.

The brain has several complex compensatory mechanisms that can help prevent neurologic injury for a limited time. In the case of an expanding intracranial hematoma, the brain cannot compensate for long.

When the brain is no longer able to compensate for the extra volume of blood it has to share intracranial space with, the pressure inside the skull increases. This is referred to as a rise in intracranial pressure.

This rise in intracranial pressure damages brain cells and is evidenced by deterioration in the patient's neurologic status. Physical findings associated with such a rise in ICP are listed in Table 21-1. It is important to remember that not all symptoms may be present with an increase in intracranial pressure.

It is crucial that the EMT recognize these signs and take appropriate measures to attempt to lower the ICP. These measures are detailed later in the chapter.

ASSOCIATED INJURIES

When considering the mechanism behind the head injury, the EMT should carefully consider the possibility of associated injury of other body parts.

Neck

Approximately 5% of patients suffering from severe head injury will also have a cervical spine fracture. A missed spinal fracture can result in serious neurologic injury and even paralysis.

It is generally accepted that if a patient suffers any significant trauma above the clavicles, injury to the cervical spine may also be present. This means that any movement of the patient should be done while keeping the cervical spine immobilized. The concepts of cervical immobilization are discussed in the next chapter.

Face

When treating the patient who has significant injuries to the face, remember that the face is a part of the head and the brain lies just behind the face. Despite the upsetting nature of facial injuries, the EMT must remain calm and remember the principles of treating the patient with potential head injury.

Patients with obvious injuries to their face should not have anything placed into their nose. The thin bones behind the nose may be easily broken, and *a nasopharyngeal airway or soft suction catheter could easily penetrate into the brain itself*. Figure 21-8 shows a patient with significant facial trauma in whom a nasopharyngeal airway would be contraindicated.

Patients with significant facial trauma should be assumed to have a head and neck injury until proved otherwise.

PATIENT PRESENTATION

It is easy to recognize that a patient has suffered a head injury when the injury is severe. Some patients may not have obvious findings. It will be up to the EMT to elicit important historical information and to observe physical findings in order to recognize the potential for serious head injury.

Mechanism of Injury

To determine whether the patient is at risk of having a significant head injury, the EMT should carefully assess the mechanism of the injury. If anyone can provide the details of the injury, the EMT should document these details carefully.

If the patient was struck with an object, the EMT should determine what type of object and how many times the patient was struck. Did the patient fall and strike the head after being struck? If there was a fall, what was the surface the patient fell upon? How great a distance did the patient fall? What part of the body struck first?

If the mechanism was a motor vehicle collision, what parts of the vehicle sustained damage? Is there evidence of damage inside the car from the patient's head? A star pattern in the windshield is a classic sign of a person's head striking the glass forcefully. Figure 21-9 illustrates this important finding.

Seat belt restraint use inside a motor vehicle has been shown to significantly reduce the severity of injury in many cases. Properly used

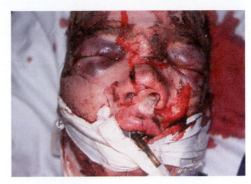

FIGURE 21-8 The presence of significant facial injuries is a contraindication to using a nasopharyngeal airway. (Courtesy of Kevin Reilly, MD, Albany Medical Center, Albany, NY.)

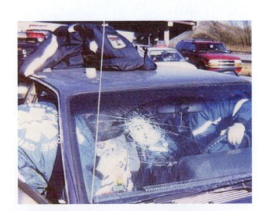

FIGURE 21-9 A starred windshield indicates that an object, likely a head, contacted it with great force. (Courtesy of Deborah Funk, MD, Albany Medical Center, Albany, NY.)

seat belt restraints prevent the person from being thrown about the vehicle in a crash. The EMT should determine whether the patient was wearing an appropriate seat belt restraint at the time of the accident.

If the patient was participating in a sport that usually requires a helmet, was a helmet used? If one was, looking at the helmet for damage can give the EMT an idea of the force of impact and the area of the head that received the force.

Signs and Symptoms

Trauma to the head is often apparent upon careful physical exam. During a detailed trauma assessment, the EMT should look for DCAP-BTLS (see Table 14-3) on the head. If any of these indications of injury are present, the EMT should consider the patient to have sustained a head injury. Careful reassessment and examination looking for other evidence of serious head injury are indicated. Figure 21-10 illustrates some physical findings associated with a head injury.

If a patient suffered an injury to the head and has physical findings consistent with head injury but is awake with no apparent neurologic injury, then the head injury may be minor. Patients who are awake upon first assessment and do not deteriorate have an excellent prognosis.

The patient who presents to emergency medical services (EMS) with signs of elevated intracranial pressure is considered to have a serious head injury. Depending upon the type of intracranial injury, the prognosis may be quite poor.

History

It is important for the EMT to gather any available history from the patient or bystanders. The usual SAMPLE (see Table 10-5) history is important to obtain, but in the case of head injury, there are additional points the EMT should attempt to elicit.

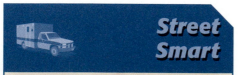

Street Smart

Remember that it often takes some time for obvious signs of trauma to develop. The EMT often must rely upon tiny abrasions to provide clues to the possibility of head injury. It pays to watch these patients carefully and reassess them frequently. Head injury patients can quickly decompensate. The astute EMT will have picked up on minor signs of injury and will be prepared for such decompensation.

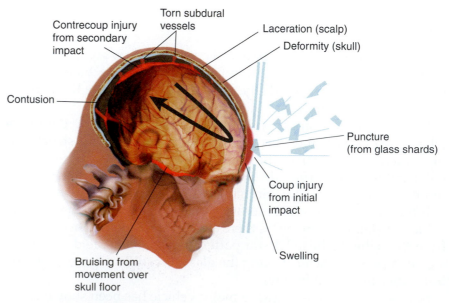

FIGURE 21-10 The EMT should look for physical findings that would indicate injury to the skull and brain.

Loss of Consciousness

In addition to the mechanism of the injury, bystanders can often provide valuable information regarding the patient's condition before the EMT's arrival.

Witnesses should be asked whether there was any loss of consciousness. It is not uncommon for a patient who has suffered an injury to the head to lose consciousness immediately after the incident. The length of the loss of consciousness should be determined if possible. The longer the loss of consciousness, the more significant the injury may be.

Seizure

Sometimes, after an injury to the head, a patient may suffer a seizure. A seizure that occurs immediately after a blow to the head is called a **post-traumatic seizure**. This type of seizure occurs in around 5% of patients sustaining blunt head injury. An immediate post-traumatic seizure does not necessarily mean that the head injury is severe. Often, the patient is awake by the time the EMT arrives.

The EMT should care for the patient in much the same way he would care for any other seizure patient, paying careful attention to the possibility of cervical spine injury. Careful reassessments and observation for deterioration are in order.

Vomiting

One sign of intracranial injury is persistent vomiting. It is not uncommon for a person who has sustained even a minor head injury to vomit; however, *persistent* vomiting is associated with more serious brain injury. Bystanders should be questioned about this symptom.

The EMT should ensure that the vomiting patient is able to clear her own airway. A backboarded patient may need to be lifted onto her side and assisted in clearing her airway with a large-bore suction catheter. Figure 21-11 illustrates this technique.

Assessment

In assessing the patient who has suffered a head injury, the EMT must pay careful attention to certain factors. The airway, breathing, and circulatory status are of key importance, as in any patient. There are also a few focused neurologic exam findings that will be useful. The EMT should become proficient in completing these.

Initial Assessment

The most important thing an EMT can do to improve the outcome of a head-injured patient is to adequately assess and manage the airway, breathing, and circulatory status. The brain needs adequate perfusion with well-oxygenated blood. If the patient's airway is in jeopardy, there is no sense in proceeding with the assessment until that problem has been remedied.

After ensuring that an adequate airway exists, the EMT must address the effectiveness of the patient's own breathing. After any issues related to adequacy of breathing have been dealt with, the EMT should turn his attention to the circulatory status.

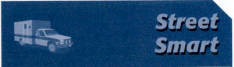

Street Smart

Bystanders often will greatly overestimate the length of time a patient was unconscious. The EMT should compare the reported time of unconsciousness with known time variables such as the time the call was dispatched and the time of arrival on the scene.

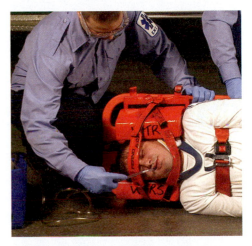

FIGURE 21-11 EMTs should be prepared to assist the head-injured patient in clearing her airway if vomiting occurs.

Doctors have learned that head-injured patients may become hypertensive. This is considered to be a protective mechanism for the brain. If the brain is not getting sufficient oxygenated blood, raising the blood pressure will theoretically provide more blood to the brain. Although this is a complicated pathway and not always effective, the effects of *hypotension* are very simple. Low blood pressure in conjunction with a head injury is lethal. The EMT must recognize and address signs of hypoperfusion and hypotension rapidly in order to attempt to improve the outcome of a seriously head-injured patient.

Rapid Trauma Assessment

For the patient who has suffered a significant injury, after the initial assessment has been completed and any life-threatening problems have been addressed, the EMT should move on to a rapid trauma assessment.

This rapid trauma assessment will include a head-to-toe search for significant injury. For a high-priority patient, this assessment will be done immediately before or during transport.

A complete set of vital signs is needed as soon as possible and should be repeated as frequently as the patient's condition requires. Every 5 minutes is appropriate for the high-priority patient, less often for patients who are not as ill.

Glasgow Coma Scale

During the initial assessment and rapid trauma assessment, the EMT should be able to gather some important information about the patient's neurologic status. The patient's level of consciousness is the most important part of this neurologic exam. A reliable way to quantify this assessment is by using the **Glasgow Coma Scale (GCS)**.

The Glasgow Coma Scale is a method used to evaluate three aspects of a patient's responsiveness: eye opening, best verbal response, and best motor response. Each category has assigned values for different responses that, when totaled, are correlated with the degree of neurologic impairment.

The lowest score is 3, allowing one point for each category. The highest score is 15. A score of 8 or less defines a severe head injury; a moderate head injury is associated with a score of 9–12. Head-injured patients whose GCS score falls between 13 and 15 are considered to have a mild, although still significant, head injury.

It is very important for the EMT to formally score the head-injured patient during the initial assessment and each reassessment. Any changes in the total score should be carefully noted and passed along to the staff at the hospital. It is not uncommon for a patient to either improve or deteriorate neurologically during prehospital care. This change can be easily measured using the GCS.

Table 21-2 outlines the point assignments in the Glasgow Coma Scale. A reproduction of this scale is useful for the EMT to keep in a pocket manual for easy reference.

Vital Signs

As he does for every other patient, the EMT should measure the head-injured patient's vital signs as often as is indicated by the condition.

TABLE 21-2

The Glasgow Coma Scale

	Best Response	Points
Eyes	Open spontaneously	4
	Open to verbal command	3
	Open to painful stimulus	2
	Do not open	1
Verbal	Oriented	5
	Disoriented	4
	Inappropriate words	3
	Incomprehensible sounds	2
	No response	1
Motor	Obeys command	6
	Localizes pain	5
	Withdraws from pain	4
	Shows abnormal flexion	3
	Shows abnormal extension	2
	No response	1
TOTAL		3–15

Certain characteristic findings may be seen with a serious head injury.

As previously discussed, the injured brain may induce an elevation in the blood pressure in an attempt to improve its own perfusion. A well-known, though incompletely understood, reflex, called **Cushing's reflex**, results in a bradycardia in serious head injuries.

Another component to this reflex that is commonly seen is an alteration in the respiratory pattern. The normal, regular pattern of the respirations is no longer present. Rather, one of several patterns of irregular respirations is noted.

Hypertension, bradycardia, and an altered respiratory pattern are referred to as **Cushing's triad**. This triad of physical findings is indicative of a very serious head injury.

Management

The priority in management of the patient with a head injury is to maintain an adequate supply of oxygenated blood to the brain without compromising the cervical spine. This goal can be achieved by following the same techniques of assessment and priorities in management that the EMT has learned in managing other high-priority patients.

The ABCs

The initial assessment will reveal any problems related to the patient's airway, breathing, or circulation. The EMT must rapidly and proficiently gain control of the airway if needed. High-flow oxygen is always indicated for the head-injured patient. Ventilatory assistance may be needed if the patient is not effectively moving air.

Keeping in mind that many patients who are involved in an incident that results in head injury may also have injury to other body systems, the EMT should identify signs of hypoperfusion and address them as appropriate. Adequate perfusion to the brain is critical to prevent worsening brain injury.

The EMT should remember to note the patient's initial mental status and, when time permits, calculate and document a GCS score. This can then be compared with scores obtained later in the management of this patient.

Spine Precautions

Because any significant trauma to the head may be associated with injury to the cervical spine, the EMT should always maintain immobilization of the spine of the head-injured patient. All management should be done with this principle in mind. A cervical collar should be applied to assist in keeping the neck immobilized. The details of this procedure are addressed in the next chapter.

Maintenance of Oxygenation

The injured brain has many compensatory mechanisms in order to maintain adequate oxygenation to itself. The EMT can assist in this effort by ensuring adequate oxygenation at all times. The use of 100% oxygen in the acute setting of a head injury will help reduce complications related to poor oxygenation.

Pediatric Considerations

Because a child's normal respiratory rate is higher than that of an adult, the rate of ventilation and hyperventilation would be higher as well. Rates of hyperventilation for a child should be at least 20 but not more than 25.

An infant's respiratory rate depends upon age. The younger the infant, the higher the respiratory rate. Tables of normal pediatric respiratory rates can be found in Chapter 8. To provide hyperventilation, the EMT should increase the rate from the normal by around 5 breaths per minute. Local protocols and medical control will dictate specific rates of ventilation and hyperventilation.

Hyperventilation

When serious brain injury exists and pressures within the skull are elevated, there are several techniques (based upon state or local protocol) the EMT can use to help temporarily decrease that intracranial pressure. One such technique is to hyperventilate the patient.

If the patient requires ventilatory assistance and has physical signs of elevated intracranial pressure as listed in Table 21-1, the EMT should assist ventilations at a higher rate than usual. If the normal rate for artificial ventilations is 12, this technique will involve ventilatory rates of 15–20.

Hyperventilation will decrease levels of carbon dioxide in the blood by increasing the rate at which it is blown off through exhalation. These decreased levels of carbon dioxide will result in vasoconstriction of the blood vessels in the brain. This vasoconstriction is roughly proportionate to the amount of carbon dioxide lost. The faster the ventilations, the lower the carbon dioxide level will go and the more the vessels in the brain will constrict. Figure 21-12 illustrates this concept.

Decreasing the amount of blood in the brain by vasoconstriction will make more room for a hematoma and will prevent an increase in intracranial pressure. Remember though, constricting the blood vessels to the brain too much would result in completely cutting off circulation to the brain! The EMT must pay careful attention to the rates of ventilation he provides to any patient, but especially to the patient with a serious head injury. The rate of hyperventilation should not exceed 20 breaths per minute in adults.

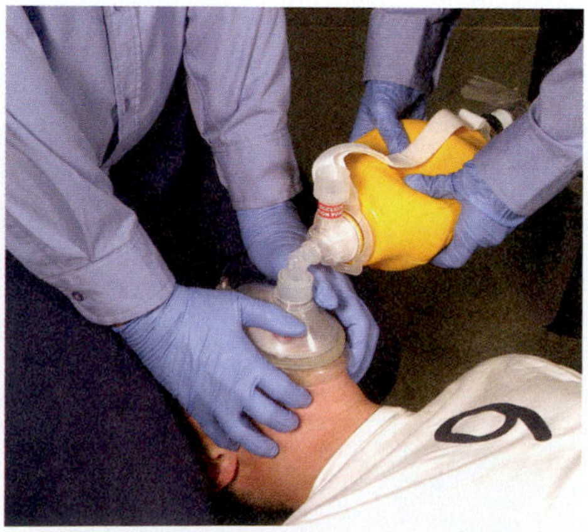

FIGURE 21-12 Hyperventilation is an important technique that can help decrease intracranial pressure when used properly.

Control of External Blood Loss

For an adequate supply of oxygenated blood to the brain to be maintained, there must be a sufficient supply of blood within the vessels. The EMT should be sure to control any external blood loss during the initial assessment.

Elevation of Head of Stretcher

One additional step during care of the patient with a serious head injury that may help decrease intracranial pressure is to elevate the head of the stretcher slightly. This elevation of the patient's head will allow gravity to participate in decreasing the pressure within the head.

Care must be taken to maintain spinal immobilization when it is indicated. A good technique is to elevate the head end of the backboard 6 inches or so with a few towels or a blanket under the board itself. Alternatively, simply raising the head of the stretcher slightly, with the patient remaining secured on the backboard, will have the same effect. This slight elevation of the patient's head will help decrease the intracranial pressure. Figure 21-13 illustrates this position.

Transport

Once a patient has been determined to have a potential head injury, transport should not be delayed. The potential for decompensation always exists, and it is the job of the EMT to get the patient to the appropriate facility as soon as possible.

Many EMS systems have the option of several different modes of transportation for seriously injured patients. A ground ambulance is the most common means of transportation for injured patients. Some areas have the ability to use a helicopter, or air ambulance, to more rapidly transport a patient to the hospital (Figure 21-14). This option is obviously reserved for the most critical patients when ground transport would take an unacceptable amount of time. The use of such services is governed by local protocols.

High-priority patients should be transported directly to a hospital that is known to have the capability to care for such injuries. Usually the regional trauma center will be the choice hospital, but the choice may depend upon local resources. The EMT should be familiar with the basic capabilities of surrounding hospitals. As with the use of helicopter transport, the EMT should always follow local protocols.

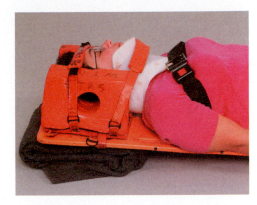

FIGURE 21-13 Slight elevation of the patient's head can help decrease the intracranial pressure.

Ongoing Assessment

Just as it is important for the EMT to note any changes in patient condition during his care, it is important to ask any witnesses to the event whether the patient seems to have changed at all in their eyes. Even untrained bystanders will be able to pick up on changes in mental status.

Any deterioration in mental status or neurologic function should be noted and considered to be an ominous sign of a serious head injury. The patient's vital signs and neurologic status should be reexamined frequently during transport. It is useful to repeat the GCS with each set of vital signs in the head-injured patient.

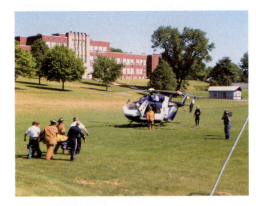

FIGURE 21-14 Helicopter evacuation may be necessary for some patients with serious head injuries. (Courtesy of Deborah Funk, MD, Albany Medical Center, Albany, NY.)

CONCLUSION

Head injuries account for many deaths and a significant amount of disability. Recognition of the potential for a serious head injury is the first step to providing appropriate care. Skilled assessment with efficient treatment provided by the EMT can help improve the outcome of head-injured patients.

TEST YOUR KNOWLEDGE

1. Discuss the relevance of head injuries to the American public.
2. Describe the anatomy of the scalp, skull, and brain.
3. Identify injuries that are commonly associated with head injuries.
4. Describe the management priorities of the patient with a scalp injury, a skull injury, and a brain injury.
5. Discuss the physical findings associated with a scalp injury, a skull injury, and a brain injury.
6. Describe the Glasgow Coma Scale.
7. Discuss the consequences of raised intracranial pressure.

8. Identify the physical findings associated with increased intracranial pressure.

9. Describe the appropriate treatment modalities used by the EMT that can help decrease intracranial pressure.

INTERNET RESOURCES

Check out the following resources for additional information related to head injuries:

- Alabama Head Injury Foundation, http://www.ahif.org
- Head Injury Hotline, http://www.headinjury.com
- Head Injury Society of New Zealand, http://www.head-injury.org.nz
- National Association of State Head Injury Administrators, http://www.nashia.org

FURTHER STUDY

Armstrong, J. (1998). Bombs and other blasts. *RN, 61*(11), 26–35.

Jastemski, C. (1998). Trauma! Head injuries. *RN, 61*(12), 40–44.

Murphy, P., & Heightman, A. (1998). Head injuries. *Journal of Emergency Medical Services, 23*(4), 66–70.

Price, D., & Burns, B. (1999). Brain injuries. *Emergency Medical Services, 28*(6), 65–71.

Schultz, R. (1997). Eggs and brains. *Emergency Medical Services, 26*(4), 29–35.

CHAPTER 22

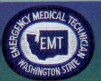

Spine Injuries

KEY TERMS

cervical spine
  immobilization device
neurogenic shock
paralysis
paraplegia
paresthesia
priapism
quadriplegia
standing takedown

OBJECTIVES

Upon completion of this chapter, the reader should be able to:

1. Describe the anatomy and physiology of the spinal column and spinal cord.
2. Describe different types of spine injuries.
3. Identify injuries commonly associated with injuries to the spine.
4. Identify the potential complications of spinal cord injuries.
5. Describe the patient presentation that would lead the EMT to suspect a spine injury.
6. Relate the mechanism of injury to potential injuries of the spine.
7. Describe the appropriate assessment techniques to use when the EMT suspects the patient has a spine injury.
8. Identify how airway management is different for patients with suspected spine injuries compared to that used for other patients.
9. Identify the priorities in management of patients with spine injuries.
10. Identify when spinal immobilization is necessary.
11. Describe how to properly apply a cervical spine immobilization device.
12. Describe how to immobilize a patient using a short immobilization device.
13. Describe how to perform a rapid extrication from a vehicle.
14. Describe how to immobilize a patient to a long spine board from the standing and supine positions.
15. Identify the situations that would require helmet removal.
16. Describe different types of helmets and the preferred method of removing them.

OVERVIEW

There are an estimated 10,000 new spinal cord injuries in the United States each year. Spinal cord injuries can leave patients with devastating neurologic injuries. The impact of these injuries on patients, their families, and on society as a whole is tremendous.

449

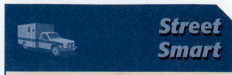

Street Smart

The EMT should be aware that a patient who is walking around at the scene of an accident may have suffered a spinal injury. An injury that does not involve the spinal cord may allow unimpeded walking, but further movement may cause spinal cord injury and therefore must be prevented.

An EMT who suspects a spinal injury should treat the patient as though one exists.

The immediate care provided to the patient with a spine injury is critical, as it can prevent further damage. An emergency medical technician (EMT) is often the primary prehospital caregiver for patients who have sustained spine injuries. The EMT must know how to recognize when spine injuries may exist and how to properly care for such patients.

ANATOMY REVIEW

To deal with injuries to the spine, the EMT needs to understand normal anatomy. Chapter 5 discusses the normal anatomy of the spinal column and the spinal cord; it should be reviewed at this time. Figure 22-1 illustrates the anatomy of the spinal cord and the protective spinal column.

Head-on Collision

Officer Shulman knew that something was seriously wrong when he approached the scene of an accident that involved a head-on collision and another rear-end collision. One car was a mess, and the driver was still sitting in the front seat. Usually by the time he arrived, all the

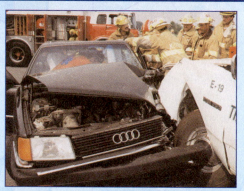

(Courtesy of David J. Reimer Sr.)

drivers would be out of their cars, or at least fumbling through their glove compartments looking for their insurance cards.

Officer Shulman approached the car and uttered, "Good evening, ma'am." The driver of the car softly responded, "I can't feel my legs." Immediately recognizing the seriousness of the situation, Officer Shulman advised the driver not to turn or move her head. He clicked his lapel mike and said, "Control, Unit five. Send EMS and a supervisor to my location, probable spinal injury from MVC, and tell them to expedite."

He then climbed into the backseat of the car and manually stabilized the patient's neck, telling her in a calm voice, "The ambulance is on the way."

- What are the priorities in the assessment of this patient?
- What special assessment considerations should the EMT use?
- What special transportation considerations should the EMT use?

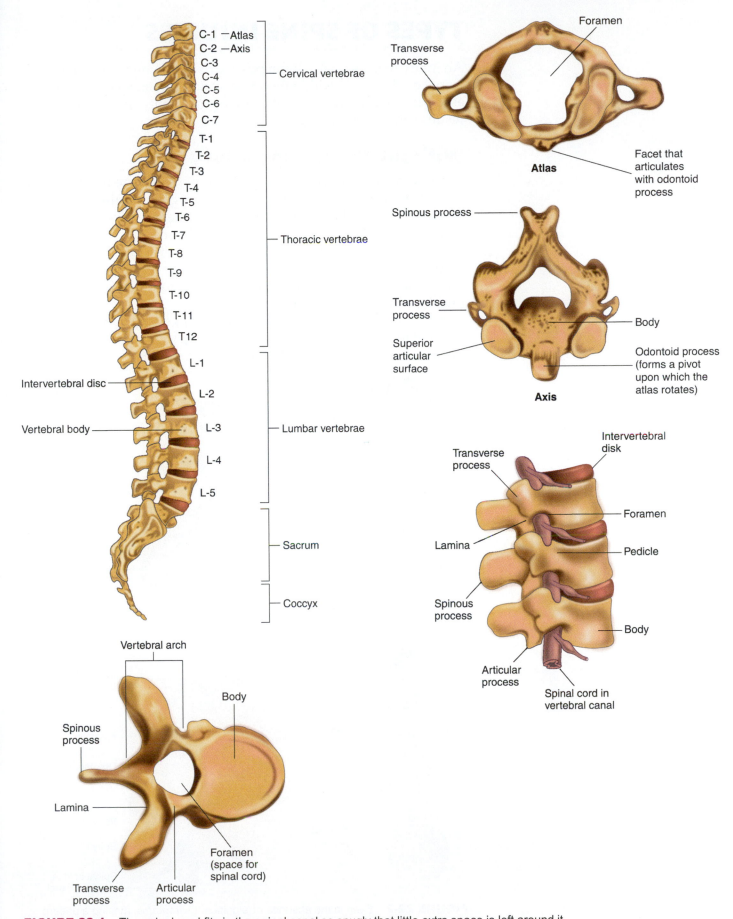

Atlas

Foramen

Transverse process

Facet that articulates with odontoid process

Axis

Spinous process

Transverse process

Superior articular surface

Body

Odontoid process (forms a pivot upon which the atlas rotates)

Intervertebral disk

Transverse process

Foramen

Lamina

Pedicle

Spinous process

Body

Articular process

Spinal cord in vertebral canal

C-1 —Atlas
C-2 —Axis
C-3
C-4
C-5
C-6
C-7
Cervical vertebrae

T-1
T-2
T-3
T-4
T-5
T-6
T-7
T-8
T-9
T-10
T-11
T12
Thoracic vertebrae

L-1
L-2
L-3
L-4
L-5
Lumbar vertebrae

Intervertebral disc

Vertebral body

Sacrum

Coccyx

Vertebral arch

Body

Spinous process

Lamina

Foramen (space for spinal cord)

Transverse process

Articular process

FIGURE 22-1   The spinal cord fits in the spinal canal so snugly that little extra space is left around it.

TYPES OF SPINE INJURIES

An injury to the spinal column poses a risk of damage to the sensitive spinal cord that lies within the spinal canal. Not all spinal injuries are associated with damage to the spinal cord, but when they are, the results can be devastating.

Without Neurologic Injury

Some spinal injuries consist only of ligament or bone injuries. If the damage to these support structures does not compromise the patency of the spinal canal or directly traumatize the sensitive cord, neurologic injury will not be present. An isolated bone injury, however, can be unstable in its position. If the bone injury disrupts the supportive nature of the spinal column, any movement of the column can cause unnatural movement of the spine and compromise the spinal canal, thus injuring the spinal cord.

A patient who has sustained a possible spinal injury should not be allowed to move at all. Any movement can potentially cause injury to the spinal cord. Figure 22-2 illustrates this concept.

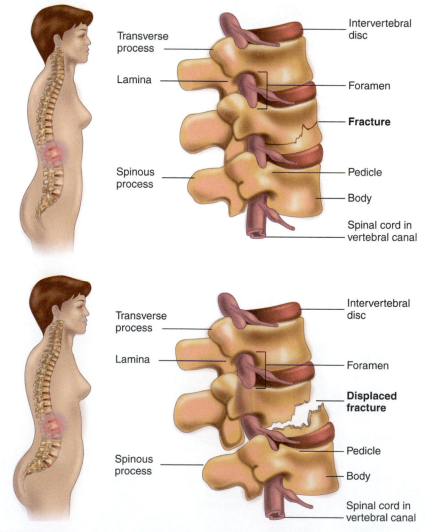

FIGURE 22-2   Even in the absence of significant symptoms, moving a patient with a spinal injury can cause damage to the spinal cord.

With Neurologic Injury

Some spinal injuries immediately cause injury to the spinal cord. Such an injury is shown in Figure 22-3. Certain signs and symptoms indicate neurologic injury. These signs and symptoms, which result from an interruption in the normal message flow back and forth between the brain and the body, is discussed later.

Region of the Spine

Each segment of the spine has its own specific features that make it susceptible to different types of injury. Although the EMT need not isolate the site of a spinal injury, an understanding of the anatomic differences is useful to the EMT.

Cervical

Of all of the spine segments, the cervical spine is of greatest concern for prehospital providers because injury to it holds the most extensive consequences for the patient. Nearly 40% of cervical fractures have associated spinal cord injury. The cervical spine is relatively isolated from the rest of the body and is directly under the head, so sometimes keeping it motionless is difficult. The EMT's job is to prevent any movement of the cervical spine when an injury is suspected. In the United States, motor vehicle crashes account for a large number of cervical spine injuries.

Thoracic

The thoracic spine is relatively immobile and therefore is not injured as often as the more mobile areas of the spine. When an injury does occur, however, it is more likely to involve the spinal cord because the spinal canal at this level is fairly narrow compared with other areas of the spine. Thoracic spine injuries most often result from a direct blow to the back.

Lumbar

Lumbar spinal cord injuries may not be as evident on physical examination as other, higher cord injuries. The EMT should consider the mechanism of injury and the presence of pain in the low back area in determining whether injuries to this area may exist. These injuries are usually caused by a flexion/extension/rotational type of mechanism.

Sacrococcygeal

The sacrum is a fairly strong collection of bones and is not often broken. Injury to this segment of the spine usually results from a direct blow. The bony tailbone, or coccyx, is commonly injured in a fall. The spinal cord does not extend as far as the coccyx; therefore, injury to these bones does not cause spinal cord injury.

PATIENT PRESENTATION

Because initial treatment of patients with spine injuries can prevent further injury, EMTs must learn to recognize when patients have

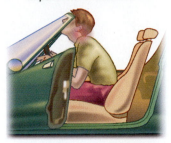
Impact with windshield

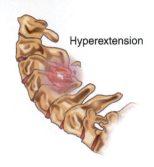
Hyperextension

FIGURE 22-3 Some spinal injuries cause damage to the spinal cord that is immediately evident.

potential spinal injuries. EMTs often treat patients for potential spine injuries when none exist, a practice that is perfectly acceptable and should be encouraged. It is much better to immobilize too many people than to fail to immobilize one who really needs it.

Mechanism of Injury

Given the stacked nature of the vertebrae and the tenuous position of the sensitive spinal cord within the spinal canal, a variety of mechanisms can result in injury to these important structures. The EMT's first clue to the possibility of a spine injury is the mechanism of the injury. Any mechanism that involved a blow to the spine or created a severe flexion, extension, or rotation of the spine should be considered suspect. In addition, any significant injury to an adjacent body part, such as the head, chest, or abdomen, should create suspicion of spinal injury. It should be noted that the large majority of spinal cord injuries, approximately 82%, occur in males between the ages of 16 and 30 and are the result of motor vehicle collisions, violence, or falls.

Motor Vehicle Crash

The forces in a motor vehicle crash often cause the neck to flex and extend forcefully as the vehicle comes to a stop. Any type of spinal injury is possible in a motor vehicle crash, but the flexion/extension type is probably most common.

Flexion/Extension/Rotation

The spinal column is designed to allow a certain amount of flexion (forward movement of the upper body), extension (backward movement of the upper body), and rotation (side-to-side movement). Figure 22-4 illustrates the motion that is normally allowed by the spinal column.

If force, such as the force of a motor vehicle crash, causes motion beyond that which is normally allowed, the spinal column may be damaged. The supporting ligaments may stretch or tear, and the vertebrae may crack or be dislocated from their normal position. When a significant disruption in the normal anatomy of the spinal column intrudes into the narrow canal, injury to the spinal cord may occur. Review Figure 22-3 for an illustration of how this can happen.

Falls

Falls also may result in injuries to the spine. A fall directly onto any bone may cause injury to either the spine or the vertebrae. A fall from any height can result in a broken bone, but falls from greater heights have a higher risk of creating such an injury.

Compression

Compression fractures are often seen in patients who have experienced a direct blow to a vertebra. A compression fracture is a crushing injury to an individual bone that causes the bone to weaken and break. A compression fracture of a vertebra weakens the support created by the spinal column and may cause injury to the spinal cord.

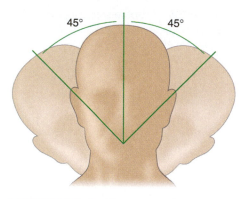

FIGURE 22-4 The extent of motion allowed by the spinal column is somewhat limited in each direction.

Figure 22-5 illustrates a compression injury to a vertebra that could potentially involve injury to the spinal cord.

Victims who fall from a height and land on their feet, a phenomenon known as axial loading, may experience spinal injuries. The force of the fall is transmitted from the feet, up through the legs, and into the spine. In this situation, broken bones in the patient's feet and injuries to the patient's lumbar spine are common. See Figure 22-6 for an illustration of this concept.

Firearms

More and more people routinely carry firearms in the United States, and the number of injuries related to them has become significant. A firearm can create a penetrating injury that directly injures a vertebra or the spinal cord itself. Because the direction of internal travel of a bullet is often difficult to discern in the field, the EMT must not dismiss the possibility of spinal injury. Every patient who has suffered a gunshot wound to the torso or neck should be treated for a potential spinal injury.

Although less common than spinal injuries from gunshot wounds, sharp objects such as knives can cause injury to the spine and spinal cord. All patients who have suffered penetrating trauma near the back or neck should be treated for a potential spinal injury. Figure 22-7 depicts a penetrating injury resulting in injury to the spine.

Recreation

Recreational sports are usually a safe way to get exercise and keep healthy, but they can result in spinal injuries. Football injuries account

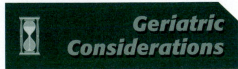

Geriatric Considerations

Older patients often have brittle bones from loss of calcium and other minerals. A fall that seems insignificant to an EMT may easily result in a broken bone for an elderly patient. The EMT should be more suspicious of bone injury, including spinal injury, when the patient is an elderly person.

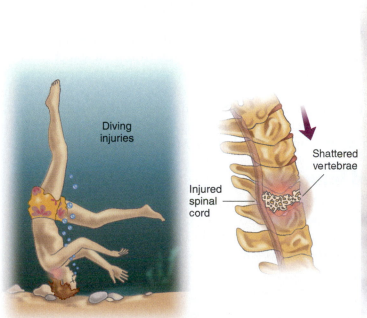

FIGURE 22-5   A vertebral compression fracture can lead to spinal cord injury.

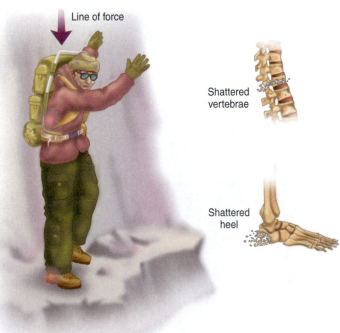

FIGURE 22-6   Axial loading after a jump from a height can cause heel fractures and lumbar spine fractures.

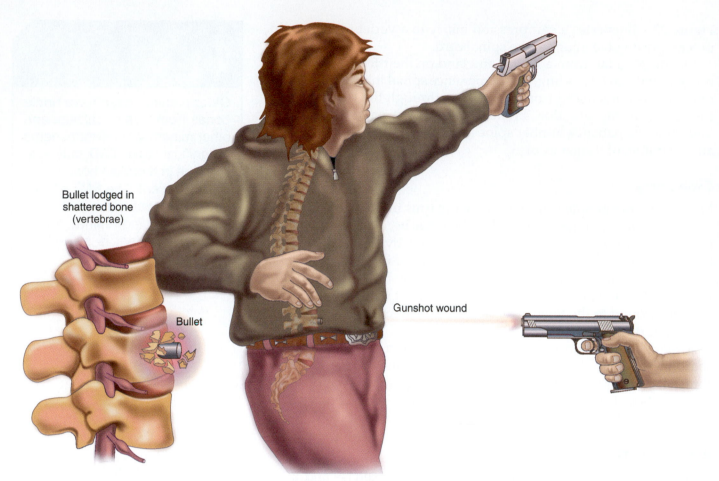

Bullet lodged in
shattered bone
(vertebrae)

Bullet

Gunshot wound

FIGURE 22-7 Penetrating injuries to the torso often cause spinal cord injury.

TABLE 22-1	
Common Types of Incidents That May Result in Spinal Injury	
	Injuries Caused
1. Motor vehicle crashes	36.0%*
2. Violence/crime	28.9%*
3. Falls	21.2%*

*Retrieved from Spinal Cord Injury Resource Center, http://www.spinalinjury.net.

for the largest number of spinal injuries during organized sports events. High-school football results in 20 to 30 permanent spinal cord injuries annually in the United States. Diving and rugby also account for a significant proportion of spinal injuries from recreational sports.

Depending upon the sport, the mechanism of the spinal injury may vary with each situation. The EMT must determine the exact mechanism of any injury from sport-related activity. If the patient may have experienced a direct blow or excessive flexion, extension, or rotation of the spine, the EMT should consider the potential for spine injury. Figure 22-8 depicts mechanisms resulting in spinal injury. Table 22-1 lists common types of incidents that may result in spinal injury.

Associated Injuries

Because the spine is located near many other body parts, an injury to other parts of the body can also cause injury to the spine. The EMT should maintain a high index of suspicion for spinal injury if any significant trauma is sustained by any part of the body that is close to the spine.

Head

Because the head rests on top of the neck, if it sustains any significant trauma, the cervical spine is also at risk of injury. A good rule to follow

Description	Diagram	Examples
A **Hyperextension** Excessive posterior movement of head or neck		Football tackler Face in windshield in MVC Elderly person falling to the floor Dive into shallow water
B **Hyperflexion** Excessive anterior movement of the head onto chest		Rider thrown off of motorcycle or horse Dive into shallow water
C **Compression** Weight of head or pelvis driven into stationary neck or torso		Dive into shallow water Fall of greater than 10 to 20 feet onto head or legs

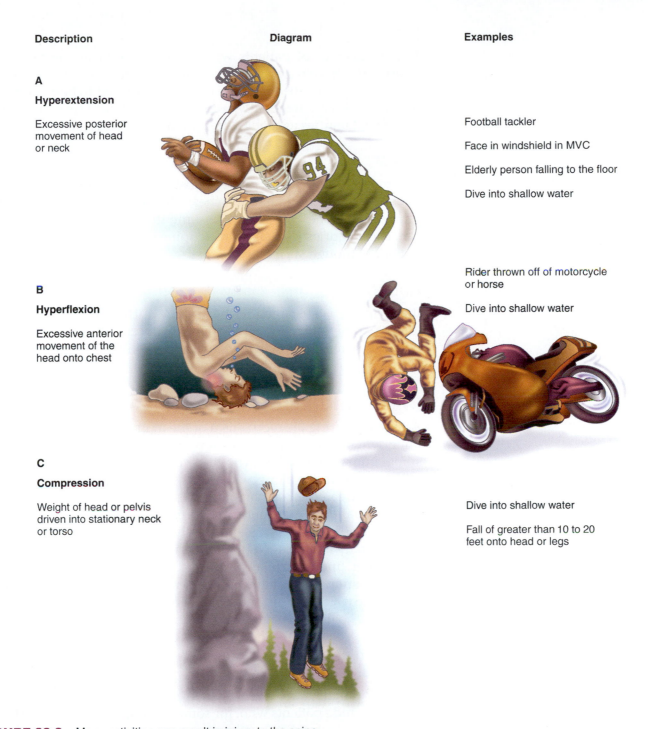

FIGURE 22-8 Many activities can result in injury to the spine.

is to assume that any significant trauma above the clavicles involves the cervical spine. It is always better to err on the side of treating for the possibility of spine injury.

An injured patient who is unconscious may have sustained a significant head injury. The EMT should always treat such patients as though there were concurrent spine injury.

Face

Twenty percent of patients who sustain significant cervical spine injuries also have facial injuries. Because the face is in such close proximity to the neck, the forces are easily transmitted to both, and coexisting injuries are frequently seen. The EMT should treat any patient with facial injuries as though the patient has a cervical spine injury.

Chest

The thoracic spine makes up the posterior support of the chest. If a patient sustains trauma to the chest, the potential for thoracic spine injury exists. The EMT should assume that any patient with significant chest injuries also has thoracic spine injuries and should treat the patient as though such injuries exist.

Abdomen

If any injury is sustained to the abdomen, the EMT should suspect lumbar spine injury as well. Proper treatment of the patient with a potential spine injury will reduce the possibility of complications and potential worsening of the injury.

Signs and Symptoms

After considering the mechanism of the injury, the EMT should determine whether the patient has any signs or symptoms of possible spinal injury. The patient who has a mechanism of injury consistent with spinal injury along with signs and symptoms of that injury should be treated for spinal injury.

Some patients may not have symptoms of spinal injury even though the mechanism is one likely to cause such injury. These patients may be managed in a different manner than other patients, depending upon regional protocols. An EMT who has any doubt should assume the patient has a spinal injury and treat the patient accordingly. Otherwise, the EMT should follow local protocol for patients who have no symptoms of spinal injury.

Limitations

Several groups of patients may not be able to notice or describe symptoms of spinal injury even if such symptoms are present. These groups include patients who, for some reason, may not be able to feel pain and patients who are otherwise distracted.

Intoxication

Patients who are intoxicated may not feel even severe pain and, therefore, cannot be relied upon to describe the symptoms of spinal injury. Intoxicated patients who have a mechanism of injury consistent with a spinal injury should be treated as though a spinal injury is present.

Distracting Injury

The presence of another painful injury may distract a patient from the symptoms of a spinal injury. For example, a patient with pain from a broken leg may be distracted from the pain of a broken vertebra, as the pain from the broken leg may be more intense. Any patient who has a significant mechanism of injury and a potentially distracting injury should be treated for a spine injury regardless of the presence of symptoms.

Altered Mental Status

An unconscious patient, or a patient with an altered mental status, cannot relay symptoms of a spine injury to the EMT; therefore, the EMT should assume the patient has a spine injury if any potentially serious mechanism exists. For example, a patient who is found unconscious on a bed and whose family denies that any fall or other trauma occurred probably does not have a spinal injury. On the other hand, the EMT should assume that a patient who has fallen down a flight of stairs and has been found unconscious at the bottom has a spinal injury. The best rule is to assume spinal injury is present unless it can be ruled out.

Neck or Back Pain

Although it seems that a patient who sustains an injury to the spine would feel pain in the back or neck, this is not always the case. If neck or back pain is present, the patient should be treated as if a spinal injury exists. If the patient has no neck or back pain but does have tenderness upon palpation of the neck or back, the EMT should assume that spinal injury exists.

Neurologic Abnormality

Several neurologic findings may be seen in the patient with a spinal cord injury. The EMT must be able to recognize these findings immediately, as they indicate the need for spinal immobilization.

When the spinal cord is injured, signs and symptoms are usually evident soon after the incident. The EMT should be aware of several complications related to failed communication between the brain and other body organs.

Respiratory Failure

The diaphragm receives orders from the brain via nerves in the cervical spinal cord. These nerves, which travel through cervical levels 3, 4, and 5, must be intact for the diaphragm to function. The diaphragm is a muscle that is necessary for breathing. A good way to remember this important connection is to say, "3, 4, and 5 keeps you alive."

When the nerve supply to the diaphragm is cut off, the patient's breathing efforts become ineffective because the main muscle of breathing is no longer functional. This may be evidenced by the patient's feeling short of breath or having obvious respiratory difficulty, or simply by apnea.

Neurogenic Shock

The nerves that control the constriction of blood vessels pass through the spinal cord. An injury to the spinal cord may interrupt this control and cause generalized dilation of the blood vessels below the area of the injury. Such dilation will cause the patient's skin to appear flushed as more blood moves closer to the skin's surface.

Normally, when blood vessels dilate, the heart rate increases in response in order to maintain an adequate blood pressure. This requires communication between the brain and the blood vessels. In a patient with a spinal cord injury, this communication may not exist. If it does not exist, the patient's heart rate will not increase despite a falling blood pressure.

The combination of hypotension with bradycardia and flushed, warm skin is called **neurogenic shock** and is indicative of a serious spinal cord injury.

Paralysis

Perhaps the most well known and easily recognized complication of a spinal cord injury is the inability to move. This is known as **paralysis** and is highly suggestive of a serious spinal cord injury.

Depending upon the location of the spinal cord injury, the areas affected by paralysis differ. The nerves to the legs come from the lower parts of the spinal cord, while the nerves to the arms come from the higher parts of the spinal cord. If the cord is injured at a high level, however, all messages flowing through that area will be interrupted, which means that everything below the affected area may be paralyzed.

A patient who has lost the use of both arms and legs has **quadriplegia**, a term that refers to the four extremities that are unable to function. A patient who has lost the use of only his legs has **paraplegia**, a term that refers to loss of function in the lower part of the body.

The nerves that relay sensation usually are damaged when the nerves that relay movement information are damaged. Patients with spinal cord injuries may not be able to move or feel their bodies below a certain level, depending upon the level of the cord injury. The EMT need not determine the exact level of the injury but should realize that a high spinal cord lesion can cause respiratory failure. The patient who is unable to move and/or feel his arms and legs should be assumed to have a high cord injury, and the EMT should very carefully monitor the patient for signs of respiratory decompensation.

Paresthesias

One of the neurologic abnormalities that the EMT may find in the patient with a spinal cord injury is an area of numbness or tingling below the level of injury. The term used to describe a sensory problem is **paresthesia**. The EMT should check the arms and the legs for paresthesia during the trauma assessment. The EMT can test for paresthesia by asking the patient whether he can feel a particular physical stimulus, such as a fingernail or pen scratching the skin.

Other

Another sign of spinal cord injury is the inability to control bowel function. If the nerves controlling the anal sphincter are injured, it will not remain closed reliably and incontinence of stool may occur.

Although incontinence can be caused by other illnesses, in the presence of symptoms or signs of spinal injury, it supports the suspicion of spinal cord injury.

Another physical sign of possible injury to the spinal cord is **priapism**. This term refers to a painful penile erection that may be present when the nerves controlling this bodily function are injured.

Table 22-2 lists some signs and symptoms that may be associated with a spine injury.

Assessment

The EMT's assessment of the patient determines whether or not spinal injury is suspected. The assessment must include an initial survey of the scene, not only for hazards, but also for the mechanism of injury. The EMT completes the remainder of the assessment just as she would for any other trauma patient, altering it if indicated by the priority of the patient's illness. Chapters 12 to 15 discuss assessment of trauma patients.

Initial Assessment

The purpose of the initial assessment is to find and treat any immediate life-threatening problems. The patient with a spinal cord injury may have serious respiratory compromise and may require ventilatory assistance. Any patient with an injury that also may have caused a spinal injury should be given high-flow oxygen during the initial assessment.

Focused History and Physical Examination

The focused trauma assessment should be geared toward finding any evidence of spinal injury or any other injury sustained during the incident. The EMT should use an organized head-to-toe approach to assessment discussed in detail in Chapter 14.

Vital Signs

The patient with a spinal cord injury may undergo generalized vasodilation below the level of the injury, which may result in neurogenic shock. This type of shock is characterized by hypotension without tachycardia and flushed, warm skin. The EMT should carefully assess the vital signs on the patient with a potential spine injury and note any changes in them.

History

A description of the mechanism of injury along with the history obtained by the EMT can be very helpful to the hospital staff who treat a patient with a spine injury. The nature of the injury is probably the most important information the EMT can obtain because hospital personnel have no way of getting this information if the EMT does not provide it.

The patient's neurologic status immediately after the incident is sometimes helpful to hospital staff, as it can reveal the type of injury sustained. If a patient has changing neurologic findings, the EMT

TABLE 22-2

Signs and Symptoms of Spinal Injury

Tenderness to spine

Pain associated with moving

Obvious deformity of spine

Soft tissue injuries in proximity to spine

Numbness, weakness, or tingling in the extremities

Loss of sensation or paralysis below the suspected level of injury

Loss of sensation or paralysis in the upper or lower extremities

Incontinence

Priapism

? **Ask the Doc**

The National Association of Emergency Medical Services Physicians has a position paper entitled "Indications for Spinal Immobilization." Some emergency medical services (EMS) systems use these indications for spinal immobilization to selectively immobilize trauma patients. An EMT should follow local, regional, or state protocols in regard to practices of spinal immobilization.

should determine what was happening at the incident site before the EMT arrived. In addition, the hospital staff needs to know about the presence of any preexisting neurologic injury; the EMT should obtain such information whenever possible.

Management

The priorities in managing the patient with a potential spinal injury are threefold: the first priority is to save the patient's life; the second priority is to protect the spinal cord; and the final priority is to deliver the patient to definitive care.

Save the Patient

Preserving the patient's life is best accomplished by following the priorities of the initial assessment. The EMT should address airway, breathing, and circulation problems in that order to prevent a bad outcome.

Protect the Cord

When the EMT suspects a spinal injury, the EMT should perform all treatment with protection of the spinal cord in mind. The EMT should immediately position the patient so that the patient's head is in a neutral position, and then should maintain in-line immobilization of the head and spine during all phases of treatment.

Because patients are found in many different positions and circumstances, the EMT must have many different means of providing in-line spinal immobilization. The exact techniques used depend on the particular situation. The most common techniques used in the field to immobilize a patient's spine are outlined here.

Cervical Spine Immobilization Device

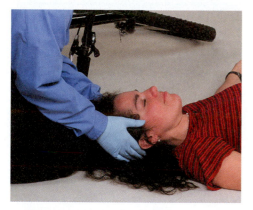

FIGURE 22-9   Manual head stabilization is the best way to keep a patient's head and neck in line.

The best way to keep a patient's head and neck in line is to manually hold stabilization. The EMT places one hand on each side of the patient's head and holds the head and neck in line as depicted in Figure 22-9. Often the EMT cannot maintain manual stabilization for long periods because other things need to be done. Tools allow the EMT to maintain spinal stabilization when the EMT cannot maintain it manually.

The **cervical spine immobilization device**, sometimes called a cervical collar, is a semirigid device that is used as an aid to immobilization. It is designed to fit around the patient's neck snugly enough to discourage movement, but not so tightly as to restrict breathing. Figure 22-10 shows several different sizes of the cervical spine immobilization device.

There are many models of the cervical collar, but all of them operate on the same principle. The EMT must measure the patient to determine the correct size of collar to use. Then one person holds the patient's head in line with the spine while another places the collar around the back of the neck and secures it. Skill 22-1 reviews the proper technique for applying the cervical spine immobilization device.

The EMT should be able to fit a collar around a patient's neck easily without moving the patient. A cervical collar that fits properly keeps the patient's head in the neutral position. If the collar allows the

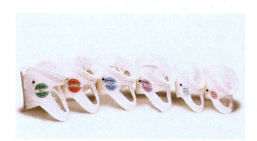

FIGURE 22-10   Several different sizes of cervical spine immobilization devices are available. (Courtesy of Laerdal Medical Corporation, Wappingers Falls, NY.)

SKILL 22-1 *Application of the Cervical Spine Immobilization Device*

PURPOSE: To aid the EMT in stabilization of the cervical spine.

STANDARD PRECAUTIONS:

☑ Assortment of cervical spine immobilization devices (collars)

☑ Personal protective equipment

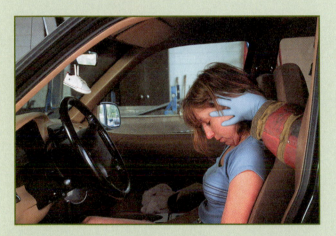

1 The EMT first moves the patient's head into neutral alignment. If the patient complains of pain or the EMT feels resistance, then the patient's neck should be splinted in position.

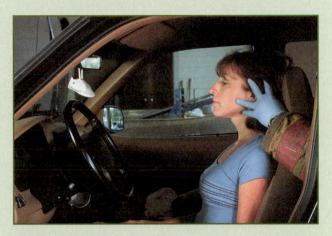

2 The EMT should maintain continuous manual stabilization of the patient's head throughout the rest of the procedure.

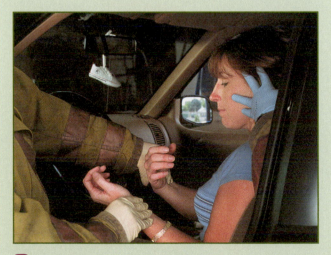

3 Next, a second EMT checks for distal pulses, movement, and sensation.

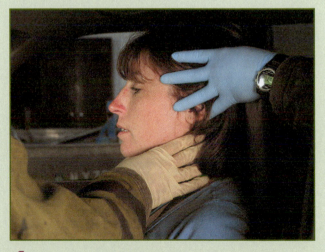

4 The second EMT then measures the patient's neck for a cervical collar, according to manufacturer recommendations.

(continues)

SKILL 22-1 *(continued)*

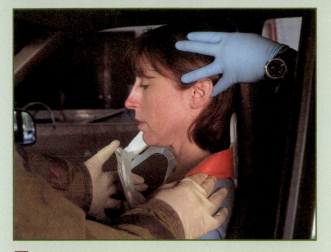

5 The second EMT then slides the posterior portion of collar in the void behind the neck.

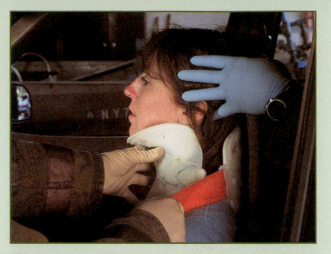

6 Cupping the chin piece in one hand, the second EMT slides the anterior portion of the collar up the chest until it captures the chin.

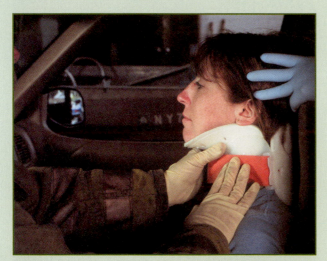

7 With collar in place, the second EMT fastens the Velcro securely.

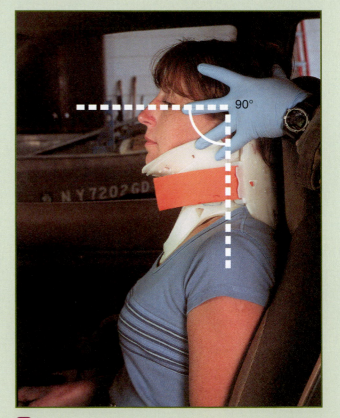

8 Checking for a proper collar fit, the second EMT mentally draws a line from the opening of the ear to the middle of the shoulder, and from the opening of the ear to the eyes. There should be a 90-degree angle imagined.

(continues)

SKILL 22-1 *(continued)*

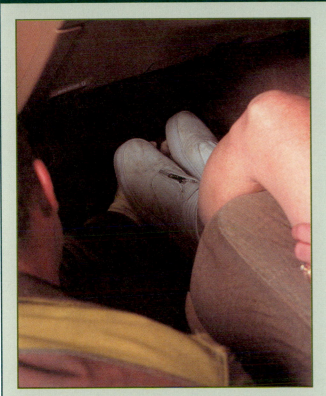

9 The second EMT finally rechecks for distal pulses, sensation, and movement.

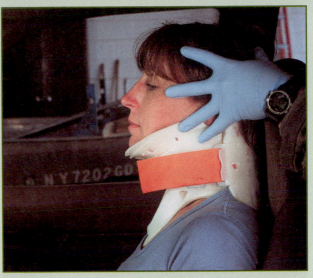

10 Continuous manual stabilization must be maintained, despite the presence of the cervical immobilization device.

patient's head to easily flex, extend, or rotate, it does not fit properly. The EMT should practice fitting and applying cervical collars until she is proficient in this technique. The EMT should follow the manufacturer's recommendation for fitting the cervical collar.

If a properly fitting cervical collar is unavailable, the EMT can improvise by wrapping a rolled-up towel around a patient's neck and shoulders as shown in Figure 22-11. Alternatively, the EMT can maintain manual stabilization throughout transport.

Because a cervical spine immobilization device is merely an aid and not a definitive means of spinal immobilization, the EMT should assign a trained assistant to hold manual stabilization even after the collar has been applied. This stabilization should be maintained until the patient has been secured in a more definitive fashion.

Short Immobilization Device

If a patient is seated and has a suspected spine injury, as would be the case in a motor vehicle crash, a short immobilization device is utilized. Several different types of short immobilization devices are available, but the purpose of all these devices is to maintain in-line immobilization of the head, neck, and back while the patient is extricated from the site and transported. Application of the short immobilization device is detailed in Skill 22-2.

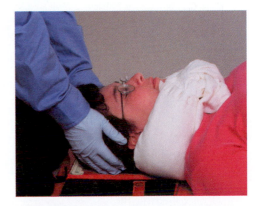

FIGURE 22-11 When a patient does not fit into a standard cervical collar, a towel may be used to help support the neck.

SKILL 22-2 *Application of the Short Immobilization Device*

PURPOSE: To further immobilize the injured patient's spine after the application of the cervical collar.

STANDARD PRECAUTIONS:

- ☑ Assortment of cervical spine immobilization devices
- ☑ Short immobilization device
- ☑ Personal protective equipment

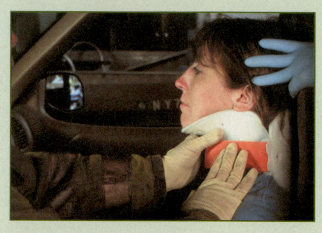

1 First, an EMT manually stabilizes the spine. A second EMT then applies a properly sized cervical spine immobilization device. Once the collar is secure, the second EMT checks distal pulses, movement, and sensation.

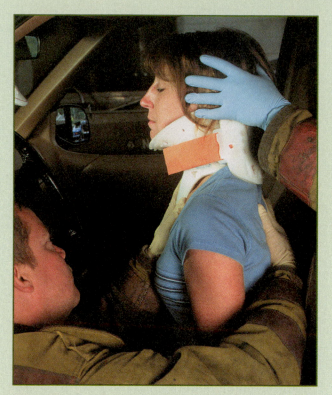

2 While a trained assistant maintains continuous manual stabilization, the EMT places his arms along the anterior and posterior thorax. The patient may now be moved forward as a unit, keeping the spine in line.

(continues)

Before placing a short immobilization device onto a patient, the EMT should place a cervical spine immobilization device on the patient to maintain in-line stabilization of the patient's neck. Once the patient is secured in a short immobilization device, the EMT should place the patient on a long spine board. The long spine board provides support and immobilization of the entire spine and body.

In applying a short immobilization device, the EMT secures the torso prior to securing the head. The torso is secured first because securing the head first could allow the head to be moved around unnecessarily as the rest of the body is secured. Also, if the patient's condition deteriorates and the patient needs to be removed from the site before the patient has been completely secured into the device, the

SKILL 22-2 *(continued)*

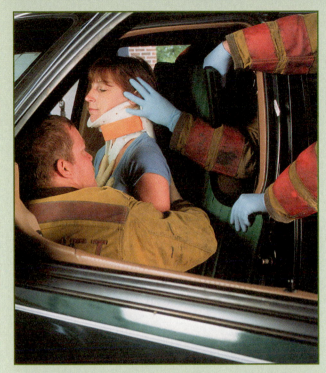

3 The device is then positioned behind the patient cautiously, and the patient is leaned back against the device.

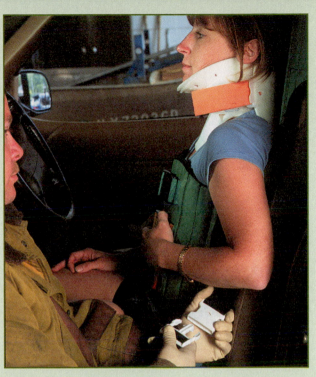

4 Next, the patient's torso, including the legs, is secured to the device.

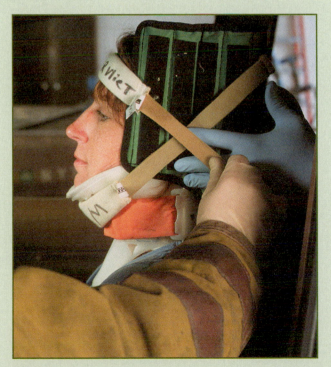

5 Finally, the patient's head is secured to the device. The EMT pads the void behind the head as needed.

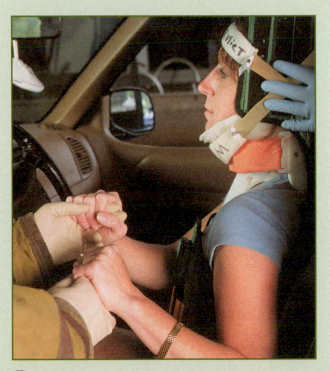

6 The EMT then reassesses distal pulses, movement, and sensory function of the patient before transferring the patient to the backboard.

heaviest part of the patient's body will already be secured. If the torso is adequately secured, an EMT can manually stabilize the patient's head during extrication.

Rapid Extrication

The process of short spine immobilization is always necessary for the seated patient who may have a spinal injury except when the patient must be removed from that position more quickly because of the severity of the patient's injuries, the EMT's need to gain access to other victims, or because of dangers at the scene. Patients in such situations should be removed rapidly, although the EMT still should be careful to keep the patient's spine in line. The EMT should provide manual stabilization while the patient is rotated and then lowered onto a long spine board as shown in Skill 22-3.

Long Spine Board

If the patient is found standing or lying down rather than sitting, a long spine board may be used for immobilization. To place a patient on this immobilization device, the EMT will need several trained assistants. The concept of maintaining in-line stabilization remains the same.

SKILL 22-3 *Rapid Extrication*

PURPOSE: To manually immobilize the spine of an unstable patient who may have a spinal injury as a result of a motor vehicle collision.

STANDARD PRECAUTIONS:

☑ Assortment of cervical spine immobilization devices
☑ Long spine board
☑ Turnout gear
☑ Personal protective equipment

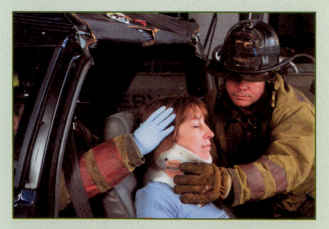

1 The EMT first checks distal pulses, movement, and sensation. Then the EMT moves the head to a neutral position and has another EMT apply a properly sized cervical collar.

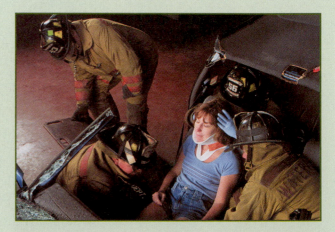

2 With an EMT on each side of the patient, the patient is gently lifted a couple of inches so that a long spine board may be inserted under the patient's buttocks.

(continues)

SKILL 22-3 *(continued)*

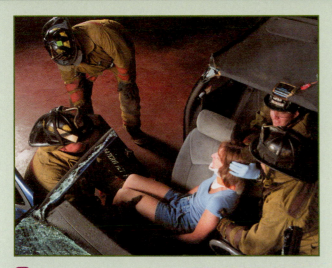

3 While an EMT continues to maintain manual stabilization of the spine, one EMT grasps the patient under the arms while another grasps the patient at the hips. Then, on command, the EMTs rotate the patient to the side about 45 degrees. At this point, the EMTs may need to switch places if the car's B post becomes an obstruction. After two or three small turns to rotate the patient, the patient should be parallel to the long spine board.

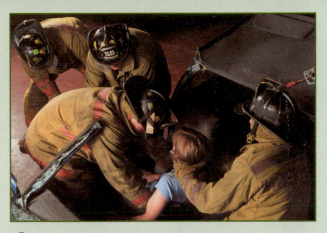

4 Once the patient is parallel to the long spine board, the patient is lowered, as a stiff unit, to the long spine board while the EMTs maintain in-line stabilization.

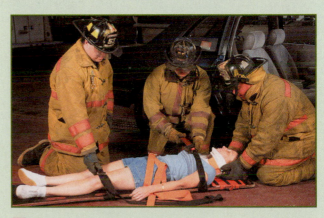

5 Once the patient is on the long spine board, first the body, and then the head, should be fastened securely, and the EMT should recheck the patient's distal pulses, movement, and sensation.

Supine Patient If an injured patient is found in a lying position, the EMT should immediately gain control of the cervical spine by holding the head and neck, and then roll the patient into the supine position. The EMT should move the patient as a unit while keeping the patient's head and neck in line with the rest of his body. In the supine position, the airway can be more adequately managed and the patient may be fully assessed.

To immobilize the supine patient, the EMT should first check pulses and motor and sensory function in all four extremities; apply a collar; and then move the patient onto the long spine board with the assistance of several trained assistants as demonstrated in Skill 22-5 and Skill 22-6.

Street Smart

The long spine board can also be used to move patients who do not have spine injuries. The board is a firm surface on which patients can be supported as they are transferred. It is useful for carrying patients over distances and provides a firm surface on which cardiopulmonary resuscitation (CPR) can be performed.

SKILL 22-4 *Long Axis Drag*

PURPOSE: To rapidly remove a patient, who is in immediate danger, from a motor vehicle with a minimum of spinal manipulation.

STANDARD PRECAUTIONS:

☑ Personal protective equipment

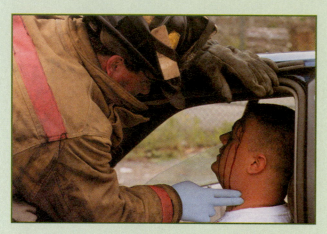

1 First, the EMT determines that the patient needs immediate extrication for some reason, for example, the patient is in cardiac arrest.

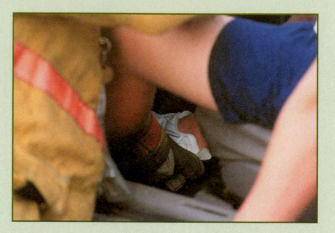

2 Opening the closest door and entering the passenger compartment, the EMT disentangles any extremities from pedals and other obstructions.

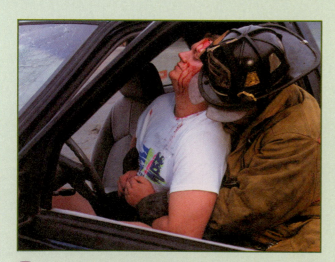

3 Then the EMT reaches behind the patient's back and under both of the patient's arms to grab the patient's wrists.

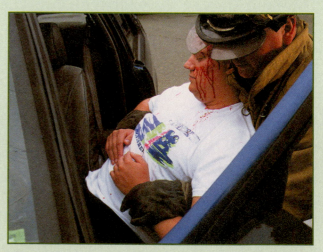

4 The EMT then rotates the patient, as a unit, and places the patient into a semi-inclined position.

(continues)

SKILL 22-4 (continued)

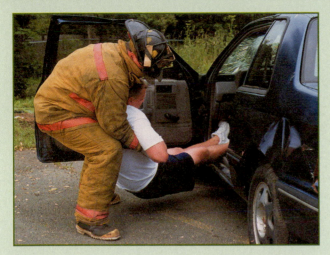

5 The EMT then drags the patient out of the motor vehicle with the patient's head resting on the EMT's forearms.

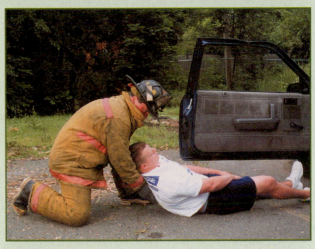

6 By dropping to his knees, the EMT can lower the patient and crawl backward with the patient, while performing a long axis drag.

SKILL 22-5 *Modified Logroll of the Supine Patient*

PURPOSE: To immobilize the spine of a supine patient who may have a spinal injury.

STANDARD PRECAUTIONS:

☑ Selection of cervical collars
☑ Long spine board
☑ Strapping system
☑ Head immobilization system

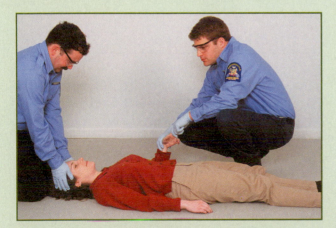

1 An EMT checks distal pulses, movement, and sensation of all four extremities while another EMT maintains manual stabilization.

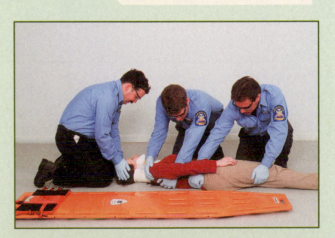

2 While one EMT holds manual stabilization, two more EMTs take positions at the patient's shoulders and pelvis, reaching across the patient and grasping the patient's shoulders and pelvis, respectively.

(continues)

SKILL 22-5 *(continued)*

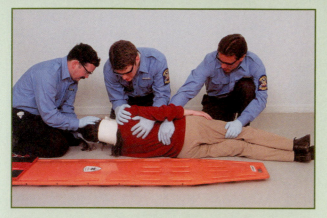

3 On command, the three EMTs roll the patient on her side. The patient's arms should be at her side.

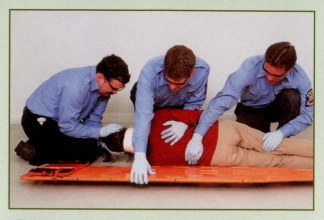

4 One EMT pulls the long spine board under the patient. The long spine board should end at the back of the patient's knees.

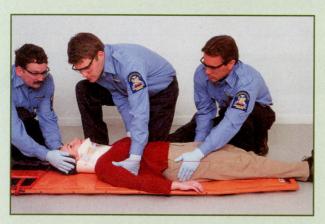

5 On command, the patient is rolled back onto the long spine board, and the patient is pulled up to the center of the board, using a long axis drag.

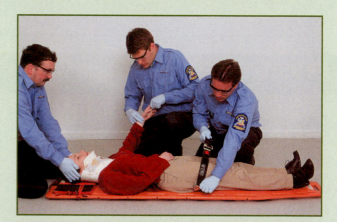

6 Once the patient is centered on the long spine board, the EMT secures the patient to the long spine board and reassesses distal pulses, movement, and sensation.

The EMT secures the patient's head to the board only after securing the torso and legs because the head is the easiest part of the body to control manually. If a patient is halfway secured and suddenly needs to be turned, for example, if he vomits, the EMT must be able to manually support the patient without compromising the spine. By securing the torso first and the head last, if the patient must be rolled, the straps will be holding the heaviest part of the patient's body and the EMT can control his head and neck.

Standing Patient Upon arrival on the scene, the EMT will often encounter patients who are standing. A good example is a motor vehicle crash; less seriously injured patients may have gotten out of their cars and may be walking around the scene when the EMT arrives. If the crash was a serious one, the EMT should suspect spinal injury and should immobilize them to protect their spinal cords.

SKILL 22-6 *Four-Person Lift*

PURPOSE: To immobilize the spine of a supine patient who may have a spinal injury.

STANDARD PRECAUTIONS:

☑ Assortment of cervical collars
☑ Long spine board
☑ Strapping system
☑ Head immobilization system

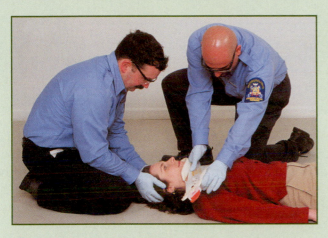

1 The first EMT kneels at the patient's head and immediately obtains manual stabilization. The second EMT checks the patient's distal pulses, movement, and sensation and applies a cervical collar.

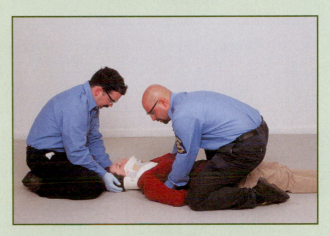

2 The second EMT then straddles the patient and drops one knee to the ground. Placing his hands under the patient's arms, he grasps the shoulder girdle.

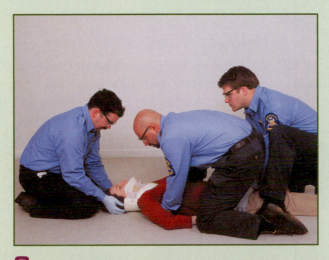

3 A third EMT straddles the patient, at the hips, and drops his opposite knee to the ground. He then grasps the patient around the hips.

(continues)

SKILL 22-6 *(continued)*

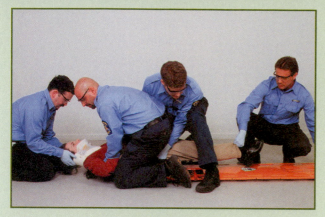

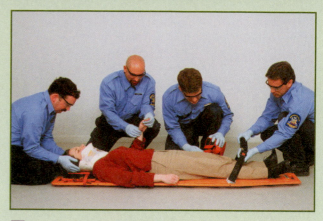

4 On command, all three EMTs gently and evenly lift the patient about 2 inches while a fourth EMT slides the long spine board under the patient.

5 Once the patient is properly positioned, the EMTs proceed to immobilize the torso, and then the head, of the patient. Then the EMT rechecks distal pulses, movement, and sensation.

Street Smart

The standing takedown procedure is a very effective way to immobilize the standing patient, but it can be quite frightening to the patient. The EMT should thoroughly explain the procedure to the patient and reassure the patient throughout the procedure that the patient will not be dropped. The patient must rest against the board as he is lowered to the ground. Patients will be able to do this with encouragement from the EMT.

Street Smart

Children playing sports often do not have custom-fit helmets; therefore, their helmets often do not fit very well. A poor-fitting helmet may allow excessive movement of the head inside it, so the EMT may need to remove such a helmet.

The best way to get the standing patient onto a long spine board is to perform the **standing takedown** maneuver as demonstrated in Skill 22-7. This technique is an easy and safe way to have the standing patient lie down without compromising the patient's spine. Asking the patient to sit or lie down would be asking for movement of the spine, but this technique requires no movement on the patient's part at all.

Special Considerations

Certain circumstances require the EMT to perform spinal immobilization in a manner that is somewhat different from the usual procedure. The priorities of maintaining in-line immobilization are still the same, however, regardless of the procedure used by the EMT.

Helmets

As some spinal injuries are sustained during recreational sports, a patient may be wearing a helmet at the time of the EMT's arrival. It is important for the EMT to know whether it is safest to take the helmet off or to leave it on.

During helmet removal, the EMT must not compromise the spine. A specific technique for removing helmets that minimizes head and neck movement is shown in Skill 22-8.

A helmet may remain in place if it fits well and does not impede the EMT's ability to assess and manage the patient's airway and breathing and to immobilize the patient. A helmet that fits poorly or creates a barrier to proper airway and breathing management must be removed. A helmet that prevents the EMT from effectively immobilizing the patient with the helmet in place also must be removed.

The EMT may encounter different types of helmets. A typical sports helmet is open anteriorly and affords fairly easy access to the airway. The full-face motorcycle helmet, on the other hand, makes assessment of the patient difficult, and it makes management of an airway nearly impossible.

SKILL 22-7 Long Spine Board Immobilization of the Standing Patient

PURPOSE: To immobilize the spine of a standing patient who has a potential spine injury.

STANDARD PRECAUTIONS:

- ☑ Assortment of cervical collars
- ☑ Long spine board
- ☑ Strapping system
- ☑ Head immobilization system

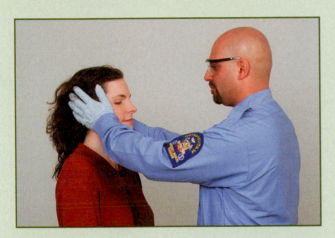

1 The EMT approaches the patient from the front and takes immediate anterior head stabilization.

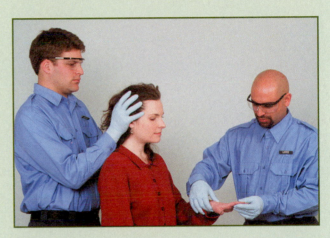

2 Another EMT takes head stabilization from the rear, while the first EMT assesses distal pulses, movement, and sensation.

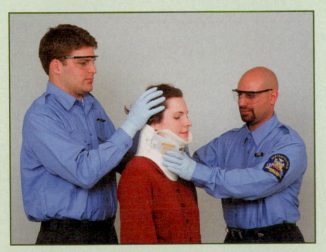

3 An appropriately sized cervical collar is applied to the patient.

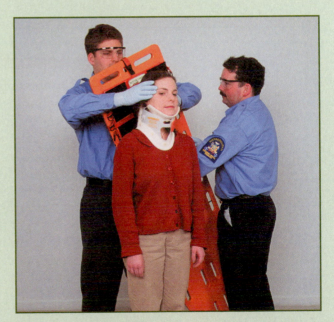

4 Another EMT places the long spine board upright behind the patient and between the arms of the EMT holding stabilization.

(continues)

SKILL 22-7 *(continued)*

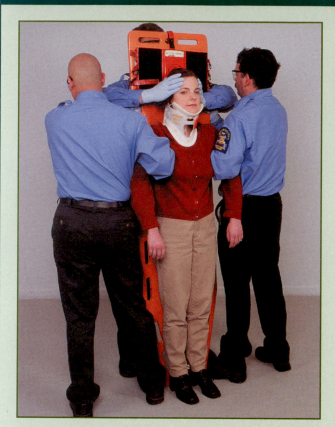

5 One EMT then stands on either side of the patient, holds the board under the patient's arms, and stabilizes the bottom of the board with a foot.

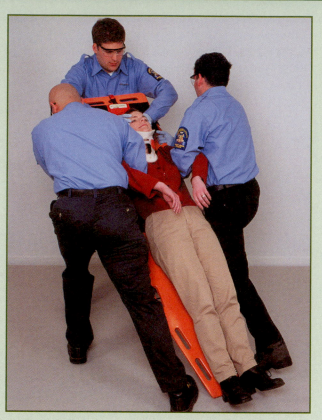

6 Slowly, the board and the patient are lowered to the ground, while the EMT at the head stabilizes the head and neck. The EMT then immobilizes the patient and rechecks distal pulses, movement, and sensation.

Transport

Usually the patient who has sustained a previous spinal cord injury not only has lost movement in the affected body part but also has lost sensation in that part. The EMT must pay special attention to handling the patient gently. Such a patient, for example, may not be able to feel his fingers get caught under the backboard, but the fingers will still be injured. The EMT also should provide extra padding to the patient's affected body parts during longer transports.

The last priority in managing the patient with the potential spinal injury is to get the patient safely to the most appropriate hospital in a reasonable amount of time. Some treatments for spinal cord injuries are very time dependent. The sooner the patient gets to the appropriate hospital, the sooner the care can be given. The EMT should follow local protocols regarding the facilities to which these patients should be transported and the appropriate way to accomplish such transports.

The ongoing assessment of patients with potential spinal cord injuries must include a repeat of the initial assessment, vital signs, as well as an assessment for any of the findings of spinal cord injury discussed in this chapter. The EMT should document any change in the patient's status and advise hospital staff of the change.

Pediatric Considerations

Children present unique challenges to the EMT who is attempting immobilization. The head of a child is relatively larger than that of an adult. As a result, when lying flat, the child's head forces the neck into a flexed position. This position compromises the in-line stabilization of the cervical spine, which cannot be allowed to happen. This flexed position is illustrated in Figure 22-12.

Pediatric immobilization boards are made specifically for smaller children to resolve this problem. These boards have a dip in the head section to make room for the child's larger occiput. Alternatively, the EMT can place padding under the child's body from the shoulders to the heels to maintain the child's neutral position on a long spine board (Figure 22-13). For older children, merely leaving out the padding that is normally on the head of the adult long spine board will likely solve the problem.

Once a child is placed on a long spine board, the EMT should carefully assess the child's position to ensure that the child's cervical spine is in an appropriate neutral position.

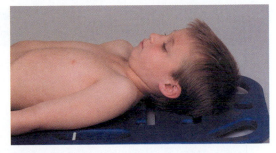

FIGURE 22-12   The prominent occiput of a child forces the neck into a flexed position when the child is lying flat.

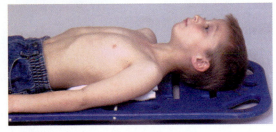

FIGURE 22-13   Padding behind the child's body from the shoulders to the heels puts the neck in a neutral position when the child is placed on a spine board.

SKILL 22-8 *Helmet Removal*

PURPOSE: To immobilize the spine of a patient who is wearing a full-face helmet and may have a spine injury.

STANDARD PRECAUTIONS:

- ☑ Backboard
- ☑ Scissors
- ☑ Assortment of cervical collars

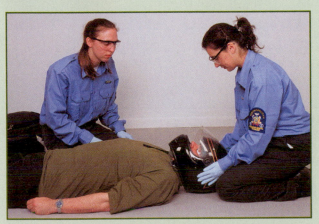

1 The first EMT manually stabilizes the head in the helmet, while the second EMT assesses distal pulses, movement, and sensation. Any glasses should be removed at this time.

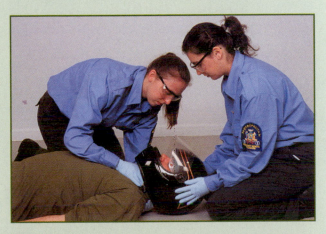

2 The second EMT then cuts or unfastens the chin strap, slides one hand under the head, stabilizing the head from below, and places her hand on the jaw, stabilizing the head from above.

(continues)

SKILL 22-8 *(continued)*

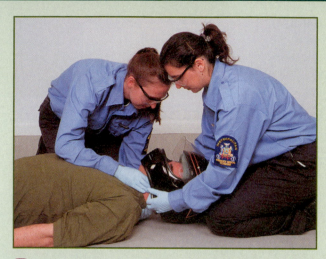

3 The first EMT then removes the helmet by spreading the helmet apart gently while moving the helmet from the back of the head.

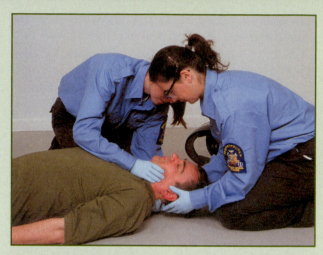

4 Once the helmet is completely removed, the first EMT assumes manual stabilization of the head. It may be necessary to pad under the head.

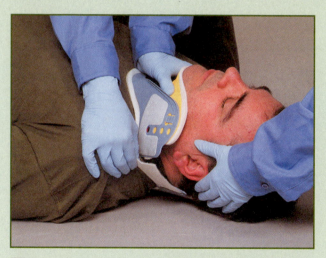

5 A cervical collar is then fitted to the patient.

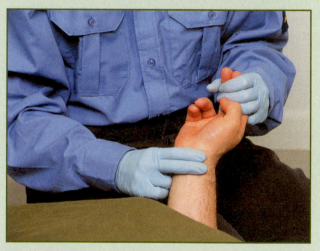

6 With the collar in place, and the head in a neutral position, the EMT rechecks distal pulses, movement, and sensation.

CONCLUSION

Many people in the United States sustain spinal cord injuries every year. The EMT's quick recognition of the potential for such an injury can help to prevent further damage from occurring to the sensitive spinal cord. Careful immobilization while maintaining in-line stabilization is key in managing the patient who has sustained a spinal injury.

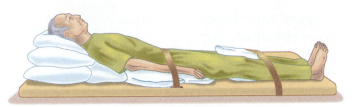

FIGURE 22-14 Padding the gaps around the elderly patient's spine makes immobilization more comfortable.

TEST YOUR KNOWLEDGE

1. Describe the anatomy and physiology of the spinal column and spinal cord.
2. Relate mechanism of injury to potential injuries of the spine.
3. Identify other injuries commonly associated with injuries to the spine.
4. Describe different types of spine injuries.
5. Identify the potential complications of spinal cord injuries.
6. Describe the patient presentation that would lead the EMT to suspect a spine injury.
7. Describe the appropriate assessment techniques to be used for the patient with a suspected spine injury.
8. Identify the differences in airway management in the patient with a suspected spine injury.
9. Identify the priorities in management of the patient with a spine injury.
10. Identify when spinal immobilization is necessary.
11. Describe how to properly apply a cervical spine immobilization device.
12. Describe how to immobilize a patient using a short immobilization device.
13. Describe how to perform a rapid extrication from a vehicle.
14. Describe how to perform immobilization with a long spine board for both the standing and supine patient.
15. Identify the situations that would require helmet removal.
16. Describe different types of helmets and the preferred method to remove them.

INTERNET RESOURCES

Visit the Web sites below to learn more about spinal injury and the impact it has on those suffering from it:

- American Spinal Injury Association, http://www.asia-spinalinjury.org
- Association for Spinal Injury, http://www.aspire.org.uk

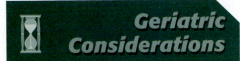

Geriatric Considerations

Some patients, especially elderly patients, have a condition in which the curvature of the spine is excessive. This condition is called scoliosis when the curvature is lateral and kyphosis when the curvature is in the anterior posterior dimension. Either condition presents a challenge for the EMT who needs to provide adequate immobilization on a long spine board.

The best way to provide immobilization for a patient with a curvature of the spine is to use a lot of padding. Placing the patient on the board and filling all the gaps with pillows, blankets, and towels for padding will accomplish the goal of immobilization and will not create too much discomfort for the patient (Figure 22-14).

- National Spinal Cord Injury Association, http://www.spinalcord.org
- Spinal Cord Injury Network International, http://www.spinalcordinjury.org
- Spinal Cord Injury Resource Center, http://www.spinalinjury.net
- Spinal Injuries Association, http://www.spinal.co.uk
- Spinal Injuries Scotland, http://www.sisonline.org

FURTHER STUDY

Bilkasley, M., & Ryder, T. (1997). The halo orthosis. *Journal of Emergency Medical Services, 22*(12), 52–58.

Blank-Reid, C. (1999). Strangulation. *RN, 62*(2), 32–36.

Brown, L. H., Gough, J. E., & Simonds, W. B. (1998, January–March). Can EMS providers adequately assess trauma patients for cervical spinal injury? *Prehospital Emergency Care, 2*(1), 33–36.

Cone, D. C., Wydro, G. C., & Mininger, C. M. (1999, January–March). Current practice in clinical cervical spinal clearance: Implication for EMS. *Prehospital Emergency Care, 3*(1), 42–46.

Meldon, S. W., Brant, T. A., Cydulka, R. K., Collins, T. E., & Shade, B. R. (1998, December). Out-of-hospital cervical spine clearance: Agreement between emergency medical technicians and emergency physicians. *Journal of Trauma, 45*(6), 1058–1061.

Murphy, P., & Colwell, C. (2000). Prehospital management of neck trauma. *Emergency Medical Services, 29*(5), 53–60.

Sahni, R., Menegazzi, J. J., & Mosesso, V. N., Jr. (1997, January–March). Paramedic evaluation of clinical indicators of cervical spinal injury. *Prehospital Emergency Care, 1*(1), 16–18.

VanStralen, D., & Goss, J. (1998). Damage control for pediatric spinal injuries. *Journal of Emergency Medical Services, 23*(3), 114.

CHAPTER 23

Chest and Abdominal Injuries

KEY TERMS

cardiac contusion

evisceration

flail segment

hemoptysis

hemothorax

occlusive dressing

paradoxical motion

pericardial tamponade

petechiae

pneumothorax

pulmonary contusion

pulse pressure

subcutaneous emphysema

sucking chest wound

tension pneumothorax

tracheal deviation

traumatic asphyxia

OBJECTIVES

Upon completion of this chapter, the reader should be able to:

1. Recognize the impact of a mechanism of injury on chest and/or abdominal trauma.
2. Recognize the signs and symptoms of the following chest injuries:
   Simple pneumothorax
   Tension pneumothorax
   Fractured ribs
   Flail segment
   Pulmonary contusion
   Cardiac contusion
   Pericardial tamponade
   Aortic injury
   Traumatic asphyxia
3. Explain the management of an open chest wound.
4. Explain the management of closed chest injuries.
5. Recognize the signs and symptoms of the following open abdominal wounds:
   Evisceration
   Impaled object
6. Explain the management of the open abdominal wound.
7. Recognize the signs and symptoms of the following closed abdominal injuries:
   Liver and spleen injury
   Pelvic fracture
8. Explain the management of closed abdominal injuries.

OVERVIEW

What do motor vehicle collisions and gunshot wounds have in common? Both of these mechanisms of injury can result in injury to the chest and the abdomen. In fact, more than one-half of all serious

481

trauma patients have chest and/or abdominal trauma. Nearly two-thirds of these patients are alive when they arrive at a trauma center.

Prehospital care provided by emergency medical technicians (EMTs) often has a positive impact on the survival of patients with chest and abdominal injuries. There are several basic principles regarding the management of these patients. This chapter reviews those principles.

ANATOMY REVIEW

Within the trunk of the body are two spaces or cavities called the thoracic cavity and the abdominal cavity. The thoracic and abdominal cavities contain some of the most important organs of the body (Figure 23-1). Vital activities, such as breathing, circulation, and digestion, occur within the chest and abdomen. Chapter 5 discusses the anatomy and physiology of the chest and abdominal organs and should be reviewed at this time.

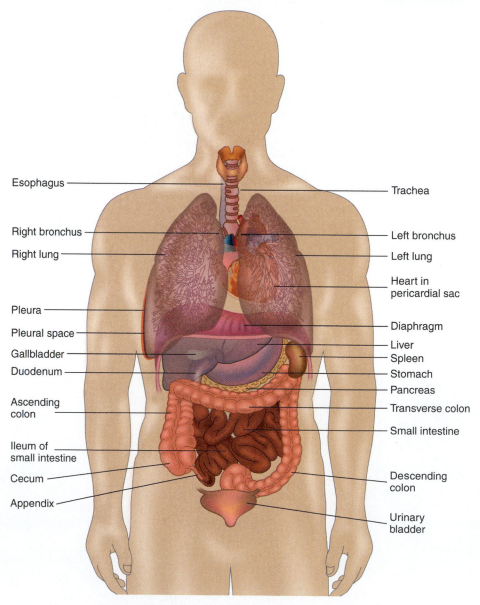

Esophagus

Right bronchus

Right lung

Pleura

Pleural space

Gallbladder

Duodenum

Ascending colon

Ileum of small intestine

Cecum

Appendix

Trachea

Left bronchus

Left lung

Heart in pericardial sac

Diaphragm

Liver

Spleen

Stomach

Pancreas

Transverse colon

Small intestine

Descending colon

Urinary bladder

FIGURE 23-1 The trunk of the body contains the majority of vital organs.

CHEST TRAUMA

Injuries to the chest result in significant numbers of deaths each year. The chest contains organs that are essential to life. When these organs are damaged, life may be threatened. The most common consequence of chest trauma from any source is hypoxia. Injuries to the chest wall or internal organs can lead to ineffective ventilation and oxygenation. The job of the EMT is to recognize the presence of chest injuries, to quickly initiate the proper management, and to facilitate expedient transport to the most appropriate hospital.

Mechanism of Injury

One of the first things an EMT will assess on the scene of an injured patient is the mechanism of injury. Knowing the forces that were applied to the patient will help the EMT to suspect and find even subtle injuries that may have significant consequences.

Blunt Chest Trauma

The most common cause of serious chest injuries is blunt chest trauma. Motor vehicle accidents, falls, direct blows, and crushing injuries are some of the ways that blunt chest trauma occurs. With this

 ## Rollover

The first sheriff's unit to arrive at the accident on County Highway 11 reported, "Possible rollover, no victim found." The deputy who sent that message knew that someone had been driving the car recently, as the engine was still warm, but he could not find the driver. When the state trooper and the county sheriff arrived, they started a search of the roads and local farmhouses while EMS staged on scene.

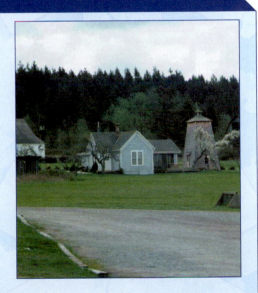

Waiting for the order to "return to service," EMT Clayton went down to inspect the car in the ditch. The crushed roof indicated that the car may have rolled, and the starred windshield indicated that someone or something had been thrown forward. The top half of the steering wheel was bent, and the directional signal was snapped in half at midshaft. Drops of blood were visible on the seat and over into the backseat. The rear window appeared to have been kicked out, and blood was evident on the trunk lid and the ground behind the car.

The radio crackled to life, "Police Unit 4, report from the Eveleigh farm, Route 11, possible prowler, man banging on the front door, appears to be bleeding. Says he needs an ambulance because he can't breathe."

- Based on the mechanism of injury, what injuries might an EMT suspect?
- What are the assessment priorities for this patient?
- What are the management priorities for this patient?
- How could this patient deteriorate?

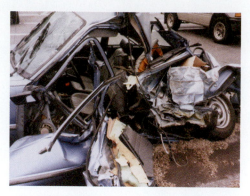

FIGURE 23-2 Major damage to a motor vehicle indicates that significant force was applied to the occupant's body during the collision. (Courtesy of Craig Smith.)

type of mechanism, the EMT may not find evidence of serious injury immediately. Many of the findings on physical examination are somewhat delayed and may not be immediately apparent to the EMT. Nonetheless, failure to recognize a chest injury can have disastrous consequences.

Blunt trauma occurs when a force is applied to the chest wall. Depending upon the size of the object applying the force and the speed with which the force is applied, the injuries may be limited to the external chest wall or may extend deeper to involve internal thoracic organs. The more force that is applied to the chest, the deeper and more significant the injuries will likely be.

The EMT should take a moment upon arrival at a scene to evaluate the forces that were applied to the patient. For example, in the case of a motor vehicle accident, the EMT should look at the vehicle the patient was in. Significant damage to the vehicle's exterior indicates high speed and a lot of force (Figure 23-2). Damage to the inside of the vehicle can further indicate the patient's potential injuries. A broken or bent steering wheel indicates that significant force was applied to the driver's chest.

The more significant the forces that were involved in the incident, the higher the EMT's suspicion should be for serious injury to the patient.

Penetrating Trauma

Penetrating injuries to the chest are becoming increasingly common in today's society. Guns, knives, and other sharp objects can penetrate the chest wall and injure the underlying heart, lungs, and great vessels. The immediate result of penetrating injury can be severe bleeding or impaired breathing.

Although some penetrating chest injuries are certainly difficult to miss, others are quite subtle and may be easily missed without careful assessment. The key to proper management of the patient with penetrating chest trauma is to recognize that any wound to the chest can have associated underlying organ injury, no matter how superficial it may look at first glance.

The EMT can easily miss a tiny bullet entrance wound or small wound from a knife, or the EMT may assume that it is a minor wound. These mistakes will delay the proper treatment of a patient with a potential time-dependent injury. Injuries to the heart, lungs, and great vessels can quickly lead to shock and cardiac arrest. The EMT must find the wounds and be highly suspicious of the possibility of internal chest injury, no matter the size of the external wound. Figure 23-3 illustrates how a small wound can result in significant intrathoracic injury.

Signs and Symptoms

The most common symptoms seen in patients with chest injuries are pain and difficulty with breathing. The pain is often centered in the area of the injury. Difficulty with breathing may be minor initially and may progress slowly or rapidly, depending upon the injury.

Signs the EMT should look for include obvious injury to the chest wall. Using DCAP-BTLS (see Chapter 14 for a review of these find-

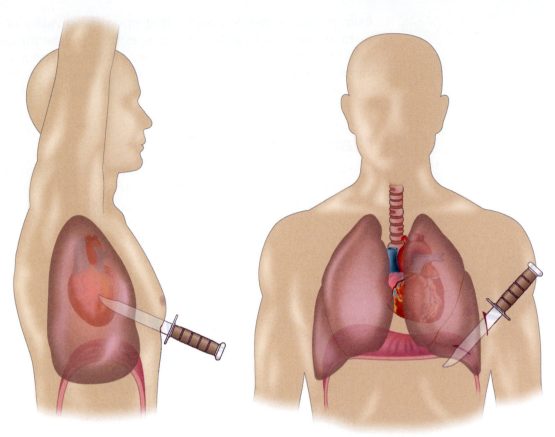

Stab wounds at nipple level or below frequently penetrate the abdomen

FIGURE 23-3   Despite small external wounds, penetrating chest trauma can be associated with serious organ injury.

ings) during the chest assessment and remembering to look at both the front and back of the chest will lead the EMT to find any injuries.

Depending upon the specific injury that is present, characteristic physical findings may be found on physical examination. When examining the patient's chest, the EMT should look specifically for any obvious deformities, contusions, abrasions, punctures, burns, tenderness, lacerations, or swelling to the chest wall. Also, during palpation of the patient's chest, the EMT should note the presence of any subcutaneous air, or **subcutaneous emphysema**. Subcutaneous emphysema is air present under the skin; this air produces a palpable feeling like Rice Krispies as the EMT presses his hands against the patient's chest wall. This feeling is also known as crepitus.

The patient with significant chest injuries may have an elevated heart rate and respiratory rate, although the absence of these findings does not exclude injury. Vital signs should be monitored carefully.

Assessment

The patient who has suffered a potential chest injury should be assessed in the manner described in Chapters 12, 13, and 14. The scene survey allows the EMT to avoid any personal dangers and provides him with information regarding the incident. The initial assessment allows the EMT to find and treat immediately life-threatening injuries. The focused history and physical will be slightly different from patient to patient, depending upon the severity of the mechanism of injury. Most patients having potential chest injuries require a rapid trauma assessment followed by vital signs and a SAMPLE (see Table 10-5) history. A detailed physical examination may follow if time allows, and ongoing assessments are performed during transport to the hospital.

Management

The management of the patient with chest trauma is centered around ensuring that the patient has adequate oxygenation and perfusion, which the EMT does by providing high-flow oxygen, ventilating when necessary, halting any obvious bleeding, supporting circulation when needed, and rapidly transporting the patient to definitive care. Treatment of specific injuries is addressed throughout this chapter.

Transport

The patient with serious chest trauma must be seen at a hospital that has the capability to diagnose and treat serious traumatic injuries. The destination hospital is often guided by local protocols. In addition, if advanced life support (ALS) is available and indicated by local protocols, the EMT should arrange to intercept the unit while the patient with serious chest injuries is being transported.

The EMT should notify the receiving hospital early in the transport so the staff can prepare for the patient's arrival. Some systems require an EMT to obtain on-line medical control during the care of the seriously injured patient. The EMT should be familiar with and adhere to local protocols.

SPECIFIC INJURIES

Although the EMT is not expected to make a definitive diagnosis in the field, the EMT can easily recognize several conditions that may impact the prehospital treatment of the patient. All EMTs should be able to recognize the signs and symptoms and understand the initial management of each of these conditions from the basic life support (BLS) perspective.

Open Chest Wounds

A sharp object that penetrates the skin on the chest wall creates an open chest wound. Determining the deepness of a wound is very difficult in the field; therefore, any wound on the chest caused by a penetrating object should be assumed to be serious, and the patient treated as though it were serious.

Beneath each rib lies an artery. The middle of the chest contains the great vessels, the aorta, and the vena cava. If any of these blood vessels is lacerated, bleeding in between the lung and the chest wall may occur. The accumulation of blood in the pleural space is called a **hemothorax**.

As much as 1,500 cc of blood can accumulate in the pleural space of each lung. The result of this massive blood loss is hypotension and shock. Eventually, the accumulation of blood can compromise breathing by crushing the air-filled lung. The EMT need not differentiate between a hemothorax and other life-threatening bleeding; instead, the EMT should concentrate on managing the hypotension and transporting the patient rapidly to the trauma center.

If a penetrating object has pierced the pleura, outside air can enter the thoracic cavity between the chest wall and the lung. As the volume of air between the chest wall and the lung expands, the lung starts to collapse. Air within the pleural space is called a **pneumothorax** (Figure 23-4).

As air passes in and out of an open chest wound, it can create a sucking-type sound. Whenever such a **sucking chest wound** is discovered, the EMT should consider the possibility of a pneumothorax.

The mechanism of injury should suggest to the EMT that a penetrating injury, and a pneumothorax, could be present. The signs of a pneumothorax include difficulty with breathing, cyanosis, and diminished breath sounds on the affected side.

After ensuring the patient has a patent airway, the EMT should proceed to examine the chest wall for holes, lacerations, or open wounds. Some chest wounds are very small, smaller than a dime; therefore, a careful inspection is needed. The EMT should look in the armpits (axilla) as well as under folds of skin.

Management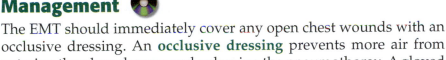

The EMT should immediately cover any open chest wounds with an occlusive dressing. An **occlusive dressing** prevents more air from entering the pleural space and enlarging the pneumothorax. A gloved hand, placed over the open wound, is an effective temporary occlusive dressing. A more effective dressing is usually prepared using clear plastic wrap or aluminum foil placed over a 4-by-4-inch Vaseline gauze dressing.

To prevent the continued buildup of air in the pleural space during each breath, the EMT must create a dressing that does not allow air to enter the chest from the outside, yet still allows excess air to exit when necessary. This type of dressing can be created by securing an occlusive dressing on only three of the four sides (Figure 23-5). The fourth side acts as a flutter valve and allows air to escape if needed. When the patient breathes in, the negative pressure of inspiration draws the dressing against the wound, sealing the wound in the process. When the patient exhales, the positive pressure of exhalation allows excess air to escape from under the dressing.

High-concentration oxygen should be administered to the patient with an open chest wound, and the patient should be transported with her unaffected side slightly elevated. Elevating the unaffected side allows the uninjured lung to inflate maximally. A bedroll or a rolled blanket under the backboard can be used to accomplish this task. The patient should then be transported as soon as possible. An advanced life support unit should intercept the ambulance if possible.

Tension Pneumothorax

Even with a flutter valve in place, air pressure can continue to build up inside the thoracic cavity, allowing a pneumothorax to enlarge.

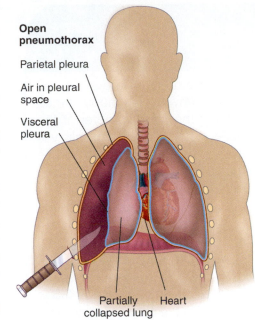

Open pneumothorax

Parietal pleura

Air in pleural space

Visceral pleura

Partially collapsed lung   Heart

- Chest wall defect
- Collapsed lung
- Ball valve effect

FIGURE 23-4 When air enters between the lung and the chest wall, *pneumothorax* is created.

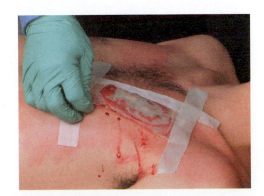

FIGURE 23-5 A sucking chest wound is covered with a 4-by-4-inch dressing that is secured on three sides; the fourth side is left open as a vent.

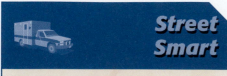

Street Smart

The area of injury around a bullet's pathway is many times greater than the diameter of the bullet. The large area of injury is the result of a concussion wave that follows in the wake of the projectile.

Because the spine extends the length of the trunk of the body, it is at great risk of injury from a gunshot wound (GSW). EMTs should implement spinal immobilization whenever a GSW is found in the chest or abdomen.

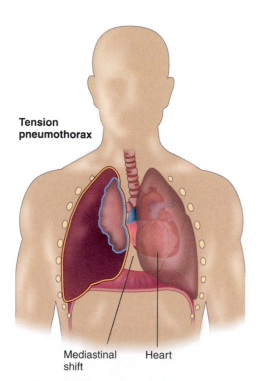

Tension pneumothorax

Mediastinal shift   Heart

FIGURE 23-6 Increasing pressure in the lung pushes the heart and great vessels to the opposite side of the chest.

The increasing pressure from the expanding air pocket can eventually collapse the lung entirely and start to push the organs in the middle of the chest, the mediastinum, to the opposite side of the chest.

When organs are pushed to the opposite side of the chest, the great vessels that empty into the heart, the vena cava, are crushed. The resultant kinking of the vena cava prevents blood from returning to the heart. In addition, the heart itself is compressed. The pressure around the heart makes effective contraction of the ventricles more difficult. Without adequate blood to fill the ventricles, and with ineffective contractions, the blood pressure falls.

This buildup of pressure in the pleural space that results in a decrease in blood pressure is called a **tension pneumothorax** (Figure 23-6). A tension pneumothorax is a potentially life-threatening condition that must be treated immediately. A tension pneumothorax can occur in both penetrating chest wounds and blunt trauma.

The signs of a tension pneumothorax include all the signs of a pneumothorax. A patient with a tension pneumothorax may also have distended neck veins, called jugular venous distension (JVD), due to a backup of blood from the compressed heart and vena cava.

When a patient has a tension pneumothorax, the patient's breathing may become so labored and rapid that the EMT is forced to assist her ventilation. When ventilations are delivered by bag-valve-mask (BVM), the EMT may note that ventilating the patient becomes increasingly more difficult. Increased difficulty with ventilation can be an indication of significant lung compression by the tension pneumothorax.

As a tension pneumothorax progresses, the organs in the mediastinum start to shift. Among these organs and structures is the trachea. Eventually the trachea shifts away from the affected side. **Tracheal deviation** is a late sign of a tension pneumothorax and may be seen by the EMT anteriorly in the neck, in the suprasternal area. The EMT may find it easier to feel than to see this movement of the trachea. The absence of tracheal deviation does not preclude the possibility of a tension pneumothorax. Signs of tension pneumothorax are outlined in Figure 23-7.

If a patient with an open chest wound becomes hypotensive, the EMT should immediately lift a corner of the occlusive dressing. Lifting a corner of the dressing may relieve the problem if the hypotension is being caused by an increase in pleural air pressure, and a tension pneumothorax. A hissing sound from escaping air is sometimes heard. After releasing the corner of the occlusive dressing, the EMT should immediately recheck the patient's blood pressure.

If the patient's blood pressure has not improved, the EMT should transport the patient immediately. An ALS unit should be contacted and met en route to the emergency room. ALS personnel have additional training with chest wound management. Table 23-1 summarizes the physical findings of pneumothorax.

Rib Fractures

The bony rib cage is intended to protect the vital organs within it. Trauma to the chest wall can result in broken or fractured ribs and injury to the underlying organs. Most rib fractures are the result of a

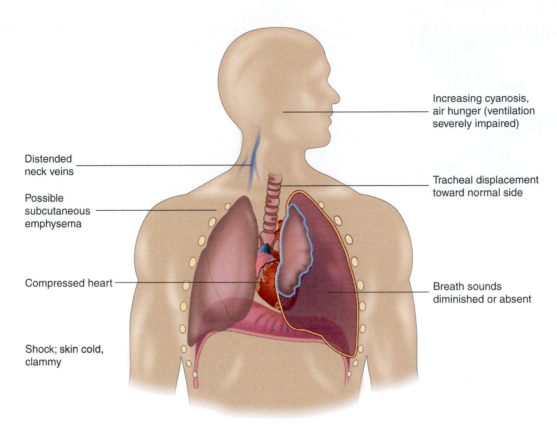

Increasing cyanosis, air hunger (ventilation severely impaired)

Distended neck veins

Possible subcutaneous emphysema

Tracheal displacement toward normal side

Compressed heart

Breath sounds diminished or absent

Shock; skin cold, clammy

FIGURE 23-7 A tension pneumothorax has all the findings of a simple pneumothorax as well as hypotension, JVD, tachycardia, and lack of breath sounds over the affected site.

TABLE 23-1

Signs of a Simple and Tension Pneumothorax*

Sign	Simple	Tension
Subcutaneous emphysema	+/–	+/–
Tachycardia	+	+
Tachypnea	+	+
Difficulty breathing (dyspnea)	+	+
Diminished breath sounds	+	+ (Absent)
Jugular venous distension	–	+
Loss of radial pulses	–	+
Decreased lung compliance	–	+
Hypotension	–	+
Tracheal deviation	–	+ (Late)

* Not all of these signs are present in every case.

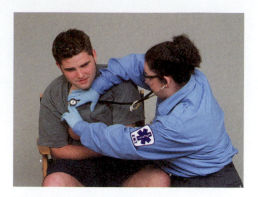

FIGURE 23-8 Breathing can be very painful with a fractured rib.

large force being distributed over a small area. Ribs are interwoven with muscles and tendons. When a rib is fractured, these muscles and tendons help to maintain the ribs in alignment. Local swelling and tenderness may be the only outward sign that a rib is broken.

Rib fractures can be very painful. Any deep breath or cough grinds the bone ends together and creates a sharp pain. When an EMT assesses a patient with a possible fractured rib, he may note shallow breathing as well as guarding of the injured area (Figure 23-8).

A rib fracture, despite being painful, is not by itself life threatening, but the EMT should be concerned about whether the broken rib has damaged the underlying lung. Ribs that are broken can be forced inward, puncture the lung, and then spring back into alignment. The EMT should carefully listen to breath sounds near any suspected rib fracture. The EMT should also be alert for signs of subcutaneous emphysema, which may indicate that the underlying lung has been injured.

Management

An EMT should move a patient with a rib fracture carefully to prevent the bone ends from puncturing a lung. Unlike other suspected bone injuries, the EMT cannot effectively splint a fractured rib. Instead, the EMT should administer oxygen and allow the patient to self-splint by assuming the most comfortable position possible. The patient should be encouraged to avoid any unnecessary movement.

Flail Segment

When three or more ribs are broken in two or more places, a segment of the rib cage may be detached from the rest. This **flail segment** of the chest is a free-floating portion of the rib cage.

When the patient inhales, the rib cage expands and is pulled outward and upward by the muscles. The flail segment does not move together with the rest of the ribs. The negative pressure created inside the thoracic cavity during inspiration draws the free-floating segment downward and inward, in the opposite direction. This movement of a section of ribs in the opposite direction of the rest of the chest wall is called **paradoxical motion** (Figure 23-9).

Paradoxical movement can significantly impair breathing and cause injury to the underlying lung as the segment moves in and out. To prevent the painful grinding of the rib ends, the flail segment must be stabilized.

Management

The EMT can quickly stabilize a flail segment by placing a gloved hand(s) over the injured area. Once manual stabilization has been done, a folded universal dressing may be placed over the segment and taped securely in place. The dressing will help to prevent the segment from moving but will not restrict the patient's breathing. The EMT should be careful not to encircle the chest wall when taping the dressing in place, as that would restrict breathing.

A large flail segment can significantly impair the patient's ability to breathe. As the patient becomes increasingly tachypneic, the EMT

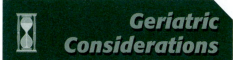

Geriatric Considerations

The bones of elderly patients are often brittle and easily broken. An elderly patient who falls from a standing position onto her side may fracture ribs. An EMT should perform a complete detailed physical examination of any elderly patient who has fallen. The EMT should take time to assess the ribs for any signs of pain, deformity, or swelling.

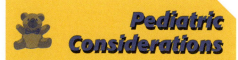

Pediatric Considerations

A child's ribs are so flexible that they can bend inward, puncture a lung, and then spring back into position without breaking. Pain on deep inspiration, point tenderness, and difficulty with breathing all may indicate that a child has injured her lung.

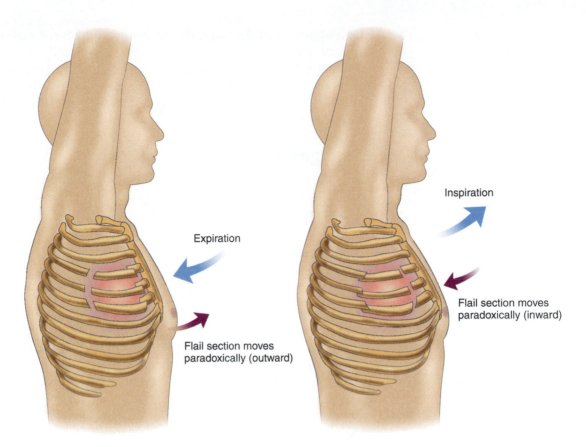

FIGURE 23-9 A flail segment impairs breathing because of its paradoxical motion.

may need to assist the patient's breathing. The positive pressure of the BVM fills the lungs equally, expanding both injured and uninjured ribs together. In a sense, the positive pressure of the BVM splints the flail segment internally.

Unless spinal precautions are needed, the patient should be transported on her side with the unaffected lung on top. Placing the patient on her injured side helps to stabilize the flail segment as well as decrease the pain the patient is experiencing from the moving bone ends.

Pulmonary Contusion

The lungs are rich with capillary beds, just like the skin. When a blunt force injures the skin, a contusion (bruise) forms. Similarly, when a blunt force injures a lung, bleeding into the lung itself results. This condition is known as a **pulmonary contusion**.

The bleeding and associated edema impair the lung's ability to exchange oxygen and carbon dioxide. If a large enough area of the lung is affected, the patient may become hypoxic and have trouble breathing. Like a bruise under the skin, a pulmonary contusion usually does not appear immediately but, rather, develops over a few hours.

Soft crackles may be heard over the site of the injury. Crackles can be an early indication of a developing pulmonary contusion. Chest pain, point tenderness, and localized swelling over the area of impact

 Safety Tip

In the past, sandbags were used to stabilize flail segments in the field. This practice has been discouraged, as the sandbags can decrease the chest wall movement and result in decreased lung volumes.

also suggest that the underlying lung might have sustained a pulmonary contusion.

When the alveoli are severely injured, bleeding can occur directly into the airway. The patient may cough up bright red, frothy blood. Coughing up blood, or **hemoptysis**, can be an indication of severe injury to the lungs.

Management

The care of pulmonary injuries revolves around supporting the patient's ventilation as needed and supplying high-flow supplemental oxygen to combat hypoxia.

Cardiac Contusion

When a significant blunt force is directed toward the sternum, the heart can be bruised. A **cardiac contusion** can impair the heart's ability to pump, just as a pulmonary contusion impairs the function of the lungs. Bleeding into the tissue of the heart can cause the heart to beat irregularly. The resulting irregular pulse should alert the EMT to the possibility of a cardiac contusion. The irregular pulse caused by a cardiac contusion rarely deteriorates into ventricular fibrillation but it can.

A massive cardiac contusion may decrease cardiac output and can result in hypotension. A large bruise forming on the anterior chest, along with chest pain and tenderness, may suggest a cardiac contusion.

Management

The patient who is suspected of having a cardiac contusion has suffered significant blunt trauma to the chest. The management priorities are similar to those of any patient in this situation: high-flow oxygen, ventilation support when needed, and support of circulation if appropriate. Because the patient with a cardiac contusion can deteriorate quickly, transport should not be delayed, and ALS should be requested.

If the patient goes into cardiac arrest, cardiopulmonary resuscitation (CPR) and/or defibrillation may be needed. The EMT should follow local protocols regarding the care and transportation of a trauma-arrested patient.

Pericardial Tamponade

Bleeding around the heart and into the pericardial sac that encloses the heart can lead to a condition called **pericardial tamponade**. This condition is usually a result of penetrating chest trauma with a laceration to the heart itself, although blunt trauma also can cause a tear in the heart and produce the same result. As with a tension pneumothorax, where air fills the pleural space and compresses the lungs, blood filling the pericardial sac during pericardial tamponade can compress the heart.

As blood accumulates in the pericardial sac, the ventricles become compressed. Blood that cannot enter the ventricles backs up into the neck veins, causing JVD. As blood continues to accumulate in the

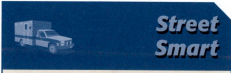

Street Smart

Contusions to the chest, heart, and lungs take time to develop. At the scene, the EMT may not have any outward indications of the injury. Careful patient assessment, using DCAP-BTLS, may reveal tenderness and reproducible pain on deep inspiration; these symptoms, along with localized swelling, may lead the EMT to suspect a chest injury.

An EMT should be even more suspicious of a chest injury if a careful assessment of the interior of the motor vehicle reveals a bent steering wheel or a locked seat belt. These are indicators that a significant force may have been applied to the patient's chest.

pericardial sac, the ventricles cannot expand and contract effectively. The difference between the pressure created by the contraction (systole) and the resting pressure (diastole) starts to narrow. The **pulse pressure**, the difference between systolic and diastolic blood pressures, may approach zero.

For the EMT in the field the most telling sign of cardiac tamponade may be the climbing heart rate, sustained above 120 beats per minute, and the weakening pulse, an indication of pulse pressure along with greatly distended neck veins.

The patient eventually becomes profoundly hypotensive and may go into cardiac arrest. Interestingly, the electrical system of the heart is usually unaffected, so although the patient may become pulseless, the electrical portion of the heart continues to function. Because this condition cannot be remedied by defibrillation, an automatic external defibrillator (AED) would likely indicate "no shock advised." Figure 23-10 summarizes the physical findings of pericardial tamponade.

Management

An EMT can do little in the field for patients with pericardial tamponade. The EMT should administer high-concentration oxygen, treat the patient for shock, and rapidly transport the patient to the emergency department. ALS personnel may have temporizing measures to offer and should be requested, but transport should not be delayed.

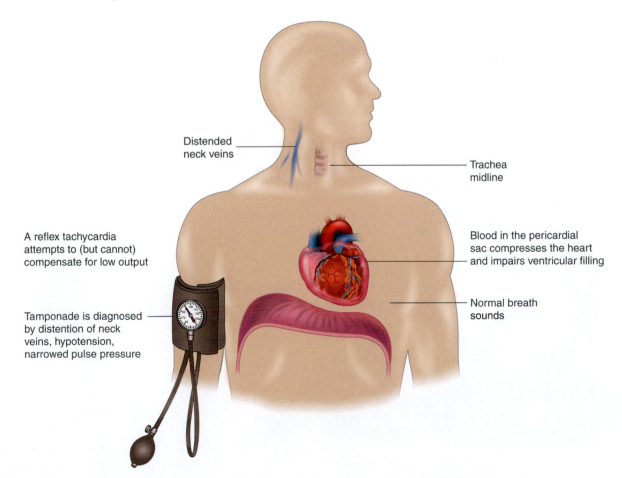

Distended neck veins

Trachea midline

A reflex tachycardia attempts to (but cannot) compensate for low output

Blood in the pericardial sac compresses the heart and impairs ventricular filling

Tamponade is diagnosed by distention of neck veins, hypotension, narrowed pulse pressure

Normal breath sounds

FIGURE 23-10   A narrowed pulse pressure and neck vein distension are signs of pericardial tamponade.

Physicians may insert a needle into the pericardial sac to remove the blood that is compressing the heart. Early notification will help the hospital staff to properly prepare for the patient.

Aortic Injury

In sudden decelerations, such as a high-speed, head-on motor vehicle collision, the organs inside the body are thrown forcefully against the front of the body. When this occurs, tears may result to various organs. The most significant of these tears is probably one in the aorta. In a sudden deceleration, the heart and aorta are thrown forward into the anterior chest wall. However, a section of the aorta is well secured into the back of the chest by a ligament. As the rest of the aorta is forcefully thrown forward, a tear can result at the site where it is held back (Figure 23-11). If the tear is completely through the aorta, the patient will die in minutes, as all of the patient's blood will be pumped out of the torn aorta into the chest. If the tear is incomplete, severe bleeding can still occur, but the patient may not die immediately.

Management

The EMT can recognize the potential for an aortic injury by identifying that a significant deceleration has occurred and noticing that the patient has chest discomfort or evidence of shock. An EMT in this situation should support the airway, breathing, and circulation as appropriate and should rapidly transport the patient to the most appropriate hospital. ALS care en route may be helpful, although transportation should not be delayed.

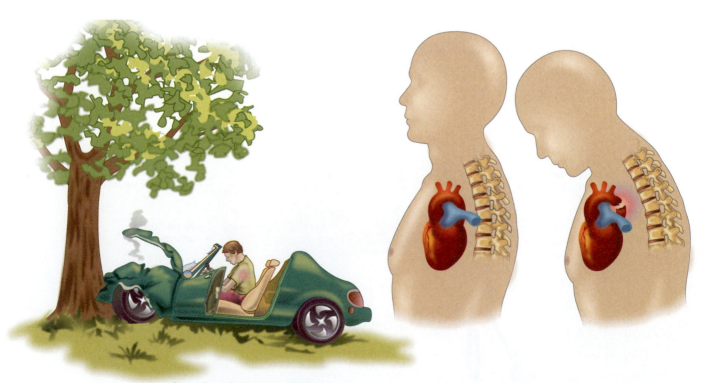

Shear force from a car accident could result in this type of injury

FIGURE 23-11 The aorta can be torn during a sudden deceleration.

Traumatic Asphyxia

When the chest is compressed rapidly, internal pressure increases dramatically, and blood is immediately forced out of the chest and into the vessels in the neck, head, and face. The neck veins instantly become distended (JVD). Cyanosis is apparent in the face, and bleeding into the sclera (white) of the eyes may occur. Small blood vessels in the cheeks and on the face may burst and bleed under the skin. These small red spots on the surface of the skin are called **petechiae**. The sudden increased blood flow to the brain also may result in brain swelling or bleeding.

Such a rapid ejection of blood and air out of the chest is called a **traumatic asphyxia**. Potential causes of traumatic asphyxia include being crushed or pinned between two objects.

Management

Crushing injuries to the chest may result in significant intrathoracic injury as well as injury to the brain, as described earlier. The injuries to the chest may result in hypotension and/or cardiac arrest. The EMT should address the airway, breathing, and circulation and should initiate rapid transport to the closest appropriate hospital.

✳ *Fall from a Roof*

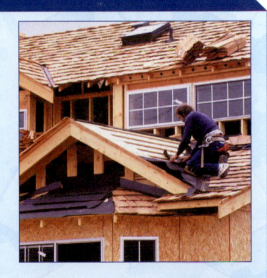

"Where's the paramedic?" asked the triage nurse. Kvar, a new EMT with Village Ambulance, answered, "His vital signs were stable on scene, so the medic thought we could take it in alone."

The triage nurse interrupted the conversation to alert the staff to the arrival of the patient needing trauma resuscitation. Then she told Kvar, "Look, he barely has a radial pulse, his heart's racing, and his belly is as hard as a rock. Even a rookie EMT could see this was going to happen!"

Kvar stammered as he replied, "We just thought it was the pain . . . but he looked like a rose!"

Just then, as the team passed the patient from the gurney to the stretcher, the ER physician interrupted and said to Kvar, "Tell me the story again."

Kvar answered, "He was replacing his roof, slipped and fell, oh, maybe 15 feet, and landed on his side. His only complaint was that his ribs hurt."

- Based on the mechanism of injury, what injuries might an EMT suspect?
- What are the assessment priorities for this patient?
- What are the management priorities for this patient?
- How could this patient deteriorate?

ABDOMINAL TRAUMA

Although many of the abdominal organs are situated so that they are protected by the lower rib cage or the pelvis, injury to intra-abdominal organs can occur as a result of blunt or penetrating trauma. The EMT should be familiar with the location of the intra-abdominal organs and the principles of management of the patient with abdominal injuries.

Mechanism of Injury

Although it is difficult to determine the exact extent of injury in the field, the EMT can expect certain types of injuries based upon the mechanism.

Penetrating Abdominal Trauma

Although not as common as blunt abdominal injury, penetrating abdominal injury is often easier to recognize. A stab wound or gun-shot wound to the abdomen, no matter how superficial it appears on the surface, can seriously injure internal organs. The EMT should gather as much information as possible regarding the mechanism to help him in identifying the injuries.

If the injury was caused by a stabbing, the EMT should attempt to determine what the patient was stabbed with. Was it a 3-inch switch-blade or a 12-inch hunting knife? If the patient sustained a gunshot wound, what was the caliber of the weapon? How many shots were fired and from what trajectory? These questions often can be answered by law enforcement personnel at the scene.

Blunt Abdominal Trauma

When the abdomen forcefully strikes an object, such as the bottom of the steering wheel, the skin starts to stretch. If the skin remains intact, a contusion may result. The energy continues to be passed on to internal organs in the abdomen.

If the steering wheel strikes the lower ribs in the upper abdomen, the liver and spleen may be injured. If the force is directed toward the lower abdominal area, some of the intestine will be crushed, spilling its contents into the abdominal cavity.

Finally, as the abdominal organs are rocked violently, veins and arteries may be torn. Shearing forces can be so great that an organ, such as the liver, can be torn in half. These injuries can cause significant bleeding. Table 23-2 summarizes the types of injuries that can result from blunt trauma to the abdomen.

Although the external signs of injury may not be as impressive in blunt trauma as in penetrating trauma, the potential for injury is just as great. The EMT must assess the mechanism of injury and determine the likelihood of an intra-abdominal injury.

The potential for injury to intra-abdominal organs exists whenever a patient has experienced impact directly to the abdomen. The EMT must determine whether such an impact has occurred or may have occurred. Information about whether the patient was punched or kicked in the abdomen or flanks is often available in the history of the

TABLE 23-2

Intra-abdominal Injuries Sustained from Blunt Trauma

Abdominal contusions

Liver laceration

Splenic rupture

Mesentery artery tears

Intestinal rupture

Kidney contusion

Bladder rupture

incident, but in the case of motor vehicle collisions, the body parts that suffered impact must be inferred from the damage to the vehicle.

If the patient slid down and underneath the steering wheel, the bottom of the steering wheel may have struck the patient in the abdomen. The EMT should lift the deflated airbag and examine the steering wheel to determine whether the bottom of it is bent. A bent steering wheel is a good indicator of serious abdominal trauma.

Although airbags, especially when coupled with use of a seat belt, have been very effective in preventing injuries and have saved countless lives, the EMT should keep in mind that in severe motor vehicle crashes, the patient may still sustain significant injuries. Also, most airbags, at present, are effective only in front-end collisions. The patient can sustain serious abdominal injuries in a lateral impact. The door can be pushed into the passenger compartment, striking the patient from the level of the hip to the level of the lower ribs.

Side airbag protection has been made available recently in certain automobile models. Until side airbag protection is available in all cars, however, the EMT must be alert to the possibility of abdominal injuries in any side collision where there is greater than 12 inches of intrusion into the passenger side (Figure 23-12).

Patients who wear seat belts improperly, for example, too high on the abdomen, may suffer injury to the abdomen in a collision. In addition, patients who do not wear seat belts at all will be thrown around the vehicle and perhaps ejected. Potential for serious abdominal injury is high in these situations.

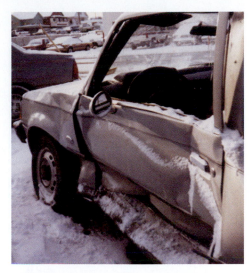

FIGURE 23-12 Side impacts can cause chest and abdominal injuries.

Signs and Symptoms

Although pain is the most commonly found symptom in patients with abdominal injuries, there are many cases in which the patient is unable to express this complaint, or just fails to notice it because of other injuries or factors. The unconscious patient or the patient with an altered mental status will not be able to provide reliable symptoms. In such cases, the EMT has to rely upon sometimes subtle physical findings and the mechanism of injury.

The EMT should assess for the following signs of abdominal injury: any evidence of deformities, contusions, abrasions, punctures, burns, tenderness, lacerations, or swelling to the lower chest, back, or abdomen.

Other signs of abdominal injury include abdominal wall rigidity, rebound tenderness, and abdominal distention. Abdominal wall rigidity can be the result of irritation of the peritoneal lining of the abdomen caused by the contents of rupture of hollow organs. This is often a late sign and may be confused with guarding, which can be involuntary tightening of the abdominal muscles or voluntary tightening (ticklishness). Rebound tenderness, another sign of peritoneal irritation, is pain that occurs as pressure is released by palpation. The EMT should focus on establishing point tenderness, the location of the discomfort, rather than establishing rebound tenderness or guarding. The third sign of abdominal injury is distention. Distention is the result of fluids, including blood, collecting in the abdominal cavity. Abdominal distention can be difficult to detect because the abdomen is so distensible. However, during a trauma assessment, any palpable

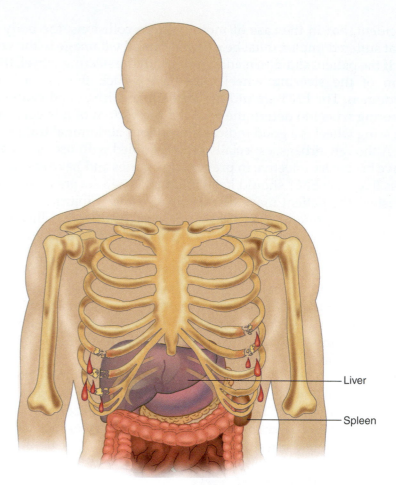

Liver

Spleen

FIGURE 23-13 Lower rib fractures can result in injury to the liver or spleen.

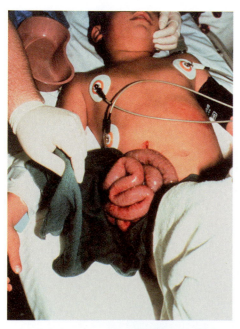

FIGURE 23-14 Penetrating trauma to the abdomen can result in evisceration of intestines. (Courtesy of Deborah Funk, MD, Albany Medical Center, Albany, NY.)

mass in the abdominal cavity should be assumed to indicate bleeding. The exact location of the mass should be noted and reported. These signs are generally less reliable in the field, and the EMT should focus on the patient's complaints of pain and assess for evidence of hypoperfusion.

The abdominal organs extend up into the lower chest, so lower rib injuries can often be associated with injury to the upper abdominal organs such as the liver and spleen (Figure 23-13).

Signs of penetrating trauma are often quite obvious to the EMT. Any puncture mark should be assumed to be associated with intra-abdominal injury. A larger opening in the abdominal wall may result in the internal organs, most often intestines, extruding out of the abdomen. The extrusion of intestines outside the abdomen as a result of penetrating trauma is called **evisceration** (Figure 23-14).

Assessment

The patient with abdominal injuries may have other injuries as well. The EMT must perform the usual assessment for a trauma patient in an orderly fashion, no matter how impressive a particular injury may seem. A scene size-up is needed to determine the safety of the area as well as the mechanism of injury. The EMT must complete the initial assessment quickly and address any immediately life-threatening conditions. The EMT also should complete the focused history and physical examination as outlined in Chapter 14, looking for evidence of serious injury. The detailed physical examination may be done during transport if appropriate.

An orderly manner of assessment of the patient with serious injuries is the best way to find and manage the patient's most life-threatening injuries.

Management

Because the diagnosis of specific abdominal injuries often is not made in the field, the EMT should treat the patient who has potential abdominal injuries with several familiar principles in mind. The pre-hospital care of an abdominal wound should focus on assessment and management of hemorrhage and hypoperfusion and on rapid transportation to a trauma center. Penetrating abdominal wounds frequently require surgical management.

The EMT should apply high-flow oxygen and support ventilation and circulation as necessary. One of the most important things an EMT can do for the patient with significant intra-abdominal injuries is to provide rapid transport to the closest appropriate hospital, usually a trauma center.

Transport

The greatest danger to the injured patient is excessive time spent on scene. The patient's best chance of survival depends on timely transport to a hospital capable of caring for the patient's injuries, along with appropriate emergency care while en route.

The EMT should continue his care of the patient during transport by completing the ongoing assessment as often as is indicated by the patient's condition. ALS should be requested to assist in the management of the seriously injured patient, and the EMT should follow local protocols regarding need for medical control.

Early notification of the destination hospital will enable the staff to make appropriate preparations to best care for the seriously injured patient.

Specific Conditions

Although the general management principles are the same, no matter the specific injury, there are several conditions that are worth addressing individually.

Liver and Spleen Injury

The liver and spleen are the most commonly injured abdominal organs. Both are very vascular organs and have the potential to bleed into the abdomen, causing shock. The EMT who recognizes such injuries can provide the appropriate therapy and warn the receiving hospital staff of the situation.

Contusions and abrasions over the lower rib cage with upper abdominal tenderness are signs of liver or spleen injury. These findings may not be present upon the first examination, so the ongoing assessment of the injured patient should include repeated abdominal examinations.

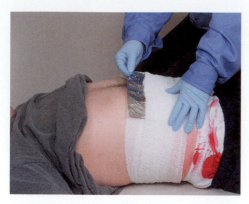

FIGURE 23-15 An evisceration should be covered with a moist sterile dressing and then a layer of aluminum foil to help retain the patient's body heat.

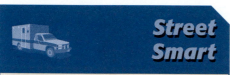

Street Smart

In the case of penetrating trauma, if a knife or any object is still impaled in the patient, the EMT should immediately stabilize the object in place with his gloved hands. The EMT should then use bulky dressings to stabilize the object and should transport the patient rapidly. Under no circumstances should an impaled object be removed from a patient's chest or abdomen.

Management

There is nothing an EMT can do in the field aside from the usual airway, breathing, and circulation support that will benefit the patient with a liver or spleen injury. Therefore, the best treatment the EMT can offer in this situation is rapid transport to the hospital.

Evisceration

A large abdominal wound may allow abdominal contents, such as the small intestine, to eviscerate through the wound opening. The EMT can recognize evisceration easily and should not let it distract him from addressing other potentially life-threatening issues.

Management

The EMT should never try to replace abdominal contents in the abdomen once they have eviscerated. Instead, the EMT should cover the protruding abdominal contents with a dry sterile dressing; some emergency medical services (EMS) authorities advocate the use of a moist dressing. A nonadherent dressing is preferred. The entire dressing should be reinforced with a large dressing, usually an abdominal or universal dressing. Frequently, EMTs cover the moist dressing with a sheet of aluminum foil (Figure 23-15). The aluminum foil helps to retain heat and protect the organs from further injury.

Pelvic Fractures

Fractures of the bony pelvis can result in injury to the underlying organs and vessels. A major problem with pelvic fractures is internal bleeding resulting in hemorrhagic shock. Fractures may be identified during the rapid trauma assessment by finding bony crepitus and tenderness during compression of the pelvic bones.

Management

If the EMT finds evidence of pelvic fractures on examination, he should consider military anti-shock trousers (MAST) use for stabilization along with rapid transport to a trauma center.

CONCLUSION

Serious trauma patients often have trauma to the chest and abdomen. Any major mechanism of injury has the potential to produce significant chest and abdominal trauma.

If the EMT suspects chest and abdominal injuries and assesses the patient with those suspicions in mind, he will have a greater chance of detecting life-threatening injuries, making the right decisions, and having a positive impact on the patient's outcome.

TEST YOUR KNOWLEDGE

1. What is the difference between blunt and penetrating trauma?
2. What differentiates a simple pneumothorax from a tension pneumothorax?
3. How does an EMT manage an open chest wound?
4. What are the signs of a fractured rib?
5. How does an EMT manage a flail chest segment?
6. What is an evisceration?
7. How does an EMT manage an evisceration?
8. What injuries can be caused by blunt trauma to the lower ribs?
9. How does an EMT manage a closed abdominal injury?

INTERNET RESOURCES

Search for articles related to chest and abdominal trauma at the following Web sites:

- eMedicine, http://www.emedicine.com
- Library of the National Medical Society, http://www.medical-library.org
- Trauma.org, http://www.trauma.org

FURTHER STUDY

Hunt, D. (1997). Thoracic park re-visited. *Emergency Medical Services, 26*(7), 47–57.

Keenan, D., & Phrampus, P. (1999). Puncture pathways. *Journal of Emergency Medical Services, 24*(9), 76–79.

Murphy, P. (1997). Gunshot wounds. *Journal of Emergency Medical Services, 22*(6), 74–79.

Phillips, K. (1997). Prehospital evaluation and care of the abdomen. *Emergency Medical Services, 26*(8), 37–40.

Rhodes, M., & Heightman, A. (1999). Retroperitoneal injuries. *Journal of Emergency Medical Services, 24*(4), 58–64.

Sahni, R. (1998). Chest trauma. *Journal of Emergency Medical Services, 23*(10), 86–90.

Stewart, C. (1999). Prehospital management of cardiothoracic trauma. *Emergency Medical Services, 28*(9), 37–45.

CHAPTER 24

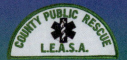

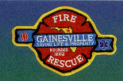

Soft Tissue Injuries

KEY TERMS

abrasion
amputation
avulsion
bandage
coagulation
cold zone
compartment syndrome
compress
conductor
contusion
cravat
crush injury
current
degloving avulsion
direct pressure
dressing
ecchymosis
elevate
embolism
Emergency Response
    Guidebook (ERG)
entrance wound
evisceration
exit wound
fasciotomy
figure-of-eight
full-thickness burn
gauze dressing
hematoma
hemorrhage

(continues)

OBJECTIVES

Upon completion of this chapter, the reader should be able to:

1. Identify different types of bleeding.
2. Describe the principles of bleeding control.
3. Describe the purpose of a sterile dressing.
4. Describe the major classification of wounds.
5. Discuss the indications and contraindications for using a tourniquet.
6. Classify the different types of bandages according to their use.
7. Explain why neck wounds are potentially lethal.
8. Explain the field care of an evisceration.
9. Explain the field care of an amputation.
10. Describe the classification of burn injuries.
11. Explain the care and management of a burn injury.
12. Explain how chemical burns are managed.
13. Describe the injuries that can occur from an electrical shock.
14. Explain the management of an electrical injury.

OVERVIEW

An emergency medical technician (EMT) seeing a pool of blood might be impressed by the apparent magnitude of the blood lost. Yet, the majority of people who are bleeding do not "bleed to death." That is not to say that bleeding cannot be fatal. Uncontrolled bleeding can lead to shock and even death. Fortunately, most external bleeding is easily controlled using some very simple maneuvers. This chapter reviews those methods as well as how to assess and treat other wounds.

ANATOMY REVIEW

The skin is a complex matrix of different cell types and specialized tissues. Together these cells protect the internal organs, regulate the internal environment, and allow us to sense our environment. The skin's cells and tissues constitute the largest organ system in the body, the **integumentary system**.

The integumentary system protects all of the internal organs of the body from the outside environment. Bacteria and other infectious agents cannot penetrate healthy, intact skin. Thus, the skin protects the body from infection. The skin is also very resilient. It withstands constant wear and tear. The skin stretches to allow movement or prevent penetration.

The skin works in the opposite way as well, that is, the skin keeps all of the bodily fluids, including blood, inside the body. A break in the skin can result in severe bleeding that can ultimately lead to death.

Injury to the Skin

If the skin is damaged, the first and immediate sensation is pain. Pain warns the body that its protective barrier has been injured. Injury also sets off internal protective responses, called **inflammation**. This complex process is the body's attempt to prevent infection and begin healing (Figure 24-1).

Imagine the skin as a dam. When the dam is breached, a river (blood) pours through the break. The alarm is sounded (pain), and rescue workers swarm to the scene to seal the breach (clotting). Provided the rescue workers have the right tools, in sufficient quantities, the dam's breach can be avoided and damage (infection) prevented. Any damage that remains will be repaired (scarring), and the dam will be as good as new.

BLEEDING

A wound is any break in the skin, and most wounds bleed. Some wounds bleed more vigorously than others. The amount of blood loss depends on how much skin is damaged and how much force is behind the bleeding. Of the two components of bleeding, the force behind the bleeding is the most important.

The blood in an artery is under a great deal of pressure when it leaves the heart. This force is called the systolic pressure. A cut to an artery can cause bright red blood to spurt across an ambulance compartment. (Oxygenated blood, on the arterial side, is generally bright red, whereas deoxygenated blood, usually on the venous side, is darker red, sometimes with a bluish hue.)

KEY TERMS

(continued)

impaled object

incision

inflammation

insulator

integumentary system

laceration

linear

Material Safety Data Sheet (MSDS)

necrotic

occlusive dressing

Occupational Safety and Health Administration (OSHA)

palmar method

partial-thickness burn

puncture

recurrent bandage

roller bandage

rule of nines

spiral bandage

stellate

straddle injury

stridor

sucking chest wound

superficial burn

tattooing

tourniquet

trauma dressing

triangular bandage

universal dressing

wound

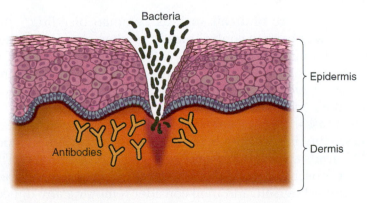

FIGURE 24-1 The body's response to injury is inflammation.

Profuse Bleeding

"Oh, that was stupid!" thought Janine. "I'm always in too much of a hurry." While dashing out of the house, Janine had reached for the door, missed the handle, and put her arm through the glass. Instinctively, she had pulled her arm back, which resulted in a long cut down the length of her forearm. Now she is bleeding profusely.

"This ought to be a trick; how am I going to do this?" Janine ponders as she holds a towel with one hand over the other arm and looks at the phone. "Maybe I can dial 9–1–1 with my nose." Janine drops the towel, dials 9–1–1, and picks up the towel, noticing that her arm is bleeding again.

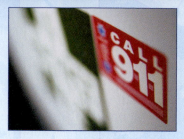

(Courtesy of PhotoDisc.)

A voice on the other end of the phone line says, "9–1–1, what is your emergency?" "EMS?" Janine asks. "Yes, ma'am," replies the communicator. "I'm bleeding," says Janine. "I cut my arm on some glass and now I'm bleeding and I can't stop it. Can you send help?"

- What are the immediate priorities in this case?
- How would an EMT control this bleeding?
- Is there a life threat here?

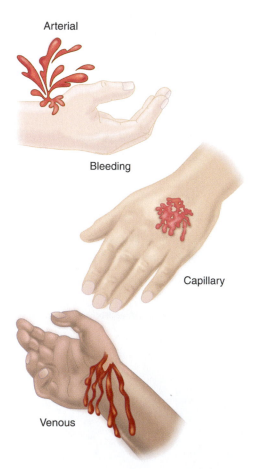

Arterial

Bleeding

Capillary

Venous

FIGURE 24-2 Arterial bleeding is bright red and spurts; capillary bleeding oozes; and venous bleeding is dark red and flows.

Capillary blood, on the other hand, is under very little pressure. This low pressure allows the blood to remain in the capillary beds while the cells extract the oxygen from the blood. As a result of this low pressure, when a capillary is cut, it oozes blood instead of spurting it.

The veins are at the end of the circulatory system. Usually a vein has been cut when serious bleeding is present. Because veins lie relatively close to the skin as compared to arteries, which usually lie next to bones, veins are at greater risk of injury. The blood returning to the heart in the veins is under low to moderate pressure. However, just because a vein does not spurt blood does not mean that a large amount of blood cannot be lost rapidly. Bleeding from a vein is usually constant, creating rivulets of blood that pour over the edge of the wound. The body's own protective mechanisms have difficulty controlling such bleeding. Figure 24-2 illustrates the different forms of bleeding.

Assessment

By the very nature of a call such as "woman bleeding," the EMT knows she will have to control bleeding when she gets to the scene. Special bleeding control supplies will be needed. The EMT should also be aware that large amounts of blood may be present, in which case the EMT will have to protect herself from possible exposure to blood and blood-borne infection.

In most cases, the EMT only has to wear examination gloves to protect herself; but in some cases, forceful bleeding can splash blood, and the EMT needs eye protection and a gown as well as gloves. The EMT should approach the scene wearing all the barrier devices she might need to protect herself, and then consider removing any unnecessary ones after the patient has been assessed.

Scene Size-Up

An EMT may feel awestruck when she sees a pool of blood next to a patient and want to immediately spring into action. Breaks and cuts in the skin, however, are usually caused by an object, such as a knife or machinery. The EMT should be mindful that the mechanism of injury can injure the EMT just as easily as it injured the patient. Therefore, the mechanism of injury should be assessed and rendered harmless before the EMT approaches the patient. Machines, for example, should be turned off and the power disconnected, and weapons should be removed from the area, before the EMT approaches the patient.

The EMT is also responsible for seeing that no one else gets hurt. This responsibility includes preventing bystanders from becoming exposed to the blood at the scene. A perimeter should be established around the patient to prevent onlookers from becoming contaminated. Sometimes just placing the "jump kit" or first aid bag in the way prevents well-meaning onlookers from trying to help.

Initial Assessment

In every case, the EMT must complete the initial assessment of the patient with a traumatic injury. The patient will be focused on the bleeding, but other problems, such as loss of the airway if the patient suddenly becomes unconscious, may be more important. The bleeding must be stopped, but the EMT must also constantly consider the patient's airway, breathing, and circulation.

In the past, ambulance drivers sometimes brought patients into the hospital with all the patients' wounds dressed perfectly, but the patients were dead. The EMT should always keep her attention on the important facts. Bleeding is not fatal; it is the hypoperfusion and resultant shock that kill the patient. Sometimes simply holding a towel over a wound while rapidly extricating the patient is more appropriate than making sure that each minor wound is dressed.

The EMT should always expose the entire length of the wounded limb. This exposure allows the EMT to better control the bleeding and to monitor the wound for further bleeding once the bleeding is controlled. Typically, the EMT uses a pair of scissors to cut pants or shirtsleeves on the seam and then moves the clothing away from the wound.

Management

Once the scene has been made safe, the EMT's first concern is to control the bleeding immediately. Fortunately, several means of controlling bleeding are available. In most cases, the EMT should begin with the easiest and safest techniques, and then progress methodically through the other techniques, always mindful of the principles of bleeding control.

Principles of Bleeding Control

When an EMT discovers severe bleeding, the first question the EMT asks herself is, "Can this bleeding lead to shock and possibly even death?" If the bleeding is not immediately life threatening, the EMT should continue with the initial assessment of the patient. If the

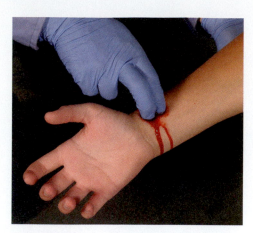

FIGURE 24-3 Firm direct pressure is very effective in stopping bleeding.

bleeding, or **hemorrhage**, is life threatening, it must be dealt with immediately. The following are some methods of controlling life-threatening bleeding.

First, the EMT should do nothing. The body does a good job of controlling hemorrhaging by itself. To stop bleeding, the body forms blood clots. Blood clots are made of clumps of cells, held together by strands of fiber. The clumps of cells eventually form an impenetrable barrier, and the bleeding stops. This process of blood clotting is called **coagulation**. For coagulation to occur, sufficient amounts of blood, with clotting factors, must be at the injury site. The process can be compared to building a dam. Without steel reinforcing rods, the concrete would crumble. Without concrete, the water would leak through the maze of rods. Together, the concrete and steel rods hold back the volume of water and create a dam.

To control active bleeding from a wound, the EMT should apply direct finger pressure to the bleeding site, exerting firm, constant force or, in other words, **direct pressure** on the wound (Figure 24-3). The EMT's actions are intended to support the body's own clotting activities. Direct pressure helps to slow the bleeding by compressing the blood vessels, allowing it to clot. As the bleeding slows, the blood's clotting elements have time to clump together and form a clot.

If bleeding continues despite direct pressure on the site itself, then the EMT should raise, or **elevate**, the wound above the level of the heart. Raising the wound above heart level helps to reduce the pressure at the wound site even more, and allows blood to pool and clot.

If bleeding continues, the EMT should apply an absorbent cloth, called a **dressing**, to the wound and continue to apply pressure (Figure 24-4).

Finally, if bleeding still has not stopped, the EMT must physically occlude the artery that is supplying blood to the wound. By applying manual pressure to the artery at a pressure point, where the artery lies next to a bone, the EMT can stop blood flow to the wound (Figure 24-5).

Any point where a pulse can be obtained is a pressure point to control hemorrhage (Figure 24-6). Pressure on the radial pulse may help control bleeding of the hand, although the ulnar artery on the anterior lateral wrist can supply collateral blood flow. Firm, direct pressure to the brachial artery can help control bleeding of the forearm, and direct pressure to the femoral artery, proximal to the inguinal area, can control bleeding of thigh.

Bleeding from the scalp or temple can be controlled by applying even, direct pressure to the temporal (temple) artery, and bleeding from a wound of the upper shoulder can be controlled by direct pressure to the subclavian artery, located immediately under the clavicle.

In some rare cases, the bleeding is so severe that direct pressure to the pressure point alone does not stop the bleeding. In those few cases, an arterial-constricting band, called a **tourniquet**, must be applied to the entire limb.

Desperate times require desperate measures. When severe bleeding that is life threatening absolutely cannot be stopped by any other means, a tourniquet must be used. This decision cannot be taken lightly. Application of a tourniquet may result in the loss of the limb. The situation, therefore, clearly must be one of "life over limb" before the EMT applies a tourniquet.

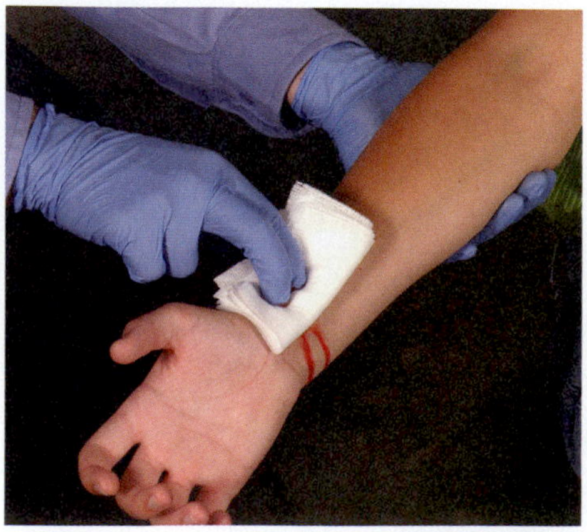

FIGURE 24-4 If bleeding continues, a dressing may be applied.

Any tight, constricting band placed over an artery will function as a tourniquet. This type of tourniquet should not be confused with the venous tourniquet that paramedics use to distend veins. An arterial tourniquet eliminates any pulses distal to the tourniquet. Without pulses, the distal bones, muscles, and skin die. Application of a tourniquet may result in the surgical amputation of the distal limb.

The EMT should choose a wide-width material, no less than 2 inches. Nylon straps also can be used to make a constricting band. The EMT places the band between the heart and the wound. The constricting band is placed about 2 inches from the wound. A small padded board may be placed under the band and above the pulse to concentrate pressure on the artery supplying blood to the distal limb. Once the band is in place, the EMT ties a knot over the artery, places a stick in the middle of the knot, and finishes tying the knot. The stick can then be used like a Spanish windlass; each rotation of the stick will apply pressure to the tourniquet and make it tighter and tighter. When the bleeding has stopped, the ends of the windlass should be tied to the extremity with another cravat.

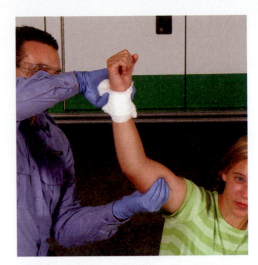

FIGURE 24-5   Manual pressure to a pressure point can limit blood flow to a wound.

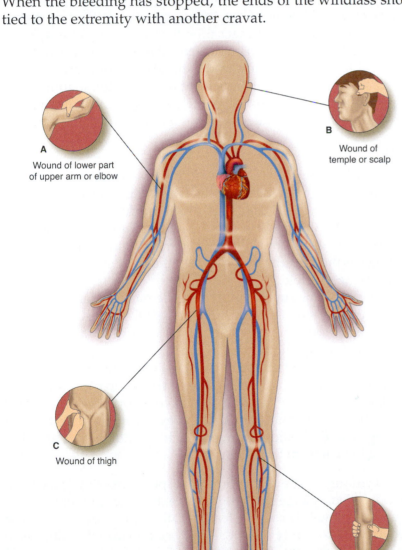

A
Wound of lower part of upper arm or elbow

B
Wound of temple or scalp

C
Wound of thigh

D
Wound of lower leg

FIGURE 24-6   Direct firm pressure to a pulse point will help to control bleeding.

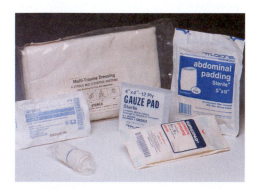

FIGURE 24-7 Varieties of dressings have been created for an even larger variety of wounds.

Once a tourniquet is in place, it should not be loosened or removed without a physician's order. If the tourniquet is prematurely released, blood clots may be liberated from the wound site to float upstream into the core circulation. The exact time that a tourniquet is applied should be noted. In some emergency medical services (EMS) systems, the practice is to write the time and the initials TK, for tourniquet, on the patient's forehead. Placing a piece of tape next to the tourniquet and noting the time on it is usually sufficient. Marking a tourniquet clearly makes the fact that the patient has a tourniquet more evident.

Dressings

Once bleeding has been controlled, wounds are covered by a dressing that is intended to protect the wound from further injury, while supporting the clotting activity that is going on inside the wound. These dressings should not introduce contamination into the wound; ideally, a sterile dressing should be used. Unfortunately, in the field, maintaining sterility is difficult. However, the EMT should apply the cleanest dressing possible.

Dressings should be furnished in a sterile package, and the EMT should keep the dressing in the original packaging as much as is practical, removing the dressing from the package only while wearing clean gloves. Dressings should never be placed on the ground, on the crew bench, or on any other "dirty" surface. Opening the packaging and laying it flat provides a sterile surface on which to place the dressing. The EMT should lift the dressing by the corners and place it directly on the wound, and then apply pressure over the outside of the dressing. The EMT should never touch the side of the dressing that is going to lie next to the wound.

Types of Dressings The most common type of dressing is a cotton weave cloth called a **gauze dressing**. Gauze dressings are remarkably flexible and absorbent. These two features allow gauze dressings to be wrapped around extremity wounds of any size. Gauze dressings also come in a variety of sizes, from the small 2-by-2-inch square (2×2) dressings, used for small puncture wounds, to the large trauma dressing (Figure 24-7). The **trauma dressing**, usually two layers of gauze with an absorbent cotton core, covers the majority of the abdomen, like a blanket.

Some dressings have a nonadherent material over the gauze to prevent the cotton from sticking to the wound's dried blood. Some are self-adherent dressings, which means the dressing sticks to the wound by itself. A Band-Aid is an example of a self-adherent dressing. Others are called **occlusive dressings**. Occlusive dressings prevent the escape of air and moisture from the wound and are often impregnated with a petroleum gel, such as the Vaseline gauze dressing, or covered with a thin plastic film. Occlusive dressings are useful in several special situations, discussed elsewhere in this book.

The **universal dressing** is a large, 9-by-36-inch dressing with several layers of absorbent cotton inside. The universal dressing can be laid flat and used like an abdominal dressing, or it can be folded into halves or smaller to make a smaller dressing. Universal dressings are very practical for mass casualty incidents when the EMT does not know what type or size of injury she may encounter.

Pressure Dressing   When bleeding continues despite direct pressure, a dressing, and elevation, then the EMT should use a pressure dressing. A pressure dressing, in effect, maintains continuous pressure over the wound edges and attempts to compress the surrounding blood vessels. In reality, the best pressure dressing that can be applied is the one that the EMT creates when she takes a dressing and applies manual pressure to the wound. It is not always practical, however, for an EMT to maintain constant pressure all the way to the hospital. When that is the case, a pressure dressing is applied to relieve the EMT of this task.

To create a pressure dressing, the EMT starts by placing a roll of Kling or a roller bandage directly against the dressing over the wound. Then using either a roller bandage or cravat, the EMT ties down the rolled bandage firmly and tightly. Often the knot is placed over the wound site to help maintain the added pressure (Figure 24-8).

Transportation

The priority of the patient's transport is not dictated by the type of bleeding, but rather by the presence or absence of hypoperfusion. Therefore, a complete set of vital signs is critically important to the EMT's decision-making process. The EMT should ask herself, "Is this bleeding life threatening? Is the patient showing signs of hypoperfusion and going into shock?" The answers to these questions will help the EMT to determine the priority and destination of the patient.

TYPES OF WOUNDS

Injuries to the skin can result from either blunt forces, like a baseball bat, or from sharp edges, like a knife. Each mechanism of injury leaves a break in the skin called a **wound**. The following is a review of common skin wounds and the mechanisms that might create them.

Abrasions

When the uppermost layer of skin is scraped away, minor capillary bleeding occurs, nerve endings are exposed, and an **abrasion** results.

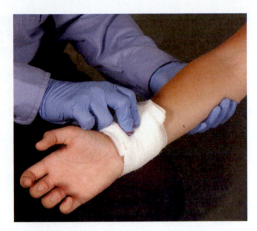

FIGURE 24-8   A pressure dressing helps to maintain constant pressure over the bleeding.

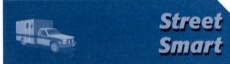

Street Smart

The body has a limited ability to clot blood. Removing old dressings and replacing them with fresh dressings disturbs clot formation and restarts bleeding. Before dressing any wound, the EMT should examine the wound carefully. The EMT should remove debris and then estimate the depth, length, and width of the wound. The exact findings should always be reported to the next provider or to the hospital staff. Making careful observations and reporting them to other providers will discourage the other providers from "breaking down the dressing" to see the wound.

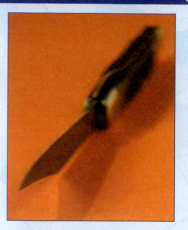
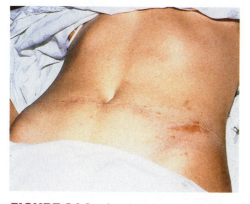

FIGURE 24-9 An abrasion usually oozes capillary blood. (Courtesy of Deborah Funk, MD, Albany Medical Center, Albany, NY.)

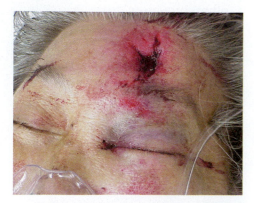

FIGURE 24-10 A blunt trauma can result in a stellate laceration. (Courtesy of Ron Straum, MD, Albany Medical Center, Albany, NY.)

Abrasions are usually the result of the skin on an arm or leg being rubbed against a solid surface (Figure 24-9). If the skin is rubbed against a carpet, for example, an abrasion may result. The rub burn, like a thermal burn, removes the upper layer of skin, and the resulting abrasion is painful.

A fall forward onto outstretched hands can create abrasions on the palms of the hands. A cyclist who is thrown from his bicycle onto the asphalt roadway may acquire an abrasion called a "road rash." A wilderness EMT who slides down a rope bare-handed may develop a "rope burn." In fact, whenever a body in motion contacts a rough surface, the chance of an abrasion is great.

Lacerations

When a large amount of force is applied to a small area of skin, the skin will tear. A skin tear that is the full thickness of the skin is called a **laceration**. Typically, the edge of a laceration is jagged and uneven. When a laceration is allowed to heal without surgical repair, the result is an irregularly shaped scar.

Because a laceration is deep, it can involve veins and arteries, as well as bones. An EMT who observes a laceration should always be concerned about the tissues underneath. For example, a bone that is broken and is forced through the skin creates a laceration. Frequently, the bone ends fall back under the skin as the limb returns to its normal anatomic position. The only evidence of this bone injury may be the laceration. All lacerations over bones should be considered evidence of bone injury and should be treated accordingly.

If the skin is struck with the straight edge of a surface, the laceration will be straight or **linear**. If the skin is struck with a blunt force, such as the ground, the laceration will take on a starlike, or **stellate**, appearance (Figure 24-10).

Incisions

An **incision** is a full-thickness injury of the skin. Unlike a laceration, an incision is usually made by a knife, which goes through the full thickness of the skin. Also unlike a laceration, the wound edges are straight and the surrounding tissue has not been stretched or injured (Figure 24-11). An incision can interrupt veins and arteries that lie immediately underneath the skin, causing potentially life-threatening bleeding.

Punctures

A **puncture** is an incision made by a sharp, pointed object. The EMT should have the same issues and concerns about a puncture wound that she should have about an incision. The severity of a puncture depends upon the depth and the location of the injury. Gunshot wounds (GSWs) are generally considered puncture wounds. Most of the damage done by a GSW is hidden under the skin and is not visible (Figure 24-12). Therefore, all GSWs should be considered serious.

A GSW typically makes an entrance wound that appears like a puncture and leaves a much larger exit wound as the blast creates an opening in the body. Every effort should be made to find all wounds associated with a GSW. If the weapon was discharged close to the patient, the entrance wound may have black speckles of partially burnt gunpowder on and around it. This phenomenon is called **tattooing**.

Avulsions and Amputations

The clean removal of a limb from the body, resulting in a clear line of demarcation, is called an **amputation**. A doctor surgically removes, or amputates, a lifeless extremity from the patient's body when there is no hope of recovery.

The forceful separation of a limb from the body because of trauma is properly called an **avulsion**. The forceful tearing of the skin leaves the wound margins ragged, and the remaining tissue may appear shredded. An avulsion can be either partial or complete.

EMTs commonly call a complete avulsion an amputation. Although not technically correct, this usage is widely accepted, and the two terms often are used interchangeably.

Assessment

A cut in the skin implies that some violence occurred. The source of that violence should be identified and neutralized whenever possible. Law enforcement officers should detain the perpetrator or establish a perimeter around the patient. In some cases, it may be wiser to move the patient to the back of the ambulance before examining him, provided he is capable of walking and no immediately life-threatening injuries are present.

Scene Size-Up

The EMT should be aware that the cause of the trauma that caused the bleeding, that is, the mechanism of injury, can cause the EMT injury.

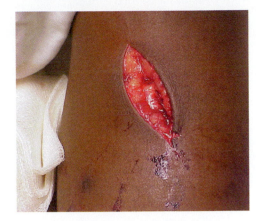

FIGURE 24-11 The small entrance wound of an incision can be deceptive. A larger area of injury can lie under the skin. (Courtesy of Ron Straum, MD, Albany Medical Center, Albany, NY.)

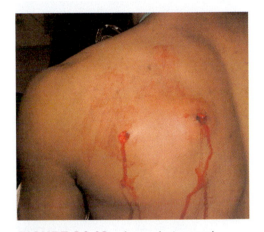

FIGURE 24-12 A gunshot wound (GSW) is a common puncture wound. (Courtesy of Deborah Funk, MD, Albany Medical Center, Albany, NY.)

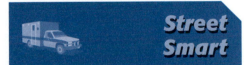

Street Smart

An entrance wound is typically smaller than an exit wound, but this is not universally true. Furthermore, a bullet may break apart and create several exit wounds, or none at all. The EMT should concentrate on finding all wounds. An EMT who is satisfied with finding two wounds may leave other wounds undiscovered.

Therefore, the EMT should identify the mechanism of injury and either render it safe by disabling it or by moving the patient away from the immediate danger to a safe location before proceeding with patient care.

It is fair to assume that if the patient is cut, then the patient also may be bleeding. Standard precautions against blood should be taken by the EMT before she approaches the scene. The EMT should carefully evaluate the scene as well as the patient for possible sources of blood contamination.

Initial Assessment

Initially, the EMT may be absorbed by the gross appearance of the wound; however, the EMT should remember that the external appearance of the wound is only part of the story. What has happened under the skin may be life threatening, and the EMT should focus on assessing for signs of hypoperfusion, such as tachycardia and tachypnea.

Rapid Trauma Assessment

Assuming that no life-threatening injuries have been identified, the EMT should proceed with a complete head-to-toe rapid trauma assessment while at the scene. The EMT should focus on the DCAP-BTLS (see Table 14-3) to identify other injuries as well as wounds.

Management

Once the bleeding has been controlled, the EMT's next priority in wound management is to protect the wound from further injury as well as contamination by applying a dressing and bandaging the wound.

Bandages

The primary purpose of a **bandage** is to hold a dressing in place. Bandages are strips of cloth or similar materials that serve this purpose. A bandage should be clean, but it does not need to be sterile as long as a dressing is against the wound. Bandages can also be utilized to apply pressure, over the dressing, to the wound site. This additional pressure can help to control bleeding.

A **roller bandage**, a cotton cloth rolled into a cylinder, is wrapped around and around the dressing until the dressing is held in place (Figure 24-13). Most roller bandages are one-headed, meaning that the bandage can be rolled in only one direction. Two-headed roller bandages are sometimes more convenient; they can be rolled in two directions at once, while still maintaining pressure on the dressing.

The military **compress** is a cotton dressing integrated into a two-tailed bandage or cravat (Figure 24-14). One provider can apply the dressing and wrap the bandage around the wound at the same time. Prepackaged for use in combat, these compresses are very convenient for use in the field by civilian EMTs as well.

Some roller bandages have elastic fibers woven into the fabric. The result is a flexible, elastic bandage that applies constant pressure to prevent swelling. The Ace bandage is an example of an elastic bandage. Ace bandages are very useful when the EMT wants to apply pressure to a wide area, such as an ankle, to prevent further bleeding and swelling.

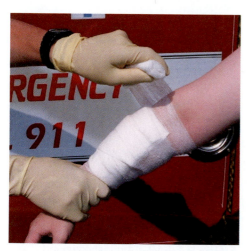

FIGURE 24-13 A roller bandage has a tail that can be anchored and then wrapped around the extremity.

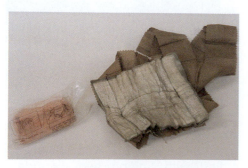

FIGURE 24-14 A military compress has a dressing integrated into the bandage, making it convenient to use in an emergency.

The alternative to a roller bandage is the **triangular bandage**. The triangular bandage is made by cutting a 36-inch- or 42-inch-square piece of muslin cloth from corner to corner (Figure 24-15). The results are two triangular bandages. Triangular bandages have been used in many ways over the years. The first "Advanced First Aiders" were extensively trained in the application of the triangular bandage to every part of the body. The triangular bandage has fallen out of favor somewhat with EMTs who prefer the shape-conforming, self-adhering gauze bandages available today.

Sometimes EMTs start at the apex of the triangle and fold the bandage into a strong belt. This belt, called a **cravat**, can be used instead of a roller bandage to tie dressings into place.

The saying "one size fits no one" often applies in EMS; sometimes the EMT must be creative with the application of EMS equipment. A cravat is often used to extend straps or adapt standard equipment, such as splints and backboards, to extremely small people, like children, and to extremely large people.

Although it is not frequently used in the field, an EMT might encounter a 12- to 18-inch-wide and 4-foot-long binder bandage. Binders wrap around the circumference of the patient's chest or abdomen to hold a dressing in place. Some binders are tied in place, while others use Velcro fasteners. Binders are usually used when trying to stabilize a large dressing. A large towel, wrapped around the abdomen like a binder, will hold several layers of abdominal dressings in place.

Principles of Wound Bandaging

Wounds can occur on the chest, on the abdomen, or on the extremities. Wounds can occur along flat skin, like the small of the back, or at joints, like the knees. All of these wounds are dressed somewhat differently. Several fundamental bandaging techniques help to reduce the confusion with wound bandaging. Whether used individually or combined, these bandaging techniques help the EMT to maintain bleeding control by effectively maintaining wound edges in close proximity, while keeping the dressing in place.

Recurrent Bandage

A **recurrent bandage** is useful when the EMT is trying to hold a dressing down over a large area. Using a roller bandage, the EMT starts by anchoring the bandage with either one hand or a wrap around the narrowest portion of the limb. Then the bandage is passed over the dressing and anchored on the opposite side. The roller bandage is then passed back and forth over the dressing. Finally, the two anchors are wrapped securely and the ends are taped or pinned (Figure 24-16).

Spiral Bandage

Using a roller bandage, the EMT starts by anchoring the bandage, with a wrap, around the narrowest part of the limb. Then the bandage is wound around the limb in a corkscrew fashion. Each wrap should cover about one-half of the previous wrap to ensure complete coverage of the dressing. When completed, the **spiral bandage** looks like a barber's pole (Figure 24-17).

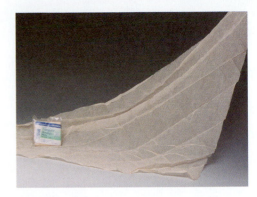

FIGURE 24-15 A triangular bandage was perhaps the most commonly used in the field before the development of roller gauze.

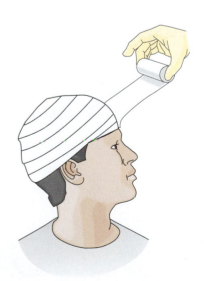

FIGURE 24-16 A recurrent bandage of the head holds a dressing in place.

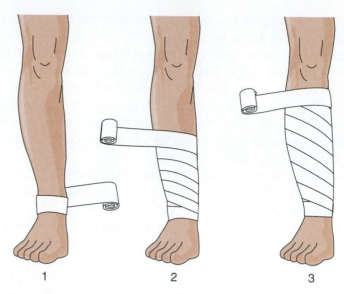

FIGURE 24-17 A spiral bandage is wrapped around the extremity, like the stripes on a barber's pole.

Figure-of-Eight

In a **figure-of-eight**, the roller bandage turns across itself like a figure-of-eight. The end of the bandage is often just "tucked in" to the preceding winds of the bandage. The figure-of-eight is particularly useful for holding dressings on wounds in the joints (Figure 24-18).

Figure 24-19 (A through M) demonstrates how these three bandaging techniques are used, individually or in combination, on a large variety of wounds. EMTs are expected to be proficient at wound dressing. The key to success in wound bandaging is practice.

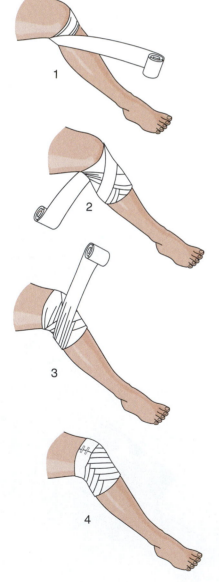

FIGURE 24-18 A figure-of-eight is anchored against itself.

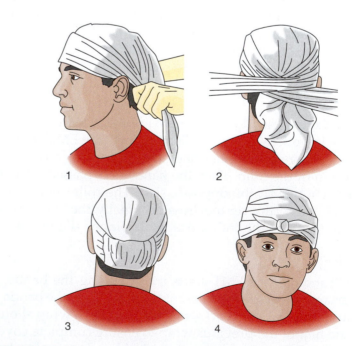

FIGURE 24-19A A. A triangular bandage has been applied over a head wound.

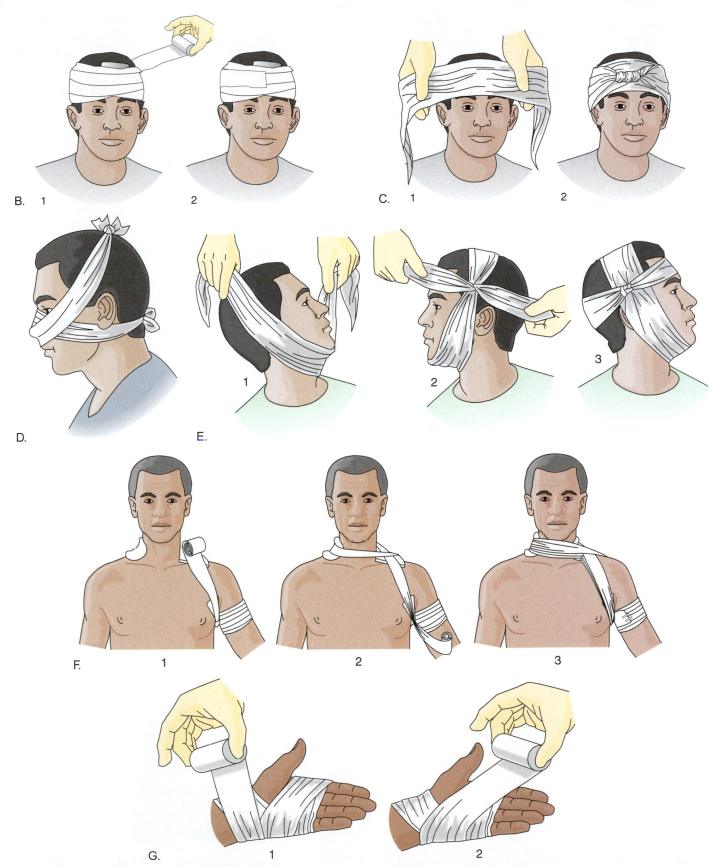

FIGURE 24-19B–G B. A roller bandage holds a dressing on a scalp wound. C. A cravat holds a dressing over a forehead wound. D. A four-tailed dressing created from two triangular bandages holds a dressing under a nose wound. E. The juxtaposition of two cravats holds a dressing onto an ear injury. F. An occlusive dressing is held in place by a roller bandage. G. A figure-of-eight bandage holds a dressing on a dorsal hand wound.

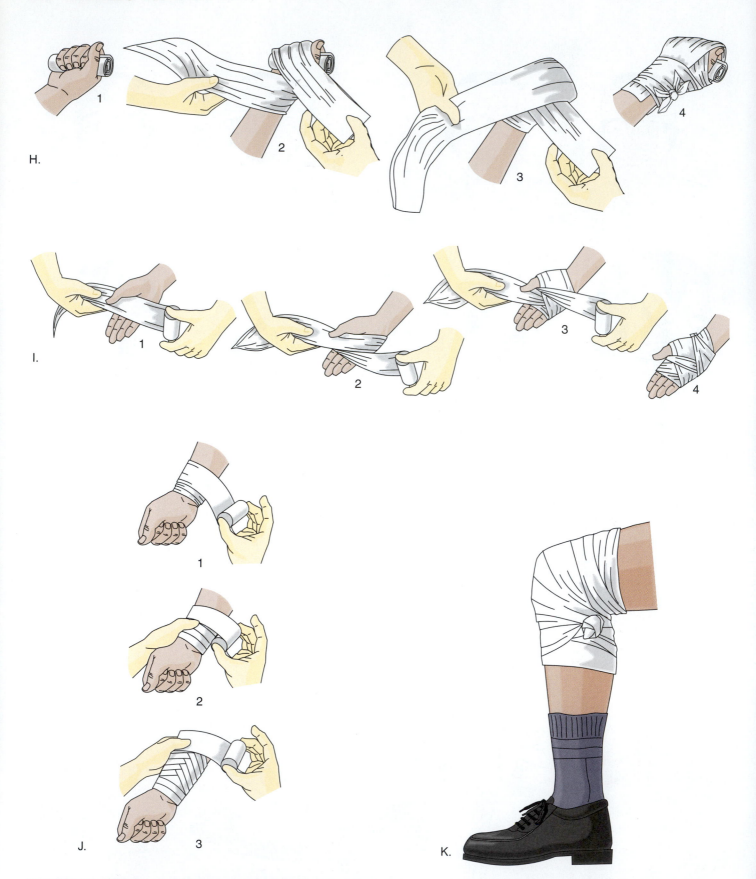

FIGURE 24-19H–K H. A triangular bandage holds a dressing over an entire hand, like a boxer's glove. I. A triangular bandage across a palmer injury holds a dressing a place. J. A reversed spiral roller bandage holds a dressing in place on a forearm. K. A triangular bandage holds a dressing in place on the knee.

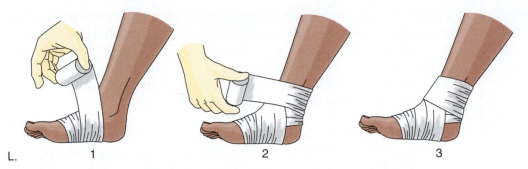

FIGURE 24-19L L. A foot wound is bandaged with a spiral roller bandage.

Special Bandages

Some wounds require special or unique bandages. The following is a review of some of those wounds and the bandages that would be used for them.

Neck Wounds A deep cut to the throat can lacerate a jugular vein. When the patient takes in a breath, negative pressure, created in the chest cavity, will draw air directly into the neck wound. This air creates a blockage, or **embolism**, that can occlude the vein and interfere with circulation.

To prevent an air embolism, an occlusive dressing must be immediately applied to any neck wound. Often a gloved hand is sufficient until a dressing can be assembled. Once the wound is properly dressed, the patient should be closely monitored for signs of hypoxia.

Sucking Chest Wound When the chest wall is penetrated, air moves in and out of the wound. This type of wound is called a **sucking chest wound**. Whatever the cause of the injury, it is important to stop air from entering the chest cavity. An occlusive dressing is used for this purpose.

An occlusive dressing is applied, and three sides are taped down while the fourth side is left unattached so that it can operate as a flutter valve. Air that is escaping will lift the fourth side, but air is prevented from entering when the dressing is "sucked" into the wound. More details about a three-sided dressing are provided in Chapter 23.

Evisceration An abdominal organ that protrudes through an open abdominal wound is called an **evisceration**. Although an evisceration may be gruesome in appearance, it is rarely immediately life threatening. Associated injuries to deeper internal organs may be more acutely dangerous.

Once any life-threatening conditions have been dealt with, the EMT should turn her attention to the evisceration. The EMT should not attempt to place the tissue back into the abdominal cavity. Any obvious gross contamination, such as glass fragments and the like, should be removed from the wound. The EMT should cover the protruding tissue with a dry, sterile dressing. The large trauma dressing was designed for this purpose. Some EMS authorities advocate the use of

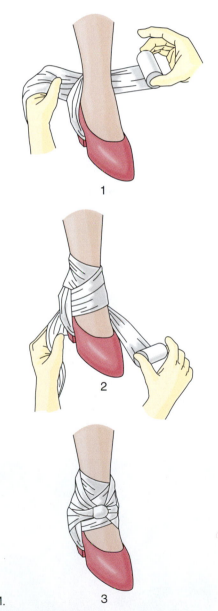

FIGURE 24-19M M. A triangular bandage holds a dressing in place on a foot.

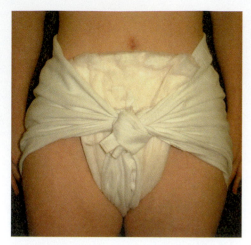

FIGURE 24-20 A diaper bandage is created to hold a trauma dressing in place in the perineal area.

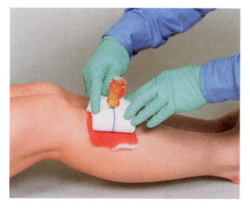

FIGURE 24-21 Two rolls of gauze can also help to stabilize an impaled object.

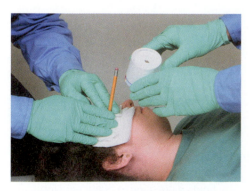

FIGURE 24-22 A cup helps hold an impaled object into the eye in place.

a moist dressing to keep the dressing from adhering to the tissue, and other EMS authorities advocate placing a layer of aluminum foil over the entire dressing to help retain heat. The EMT must follow the local medical protocols for the treatment of an evisceration. If the patient does not have any lower extremity injuries, having the patient flex his legs helps to relieve tension on the abdominal wall.

Straddle Injury While riding a motorcycle, a bicycle, or a horse, the rider may be thrown forward and strike his genitals against a post or other fixed object. The resulting soft tissue injury is called a **straddle injury**. Cuts and injuries to the perineal area or the genitals can bleed profusely. The EMT should place an abdominal dressing or a universal dressing against the perineum first; then, using a cravat, the EMT should create a belt and tie it around the waist. Taking a second triangular bandage, the EMT should place it, apex forward, between the patient's legs. The EMT then secures the three corners of the triangular bandage to the belt/cravat in diaperlike fashion (Figure 24-20). This type of bandage effectively holds the dressing in place and helps to control the bleeding.

Impaled Objects Any object that is discovered embedded in the patient is called an **impaled object** and should be stabilized in the position in which it is found. It is impossible to determine, in the field, the depth that the object may have penetrated and the internal organs that may have been injured. Therefore, the EMT would be imprudent if she removed the object. Rather, careful surgical extraction, with attention to bleeding control, is required; and this can be performed adequately only in the hospital.

The EMT should first manually stabilize the object to prevent further tissue injury. Then the EMT should carefully expose the wound by cutting any clothing from around the object. The EMT should be careful *not* to cut through the hole, if possible. Law enforcement officers may need the clothing, including the intact hole, for evidence.

If copious bleeding is present, it can be controlled by applying direct pressure to both sides of the object at once. The EMT should avoid applying any lateral pressure to the penetrating object, as that could cause further tissue injury.

If the object is still part of a larger assembly, for example, a fence post, the EMT may need to separate the impaled section from the larger assembly. Once the patient and the impaled object can be transported safely, the EMT should secure the impaled object with a large bulky bandage. A cravat can be rolled into a ring and placed around some narrow objects. Analogously, two rolls of gauze bandage can be placed on each side of the object to support it, and then a figure-of-eight bandage can be wrapped around the object and the extremity (Figure 24-21). Finally, a column of 4-by-4-inch (4 × 4) gauze pads, cut to the middle, can be stacked around the object to provide support as well as protection. Again, a figure-of-eight bandage is wrapped around the dressing to hold it in place.

If an object, like a pencil, is in the eye, a paper cup may be placed over the eye to stabilize the object (Figure 24-22). The EMT should puncture a hole in the bottom of the paper cup and slide the cup over the object, then tape the cup securely in place.

Street Smart

The exception to the rule "never remove an impaled object" occurs when the object is impaled in the cheek. Bleeding from an impaled object can create problems in the airway. Because pressure can be applied to both sides of the cheek to control bleeding, an impaled object in the cheek can be safely removed. Vigorous bleeding can occur after the object is removed. Suction needs to be ready in case the patient's mouth fills with blood.

Alternatively, if there is no bleeding into the mouth and no threat to the airway, the object can be safely left in place. In that case, the EMT should consider stabilizing the impaled object and preparing the patient for transportation.

Avulsions and Amputations   A partially avulsed limb should be reaffixed to its natural position. Areas of the body that are commonly partially avulsed include the nose, toes, ears, fingers, and the penis. The flap of skin holding the limb to the body may be supplying vitally needed blood to the avulsed limb.

Although amputations often stop bleeding spontaneously because the blood vessels contract into the stump and stop bleeding, avulsions tend to bleed vigorously because the blood vessels were torn, and not cut. The first priority, in every case of amputation or avulsion, is to control the bleeding. Poor control of bleeding by the EMT may lead to life-threatening blood loss.

The EMT's first action, after stabilizing the cervical spine, is to lay the patient down and elevate the stump above the level of the heart. Putting the patient in a modified Trendelenburg position will accomplish this.

If the bleeding persists, the EMT should take a moistened dressing and place it directly against the end of the stump. It is important that the EMT maintain constant pressure on the dressing and not release the dressing. Premature release of a dressing can lead to further, perhaps uncontrollable, blood loss.

Once the bleeding is controlled, several layers of dressings, as well as pressure on a pressure point, may be needed to maintain control. The EMT uses a triangular bandage to secure the dressings in place. First, the EMT places the stump and dressing in the middle of the triangular bandage. The two corners along the base are then wrapped around the stump and tied on the opposite side. The remaining corner, or the apex of the triangular dressing, is then tucked into the band that has been created (Figure 24-23).

While transporting the patient, keep the stump above the level of the heart. The EMT should administer oxygen, as per protocol, and monitor for signs of shock. The hospital should be alerted as soon as possible; surgeons should be on standby for the patient's arrival.

When the amputated part is found, it should be wrapped in moistened sterile gauze and placed in a plastic bag. A moist, but not wet, dressing is created by pouring sterile water over the sterile gauze dressing, and then squeezing out the excess water. A moist dressing does not drip water when it is squeezed.

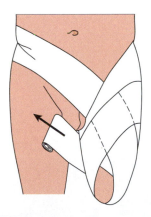

FIGURE 24-23   A roller bandage is applied to the stump remaining after an amputation, then held in place by a dressing.

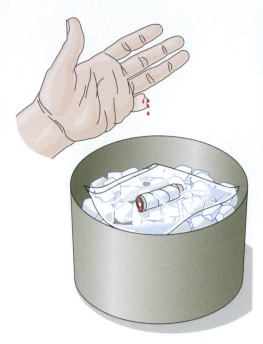

FIGURE 24-24 An amputated body part should be wrapped in moist gauze, placed in a plastic bag, then placed on an ice pack.

Street Smart

The EMT should not delay transportation of the patient with life-threatening injuries while searching for an amputated part. Life comes before limb. The EMT should transport the patient immediately, leaving personnel behind to search for the amputated part.

Personnel left behind to search for an amputated body part should organize a careful search of the area and take the time to find the amputated part. Snow blowers, chainsaws, and similar gas-powered devices can throw a body part a surprising distance; therefore, the search area should be generous.

When the body part is finally retrieved, it should be packaged and taken to the hospital quickly. Often a law enforcement officer can be enlisted to assist with transporting the body part to the hospital. The hospital should be advised immediately of the recovery and the impending arrival of the body part so that preparations can be made for reimplantation.

The EMT needs to keep the amputated body part cool, but not cold (Figure 24-24). Contact with ice, for example, can freeze the tissue. Frozen tissue cannot be reimplanted. Ice packs usually provide sufficient cooling.

Amputations of arms, hands, legs, and feet, unlike amputations of digits, are considered serious, and the patient with this type of amputation is high priority. Early notification of the hospital is important.

Degloving Avulsions Certain mechanisms, often high-speed spinning shafts, can rip the skin from the bone. For example, the power takeoff on a farm tractor can tear the flesh off a leg in seconds. When skin is completely torn from the shaft of an arm or leg, the wound is called a **degloving avulsion** (Figure 24-25).

Degloving avulsions should be treated in the same manner as any large wound. Great care should be taken in handling the extremity, as bone fractures often accompany a degloving avulsion.

Transportation

A wound can be very painful; rough handling and even rougher roads can make even the most stoic patient cry out in pain. The EMT should carefully consider whether any true threats to the patient's life exist, based on the EMT's assessment of the patient's perfusion. Often large wounds appear life threatening but in reality are not. If the patient does not have a life-threatening injury, the EMT should focus on caring and comforting the patient, including driving carefully to the hospital.

Ongoing Assessment

All bandages must be carefully monitored. Often a bandage becomes slack and loosens its hold on the dressing. Subsequently, the bleeding may begin again. On the other hand, swelling under the bandage may cause the bandage to act like a tourniquet. If this effect is not desired,

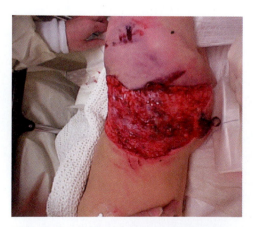

FIGURE 24-25 A degloving injury is seen most commonly around machinery. (Courtesy of Kevin Reilly, MD, Albany Medical Center, Albany, NY.)

the EMT must frequently, every time she takes a set of vital signs, for example, check the distal pulses. If the pulses have become weaker or are absent, the EMT may have to loosen the bandage, after checking the patient's perfusion status.

BRUISING

When a force is distributed over a large area, the skin may remain intact, but bleeding can occur immediately under the skin, in which case a bruise will form. The medical term for a bruise is a **contusion**.

Contusions imply that there can be damage to deeper tissues and organs. When an EMT discovers a contusion over the right lower ribs, for example, she must suspect that the liver underneath also may be injured. Although an EMT cannot see internal injury, she can have a high index of suspicion that certain organs are injured, based on the location of the contusion.

Hematoma

At various points on the body surface, arteries and veins run close to the skin. If a force, from hitting the floor during a fall, for example, impacts on one of these points, the blood vessel can tear. Bleeding can quickly form a swelling under the skin called a **hematoma**. A hematoma on the forehead is often called an "egg" by laypeople. A considerable amount of blood can be lost in a hematoma that is the size of an egg. A hematoma that is the size of the person's fist can mean that as much as 250 cc of blood have been removed from circulation.

✳ *Construction Accident*

"Help, I'm trapped," yells Fred. Fred had been working in a ditch when the shoring gave way and tons of sand and rock poured over and around him like an angry river. Now Fred can hardly breathe and is yelling for help.

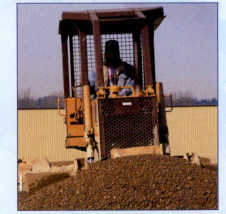

Fortunately, nearby workers call the local Emergency Services Department immediately. The EMTs in the rescue squad that arrives have just received training in confined space rescue. The rescue squad quickly and efficiently frees Fred from his entrapment and delivers him to the waiting ambulance in a Stokes basket.

Aboard the ambulance is Theola, a new EMT, and her field training officer, Sam. "Go ahead, Theola, check him out," Sam directs while he prepares to call for a paramedic intercept from the county.

- What potential harms could have befallen this patient while he was trapped?
- What assessment findings can the EMT expect to find when examining the patient?
- What are the EMT's priorities for managing the patient?

TABLE 24-1

Mechanisms of Crush Injury/Compartment Syndrome

1. Prolonged immobilization
   Falls
   Alcohol
   Drug overdose
   Stroke
   Broken hip

2. Entrapment
   Building collapse
   Mud slides
   Trench collapse

3. Prolonged extrication
   Airplane crash
   Extensive driver compartment intrusion
   Vehicle rollover
   Entrapment under vehicle

CRUSH INJURY

Prolonged pressure on the skin and underlying tissue, from the weight of a body, for example, will eventually cut off circulation, compromise nerve function, and cause the tissue to die or become **necrotic**. The result of this sustained pressure is called a **crush injury**.

When tissues are crushed, they release toxic chemicals, including acids, from within the cells into the surrounding tissues and into the bloodstream. Some of these chemicals are toxic to the body, especially to the kidneys. Often these chemicals can cause kidney failure hours or days after a crush injury.

Occasionally, when large amounts of acid are washed out from a crushed limb, the body's chemistry changes. The increased amount of acid in the blood, or acidosis, is very irritating to the heart. If the heart becomes too irritated, it can go into ventricular fibrillation and cause sudden cardiac death.

Compartment Syndrome

Muscles are enclosed and divided by thin sheets of fibrous tissue, called fascia, into individual compartments. If a limb is crushed under a large weight for a prolonged period, such as may occur in a cave-in, swelling within these muscular compartments results. As the swelling steadily worsens, the pressure within these compartments increases and compresses nerves and blood vessels. The result of compressed nerves and blood vessels is a loss of feeling, called paresthesia; a loss of motion, called paralysis; and a loss of circulation, or pulselessness. Together these three signs—paresthesia, paralysis, and pulselessness—indicate that the patient is experiencing **compartment syndrome**. Table 24-1 lists the mechanisms of injury that may result in compartment syndrome.

Compartment syndrome is a true surgical emergency. Treatment for compartment syndrome includes cutting through the skin and into the fascia to relieve the pressure. This surgical procedure is called a **fasciotomy**. In the field, treatment of the affected extremity includes

Street Smart

When a person is trapped under a heavy object, the weight applied to the limb acts like pressure on a pressure point. In other words, further bleeding is prevented, and the patient is in no immediate danger. When the object is lifted off the patient and the pressure is released, however, the patient's wounds may begin to actively bleed again. In some cases, the blood loss can be so massive that the patient quickly goes into shock and may even go into cardiac arrest.

When prolonged extrication is anticipated, advanced life support personnel, or even an emergency physician, should be called to the scene. Advanced care, such as intravenous (IV) solutions, medications, and special surgical techniques, can improve the patient's chance of survival.

splinting and transportation to the closest appropriate facility. En route to the hospital, the EMT also treats the patient for hypoperfusion.

Assessment

A contusion is slow bleeding under the skin. A visible bruise under the skin may take up to an hour to form. Therefore, an EMT must depend on other signs of injury to predict bleeding into soft tissues. Some of those signs include abrasion marks, left by a seat belt, for example, and localized swelling. As the bleeding continues and the contusion enlarges, blood fills the spaces between the tissues, making the soft tissue feel more dense. Using the uninjured limb for comparison, the EMT will note that a contused limb is slightly larger, asymmetrical, and firmer to the touch than the other limb.

This assessment is important. Bleeding into the thigh from a femur fracture, for example, can be serious. One liter of blood can be lost in each thigh. Similarly, bleeding from a pelvic fracture can be life threatening.

Bleeding from ruptured capillaries also may produce a large, irregularly shaped pool of blood under the skin that is larger than the margins of the point of contact. This skin injury is called **ecchymosis** (Figure 24-26). These ecchymotic areas, like contusions, have a bluish tinge from the deoxygenated blood under the skin. Over time, the ecchymosis will turn black as the blood coagulates. (This is the origin of the term *"black and blue" mark*.) Finally, a couple of weeks later, the ecchymosis will appear greenish-brown or yellow as the clot dissolves and the skin heals.

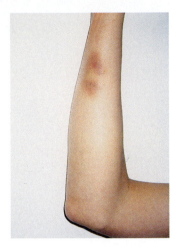

FIGURE 24-26 A wide area of capillary bleeding under the skin is called an ecchymosis.

Scene Size-Up

A confined space rescue is, by definition, a technical rescue that requires specialized equipment and specialized training. In many cases, however, the rescue team either consists of EMTs or is supported by a team of EMTs who can care for the patient once the rescue has been achieved.

An untrained and unequipped EMT should never enter into a potentially lethal confined space rescue. Instead, the EMT should stage in a convenient location that is proximal to the scene and observe the rescue, while asking herself, "What injuries could the patient have sustained?"

Confined space rescue is frequently a high-interest event, and onlookers tend to swarm around the rescuers. The incident commander ensures that an adequate perimeter is established, but every EMT is responsible for maintaining that perimeter, ever mindful of the dangers on the scene to onlookers.

Initial Assessment

The priorities in a confined space rescue are the same as those used in other trauma cases. Patients who experience trauma need spinal immobilization and rapid initial assessment. The EMT needs to assess and treat any life-threatening injuries that the patient may have developed while entrapped, and also should be mindful that hypothermia often occurs in these situations. The injury to the patient may not be

Street Smart

Seldom does an EMT appreciate the extent or severity of a patient's injuries unless she sees the patient 24 hours later. By that time, the bruises and contusions are clearly visible. The patient's eyes may be swollen almost shut and blackened by old blood that has collected, or his legs and arms may be covered with contusions that were not evident at the scene.

In the field, telltale signs like abrasions from seat belt burns or minor localized swelling may be the EMT's only indications that bleeding is occurring in the soft tissues under the skin.

clearly evident initially, so the EMT must be prepared to reassess the patient immediately if conditions change.

Rapid Trauma Assessment

It is critically important that the EMT completely assess the patient. No skin surface should remain untouched; every minor defect should be noted. A small hard area on the thigh may later turn into a large, swollen deformity.

Management

The management of the patient revolves around the ABCs of the initial assessment and the provision of advanced life support (ALS). The EMT should ensure that the patient is cared for by an advanced EMT as soon as possible. As most of the injuries are internal, the patient should be promptly packaged for transportation. The EMT should spend little time at the scene trying to immobilize potential fractures; instead, the patient's entire body should be splinted on a backboard, and the patient transported immediately.

Transportation

These patients should be transported to a trauma center, where the patient's internal injuries can be properly assessed and treated. The decision of where and how to transport the patient should be made in compliance with local protocols as well as consultation with medical control.

Ongoing Assessment

The EMT should be prepared for the possibility of the patient going into shock. Repeated assessment of the vital signs, at least every 5–10

 ## Man Down

Josh is sitting on a picnic table watching the firefighters do their thing. He has been assigned to an aid post on the far side of the building while the rest of the crew is busy setting up a rehab station. Bored out of his wits, Josh is starting to wonder if he should ask for relief at his post when the radio crackles, "Firefighter down! Exposure B."

"Exposure B?" Josh thinks, "That's around the corner!" Josh grabs his aid bag and the oxygen and runs to the other side of the building. On the ground is a firefighter. Other firefighters are already busy stripping the turnout gear off the injured firefighter as smoke rolls off his coat. As Josh approaches the patient, it hits him—that smell, the smell one never forgets, the smell of burnt flesh.

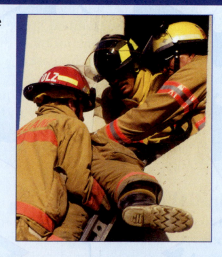

- What are the priorities in the assessment of this patient?
- What special assessment considerations should be made by the EMT?
- What special transportation considerations should be made by the EMT?

minutes, as well as assessment for hypoperfusion will ensure that the EMT identifies the impending shock and reacts correctly.

BURNS

Two million Americans suffer burn injuries annually. These burns result in more than 100,000 hospitalizations and approximately 8,000 deaths. Although the median age of a burn victim is 22 years old, those most in danger of dying are the elderly and the extremely young.

Over the short term, burns are painful and potentially life threatening. Over the long term, burns can be physically disfiguring and psychologically damaging. Prompt intervention by an EMT can decrease the patient's pain and suffering and increase the patient's chances of a full recovery.

There are four sources of burns. The majority of burns are caused by thermal energy or flame. Electrical burns, chemical burns, and radiation burns, however, make up a significant percentage of burns as well.

Burn Trauma

Open flame can be a source of a burn. A child pulling a pot of scalding hot water off the stove will be burned. Prolonged contact with a house radiator will create a burn. Superheated steam from a car's radiator can cause a burn. There are numerous sources of burn injury. They all have the same impact, the destruction of the skin.

The skin provides protection against infections as well as protection and insulation of the body from the environment. The skin aids in the regulation of body temperature. Without skin, the patient is at risk for infection and hypothermia.

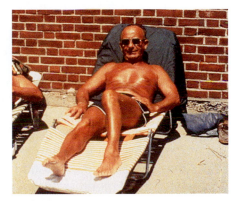

FIGURE 24-27 Sunburn is an example of a superficial burn. (Courtesy of Phoenix Society for Burn Survivors, Inc.)

Classifications of Burn Injury

Skin can be divided into three layers. The topmost, or superficial, layer is called the epidermis. The epidermis is largely dead cells that act as a barrier between the outside world and internal organs of the body. The middle layer, the dermis, contains *live* skin cells as well as nerve endings. Just below the dermis is the subcutaneous layer. The subcutaneous layer contains muscles, fat, and some shallow veins visible through the skin. For a more detailed description of the skin, refer to Chapter 5.

Burns also can be divided into three classifications, each according to the layer of skin involved. A burn to the topmost, or epidermal, layer is called a **superficial burn**. Because most of the epidermis is dead, little physical damage is done. However, nerve endings just under the epidermis make the reddened skin feel very painful. Sunburn is a classic example of a superficial burn (Figure 24-27).

A **partial-thickness burn** involves the dermal layer. Burn injury to the tissue causes swelling, blister formation on the surface, and vasodilation, which causes the skin to appear flushed (Figure 24-28). Severe scalds create a partial-thickness burn. The danger of secondary infections is greater in a partial-thickness burn than a superficial burn.

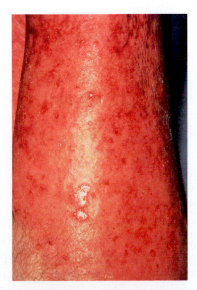

FIGURE 24-28 Blisters are the hallmark of a partial-thickness burn. (Courtesy of Phoenix Society for Burn Survivors, Inc.)

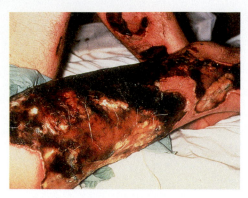

FIGURE 24-29 Full-thickness burns are frequently painless. (Courtesy of Phoenix Society for Burn Survivors, Inc.)

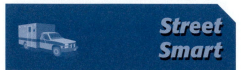

A **full-thickness burn** involves all the layers of skin. The greatest risk presented by a full-thickness burn is the loss of the body's protective barrier. The skin acts as a barrier to keep bacteria out of the body and bodily fluids in the body. When the skin is no longer able to protect the patient from external contamination by bacteria, the patient is at risk for massive life-threatening infections that can lead to septic shock and death. When the skin can no longer keep bodily fluids from leaking out of the body, the patient is at risk for massive fluid loss, which can lead to hypoperfusion, hypovolemic shock, and death.

These consequences of burns, however, are seldom seen in the field. It takes hours for an infection to set in or for a sufficient amount of body fluid loss to cause hypoperfusion. The more immediately pressing problems that occur along with the burn, such as inhalation of superheated air, are usually the cause of immediate death in the field.

With a full-thickness burn, nerve endings are all destroyed, creating a so-called *painless* burn. Muscle and fat also are destroyed, resulting in reduced movement and function in the affected area. The surface of a full-thickness burn quickly becomes hardened, inelastic, and almost leatherlike and appears black, like charcoal, and burnt (Figure 24-29).

Burn Severity

A significant burn seldom has just one type of burn. A large area of superficial burn may be combined with areas of partial-thickness burn. Alternatively, an area of full-thickness burn, at a point of contact, may have concentric rings of partial-thickness burn around it.

A formula for estimating the percentage of burns over the body surface area has been developed. Called the **rule of nines**, the formula provides the EMT with a quick percentage of burn area. In an adult, each arm represents 9%, each leg 18%, the upper back and lower back are 18%, and the chest and abdomen are 18%. There are 11 areas that, when totaled, equal 99%. Refer to Figure 24-30 for a representation of all 11 areas in the rule of nines. The remaining 1% is assigned to the genitals.

The rule of nines is useful for large burns but is difficult to use with small burns or with burns that are spread across the body. (A splash pattern from a scald injury can leave multiple small burns, for example.) In those cases, the **palmar method** is more accurate. The palm of the patient's hand is estimated to be about 1% of the patient's body surface area. Therefore, the EMT can use the patient's palm to estimate the total percent of burn trauma.

Critical Burns

Some patients with full- and/or partial-thickness burns would benefit from the care that they could receive at a burn center. These patients, who are said to have critical burns, should be transported, by air or by ground, to the closest burn center. The EMT should refer to local protocol for guidance with this decision while in the field.

A full-thickness burn or a partial-thickness burn that is 10% or greater is considered to be critical.

Certain burns, regardless of area of body surface involved, are considered critical. A patient with such burns should be considered high priority, and transportation to a burn center should be considered.

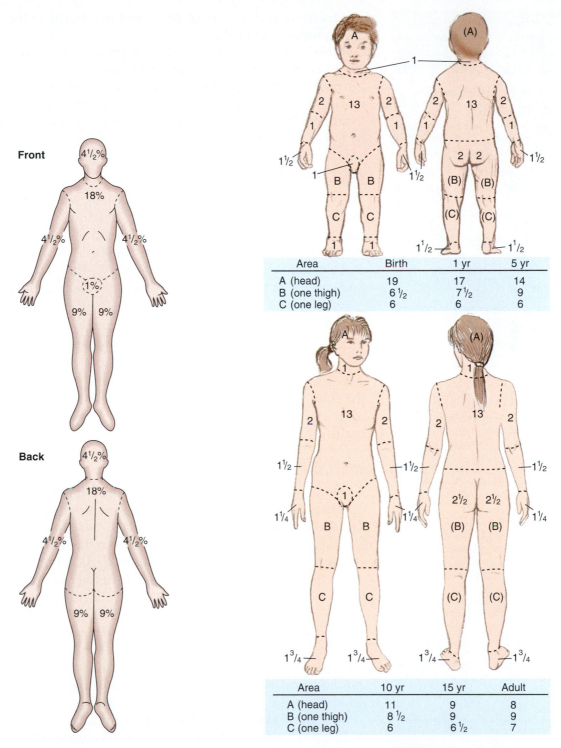

Area	Birth	1 yr	5 yr
A (head)	19	17	14
B (one thigh)	6 ½	7 ½	9
C (one leg)	6	6	6

Area	10 yr	15 yr	Adult
A (head)	11	9	8
B (one thigh)	8 ½	9	9
C (one leg)	6	6 ½	7

FIGURE 24-30 The rule of nines is used to estimate the percentage of body surface area burned.

Burns to the face are always considered critical. Burns of the upper or lower airway are one of the major causes of death from burns. If the patient experiences a loss of the airway in the field, immediate transportation to the closest facility, or advanced life support (ALS) intercept, takes priority over transportation to the burn center.

Burns of the hands or feet also are considered critical. Burns of the hands or feet have significant long-term ramifications to the patient's

TABLE 24-2

Burn Unit Referral Criteria

A burn unit may treat adults or children or both.

Burn injuries that should be referred to a burn unit include the following:

1. Partial-thickness burns greater than 10% total body surface area (TBSA)

2. Burns that involve the face, hands, feet, gentailia, perineum, or major joints

3. Third-degree burns in any age group

4. Electrical burns, including lightning injury

5. Chemical burns

6. Inhalation injury

7. Burn injury in patients with pre-existing medical disorders that could complicate management, prolong recovery, or affect mortality

8. Any patients with burns and concomitant trauma (such as fractures) in which the burn injury poses the greatest risk of morbidity or mortality. In such cases, if the trauma poses the greater immediate risk, the patient may be initially stabilized in a trauma center before being transferred to a burn unit. Physician judgement will be necessary in such situations and should be in concert with the regional medical control plan and triage protocols.

9. Burned children in hospitals without qualified personnel or equipment for the care of children

10. Burn injury in patients who will require special social, emotional, or long-term rehabilitative intervention

Source: Committee on Trauma, American College of Surgeons, "Guidelines for the Operations of Burn Units," *Resources for Optimal Care of the Injured Patient: 1999, 1998,* 55.

productivity and quality of life. Similarly, burns to the genitals also are considered critical burns.

Table 24-2 lists the classification of patients with critical burns who may benefit from burn center management. Patients with critical burns should be transported to a regional burn center whenever possible. Local protocols may dictate that the patient be transported to a local hospital or regional trauma center, stabilized, and then transferred to the burn center.

Assessment

The assessment of the burn patient in many ways is no different than the assessment of any trauma patient. Yet, fires create special impacts that are not typically seen with other trauma patients. For example, carbon monoxide poisoning makes the task of providing oxygen to these patients problematic. Still, the EMT should focus on the basics and care for the patient as if he were any other trauma patient.

Scene Size-Up

The fire scene is inherently dangerous. The EMT must carefully assess the scene to ensure that an enlarging fire does not engulf her. Consideration must be rapidly given to the nature of the trauma and the ultimate destination to which the patient will travel. Early requests for assistance, an aeromedical mission, for example, can literally save a patient's life.

Initial Assessment

Burns of the face are considered critical. Although the eyes and appearance are important, the loss of the upper airway can be fatal. The EMT must assess all facial burns for involvement of the airway. Singed nose hairs, circumferential burns of the mouth, and soot in the sputum are all signs of burns to the upper airway.

The EMT should examine the inside of the mouth, the oropharynx, for swelling. A hoarse voice may also indicate burns to the upper airway. Then the EMT should listen to the breathing by putting the stethoscope on the patient's throat. A narrowed airway in the throat makes a low-pitched inspiratory sound called **stridor**. This low-pitched sound is usually heard best during inspiration. A stridor that can be heard without the aid of a stethoscope indicates an airway about to close. Any audible stridor is a dangerous sign, and the patient should be transported immediately.

The EMT also should listen to, or auscultate, the lungs with the stethoscope at the apices of the lungs. Wheezes indicate narrowed airways, possibly secondary to inhalation of toxic or superheated gases.

Rapid Trauma Assessment

The burn trauma patient must have a complete head-to-toe examination. The intense pain from the burn may divert the patient's attention away from other more life-threatening injuries. The EMT must be aware that a burn is a distracting injury and that she will have to depend on her assessment skills, and not the patient's responses, to discover other injuries.

Management

The EMT's first priority is to stop the burning. Smoldering clothing, grease, wax, and tarlike substances can continue to burn the skin, long after the fire is out. The EMT should cool the area with sterile water and wash away excess debris, but should not attempt to remove material that is stuck to the wound. The EMT should then expose the burned area and examine the wounds, taking care not to break any blisters that have formed.

Burn Field Dressing

The EMT first prepares the dressing materials, as needed. Universal dressings work well for large areas. Roller gauze works well for extremities. The EMT should never apply any ointments or antiseptic lotions to either the bandages or the patient. If hands or feet are involved, the digits need to be separated with gauze dressings. Some medical authorities advocate dry dressings for all burn patients. Follow local medical protocols regarding proper burn care.

If the burn involves less than 10% of the body surface area and local protocols allow it, a wet dressing may be used. The EMT wets a gauze dressing, a 4 × 4, for example, with sterile water. After squeezing out excess water while the dressing is in the wrapper, the EMT then lifts the dressing by one corner and places the moist dressing(s) on the wound. Then the EMT wraps the dressing with a dry sterile bandage (Figure 24-31).

If the burn involves more than 10% of the body surface area, the EMT should apply dry sterile dressings only (Figure 24-32). Dry dressings have been used for major burns since 1957, when the American Red Cross's first aid manual advocated dry dressings for major burns.

Hypothermia is a significant hazard to a major burn patient. Without skin, the body's heat escapes rapidly. The use of wet dressings only contributes to heat loss and hypothermia. Therefore, the EMT should minimize wet dressings, cover the patient, and use passive warming methods to treat the hypothermia.

Transportation

Patients with critical burns should be transported to the closest appropriate facility. Specialized burn centers have been established for these patients. These facilities have specially trained physicians and

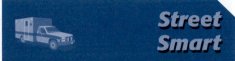

Street Smart

Many plastics, acrylics, and compounds release carbon monoxide, cyanide, and other potentially lethal toxins. Every patient suspected of smoke inhalation should be carefully monitored and transported for medical evaluation. Many of these patients will not manifest symptoms of poisoning on the scene. The EMT should contact medical control, explain the situation, and ask for further instructions on how to proceed with patient care.

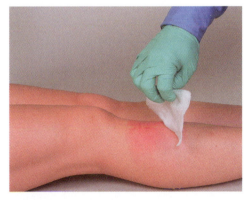

FIGURE 24-31 A wet dressing can be applied to a small burn.

Cultural Considerations

Although it is important to remove clothing from a burn patient, the EMT must keep the patient's dignity in mind. Even a semiconscious patient realizes that he is being disrobed. The EMT should explain to the patient what she is doing and why, and offer to cover the patient immediately after the assessment. A simple pillowcase over the groin, or a clean sheet over the body, can be a tremendous source of comfort to the patient.

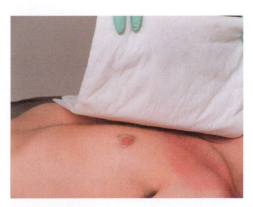

FIGURE 24-32 A dry sterile dressing should be applied to a large burn.

Street Smart

Burn patients represent a challenge to the EMT. Beyond issues of wound management, the EMT is subjected to human disfigurement and witnesses much pain and suffering. Many EMTs complain of nightmares after a call to a burn patient. A call for a burn victim may be one of the most stressful calls in an EMT's career.

Critical incident stress debriefing (CISD) can help EMTs to deal with concerns and issues around the call. CISD can help prevent post-traumatic stress disorders.

special equipment to properly treat the patient. Air medical evacuation, in the field or from a local designated hospital's landing zone (LZ), provides rapid transportation to these regional burn centers.

CHEMICAL BURNS

Mishandling of chemicals and failure to wear proper protective apparel are frequent causes of chemical burns. Chemical burns can result from direct contact with strong acids or strong alkalis or from exposure to fumes. The injuries from chemical burns are similar to those from thermal burns. Chemical reactions between the skin and the acid/alkali can create heat as well. The depth of the burn is dependent on the amount of chemical spilled and the length of time that the chemical remains in contact with the skin. Removing the chemical from the skin quickly reduces the depth and percentage of burn.

Scene Size-Up

By definition, a chemical spill is a hazardous materials incident. Specially trained personnel must respond to the spill. Routine protective equipment used by EMTs will not provide the level of protection needed. Further details regarding hazardous materials response is provided in Chapter 44.

The hazardous materials team delivers the patient to the EMT in a safe area, called the **cold zone**, at the end of a decontamination corri-

Chemical Exposure

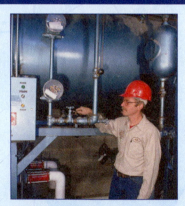

Thatcher was checking the valves and gauges in the plant as a part of his regular duties. "High-pressure gauge check, steam release valve tight and check, drainage tube valve tight." As soon as he had spoken the words, the valve over his head blew off, and the hot, steamy chemical solution bathed him from above. Screaming out in pain, Thatcher clawed his way on all fours to the wall. Running his hand across the wall, he found the alarm and yelled into the PA system, "I've got something in my eyes!" Then he reached out and pulled the shower handle, and 50 gallons of water began pouring over his head.

- What are the priorities in the assessment of this patient?
- What special assessment considerations should be made by the EMT?
- What special transportation considerations should be made by the EMT?

dor. The EMT should be wearing protective apparel, including gloves, mask, an impenetrable gown, and eye protection.

A victim of a very small chemical spill may be treated by an EMT, but caution is advised; the EMT should wear, at a minimum, eye protection and gloves. First the EMT removes the patient from the immediate vicinity of the spill, and then treats the patient according to guidelines. If the EMT has any doubt about procedures, the EMT should call the hazardous materials spill response team. Unless an EMT is trained for a hazardous materials incident, she should alert the appropriate authorities and remain out of immediate danger. Table 24-3 outlines some chemicals related to minor hazardous materials injuries.

Initial Assessment

The initial assessment of the patient should focus on injuries to the airway and difficulty with breathing that could be life threatening. Seldom is there a problem of circulation and perfusion in these cases.

Management

Although there are literally thousands of types of chemicals, treatments for chemical burns are relatively similar. Once the patient has been decontaminated, basic medical care can begin. The first task is to identify the offending chemical. If a label is visible, the EMT can read the instructions on the label. If the patient is inside a storage or manufacturing facility, the EMT can refer to the **Material Safety Data Sheet (MSDS)**. Federal safety regulations from the **Occupational Safety and Health Administration (OSHA)** require that employers keep copies of the MSDS readily available in case of emergency. The MSDS contains information about specific chemicals and how to treat an accidental exposure (Figure 24-33).

If the patient is transporting the chemical at the time of exposure, the shipping papers, called the manifest, will list the name of the chemical(s). If the manifest is not available, the EMT should look for a diamond-shaped placard on the side of the truck and record the number that is on the placard. Then, using the **Emergency Response Guidebook (ERG)**, a free publication of the federal Department of Transportation (DOT) that is available to all emergency response agencies, the EMT can cross-reference the chemical's number, or name, to the guide number (Figure 24-34). The guide provides detailed instructions on how to handle a chemical spill, including first aid.

If the hazardous materials (chemicals) that the patient is exposed to are being transported by air, rail, or road it may be helpful to call CHEMTREC. CHEMTREC is a 24-hour emergency telephone number created by the American Chemistry Council (formerly known as the Chemical Manufacturers Association) that provides information on the materials and substances that manufacturers have in transit to firefighters, EMS, and other emergency responders. The information provided includes first aid procedures in the event of accidental exposure. The toll free number for CHEMTREC is 800-424-9300.

TABLE 24-3

Minor Chemical Spills

Chemical	Source
Hydrochloric acid	Exploded battery
Lime	Dry cement
OCR	Pepper spray
Organophosphate	Garden fertilizers
CN/CS gas	Mace
Dry chemical	Fire extinguisher

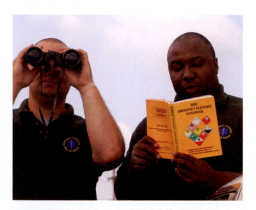

FIGURE 24-34 The *Emergency Response Guidebook* provides the EMT initial instructions at a hazardous materials incident.

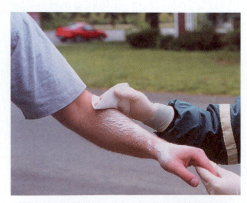

FIGURE 24-35 Dry chemicals should be brushed off first, then large volumes of water used to rinse the residue off the patient.

AIR PRODUCTS

Material Safety Data Sheet
Version 1.7
Revision Date 05/16/2004

MSDS Number 300000000110
Print Date 07/28/2004

1. PRODUCT AND COMPANY IDENTIFICATION

Product name	: Oxygen
Chemical formula	: O2
Synonyms	: Oxygen, Oxygen gas, Gaseous Oxygen, GOX
Product Use Description	: General Industrial
Company	: Air Products and Chemicals,Inc 7201 Hamilton Blvd. Allentown, PA 18195-1501
Telephone	: 800-345-3148
Emergency telephone number	: 800-523-9374 USA 01-610-481-7711 International

2. COMPOSITION/INFORMATION ON INGREDIENTS

Components	CAS Number	Concentration (Volume)
Oxygen	7782-44-7	100 %

Concentration is nominal. For the exact product composition, please refer to Air Products technical specifications.

3. HAZARDS IDENTIFICATION

Emergency Overview

High pressure, oxidizing gas.
Vigorously accelerates combustion.
Keep oil, grease, and combustibles away.
May react violently with combustible materials.

Potential Health Effects

Inhalation	: Breathing 75% or more oxygen at atmospheric pressure for more than a few hours may cause nasal stuffiness, cough, sore throat, chest pain and breathing difficulty. Breathing pure oxygen under pressure may cause lung damage and also central nervous system effects.
Eye contact	: No adverse effect.
Skin contact	: No adverse effect.
Ingestion	: Ingestion is not considered a potential route of exposure.

Exposure Guidelines

1/7

Air Products and Chemicals,Inc   Oxygen

FIGURE 24-33 The Material Data Safety Sheet (MSDS) contains a great deal of information important to an EMT. (Courtesy of Air Products and Chemicals Inc.)

Dry Chemicals

Typically, dry chemicals have to be brushed off the patient and clothing has to be removed before decontamination may begin (Figure 24-35). The EMT must, at a minimum, wear a dust/mist mask. Dry chemicals can become airborne and enter the EMT's airway. The EMT should flush the chemicals off the patient with copious amounts of water only if the MSDS, ERG, or similar authority indicates that this is the correct procedure. Some dry chemicals must be neutralized with oils or other substances. Other dry chemicals can react violently upon contact with water.

Wet Chemicals

Typically, wet chemicals have to be washed off the patient after the patient's clothing has been removed. The EMT must wear a gown and eye protection. Splash from the patient can make the EMT a secondary victim.

When flushing chemicals off a patient with copious amounts of water, as indicated by the MSDS, ERG, or other hazardous materials information source, the EMT should monitor the patient constantly. While many experts advocate 20–30 minutes of flushing, continuous irrigation for as long as possible is preferred. Transportation, however, should begin within 20 minutes, with continuous irrigation while en route.

A gentle irrigation is preferred to a forceful jet. Burned tissues are delicate, and further injury can occur when streams of water are used. The EMT should monitor the patient for hypothermia. Review the treatment of the mildly hypothermic patient in Chapter 34.

The EMT should carefully control runoff. If the patient is lying in a pool of runoff, he may experience secondary burns to his back and buttocks. The EMT needs to position the patient so that runoff does not flow into the patient's uninjured body areas.

Eye Injury

Chemical burns to the eyes can be particularly distressing to the patient. The EMT needs to begin irrigation of the eyes, if indicated, as soon as possible. Irrigating an eye is difficult. The eye's protective reflexes want to close the eyelids. Often another EMT has to help keep the patient's eye open. Once the patient's eye is open, the EMT should keep the irrigation stream running continuously. Eventually, the eye becomes desensitized and will stay open on its own.

A simple IV solution and tubing setup allows the EMT to irrigate one eye continuously for 20–30 minutes (Figure 24-36). The EMT must ensure that the drainage is running away from the unaffected eye. If both eyes need irrigation, the EMT can use an IV setup attached to a nasal cannula. The nasal prongs can be directed into each eye, and the drainage will be away from the other eye. Once both eyes have been sufficiently irrigated or the irrigation solution is gone, the EMT should bandage both eyes and notify the hospital early.

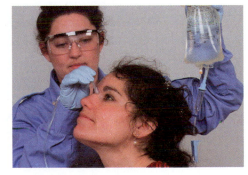

FIGURE 24-36 IV solution can be used to provide continuous eye irrigation.

Once the patient has been properly decontaminated, the EMT's attention should turn to a complete assessment. Frequently, the chemicals on the skin are absorbed by the patient's body. The result is that the patient is poisoned as well as contaminated.

The EMT should monitor the patient's level of consciousness. Early contact with medical control can provide the EMT with much-needed instruction. All patients are routinely administered high-concentration oxygen. The EMT should complete a detailed physical examination,

 Street Smart

While awaiting the arrival of a hazardous materials team, the EMT should start the decontamination process. The EMT begins by having the patient remove all clothing; modesty has no place at a chemical spill. Spilled chemicals held in underwear material or against the skin by elastic bands will continue to burn. The patient needs to remove all watches, rings, and any other jewelry that could react with the chemical(s).

Following the instructions on the Material Safety Data Sheet or in the *Emergency Response Guidebook*, the EMT should encourage the patient to self-decontaminate. Garden hoses, emergency showers, and sinks all provide readily available water. If limited resources are available, the EMT should have the patient concentrate on decontaminating the eyes first.

concentrating on hidden or concealed chemical burns in the folds of the skin. The pain from the burning chemicals may mask other injuries that the patient has sustained. The EMT must be alert to the possibility of concurrent injury from falls, explosions, and fire. The EMT may need to protect the patient's spine, using a backboard and cervical immobilization device.

The EMT should cover any burned areas with a dressing, keep the patient warm, and transport the patient to an appropriate facility. The hospital needs early notification of a potential hazardous materials exposure. Early notification allows the hospital time to prepare for the patient and prevents secondary contamination of the emergency department.

ELECTRICAL BURNS

For electricity to pass through an object, or make a **current**, there must be a source and a ground. The source can be a high-powered electric line from a power pole. Ordinary house current, however, is sufficient to kill or injure a patient.

Some materials allow electricity to pass through them without any resistance. These materials are **conductors**. Water is an excellent conductor of electricity. Materials that resist the flow of electricity are called **insulators**. Skin and bones are excellent insulators. When electricity meets resistance in an insulator, heat energy is the by-product.

Finding a break in the skin, the electricity enters the body through an **entrance wound**. The electricity then flows through the path of least resistance toward a ground (Figure 24-37). The bloodstream

Street Smart

When the entire body is immersed in a conductive medium, such as a bathtub full of water, and a source, a hairdryer, for example, is introduced, there may not be any entrance or exit wounds.

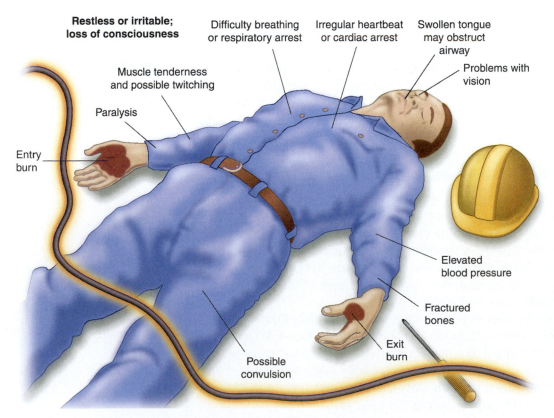

FIGURE 24-37 An electrical shock can cause a large number of injuries inside the body.

offers the least resistance to electrical current. Therefore, electricity generally follows the blood vessels, looking for a ground.

Eventually electricity finds a ground. Once enough energy accumulates to overcome the resistance of the skin, the electricity literally explodes out of the body. This explosion creates an **exit wound**. Some exit wounds can be very deep, exposing bones and tendons.

Scene Size-Up

Utility poles represent a serious hazard to all emergency responders. They line many of America's highways and are frequently involved during motor vehicle collisions. Some poles are broken, or even sheared off, at the base, and the only thing holding them is the power line. An average utility pole weighs between 800 and 1,200 pounds. That weight can quickly overcome the tensile strength of the power line.

Utility poles may drop power lines onto the ground. If the wire strikes the road surface, the asphalt may act as an insulator, preventing breakers down the line from tripping and keeping the line energized. If the line falls across a guy wire, or a telephone line, it may energize those as well. The EMT should consider that all downed utility pole lines are dangerous until proved otherwise.

Many planned housing developments bury power lines underground. Often the only visible sign of a buried cable is the green splice box. Many homeowners conceal these splice boxes behind low bushes and shrubbery. When a motor vehicle travels across the lawn, it can come to rest on top of a splice box. The vehicle may become energized. Always look under, as well as above, a vehicle for electrical dangers.

While a power line may appear to have insulation around it, the wrap on the line is primarily intended to prevent corrosion. An EMT

Electric Shock

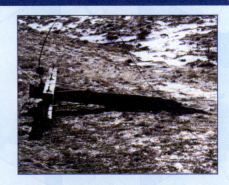

As the EMS crew disembarks from the ambulance, the power company foreman approaches them, saying, "He's over there, got blown clean off the pole. He's got a pulse and is breathing, but he looks pretty shook up." The EMT looks in the general direction in which the foreman is pointing. "Boy, I'll bet that tingled," the EMT says. Then the EMT asks the foreman, "Hey, are the lines safe? I mean, is the power shut down?" "Yeah," the foreman replies, "We shut it down the moment it happened. I called the main switch and told 'em to keep it shut down 'til you boys get out of here."

Picking up the ready bags, the EMS crew approaches the patient. Another lineman is already at the patient's head, holding manual stabilization of the patient's neck. The patient looks a little pale but is obviously awake and alert. "What hurts you the most?" asks the EMT.

- What are the priorities in the assessment of this patient?
- What special assessment considerations should be made by the EMT?
- What special transportation considerations should be made by the EMT?

When approaching a scene, if an EMT starts to feel a tingling sensation in her legs, the EMT should immediately stop. The EMT has entered an *electric field*. The tingling sensation indicates that the area is energized. Electricity fans out in ever-widening circles called *gradients*. The tingling sensation indicates that the EMT is on the edge of the first gradient.

Backing out of the danger can be more dangerous than standing still. By lifting one leg and then setting it down, the EMT creates a circuit. If possible, the EMT should wait until the all-clear sign indicates that it is safe to move. Otherwise, the EMT should shuffle backward, keeping both feet on the ground firmly, or hop out of the area. Whatever the EMT does, she should never run.

should never touch a downed line or attempt to remove a charged power line with blocks and rope, "hot sticks," or any other apparatus. Instead, the EMT should call for assistance from the power company or fire department and leave the removal of power lines for the experts.

Assessment

Injuries from an electrical shock can be compared to an iceberg. While the tip of the iceberg is visible, the majority of the iceberg is under the surface. Similarly, the entrance wound can be small, but the internal damage created by the heat energy can be substantial.

The single most important factor in determining the degree of electrical burn injury is the duration of contact. At about 1.1 milliamperes (mA), the patient starts to feel an uncomfortable tingling. If the patient is holding the source, a wire, for example, he usually drops the wire immediately.

When the energy increases to about 15 mA, the alternating current of the electricity paralyzes the patient, preventing him from dropping the wire. This is called the let-go energy threshold. Below that energy level, the patient can let go of the source, but above that energy level, the patient's muscles spasm and the patient is "frozen" to the electric source.

When a patient is unable to let go of the source, the electricity has ample time to create tremendous internal injuries. Frequently the diaphragm, the muscle that controls breathing, becomes paralyzed and the patient stops breathing. If the current continues to pass through the patient, the heart may fibrillate, and the patient may suffer a cardiac arrest. If the current stops, because of a circuit-breaker trip, for example, the patient may have a chance for recovery.

Management

Electrical burns should be treated like any trauma, starting with spinal precautions. The EMT should immediately check the airway, breathing, circulation (ABCs) and start cardiopulmonary resuscitation (CPR) as needed. The heart, stunned by the electrical shock, may respond quickly to CPR (Figure 24-38). Defibrillation should be performed, using an automated external defibrillator (AED), as indicated.

If the patient is breathing adequately, the EMT can administer high-concentration oxygen via a non-rebreather mask. The EMT should carefully monitor the patient's breathing. If the patient's breathing is erratic, the EMT should consider assisting the patient's ventilation with a bag-valve-mask. All entrance and exit wounds should be covered, and the electrical burns treated in the same manner as thermal burns.

All patients suffering an electrical shock require rapid transportation and evaluation by an emergency physician. The EMT should attempt to ascertain and report the energy (amperes and volts) encountered as well as the duration of the contact.

Transportation

All electrical burns can create potentially serious internal injuries. Some EMS systems routinely transport all electrical burn patients to

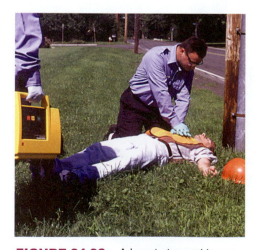

FIGURE 24-38 A heart stunned by an electrical shock may respond to CPR.

the regional burn or trauma center. The EMT should always refer to and follow local protocols.

Ongoing Assessment

The heart of the patient who has suffered an electrical shock can be very irritable, occasionally resulting in a "skipped beat." The EMT should constantly monitor the patient's pulse, particularly its rhythm, for these skipped beats and report them to either an ALS provider or the hospital staff. In rare circumstances, the heart may stop beating, and the patient may go into cardiac arrest. If this occurs, the EMT should follow standard cardiac arrest protocols. Nothing in the patient's condition prevents an EMT from using an AED to restart the heart of a patient who has suffered an electrical shock.

CONCLUSION

The EMT's first job is to prevent any further injury to the patient. After the EMT protects the patient, the EMT must prepare expedient transportation of the patient to the most appropriate facility.

While each type of tissue trauma is different, most are managed in the same, or a similar, way. Thus, the EMT can apply his knowledge of wound care in unique ways.

TEST YOUR KNOWLEDGE

1. What are the principles of bleeding control management?
2. What are the types of bleeding?
3. What is the purpose of a dressing?
4. What are the indications and dangers of using a tourniquet?
5. What are the different bandages used?
6. What is the special danger of neck wounds?
7. What are the different types of wounds?
8. What is the field care of an evisceration?
9. What is the field care of an amputation?
10. What are the levels of burn injury?
11. What is the field care of a burn?
12. What danger do chemical burns represent to the EMT?
13. What injuries can occur from an electrical shock?
14. What is the field care of an electrical injury?

INTERNET RESOURCES

Look for additional information on soft tissue injuries at these Web sites:

- eMedicine, http://www.emedicine.com
- International Society for Burn Injuries, http://www.worldburn.org

- World Wide Wounds, http://www.worldwidewounds.com
- Wounds UK, http://www.wounds-uk.com

Do a key word search using the various types of injuries discussed in this chapter to look for additional information related to the emergency care of those injuries.

FURTHER STUDY

Bozinko, G., Lowe, K., & Reigart, C. (1998). Burns. *RN, 61*(11), 37–40.

Carroll, P. (1999). Chest injuries. *RN, 62*(1), 36–42.

Hansen, S., Paul, C., & Voigt, D. (1999). Chemical injuries. *Journal of Emergency Medical Services, 24*(8), 82–88.

Shellenbarger, T. (2000). Nosebleeds: Not just kid's stuff. *RN, 63*(2), 50–54.

Wiebelhaus, P., & Hansen, S. (1999). Burns: Handle with care. *RN, 62*(11), 52–58.

CHAPTER 25

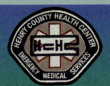
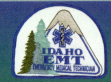
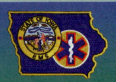

Bony Injuries

KEY TERMS

acromioclavicular (A/C) dislocation

appendicular skeleton

axial skeleton

bipolar traction splint

calcaneus

closed fracture

Colles' fracture

crepitus

direct force

dislocation

dorsiflexion

false motion

flexible splint

footdrop

fracture

guarding

indirect force

ligament

locked

motor nerves

open fracture

osteoporosis

paralysis

paresis

paresthesia

patella

pelvic girdle

pelvic wrap technique

pneumatic splint

(continues)

OBJECTIVES

Upon completion of this chapter, the reader should be able to:

1. List the three mechanisms of force that can cause injury to a bone.
2. Describe a ligament and a tendon.
3. Describe and differentiate between a closed and open fracture.
4. Define when a dislocation becomes an emergency.
5. Describe the common signs and symptoms of a bone injury.
6. List the principles of splinting.
7. Describe the different techniques of splinting.
8. Describe a splinting technique for the following bone injuries:
   a. Collarbone
   b. Shoulder blade
   c. Acromioclavicular dislocation
   d. Shoulder
   e. Upper arm
   f. Elbow
   g. Forearm
   h. Wrist and hand
   i. Hip
   j. Proximal femur
   k. Midshaft femur
   l. Patella
   m. Knee
   n. Lower leg
   o. Ankle
   p. Foot
9. Discuss the importance of differentiating a knee dislocation from a kneecap dislocation.
10. Describe when an EMT can straighten a fracture or dislocation.

KEY TERMS

(continued)

point tenderness
position of function
range of motion (ROM)
rigid splint
sciatic nerve
self-splint
sensory nerves
shoulder dislocation
shoulder girdle
sling and swathe (S/S)
spontaneous reduction
sprain
symphysis pubis
tendon
traction
traction splint
twisting force
unipolar traction splint

OVERVIEW

Many patients complain bitterly about the pain they are experiencing, which may alarm the inexperienced emergency medical technician (EMT), but most bone injuries are not life threatening. The EMT, however, should carefully and methodically manage the injury. When mistreated, bone injuries can result in permanent, lifelong disabilities. Therefore, careful attention by an EMT to the treatment of bone injuries is important; it can lead to reduced suffering and prevention of further injury, and ultimately assist the patient to her return to health.

ANATOMY REVIEW

As discussed in Chapter 5, the body has three types of muscles: involuntary muscles, cardiac muscles, and voluntary muscles. This chapter focuses on the voluntary muscles, those muscles that are under the patient's conscious control. Voluntary muscles cause movement of bones that permit locomotion. When a traumatic force is applied to a bone or a muscle, movement can be impaired, and an injury may result.

The bones of the body make up the skeletal system. The skeletal system can be divided into two subsystems. The bones of the spine and cranium are called the **axial skeleton**. The axial skeleton provides support for the muscles of the trunk and protection of the core organs, including the heart, lungs, and brain. The axial skeleton also allows movement, such as bending and lifting. Injuries to the head and spine have been discussed in earlier chapters.

✴ *Football Injury*

It was fourth down and a yard to go. There was the snap and the run and another snap, only this time the second snap came from the quarterback's leg. The referees ran to the downed player, then waved EMS onto the field.

The two EMTs followed the athletic trainer who pulled a stretcher loaded with gear and a backboard. Once they were at the patient's side, an EMT maintained manual stabilization of the player's helmet while the trainer asked, "Roger, where do you hurt?"

"It's my leg," the patient replied, "I think I broke my leg." After a few more questions, both the EMT and the trainer were satisfied that the patient's only injury was in his left leg. The second EMT immediately cut the pant leg off the injured leg, using a trainer's angel. There was blood at the site of the deformity.

- Based on the mechanism of injury, what injuries might an EMT suspect?
- What are the assessment priorities for this patient?
- What are the management priorities for this patient?
- How could this patient deteriorate?

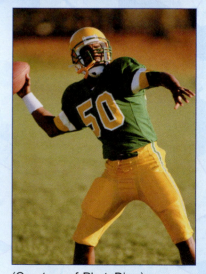

(Courtesy of PhotoDisc.)

The other bones, the bones of the extremities, form the **appendicular skeleton** (Figure 25-1). The appendicular skeleton allows the body to run, to shoulder a load, or to stand erect.

The bones of the appendicular skeleton can be further subdivided into two more groups of bones. The bones of the shoulder and arms make up what can be loosely called the **shoulder girdle**. The bones of the pelvis make up the **pelvic girdle**.

The advantage of putting these bones into groups is that it aids in understanding that force transmitted to one bone may be transmitted to adjacent bones as well. These bones work together, as a group, to effect motion; when one bone is injured, the range of motion of the bones in that group may be reduced.

INJURY

Injury to bones, and muscles, can occur from either a direct or an indirect force. A **direct force**, such as a blow from a baseball, delivers energy immediately to the bone. An **indirect force** transmits energy, through either the shoulder or pelvic girdle, to a bone that is not in contact with the force. For example, when a person falls upon an outstretched hand and injures the shoulder, the shoulder is injured by an indirect force.

Some forces, direct and indirect, can rotate along the axis of the bone. The result of this **twisting force** can be injury to both muscles and bones. The bones that are twisted may stay straight and inline, whereas the other mechanisms of injury often produce deformity. These three forms of force are illustrated in Figure 25-2.

Muscular Injuries

Muscles can be torn, crushed, bruised, and cut. Because of the attachment of muscles to bones, when a bone is injured, a muscle also may be injured. The connective tissue that attaches the muscle to the bone is called the **tendon**. Similarly, two bones are connected to each other at joints. These joints are held together by sinewy bands of connective tissue called **ligaments**.

These connective tissues provide stability to a joint. Tendons and ligaments in a joint allow a bone to move in certain directions within the joint's **range of motion (ROM)** (Figure 25-3). The tendons and ligaments also prevent the joint from moving beyond its normal ROM.

A violent force to a joint may force the joint beyond its normal ROM. When a joint is forced beyond its ROM, the tendons or ligaments can become stretched, torn, or **sprained**, resulting in tissue injury. For example, the knee normally moves forward and backward; that is the direction of the knee's normal ROM. When a severe force makes the knee twist laterally, the ligaments and tendons stretch, the knee fails (or buckles), and the knee is injured.

Because the tendons and ligaments are inserted into the bone itself, a tendon injury can also pull a piece of bone from the shaft. The EMT cannot determine whether the underlying bone has or has not been injured; therefore, the EMT must treat all suspected sprains as though a bone injury is present as well.

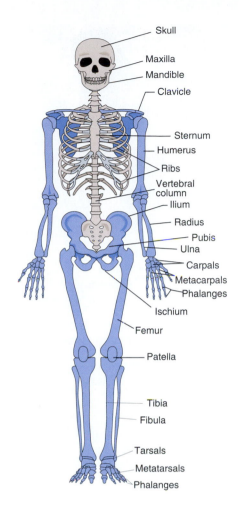

Appendicular skeleton (blue)
Axial skeleton (gray)

FIGURE 25-1 The appendicular skeleton consists of all bones outside of the axial skeleton.

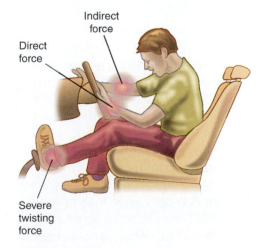

FIGURE 25-2 Direct, indirect, or twisting forces create bone injuries.

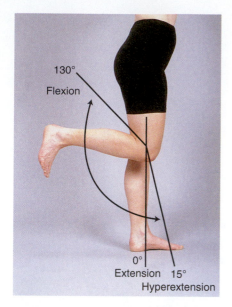

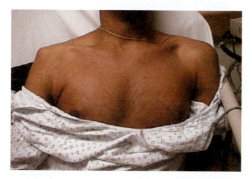

FIGURE 25-3   An injury to a joint can limit the patient's range of motion in that joint.

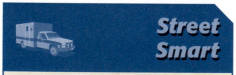

FIGURE 25-4   A dislocation is when a bone is forced out of a joint. (Courtesy of Kevin Reilly, MD, Albany Medical Center, Albany, NY.)

Street Smart

It is not always practical to transport a patient in the wilderness. In certain cases, a specially trained EMT, a Wilderness EMT (WEMT), will attempt a reduction in the field. A WEMT must have training in the treatment of orthopedic injuries before attempting a reduction in the field.

In some special cases, where there is a danger of loss of limb, an EMT may attempt a reduction in the field. This is explained more fully later in the chapter.

Street Smart

Injuries may occur during sporting events, such as football, soccer, and baseball games. EMTs are often called to respond to or stand by at athletic events. On the scene, the EMT may encounter a certified athletic trainer (ATC). Certified athletic trainers have undergone training in sports medicine. Sports medicine is the application of medicine to treat athletic injuries.

The athletic trainer is responsible for the care of the athletes and will request assistance from an EMT only when the trainer is unable to provide appropriate care on the scene. An ATC should be viewed as a fellow health care provider who is highly trained to treat athletic injuries.

An EMT working at a sporting event should identify the athletic trainer, and verify his credentials, before an athlete is injured. The EMT and the trainer must work together in the patient's best interest; cooperation, not competition, will ensure that an injured athlete gets the proper medical attention.

Joint Injuries

A joint is usually stable as it moves through its normal range of motion. When a person overextends the joint beyond the normal range of motion, the bone ends can slip out of joint. When a bone slips out of joint and out of alignment, adjacent structures, including arteries, nerves, and veins, can be injured. The displacement of any bone from its normal position in a joint is called a **dislocation** (Figure 25-4).

When a dislocation occurs, adjacent muscles struggle to return the bone to the joint. A bone returning to its natural position within the joint without assistance is called a **spontaneous reduction**. If the bone is **locked**, prevented from returning to the joint, then the muscles around the joint start to spasm from the stress. This spasm can be very painful.

A dislocation can lock for a number of reasons. The bone's end may be broken. Tendons and ligaments may be torn or injured. The bone may be physically obstructed from returning to the joint.

A dislocated joint means that nerves, arteries, and veins may be injured. Arteries can be pinched in the joint, compromising distal circulation. Nerves can stretch beyond their physical limits, snapping and creating paralysis. Bleeding can compress surrounding soft tissues, further compromising distal function and movement.

The EMT must stabilize the joint, to prevent further injury, and transport the patient to the hospital. At the hospital, doctors can attempt to manually reduce the dislocation. In some cases, the patient may require surgery to have the reduction performed.

Broken Bones

When a great force is applied to a bone, the bone may break or **fracture**. Although an EMT usually cannot see the fracture, indirect signs of injury tell the EMT that the bone may be broken.

Fractures can be divided into two categories. If the force moves the bone out of line, the bone ends may erupt through the skin, lacerating the skin and creating an **open fracture** (Figure 25-5). If the bone ends remain roughly in line and do not break the skin, the fracture is called a **closed fracture**. Most fractures are closed fractures.

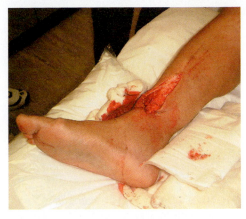

FIGURE 25-5 An open fracture occurs when the bone ends break through the skin. (Courtesy of Deborah Funk, MD, Albany Medical Center, Albany, NY.)

Assessment

By its nature, a bone injury implies that a great deal of violence and resultant trauma has occurred. Although the appearance of a grotesquely deformed leg may be sensational, the EMT must keep in mind that if there was enough force to break bones, then softer tissues are also likely to be injured.

Scene Size-Up

The key to discovering bone injuries is a high index of suspicion that a bone injury may exist in the first place. The EMT should first consider carefully the mechanism of injury.

The mechanism of injury tells the EMT where the injury is likely to be found. By following the line of force, the direction of the violence, and the points of impact on the body, the EMT can suspect certain injuries. For example, a "jumper," a person who attempts suicide by leaping from a tall building, usually will land on her feet, and the line of force, through her body, will compress and crush bones in a predictable pattern, starting at her heels and proceeding up the axial skeleton.

General Impression

The EMT should carefully consider the patient next, stopping to listen to the patient. Bone injuries are very painful. Often the patient's yelling will alert the EMT to the possible presence of a bone injury. Next the EMT should look at the patient's posture and demeanor. Patients often protect and even splint an injured limb rather than endure more pain. The patient's stance can say a lot about the patient's injuries.

Initial Assessment

Because of the proximity of bones and blood vessels, if one is injured, the other can be injured as well. An EMT who is assessing a patient should always remain focused on his priorities and not be distracted by the gross injury. Rarely does a broken bone cause death; however, bleeding from a broken bone, either internal or external, can lead to life-threatening consequences.

Focused Physical Examination

While individual bone injuries can have specific physical findings, an EMT can detect most bone injuries by simply focusing his attention on assessing DCAP-BTLS (see Table 14-3).

Signs and Symptoms

Next to most long bones lie an artery, a nerve, and a vein. Surrounding these bones are muscles, tendons, and other soft tissues.

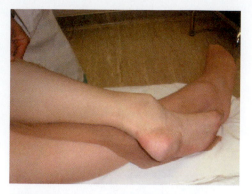

FIGURE 25-6 The area around a closed fracture may be painful, swollen, or deformed. (Courtesy of Deborah Funk, MD, Albany Medical Center, Albany, NY.)

Covering all this is the skin. When a bone is broken and moves out of alignment, the bone ends can damage these tissues. Rarely does an EMT see a broken bone unless the bone ends stick out of the skin. However, an EMT who is assessing a patient can detect the indirect signs of a broken bone and make an assumption, based on these findings, that the bone may be broken (Figure 25-6).

If the artery is pierced by sharp shards of bone, severe bleeding can occur. For example, if the femoral artery, which lies next to the femur, is cut by broken bone ends, the artery will bleed into the thigh. The soft tissues of the thigh will quickly become painful, swollen, and deformed. As the thigh fills with blood, as much as a liter in some cases, the thigh will feel firm to the touch.

If the artery is severed, distal circulation to the affected limb may be compromised. Distal pulses may become weak or absent. The limb may become bluish or cyanotic as well as pulseless.

Pulselessness and cyanosis to any injured extremity constitute a medical emergency. Without medical treatment, the limb may have to be amputated. The EMT should promptly splint the limb and transport the patient to the closest appropriate facility.

A contusion, the blue-gray discoloration under the skin from bleeding, indicates that soft tissue injury may have occurred. Whenever a significant contusion is discovered overlying a bone, the EMT should suspect a bone injury.

Nerves provide pathways for signals to and from the brain. Some nerves, the **motor nerves**, affect muscles, causing them to contract and move. Other nerves, the **sensory nerves**, transmit feelings of pain and pressure to the brain.

If the sensory nerve is injured, the patient may complain of severe pain or no pain at all. A sensation of numbness or tingling, called **paresthesia**, may indicate that the sensory nerve has been injured (Figure 25-7).

If a motor nerve is injured, the patient may complain of weakness in the affected extremity. This weakness, called **paresis**, may be difficult to assess on the scene. An EMT should use extreme caution when asking the patient to move her hands or feet; one wrong move can move bone ends, causing more injury.

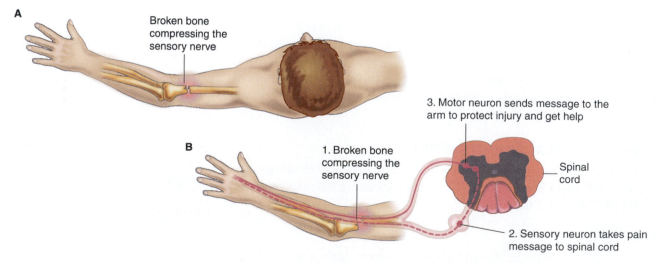

FIGURE 25-7 Broken bone ends can cut sensory and motor nerves, creating weakness or numbness below the injury.

If the patient cannot move one of her extremities, a condition called **paralysis**, the EMT should quickly check the other extremity. If the patient cannot move either extremity, the EMT should suspect a possible spinal injury.

An elevated bone end may tent the skin. The EMT should carefully stabilize this injury. Sudden or improper movement of the limb may change a closed fracture into an open fracture. Open fractures frequently require surgical repair and a longer recovery time.

If the bone breaks the skin, bone ends may be visible. The first priority is to control any bleeding. The EMT should cover any exposed bone ends with a dry sterile dressing, and then splint the limb in the position found. The EMT should never push exposed bone ends back into the wound. If the bone ends fall back into the wound, the EMT needs to report and record this finding.

If the patient moves the injured extremity, a grating sound, called **crepitus**, may be heard. Crepitus is created when two bone ends grind against each other. An EMT should never move an injured extremity to try to hear crepitus.

When an EMT runs his fingers down the length of the shaft of the bone, feeling for injury, and he contacts an injury, the patient may complain of sudden pain. This sudden pain is called **point tenderness**. Once point tenderness has been established, the EMT need not repeatedly touch the area. The EMT should report point tenderness to the emergency department.

Often a patient uses her own body to immobilize an injured extremity, to **self-splint** the injured bone (Figure 25-8). When the EMT attempts to assess the patient, the patient will try to prevent the EMT from touching the injury. This behavior is called **guarding**.

In extreme cases, a patient may try to walk on a broken leg, to escape a fire, for example, and the bone will bend at an unnatural point. This new joint, or unnatural movement of the bone, is called **false motion** and is an indication of a severe fracture.

In a nutshell, DCAP-BTLS essentially covers all the physical findings that are typically found with a bone injury. Injuries to the muscles, tendons, ligaments, and dislocations of a joint can all present with the signs and symptoms of a fractured bone, which are summarized in Table 25-1. Therefore, any painful, swollen deformity is assumed to be a fractured bone until proved otherwise.

Management

An EMT's first priority is always safety. If the injury is an open wound, the EMT must take body substance isolation. Caution should be exercised when dressing the wound. Sharp bone ends can pierce the EMT's gloves and puncture the skin. A lacerated artery can spurt blood into an unsuspecting EMT's eyes. The EMT should wear eye protection if blood is present.

After performing an initial assessment and controlling any bleeding found, the EMT should perform a focused history and physical examination. The EMT should concentrate on looking for DCAP-BTLS.

When a swollen, painful deformity is found, an EMT should immediately stabilize the injury. This is accomplished by placing a hand

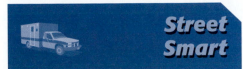
Street Smart

Any laceration near the site of a suspected broken bone may indicate that an open fracture was present earlier. The EMT should treat all wounds near a suspected broken bone as if an open fracture exists.

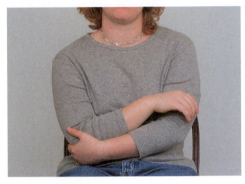
FIGURE 25-8 The patient may "self-splint" in an attempt to prevent further pain and injury.

TABLE 25-1

Signs and Symptoms of a Suspected Fracture

Swelling

Pain

Deformity

Paralysis

Paresthesia

Pulselessness

Cyanosis

Crepitus

Point tenderness

Guarding

Self-splinting

above and below the injury to prevent any further movement. The EMT should *not* release stabilization of the bone until *after* the limb has been properly immobilized.

Then a second EMT should expose the injury, cutting clothing away carefully, and control any bleeding. This EMT should then cover any protruding bone ends with a dry sterile dressing and proceed with splinting the limb.

Several different splints may be used on the same limb, depending on the location of the injury on the limb. Several different splinting techniques can be used for an injury in the same place on the same limb.

Splinting

Normally, a bone provides structure and support to a limb. A splint is designed to provide support to a limb where the bone is injured. In a sense, the splint is an external skeleton that takes the place of the internal skeleton.

A splint prevents movement and, therefore, further injury to the bone and surrounding soft tissues. Splints also reduce pain, as movement of bone ends against one another can be very painful. By preventing such movement, a splint reduces the pain the patient is experiencing.

Finally, splints help to control bleeding. A splint prevents bone ends from cutting soft tissues and blood vessels surrounding the injury site.

Principles of Splinting

There are more than 200 bones in the body. Each bone can be fractured and each bone can be splinted in several different ways. The number of techniques used to splint fractures seems almost endless, yet several basic principles provide a foundation for the application of all splints.

The first principle is life before limb. The EMT must never compromise a patient's survival just to splint an injured extremity. Life-threatening injuries must be dealt with first. If the patient needs immediate transportation and the possibility of bone injuries exists, the EMT should immobilize the entire body to a backboard.

The EMT should immediately stabilize the limb to prevent further injury. The EMT should take a firm handhold above and below the injury and manually hold the bone in place until another EMT has a splint in place. The second EMT should always expose the wound and investigate the possibility of an open fracture. Bleeding control usually takes priority over fracture management. The techniques used to stop severe bleeding are described in Chapter 24.

The second EMT should check for distal pulses, movement, and sensation before applying a splint. Pulselessness is a medical emergency. Surgical intervention may be necessary. The EMT should contact medical control immediately for further instructions.

Some patients may want to try to walk (weight-bear) on the injured limb. The EMT should never allow the patient to walk on or use the extremity. Weight bearing can further aggravate the injury.

The EMT should attempt to splint the bones in the position found, if possible. Joints should never be straightened unless distal pulses are absent. Long bones should be straightened only when application of the splint in the position the bone was found is impractical. More information about straightening an extremity fracture is provided later in the chapter.

The splint should immobilize the joints above and below the injury site. Movement of these joints can create movement of the bone ends. A splint should be chosen that is long enough to immobilize all three places.

Whenever possible, the patient's hands or feet should be placed in a natural position called the **position of function**. The position of function for the ankle is relaxed at a 90-degree angle. The hand should be splinted in a slightly closed position, as if the patient were holding an egg.

The EMT should pad the voids between the splint and the limb. This padding makes the splint more comfortable and improves stabilization by providing support along a wider surface. Towels, universal dressings, and foam are excellent materials to use for padding.

The EMT should avoid placing straps over the injury site. Pressure from a strap may displace bone ends and cause further injury. If pressure is needed at the site to control bleeding, a pressure bandage should be applied, and then the limb should be splinted.

The limb should be elevated above the level of the heart. Elevation of an injured limb helps to reduce swelling and pain. Application of ice or cold packs to the injury is also recommended.

Finally, the distal pulses, movement, and sensation should be reassessed and documented. Any change in the patient's condition should be noted. Loss of pulses may be caused by tight bandages. The EMT should loosen the bandages and recheck the pulses; if the pulse is still absent, the patient should be packaged and transported. Table 25-2 summarizes the principles of splinting.

Distal Pulses

Distal pulses should be assessed whenever a bone injury is suspected. The radial pulse is the distal pulse point for an arm. The radial pulse is located on the lateral wrist, proximal to the thumb.

The feet have several pulses an EMT can use to assess distal circulation. The pedal pulse (dorsalis pedis) is on the anterior surface of the foot, midline and midway between the toes and the ankle. Figure 25-9 shows an EMT checking a pedal pulse.

At the distal tibia, on the inside of the ankle where the bone meets the ankle, is a bony protrusion called the medial malleolus. The posterior tibial artery runs just behind the malleolus, and a pulse usually can be palpated at that point. Figure 25-10 shows an EMT checking a posterior tibial pulse.

Realigning Bones

Pulselessness in an injured extremity is an ominous finding. If pulses do not return, tissue death may necessitate an amputation. In cases in which pulses are absent, the EMT should consider making one attempt to realign the bones and relieve pressure on the impinged

TABLE 25-2
Principles of Splinting

1. Always consider life before limb.

2. Manually stabilize a suspected fracture.

3. Expose the injury.

4. Control bleeding. (Any life-threatening bleeding would have been dealt with during the initial assessment.)

5. Check for pulses, movement, and sensation distal to the injury.

6. Never allow the patient to bear weight on the injured limb.

7. Splint the injury in the position found.

8. Immobilize the joints above and below the injury. (If a joint is injured, then immobilize the bones above and below the joint.)

9. Elevate the injury above the level of the heart.

10. Pad the voids between the splint and the limb.

11. Avoid placing straps directly over the injured area.

12. Recheck distal pulses, movement, and sensation after the splint is applied.

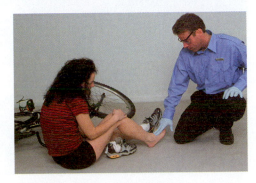

FIGURE 25-9 A pedal pulse is a positive sign of distal circulation.

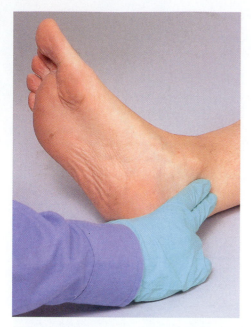

FIGURE 25-10 The posterior tibial pulse may be easier to palpate.

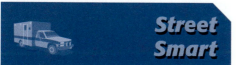

Often it is difficult to obtain a distal pulse in the feet. The patient may have poor peripheral circulation due to age, disease, or the cold. Many EMTs try to find the posterior tibial pulse because the landmark, the malleolus, is easy to identify. When a distal pulse is found, the EMT can lightly mark the pulse point with a pen. Pen ink can be easily washed off later, and the mark can save time when pulses are rechecked.

Street Smart

A splint that was applied correctly on the scene can loosen with movement during transportation. The EMT should recheck the splint frequently, at least as often as he checks the vital signs, to ensure that the splint is doing what it was created to do, that is, splinting the injury. Failure to constantly monitor a splint can mean movement of bone ends, which can cut blood vessels and cause bleeding.

artery. The EMT can call medical control for advice and direction, and should always follow local medical protocols.

In attempting to realign the bones, the EMT grasps the limb firmly and exerts a continuous gentle pull, called **traction**, along the long axis of the bone. Slight rotation, back to a natural alignment, is sometimes needed as well. The EMT should stop applying traction once the bone is in line or resistance is met.

If pulses have not returned after the EMT's attempt to realign the bones, the patient should be packaged and transported immediately to the closest appropriate facility.

Splinting Devices

A large assortment of splinting devices and materials is on the market, but all of them serve the same purpose, to provide external support to an injured bone. These splinting devices can be grouped into five general classifications.

The **sling and swathe (S/S)** was probably the first splint ever used. An injured arm is first suspended in a triangular bandage made into a sling, and then firmly anchored to the body's side using a cravat called a swathe (Figure 25-11). The body provides the external support and rigidity needed.

A **flexible splint** can be made from any material that can be formed to fit any angle and then made to be rigid. Aluminum ladder splints and structural aluminum malleable (SAM) splints are examples of flexible splints. Flexible splints are particularly useful for injuries in joints, including the joints in the hands and feet (Figure 25-12).

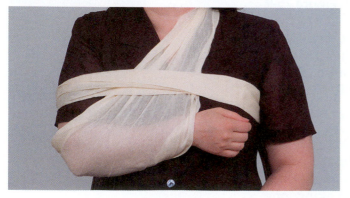

FIGURE 25-11 The sling and swathe, using triangular bandages, is commonly used to splint upper extremity injuries.

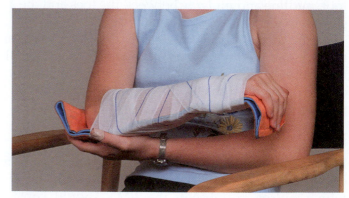

FIGURE 25-12 A flexible splint, like the SAM splint, is convenient for splinting a deformed extremity.

A **rigid splint** is made of any firm material that can be placed next to the limb to provide support. A padded board splint is commonly used as a rigid splint. Rolled newspapers and magazines, wooden spoons, and salad forks have all been used as rigid splints in an emergency. Some rigid splints are manufactured with an inflexible metal or wooden splint inside and a flexible canvas or plastic sleeve that can be closed with Velcro fasteners on the outside. Rigid splints are used whenever an injury occurs along the midshaft portion of the bone.

A splint that allows air to be pumped in or suctioned out of it is a **pneumatic splint** (Figure 25-13). The splint is placed around the limb and inflated/deflated until it becomes rigid. The military anti-shock trousers/pneumatic anti-shock garment (MAST/PASG) used in the stabilization of pelvic fractures is an example of a pneumatic splint.

Femur fractures are stabilized with a splint that can maintain a continuous positive force, or traction, on the femur. **Traction splints** decrease muscular spasm and pain as well as prevent bone ends from overriding.

Some traction splints use just one pole for external support of the injured leg and therefore are referred to as **unipolar traction splints**. Skill 25-1 demonstrates the use of this type of splinting device.

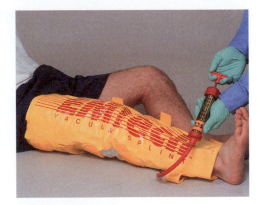

FIGURE 25-13 A vacuum splint is a type of pneumatic splint.

SKILL 25-1 *Application of a Unipolar Traction Splint*

PURPOSE: To apply a traction device to a possible mid-shaft femur fracture.

STANDARD PRECAUTIONS:

☑ Scissors
☑ Unipolar traction device
☑ Personal protective equipment

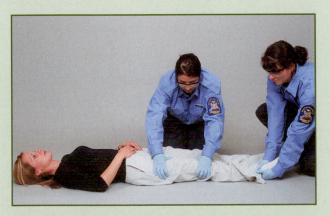

1 The EMT should manually stabilize the limb while instructing a trained assistant to grasp the leg and apply manual stabilization of the affected leg.

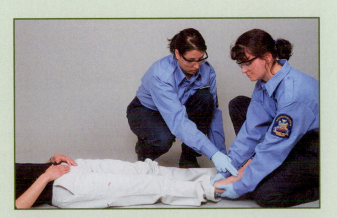

2 The EMT checks distal pulses, movement, and circulation in the affected leg.

(continues)

SKILL 25-1 (continued)

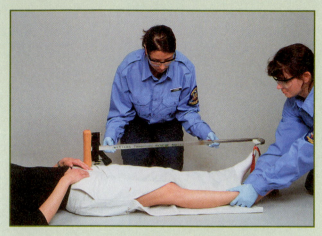

3 The EMT then prepares the traction device, adjusting it to about 3 to 4 inches past the leg.

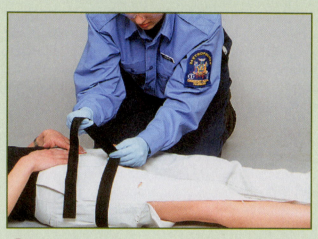

4 The EMT slides the traction splint between the legs and secures the ischial strap across the thigh.

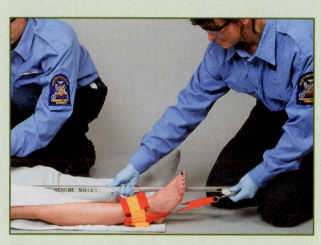

5 Next, the EMT applies the ankle hitch to the ankle and applies traction of the leg.

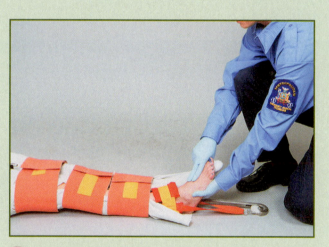

6 The EMT then puts the straps in place and rechecks distal pulses, movement, and sensation.

Another type of traction splint is the **bipolar traction splint**. The bipolar splint uses two external poles, one on each side of the leg, to provide external support for the injured leg. The bipolar splint is a direct descendant of the Thomas half-ring splint that was originally put into service in World War I. Skill 25-2 demonstrates the use of this type of splinting device.

Transportation

The EMT makes a mistake when, instead of focusing on the more important patient problems such as hypoperfusion, he focuses on the grievous bony injuries that the patient has sustained. The EMT's first

SKILL 25-2 *Application of a Bipolar Traction Splint*

PURPOSE: To apply a traction device to a possible mid-shaft femur fracture.

STANDARD PRECAUTIONS:

- ☑ Bipolar traction splint
- ☑ Personal protective equipment
- ☑ Scissors

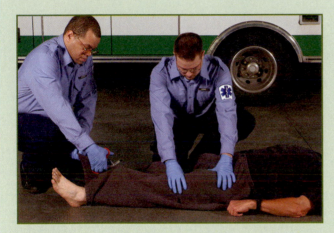

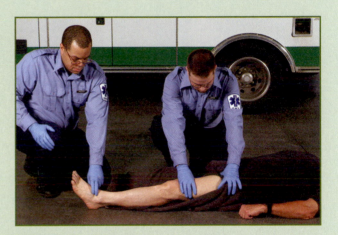

1 One EMT should manually stabilize the limb as another EMT exposes the wound.

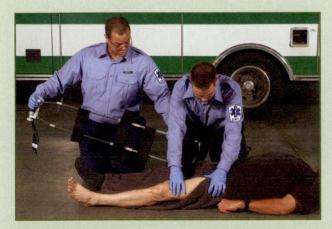

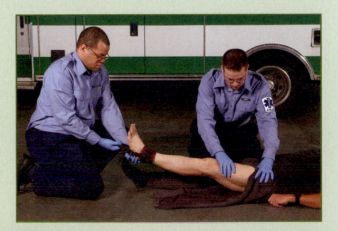

3 The EMT then prepares the traction device, adjusting it beyond the length of the uninjured leg, and moves the straps into place.

4 Next, the EMT applies the ankle hitch to the ankle and assumes traction of the leg.

(continues)

SKILL 25-2 (continued)

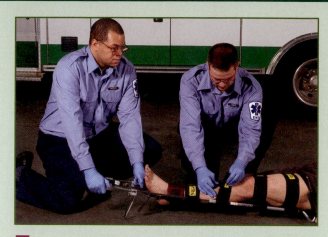

5 Then the EMT slides the traction splint under the legs and secures the straps.

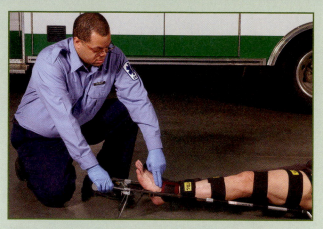

6 In the last step, the EMT applies the ankle hitch to the ratchet and applies mechanical traction. With the straps in place, the EMT rechecks distal pulses, movement, and sensation.

priority is always life over limb. Sometimes a broken bone will not be individually splinted; rather, the patient's entire body will be splinted and the patient transported immediately. The EMT must make a careful, considered decision on when, where, and how to transport a trauma patient. A wrong decision may mean the difference between life and death.

In almost every case, from serious multisystem trauma with multiple broken bones to the simple twisted ankle, the patient is going to be in pain. In many cases, advanced life support (ALS) can provide the patient with some relief from the oppressive pain. Pain management, using pain medicines such as narcotics, is a part of the expertise that an ALS provider can bring to the scene. The EMT should consider calling for ALS early during patient care.

Ongoing Assessment

Soft tissue injury almost always occurs with bone injury, resulting in tissue swelling that can cause bandages to become so tight they act like a tourniquet. For this reason, whenever an EMT checks the patient's vital signs, he also should reassess the distal circulation of any extremity that is splinted.

INJURIES TO THE SHOULDER GIRDLE

Whenever an EMT is assessing for possible bony injury, he must be mindful of the possibility of secondary associated injury. A fractured forearm, for example, as well as an injured wrist is common in patients who have taken a fall.

Climbing Accident

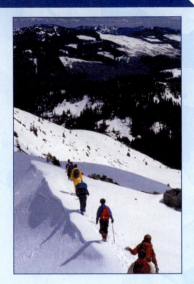

It was Ranger Fish's last winter on the job before he retired. He had seen it all—campers mauled by bears, campers burnt by campfires, campers infected with "beaver fever"—but what made him nervous were the ice climbers.

Recently, the Trap Dike, next to the slides of Mount Colden, had become a new sensation for ice climbers, and it seemed like busloads of them were trekking in for a weekend and a shot at glory. There had already been three major rescues this season, and Ranger Fish was carefully watching the newest group of climbers ascend over the waterfalls.

Then it happened. A misstep or a lost point, it did not matter. The climber made a short slide, then fell backward for what seemed like forever. Finally an ice screw grabbed hold and the climber hung in midair, upside down, yelling.

As Ranger Fish made his way across the frozen lake, he could not help but think, "Darn fool kids." The other climbers had already managed to get the injured climber off the ice and onto the ground as Ranger Fish approached. "Hi, kid. What's your name? Where do you hurt?" he asked.

"Steve, and I think I hurt my shoulder," replied the climber. "Do you think you can walk?" asked the ranger. "Sure," Steve replied. "Well, let me check you out," the ranger said, "and then we'll get back to the station." The ranger unslung his backpack and removed the necessary first-aid gear.

- Based on the mechanism of injury, what injuries might an EMT suspect?
- What are the assessment priorities for this patient?
- What are the management priorities for this patient?
- How could this patient deteriorate?

Injury of the Clavicle

The collarbone, or clavicle, is a long S-shaped bone located in the upper anterior chest wall. It is a part of the shoulder girdle. The clavicle, at its distal end, joins the shoulder blade, or scapula. Many of the accessory muscles of breathing are attached to the clavicle.

The clavicle is very prone to injury because of its relatively exposed location. For example, any force on the arm may be transmitted to the clavicle, causing a fracture. An example of indirect trauma creating an injury of the clavicle would be when a child falls off a bicycle onto an outstretched hand, and a clavicular fracture occurs.

A direct force, such as a blow to the shoulder, can also fracture the clavicle. Likewise, compression of the thoracic cage and the shoulder girdle can produce a clavicular fracture. In fact, the clavicle is one of the most commonly fractured bones in the body.

Under the clavicle lie several major blood vessels, including the subclavian artery. For this reason, neurovascular injury may accompany a clavicular fracture.

Signs and Symptoms

The presentation of a patient with a clavicular injury is classic. At the site of the fracture, the skin is often tented, since the clavicle is just

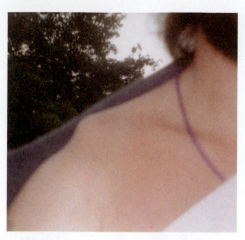

FIGURE 25-14   A fractured clavicle often has a classic handlebar shape that tents the overlying skin.

below the skin (Figure 25-14). Often the bone ends are displaced, leaving a distinctive "stepped off" appearance, like a bicycle's handlebar. Finally, the patient often holds the injured arm across the front of her body in an effort to self-splint the injury.

The shoulder girdle and the clavicles are proximal to the rib cage and the lungs. A displaced bone can easily puncture a lung and cause a pneumothorax. (See Chapter 23 for signs and symptoms of a pneumothorax.) The EMT should follow the standard order of assessment while remembering that a life-threatening injury to the lung may have occurred. Once the EMT is satisfied that no immediate life threats exist, the EMT should continue with his focused physical examination, looking for the general signs and symptoms of a bone injury as previously described.

Management

Before splinting a clavicle, the EMT must carefully assess the patient for any associated injury to adjacent scapula and humerus. Then, supporting the patient's efforts to self-splint, the EMT should use a sling and swathe. The sling supports the weight of the arm, while the swathe binds the arm to the body to prevent further movement. The EMT should keep the patient in a sitting position during transport.

Injury of the Scapula

The scapula is a broad, triangular-shaped bone located in the upper portion of the back. Fractures of the scapula are rare. Thick, flat muscles overlying the scapula and elastic ribs underneath the scapula permit the scapula to absorb a great deal of force without breaking. Consequently, when an EMT discovers a potential scapular fracture, he should have a high index of suspicion that other injuries also may be present.

Signs and Sypmtoms

The bone ends seldom displace in a scapular fracture; therefore, the classic "deformity" is not found. Often the only outward signs of a scapular fracture are point tenderness and a contusion at the site of injury.

Management

The patient's arm should be secured to the chest with a sling and swathe to prevent movement of the shoulder on the affected side.

Injury of the Acromioclavicular (A/C) Joint

The acromion process of the scapula and the clavicle join to form the shoulder joint. Inserted into this shoulder joint is the humerus. When the clavicle is forced downward, the tendons are torn. This movement of the clavicle out of the joint is called an **acromioclavicular (A/C) dislocation**.

A common mechanism that creates A/C dislocations is a blow from above directly onto the clavicle. Again, the patient will frequently self-splint to protect the injury. The EMT should apply a sling and swathe to prevent further movement of the bone.

Injury of the Shoulder

The shoulder has a great range of motion. When an arm is held overhead, or outreached, and a sudden force strikes it, the humerus can literally "pop" out of joint, resulting in a **shoulder dislocation**. The shoulder is one of the most commonly dislocated joints in the body.

Signs and Symptoms

A shoulder dislocation can be very painful. The powerful shoulder muscles spasm while trying to get the humerus back into the joint. Any movement, even the vibration of the ambulance, can create severe pain.

The injured shoulder will appear "squared off," lacking its naturally rounded contour. The injured shoulder also will appear different, asymmetrical, when compared to the uninjured shoulder.

The majority of shoulder dislocations are anterior dislocations. The arm has been forced away from the body and is unable to return to its natural position. The patient, in an attempt to prevent further pain, will hold the arm out away from the body.

Management

A shoulder injury could be managed with a sling and swathe, but any attempt to move the patient's arm closer to her body usually elicits a loud protest from the patient. In addition, a nerve bundle runs over the top of the humerus, and the nerves occasionally become entrapped in the socket of a dislocated shoulder. Consequently, the patient may complain of numbness along the upper arm, near the deltoid muscle, or in the hands. Therefore, the EMT must be extremely cautious when splinting a possibly dislocated shoulder.

To splint a dislocated shoulder, the EMT may place either a pillow or a bedroll under the arm and secure the cushion in place with a cravat around the chest (Figure 25-15). Once the cushion is secured, the elbow may be flexed to a 90-degree angle and a sling and swathe applied. The EMT should carefully reassess distal pulses, movement, and sensation of the injured limb, and should place the patient in a seated position for transport.

Injury of the Upper Arm

The humerus is the long straight bone in the upper arm. Most injuries to the humerus occur after a large force has been applied to a small portion of the bone. Consequently, the bone ends may be displaced, and the injury appears swollen and deformed.

Management

In most cases, a fracture of the humerus can be splinted in the position found. In rare cases in which there is neurovascular compromise, the EMT may need to straighten the humerus before applying the splint.

After assessing distal pulses, sensation, and movement, the EMT would grasp the patient's arm at the elbow and the shoulder. Placing the thumb of one hand at the midline of the shoulder, the EMT would then firmly grasp the upper arm. The EMT's other hand would grasp the elbow. By applying continuous downward pressure along the axis

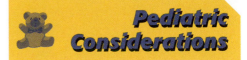

Pediatric Considerations

A child often has difficulty explaining exactly where the pain is located. Often the child will complain that an entire arm hurts. Observing the mechanism of injury may provide a clue to the injury. Falls from bikes, trees, and so forth can cause wrist, elbow, shoulder, and clavicle injuries. If a clavicular injury is present, assessment of the child's clavicle will reveal point tenderness, swelling, and deformity of the clavicle.

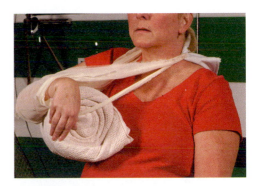

FIGURE 25-15 A bedroll, secured around the body by a cravat, maintains the arm in the position found.

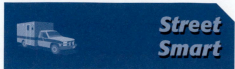

Street Smart

Once injured, the shoulder is prone to injury again. The weakened ligaments allow the head of the humerus to "slip out of joint" easily. Many patients learn to reduce their own fractures. Eventually this approach fails, often after several dozen dislocations, and the shoulder becomes locked into position. When that occurs, the patient will elect to call emergency medical services (EMS).

of the bone, the EMT may be able to realign the bone ends. The EMT should stop, however, if the patient complains loudly about the pain or resistance is met.

Once the arm is grossly in line, another EMT should place a padded board splint along the length of the upper arm and secure it. A sling and swathe can then be applied. The EMT should follow local protocols regarding straightening bone injuries or consider calling medical control for advice.

Injury of the Elbow

At the juncture of three bones, the ulna, the radius, and the humerus, is the elbow. Force applied to any or several of these bones can either fracture a bone or dislocate the elbow itself.

Signs and Symptoms

Typically, the elbow becomes locked into position and the patient complains of severe pain. The elbow will appear out of line and severely deformed.

Management

Blood vessels and nerves run through the elbow, as they do through the shoulder. Any movement puts these blood vessels and nerves at risk for further injury. For this reason, the elbow is usually splinted in the position that it is found.

The EMT begins by assessing the distal pulse, movement, and sensation. Weak or absent pulses may indicate that a blood vessel has been crimped or severed. The EMT should contact medical control immediately for further instructions. Immediate transportation of the patient may be ordered. The EMT also should follow local medical protocols regarding procedures for pulseless limbs.

If a pulse is present, the EMT places one padded board splint under the arm so that the ends are at the wrist under the forearm and at the shoulder. Then another padded board splint is placed on top of the first padded board splint. The EMT firmly secures the two ends of the board splints to each other. The elbow should be firmly immobilized between the two boards. A sling may be used to support the entire arm.

Flexible splints, like the wire ladder splint and the SAM splint, can be shaped to conform to the length of the limb (Figure 25-16). Once in place, the flexible splint should be secured with a roller bandage. A sling will help support the arm and relieve pressure on the elbow.

Injury of the Forearm

Children commonly injure the forearm. Sports, horseplay, and falls account for a large number of these injuries. Typically, both the radius and the ulna are fractured. Without any bony support, the limb may move where there is no joint.

Management

Rigid splints, flexible splints, and pneumatic splints all can be used to splint the forearm. Before any splint is applied, the EMT must first manually stabilize the forearm.

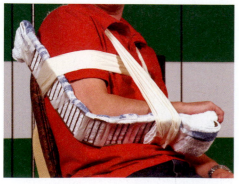

FIGURE 25-16 A ladder splint is very effective when trying to splint a joint.

Typically, a rigid board splint is applied to the underside of the forearm, and then the arm is secured, past the wrist to the fingertips, to the board splint with cravats (Figure 25-17). A sling and swathe is then applied to the patient's entire arm. The patient's fingers should be exposed so the EMT can easily access them for assessment, and the patient's hand should be elevated above the level of the heart.

Injury of the Wrist and Hand

The wrist and hand contain a complex collection of small bones that allow a deal great of motion. These bones are also prone to a great number of injuries.

Signs and Symptoms

When the distal radius bone is involved, the wrist takes on a characteristic deformity that looks like a silver fork. This silver fork fracture is also called a **Colles' fracture** (Figure 25-18).

Other injuries can result in rapid swelling, pain, and loss of function. The importance of properly caring for a wrist and hand injury cannot be overemphasized. Often the patient's ability to make a living is dependent on the hands. Serious hand injuries can lead to permanent disabilities. Any injury, whether it is a simple laceration or a possible bone injury, should be treated as serious.

Management

The EMT should first attempt to place the hand in the position of function. A 3-inch roller bandage placed in the palm of the hand works well. Then the EMT should place the entire forearm onto a padded board splint. Flexible splints, such as the wire ladder splint, can be useful for a severely deformed wrist.

When wrapping the forearm with a bandage, the EMT needs to make sure that the fingers remain out in the open. The usual distal pulses will be covered by the bandage, so the EMT must depend on the presence of good capillary refill to verify distal circulation.

The entire forearm should be placed in a sling and swathe, with the hand positioned above the heart. If this is not practical, then the forearm should be placed on a pillow to elevate it above the heart.

INJURIES TO THE PELVIC GIRDLE

The pelvic girdle contains some of the largest bones in the body. The pelvic girdle also accommodates some of the largest blood vessels in the body. When an injury occurs anywhere in the pelvic girdle, the possibility of serious internal bleeding must be considered.

The initial assessment must always be completed in order. If the EMT has a high index of suspicion, based on the mechanism of the injury, that the patient may have sustained a pelvic girdle injury, the EMT should always keep in mind the possibility of internal bleeding and resultant systemic hypoperfusion.

Injury of the Pelvis

The pelvis itself is made up of several flat bones that form a ring. A ring, by its physical nature, is very strong. For this reason, it takes an extreme

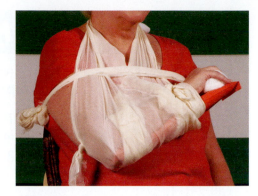

FIGURE 25-17 A padded board splint secures a forearm, and the sling and swathe stabilizes the joint above and below.

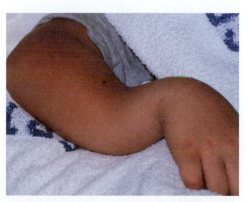

FIGURE 25-18 A Colles', or silver fork fracture, is very distinctive. (Courtesy of Deborah Funk, MD, Albany Medical Center, Albany, NY.)

Fall from a Horse

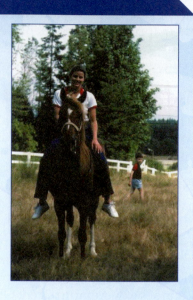

The horse was galloping along when suddenly its front leg went into a hole. The horse fell sideways, right on top of its young rider, Carolyn.

Realizing immediately what had happened, Katie, the trainer at Three Pines Stables, ran to Carolyn and immediately pulled her from underneath the horse. Carolyn, not comprehending what had happened, tried to stand up but could not. So she remained on her back while Katie ran to the barn to call 9-1-1.

The engine company arrived quickly; the officer-in-charge ordered two men to get the basket, while the EMT on the crew, Stanley, went to the patient's side.

"Please don't move," Stanley advised his young patient. "My name is Stanley, and I am with the fire department. The ambulance is coming from the city, but it might be a few minutes. Can you tell me what hurts?"

Carolyn, who was starting to feel the pain, said, "My hip hurts." Stanley started to take a set of vital signs, looked at the horse, and then decided he had better have an ALS unit respond to the scene.

- Based on the mechanism of injury, what injuries might an EMT suspect?
- What are the assessment priorities for this patient?
- What are the management priorities for this patient?
- How could this patient deteriorate?

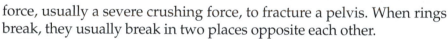

force, usually a severe crushing force, to fracture a pelvis. When rings break, they usually break in two places opposite each other.

The broad wings, or crests, of the pelvis protect a large number of important organs. The bladder, the intestine, the uterus, the iliac arteries, and the sciatic nerve, to name a few, all reside within the pelvis. Injury to the pelvis may cause injury to those organs.

Open fractures of the pelvis are rare because the pelvis is surrounded by layers of large muscles and fat. The majority of bleeding from a pelvic fracture is internal, usually bleeding into the pelvis and the retroperitoneal cavity. The retroperitoneal cavity is found behind the abdominal cavity and contains the kidneys, the aorta, the vena cava, and other organs.

Bleeding into the retroperitoneal space is often obscure, and thus goes undetected. Internal bleeding from a pelvic fracture into the retroperitoneal space can be life threatening. Over time significant retroperitoneal blood collection can be seen as bruising at the flank (Figure 25-19). Several liters of blood can be lost, resulting in hypoperfusion and hypotension.

Signs and Symptoms

Any patient who has been involved in a high-speed motor vehicle collision, a fall from a great height, or other similar high-velocity mechanism of injury, or who has been crushed between two objects, should

FIGURE 25-19 Significant retroperitoneal blood collection can be seen as bruising at the flank.

be suspected of having a pelvic fracture. Likewise, a patient who, after sustaining a serious trauma, complains of an ache or pain in the lower back should be suspected of having a pelvic fracture. The danger of serious life-threatening bleeding is so high that any patient involved in a significant trauma should be suspected of having a pelvic injury.

Perhaps the best indication of a pelvic fracture is a sharp pain or diffuse tenderness when the pelvic ring is lightly compressed. Gentle compression of the pelvis should be a part of every detailed physical examination. The **symphysis pubis**, the union of the two pubic bones found above the genitalia, also should be gently compressed, although this step should be avoided if the patient complains of pain, no further assessment is needed, or a pelvic fracture can be safely assumed. The proper methods of assessing the pelvis are covered in Chapter 15 and should be reviewed.

If sharp pain or point tenderness is noted upon gentle compression, a pelvic fracture should be suspected, and the EMT should assess for signs of hypoperfusion and shock.

Management

Fractures of the pelvis, also known as the pelvic ring, have been associated with a higher mortality. In any case of suspected pelvic instability, the fractured bones need external support. The EMT may elect to use the **pelvic wrap technique**. The pelvic wrap consists of a wide swath of material, generally cotton, that can be placed around the circumference of the pelvis and secured tightly.

The pelvic wrap, very similar to an abdominal binder that is used postoperatively to hold abdominal dressings in place, provides a gentle, circumferential pressure that keeps all of the bones of the pelvic ring in alignment. Keeping these bones in place helps to prevent lacerations of major blood vessels such as the femoral artery, puncture of the bladder, or perforation of the colon and rectum.

The use of PASG has been somewhat controversial over the past several years, yet this device provides immobilization for unstable pelvic fractures.

There are several methods of applying PASG. One method is to open the PASG and lay the PASG on top of a board. The patient can be logrolled onto the PASG, although this can be very painful and potentially cause further injury. Use of the orthopedic stretcher, also called the scoop stretcher, to lift and place the patient on the PASG and backboard is less traumatic to the patient (Figure 25-20).

Another technique of applying PASG involves placing the patient on the long backboard, then slipping the PASG onto the patient like a pair of pants. One EMT runs his hands up the pant legs of the PASG and grabs the patient's ankles, then another EMT pulls the PASG onto the patient.

The top of the PASG should be at the bottom of the lowest rib. Occasionally, the abdominal section needs to be folded in half to prevent the abdominal section from overriding the ribs. The legs of the PASG also may be adjusted, folding small sections underneath and inside the pant leg. The PASG should be properly fitted to the patient before inflation starts.

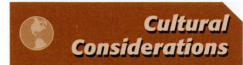

Cultural Considerations

Some patients may be uncomfortable with an EMT pressing on their symphysis pubis because of its relative proximity to the genitals. To increase the patient's comfort with this important aspect of the physical examination, the EMT may take the patient's uninjured hand and place it over the pubic bone, then place his hand on top of the patient's hand and gently compress the pubis.

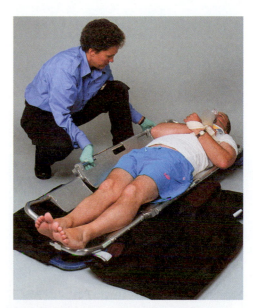

FIGURE 25-20 The orthopedic stretcher may be used to move a patient whose pelvis is unstable onto a long backboard with the PASG.

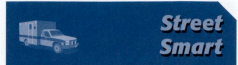

The PASG should be inflated to about 60 mm Hg, if the PASG has gauges, or until an indentation can be created with the thumb, as with an air splint. In fact, the PASG is just one massive air splint that completely pads all the surfaces of the patient's lower extremities.

If the patient's condition starts to deteriorate, the PASG can be rapidly inflated. Chapter 9 provides specific steps to follow in applying the PASG, as well as a photo procedure guide.

Pelvic fractures can cause massive bleeding. The abdominal cavity and the retroperitoneal space can obscure and hide massive bleeding. Unfortunately, it is often late when an EMT discovers that the patient is experiencing massive internal bleeding from the pelvic injury. The EMT often attributes the sustained tachycardia and other signs of hypoperfusion that the patient is exhibiting to the pain that the patient is experiencing.

The key to early detection lies in careful reevaluation of the patient's vital signs and an analysis of the trend that is created. If the patient's heart rate is increasing steadily, instead of decreasing after splinting, and the blood pressure is starting to fall, the EMT should suspect internal bleeding and request an ALS intercept or rapid transportation to a trauma center.

Injury of the Proximal Femur

The femur, the strongest bone in the body, provides the foundation for the muscles of the legs so that people can walk. Without an intact femur, walking is almost impossible.

When a powerful force is applied to the femur, either at the insertion of the femur into the pelvis or at the end of the femur proximal to the knee, the femur can either dislocate or break. The femur tends to break at the thinnest portion of the femur, called the surgical neck. The surgical neck is proximal to the head of the femur, which inserts into the pelvis.

Signs and Symptoms

Injury of the femur can be caused by indirect violence, such as when the knee is struck, which can drive the femur backward and dislocate the femur from the pelvis. The femur can be injured from direct trauma as well, for example, if the door of a car is driven into the hip of a patient in a motor vehicle collision. Regardless of the mechanism of injury, a hip injury can have serious complications.

The nerve that provides sensation and movement to the legs, the **sciatic nerve**, runs adjacent to the femur. A hip injury can injure the sciatic nerve, leaving the patient's leg numb (paresthesia) or unable to move (paralysis).

A subtle, yet easily detected, sign of sciatic nerve injury is **footdrop**. The sciatic nerve controls the elevation, or **dorsiflexion**, of the foot. A foot that cannot be lifted (dorsiflexion) is a sign that the patient's sciatic nerve, and the hip, may be injured.

The most dependable sign of a hip injury is severe pain with gentle compression upon the femur's point of insertion into the pelvis. The EMT should place his hands on each side of the hip, with his palms on the firm portion of the lateral buttocks, and press gently. If the femoral head is broken or the hip is dislocated, the patient should protest loudly.

Typically, when the hip is fractured, one leg will be shortened, compared to the other, and externally rotated (pointing away from midline) (Figure 25-21). If the hip is dislocated, the injured hip will be flexed, and the leg internally rotated (pointing toward the midline).

Management

The EMT does not need to distinguish a hip fracture from a hip dislocation in the field. In both cases, the hip must be handled carefully to avoid further injury. The EMT should support the affected limb by putting either pillows or blankets between and under the legs. The patient's hip and leg should be securely fastened to a long backboard.

The EMT also must consider the possibility of concurrent spine injury. If the force was great enough to break a hip, it may have broken the neck as well. A detailed physical examination, with attention to peripheral pulses, movement, and sensation, should be performed before and after immobilization.

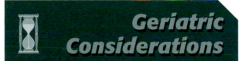

FIGURE 25-21 Often the leg of a broken hip will be shortened and rotated externally. (Courtesy of Deborah Funk, MD, Albany Medical Center, Albany, NY.)

Injury of the Midshaft Femur

The femur is the longest bone in the body, almost 18 inches long in the average 6-foot-tall person. Powerful muscles in the thighs attach to the femur and, by contraction, move the leg forward, propelling the body along with it.

The middle portion of the femur, or the midshaft, is very strong and can resist injury. However, enough force, a fall from a height, for example, can shatter even the strongest femur.

Street Smart

A patient involved in a motor vehicle collision may complain that she simply "cannot get out of the car." When the femur is driven backward and the hip becomes dislocated, the patient's hips will be locked into the seated position.

Careful examination of the crash bar under the dashboard may reveal damage from the patient's knee striking the crash bar. Palpation of the patient's knee may reveal swelling and tenderness over the kneecap, or patella. If the EMT palpates the posterior buttocks, he may discover a lump, which would be the head of the femur.

A hip dislocation is very painful, and the patient may resist any attempts at moving the hip. For this reason, the patient must be moved as a unit. Frequently, the car has to be dismantled before the patient can be lifted out. Heavy rescue and EMS must work together to create the easiest means of access to and exit for the patient.

Geriatric Considerations

Osteoporosis, a softening of the bones from calcium loss, frequently occurs with old age. Osteoporosis occurs more commonly in women than men, usually starting after the woman has completed menopause.

Softened bones are more prone to fractures. Very little violence is necessary to break the surgical neck of the femur in an elderly woman. A careful history taken from the patient may reveal that the patient heard a crack (the sound a bone makes when it breaks), and then fell, instead of falling and then hearing a crack. These spontaneous fractures can occur with little or no pain. The detailed physical examination generally uncovers the injury.

Signs and Symptoms

When the middle section of the femur is broken, the muscles contract and drive the bone ends together. The resulting spasm, as the muscle ineffectually strives to move the leg, is very painful.

Nearby blood vessels, as well as muscles, can be lacerated by the sharp bone shards. The result is significant bleeding into the thigh. As much as 1 liter of blood can be lost into each thigh from internal bleeding.

The effect of the muscles in spasm tends to cause the bone to become distorted and deformed. Severe deformity can result in an open fracture of the femur. If this occurs, the EMT should immediately control the bleeding and cover the wound with a dry sterile dressing.

Management

During World War I, Dr. Thomas, a noted orthopedic surgeon, realized that applying a gentle counterpressure against a muscle spasm relieved the spasm and prevented bones from lacerating blood vessels, and thus prevented further bleeding. This finding was very significant. At that time, there was a 50% mortality rate associated with a midshaft femur fracture. The Thomas half ring was an early medical device that provided the foundation for gentle counterpressure, or traction, to be applied to a broken femur.

Modern traction splints are easier to apply and operate than the early Thomas half ring with Spanish windlass. Some traction splints depend on two parallel bars, much like the early Thomas half ring. At the bottom of the device is a ratchet attached to an ankle hitch. When the ratchet is tightened, traction is applied to the ankle hitch and thus to the leg. (See Skill 25-2).

Another adaptation of the same idea uses a single pole, usually placed between the patient's legs, and a spring-loaded device that applies the traction. The advantage of the unipolar traction device is that the force is measurable, and it can easily be placed inside the PASG. (See Skill 25-1).

When the traction device is applied and the traction is in effect, the leg spasms less often, and the patient usually obtains noticeable relief of symptoms. The patient must be continually monitored for signs of hypoperfusion and transported to the closest appropriate facility.

Injury of the Patella

The kneecap, or **patella**, is a flat triangular bone that is found anterior of the knee. It primarily protects the knee joint from injury, for example, when a person kneels on one knee.

Signs and Symptoms

Typically, the kneecap is injured when the knee is twisted. When the knee twists, the kneecap often shifts laterally and is then dislocated (Figure 25-22). Although a dislocated kneecap can be very painful, it is not dangerous. Unlike other bones, there are no veins, arteries, or nerves near the kneecap.

A larger problem exists when the kneecap is actually fractured. Gentle palpation of the borders of the kneecap should reveal a single

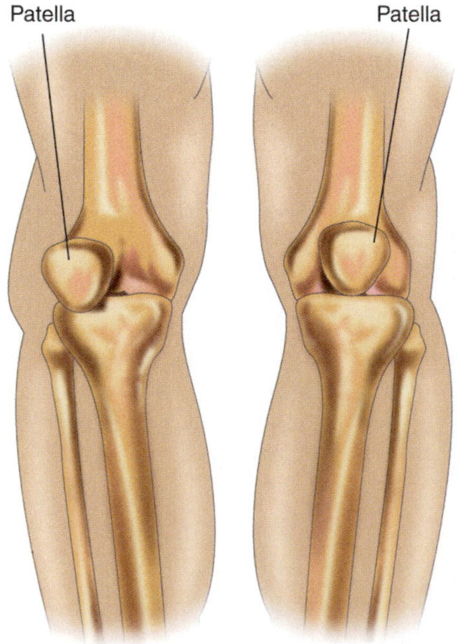

Patella   Patella

FIGURE 25-22 Kneecap dislocations usually shift laterally, appearing as a lump on the outside of the knee.

triangular-shaped bone. If the force against the kneecap was great enough, the kneecap may split into two pieces.

Management

An isolated injury to the kneecap should be treated with stabilization, immobilization, and transportation. Often the patient has already manually stabilized the knee by placing one hand on each side of the knee.

Immobilization can be accomplished with a pair of padded board splints in a manner similar to the way the elbow is immobilized. Immobilization also can be accomplished with a pillow placed under the knee and secured around the knee with cravats.

Local tissue swelling can be impressive. Ice or ice packs should be applied to the injury and the patient transported as soon as possible.

Injury of the Knee

As a joint, the knee consists of the femur, in the thigh, meeting the two bones of the lower leg, the tibia and the fibula. When a significant force is applied to either the femur or the tibia, the bone may move out of alignment. Frequently, the patient is unable to move her leg; the knee is said to be locked. The patient also may complain of severe pain. The knee is surrounded by many ligaments that are painful when injured. The leg also may appear grossly deformed, often with a distinctive drop, or "step off," in the skin's surface (Figure 25-23).

Behind the bones in the knee lie the major arteries of the lower leg. A disruption in the alignment of the bones may mean that distal circulation is disrupted. The EMT should check carefully for distal pulses. Pulselessness in the affected leg is a true medical emergency. Signs and symptoms of patella and knee dislocation are summarized in Table 25-3.

Management

In certain instances, medical control may advise the EMT to straighten the leg in an attempt to get pulses to return. The EMT should make only one attempt, being careful to monitor the pulses in the process. If pulses do not return after the leg has been straightened,

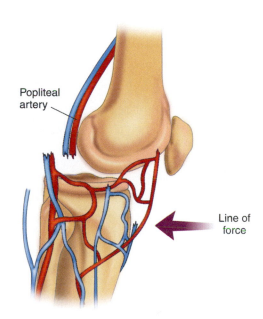

Politeal artery

Line of force

FIGURE 25-23   A knee dislocation has a characteristic "stepped off" appearance.

TABLE 25-3		
Comparison of a Kneecap and a Knee Dislocation		
Finding	**Patella or Kneecap**	**Knee**
Mechanism	Usually a fall or misstep	Major trauma
Deformity	Lateral	Anterior
Distal pulses	Present	May be absent
Severity	Low priority	High priority
Surgery	Rare	Common

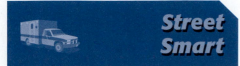

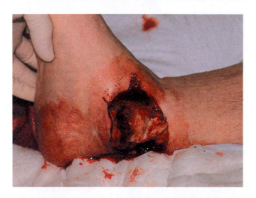

FIGURE 25-24 A tibia fracture is often an open fracture. (Courtesy of Deborah Funk, MD, Albany Medical Center, Albany, NY.)

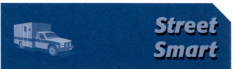

the EMT should quickly package the patient for transportation. The EMT should call the hospital and advise the emergency department of the situation so that proper preparations can be made. In every instance, the EMT should follow local medical protocols.

Injury of the Lower Leg

The bone that is found just under the skin of the anterior leg is called the tibia; the lay term is *shinbone*. This bone is responsible for weight bearing. The smaller bone behind the tibia, the fibula, is fractured more frequently than the tibia. A fracture in the fibula has fewer consequences for the patient.

Management

Because the tibia is so close to the skin, open fractures of this bone are common (Figure 25-24). The EMT should first control the bleeding, and then bandage the injury with a dry sterile dressing.

The tibia and the fibula can be immobilized using padded board splints or a vacuum splint. Keeping the principles of immobilization in mind, the EMT can effectively splint this injury.

Injury of the Ankle

Ankle injuries frequently occur, whether from sports injuries, falls, or just stepping off a curb. The ankle, like the hand, is a collection of small bones. While the majority of ankle injuries are sprains of the ligaments, each bone is capable of being fractured.

Management

It is best if an ankle injury is treated like an ankle fracture. The ankle should be immobilized with an air splint, pillow splint, or a padded board splint (Figure 25-25).

Injury of the Foot

The heel is the most commonly fractured bone in the foot. The heel, or **calcaneus**, absorbs all the force of impact in a fall or a jump. If the force is great enough, the calcaneus usually swells immediately, and the heel becomes ecchymotic.

Management

A simple pillow splint is usually sufficient to immobilize the foot. The EMT should remember to leave the toes exposed so that distal circulation and capillary refill may be assessed.

The foot is very vascular, and swelling can be rapid. The EMT should place the foot on a pillow that elevates the foot above the level of the heart. Application of ice may also decrease swelling.

The EMT should be sure to assess all the joints immediately superior to the ankle. Injury from indirect trauma can impact the knee, and even the hip as well.

CONCLUSION

A large number of bony injuries can occur to a patient. After all, there are more than 200 bones in the human body. Each bone injury is treated somewhat differently from the others, but overall, treatments for all bony injuries are similar if the EMT keeps a few principles in mind. By keeping these basic principles in mind, and often with a little inventiveness to accommodate the different patients to the limited number of splints, the EMT can overcome any problem, safely immobilize the patient's injury, and then safely transport the patient for further treatment.

TEST YOUR KNOWLEDGE

1. What are the three forces that can cause injury to a bone?
2. What are ligaments and tendons?
3. When does a dislocation become an emergency?
4. What is the difference between a closed and open fracture?
5. What are the common signs and symptoms of a bone injury?
6. What are the 12 principles of splint application?
7. What are the different techniques of splint application?
8. What are some splint application techniques for the following bone injuries:
   a. Collarbone
   b. Shoulder blade
   c. Acromioclavicular dislocation
   d. Shoulder
   e. Upper arm
   f. Elbow
   g. Forearm
   h. Wrist and hand
   i. Hip
   j. Proximal femur
   k. Midshaft femur
   l. Patella
   m. Knee
   n. Lower leg
   o. Ankle
   p. Foot
9. What is the importance of differentiating a knee dislocation from a kneecap dislocation?
10. When can an EMT straighten a fracture or dislocation?

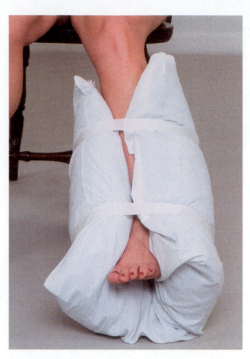

FIGURE 25-25   A pillow can serve as a splint for an ankle injury.

INTERNET RESOURCES

Conduct a search using the various types of bone injuries discussed in this chapter and key terms. What additional information can you find on the emergency treatment of these injuries? Share information with your colleagues.

FURTHER STUDY

Payne, B. (1997). Knee trauma. *Journal of Emergency Medical Services,* 22(10), 72–78.

Schultz, C., & Koenig, K. (1997). Preventing crush syndrome. *Journal of Emergency Medical Services, 22(2),* 30–38.

Stewart, C. (1999). Lower extremity trauma part I. *Emergency Medical Services, 28(4),* 43–46.

Stewart, C. (1999). Lower extremity trauma part II. *Emergency Medical Services, 28(5),* 57–59.

Stewart, C. (1999). Prehospital management of crushing injuries. *Emergency Medical Services, 28(7),* 51–55.

Suter, R. (1997). Nontraumatic extremity complaints. *Journal of Emergency Medical Services, 22(2),* 52–58.

Ward, B., & Godbout, B. (1999). Foul play. *Journal of Emergency Medical Services, 24(7),* 66–69.

Wood, S. (1998). Hip fractures and dislocations. *Journal of Emergency Medical Services, 23(11),* 154–158.

EMS in Action

As EMTs making assessments, we look for the obvious and rule out as we move forward. Successful EMTs piece together the environment, what they see, and what the patient and observers tell them to reach a correct assessment and treatment plan. However, sometimes we get thrown a curve ball and fail to see the obvious in light of logic.

One hot and humid August morning, we received a 3:00 A.M. dispatch to a bar on the southern end of Guam, where an intoxicated male had fallen down a hill and couldn't move. According to his friends, he stepped out of the bar approximately three hours earlier to "relieve" himself in the jungle.

We rappelled down a steep 50-foot embankment where the patient was upright, waist high in fresh water, leaning against the embankment. He had evidently lost his footing at the top of the embankment and slid or fell to the bottom. He was oriented to time, place, and person but his speech was slurred and he had transient lapses in consciousness. Blood pressure, pulse, and respirations were within normal limits, and on physical examination he complained of paresthesia below the waist and couldn't move his feet. Pupils were equal and reactive to light and motor function in the upper extremities was bilaterally strong. No skeletal deformities were found above the knee and assessment below the knee was prevented by thick mud and waist-high water.

Suspecting lumbar spinal trauma, we attached a backboard and hoisted the patient to the top of the embankment, where we completed our physical assessment. The victim continued lower extremity paresthesia but was able to move his toes on command. While the movement of the lower extremities was a relief, I was still concerned about a spinal injury. We packaged the patient and repeated vital signs in the ambulance, where the patient's temperature was 96.3. Then the light in my head came on; I was dealing with hypothermia.

In 10 years of EMS, some in the harshest of cold weather environments, I had never treated a patient for hypothermia. Yet in Guam, near the equator, I was sandbagged by the hot ambient temperatures not thinking about hypothermia.

James Reimer, MEd, RN
Medtronic Clinical Consultant
Medtronic Emergency Response Systems, Redmond, Washington

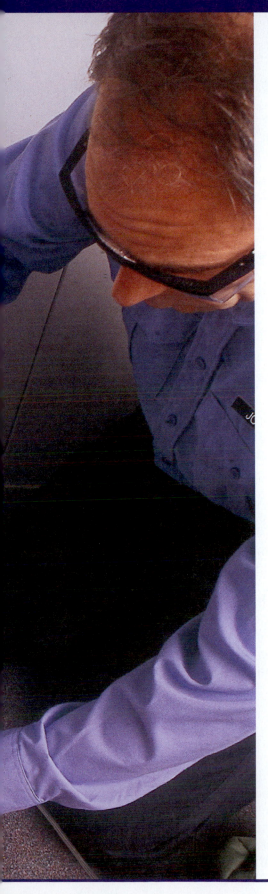

Emergency Medical Care

Often, patients call EMS because they are suffering from an illness, sickness, or affliction. It is the EMT's responsibility to determine the nature of the illness and offer the patient some symptomatic relief. The EMT's treatment is therefore based upon assessment of the patient's condition.

The diagnosis of illness could fill a library, but the EMT focuses on only a few of the more common complaints. Chest pain and shortness of breath are two complaints the EMT can often positively affect.

This section is an overview of the medical emergencies an EMT would be expected to assess, treat, and transport to an emergency department.

CHAPTER 26

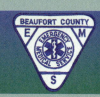

Medication Administration for the EMT

KEY TERMS

- action
- activated charcoal
- angina
- bronchodilator
- dose
- epinephrine
- expiration date
- generic
- glucose
- hypoglycemia
- intramuscular
- intravenous
- metered dose inhaler
- nebulizer
- nitroglycerin
- oral
- oxygen
- pharmacology
- side effect
- subcutaneous
- sublingual
- suspension
- topical
- trade name

OBJECTIVES

Upon completion of this chapter, the reader should be able to:

1. Discuss the importance of basic pharmacology to the EMT.
2. Explain the difference between the generic name and the trade name for medications.
3. Define the terms *indication* and *contraindication*.
4. List the different forms that medications may come in.
5. List at least three routes of drug administration used by the EMT.
6. Review the "five rights" verified before drug administration.
7. Discuss the importance of reassessment after drug administration.
8. Explain how drug administration is documented.
9. Explain the importance of the role of medical control in the administration of medication by the EMT.
10. Describe the indications, contraindications, actions, side effects, dose, and route of the following medications: activated charcoal, oral glucose, oxygen, prescribed inhaler, nitroglycerin, epinephrine.
11. Discuss the difference between an EMT's administering a drug and an EMT's assisting a patient to take a previously prescribed medication.

OVERVIEW

The emergency medical technician (EMT) will encounter many patients who are in need of a medication for one reason or another. Some patients may require a medication the EMT routinely carries, whereas others may simply need help in using their own prescribed medicines. Regardless of the particular situation, the EMT is responsible for knowing some basic information about commonly encountered medicines.

The study of medications and their interactions is called **pharmacology**. This chapter provides the information that an EMT will need to safely administer medications that are commonly used by the EMT during an emergency.

TERMINOLOGY

As does the rest of medical practice, pharmacology involves terms that must be learned. It is important for the EMT to be familiar with a few key pharmacological terms when caring for patients requiring medications.

Drug Names

No terminology will be as complex or difficult to remember as a book full of medication names! It is important for the EMT to be familiar with the names of medications commonly seen in the field, and certainly those approved for use by the EMT.

No single person can be expected to remember every name of every medication. Even physicians carry pocket reference books to look up medications. It is not a bad idea for the EMT to also carry a similar handbook that includes some basic medication information for prehospital use.

Generic

When a medication is developed, it is given a name that will appear in a governmental publication listing all drugs in the United States, called the *U.S. Pharmacopoeia*. This initial name is often a short form of the chemical name and is referred to as the **generic** name. The generic name is often longer and more difficult to pronounce than the more showy names given to the medications later when they are marketed by different companies.

Trade

The brand name that is given to a medication by the manufacturer is called the **trade name**. The trade name is often shorter, more eye catching, and easier to pronounce than the initial generic name. This trade name is used in marketing the medication.

Because some medications are manufactured by several different companies, *one medication may be given several different trade names*. This multitude of names may seem confusing, but when looked up in a drug handbook, the trade names will refer to the generic name and medication information. For this reason, some health care providers choose to learn and remember the generic names for the most common medications. Table 26-1 lists some common medications by both their generic and trade names.

Indication

The reason for giving a medication is called the indication. If an EMT is going to be allowed to administer medications, it is important to know the most commonly encountered indications for medications.

TABLE 26-1

Common Medications by Generic and Trade Names

Generic Name	Trade Name
acetaminophen	Tylenol
ibuprofen	Motrin, Advil
albuterol	Ventolin, Proventil
pseudoephedrine	Sudafed
diphenhydramine	Benadryl

An example of an indication for a medication the EMT student may be familiar with is use of acetaminophen for fever. Indications for medications that are used by the EMT are covered in detail later in this chapter.

Contraindication

There are certain circumstances in which a particular medication should not be administered because it may cause more harm than good. These instances are considered contraindications.

A good example of a contraindication is an allergy to the medication. If a patient states he is allergic to penicillin, then penicillin is contraindicated for that patient. An allergy to a medication is always a contraindication to that medication.

In some cases the patient, or the EMT, may be uncertain if a patient truly has an allergy to a medication or has experienced an unpleasant side effect to the medication. In those cases, the EMT should contact medical control for further instructions and guidance.

Actions

The effects of a medication on the person who takes it are also known as the **actions** of the medication. An example of a medication's action is the antipyretic (fever-reducing) effect of acetaminophen. The EMT must be familiar with the actions of the medications she has been approved to administer so that she knows what to expect once the medication has been given.

Side Effects

Perhaps even more important for the EMT to know are the side effects of a medication. A **side effect** is an effect of a medication that was not the intended effect. It may be unpleasant or harmful to the patient.

An example of a side effect that is discussed in more detail later in the chapter is one that is seen with nitroglycerin, a medication an EMT may administer to a patient complaining of chest pain. Nitroglycerin is intended to open up the blood vessels supplying the heart with oxygenated blood and to decrease chest pain. Nitroglycerin also tends to cause a fall in blood pressure, sometimes quite significantly. This fall in blood pressure is not the intended action of the medication but is a side effect. Not everyone who uses a medication experiences every reported side effect; therefore, not every patient who receives nitroglycerin will experience a decrease in blood pressure. If a patient's blood pressure falls after nitroglycerin administration, the EMT should be prepared for it and ready to effectively manage the situation.

It is useful for the EMT to be aware of potential side effects from medications that may be encountered during patient care in order to be ready to deal with their consequences.

Prescribing Information

When prescribing medications, physicians use several common abbreviations to instruct the patient on how to take the medicine

H-90050 (REV. 10/91)

Physician's Order Sheet

INSTRUCTIONS:
1. Imprint patient's plate before placing in chart.
2. After each medication order is written, remove first copy and fax to PHARMACY.
3. "X" out remaining unused lines after last copy is used.
4. Imprint new set and place in chart.
5. Each order must be dated, timed and signed by the ordering physician.

MR 65029
SERIAL 202798474
HOLMS, MARY
DOB 02/07/1949 SEX F
ATT BOCK MD, George 640

PATIENT IDENTIFICATION PLATE

ALLERGIES:

Date Ordered	Time Ordered	USE BLACK BALL POINT PEN ONLY - PRESS FIRMLY
		Present Weight _____ lbs. _____ kg.
1/15		Tagamet 800mg po @ HS
		Sinemet 25mg PO TID
		Procan SR 500mg po q 3h
		K. Mach MD

THE PRESCRIBER AUTHORIZES THE USE OF GENERIC EQUIVALENTS AND AUTOMATIC INTERCHANGE OF APPROVED THERAPEUTIC EQUIVALENT DRUGS UNLESS OTHERWISE NOTED.

FIGURE 26-1 The EMT should be able to recognize the abbreviations commonly used to describe medication dosing.

TABLE 26-2

Common Prescribing Abbreviations

Abbreviation	Meaning
bid	Twice daily
IM	Intramuscularly
IV	Intravenously
PO	By mouth
PR	Per rectum
Prn	As needed
qd	Every day
qhs	At bedtime
qid	Four times daily
qod	Every other day
SC	Subcutaneously
SL	Sublingually
tid	Three times daily

(Figure 26-1). These abbreviations are helpful for the EMT to know and are listed in Table 26-2 just as they may be found on prescription labels.

FORMS OF MEDICATIONS

Medications come in many different physical forms. Some may be liquids; others may be solid tablets or powders. The EMT should be familiar with all the possible medication forms encountered during patient care.

Compressed Powders and Tablets

Some medications are produced as a powder and are easily compressed into a tablet shape for ease of measurement and administration. Tablets are usually placed in the mouth to be either swallowed or dissolved and absorbed. Nitroglycerin is an example of a tablet meant to be placed under the tongue to dissolve (Figure 26-2).

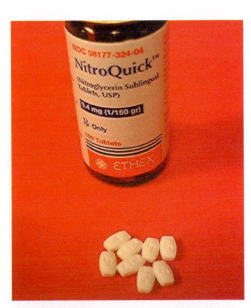

FIGURE 26-2 Some medications are produced as a powder and are compressed into tablet shape for administration.

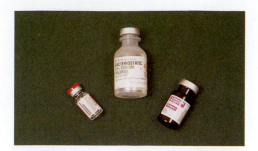

FIGURE 26-3 Medications may come in a liquid meant for injection.

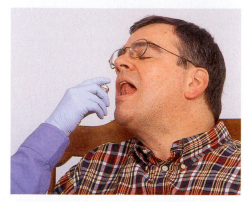

FIGURE 26-4 The EMT will sometimes assist a patient to take nitroglycerin.

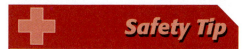

Safety Tip

If an EMT is using medications in a liquid form for injection, she must be familiar with the proper handling of needles. There are important rules that every health care provider must abide by when handling needles to avoid inadvertent injury. Great care should always be taken to properly handle and dispose of sharp instruments such as needles. Chapter 6 reviews these principles.

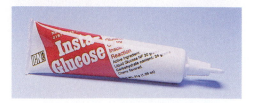

FIGURE 26-5 Oral glucose is a medication that is commonly marketed in a gel form for ease of administration.

Liquids

Medications such as epinephrine come in a liquid form that must be injected into a muscle in order to be absorbed and be effective (Figure 26-3).

Some medications are in a liquid form that can be absorbed under the tongue into the many blood vessels located there. **Sublingual** is a term used to describe the space under the tongue. Nitroglycerin also comes in a liquid form for placement under the tongue (Figure 26-4).

Gels

Oral glucose is an example of a medication commonly formed as a gel for ease of administration and absorption (Figure 26-5). Gel medications are most often designed to be administered orally because they can be easily absorbed through the well-vascularized mucous membranes of the mouth.

Suspensions

Some medications are initially in a powder form, but to make them more palatable to the patient, they are suspended, or mixed, in a liquid. This powder suspended in a liquid is referred to as a **suspension** and can be offered to the patient to drink.

An example of a suspension the EMT may have occasion to use is activated charcoal (Figure 26-6). Patients are given an activated charcoal suspension to drink if they have ingested certain harmful substances.

Powder for Inhalation

Certain medications must be inhaled into the lungs to act directly on the airways. These medicines may be in a powder or liquid form and must be aerosolized for inhalation. Some inhalers contain powdered medications that are aerosolized and may be inhaled directly into the airways.

Gases

An example of a medication in a gas form is oxygen. Special administration systems are often required to administer a gas to a patient while avoiding excess leakage into the environment, where it can be inhaled by the health care providers. Most often, a pressurized tank will be attached to a mask, which can then be applied to the patient's face (Figure 26-7).

Aerosols

Liquid medications may also be inhaled and absorbed directly into the airways. Examples of inhaled liquid medicines are bronchodilating medicines that are often used for asthma.

These liquids can be placed in a device that will be attached to an air source and aerosolized into the air so that the liquid is broken up into tiny particles and can easily be inhaled. This device is called a **nebulizer** and is commonly used by asthma patients (Figure 26-8).

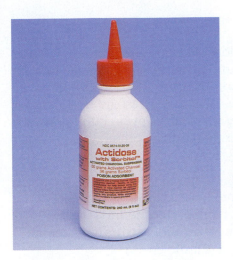

FIGURE 26-6 Some medications are prepared as a powder suspended in a liquid, called a suspension.

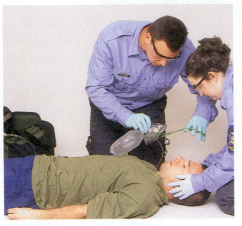

FIGURE 26-7 The EMT commonly administers oxygen.

ROUTES OF ADMINISTRATION

Just as there are many forms of medication, there are many ways to administer these drugs. The EMT must be familiar with the many routes of drug administration.

Inhalation

Liquid, powdered, or gaseous medicines may be inhaled into the lungs, where they will come into direct contact with airways. Most often, these medicines are meant to act on the airways directly; therefore, applying them directly makes sense. The EMT will learn to assist a patient in taking specific previously prescribed inhaled medicines.

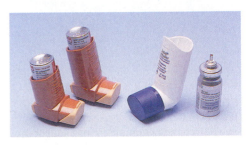

FIGURE 26-8 A metered dose inhaler (MDI) allows aerosolization of a liquid medication for inhalation.

Sublingual

The space under the tongue has many blood vessels very close to the surface. If a medication is allowed to dissolve in this sublingual space, it will be well absorbed into these blood vessels. Sublingual administration is a very effective route for medicines that require rapid absorption, such as nitroglycerin.

Injection

Some medications are not effective unless they are injected with a needle directly into or very near a blood vessel. There are several means of injecting liquid medicines.

Subcutaneous

Injecting the medicine just under the skin in the **subcutaneous** tissue allows gradual absorption of the medicine into a blood vessel (Figure 26-9). This subcutaneous space is made up of fat and tiny blood vessels, and the medicine will be slowly absorbed into the tiny blood vessels. Insulin is a medicine that is used by diabetic patients that must be injected subcutaneously.

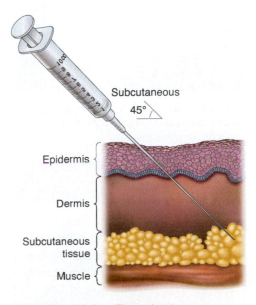

FIGURE 26-9 The subcutaneous space is just under the skin.

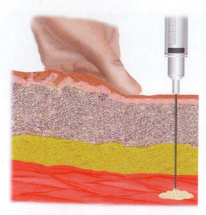

FIGURE 26-10 Epinephrine is commonly administered into the intramuscular space in an emergency.

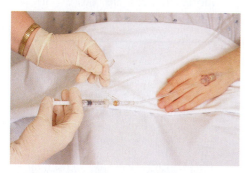

FIGURE 26-11 Advanced-level providers can access the intravenous space to directly administer medications into the bloodstream.

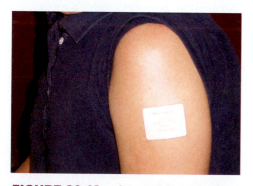

FIGURE 26-12 A transdermal patch allows medication to be applied topically to the skin for absorption.

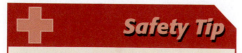

Safety Tip

Because the medication on a topical patch is absorbed through the skin, the EMT should handle these patches only while wearing gloves to avoid any absorption of the drug into herself.

Intramuscular

If the medicine must be delivered closer to a larger blood vessel, but it is not desirable to inject it directly into a vessel, the medicine may be administered into a muscle, or **intramuscularly** (Figure 26-10).

Medicines such as epinephrine may be given in this manner because it is desirable to have fairly rapid absorption into the bloodstream, but direct intravenous injection may be potentially harmful.

Intravenous

If a medication is injected directly into a blood vessel, it is being given **intravenously**. This route will not be used by the EMT-Basic but is used regularly by more-advanced-level providers to administer medications directly into the bloodstream (Figure 26-11).

Oral

Perhaps the most familiar route of medication administration is by direct oral consumption. When a medication is swallowed, it is being given by the **oral** route. Most medicines are prescribed for oral use. Although the EMT will not often have occasion to administer a drug orally, an example of an orally administered drug is activated charcoal.

Topical

It is sometimes desirable to allow a medication to be absorbed very slowly and gradually over the course of a day or more. Some medications can be made into a paste or gel-like material that can be applied to the skin under a patch of waterproof material (Figure 26-12). This method of drug administration is called **topical**.

This topical application of a medication is a way to allow slow absorption through the skin over time. Nitroglycerin is made in the form of a topical patch.

MEDICATION ADMINISTRATION PROCEDURE

Before administering medications, the EMT must assess the patient and determine whether a medication is appropriate for the given condition. It is imperative for the EMT to thoroughly assess the patient and the need for the medication as well as the presence of medication allergies. After medication administration, the EMT also must continually reassess the patient to see whether the drug had its desired effect or any unwanted side effects.

Patient Assessment

The EMT should accomplish a complete patient assessment as appropriate for the individual patient. The assessment should include the initial assessment and then the appropriate focused history and physical examination. A complete medication history is needed if a medication is to be administered.

The "Five Rights" of Drug Administration

There are a number of questions the EMT must address each time a medication is administered, no matter how routine it may seem. These questions address whether the medication is safe and appropriate for the given situation (Figure 26-13).

The Right Patient

The EMT must determine whether the medication in question is indicated for that particular patient. If it is a prescribed medicine, does the prescription label have that patient's name on it? It is never advisable for the EMT to administer medication that belongs to someone other than the patient.

If the medication does not have a prescription label on it, the EMT must use her judgment to determine whether the drug is actually prescribed to the patient. If there is any question about who is actually prescribed the medicine, the EMT should speak with a medical control physician and get his advice on the situation. When in doubt, the safest course to take is to withhold the medication.

The Right Medication

In addition to ensuring that the medication in question belongs to the patient in question, the EMT must be certain that she is administering the correct drug. The name of the drug should be clearly labeled on the packaging. If the medication is not clearly labeled, it should not be administered to the patent.

The Right Route

Once the EMT is certain of the right patient and the right drug, the right route of administration must be determined. Most prescription labels will state which route—oral, intramuscular, and so on—should be used.

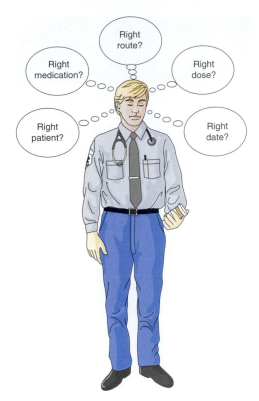

FIGURE 26-13 Before administering medication, the EMT must ensure the right patient, medication, route, dose, and date.

Street Smart

Just as patients sometimes will carry medications without prescription labels on them, some people also tend to carry medicines not in their original containers. If a medication is not in its labeled container and the EMT cannot be sure of what the drug actually is, it should not be administered. The potential for significant harm exists if an inappropriate medication is inadvertently given to a patient.

Street Smart

Some medications, such as prescribed inhalers and nitroglycerin, are frequently carried around by the patient and may not have a prescription label on the medication itself. Often, the prescription label was placed by the pharmacist on the cardboard box that the drug was initially dispensed in.

The box is inconvenient to carry around, so the patient will usually take the inhaler or bottle of medicine out of the box and carry it individually. An EMT is left to wonder whether the prescription actually belongs to the patient or to someone else.

A good rule of thumb is to trust the patient in this matter. If he claims that the medication is his own, it is usually safe to believe him. Of course, if there is any question in the EMT's mind, the drug should not be given.

If any doubt exists, the EMT should ask the patient how he normally takes the medicine. If asking the patient does not clear things up, the EMT should speak with a medical control physician. The use of on-line medical control is discussed in detail in Chapters 18 and 19.

The Right Dose

Medications are prescribed in a particular **dose**, or amount. When administering a medication, the EMT must be certain that the correct dose is given. The prescription label of a prescribed medication will specify how many tablets, sprays, or units of drug to use.

If administering a medication such as oxygen, oral glucose, or activated charcoal, the EMT should follow local protocols. The usual doses of medications the EMT will commonly utilize will be reviewed.

The Right Date

When medications are made, they are not guaranteed to remain in the same form, or at the same strength, over an indefinite period of time. Usually, the manufacturer will guarantee the medication to be safe and effective for a certain period of time after its production. Beyond this guaranteed time frame, the medication may be less potent or may even degenerate into a potentially harmful compound.

All medications have what is known as the **expiration date**. This expiration date identifies the length of time that a medication is good for. Medications should never be used past their expiration date.

The EMT must always check the expiration date on any medication to ensure that it has not expired. An expired medication should *never* be administered.

Reassessment

After any intervention has been provided to a patient, including medication administration, the EMT must perform a thorough reassessment. A reassessment should be done and documented within 5 minutes after the medication has been given. The reassessment findings should also be recorded. The initial assessment should quickly be reviewed, then the relevant parts of the focused exam should be reviewed. The patient should be questioned as to any changes in symptoms, and a complete set of vital signs should be obtained. The results of the reassessment should be noted, with special attention paid to any changes.

DOCUMENTATION

As with any other aspect of patient care, when it comes to medication administration, it is not over until the paperwork is done. It is critically important that the EMT completely document the patient interaction.

Documentation should include the findings on the patient assessment and the history that led the EMT to administer a medication. The EMT should carefully consider local protocols when deciding to administer a medication for a particular problem.

The exact name of the medication, dose, and route should be carefully documented, as well as the time it was administered and by whom.

The symptoms and signs that led the EMT to administer the medication should be addressed in the reassessment. Any contact with medical control should be accurately documented in the Prehospital Care Report as well. Figure 26-14 illustrates the appropriate documentation of nitroglycerin administration.

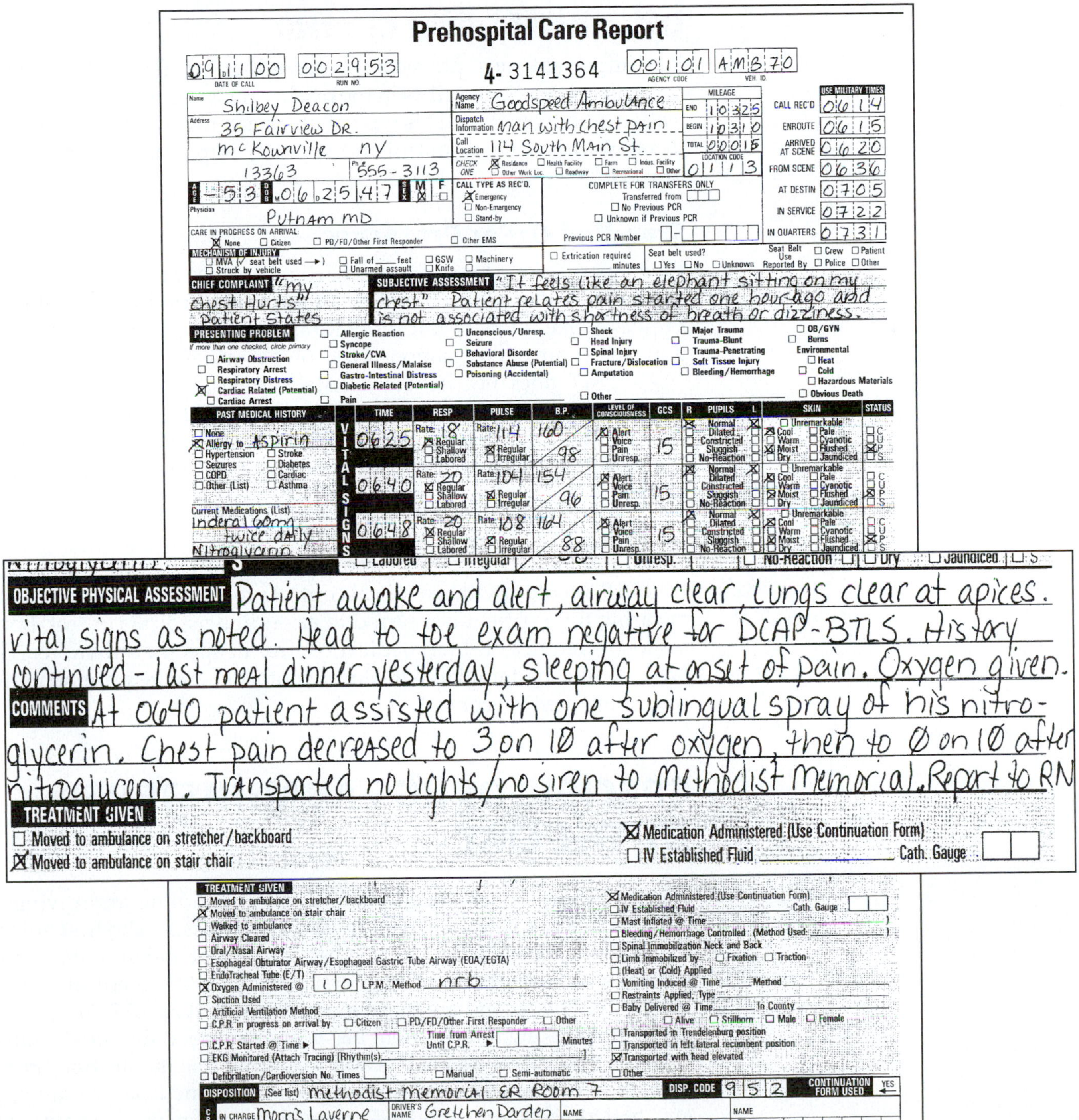

Prehospital Care Report

09/11/00 (DATE OF CALL) 002953 (RUN NO.) 4-3141364 00101 (AGENCY CODE) AMB70 (VEH ID)

Name: Shilbey Deacon
Address: 35 Fairview DR. mcKownville ny 13363 Ph 555-3113
Agency Name: Goodspeed Ambulance
Dispatch Information: man with chest pain
Call Location: 114 South Main St.
CHECK ONE: ☒ Residence
Mileage: END 10325 BEGIN 10310 TOTAL 00015 LOCATION CODE 01113
AGE 53 DOB 06/25/47 SEX M
Physician: Putnam MD
CALL TYPE AS REC'D: ☒ Emergency
USE MILITARY TIMES: CALL REC'D 0614; ENROUTE 0615; ARRIVED AT SCENE 0620; FROM SCENE 0636; AT DESTIN 0705; IN SERVICE 0722; IN QUARTERS 0731
CARE IN PROGRESS ON ARRIVAL: ☒ None

CHIEF COMPLAINT: "my Chest Hurts" patient states
SUBJECTIVE ASSESSMENT: "It feels like an elephant sitting on my chest." Patient relates pain started one hour ago and is not associated with shortness of breath or dizziness.

PRESENTING PROBLEM: ☒ Cardiac Related (Potential)

PAST MEDICAL HISTORY: ☒ Allergy to Aspirin
Current Medications (List): Inderal 60mg twice daily, Nitroglycerin

TIME	RESP	PULSE	B.P.	LEVEL OF CONSCIOUSNESS	GCS	PUPILS	SKIN	STATUS
0625	Rate 18, Regular	Rate 114, Regular	160/98	Alert	15	Normal	Cool, Moist	P
0640	Rate 20, Regular	Rate 104, Regular	154/96	Alert	15	Normal	Cool, Moist	S
0648	Rate 20, Regular	Rate 108, Regular	164/88	Alert	15	Normal	Cool, Moist	P

OBJECTIVE PHYSICAL ASSESSMENT: Patient awake and alert, airway clear, Lungs clear at apices. vital signs as noted. Head to toe exam negative for DCAP-BTLS. History continued - last meal dinner yesterday, sleeping at onset of pain. Oxygen given.

COMMENTS: At 0640 patient assisted with one sublingual spray of his nitroglycerin. Chest pain decreased to 3 on 10 after oxygen, then to 0 on 10 after nitroglycerin. Transported no lights/no siren to Methodist Memorial. Report to RN

TREATMENT GIVEN
☐ Moved to ambulance on stretcher/backboard
☒ Moved to ambulance on stair chair
☒ Medication Administered (Use Continuation Form)
☐ IV Established Fluid ____ Cath. Gauge
☒ Oxygen Administered @ 10 L.P.M., Method nrb
☒ Transported with head elevated

DISPOSITION: Methodist Memorial ER Room 7 DISP. CODE 952
CREW: IN CHARGE Morris Laverne, ☒ EMT 028453; DRIVER'S NAME Gretchen Darden, ☒ CFR 306222

FIGURE 26-14 Thorough documentation of medication administration is imperative.

MEDICAL CONTROL

There is perhaps no place in the EMT's practice in which it is more necessary to have physician input than in the administration of medications. Medications are prescribed by a licensed physician or by the physician's designee. When the EMT administers a medication, she is acting as the designee and therefore must follow the physician's instructions in this matter.

Off-Line Medical Control

It is important for a physician to have input in the preparation of guiding protocols as well as in the quality review of instances of medication administration. This type of physician involvement is referred to as off-line medical control and is of key importance in the EMT's practice.

Standing Order Protocols

When instructions for caring for particular types of patients are written down and made into a policy, they are referred to as protocols. Protocols that allow medication administration or procedures to be done in certain circumstances are known as *standing orders*.

An EMT does not have to contact medical control to perform procedures allowed under standing orders. Of course, if there is ever a question about the appropriateness of the procedure or medication administration, the EMT should contact medical control and discuss it.

On-Line Medical Control

An EMT's contact with a medical control physician during the course of caring for a patient is referred to as on-line medical control. Local protocols require on-line medical control in specific situations. The EMT should be familiar with local protocols and requirements for contacting medical control.

SPECIFIC DRUGS ADMINISTERED BY THE EMT

When we speak of medications an EMT is handling and giving to patients, we can consider them in two main classes. The first are the medications the EMT can carry in her equipment and administer to a patient who has not necessarily been prescribed that medication by a physician. The second are those medications that an EMT may assist a patient in taking if the patient has been prescribed that medication.

In the first class, the EMT is administering this medication on the basis of her local protocols. Examples of these medications are oxygen, oral glucose, and activated charcoal. Some agencies may include other medications on this list. As usual, the EMT should be familiar with regional protocols.

Firefighter Down

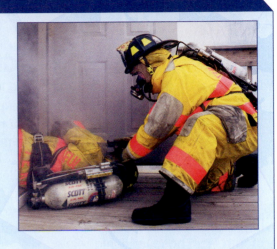

Bill, a firefighter in his 40s, was dragged out of the fire by two fire-fighters. They dropped him on the front lawn. One firefighter, pulling his facemask up, yelled "Medic!" Turning about-face, the two firefighters walked back into the smoke and disappeared from sight.

Greg, the first EMT on scene, helped half-carry, half-drag Bill to the back step of the pumper. Bill was coughing vigorously and spitting out soot-laden sputum. Apparently, his facemask had blown off his face when the fire flashed over his head and knocked him backward.

Bill yelled out, "Somebody got a cigarette?" while Greg started his assessment.

- What are some indications for oxygen administration?
- What is the dose of oxygen that would be appropriate for this patient?
- Are there any contraindications to oxygen administration?

Oxygen

Oxygen is a colorless gas that the body needs in adequate amounts to function normally. It is used to produce energy by all of the tissues of the body. Without appropriate amounts of oxygen, many systems in the body will malfunction.

When an organ is not getting sufficient oxygen, the patient may feel pain in that area of the body. Without adequate oxygen in the blood, the person may also feel short of breath. The body may stimulate rapid respirations in order to try to bring in more oxygen.

An EMT should administer oxygen to any patient who complains of respiratory difficulty or has any potentially cardiac-related complaint. Patients who show evidence of poor oxygen supply to the brain, as seen in stroke patients, seizure patients, or patients with an altered mental status, would also benefit from oxygen administration. Patients suspected to be in shock should also be given oxygen in order to try to increase the oxygen content of the blood. Each of these conditions will be discussed in detail later in this text.

Administration Procedure

As discussed in Chapter 8, oxygen may be administered in a variety of ways depending on the patient's condition. If the patient is not breathing, the oxygen must be administered with positive pressure ventilations as given by a bag-valve-mask, pocket mask, or oxygen-powered ventilation device.

If the patient is ventilating adequately on his own, the EMT should apply supplemental oxygen to allow the patient to breathe in a higher concentration of oxygen than is in the ambient air. A non-rebreather

Street Smart

It is useful to use pulse oximetry to follow the oxygen saturation of the blood. The EMT must realize, however, that if a patient has an indication for oxygen administration, the medication should be administered regardless of the oxygen saturation. This is because it is possible to cause more oxygen to dissolve into the bloodstream even when the pulse oximeter indicates a normal value. Patients with evidence of inadequate oxygenation should receive supplemental oxygen regardless of the oxygen saturation.

mask is the most appropriate device used to administer high-concentration oxygen to a patient in need of this medication. If the patient does not tolerate this mask or does not need such a high concentration of oxygen, a nasal cannula may be used.

Glucose

Glucose is a substance used by the body for fuel. All the body organs, especially the brain, are dependent upon this important carbohydrate for energy. The body regulates the blood glucose levels carefully with special hormones.

Insulin is a hormone that helps the body use glucose effectively. Because insulin assists the body in using glucose, it lowers the blood glucose level. Most people have the ability to release glucose from stored supplies if the blood level gets too low. People with a condition called diabetes may not be able to do this.

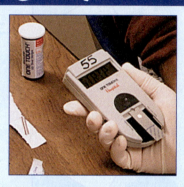

People with diabetes take medicines, such as insulin, that help them use their glucose and keep the blood level balanced. Sometimes their glucose level gets out of balance and becomes either too high or too low. A person with a very low blood glucose level will become ill. Low blood glucose is called **hypoglycemia**. Signs and symptoms of hypoglycemia include shakiness, tremulousness, tachycardia, moist skin, dizziness, and confusion. If hypoglycemia is allowed to progress to the point where the glucose levels are so low that the brain no longer has enough fuel to function, the patient may become unconscious or may suffer a seizure.

If an EMT is treating a patient who has symptoms as described above and a low blood glucose level is suspected, oral glucose is indicated. When oral glucose is administered to a patient with low blood glucose, the glucose level in the blood will rise and the patient's symptoms should rapidly resolve.

The one condition for oral glucose administration is that the patient must be capable of swallowing the gel-like material. If the patient is unconscious or otherwise unable to swallow, it is dangerous to put any substance in his mouth because it may create an airway obstruction.

If the EMT is unable to administer oral glucose, yet believes that the patient suffers from hypoglycemia, then the EMT must make every effort to intercept with an advanced-level provider who can give glucose intravenously. If a hospital is closer than the advanced life support (ALS) intercept, then the EMT should bring the patient immediately to the closest hospital.

Administration Procedure

Once the EMT has determined that it is safe to administer oral glucose, she should check the "five rights" as discussed earlier, then open the medication container. The patient will often be able to hold the tube of glucose on his own and suck the sweet gel out. The EMT may have to help by squeezing small amounts of the glucose material into the patient's mouth (Figure 26-15).

If at any time the EMT becomes concerned that the patient is not swallowing effectively or the patency of the airway becomes questionable, she should immediately stop administration of the medication and suction out any remaining material.

When documenting oral glucose administration, as with any medication administration, the EMT should take care to note the patient's condition before and after its administration.

Even if the patient's condition has completely resolved after oral glucose administration, the patient should be evaluated by a physician. If the patient resists being transported, the EMT should contact a medical control physician, explain the situation, and ask for instruction.

Activated Charcoal

Activated charcoal is a suspension of charcoal in a liquid, often prepared with sorbitol. This concoction has the ability to bind most ingested toxins and prevent their absorption. It is therefore very useful to use for patients who have intentionally or unintentionally ingested a harmful substance.

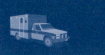

Street Smart

A good rule of thumb in oral glucose administration is that if the patient is awake and swallowing his own secretions, he can safely be given oral glucose. If he is not awake or is drooling profusely, then it is not safe to give anything by mouth for fear the patient may aspirate the glucose into the lungs.

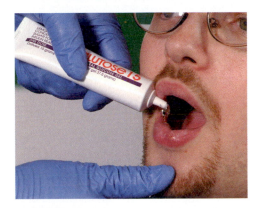

FIGURE 26-15 Oral glucose is given to the conscious patient suffering a diabetic emergency.

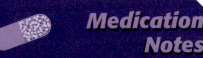

Medication Notes

Generic name: Oral glucose

Trade name: Insta-Glucose, and others

Indications: Suspected low blood glucose

Contraindications: Patients who cannot control their own airway and swallow their own secretions should *not* be given oral medications.

Dose: One tube, or container

Route: Oral only

Possible Poisoning

Putting the phone down, Alisha went to see what her 3-year-old daughter, Desiree, was doing. Looking in the bedroom, then in the family room, she couldn't find the child. Calling out "Desiree," she heard a faint call from the bathroom: "Mommy." Rushing into the bathroom, Alisha found Desiree sitting on the floor, with pill bottles strewn around her and a hand full of pills.

Quickly, Alisha knocked the pills from the little girl's hand and swept out her mouth with her fingers. Pill fragments fell to the floor. Scooping the child up in her arms, the young mother ran to the kitchen and called poison control. While speaking to poison control, Alisha pulled the poison kit from the kitchen cabinet. Poison control proceeded to ask Alisha a series of questions.

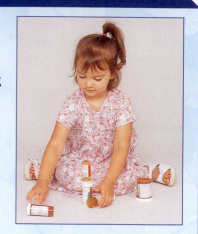

- What are indications for activated charcoal administration?
- What are contraindications to giving any medication by mouth?
- Are there any issues surrounding the administration of an activated charcoal suspension?

Because the charcoal has to come into contact with the offending substance in order to bind it, it is useful only if the poison is still in the patient's stomach. With a few exceptions, if the ingestion occurred more than 1 or 2 hours before contact with a health care provider, the poison is no longer in the stomach and is not susceptible to binding by charcoal. Activated charcoal is therefore indicated when a patient has recently (within 1–2 hours) ingested a toxin that can be bound by charcoal. Most commonly ingested toxins are able to be bound by this agent.

As with any orally administered medication, activated charcoal should not be given to any patient who cannot maintain his own airway and swallow on his own. The EMT must be clear that the patient is capable of maintaining his own airway at the time of charcoal administration and for the next 30–60 minutes.

Some poisoned patients have the potential to lose consciousness or have a seizure due to the effects of the ingested substance. An unconscious or seizing patient cannot reliably maintain an airway. If a patient is given charcoal and soon after loses his airway reflexes, he may regurgitate the charcoal and aspirate some into his lungs. Charcoal is very harmful if aspirated and should therefore be given with great caution to patients who have ingested substances that may cause unconsciousness or seizure.

The EMT should be familiar with and follow local protocols regarding the use of activated charcoal. If ever in doubt as to the appropriateness of this medication, the EMT should contact medical control immediately for advice.

Administration Procedure

Activated charcoal must not be stored at extremes of temperature because it will not mix properly if too cold or too hot. Before opening the container, the EMT must thoroughly shake the bottle in order to suspend the charcoal particles in the liquid base. A straw may then be placed in the container, or the liquid may be poured into another container for administration (Figure 26-16).

The EMT should give the suspension to the patient and have him drink it. Under no circumstances should an EMT pour this liquid into the mouth of a patient who cannot drink it under his own volition.

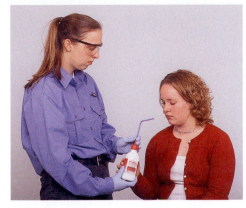

FIGURE 26-16 The EMT should be familiar with administration of activated charcoal in the setting of a toxic ingestion.

Street Smart

On the warning labels of many chemicals and over-the-counter medications are the instructions to induce vomiting in cases of accidental ingestion. Many families keep syrup of ipecac, an emetic that causes vomiting, in the medicine cabinet for just such emergencies. If the patient has been given syrup of ipecac, then the EMT should first contact medical control for further instructions and guidance before administering activated charcoal. Syrup of ipecac may take as long as 30 minutes before it stimulates vomiting. If the patient has swallowed activated charcoal in the interim, he may vomit, and potentially aspirate, the activated charcoal.

Street Smart

As you can imagine, activated charcoal neither looks nor tastes very appealing. For this reason, it is often useful to leave the material in a container that does not allow the patient to see it easily. Many manufacturers sell the product in such a container. After shaking the container for suspension, the EMT can merely place a straw in the container and have the patient drink the liquid.

Some manufacturers produce the suspension with a sweet taste, such as cherry. If this is not the case, or if the taste is unpalatable for the patient, an alternative flavor enhancer may be utilized. Chocolate syrup is a favorite for some providers.

Safety Tip

The EMT should be careful when handling activated charcoal because it invariably splashes or spills during administration, and it will stain many fabrics it contacts. Proper personal protective equipment must always be used.

Medication Notes

Generic name: Activated charcoal

Trade name: Acti-Dose, Super-Char, and others

Indications: Recent ingestion of susceptible poison

Contraindications: Patients who cannot control their own airway and swallow their own secretions should *not* be given oral medications.

Dose: 1 gram/kilogram (g/kg) (50–100 g for typical adult)

Route: Oral

Pediatric Considerations

When giving activated charcoal to a child, the EMT should be sure that the formulation does not have sorbitol in it. Many forms of this adsorbent material are packaged with sorbitol. This will act as a laxative and result in rapid movement of the charcoal through the patient's gastrointestinal tract. Sorbitol can result in serious diarrhea and dehydration in a small child and should be avoided for that reason.

SPECIFIC ASSISTED MEDICATIONS

The second group of medications EMTs must be familiar with are those that they may help a patient use if the patient has been previously prescribed that medication by a physician. Before considering giving such assistance, the EMT should confirm that the medication has been prescribed for that patient for the exact symptom or disease process that the patient is complaining of at the time of evaluation.

The EMT is relying upon the fact that the patient has been diagnosed by a physician with a condition that could benefit from the medication in question. Perhaps more important, the physician has determined that the risk to using the medication for that patient is low. An EMT does not have the training or licensure to allow diagnosis of diseases or assessment of the risk of administering controlled substances to individuals.

Definitions

There are several terms that may be difficult to define in this text and should probably be left up to local and state agencies to define. EMTs should clarify in their own region what specifically is expected of them when dealing with prescribed medications. Local protocols will likely provide this clarification.

One of the terms that may differ in interpretation from state to state is the term *assist*. What exactly does allowing an EMT to assist a patient in taking his own medication mean? Each locale must decide and clarify in its protocols whether an EMT may hand the patient the medication, help the patient place his hand to his mouth to take the drug, or simply give the patient the substance if he is unable to take it himself. The definition of *assist* must be clear to every EMT.

Prescribed Inhalers

Many patients with lung diseases such as asthma, emphysema, and bronchitis use inhaled medications to help keep the airways open and ease their breathing. These medications may come in the form of a metered dose inhaler.

Metered dose inhalers are handheld devices that carry a form of medication that may be aerosolized upon discharge of the inhaler device. The device expels a specific amount of medication with each puff; therefore, these types of medicines are often dosed in numbers of puffs rather than in milligrams. This aerosolized medication can then be inhaled by the patient, allowing the medication to directly contact the constricted airways. It is this direct contact that allows this medication to exert immediate effects of relaxing the constricted airways. Figure 26-17 illustrates how these devices work to get medication into the airways.

Bronchodilator Inhalers

Opening of constricted airways is referred to as bronchodilation. The medications that open airways are therefore called **bronchodilators**. It is important for the EMT to realize that not all inhaled medicines are bronchodilators. Patients may use other medicines in an inhaled form

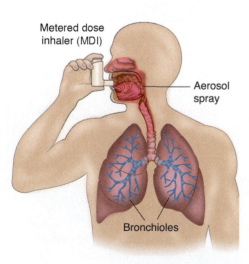

Metered dose inhaler (MDI)

Aerosol spray

Bronchioles

FIGURE 26-17 The metered dose inhaler aerosolizes medication for inhalation directly into the airways.

Asthma Attack

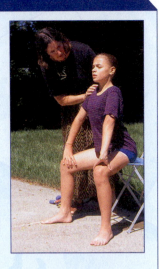

"Squad 23 out, Pinebush School." EMT-Firefighters Seigel and Sorenson step off the pumper and proceed to the school nurse's office. After being ushered into the room, the firefighters note a teenaged girl with apparent shortness of breath. The nurse explains that the girl's wheezing started right after gym class. The nurse had called the girl's mother, but the girl was getting progressively worse, even after one treatment with her prescribed inhaler. So the nurse decided to call emergency medical services (EMS).

- What are indications to assist a patient to use her own prescribed inhaler?
- What are contraindications to prescribed inhaler use?

also. However, it is only the bronchodilators that will be quickly helpful to the patient with constricted airways.

The EMT should review local protocols regarding which specific medications are approved for EMT assistance. An example of a commonly used bronchodilator is albuterol (trade names, Proventil and Ventolin), but there are certainly more.

The EMT may assist a patient to use a prescribed bronchodilator inhaler if the patient complains of shortness of breath and has been instructed by a physician to use that specific medication for such a complaint. After administration of this medication, of course, the EMT should reassess the patient and document any changes in condition, complaint, or vital signs.

Administration Procedure

If the EMT is to assist a patient in using an inhaler, she must be familiar with the administration procedure. However, it is important for the EMT to complete an initial assessment before assisting the patient with any medications.

If the patient has a decreased level of consciousness and cannot cooperate with the inhaler use or if the patient requires ventilatory assistance, the EMT should not administer the inhaler because it will not be effective.

Once it has been decided that a metered dose inhaler is needed, the EMT should confirm the "five rights" as previously discussed, then prepare the inhaler for use. An inhaler comes with a cover over the mouthpiece that must be removed. The container must be shaken several times to suspend the medication inside it.

The oxygen mask should then be removed from the patient's face and the patient should be instructed to exhale, then inhale deeply. As the patient begins to inhale, the inhaler device should be held up to

Pediatric Considerations

Children (and some adults) may use a device called a spacer between the inhaler and their mouth to assist in coordination (Figure 26-18). This device reduces the coordination of breathing necessary to effectively administer the medication. The EMT should definitely utilize this device if it is available with the inhaler.

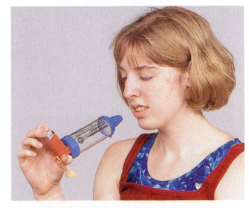

FIGURE 26-18 A spacer is a device that is commonly used in conjunction with an inhaler, especially by children.

the mouth and a puff should be administered during the inhalation. The patient should continue the inhalation as long as possible, then should hold his breath as long as possible. This procedure allows a maximal amount of medication to enter the lungs and settle into the smaller airways, where it will have the greatest effect.

After holding his breath for a few seconds, the patient should be instructed to breathe normally for a minute while oxygen is reapplied. After 1 minute, the procedure is repeated a second time to administer a second puff of medication. The typical dose is two puffs. This skill can be reviewed in Skill 26-1.

SKILL 26-1 *Assistance with a Metered Dose Inhaler*

PURPOSE: To assist the patient with the use of a prescribed metered dose inhaler.

STANDARD PRECAUTIONS:

☑ Appropriate pre-scribed metered dose inhaler

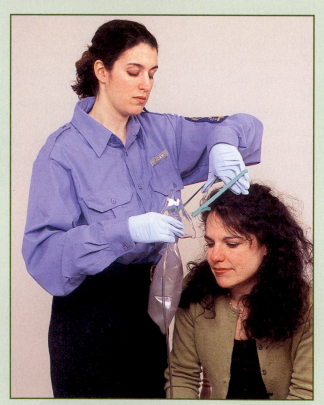

1 The EMT assesses the patient and applies oxygen as appropriate.

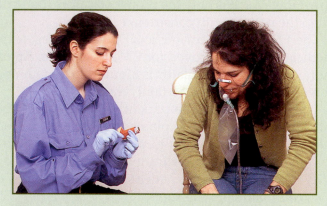

2 The EMT next confirms that the inhaler is the patient's prescribed inhaler and checks the expiration date.

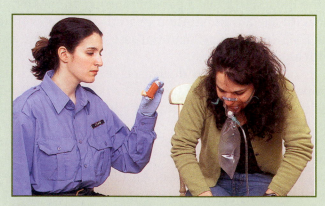

3 The EMT then vigorously shakes the inhaler and removes the mouthpiece.

(continues)

SKILL 26-1 *(continued)*

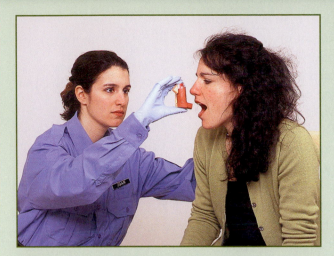

4 After removing the oxygen mask, the EMT asks the patient to exhale, then inhale slowly and deeply, as the EMT depresses the inhaler for one puff.

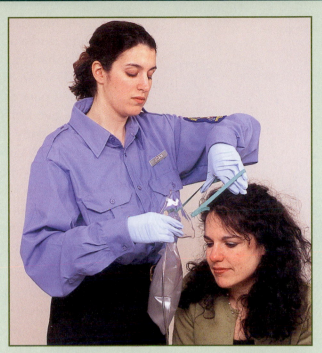

5 The EMT then removes the inhaler from the patient's mouth and reapplies oxygen while instructing the patient to continue to hold her breath for several seconds. The EMT then reevaluates the patient and considers whether a second dose of medicine is needed.

 Street Smart

In some areas, an EMT may be trained to administer albuterol in a nebulized form in specific circumstances. This may be useful if a patient is unable to cooperate enough for coordination of the metered dose inhaler. Further training should be provided to the EMT who will be administering albuterol by nebulizer.

Nitroglycerin

Nitroglycerin is a medication that dilates, or opens, blood vessels. It specifically dilates the blood vessels that supply the heart with oxygenated blood, the coronary arteries. Widening these vessels is useful when they are narrowed as in a heart attack.

Sudden narrowing or blockage of a coronary artery will cause decreased blood supply to the heart. This decreased blood supply translates into pain as the heart is without oxygen for a short period of time. Pain as a result of such lack of blood supply to the heart is known as **angina**. The details of cardiac disease will be discussed in detail in Chapter 28.

 Medication Notes

Generic name: Albuterol

Trade name: Ventolin, Proventil

Indications: Signs and symptoms of respiratory distress in a patient who has a physician-prescribed handheld inhaler

Contraindications: The nonalert patient who cannot cooperate with administration of an inhaler

Dose: Two puffs given 1 minute apart

Route: Inhalation

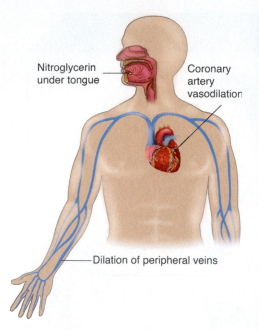

FIGURE 26-19 Nitroglycerin dilates blood vessels.

Nitroglycerin under tongue

Coronary artery vasodilation

Dilation of peripheral veins

Repeat Attack

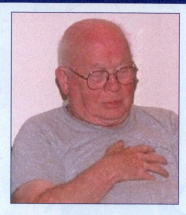

Mr. Moon, an older man living alone in a studio apartment on Manhattan's Upper West Side, calls EMS when he starts to feel a bout of chest pain coming on. He relates to the two EMTs, Matt and Forrest, that he recently had a heart attack and that he is currently experiencing feelings in his chest just like that, only worse. He has been prescribed nitroglycerin but is not sure if he should use it. When Matt asks where the medicine is, Mr. Moon points to the cabinet over the kitchen sink.

Matt, opening the cabinet, finds a little brown bottle with the label marked "Nitroglycerin" but no prescription. He carries the bottle over to Mr. Moon, and asks him if this is his medicine. "Yes, that's my medicine," Mr. Moon can be heard to say through the oxygen mask.

- What are the indications for using nitroglycerin?
- What are the contraindications?
- What are some of the more common side effects from the medication?

Safety Tip

Knowing that hypotension can occur after administration of nitroglycerin, the street-smart EMT will ensure that the patient is seated or even semireclined on the stretcher before helping him take this medication. In this position, if the patient's blood pressure should fall significantly, he is less likely to become dizzy or to fall down. Having him seated or reclining will protect the patient from being injured and will save the EMT the work of having to pick him up! In this situation, as in many faced by the EMT, it pays to be prepared for the worst possibility.

Nitroglycerin can sometimes help to open narrowed coronary arteries, improving blood flow to the heart and decreasing symptoms of angina (Figure 26-19). This medication can be an important adjunct to the EMT's care of the heart attack victim.

Unfortunately, the use of nitroglycerin is not without risk. As it dilates the coronary arteries, it also dilates many other vessels in the body, resulting in a fall in blood pressure. Sometimes this drop in blood pressure is insignificant; at other times it can be devastating. Whether any one patient will experience a drop in blood pressure cannot be predicted, so the EMT should be prepared to see it happen in any patient being given nitroglycerin.

To avoid hypotension, the EMT should not assist a patient to take nitroglycerin if the patient has a low blood pressure at the time of assessment. Local protocols will dictate what constitutes a "low blood pressure," but many locales will require a patient to have a minimal systolic blood pressure of 100 or 120 millimeters of mercury (mm Hg) in order for nitroglycerin to be considered.

Some regions will not permit nitroglycerin administration without intravenous access having been established. This practice is to allow for rapid fluid administration in the event of a significant drop in blood pressure. The EMT should take this requirement into consideration if she practices in a system that has ALS readily available.

Another bothersome side effect that nitroglycerin commonly has is that of headache. This effect is also thought to be related to the dilation of blood vessels, those in the head. This effect is rarely serious and can be relieved with a dose of acetaminophen (Tylenol) or other mild analgesic once the patient arrives at the hospital.

Nitroglycerin is administered in the form of a small tablet under the tongue, or via a spray sublingually. The dose of a single tablet is 0.4 milligram and is often repeated every 5 minutes if the chest pain continues, as long as the blood pressure remains high enough to allow repeated administration. Usually, no more than three doses are used without consultation with a doctor.

The EMT must thoroughly assess the patient before medication administration as well as 2–5 minutes after. Any changes in condition, symptoms, or vital signs should be recorded.

Local protocols may differ significantly in the regulations and requirements for nitroglycerin administration by the EMT. It is the responsibility of the EMT to be familiar with her own protocols. If there is ever any question about the administration of nitroglycerin, as with any medication, the EMT should contact medical control for advice.

Patients who call an ambulance and who require nitroglycerin may be suffering from a life-threatening condition. The EMT should never delay transport to administer nitroglycerin and should always attempt to intercept with an ALS agency if it is available so that further treatment may be given to the patient.

Administration Procedure

When considering assisting a patient to take nitroglycerin, the EMT must ensure that several things have first been accomplished. An initial assessment should have been completed, including initiation of oxygen as appropriate. The focused history and physical examination should be completed, and transport decisions should be made.

The patient suffering from cardiac chest pain requires timely transport to an appropriate hospital with an ALS intercept along the way if it does not delay arrival at the hospital. The EMT should consider nitroglycerin administration to the patient who is having chest pain that is known to be cardiac in nature and who has been prescribed nitroglycerin.

The EMT should *never* assist a patient to use someone else's prescription for nitroglycerin. An EMT does not have sufficient training or licensure to diagnose cardiac disease or to prescribe medications for it. There are significant risks to using nitroglycerin inappropriately.

After completing the assessment, the EMT should be sure that the patient is comfortably seated, preferably on the stretcher. She should confirm that the patient's systolic blood pressure is at least 100 mm Hg (or whatever minimum number is dictated by local protocols). If it is and the patient states that he is having symptoms for which nitroglycerin has been prescribed, the EMT should assist the patient in taking nitroglycerin according to local protocols.

After the medication has been administered, the EMT should carefully recheck the patient's vital signs and ask whether the discomfort has subsided, using the 0–10 scale. Medical control can play an important role in assisting the EMT to make a wise treatment plan for the cardiac patient.

Safety Tip

Nitroglycerin comes in many forms such as tablets, metered dose sprays, slow release patches, or paste that is meant to absorb through the skin slowly. Because of the potential for nitroglycerin to absorb through the skin, the EMT should always wear gloves when handling this medication to avoid unnecessary exposure and potential side effects.

Medication Notes

Generic name: Nitroglycerin
Trade name: Nitrostat
Indications: Cardiac-related chest pain or angina
Contraindications: Hypotension patients, infants and children, who have already taken the maximum dosage before EMS arrival
Dose: 0.4 mg tablet or metered dose spray
Route: Sublingual

Street Smart

Nitroglycerin has a "limited shelf life." Light, heat, and especially moisture can "denature" nitroglycerin; to denature a drug is to render it impotent and therefore ineffective. An opened container of nitroglycerin tablets may only be potent for as little as 30 days. If the patient has self-administered nitroglycerin that is outdated or stored in packaging other than the original packaging, it may not be potent and therefore may not relieve the patient's symptoms.

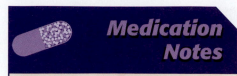

Aspirin

After calling 9-1-1, the American Heart Association advocates that patients who can should take aspirin. Aspirin, given early, has been shown to significantly improve the patient's chances of survival from an acute coronary event, such as acute myocardial infarction. Some EMS systems permit an EMT to either administer aspirin to a patient with symptoms of an acute coronary event or to assist the patient with self-administration of aspirin.

Aspirin, a 100-year-old drug, prevents platelets in the blood from sticking to one another and causing a blood clot. This can be useful in preventing clot formation or for preventing a clot from enlarging.

However, aspirin is not without its risks. Aspirin should not be given to a patient with active bleeding or to those with a bleeding disorder such as hemophilia. Similarly, aspirin should not be given to patients who are allergic to aspirin or who have aspirin-induced asthma.

Aspirin is usually given in doses from 81 milligrams (mg) to 325 mg immediately following the onset of symptoms associated with an acute coronary event. Often one to four chewable baby aspirin are used, making administration simpler and easier.

In some cases, the patient may already take aspirin daily as part of a medical regimen to prevent an acute coronary event. Those patients may take another dose of aspirin without risk of harm.

Epinephrine

Epinephrine is a medication that dilates the airways and constricts the blood vessels. It is used commonly for a condition called anaphylaxis. Anaphylaxis is a form of severe, life-threatening allergic reaction that can cause airway swelling, bronchoconstriction, dilation of blood vessels with hypotension, and a type of rash called hives. This type of allergic reaction can come on within minutes; therefore, speed of administration of this medication is crucial. More about anaphylaxis is discussed in Chapter 34.

Epinephrine is an effective antidote for this severe allergic reaction and is often prescribed to patients in the form of an easily used preloaded syringe for intramuscular injection. It is this preloaded syringe that the EMT should become familiar with in order to assist patients in its use should the need arise.

As do many medications, epinephrine has many potentially significant side effects. In addition to its beneficial effects of bronchodilation and vasoconstriction, epinephrine can cause a significant rise in heart rate. In addition, the heart is forced to work much harder after epinephrine administration. These effects will likely cause the patient to feel as if his heart is pounding very quickly and may cause some tremulousness. They are the same effects as seen when epinephrine is secreted by the body itself during a fight or flight response (Figure 26-20).

In the young patient with a healthy heart, these effects likely will not have any harmful result. In the older patient, or the patient with underlying cardiac disease, this increased workload on the heart may have life-threatening consequences. Epinephrine has been known to

Bee Sting

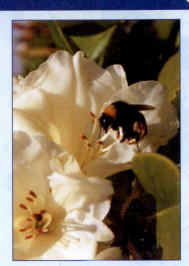

Eric dutifully climbs up the ladder and starts to clean out the leaves in the rain gutter, thinking to himself what a pain this chore is, when suddenly a swarm of bees arises. Scrambling down the ladder, Eric runs away from the bees.

Too late, Eric is stung by one of the bees on the back of the neck. Recalling his nearly fatal reaction the last time he was stung, he yells for his wife Bette to call 9-1-1. "Tell them to hurry. I've been stung by a bee!" Bette grabs the portable phone, dials 9-1-1, and starts talking to the communicator, while looking through the medicine cabinet. She remembered that Eric's doctor had prescribed an EpiPen just in case an emergency like this arose.

Finding the EpiPen in the back of the cabinet, she grabs it and starts to run outside. The rescue squad crew is already with Eric, loosening his shirt and listening to his lungs. His chest is bright red with a rash, and Eric's speech sounds like he's drunk, it's so thick. Bette thrusts the EpiPen into an EMT's hands and says, "Use this!"

- What are the indications for epinephrine injection?
- Are there any contraindications?
- What are some special concerns the EMT should have about handling needles after injections?

cause heart attacks or cardiac arrest in patients with preexisting heart disease.

The potential severe nature of the side effects associated with this drug's use requires the EMT to use special care in determining its necessity. There must be clear indications for its use, and local protocols must be followed to the letter.

Under *no* circumstances should an EMT assist someone to use an epinephrine injector that has not been prescribed to the person by a physician unless doing so is specifically allowed by local protocol. A physician can help determine whether the helpful effects of the drug are worth the potential risks of its use. If any question arises, medical control should be consulted immediately.

Administration Procedure

The initial assessment of the anaphylaxis patient must be done very quickly and must include administration of high-flow oxygen. If it is determined that a prescribed epinephrine injector is indicated and it is present on the scene, the EMT should assist the patient to use it (Figure 26-21).

The most common site for injection of this medication is the thigh because it is the largest muscle that is easily accessible to a patient who is self-administering the medication. If possible, the side of the leg should be bared, although most of the auto-injectors are designed to be able to go through a single layer of clothing. Skill 26-2 depicts this procedure in detail.

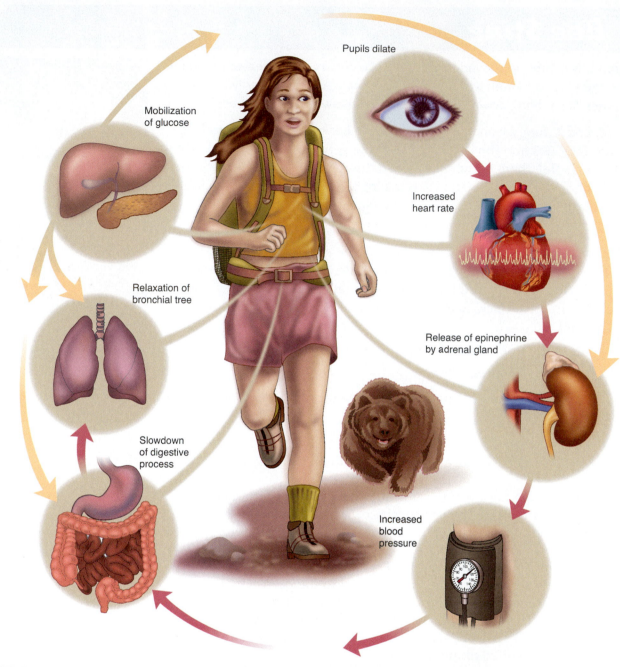

Mobilization
of glucose

Pupils dilate

Increased
heart rate

Relaxation of
bronchial tree

Release of epinephrine
by adrenal gland

Slowdown
of digestive
process

Increased
blood
pressure

FIGURE 26-20 Epinephrine administration mimics the fight or flight response.

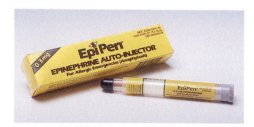

FIGURE 26-21 Epinephrine may be packaged in a preloaded syringe for ease of administration.

Safety Tip

When assisting a patient to use an epinephrine auto-injector, the EMT should take care to properly handle and dispose of the needle. Proper disposal includes placement into an approved sharps container, as discussed in Chapter 6.

Most epinephrine auto-injectors have a safety function that will withdraw the needle after the drug has been injected. If this is not the case, the EMT should never attempt to force the needle to retract. She should simply dispose of the entire unit in an appropriate manner.

As with any other medication administration, the EMT should take care to reassess the patient and carefully document any changes. The patient with anaphylaxis who receives epinephrine should begin to improve within minutes after its administration if it is going to be effective.

The potential does exist for the patient to decompensate, even after epinephrine administration. Because of this possibility, the EMT should initiate transport as quickly as possible and arrange for ALS intercept if available.

Medication Notes

Generic name: Epinephrine
Trade name: EpiPen, EpiPen Jr.
Indications: Life-threatening allergic reaction
Contraindications: None in the presence of an indication
Dose: 0.3–0.5 mg for adults; 0.15–0.3 mg for children
Route: Intramuscular

Pediatric Considerations

Children are also susceptible to life-threatening allergic reactions and may be prescribed epinephrine auto-injectors. The pediatric dose is smaller than the adult dose, often 0.3 mg, and will be indicated on the injector device. EpiPen Jr. is a common trade name for the pediatric dose of the medication.

SKILL 26-2 *Assistance with an Epinephrine Auto-Injector*

PURPOSE: To assist the patient in administration of prescribed epinephrine, using the auto-injector.

STANDARD PRECAUTIONS:

- ☑ Oxygen
- ☑ Prescribed epinephrine auto-injector
- ☑ Scissors
- ☑ Sharps container

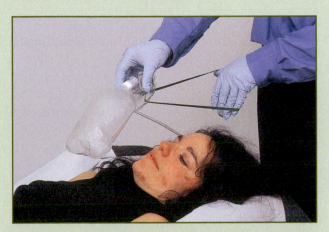

1 The EMT assesses the patient and applies oxygen as appropriate.

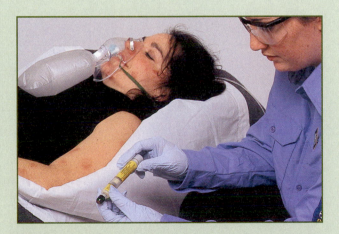

2 The EMT confirms that the auto-injector is the patient's prescribed auto-injector and checks the expiration date.

(continues)

SKILL 26-2 *(continued)*

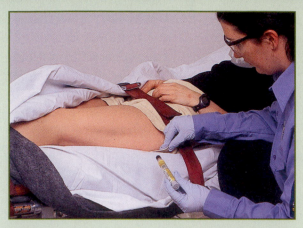

3 The EMT bares the patient's lateral thigh (using scissors to cut away clothing if necessary) and then removes the safety cap on the auto-injector.

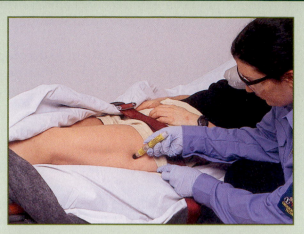

4 Pressing the auto-injector firmly against the patient's lateral thigh, midway between the knee and the hip, the EMT allows about 10 seconds for the medication administration.

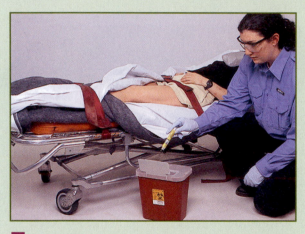

5 The EMT removes the auto-injector and properly disposes of the auto-injector in a sharps container at the patient's side.

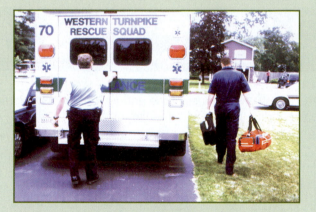

6 The EMT reassesses the patient and initiates transport as soon as possible. The EMT should arrange for an ALS intercept if possible.

Glucagon

Families of patients with diabetes may be prescribed glucagon for use if the patient experiences low blood sugar and cannot take glucose by mouth.

Glucagon works by releasing stored glucose from the liver to go into the bloodstream. Glucagon is only effective if the liver has a store of glucose available for use. Once the glucagon has been administered, it will start to take effect within 8–10 minutes and may last up to 30 minutes.

Some EMS systems may permit an EMT to assist the family or the patient with administering the glucagon. After the glucagon has been given, the EMT should not delay transport waiting for the glucagon to take effect but should immediately transport the patient to the closest advanced-level care, either an emergency department or advanced EMT.

Administration Procedure

Glucagon has a limited shelf life when it is in liquid form. For this reason glucagon comes packaged in two vials inside an "emergency kit." The first vial has the powdered glucagon. The second vial has a liquid, called a diluent, that is drawn out of the vial by syringe and then injected into the second vial.

Once the liquid diluent is in contact with the glucagon powder, it should be mixed by gently rolling the vial in the palm of the hand until it is completely mixed and no powder residue is evident. Then the EMT should draw up the glucagon liquid, displace any air in the syringe, and then inject the drug into the muscle at the lateral thigh.

After injecting the glucagon, the syringe and needle should be discarded into a sharps container and the patient monitored for the effect of the drug.

This procedure requires an EMT take additional training and to practice drawing up the medications and injecting them in order to be proficient during an emergency.

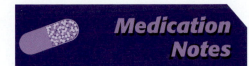

Medication Notes

Generic Name: Glucagon
Trade Name: Glucagon Emergency Kit
Indications: Low blood sugar
Contraindications: Rare, if used to treat low blood sugar
Dose: 1 mg
Route: Intramuscular

CONCLUSION

The EMT will often have occasion to care for patients who have potentially life-threatening conditions. Some of these conditions may require the administration of medication, so the EMT must be familiar with some basic pharmacology.

EMTs must be thoroughly familiar with the medications that they are responsible for carrying and administering, such as oxygen, oral glucose, and activated charcoal. In addition, the EMT must be familiar with a few prescribed medications for patients who have serious medical problems and may require assistance in administration. These medications include bronchodilator inhalers, nitroglycerin, and epinephrine auto-injectors.

This text provides an overview of the common use of these medications. Each EMT must be responsible for investigating the local regulations pertaining to these medications and the protocols governing their use. These protocols may differ significantly from one locale to another. The involvement of medical control physicians in the decision to administer medications by the EMT-B is often helpful and sometimes even required by the local protocols.

TEST YOUR KNOWLEDGE

1. Discuss the importance of basic pharmacology to the EMT.
2. Explain the difference between the generic name and the trade name for medications.
3. Define the terms *indication* and *contraindication*.
4. List the different forms that medications may come in.
5. List at least three routes of drug administration used by the EMT.
6. Review the "five rights" that must be verified before drug administration.
7. Discuss the importance of reassessment after drug administration.

8. Explain how drug administration is documented.

9. Describe the indications, contraindications, actions, side effects, dose, and route of the following medications: activated charcoal, oral gulcose, oxygen, prescribed inhaler, nitroglycerin, epinephrine.

10. Discuss the difference between an EMT's administering a drug and an EMT's assisting a patient to take a previously prescribed medication.

INTERNET RESOURCES

- Conduct a search using the drugs discussed in this chapter as key terms. What additional information can you find related to the use of these drugs in emergency care?

- Do a search looking for research that may be in process for allowing the EMT-B to administer more drugs in the prehospital setting. Is any such research underway?

FURTHER STUDY

Gonsoulin, S., & Raynovich, W. (2000). *Prehospital drug therapy*. Philadelphia: Mosby.

CHAPTER 27

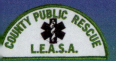

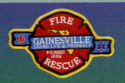

Shortness of Breath

KEY TERMS

alveolar-capillary gas exchange

asthma

bronchospasm

cellular respiration

chronic obstructive pulmonary disease (COPD)

congestive heart failure (CHF)

crackles

croup

diffusion

epiglottitis

hypoxic drive

pulmonary embolus

rhonchi

wheezing

OBJECTIVES

Upon completion of this chapter, the reader should be able to:

1. List the structures and functions of the respiratory system.
2. State the signs and symptoms of a patient with difficulty breathing.
3. Describe the emergency medical care of the patient with difficulty breathing.
4. Recognize the need for medical direction to assist in the emergency medical care of the patient with difficulty breathing.
5. Recognize the patient in need of airway management and ventilatory assistance.
6. List the signs of adequate air exchange.
7. Identify when administration of a prescribed inhaler is indicated.
8. Identify the key elements in management of patients with epiglottitis, croup, asthma, COPD, and CHF.

OVERVIEW

Difficulty breathing can be caused by many different problems. Each of these problems may result from a different disease; however, each causes dysfunction of the respiratory system.

The respiratory system is a vital organ system responsible for providing oxygen to the body and removing the metabolic waste product carbon dioxide. The body has backup systems for times when the respiratory system is not functioning ideally; however, if the problem goes on long enough, these backup systems can also fail.

Emergency medical technicians (EMTs) are often called to assist patients whose respiratory system is not functioning normally, causing them to feel as though they cannot breathe. *Dyspnea* is a term that means difficulty breathing. Dyspnea, a Latin word, comes from "dys," difficulty, and "pnea," breathing. It is one of many medical terms that have Latin or Greek origins for their meanings. These roots can also be used in other combinations; for example, *apnea* comes from "a," without, and "pnea," breathing, and is the medical term for lack of breathing. EMTs encounter many medical terms in their practice.

This chapter reviews the normal anatomy of the respiratory system and why it can fail. The common signs and symptoms and the appropriate history and physical examination are outlined. In addition, the appropriate management of the patient who is short of breath is discussed.

ANATOMY REVIEW

The respiratory system is made up of airways, lungs, and blood vessels. Each will be reviewed separately, and their interaction with the muscular diaphragm and the muscles of the chest wall to take in oxygen and get rid of carbon dioxide will also be reviewed. Additional discussions of respiratory anatomy and physiology are found in Chapter 5.

Upper Airway

Air enters the lungs through the nose and mouth, where it is warmed and humidified. The warm, moist air then moves through the pharynx, where it passes the epiglottis and the larynx to enter the trachea.

Respiratory Tree

The trachea is made up of cartilaginous rings and branches into two main bronchi (the left and the right). The bronchi branch further into smaller airways called bronchioles, which eventually empty into small grapelike clusters of tiny air spaces, called alveoli.

The alveoli are surrounded by tiny blood vessels called capillaries. These capillaries carry all of the deoxygenated blood from the body to be reoxygenated at the alveoli. Figure 27-1 reviews the anatomy of the respiratory system, illustrating the branching of the airways and the movement of air into and out of the alveoli.

Musculature

There are multiple muscles that are actively involved in ventilation. Ventilation refers to the movement of air into and out of the lungs. These muscles are generally controlled by the nervous system without conscious effort.

Diaphragm

The diaphragm is a large muscle inside the bottom of the chest. It contracts during inspiration and relaxes to allow exhalation. Nerves from the cervical spinal cord in the neck control this large muscle.

Chest Wall Muscles

Within the chest wall itself are many other smaller muscles that assist in breathing. These are muscles between the ribs, in the neck, and other external chest muscles. This muscular system helps to raise the chest during inspiration and is especially important when the diaphragm is unable to work efficiently. These muscles are commonly referred to as the accessory muscles of respiration.

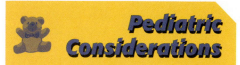

Pediatric Considerations

The respiratory system of infants and children functions essentially the same as that of adults, but the airway anatomy is somewhat different in relation to size. The pediatric patient has a relatively smaller airway and relatively bigger tongue and epiglottis. This difference allows for much easier obstruction of the airway because it would take a smaller amount of blockage to completely occlude a small airway.

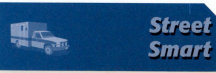

Street Smart

Some patients who have sustained serious injury to their neck may have damage to the nerves controlling the diaphragm. These patients may have difficulty breathing or may not be able to breathe at all. The EMT should carefully observe the breathing of patients with neck injuries.

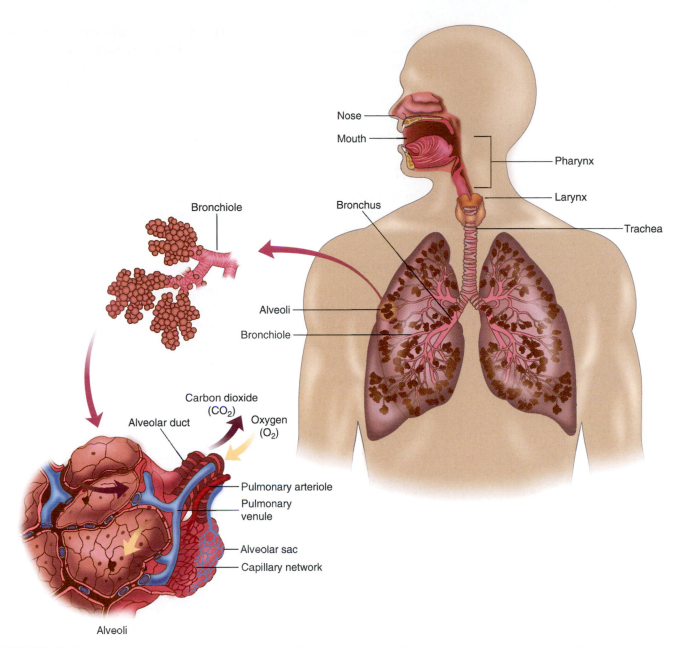

FIGURE 27-1   The respiratory system is composed of branching airways that get progressively smaller as they get farther away from the trachea.

PHYSIOLOGY REVIEW

It is important for the EMT to understand how normal breathing occurs to better understand what is going on when there is a problem.

Respiratory Drive

The brain monitors many things within the body. One of the things the brain monitors carefully is the pH, or acid levels, in the blood. The blood level of carbon dioxide directly influences this acid level. When carbon dioxide levels are too high, the acid level rises and the body reacts in a number of ways.

One response to this abnormality is to try to lower the carbon dioxide level. It can be lowered by breathing faster, as each exhalation gets rid of more of this waste product. Therefore, the normal person's respiratory rate is determined by the person's carbon dioxide levels. The higher the level, the more stimulation to breathe. It is important to realize that it is not the *oxygen* level that normally stimulates a person to breathe.

Ventilation

Once the brain indicates to the respiratory system that breathing should occur, some muscular work needs to be done in order for breathing to be accomplished.

Inhalation

A breath begins when the diaphragm contracts and pulls down toward the abdomen and the ribs rise. This action generates a negative pressure within the chest, similar to a vacuum. Air is pulled into the chest through the mouth and nose and the rest of the airways until the air spaces are full. This concept of negative pressure generating inspiration can be visualized in Figure 27-2.

Exhalation

After enough time has been allowed for gas exchange between the alveolar sacs and the capillaries, exhalation occurs. The diaphragm relaxes and allows the air to rush back out of the airways and the mouth and nose into the surrounding environment, ending the breath.

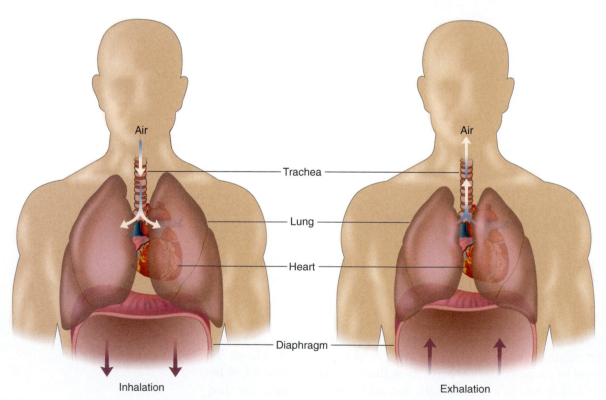

	Trachea	
	Lung	
	Heart	
	Diaphragm	

Inhalation Exhalation

FIGURE 27-2 Air is drawn into the chest during inhalation by a negative pressure created by diaphragmatic contraction. As the diaphragm relaxes, air is passively released during exhalation.

Respiration

The EMT should remember that the term *respiration* actually refers to the gas exchange that occurs in the lungs and in the peripheral tissues, not to the act of moving air into and out of the lungs. Recall that the mechanical act of breathing can be accurately referred to as ventilation.

Pulmonary Respiration

As the capillaries pass between the air-filled alveoli, a process called **diffusion** occurs. This means that the oxygen passes from the air space into the blood, where the concentration of oxygen is lower, and the carbon dioxide passes from the blood into the air space, where the concentration of carbon dioxide is lower. This **alveolar-capillary gas exchange** occurs passively since the natural preference of these molecules is to be in balance, or in equal amounts on both sides.

The success of this exchange relies upon several factors. The air in the air space must be rich in oxygen, the blood must pass closely to the alveoli, and the wall between them must be very thin (one cell layer, in fact!).

Cellular Respiration

After oxygenated blood is pumped out of the heart, it must be delivered to the peripheral tissues. It is in the peripheral tissues where carbon dioxide is picked up for delivery back to the lungs, where it is exhaled.

The process that allows the exchange of gases in the periphery is called **cellular respiration**. This process uses the similar process of diffusion, this time between the oxygen-poor tissue and the oxygen-rich blood in the peripheral capillaries. The process of pulmonary and cellular respiration is illustrated in Figure 27-3.

NORMAL BREATHING

Breathing normally takes minimal effort. The breathing rate is set by the brain as determined by blood levels of carbon dioxide, as previously discussed. Problems affecting the respiratory system will be evident in several ways.

Patient Appearance

A person breathing normally appears comfortable during both inhalation and exhalation. The diaphragm and other chest muscles of respiration smoothly contract to pull air into the chest, then easily relax and allow air to exit the airway.

Respiratory difficulty is often obvious upon looking at the patient. The patient may appear to be exerting an abnormal amount of effort in breathing and may actually get to the point at which she looks tired of that effort.

Lung Sounds

All of this air movement into and out of the lungs creates a characteristic sound that can be heard with a stethoscope held to the chest. Any

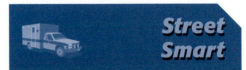

Street Smart

A patient who has been having respiratory difficulty and who begins to look tired is probably not getting ready for her afternoon nap. She may have become physically exhausted from the extra respiratory effort. This patient is in danger of respiratory arrest and will need ventilatory assistance. The EMT should learn to recognize this warning sign and act appropriately.

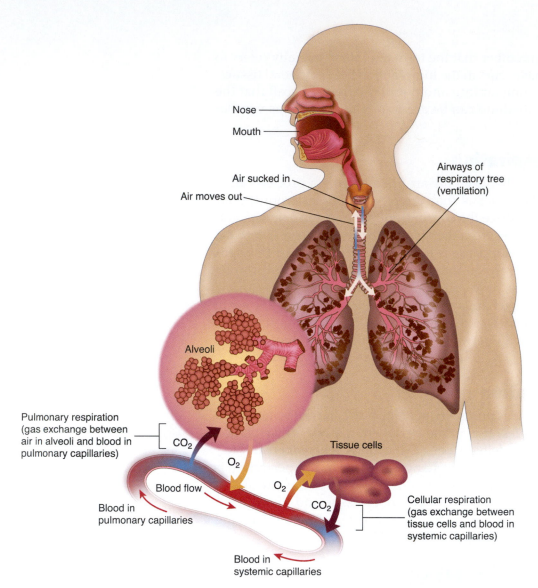

FIGURE 27-3 Oxygen and carbon dioxide are exchanged between the alveoli and the pulmonary capillaries surrounding them. Oxygen is delivered to the tissues and carbon dioxide is removed in a process called cellular respiration.

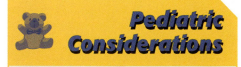

Pediatric Considerations

A child must breathe 15–30 times per minute. Infants have smaller lungs and therefore must breathe 25–50 times each minute.

alteration in this normal pattern of airflow can create abnormal sounds as air rushes into and out of the chest.

A high-pitched, whining sound may be heard as air passes through abnormally narrowed airways. This sound, called **wheezing**, is usually heard during exhalation but may be heard during both phases of ventilation.

If mucus or other foreign material accumulates in the larger airways, the air passing through the airway may cause a coarse sound that can be easily heard on both inspiration and exhalation. This rough sound is called **rhonchi**.

The next common sound heard when auscultating lungs is a sound referred to as **crackles**. This term is used to describe a crackling sound, like Rice Krispies being crushed, that is created as tiny air spaces that were stuck together by abnormal fluid accumulation pop open. Fluid in the alveoli creates the inspiratory sound of crackles.

The diseases that cause these common abnormal lung sounds will be reviewed later in this chapter.

Rates and Patterns

To maintain normal oxygen and carbon dioxide levels, the body must repeat the respiratory cycle completely 12–20 times each minute (the normal respiratory rate).

Respiratory rates lower than normal will be inadequate and result in problems. Abnormally high respiratory rates indicate some abnormality affecting the respiratory system and should not be ignored when noted.

Vital Signs

As mentioned previously, a smoothly running respiratory system requires minimal conscious effort. The vital signs reflect this relaxation with a normal heart rate and blood pressure. Any extra effort in breathing may be reflected in an abnormally high heart rate and sometimes in a higher-than-normal blood pressure.

Color

When adequate gas exchange occurs, the mucous membranes have a pink color. If the blood is poorly oxygenated because of inadequate gas exchange, the mucous membranes may take on a bluish color, especially in the lips. This blue to gray color is called cyanosis and is a sign of serious respiratory disease.

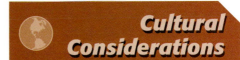

Cultural Considerations

The pink or bluish color may be difficult to visualize on darker-skinned patients. It is useful to pay careful attention to the lips and oral mucous membranes of these patients and to note any changes in color there.

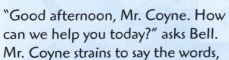

Breathing Difficulty

EMTs Bell and McCall arrive on scene to find an approximately 70-year-old, thin male sitting hunched over at a small table. His eyes are half open. A half-empty cup of coffee, an ashtray overflowing with cigarette butts, and about a half dozen prescription medicine bottles as well as two inhalers are on the table.

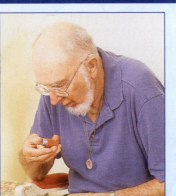

"Good afternoon, Mr. Coyne. How can we help you today?" asks Bell. Mr. Coyne strains to say the words, "Trouble . . . breathing." Looking more closely, the EMTs note that Mr. Coyne's lips are bluish.

- What signs of respiratory distress are present?
- What environmental clues may suggest respiratory disease?
- What assessment findings would the EMTs likely find?
- What are the treatment priorities?

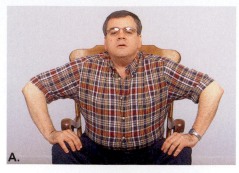

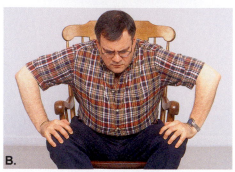

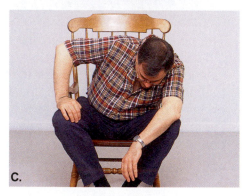

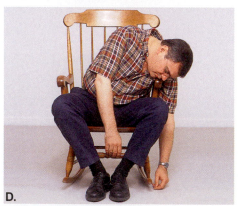

FIGURE 27-4 A. The patient with respiratory distress will often be found sitting bolt upright in the tripod position, using accessory muscles to assist in breathing. B. As hypoxia worsens, the patient will often become very anxious. C. The dyspneic patient may become very tired, as working to breathe has been very taxing. This is an ominous sign. D. The patient who is cyanotic and not alert is very sick and in need of immediate ventilatory support.

RESPIRATORY DISTRESS

The patient who has a problem within the respiratory system will often present with classic signs and symptoms that the EMT must be able to recognize. The ability to recognize the patient in respiratory distress will enable the EMT to initiate the proper treatment quickly. Without rapid treatment, some patients with respiratory distress will deteriorate and completely stop breathing. This outcome is to be avoided at all costs.

Signs and Symptoms

Patients who are having respiratory difficulty may describe their symptoms differently. Some patients say they can't breathe or are having trouble breathing. Others may describe an inability to catch their breath or say they are short of breath.

Some very sick patients may not be able to talk or describe their problem at all. The EMT may have been called by friends or family members who noted the patient's distress. In this situation, the EMT must elicit the symptoms from the people who called.

When the dyspneic patient is working very hard to breathe, the respiratory rate is usually notably higher than normal. The heart rate also is elevated just as is seen in other circumstances of exertion. As the respiratory system fails and tissues are no longer receiving oxygen, the patient's skin may become cyanotic.

Eventually, if not treated effectively, the patient will no longer be able to compensate for the abnormality in the respiratory system and will become tired. The respiratory rate may drop, and the patient will take on a more slumped, tired position. Finally, if the condition worsens, the patient may completely stop breathing. Figure 27-4 illustrates the progression of respiratory distress that may be seen without proper treatment.

Assessment

The EMT must use skills of observation and note the environment the patient is in and how the patient looks upon initial approach. This general impression of the severity of the patient's illness comes within the first 30 seconds and is often quite accurate.

The history and physical exam of the patient with difficulty breathing can be focused on the respiratory system. As always, the airway, breathing, circulation (ABC) are the crucial initial exam points. This exam should include ensuring that the patient is maintaining her own airway, is breathing spontaneously, and has a pulse.

Initial Assessment

The initial assessment is done very quickly and is meant to briefly assess the patient's mental status, airway patency, breathing, and circulation.

The conscious patient who is speaking easily may have no immediately life-threatening issues. If life-threatening problems are found during the initial assessment, such as the need for airway maintenance or ventilatory assistance, they should be taken care of as soon as they are identified.

Focused History and Physical Examination

The focused history and physical examination will be completed after the initial assessment and any life threats have been appropriately managed. If the patient is considered to be critically ill or unstable, the focused exam will likely be done in the ambulance while en route to the hospital.

If the patient is stable, the EMT can spend a few moments gathering relevant history and performing a focused physical exam before transport.

Responsive Patient

The patient who is responsive and able to speak well enough to provide the EMT with a history should be asked questions regarding the nature of the illness.

History   Every patient should be asked the SAMPLE (see Table 10-5) history questions to gather information relating to signs and symptoms, allergies, medications, pertinent past history, last oral intake, and the events leading up to the illness.

A good mnemonic to remember when obtaining further history from a medical patient is OPQRST This prompts the EMT to ask about onset, provocation, quality, radiation, severity, and time. Also important to note are any interventions the patient may have tried and any other symptoms associated with the original complaint. The details of the history of the medical patient can be reviewed in Chapter 14.

Focused Physical Examination   Once the history has been obtained in the responsive patient, it is then appropriate to continue the respiratory assessment by noting lung sounds as heard by listening through a stethoscope. The EMT should carefully observe the patient's breathing and note any irregular patterns or sounds or any extra effort. Remember that normal breathing is very regular, effortless, and quiet.

The presence of jugular venous distension (JVD) and swelling of the legs should be noted because both are associated with the backup of fluids seen in congestive heart failure (CHF), which will be discussed later in this chapter. These physical findings can be seen in Figure 27-5. The patient's skin should be briefly examined for a rash or hives, which may indicate an allergic reaction. Any abnormal skin colors, such as cyanosis, should also be noted.

Vital Signs   The remainder of the exam of the responsive patient who is short of breath should include a full set of vital signs, including blood pressure, pulse rate and quality, respiratory rate and quality, and pulse oximetry when available.

Unresponsive Patient

The EMT will alter his assessment somewhat for the unresponsive patient. The priorities will be to complete a rapid physical examination, obtain vital signs, and then obtain relevant history from any family or bystanders.

Rapid Physical Examination   After completing the initial assessment, the EMT should perform a rapid physical examination. The

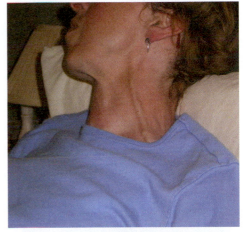

A.

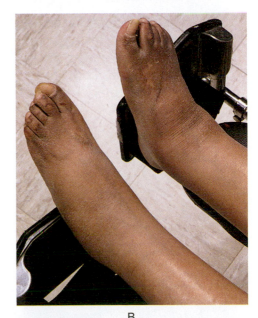

B.

FIGURE 27-5   A. Jugular venous distension is a sign of excess fluid buildup, often seen in the patient with chronic congestive heart failure. B. Edema is often seen in the ankles and legs of patients with chronic congestive heart failure.

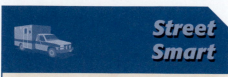

Street Smart

Pulse oximetry should improve if treatments provided are effective. A falling pulse oximetry is a sign of deterioration in the patient with a respiratory illness.

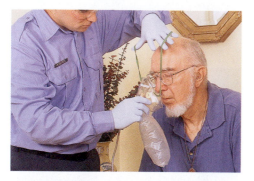

FIGURE 27-6 No matter the cause of shortness of breath, supplemental oxygen is always indicated.

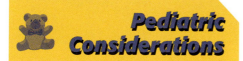

Pediatric Considerations

Children often will not allow either a mask or a cannula to be placed on their face. In this case, a blow-by technique can be used. This is described in Chapter 8 and is shown in Figure 27-7.

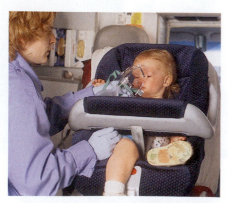

FIGURE 27-7 Some children will not tolerate having an oxygen mask placed on their face. Oxygen may be administered by a blow-by technique.

point of this quick head-to-toe survey is to find any abnormalities that may help the EMT to understand what has happened to the patient.

For example, the patient who was complaining of shortness of breath who is now unconscious may have a stab wound to the back of the chest. This injury is relevant to the patient's condition and will likely affect the EMT's priorities and management. Without looking for them, the EMT may not find important clues to the patient's illness.

Vital Signs After the initial and rapid physical exams, the next priority is to obtain a complete set of vital signs. The rate and quality of respirations and pulse should be measured. Blood pressure should be measured. Pulse oximetry is a useful tool in caring for the patient who has a respiratory problem because it can be used to follow the effectiveness of treatment provided.

History from Others An unresponsive patient is unlikely to provide the EMT with much useful history. It is important that the key parts of the history be obtained from friends, family, or bystanders. These people may be able to provide important information that may be relevant in patient care. A SAMPLE history and as much of the OPQRST history as is available from these sources should be quickly elicited by the EMT.

Management

The management of the patient with difficulty breathing should begin during the initial assessment. No matter the cause of the problem, oxygen is always appropriate since most of the diseases resulting in difficulty breathing involve lack of oxygen to the body tissues.

Other specific treatments, such as inhaled medications, may be indicated depending on the cause of the problem. It is not important for the EMT to diagnose the underlying cause of the shortness of breath. It *is* important to treat the patient on the basis of her symptoms and history.

Oxygen

Because shortness of breath is often associated with, if not due to, low oxygen levels, a crucial part of the management of the dyspneic patient is providing high-flow oxygen in whatever manner is appropriate (Figure 27-6).

Spontaneously Breathing Patient

If the patient is moving air well on her own but feeling short of breath, a non-rebreather facemask with 10–15 liters per minute of oxygen is appropriate. If the patient cannot tolerate the mask, a nasal cannula is a reasonable alternative. Although it delivers less oxygen than a mask, a little is certainly better than none at all!

Assisting Ventilations

The patient who cannot maintain an airway or whose respiratory effort is inadequate must be assisted by manual ventilation. Adequate respiratory effort can be judged by several factors. A patient whose color is pink, who has a respiratory rate within the normal range for her age and size, and whose chest is moving up and down with each breath is ventilating adequately for the time being.

If the patient becomes cyanotic or the respiratory rate becomes too fast to be efficient or too slow to be adequate, the patient may need ventilatory assistance. Using a bag-valve-mask attached to 100% oxygen to assist respiratory effort is appropriate (Figure 27-8).

Intubation

In some states, the EMT is trained to perform endotracheal intubation. If a patient requires prolonged ventilatory assistance, the EMT may choose to intubate the patient to better protect the airway and more effectively ventilate the patient. This procedure is discussed in detail in Appendix A.

Positioning

It is important for the EMT to pay attention to the position he places the patient in. Most patients who are short of breath will prefer to sit upright. In the upright position, breathing may be more effective and easier.

If the EMT finds the patient lying down, it may be worthwhile to sit her up to see if sitting helps ease her breathing. In all cases, the EMT should allow patients to be in whatever position they feel is most comfortable.

Prescribed Medications

If a medication such as an inhaler is prescribed to the patient, the EMT may contact a medical control physician and request an order to assist the patient in using the medication. Only medications prescribed specifically for that patient should be used and only if the patient is able to self-administer the drug with only *assistance* from the EMT (Figure 27-9).

Bronchodilator Inhalers

If a patient who is prescribed a bronchodilator inhaler is having trouble breathing and would normally use the medication, then the EMT should consider assisting the patient to use this medication according to local protocols.

These medicines are meant to be inhaled directly into the airways. Upon contact with the bronchioles, the medications should help relieve the spasm and allow easier passage of air. An example of such medications is albuterol (trade names: Ventolin and Proventil), although there are other names. The EMT should be familiar with these names and should refer to local protocol for regulations on which are allowed to be used. Important details regarding the use of these medications are discussed in Chapter 26.

Transport

The EMT should initiate transport as soon as he has determined the patient is a high priority. If after completing the initial assessment the EMT finds that the patient has a potentially life-threatening problem, transport should be initiated immediately.

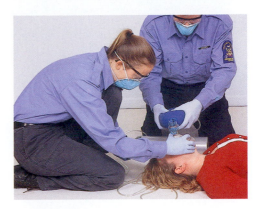

FIGURE 27-8 The EMT should be prepared to assist a patient's ventilations if necessary.

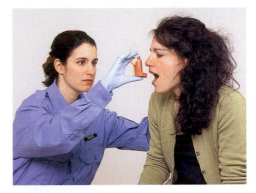

FIGURE 27-9 The EMT should be familiar with the use of an inhaler so that she may assist a patient with its use.

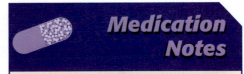

Medication Notes

Generic name: Albuterol

Trade name: Ventolin, Proventil

Indications: Signs and symptoms of respiratory distress in a patient who has a physician-prescribed handheld inhaler

Contraindications: The nonalert patient cannot cooperate with administration of an inhaler.

Dose: Two puffs given 1 minute apart

Route: By inhalation

A quick history should be obtained from the family or friends present while the patient is being prepared for transport. The remainder of the exam should be provided in the ambulance while en route to the hospital.

Destination Decisions

The patient should be transported to an appropriate facility, and the EMT must notify that facility as far in advance of arrival as possible. The unstable patient may require transport to the closest facility rather than to her preferred hospital. The EMT should be familiar with local protocols regarding destination determinations for unstable patients.

Advanced Life Support

When the patient is considered unstable or is still in distress upon initiation of transport, a basic life support (BLS) agency should make arrangements to intercept with an agency that provides a higher level of care when possible. The EMT, however, should never delay transport to wait for such care. It is sometimes necessary to intercept with an advanced life support (ALS) unit while en route to a hospital.

It may also be appropriate, depending upon local protocols, for the EMT to establish on-line medical control to ask the physician for advice. Physicians provide guidance to the EMT in the form of general protocols. If the patient is not improving despite management according to those protocols, a medical control physician may instruct the EMT to provide different or additional therapies.

Ongoing Assessment

It is important for the EMT to remember that the physical assessment is not static but ongoing. Key elements of assessment must continually be reassessed because a patient may quickly deteriorate.

Choking

The public safety officer was using the security camera and panning the lunchroom for activity when he noticed a crowd of people around someone on the floor. The person on the floor appeared to be unresponsive to the people shaking her. While keeping the camera trained on the crowd, he called 9-1-1 for an "unknown, woman down." Shortly afterward, a call came into the security office, "Listen, we need an ambulance. Some woman passed out. She appeared to be choking, then passed out." The security officer responded, "Sir, an officer has been dispatched and should be here any minute now, and I have called for an ambulance."

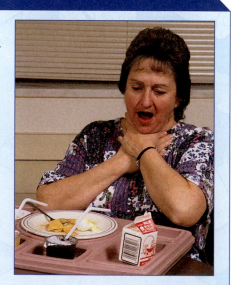

- On the basis of the limited information provided, is this patient a high- or a low-priority patient?
- What is the first priority in this patient's assessment?
- What techniques could be used to manage this situation?

To provide appropriate emergency care, continue to reassess and recognize significant changes in the patient's condition. The initial assessment should be repeated frequently, as should vital signs. Any significant changes should be relayed to the receiving hospital.

Reassessment

After any treatment has been provided to the patient who is short of breath, the EMT should perform a careful reassessment. The initial assessment, vital signs, and focused physical exam all should be repeated after any therapy. The patient should also be asked how she feels in relation to how she felt before the therapy. The EMT should always be prepared for the dyspneic patient to decompensate and need ventilatory assistance.

CAUSES OF SHORTNESS OF BREATH

Problems can arise within any part of the respiratory system, all of which may result in inadequate respiration or poor oxygenation of the blood. This section briefly describes some of the disease processes that may affect each component of the respiratory system. It may be helpful to separate these illnesses into whether they primarily originate from the airway, breathing, or circulation.

Airway

The airways cannot adequately transmit oxygen from the environment into the alveoli for gas exchange if they are obstructed. Airways can be obstructed by many things. Foreign bodies are probably the most common, although it is not unusual for parts of the airway itself to cause partial or even complete obstruction.

Foreign Body Obstruction

If a foreign body such as a large piece of poorly chewed meat becomes lodged in the trachea or one of the bronchi, air cannot pass beyond it. If air cannot get to the alveoli to deliver oxygen, the body organs cannot function properly and may even suffer permanent damage. Figure 27-10 illustrates an airway foreign body obstruction.

The brain and heart suffer permanent damage in as little as 4 minutes when deprived of oxygen. This situation requires rapid attention by the EMT. In the case of a complete obstruction, in which the patient cannot move any air or speak at all, the EMT should perform the Heimlich maneuver. The techniques for removal of airway foreign bodies are taught in a cardiopulmonary resuscitation (CPR) class.

The upper airways can also be partially occluded by a foreign body or even by excessive secretions seen in upper respiratory infections.

Epiglottitis

Another possible source of partial or complete obstruction of the upper airway is the airway structures themselves. The structure called the epiglottis sits above the opening to the trachea and normally easily flaps open and closed to protect the trachea from foreign bodies as we swallow. This structure can become inflamed and swollen in a bacterial

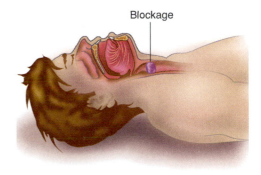

Blockage

FIGURE 27-10   A complete airway obstruction will cause death in a matter of minutes if not relieved.

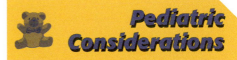

Pediatric Considerations

Airway obstruction by secretions or swelling is especially relevant in pediatric patients because their airways are relatively smaller and would require fewer secretions to significantly narrow the air passages.

infection called **epiglottitis**. The enlarged epiglottis can completely occlude the airway very quickly in this aggressive disease.

Although this condition can be seen in a patient of any age, the patients at risk for the most severe complications from epiglottitis are those with smaller airways—that is, pediatric patients.

Signs and Symptoms

The child with epiglottitis will appear frightened owing to the difficulty in air movement. The classic history is that of a sudden-onset fever, cough, and now difficulty breathing. The child will most often be seated bolt upright with her head held forward, often drooling. The inability to swallow even saliva indicates severe upper airway narrowing.

Management

The best thing to do for a child who presents in this way is to remain calm while moving the child out to the ambulance for a quick ride to the hospital. The parents should be encouraged to remain calm and to comfort the child. If tolerated, humidified oxygen can be blown by the child's face. Under no circumstances should the EMT attempt to examine the child's mouth or throat because doing so could precipitate rapid and complete airway obstruction.

Early notification of the destination hospital is helpful so the emergency department staff can prepare necessary equipment and call in any needed specialists.

If the child's airway becomes completely occluded with no air movement, and she develops cyanosis, the EMT should use a bag-valve-mask to ventilate the child with 100% oxygen. Still, no probing of the airway should be attempted because it may worsen the condition.

Croup

Croup (laryngotracheobronchitis) is a viral infection usually in young children, causing irritation and swelling of the larynx, trachea, and bronchi. This disease is not as aggressive as epiglottitis and tends to cause a partial airway obstruction only. Croup can progress to complete obstruction; however, this is a rare occurrence.

Signs and Symptoms

The child with croup classically presents after several days of upper respiratory congestion and mild fevers. The irritation of the larynx produces a characteristic barking sound when the child coughs. The sound has been likened to the barking of a seal and is almost diagnostic of croup.

In addition, if the inflammation is severe, the airway may be narrowed to the point where stridor is heard on inspiration. You will recall that stridor is a low-pitched inspiratory sound as a result of partial upper airway obstructions.

Management

The child with croup should be managed similarly to children with epiglottitis. It is sometimes very difficult to tell these two illnesses apart. The priorities are to make the child as comfortable as possible, remain calm, and move quickly to the hospital. Cool, humidified oxygen is often helpful in relieving some of the child's discomfort and should be offered if tolerated.

The EMT has several methods of delivering humidified oxygen to the patient, such as utilizing an in-line humidifier or a small volume nebulizer (SVN). The advantage of the SVN is that it can be started in the field and continue while the patient is being transferred to the ambulance. However, an SVN lasts for only about 15 minutes, whereas an in-line humidifier can last for hours.

To use an in-line humidifier the EMT would open a pre-packaged humidifier and follow the manufacturer's instructions for setting the humidifier up, or use a component system humidifier. The components of the in-line humidifier consist of the adapter that attaches to the oxygen regulator of the on-board oxygen system, a clean bowl that holds the fresh sterile water, and the tubing system that goes to the patient. The most effective in-line humidifiers use large diameter corrugated tubing that attaches to the bottom of a facemask. Systems that try to supply humidification to oxygen supply tubing are generally ineffective and deliver little moisture to the patient.

Alternatively, the EMT may elect to use the SVN, the same one patients use to administer medications such as albuterol, although in this case no medicine is added. Like the in-line humidifier, the nebulizer has several components. The nebulizer has a bowl, sometimes called an acorn, in which approximately 3 milliliters (ml) of sterile saline is added. The sterile saline can come from a larger bottle, or more conveniently, from a small prepackaged ampule of saline flush, referred to as a pearl of saline, that is commercially available. Then the T-piece portion of the nebulizer is screwed into place, oxygen tubing is connected to the portable oxygen regulator, and the regulator is set at 8 liters per minute (Figure 27-11). The other end of the T-piece can either attach to a non-rebreather mask by removing the reservoir and replacing it with the nebulizer, or handheld to blow mist over the patient's face.

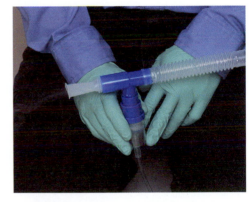

FIGURE 27-11 Humidified oxygen can be administered via a nebulizer.

Breathing

As expected, many illnesses that cause a patient to feel short of breath originate from the lungs themselves. A problem with air exchange is evident and results in shortness of breath.

Bronchospasm

One of the most common causes of shortness of breath is bronchospasm. **Bronchospasm** refers to constriction of the lower airways in the lungs. This can occur as a part of several disease processes, the most common of which will be discussed here.

Asthma

The lower airways can be affected by disease processes causing partial obstruction just as diseases such as croup and epiglottitis affect the upper airways. Hyperreactive airways found in some individuals respond to certain irritants (cigarette smoke, pollen, and cold air) by going into spasm and producing secretions. Both spasm and production of secretions can cause narrowing of the air spaces. This narrowing

Shortness of Breath

Practice was going as usual until one of the swimmers appeared to be having some trouble with her strokes. The coach advised her to rest for a minute. She stopped her practice, went to take her medicine, and then resumed her swimming. Shortly after resuming swimming, she started to experience even greater difficulty breathing and she had to be helped out of the pool. Her coach immediately sent two swimmers to the coach's office to get more help and to call 9-1-1.

After what seemed hours, but was actually only a few minutes, EMS arrived. The coach gave the EMT a quick description of what had happened and then left to call the swimmer's parents.

- What are the patient care priorities?
- On the basis of this limited information, what is the likely cause of her shortness of breath?
- How should an EMT proceed with treatment?

in the bronchioles causes a characteristic musical sound, known as wheezing, when air passes through them.

This disease process characterized by hyperreactive airways is known as reactive airway disease, or **asthma**. Chronic exposure to certain irritants (such as cigarette smoke) and other factors not completely identified can cause previously normal airways to become hyperreactive.

The patient with shortness of breath as a result of asthma will often describe some precipitating factor such as a respiratory infection, exposure to some airway irritant (smoke, animals, cold air), or sometimes even just exercise. This exposure will lead to a feeling of shortness of breath as bronchospasm occurs and it becomes more difficult to move air into and out of the chest. Figure 27-12 illustrates the basic problem in the airways in an asthma attack.

Signs and Symptoms   The patient will often look distressed, may be sitting upright, and will have an elevated respiratory rate. When the lungs are auscultated, wheezes may be heard.

Management   Patients who suffer from asthma are often prescribed medications that are meant to relieve the bronchospasm that causes the difficulty breathing. In certain circumstances, the EMT will assist the patient to use these medications in an attempt to relieve the patient's symptoms.

For all patients who complain of difficulty breathing, the first priority in management is to ensure an adequate airway and to be sure that they are adequately ventilating themselves. Oxygen should be applied immediately, and ventilations should be assisted if the patient is not managing well with her own respiratory effort.

Chronic Obstructive Pulmonary Disease

Another group of diseases that can lead to bronchospasm is **chronic obstructive pulmonary disease (COPD)**. Emphysema and chronic bronchitis make up a majority of this group.

Street Smart

If severe bronchospasm is present and no air can pass, the EMT may not hear wheezing when auscultating the chest. Remember that air movement must be present to hear wheezing. If there is no air movement, then no wheezing will be heard. No breath sounds will be heard either, and the EMT should identify this patient as being very sick, indeed.

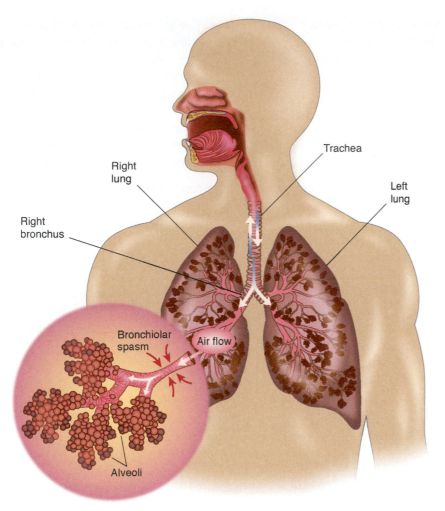

Right lung

Right bronchus

Trachea

Left lung

Bronchiolar spasm

Air flow

Alveoli

FIGURE 27-12 Asthma is a disease that involves bronchospasm and excessive airway secretions.

COPD, as the name suggests, is a chronic disorder involving obstruction of the airways in the lungs. This obstruction is a combination of bronchospasm and inflammation as seen in asthma but also includes other *nonreversible* causes of airway narrowing such as scarring and alveolar destruction.

Over the long term, the chronic airflow obstruction causes degenerative changes in the alveoli, making them less efficient. This chronic disease is often seen in older adults and results in many calls to emergency medical services (EMS).

COPD is a disease process that is still poorly understood. It is known that something causes the patient's airways to become hyperresponsive and over time become permanently damaged. Cigarette smoking is highly correlated with this disease. People who suffer from COPD have chronic bronchospasm.

Patients with COPD are treated with medications aimed at decreasing the amount of bronchospasm and the amount of secretions present in the airways. Sometimes doctors will prescribe oxygen to be used at home by these patients. Even when compliant with their medication regimen, COPD patients can suffer exacerbations (acute worsening of the disease) due to many different causes.

Pediatric Considerations

Children who suffer from asthma are very often prescribed bronchodilator inhalers. In children, frequent coughing is often a sign of airway narrowing. The EMT should carefully observe the child's respiratory effort. Children will often exhibit intercostal retractions as a sign of accessory muscle use. Cyanosis is a very late sign of respiratory decompensation in children.

Street Smart

Keep in mind when initiating transport for the patient with hyperresponsive airways that cold air can worsen the problem. Always adequately bundle up the patient who must be transported outside, even for a short time, to prevent worsening of the condition.

Signs and Symptoms   A common cause for an exacerbation is a respiratory infection. The already tightened airways become even smaller when plugged by increasing secretions found in these infections. People with severe COPD cannot tolerate even small changes in their airway size without becoming severely short of breath. This is the time that EMS will often be called to assist.

When treating a patient with COPD and shortness of breath, the EMT should try to determine the relevant historical information such as recent fevers, coughs, or other symptoms of a respiratory infection.

Hypoxic Drive   Because of their chronic respiratory insufficiency, some patients with COPD may breathe on a **hypoxic drive**. *Hypoxia* means low oxygen levels. A hypoxic drive means that the stimulus to breathe is low oxygen levels in the blood. The normal stimulus to breathe in healthy individuals is a high carbon dioxide level.

The patient with chronic airway obstruction has an inability to clear much of the carbon dioxide and will therefore have higher levels in the blood all the time. Some of these patients will adapt to that condition and begin to breathe on the basis of the oxygen levels instead, or with a hypoxic drive. Although this occurs very rarely, the EMT should be aware of the possibility of its presence.

If a patient who breathes with a hypoxic drive is given 100% oxygen, the body may see the additional oxygen as an overabundance and decrease the respiratory efforts, sometimes even allowing breathing to stop altogether. EMTs must therefore pay very close attention to the respiration of the COPD patient who is breathing 100% oxygen and assist the patient's respiration if needed.

However, oxygen should never be withheld from someone who is short of breath. Understanding the importance of providing oxygen to the body organs is key to this concept.

Management   If the patient is unable to get enough oxygen into the blood by her own respiratory efforts, it is the job of the caregiver to provide more oxygen, by whatever method it must be given. It is also appropriate to assist a patient in using prescribed medications when authorized to do so by medical control.

Respiratory Infection

Just as a respiratory infection such as pneumonia can cause bronchospasm in the patient with asthma or COPD, it can also cause a patient with previously healthy lungs to become short of breath. Pneumonia, bronchitis, and other respiratory infections cause inflammation and excess secretions in the lower airways within the lungs. These may result in lower airway narrowing, even in the patient with healthy lungs.

Signs and Symptoms

Lower airway narrowing along with the buildup of secretions in the lungs can impair oxygen exchange and lead to shortness of breath. Fever and productive cough are common complaints in the presence of a pulmonary infection.

Management

Oxygen administration is indicated for the patient with a respiratory infection causing shortness of breath. Allowing the patient to stay in a position that is most comfortable, usually sitting upright, may also help the patient to feel less short of breath during transport.

Chronic Lung Diseases

In addition to those we have discussed so far, there are many other chronic lung diseases, all of which usually create a problem with oxygenation of the blood. If a patient is short of breath and has a chronic lung disease, the EMT should find out exactly what medications are taken and how this problem is related to the usual disease. Administration of oxygen is always the right treatment in management of the patient with shortness of breath, no matter what the underlying disease is.

Circulation

Because the function of the lungs is so closely related to the function of the heart and the blood vessels, a problem with one system will often result in a problem with the other.

Pulmonary Embolus

If the airways are functioning efficiently and delivering oxygenated air to the alveoli, but there is no blood for the oxygen to diffuse into, the system fails. This condition occurs when blood flow to the alveoli is blocked by a blood clot, or embolus. This is known as a **pulmonary embolus** and is seen in people who are at risk for developing clots in their blood. Table 27-1 lists disease states or conditions that result in an increased risk of developing blood clots.

If the blood is prevented from being oxygenated, the organs do not get this necessary fuel and do not function properly. Figure 27-13 illustrates this sometimes-fatal condition.

TABLE 27-1
Disease States or Conditions That May Increase the Risk of Developing Blood Clots
Cancers

Prolonged immobility
    Casts
    Splints
    Bedbound
    Long car or plane trips

Smoking
Oral contraceptive use (birth control pills)
Prior history of blood clots
Recent surgery

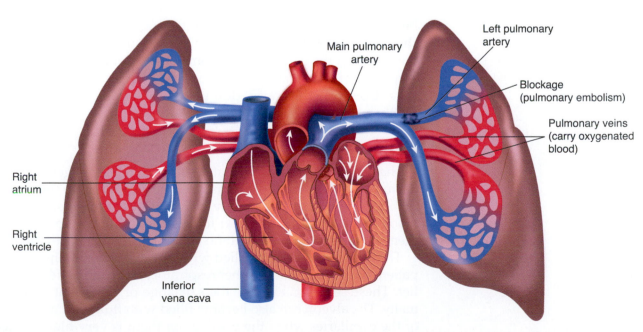

FIGURE 27-13   A blood clot in the pulmonary vessels will block oxygenation of the blood, resulting in hypoxia and shortness of breath.

Heart Problems

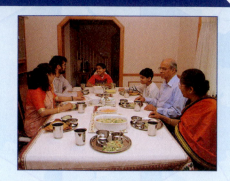

The family had just finished the holiday dinner and were sitting down to watch the football game on television. Grandma was busy washing the dishes in the kitchen when she suddenly became short of breath. Sitting down at the kitchen table to rest, she called out to Junior. Junior had seen Grandma like this before and immediately called to the fire station.

"Grandma's having troubling breathing again, you'd better get up here. She's got heart problems you know." Junior reported to the emergency hot line operator, "End of Canyon Road, second farmhouse on the right past the bridge, we'll turn the porch light on for you."

- What are the priorities in this patient's assessment?
- What physical findings might be expected?
- What are the treatment priorities?
- What differs between the treatment of this patient and the treatment of an asthmatic patient?

Signs and Symptoms

The patient with a pulmonary embolus will often complain of the sudden onset of shortness of breath. Sometimes these patients will also complain of a sharp chest pain or a dry cough. A patient who has had a pulmonary embolus or any type of blood clot before is at high risk of developing this problem again.

Because there is no problem with airflow, the patient's lung sounds will be clear. The respiratory rate will be elevated as the patient tries to increase the amount of oxygen breathed in.

Management

Because the problem is a decrease in oxygen in the blood, the EMT should apply 100% oxygen if he suspects pulmonary embolus to be the source of the patient's symptoms. If the clot is extensive, the oxygen may not significantly improve the patient's symptoms or appearance. Continued cyanosis despite 100% oxygen administration is highly worrisome.

Pulmonary Edema

We have described diseases that result in difficulty in getting air past narrowed airways and problems with getting blood to the alveoli to pick up the oxygen. A slightly different situation arises when the blood is in the capillaries next to the alveoli but the space between them is thickened. This condition can occur in several situations.

The alveoli can become filled with infectious secretions as when a patient has pneumonia or other respiratory infection as described earlier. These secretions hinder the exchange of gases that occurs normally. The alveoli can also become filled with fluid that may leak out of the capillaries when the pressure in them is very high as seen in **congestive heart failure (CHF).**

This condition occurs when the left side of the heart is not strong enough to pump the blood out of the pulmonary circulation as quickly as it enters. This delay results in a backup of pressure in the small pulmonary vessels and leakage of part of the blood into the alveoli, making gas exchange difficult. Figure 27-14 illustrates this disease process.

Signs and Symptoms

Any condition that results in fluid accumulation results in crackles being heard upon auscultation of the lungs over the fluid-filled area. Whereas pneumonia will result in crackles over the area affected by the infection, CHF will result in diffuse crackles, most often beginning at the bases of the lungs and progressing upward as the condition worsens. Severe CHF is associated with crackles heard throughout the lungs.

The patient suffering from congestive heart failure often has a history of heart trouble, hence the poor function of the left ventricle. These patients will often complain of shortness of breath that has gotten progressively worse over several days.

Their symptoms are often aggravated by lying down because the excess fluid redistributes and spreads throughout the lungs in this position. Any exertion will usually create worsening symptoms as well. Chest pain may be present in some patients.

Management

Because the problem is inadequate oxygen delivery to the blood, the appropriate treatment is to increase the oxygen content in the air in the alveoli. The more oxygen that is there, the more oxygen can diffuse across into the bloodstream. The EMT should provide the patient with CHF and shortness of breath with 100% oxygen. Allowing the patient to sit completely upright will also help to minimize the symptoms.

Shock

As we discussed in Chapter 9, one of the body's reactions to hypoperfusion is to increase the respiratory rate. This increase will bring more oxygen into the body to distribute to its hypoperfused tissues. The elevated respiratory rate may cause the patient to feel short of breath. In this case, the EMT should treat the patient according to the priorities outlined in Chapter 9.

CONCLUSION

There are many disease processes that may cause difficulty breathing, all of which result in inadequate tissue oxygenation or inadequate blood detoxification of carbon dioxide, or both. The EMT must be proficient in quickly assessing these patients and providing emergency care to them.

An EMT's treatment of a patient with difficulty breathing should always include oxygen and appropriate ventilatory assistance. Specific other medications may be indicated, depending on the most likely diagnosis and the patient's history.

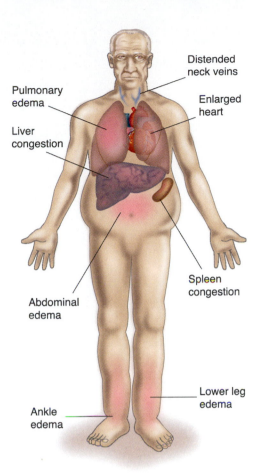

Pulmonary edema

Liver congestion

Abdominal edema

Ankle edema

Distended neck veins

Enlarged heart

Spleen congestion

Lower leg edema

FIGURE 27-14 A poorly functioning left ventricle will result in a backup of fluid pressure in the pulmonary circulation. Leakage of fluid into the alveoli will result.

It is always appropriate to call for ALS assistance if the patient continues to have difficulty breathing despite BLS measures. Appropriate decisions regarding transport and constant reassessment are also important in good prehospital management of the patient with difficulty breathing.

TEST YOUR KNOWLEDGE

1. List the structures and functions of the respiratory system.
2. State the signs and symptoms of a patient with difficulty breathing.
3. Describe the emergency medical care of the patient with difficulty breathing.
4. Why is medical direction important to the EMT when caring for the patient with difficulty breathing?
5. Describe a patient in need of airway or ventilatory support.
6. List the signs of adequate air exchange.
7. Identify when administration of a prescribed inhaler is indicated.
8. Identify the key elements in management of patients with epiglottitis, croup, asthma, COPD, and CHF.

INTERNET RESOURCES

Listen to lung sounds at the R.A.L.E. Repository Web site, http://www.rale.ca. Can you find other sites with audio of lung sounds?
For additional information on asthma, visit these Web sites:

- Allergy and Asthma Network Mothers of Asthmatics, http://www.aanma.org
- American Academy of Allergy, Asthma & Immunology, http://www.aaaai.org
- Asthma and Allergy Foundation of America, http://www.aafa.org

Search http://www.emedicine.com and MedLine Plus at http://medlineplus.gov for additional information on the disorders discussed in this chapter.

FURTHER STUDY

Beebe, R. (2002). *Functional anatomy.* Clifton Park, NY: Thomson Delmar Learning.

CHAPTER 28

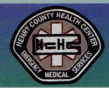
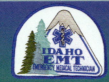
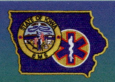

Chest Pain

KEY TERMS

acute coronary syndrome(ACS)

acute myocardial infarction (AMI)

angina

atherosclerosis

bradycardia

coronary arteries

diaphoretic

hypertension

myocardium

pulmonary edema

sudden cardiac death (SCD)

tachycardia

unstable angina

OBJECTIVES

Upon completion of this chapter, the reader should be able to:

1. Describe the importance of early cardiac care.
2. List the risk factors of heart disease.
3. Describe the circulatory system in terms of systemic and pulmonary circuits.
4. Describe the disease process that causes coronary artery disease.
5. List the signs and symptoms of cardiac-related disorders.
6. List important historical questions to ask the patient with chest pain.
7. Describe the focused physical examination of the patient with chest pain.
8. List the appropriate prehospital treatments for chest pain.
9. List the indications, contraindications, side effects, and precautions that are taken when administering nitroglycerin.
10. Describe the transportation considerations for a patient with chest pain.

OVERVIEW

Chest pain is often a symptom of heart disease. Emergency medical technicians (EMTs) are frequently called to the scene of a patient complaining of chest pain. Although only 1 in 12 of these patients is actually experiencing a heart attack, in those cases the patient is at risk for heart failure or even death.

Despite the great strides made in medicine over the past several decades, heart disease remains the number one cause of death among Americans. The prevalence of cigarette smoking and obesity likely contributes to this statistic. Moreover, Americans are at greater risk for a heart attack if they have a family history of diabetes or heart disease. Some risk factors, such as cigarette smoking, are controllable, but others, such as diabetes, are not. These risk factors, controllable and uncontrollable, leave Americans prone to heart disease. In fact, heart disease strikes one in three Americans.

The accurate assessment and quick management of the patient with chest pain are the keys to survival. This chapter reviews the care of the patient with the complaint of chest pain.

ANATOMY AND PHYSIOLOGY REVIEW

Before learning about heart disease, the EMT must have a basic knowledge of cardiac anatomy. The following is a review of cardiac anatomy. The student should review Chapter 5 as well.

The Left Heart

The heart can be thought of as a pair of pumps separated by a common wall. This anatomic arrangement allows the two pumps to work in unison. Each half of the heart pumps blood around its own circuit, or circular pathway.

The left ventricle pumps blood around the systemic circuit. The systemic circuit encompasses the entire circulatory system outside of the lungs. Left ventricular failure can lead to cardiogenic shock and, ultimately, to death. This principle was previously defined in Chapter 9.

The function of the left ventricle can be grossly estimated by blood pressure. The systolic blood pressure represents the pressure in the arteries during contraction of the heart. If the left ventricle is not pumping adequately, the systolic blood pressure will be low. The diastolic pressure represents the pressure remaining in the circulatory system during the relaxation phase of a heartbeat.

Increased resistance to the blood ejected from the left ventricle, sometimes caused by narrowing of blood vessels, forces the heart to beat harder to overcome the resistance. The result is a higher blood pressure than normal, or **hypertension**. Hypertension can contribute to heart disease.

The Right Heart

Compared with the left ventricle, the right ventricle has a relatively easy job. The right ventricle pumps the same amount of blood as the left, except exclusively to the lungs. Because the resistance is relatively low in the pulmonary circuit, the right ventricle need not work very hard to circulate the blood through the lungs. Figure 28-1 illustrates the pulmonary and systemic circuits.

Coronary Circulation

The heart's circulation is derived from the first two arteries that arise from the base of the aorta. These vessels that supply the heart with oxygenated blood are the **coronary arteries**. There are two main coronary arteries (the right and left) that branch off into several smaller vessels (Figure 28-2).

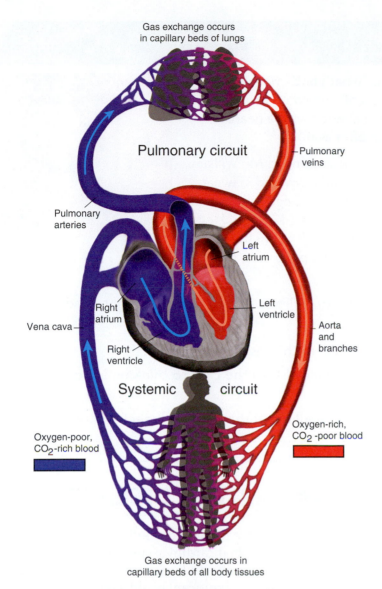

Gas exchange occurs
in capillary beds of lungs

Pulmonary circuit

Pulmonary
veins

Pulmonary
arteries

Left
atrium

Right
atrium

Left
ventricle

Vena cava

Aorta
and
branches

Right
ventricle

Systemic   circuit

Oxygen-poor,
CO_2-rich blood

Oxygen-rich,
CO_2 -poor blood

Gas exchange occurs in
capillary beds of all body tissues

FIGURE 28-1   The left heart pumps blood to the entire systemic circuit, while
the right heart pumps blood through the short pulmonary circuit.

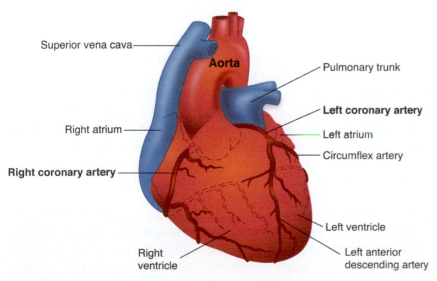

Superior vena cava

Aorta

Pulmonary trunk

Left coronary artery

Left atrium

Right atrium

Circumflex artery

Right coronary artery

Left ventricle

Right
ventricle

Left anterior
descending artery

FIGURE 28-2   The right and left coronary arteries supply oxygenated blood to
the heart.

Heart Attack

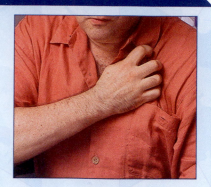

Sandy kneels in front of Mr. Williams and asks, "What's bothering you today, sir?" "It's my wife," Mr. Williams replies. "She got all nerved up and started saying that this could be a heart attack. Look, I'm not having a heart attack. It's just a little indigestion. It'll go away after awhile."

While Mr. Williams is talking, Sandy is doing a quick assessment. Mr. Williams is in his 40s and is overweight. He appears anxious and is covered in sweat. "Can you tell me the kinds of symptoms you are experiencing?" Sandy asks. Mr. Williams relates that he has had indigestion for the past 12 hours. He took some antacids, Pepto-Bismol, he thinks, but it didn't get better. When he started to get a little light-headed and could feel his pulse race, his wife, Dianne, called 9-1-1.

Just as he says, "Look, I really don't need any help," Mr. Williams appears to become light-headed and passes out.

- What immediate actions should the EMT take in this case?
- What risk factors does Mr. Williams have that might lead the EMT to think he is a candidate for heart disease?
- What symptoms does Mr. Williams have that would lead the EMT to suspect a heart attack?
- What treatments would be in order for Mr. Williams?

CORONARY ARTERY DISEASE

Cardiovascular disease is the number one killer of Americans who are over the age of 35. The fact that cardiovascular disease is so common, and is becoming more common as a large segment of the U.S. population is passing 35, makes it a significant health concern in this country. EMTs are more and more frequently getting calls to the house of a person having chest pain.

Pathophysiology

As blood circulates oxygen and nutrients to all the organs of the body, it also carries foodstuffs called fats. Small amounts of these fats, called lipids, are important for the function of cells and hormones. When too much fat is in the bloodstream, it is deposited on the walls of the blood vessel in fatty streaks. These fatty streaks build up over time in a process called **atherosclerosis**. At any place where the bloodstream slows, such as a bend in the vessel, the fat, like sand in a river, is deposited. These deposits of fat, called plaques or atheromas, can restrict the passage of blood flow (Figure 28-3).

A blood vessel, when narrowed by a plaque, is prone to blockage, or occlusion. Occasionally a piece of the plaque itself breaks off and can plug the blood vessel. Alternatively, a blood clot, called a thrombus, can form in the already narrowed vessel and completely occlude the flow of blood. The result in either situation is that all tissue beyond the occlusion is deprived of oxygen-enriched blood.

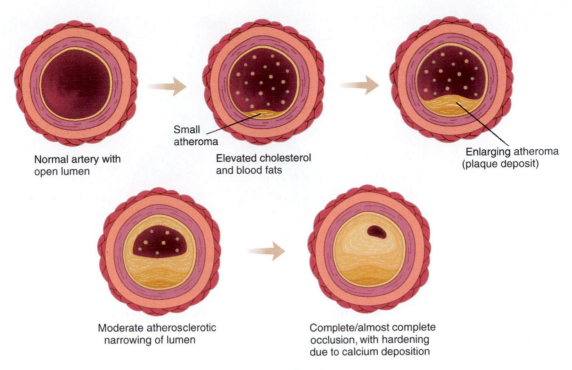

Small
atheroma

Normal artery with
open lumen

Elevated cholesterol
and blood fats

Enlarging atheroma
(plaque deposit)

Moderate atherosclerotic
narrowing of lumen

Complete/almost complete
occlusion, with hardening
due to calcium deposition

FIGURE 28-3   Atherosclerosis narrows arteries and impedes blood flow.

When the coronary arteries become narrowed, the heart muscle, or **myocardium**, receives less oxygenated blood. If the amount of oxygen supplied to the heart is insufficient for the needs at that time, the patient may experience chest pain or other symptoms. This condition is referred to as **angina**. Angina often occurs in patients with narrowed coronary arteries during exertion. This is when the oxygen requirements of the heart are increased.

If the coronary arteries become more narrowed, the person may experience angina with less exertion than previously or even at rest. This is referred to as **unstable angina** and is reflective of more serious disease.

At some point, the coronary arteries may become so narrowed, either due to atherosclerosis, spasm of the vessel, or blockage due to thrombus formation, that no oxygenated blood gets through to the myocardium, and death of myocardial cells occurs. This extreme situation is called an **acute myocardial infarction (AMI)** (Figure 28-4).

An AMI interferes with the heart's ability to effectively pump blood. It causes the injured tissue around the infarction site to become irritable. This irritability may result in inadequate pumping action, leading to cardiogenic shock (Chapter 9), or it may cause the heart to beat erratically, resulting in **sudden cardiac death (SCD)** (sudden death related to an arrhythmia) (Chapter 29).

A term that is often used to describe this continuum of conditions affecting blood flow to the heart is **acute coronary syndrome (ACS)**. An EMT will not know the extent of the injury to the heart muscle when caring for a patient with chest pain or other cardiac related symptoms. As with most other conditions an EMT will treat, the wisest course of action is to provide whatever treatment would be

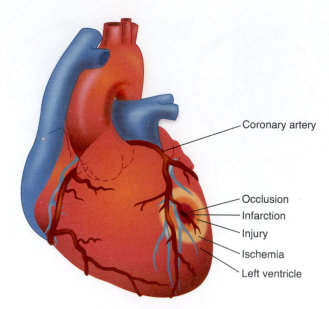

FIGURE 28-4 When a coronary artery is occluded, the heart muscle, the myocardium, dies.

appropriate for the worst possible situation. The treatment an EMT can provide for a patient with an ACS is discussed later in this chapter.

Risk Factors

Cardiovascular disease has been associated with several risk factors. Identifying these risk factors in ourselves, and in our patients, provides an opportunity to identify and come to terms with them.

Some risk factors of cardiovascular disease are a result of voluntary behaviors that can be eliminated. These *modifiable* risk factors include smoking and drug use (particularly cocaine) and lack of exercise. Other modifiable risk factors include a diet that is high in cholesterol, or a diet that leads to obesity.

Other factors are characteristics of the person. These risk factors are *nonmodifiable*. Males are more likely to have a heart attack than females, whereas females are more likely to die if they do have a heart attack. Family history plays an important role in cardiovascular disease. If the patient's parent or sibling had a heart attack, the patient is at increased risk of having cardiovascular disease.

Nonmodifiable risk factors that may be controlled somewhat include chronic hypertension and diabetes. Medications are available to control both these conditions, although controlling them will not eliminate the increased risk of cardiac disease. Table 28-1 lists both modifiable and nonmodifiable risk factors of cardiovascular disease.

Signs and Symptoms

When an acute myocardial infarction affects the heart muscle, impeding its ability to pump, the rest of the heart muscle has to compensate. The result is that the heart tends to beat more rapidly. The normal heart rate is 60–100 beats per minute. A rate of over 100 beats per minute means the heart is beating faster than normal, called **tachycardia**. Profound (greater than 150) tachycardia can result in hypotension.

TABLE 28-1

Risk Factors for Cardiovascular Disease

Modifiable risk factors

- Smoking
- Cocaine use
- Diet
- High cholesterol
- Obesity
- Lack of exercise

Nonmodifiable risk factors

- Sex
- Age
- Heredity
- Diabetes
- Hypertension

Street Smart

About 20% of the U.S. population, particularly diabetics, the elderly, and women, may not experience any chest pain despite an active AMI. These patients may present with atypical symptoms such as shortness of breath, weakness, or simply nausea.

When confronted with a patient with shortness of breath, for example, the EMT should ask herself, "Is the shortness of breath from an AMI or from another cause?"

An EMT is not expected to be able to make that distinction in the field. Fortunately, the treatment for shortness of breath is very similar to the treatment for an AMI. The assessment and treatment of shortness of breath are discussed in Chapter 22. The key to recognition of the possibility of an AMI even without the presence of chest pain is to identify that the patient has risk factors and has *any* of the classic associated symptoms listed in Table 28-2.

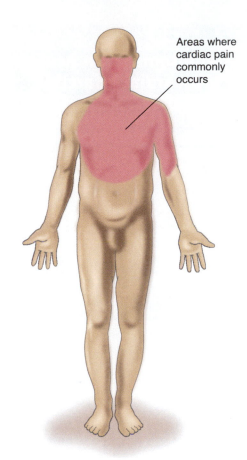

Areas where cardiac pain commonly occurs

FIGURE 28-5 Any pain from the "nose to the navel" is cardiac until proven otherwise.

A percentage of AMIs affect the electrical conduction of the heart, causing the heart to beat more slowly than usual, sometimes as slowly as 20–30 beats per minute. A heart rate that is slower than 60 bpm is called **bradycardia**. Severe bradycardia may be associated with hypotension.

A feeling of general weakness and nausea may also accompany an AMI. The patient often appears very ill, being pale and sweaty, or **diaphoretic**.

When the layperson hears the words *chest pain*, he thinks of a heart attack (AMI). Many people experiencing an AMI have chest pain as their initial presenting symptom. Chest pain is a broad, sweeping complaint that has a number of descriptors. Some patients say the discomfort is "a dull ache" or "stabbing," while others describe it as crushing and oppressive, "like an elephant is sitting on my chest."

All of these complaints may be an accurate description of the chest pain experienced by a person who may be having an AMI. Every patient experiences pain a little differently and, therefore, may describe chest pain differently.

While the complaint "I'm having chest pain" is common, particularly among males, it is common for other complaints to represent cardiac disease pain (Figure 28-5). For example, some patients complain of lower jaw pain or neck pain. Other patients may complain of indigestion or shortness of breath. Significant groups of patients complain of left shoulder or arm pain.

Noncardiac Chest Pain

Chest pain may be due to many disorders other than an AMI. Injury or disease of the lungs, or of the muscular chest wall surrounding the lungs, can give rise to a complaint of chest pain. Stomach disorders, such as ulcers, can create a similar sort of pain. Because of the proximity of the stomach to the heart, this pain can be mistaken for cardiac pain.

Table 28-3 lists several common disorders that create chest pain. There are a large number of disorders that can mimic a heart attack.

TABLE 28-2

Symptoms of an Acute Myocardial Infarction

Symptom	Common Description
Chest pain	"Pressure" "Elephant sitting on my chest" "Viselike"
Left arm pain	"Dull ache" "Numbness"
Left shoulder pain	"Ache"
Lower jaw pain	"Toothache"
Throat pain	"Burning"
Epigastric discomfort	"Indigestion" "Heartburn"
Shortness of breath	"Trouble catching breath" "Not enough air"
Sudden unexplained weakness	"No energy"
Nausea	"Sick to my stomach"
Diaphoresis	"Sweaty"

Cultural Considerations

Pain is a very subjective feeling. Pain means something different for every person. Some people will deny they are having chest pain despite the fact that it is obvious that they are. To admit, in public, that they are having pain might be seen as a sign of weakness. They may deny pain to avoid frightening loved ones. Whatever the reason, some patients will not admit to having chest pain.

By carefully choosing words, the EMT can often get the patient to concede that he is having some difficulty and that he needs medical attention. Instead of asking the patient, "Are you having chest pain" the EMT would do better to ask, "Are you having any chest discomfort." This wording provides the patient an opportunity to answer the question positively without loss of face.

TABLE 28-3

Noncardiac Chest Pain, by Organ System

Esophageal spasm	A paroxysmal difficulty in swallowing often associated with a feeling of constriction, or tightness, in the chest.
Pleurisy	An inflammation of the lung's external lining resulting in severe localized chest pain, worsened by deep inspiration.
Pneumonia	Inflammation or infection of the lungs caused by bacteria, viruses, or chemical irritants. Chest pain, chills (shaking fever), and a cough are symptoms associated with pneumonia.
Pneumothorax	A puncture of the lung that leads to air filling the pleural space. The onset of a sharp chest pain is sudden and associated with marked difficulty breathing.
Rib fractures	A swollen, painful deformity of the rib cage indicating a broken rib. Pain increases with deep inspiration.
Gastric ulcer disease	An open sore, or lesion, of the stomach lining often associated with epigastric pain.

Assessment

A broad array of chief complaints may indicate an AMI in progress. The EMT is not expected to differentiate whether the patient's chest pain is cardiac or noncardiac in origin. A common rule of thumb states, "*Any pain from the nose to the navel is cardiac until proven other-*

wise." Failure of the EMT to assess and treat all chest pain as a potential cardiac event may result in an unfortunate outcome for the patient.

The EMT should always err on the side of safety. Assess the patient with chest pain as if he were having a heart attack.

Initial Assessment

The all-too-common result of an AMI is death. The EMT must act quickly and decisively to protect the patient from further injury as well as to transport him rapidly to definitive care.

After establishing that the scene is safe, the EMT should form a general impression of the patient's condition and mental status, then assess and manage the airway, breathing, and circulation. Further assessment techniques are determined by the patient's general mental status. Chapter 13 addresses the initial assessment in detail, and Chapter 16 describes the focused assessment of the medical patient.

Unresponsive Cardiac Patient

A quick check for breathing and circulation should confirm whether the patient is in cardiac arrest. If no pulse or no breathing is found, cardiopulmonary resuscitation (CPR) must begin immediately. Chapter 29 reviews the care of the unresponsive cardiac patient.

Responsive Cardiac Patient

For the responsive patient with potential cardiac complaints, after performing an initial assessment, the EMT should proceed to a history of the present illness and a focused physical examination.

Focused History

Using the mnemonic SAMPLE (see Table 10-5), the EMT can gather a quick past medical history (Chapter 10). The mnemonic OPQRST is also helpful in trying to elicit details regarding the patient's current symptoms.

Onset

An EMT should ask the question, "What were you doing when you first noticed the discomfort?" It is important to know what the patient was doing when the symptoms started.

More than half of heart attacks occur while the patient was resting or sleeping. However, a significant number of heart attacks occur during times of high emotional or physical stress. The death of a loved one or the excitement of a surprise party can induce an AMI. The EMT would report that the chest pain was preceded by some specific stressor.

Provocation

The EMT should determine whether anything makes the discomfort better or worse. For example, does the pain subside when the patient is sitting up or lying down? Does the discomfort change at all with deep inspiration? These types of descriptors can help the physician determine the cause of the chest pain.

Safety Tip

It is not the function of an EMT to differentiate the cause of the patient's chest pain. Although there are many noncardiac causes of chest pain, one mistake made deciding that a patient's chest pain is noncardiac can result in the patient's death. All chest pain is treated as if it were a heart attack while in the field. This is the safest decision for all involved.

Street Smart

As discussed earlier, an AMI makes the heart muscle irritable. An irritable heart beats irregularly. This irregularity leads to a sudden drop in blood pressure, causing the patient to faint or lose consciousness. Loss of consciousness is frequently attributed to an irregularly beating heart. Therefore, all patients who have a loss of consciousness should be treated as potential cardiac patients.

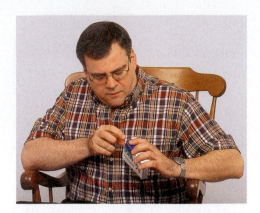

FIGURE 28-6 Many patients deny that they are having a heart attack, thinking that it's "only indigestion."

Ask the patient whether he has taken any over-the-counter (OTC) medications. Often an AMI is mistaken for indigestion. Many patients will self-treat with antacids (Figure 28-6). Ask the patient whether the medications affected the chest pain.

Quality

Patients will have many descriptions of their chest discomfort. Try to have the patient describe the discomfort in his own words. Ask open-ended questions such as, "How would you describe the pain?"

If the patient is unable to arrive at an answer, it is acceptable to give the patient a list of descriptive terms. "Is the discomfort sharp, dull, heavy, or tight?" The EMT should be cautious when providing terms so as not to "put words into the patient's mouth."

Radiation

The same nerves that convey chest pain to the brain are shared by the left shoulder. For this reason, some patients suffering from an AMI may complain of left shoulder or left arm pain, without having any history of injury to that limb. Similarly, neck or jaw pain is also associated with cardiac chest pain.

Severity

Although it is useful for an EMT to ask the patient to gauge his chest pain on a scale of 0 to 10, no amount of discomfort should be dismissed. The therapeutic goal for the cardiac patient is zero chest pain.

Time of Onset

The time of onset takes on critical importance when the EMT realizes that most patients will initially deny that their chest pain is cardiac in origin. This denial often results in a significant loss of time before medical assistance is sought.

A significant number of heart attack victims will die within the first 2 hours from onset of chest pain. Some therapies offered in the hospital are dependent upon the length of time the symptoms have been present. Therefore, it is essential that the EMT know the symptoms of a heart attack and the exact time of onset of those symptoms (Figure 28-7).

Focused Physical Examination

The physical changes the patient will demonstrate are the result of hypoperfusion to the heart and the body's efforts to compensate, using adrenaline (epinephrine).

The pupils are typically dilated as a result of the body's circulating epinephrine. Sluggish pupils may suggest that the patient is hypoxic. Note any distension of the jugular neck veins in a seated patient. Swollen neck veins, jugular venous distension (JVD), often occur when the heart fails as a pump, and blood backs up from the right side of the heart into the veins seen in the neck.

Blood backing up from the left heart also swells blood vessels in the lungs, resulting in **pulmonary edema**. After a time, this excess fluid in the vessels in the lungs will cause narrowing of the airways. Air mov-

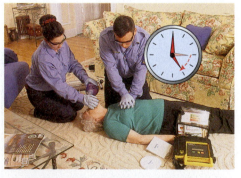

FIGURE 28-7 Time is crucial. Many AMI patients die within the first 2 hours from the onset of chest pain. Note: Normally the chest is bare in order to expose landmarks for proper hand placement.

ing through narrowed airways makes a high-pitched squeaking sound called *wheezes*. Eventually fluid leaks into the airways, and the air passing through this fluid *crackles* with each inspiration. Breath sounds often reveal the degree of failure the heart is experiencing and should be assessed by the EMT on every patient.

Baseline Vital Signs

It is important to get an accurate baseline set of vital signs. Cardiac patients can change rapidly, and a baseline helps determine the speed at which the patient's condition is changing. If pulse oximetry is available, a reading should also be obtained at this time.

Management

The patient should be immediately placed in a position of comfort. If the patient is standing, then assist him to a seated or lying position, whichever is more comfortable. The EMT should bring the stretcher or a chair to the patient to avoid unnecessary exertion in walking. This treatment is more than a mere courtesy. By resting the patient, the EMT is also helping to rest the heart.

Loosen constricting clothing, particularly around the neck. Reassure the patient that everything that can be done is being done. Maintain a calm but deliberate demeanor. High-flow oxygen via non-rebreather facemask should be applied at this time, if it is not already in place.

Nitroglycerin

If the patient has been prescribed nitroglycerin, and the EMT is trained in its administration, then the patient's nitroglycerin may be given according to local protocols (Figure 28-8). Before assisting with the administration of any patient medications, the EMT must review any precautions that should be taken.

Transport

Never allow the patient to walk to the ambulance or even to the stretcher. The resulting strain to the heart creates more work for an

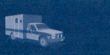

Street Smart

Some emergency medical services (EMS) system protocols allow EMTs to administer oxygen via nasal cannula, usually at 2–4 liters per minute. Some patients feel the mask is restrictive and are more comfortable with the "nose prongs."

Although there are a number of advantages to using a nasal cannula, an EMT should carefully weigh the patient's need for oxygen against the patient's desire for comfort. Never deprive a patient of much-needed oxygen when he is hypoxic. Lean toward giving high-flow oxygen via a non-rebreather facemask rather than not giving enough using a nasal cannula.

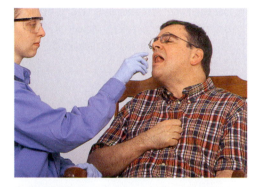

FIGURE 28-8 Nitroglycerin, a potent vasodilator, is used to relieve some of the work of the heart.

Street Smart

Be sure that the nitroglycerin the patient has is his own. Well-meaning family members and close friends may offer their prescription medications to a patient, hoping to help the patient.

Doctors are cautious when they prescribe medications. A patient who has never taken nitroglycerin before may have a dangerous drop in blood pressure. The result is the patient is worse off than if he had taken nothing.

The nitroglycerin bottle is too small to affix a prescription label to in most cases. Therefore, the EMT must ask the patient, "Is this your prescription?" If in doubt, do not administer the medication and thereby do no harm to the patient.

Medication Notes

Generic name: Nitroglycerin

Trade name: Nitrostat, Nitro-Bia

Indications: Cardiac-related chest pain or angina

Contraindications:
Hypotension, infants and children, patient had already taken maximum dosage before EMS arrived

Dose: 0.4 mg tablet or metered dose spray

Route: Sublingual

Safety Tip

Nitroglycerin can drop a patient's blood pressure very quickly. The result is the patient may feel faint and may even pass out. The patient must always be sitting or, preferably, lying down when nitroglycerin is administered.

already strained heart. Carry the patient, using any of the techniques discussed in Chapter 11.

Ensure that the patient is in a comfortable seated position before beginning transport. Continuously monitor the patient during this time.

The blare of the siren and the flashing red lights may increase the stress the patient is experiencing. It is rarely necessary to use the flashing lights and siren for the cardiac patient. Transport the patient quickly, without lights and siren, to the emergency department or appropriate facility.

Aeromedical Transportation

The advantages of modern medicine are not available to the cardiac patient if transportation delays arrival for several hours. This is a serious concern in some rural or remote areas of the United States. Residents of remote or rural areas may be better served if EMS intercepts with an air medical service.

However, some urban areas can see substantial delays in transportation owing to traffic tie-ups and gridlock. Air medical services, which have the ability to fly over traffic, may markedly improve transportation times in a large city.

ALS Intercept

Advanced life support (ALS) personnel can add a great deal to patient care. Utilizing the newest technology, advanced providers may perform many traditional emergency department functions while in the field. These skills and procedures have demonstrated a significant benefit to the cardiac patient. ALS care is an important addition to patient care (Figure 28-9).

Ongoing Assessment

The EMT should repeat vital signs as often as the patient's condition requires. Minimally, a set of vital signs is needed before and after the administration of nitroglycerin.

The EMT should review the history, paying close attention to the history of the present illness. Did the pain lessen after the oxygen was

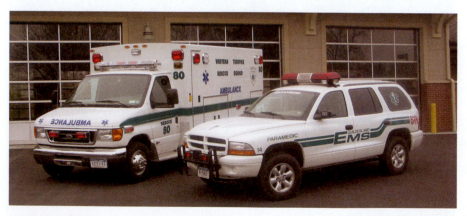

FIGURE 28-9 Advanced life support personnel bring an added level of care and safety to the patient.

given? Did the nitroglycerin help relieve the pain at all? What is the pain, on a scale of 0 to 10, now?

The EMT must be alert to the possibility of SCD and the need to do CPR (Figure 28-10).

Fibrinolytics

Medical science has created a class of drugs called fibrinolytics, formerly called thrombolytics. Most AMIs, about 70%, are caused by fibrin, a blood clot. ("Fibrinolytic" literally means to divide the fibrin.) With these new fibrinolytics, the emergency physician can attempt to open blocked arteries and reestablish blood flow to damaged heart muscle.

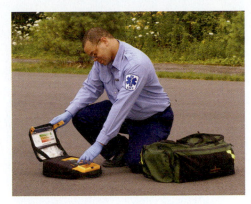

FIGURE 28-10 The EMT is always prepared for the emergency so that he can react quickly and effectively.

Fibrinolytics are most effective within the first few hours after the onset of symptoms. For this reason, it is important that the EMT quickly transport the AMI patient. The goal of EMS is to decrease the time that it takes to get the patient to the treatment. "Time is muscle" accurately describes the problem that EMTs face. The key to appropriate management of the cardiac patient involves getting the patient to definitive care, safely and with a minimum of interruptions.

In some rural areas of the country, ALS personnel are using thrombolytics to treat heart attack victims in the field under the close direction of a physician.

Interventional Cardiology

Perhaps a more direct way to open a blocked vessel is to mechanically remove the blockage. Using special catheters, the cardiologist will advance the catheter into the center of the blockage and then expand a balloon on the tip of the catheter. This procedure, called angioplasty, has made remarkable progress in reducing the incidence of permanent damage to the heart, by allowing "reperfusion." Sometimes a tiny tubelike **stent** is left in the lumen of the vessel to hold it open after the balloon and catheter are removed.

There are ongoing advances in the field of interventional cardiology that utilize different combinations of tools and medications to try and obtain the highest success rate for opening the occluded vessel and to prevent reocclusion for the greatest amount of time.

The most recent literature regarding the management of the patient with an AMI supports the use of interventional cardiology techniques when rapidly available rather than thrombolytic medications to open blocked coronary arteries. It is felt that angioplasty may be more successful with fewer side effects than the thrombolytic medications alone. The bottom line is that no matter which therapy is chosen, the blocked vessel must be opened as quickly as possible. Sometimes, the technique that is chosen is dependent upon what services are available to the patient in the most rapid fashion. Not infrequently, a combination of both techniques is used if felt to be appropriate for an individual patient.

Only certain hospitals, designated *heart centers*, have the capabilities to perform interventional cardiac procedures. Some EMS systems direct EMTs to transport all cardiac patients to a heart center. Follow your local protocols when making the decision on the transportation destination.

CONCLUSION

The complaint of chest pain is one of the most common reasons that EMS is called. The ever-present possibility of sudden cardiac death makes these EMS calls challenging. The EMT's skills and knowledge are put to the ultimate test in caring for these critically ill patients. Thoughtful consideration of the patient's situation, and deliberate action on the part of the EMT, will improve the patient's overall chance for survival.

TEST YOUR KNOWLEDGE

1. Why is early cardiac care important?
2. What are the risk factors of heart disease?
3. Describe the path a drop of blood would take to get from the left ventricle back to the left ventricle.
4. What are the signs and symptoms of a heart attack?
5. What are the treatments an EMT should give a heart attack victim?
6. What are the side effects of nitroglycerin?
7. How should an AMI patient be transported?
8. What are thrombolytics, and how have they affected EMS?

INTERNET RESOURCES

For additional information related to chest pain and heart attack, visit these Web sites:

* American Heart Association, http://www.americanheart.org
* Chest Pain Perspectives, http://www.chestpainperspectives.com
* HeartInfo, http://www.heartinfo.org
* HeartPoint, http://www.heartpoint.com

Look for additional research at http://www.emedicine.com and MedLine Plus at http://medlineplus.gov.

FURTHER STUDY

Criss, E. (1997). An unrecognized epidemic: Women and heart disease. *Journal of Emergency Medical Services, 22*(5), 58–63.

Dernocoeur, K. (1997). A page from history: Prehospital use of aspirin. *Journal of Emergency Medical Services, 22*(9), 42–48.

Henry, M., & Stapleton, E. (1998). A voyage to chest pain. *Journal of Emergency Medical Services, 23*(5), 74–79.

Wilcox, D. (1997). Angina: Improving the outcome. *RN, 60*(7), 34–40.

CHAPTER 29

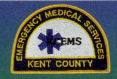

Cardiac Arrest

KEY TERMS

all clear

artificial pacemaker

asystole

automated external defibrillator (AED)

automatic implantable cardioverter/defibrillator (AICD)

automaticity

cardiac standstill

chain of survival

defibrillation

defibrillator

dysrhythmia

electrocardiogram (ECG)

escape rhythm

hypothermia

motion artifact

normal sinus rhythm (NSR)

premature ventricular complex (PVC)

public access defibrillation (PAD)

pulseless electrical activity (PEA)

rhythm

ventricular fibrillation

ventricular tachycardia

OBJECTIVES

Upon completion of this chapter, the reader should be able to:

1. Describe the assessment of the patient in cardiac arrest.
2. Describe the importance of early defibrillation.
3. Describe the importance of CPR to cardiac arrest survival.
4. List the indications for AED.
5. List the contraindications for AED.
6. Differentiate between a semiautomated and a fully automated defibrillator.
7. Describe the fundamentals of AED operation.
8. Describe the safety considerations for AED use.
9. Describe the importance of advanced life support to patient survival.
10. Discuss postresuscitative care of the arrested patient.
11. Discuss the function of the physician and AED use.
12. Discuss the importance of quality improvement for AED programs.

OVERVIEW

One of the most challenging emergency medical services (EMS) calls is for "man down, possible cardiac arrest." Adrenaline surges through the emergency medical technician's (EMT's) body, while preparing for the mental and physical challenges of providing emergency medical services (EMS) in a life or death situation.

In the not too distant past, a cardiac arrest was a death sentence. The introduction of cardiopulmonary resuscitation, or CPR, in the late 1960s, improved survival somewhat. CPR, a combination of mouth-to-mouth ventilation and chest compression, gave some hope to an otherwise grim prognosis. Even with CPR, the chances of restoring a heartbeat, "reversing" a cardiac arrest, were bleak.

CPR in Progress

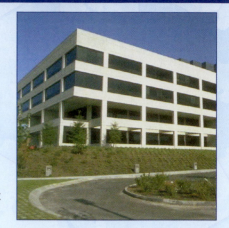

"Unit 24, man down, CPR in progress, Eagle Hills Office, Tower Lobby, time out 16:45." As he put the ambulance in gear and turned on the lights and siren, Tony thought, "The timing couldn't be worse, five o'clock traffic is a mess and we are at least 15 minutes from the scene." As Tony passed by stopped cars on the road, he thought of the minutes that were flying by for the patient.

As he pulled up to the curb in front of the tower building, Tony looked in the window. Clearly CPR was in progress. One security officer was using a pocket mask to ventilate while another was doing compressions. Then he saw it—an AED was attached to the patient. "Maybe the patient has a chance after all," he thought. Tony quickly grabbed the quick response kit and ran in the front door.

- What factors are working against this man's survival?
- What factors are working for this man's survival?
- Why is time important to this patient's survival?
- What can an EMT do to reverse the cardiac arrest?

Advances in medicine and new technology have made prehospital cardiac arrest reversal more likely. EMTs, carrying special devices called defibrillators, are able to provide definitive care to the cardiac arrest victim. This chapter focuses on defibrillation, which is a procedure that can enable an EMT to save a life.

THE HISTORY OF DEFIBRILLATION

One of the most common causes of cardiac arrest is **ventricular fibrillation**, a chaotic, unorganized electrical malfunction of the heart that results in no useful heartbeat. This chaotic electrical activity can be stopped only by applying an electrical countershock. Once the ventricular fibrillation is halted, the heart can then begin normal organized beating.

During open chest surgery, surgeons have successfully been "shocking" fibrillating hearts back to life for many years. The machines that are used to deliver this shock are called **defibrillators**, and the process of delivering a shock to the heart is called **defibrillation**. The difficulty was that early machines were large and were restricted exclusively to the operating room. Furthermore, defibrillation required that the patient's chest be opened and the heart exposed. These facts made it impractical for emergency use.

In 1956, Dr. Zoll created the first external defibrillator. Although somewhat cumbersome, it allowed defibrillation outside of the operating room. At about the same time, 1960, Dr. Kouwenhoven published a paper on closed chest compressions interposed with manual ventilations, now known as CPR.

CPR quickly became popular among emergency services personnel, but the defibrillator remained in the hospital. The advent of transistors and microprocessors brought with them the development of a smaller defibrillator capable of being used in the prehospital environment.

In 1980, Dr. Eisenberg of Seattle, Washington, started a prehospital defibrillation program using these new smaller defibrillators. His hypothesis was that properly trained EMTs using defibrillators could save many lives.

These EMTs used a defibrillator that could "read" the **electrocardiogram (ECG)**, using a logic algorithm stored in a microprocessor, advise the EMT to "shock," or defibrillate the patient, then deliver the shock. These were among the first **automated external defibrillators (AEDs)**.

Chain of Survival

Using an AED on the patient in cardiac arrest is only part of the formula for a successful cardiac arrest *reversal*. Because ventricular fibrillation quickly degenerates from active, yet chaotic, electrical activity to minimal electrical activity and then no activity at all, time is of the essence when treating the cardiac arrest victim. Every minute of delay calling EMS or getting a defibrillator to the patient decreases the chance that the heart will respond to the shock.

The American Heart Association realized the importance of speed and started to advance the concept of the **chain of survival**. Simply, the chain of survival links all the elements of a cardiac arrest reversal together. The chain of survival depicts the important steps that must be taken to improve cardiac arrest survival.

Early Access

Quick notification of EMS is key to getting EMTs trained in the use of an AED to the patient. Typically, EMS is accessed by calling 9-1-1. Unfortunately, 9-1-1 service is still not universally available in the United States.

One of the attractions of 9-1-1 is that it can provide the communications specialist the location of the call (Figure 29-1). Underlying this ability to locate a call is the assumption that the call is being placed from a stationary *landline*.

Although cellular telephones have made it easier for callers to make calls from the scene of an incident, location identification has been lost. Future cellular telephones will have this capacity.

Early CPR

CPR saves lives. There are some documented cases in which CPR alone reversed a cardiac arrest, although CPR alone is often not sufficient. Once EMS has been called, CPR helps *preserve* the brain until the EMT and AED are at the patient's side. Therefore, citizen CPR is still very important to patient survival in a prehospital cardiac arrest (Figure 29-2).

Early Defibrillation

The definitive treatment for cardiac arrest due to ventricular fibrillation is defibrillation. The AED is an easy tool to use and allows rapid application of defibrillation to the cardiac arrest victim. EMTs have been targeted to learn AED use because they are the largest group of prehospital care providers (Figure 29-3).

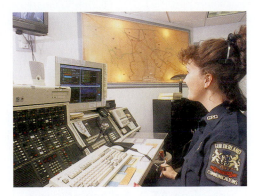

FIGURE 29-1 Early notification using 9-1-1, the first link in the chain of survival.

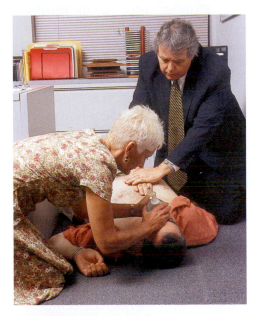

FIGURE 29-2 Early CPR buys time for the arrival of the AED.

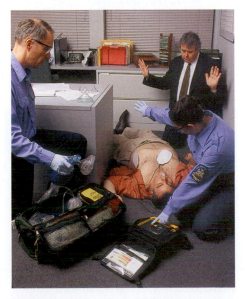

FIGURE 29-3 Early defibrillation saves lives.

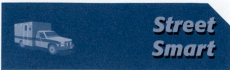

Street Smart

Do not be surprised if an AED has already been used before EMS is on scene. AEDs have so improved in simplicity and dependability that certain segments of the public are being trained in the use of an AED. Airlines now routinely train flight attendants in the use of the AED.

Public access defibrillation (PAD), the availability of a defibrillator to the lay public, is rapidly becoming commonplace in the shopping mall, on the factory floor, and in the business office. CPR courses now routinely include AED training for rescuers.

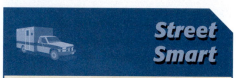

Street Smart

Large public gatherings, such as county fairs or sporting events, are often scenes of cardiac arrests. EMTs assigned to stand by at these events should have an AED readily available. The AED left in the ambulance is of no value to the patient who is in the middle of the bleachers in cardiac arrest.

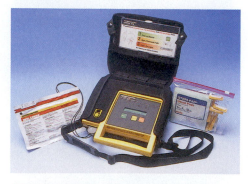

FIGURE 29-4   The automated external defibrillator, or AED.

Early Advanced Cardiac Life Support

Although an AED can reverse the fibrillation that led to the cardiac arrest, it does not address the cause of the fibrillation, and recurrence of the fibrillation is likely. Advanced life support (ALS) providers trained in advanced cardiac life support (ACLS) have the skills and knowledge to help protect the patient from further episodes of cardiac arrest. These ALS providers can help to stabilize the patient before and during transportation to the hospital.

Survival from Cardiac Arrest

Any chain is only as strong as its weakest link. If CPR is provided in less than 4 minutes and defibrillation is provided in less than 8 minutes, the patient potentially has a 43% chance of survival. For every minute that defibrillation is delayed to the victim of ventricular fibrillation, the chances of survival decrease by at least 10%. In the situation of cardiac arrest, every minute counts.

THE AUTOMATED EXTERNAL DEFIBRILLATOR

The AED consists of two large electrodes (pads that are placed on the patient's chest) and cables (leads) that connect the patient to the machine. A battery power source is also necessary to generate the electricity that is used to perform the defibrillation. Figure 29-4 shows the components of the AED.

The AED has an internal computer that samples the heart's electrical rhythm through sensors in the electrodes. The computer measures the waves in the heart's electrical activity against a logic formula. If the computer analysis indicates that the rhythm is ventricular fibrillation, or any other rhythm that will potentially respond to defibrillation (which will be discussed later in the chapter), then an audible or visual warning advises the operator (EMT).

The single largest advantage of an AED is that it does not require the EMT or operator to learn the complex rules of ECG interpretation. The ECG is the record of the heart's electrical activity. There are many different patterns of electrical activity the heart can exhibit, each of which requires a different management strategy. Some of these different patterns are discussed briefly later in this chapter, although the EMT is not expected to interpret the rhythms after reading this chapter. Much more training is required to learn the technique of ECG interpretation. The EMT can allow the AED to interpret the rhythm and advise him to shock if appropriate.

Use of the AED

At the beginning of every shift, the EMT must ensure that the AED is properly prepared for use. An overall inspection should be performed. The case should be intact. Cases may be broken when an AED is accidentally dropped. A broken case is a potential electrical hazard, and the AED should be taken out of service. Next, check the cables. Like the case, the cables should be intact. Frayed cables and bare wires are dangerous and should be replaced. Finally, check the electrodes. All electrodes should be sealed within a protective wrapper. Check the expiration date on the electrode package. Old electrodes become dried out and useless.

Batteries

The AED uses a battery for its power source. Batteries have a tendency to stop working when they are needed most. Every AED should be equipped with a backup battery. The EMT should always ensure that the primary battery and backup battery are adequately charged.

Some types of batteries require regular recharging; others have a charge that lasts for years without a need for a recharge (Figure 29-5). The EMT should familiarize himself with the type of battery his agency uses in its AED.

Supplies

In every routine equipment check, the EMT should ensure that the proper accessory supplies are with the AED. Most AEDs used by EMTs are equipped with a case that has several pockets used to hold additional supplies that may be needed.

It is always advisable to have a spare set of electrode pads as well as a spare battery on hand. Because an AED is used in life or death situations, it is important to have redundancy in critical supplies. Families of patients have successfully sued EMS providers that responded with an AED that had dead batteries.

The electrode pads must tightly adhere to the chest wall for optimal delivery of the electrical energy. Moisture prevents proper adhesion. A gauze 4-by-4 pad or a towel should be immediately available to wipe down the chest before applying the electrodes.

Excessive chest hair can also interfere with adhesion of electrodes. A pair of bandage scissors may be used to quickly shear hair. A razor may also be used to shave hair from the chest for ideal electrode adhesion; however, it is often not necessary and may waste precious time. A safety razor should, however, be available so that if it is necessary to shave a portion of the patient's chest, it can be done quickly.

After completing an AED equipment check, always document the inspection and testing of the AED (Figure 29-6). Failure to document an inspection leaves the EMT vulnerable should a lawsuit occur owing to equipment failure. Be sure to report malfunctions and take the faulty AED out of service until it can be serviced by a qualified biomedical engineer.

CARDIAC ARREST

A common consequence of acute myocardial infarction (AMI) is cardiac arrest and clinical death. This event, defined as the unexpected cessation of heartbeat within 2 hours of the onset of chest pain, is called sudden cardiac death (SCD).

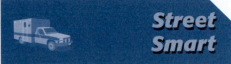

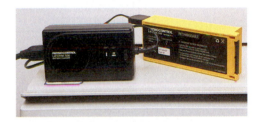

FIGURE 29-5   The rechargeable battery is the power source for the AED.

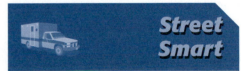

Automated External Defibrillator Maintenance Checklist

Date _____ Location _____

Inspection Performed by _____

Criteria	Status	Corrective Action / Comments
AED		
Placement visible, unobstructed and near phone		
Verify battery installation		
Check the status/ service indicator light		
Note absence of visual/ audible service alarm		
Inspect exterior components and sockets for cracks		
Supplies		
Two sets of AED pads in sealed package		
Check expiration date on pad packages		
Pocket mask with one-way valve		
Examination gloves		
Razors		
Absorbent gauze or hand towels		

Please refer to manufacturer's User's Manual for more information and proper annual maintenance procedures.

FIGURE 29-6 A precall AED checklist. (Reproduced with permission, © 2004, American Heart Association, *www.americanheart.org*)

More than 50% of the cases of sudden cardiac death occur outside of the hospital. Therefore, it is imperative for the EMT to understand why cardiac arrest occurs and how to respond to it.

Signs and Symptoms

When a patient experiences chest pain or any of the other cardiac-related symptoms described in Chapter 28, she may be experiencing an AMI. Without prompt treatment, the AMI can lead to complications such as congestive heart failure (Chapter 27), cardiogenic shock (Chapter 9), or SCD. Why does SCD occur? To understand the cause of SCD, the EMT must first understand the heart's normal electrical activity.

Normal Sinus Rhythm

To review, the heart is a pump. Pumps essentially have two interrelated components; an electrical system triggers the mechanical portion to do its job. The human heart is such a pump. It has an electrical system that triggers the ventricles, the mechanical portion, to pump blood.

The electrical impulse begins at the *sinoatrial node (SA node),* a group of specialized cells located high in the right atrium. The impulse then proceeds through the atria to the *atrioventricular node (AV node),* another specialized group of cells that is situated between the atria and the ventricles. From the AV node, the spark travels through a defined bundle of muscle fibers, called the *bundle of His.* This bundle of conductive fibers then splits into several branches known as *bundle branches.* These bundle branches carry the electrical impulse to the ventricular muscle. Within the ventricular muscle are additional specialized conductive fibers called *Purkinje fibers,* which will then stimulate the remainder of the ventricular muscle. For a review of these structures, see Chapter 5.

As the electrical impulse is carried in this organized fashion through the heart, the muscle is stimulated to contract in a coordinated fashion. Because the atria are stimulated by the electrical impulse first, they will contract first, moving blood into the ventricles.

The ventricles will contract after they have been stimulated by the electrical impulses received by the bundle branches and Purkinje fibers. When the ventricles contract in an organized fashion, the effect is for blood to be ejected out through the aorta. Figure 29-7 depicts the path of the heart's electrical stimulation.

Every heartbeat has an electrical event that precedes the mechanical event. The normal electrical event within the heart is the propagation of electrical impulses from the SA node to the ventricles as

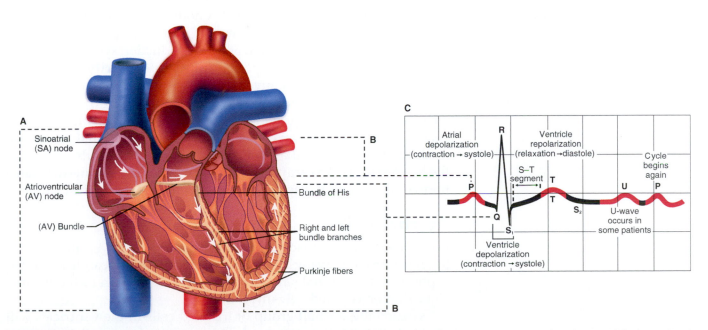

FIGURE 29-7   An electrical impulse from the SA node travels to the AV node and the ventricle, causing the ventricle to contract and creating a pulse.

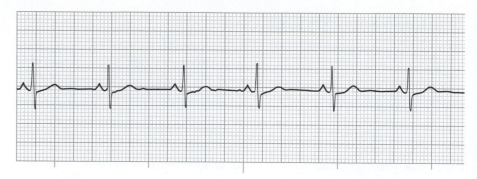

FIGURE 29-8   Normal sinus rhythm.

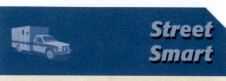

Street Smart

Normally when a patient's blood pressure drops, for whatever reason, the heart races to compensate for the loss. This reflexive tachycardia is a hallmark of shock.

When an EMT determines that the patient has a low blood pressure, he naturally assumes that the heart will be tachycardiac. This is not always the case. If the electrical system of the heart is damaged by an AMI, then an escape pacemaker will take over and the result will be a bradycardiac escape rhythm.

When an EMT sees both hypotension and bradycardia in a medical patient, he should be thinking about a possible AMI.

outlined. This electrical activity from the heart can be detected by an ECG machine and graphically displayed on an oscilloscope or printed on paper. This display is called an electrocardiogram.

An ECG normally displays a pattern of grouped waves, called complexes. These regularly repeating complexes are seen as a **rhythm** (a regularly reccurring or repeating pattern) on the ECG. The natural source of a normal cardiac complex is the SA node. Therefore, the electrical rhythm that is seen when the heart's electrical system is functioning properly is called a **normal sinus rhythm (NSR)**. A normal sinus rhythm is the predominant natural rhythm of the heart.

Although it is not important for an EMT to be able to interpret an ECG, the concept is helpful in understanding the physiology of cardiac arrest. Figure 29-8 shows an example of a normal sinus rhythm.

Escape Pacemakers

The normal source of a heartbeat is the SA node. The SA node is therefore referred to as the heart's pacemaker because it establishes the rate of stimulation and, therefore, contraction.

Heart muscle, or myocardium, has a unique ability to be its own pacemaker. If for some reason the SA node or AV node fails to function properly, the ventricles have the ability to pace themselves, although not as efficiently as the normal conduction system. This ability of the myocardium to self-pace is called **automaticity**.

The special ability of the myocardium to function independently is valuable when the electrical system fails. The resulting rhythm, called an **escape rhythm**, may provide the patient with enough blood flow to stay alive until a physician can insert an **artificial pacemaker** (a manmade electronic device that will create an electrical impulse signaling the heart to beat). An escape rhythm is slower and less efficient than a normal sinus rhythm. Pacemakers are discussed later in the chapter.

Dysrhythmia

When the heart's muscle is injured during an AMI, the muscle becomes irritable, firing chaotically. This irritability can lead to disruptions in the normal sinus rhythm. Any disruption of the normal sinus rhythm is called a **dysrhythmia**.

Occasionally, a small group of irritated cells in the ventricles will start to fire earlier than expected. This unnatural pacemaker creates a **premature ventricular complex (PVC)** (Figure 29-9). A PVC interrupts the regular sinus rhythm and is therefore a dysrhythmia. PVCs can disturb blood flow and are felt as an irregular pulse. PVCs can be an indication of ventricular irritability.

If the signal from this small group of cells in the ventricles is fast enough and strong enough, it can take over the heart's own inherent pacemaker. The ventricles often race at rates from 100 bpm to 250 bpm. The resulting ECG rhythm is called **ventricular tachycardia**. Ventricular tachycardia creates a distinctive ECG, similar to a sine wave pattern (Figure 29-10).

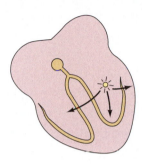

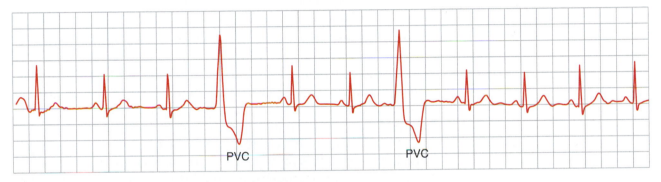

FIGURE 29-9   Unnatural pacemakers, created by an AMI, interrupt the normal sinus rhythm.

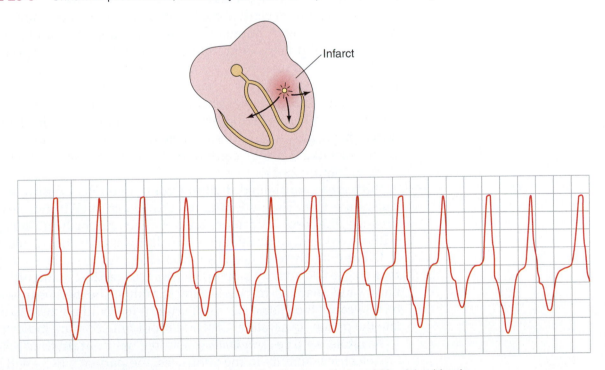

FIGURE 29-10   Ventricular tachycardia robs the heart's coronary arteries of life-giving blood.

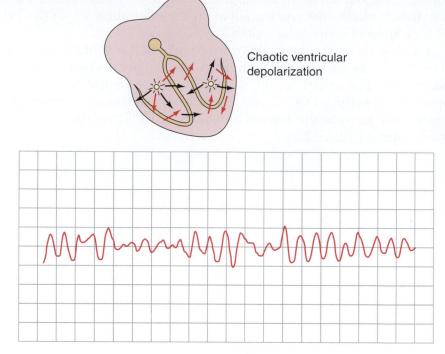

Chaotic ventricular depolarization

FIGURE 29-11   Lethal ventricular fibrillation has no discernible rhythm.

Racing ventricles with a heart rate over 150 bpm do not have enough time to fill with blood and then empty. The result is little or no blood flow to the body, particularly to the coronary arteries. Pulses are quickly lost, and the patient loses consciousness. If a normal heartbeat does not resume quickly, the patient eventually dies. Defibrillation can help to halt this rapid firing of irritable ventricular cells.

If the area of damage from an AMI is extensive, a large group of cells in the ventricle becomes irritable. These irritable cells misfire and can lead to sudden cardiac death. This process can be compared to a nuclear explosion. A pound of uranium is dangerous and potentially lethal. Several pounds of uranium are enough to create a spontaneous nuclear reaction and even a nuclear explosion. Similarly, if enough irritable ventricular myocardial cells fire prematurely, they can result in ventricular fibrillation, a chaotic firing of multiple ventricular cells resulting in no organized rhythm. During ventricular fibrillation, the heart simply quivers and does not create any forward blood flow. The ECG looks like a chaotic collection of waves that have no discernible rhythm (Figure 29-11).

Without a coordinated rhythmic contraction, blood flow stops and pulses are lost. The patient is in cardiac arrest. Without any blood pressure, the coronary arteries are not filled and the heart muscle goes without oxygen. Defibrillation can halt this chaotic firing of cells.

Eventually, the damage is so extensive, and the cells so damaged, that all cardiac activity stops. The heart, in **cardiac standstill**, will lie flaccid and unable to respond to any stimulus. The inert heart is in **asystole**. Because there is no electrical activity, it would not help to defibrillate the patient in asystole. CPR and rapid transport are indicated.

Asystole is a true *arrhythmia* (meaning "without rhythm"). Without any electrical activity in the ventricles, the patient's ECG will be flatline, or asystolic (Figure 29-12).

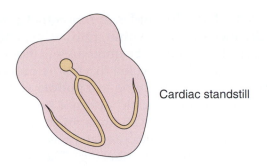

Cardiac standstill

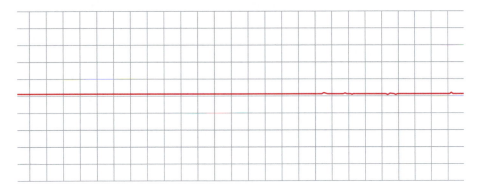

FIGURE 29-12 Asystole, a true arrhythmia, occurs in cardiac standstill.

Pulseless Electrical Activity

There are certain conditions, such as severe blood loss, that will result in no forward blood flow from the heart despite adequate electrical activity. This is called **pulseless electrical activity (PEA)**. It is important for the EMT to realize that despite normal-appearing electrical activity on an ECG, the patient may have cardiac compromise. The best bet is to pay close attention to the patient and not to the monitor. If the patient has no pulse, CPR should be begun, despite the ECG findings.

PEA is not treated with a shock, because there is nothing wrong with the electrical activity. The proper course of action is CPR, 100% oxygen, and rapid transport to the closest appropriate hospital where the cause can be determined and treated.

Assessment

The assessment of the cardiac arrest victim is done similarly to the assessment of any other unresponsive medical patient. Beginning with a scene size-up, the EMT moves through the initial assessment quickly, providing airway, breathing, and circulatory (ABC) support, in that order. Because cardiac arrest requires significant work before the completion of even the initial assessment, the EMT may never get to a focused history and physical exam. It is, however, important that the EMT gather any known history from the patient's family while care is being provided to the patient. Such historical information will be useful to both advanced providers and hospital personnel.

Scene Size-Up

As discussed in Chapter 12, scene safety must always be addressed. Fluids present a hazard to the EMT using an AED. Fluids can transmit the electrical energy to the EMT instead of to the patient, resulting in

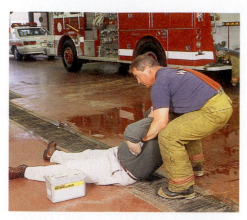

FIGURE 29-13 Before using the AED, make sure the scene is safe.

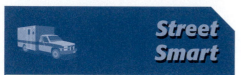

Street Smart

The AED should be a part of the standard *first-in* gear for all medical calls. It is of no use in the ambulance when it is needed immediately on scene. The few minutes lost retrieving the AED from the ambulance might cost the patient her life.

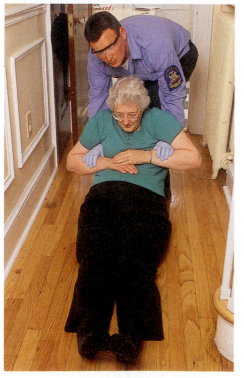

FIGURE 29-14 Quickly move the patient to a large enough area for CPR.

injury to the EMT. Examples of fluids that can potentially transmit electricity include snow, vomit, rain, urine, and pooled water. If the patient is wet, she should be immediately moved to a dry place. Then the patient should be toweled dry before proceeding. *Never* defibrillate a patient who is still lying in a puddle of liquid.

The patient's body should also not be in contact with any metal objects. Again, the metal can transmit the energy to the EMT instead of to the patient. Examples of metal objects include sidewalk grates, catwalks, and aluminum flooring. The patient should be moved immediately, in an emergency carry, to a safe location before an AED is used (Figure 29-13).

General Impression

The initial dispatch information may have been for a cardiac arrest. CPR may already be in progress when the EMT arrives. In those cases, the EMT enters the scene prepared.

In some cases, the dispatch information does not match the patient's situation. The call may have been received for a "person passed out" or, commonly, for a "person seizing." The EMT walks into those calls unaware of the situation.

Stop and look around the scene first. Get the global picture. Tables or lamps that are knocked over indicate a sudden collapse. If the telephone is off the hook, the patient may have been calling for help. Medications, both over-the-counter and prescription, left out may give a clue to the patient's condition.

Gather a quick impression from the patient's overall appearance. Whether the patient is on the ground, sitting in a chair, or lying in a bed, she will be unconscious if in cardiac arrest. Without blood circulating, the patient will be grossly cyanotic.

Try to obtain a chief complaint from any available family member or bystanders. Ask whether anybody witnessed the patient's collapse. If the patient fell, ask whether the head struck anything on the way down. If no one is available, or the answers are questionable, assume spinal trauma.

Position the patient for further assessment. If the patient is unconscious, and CPR is likely to be needed, then the patient needs to be on a firm surface. Move the patient out of the bed or chair and onto the floor. If the room is small, such as a bathroom or a cramped bedroom, consider quickly moving the patient to a larger room, such as the hallway or living room (Figure 29-14).

If the patient is unconscious, or is in cardiac arrest, the assistance of ALS personnel is required. If ALS is available, then request assistance to the scene right away.

Initial Assessment

After completing the scene size-up, the EMT should immediately determine the patient's level of consciousness. If trauma is suspected, an EMT should take manual stabilization of the head and spine first.

If the patient is unconscious and unresponsive to pain, the EMT should immediately open the airway. After the airway has been opened, the EMT should assess for the presence of breathing. If the patient is not breathing, the EMT should deliver two rescue breaths using an appropriate ventilation device. After these breaths have been given, the EMT should check for a carotid pulse.

If the patient is pulseless, the AED must be immediately prepared. If sufficient personnel are available, or if there is a delay in getting the AED to the patient's side, CPR should be begun. Think of the assessment priorities as changing from ABC to ABCD: airway, breathing, circulation, and defibrillation.

A detailed description of CPR can be reviewed in Appendix B.

Management

If an AED is immediately available, the EMT should quickly attach the electrodes on the patient's chest. First, attach the electrode pads to the cables. Then place one pad under the patient's right clavicle and the other pad on the patient's lower left rib cage. Alternatively, one pad may be placed on the anterior chest and one on the posterior chest as indicated in Figure 29-15.

A diagram for electrode pad placement is often found either on the electrodes or on the AED. The cables are also color coded. The white cable and pad are attached under the clavicle on the right. The red cable and pad are attached to the lower left rib cage (see Figure 29-15).

Once the AED has been attached to the patient, the power should be turned on. Usually the "power on" switch is prominently displayed. Every EMT should take a moment *before the call* to review the operational features of the AED before using it.

Once the AED is operational, press the analyze button to activate the AED. Often a voice prompt will advise the EMT or operator that the AED is analyzing.

If CPR is in progress, the EMT or operator should instruct everyone to stop. The usual command to the rest of the team is "**all clear**." *All clear* means that nothing, not even the bag-valve-mask, should touch the patient. Motion from CPR can create **motion artifact** (a false ECG reading created by vibration), causing the AED to mistakenly identify the ECG as ventricular fibrillation (Figure 29-16).

Street Smart

The definition of the term *dead weight* is never clearer than when an EMT has to move a patient to the floor. If a backboard is available, consider sliding the seated patient onto the backboard. Place the backboard under the patient's feet and then slide the patient down the ramp. Once the patient is on the backboard, move the backboard to the floor. If the patient is in bed, consider logrolling the patient onto the backboard and then lifting the board onto the floor.

Street Smart

A useful way to remember where the colored electrodes are placed is to say "white-right, red-ribs." The rhyme and letter coordination may make placement easier to recall.

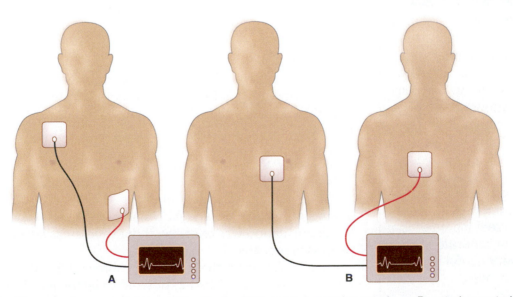

FIGURE 29-15   There are two acceptable positions for the AED pads: A. anterior-anterior or B. anterior-posterior.

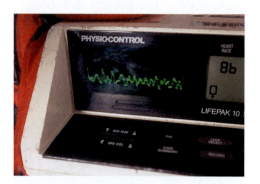

FIGURE 29-16 Motion, from road vibrations or CPR, creates ECG motion artifact.

If the patient is already aboard the ambulance when she arrests, and the ambulance is moving, instruct the driver to stop the vehicle. Road vibrations can also create motion artifact that the AED could misinterpret as ventricular fibrillation.

The AED may take a few seconds, after the analyze button has been pressed, to determine whether the ECG is a *shockable rhythm*, a rhythm that will respond to defibrillation. If a shockable rhythm is identified, the AED will start to automatically charge. Most machines create an audible warning or a verbal prompt or both. The audible warning indicates that the AED is energizing. The verbal prompt typically states "shock advised" or a similar statement.

While the AED is charging, call *all clear* again. Be sure that nothing is touching the patient. The danger of an accidental shock, and the safety of the team, cannot be overstressed. An EMT accidentally shocked could potentially go into ventricular fibrillation, making a bad situation worse by creating a second patient.

For the third and final time, the EMT or operator should call *all clear*. Some EMTs use the mantra "I'm clear, you're clear, we're all clear" while making a visual sweep of the patient before actually defibrillating the patient.

Always perform a head-to-toe visual sweep with every defibrillation. Make a habit of looking at the patient's nose, then looking at her toes, and looking again at her nose, before pressing the button to activate the defibrillator. Defibrillation should never become so routine that the EMT becomes complacent about safety.

Once all team members are physically clear of the patient, the EMT or operator then presses the *shock* button. The shock button will deliver the defibrillation from the AED to the patient.

The EMT or operator should *immediately* press the analyze button, again stating *all clear*. The AED will analyze the ECG to see whether the defibrillation was effective. If the shock was *not* effective, then the process is repeated.

Shocks are administered in sets of three repeated, or *stacked*, shocks. Each successive shock breaks down the electrical resistance in the chest wall until a current flows through the heart and breaks the fibrillation.

The goal of the EMT or operator is to deliver the three stacked shocks within 1 minute. It is *not* necessary to check for a pulse between shocks. Pulses should be checked at the beginning and at the end of the stacked shocks. The AED automatically alters the energy used in each shock according to a setting entered in its programming.

Some EMTs may be taught to use a manual defibrillator. In those cases, the first shock should be set at 200 joules, the second at 200 or 300 joules, and the final shock at maximum joules, usually 360 joules or equivalent biphasic energy setting. Always follow the manufacturer's recommendations regarding the use of a manual defibrillator.

Once the defibrillation sequence has ended, the EMT should again check for pulse and breathing. If none is present, CPR should be resumed. The AED can be used again in 1 minute to analyze the heart's rhythm to see whether a shockable rhythm is present. Remember that there are several rhythms that will result in cardiac arrest yet are not amenable to defibrillation; therefore, the machine will say "no shock advised." If the patient does not have a pulse, however, CPR must be done and the patient should be transported quickly to the closest appropriate hospital. Skill 29-1 describes the operation of an AED.

The obvious problem in a cardiac arrest is that no blood flows from the heart to the body. Although CPR provides some blood flow, CPR cannot sustain the body for a long period. The best CPR provides only about 30% of the normal cardiac output. The preferred option would be to have the heart beat naturally.

If an electrical current is passed through the fibrillating heart muscle, the electrical current will stun, or shock, the heart. All uncoordinated contractions of the heart will immediately stop simultaneously. Then natural sinus pacemakers can assume dominance over the heart and a normal sinus rhythm can begin again.

For defibrillation to work, there must be some muscular activity in the heart. Ventricular tachycardia and ventricular fibrillation are two examples of shockable rhythms.

Asystole is an example of a nonshockable rhythm. Without any muscular activity, the heart will not respond to the defibrillation. In those cases, CPR should be continued until ventricular fibrillation appears.

Special Situations

There will be several situations that may require slight deviation from the usual protocol in assessing and managing the patient in cardiac arrest. The EMT should be familiar with these few situations.

Artificial Pacemakers

When the electrical system of the heart fails, causing bradycardia, a cardiologist will place an artificial pacemaker into the patient. The artificial pacemaker will create the impulse that signals the heart to beat, ensuring a heart rate that will support a normal blood pressure.

An artificial pacemaker has a pulse generator and a set of wires that lead to the heart. The pulse generator is usually placed in a pocket under the skin, usually below the right clavicle, and the pocket is sewn shut.

Safety Tip

If the patient is on the gurney, be sure that no one's foot is touching the metal carriage. It is common for an EMT to rest his feet on the lower bar of the gurney, out of sight of the EMT or operator handling the AED. Because the hard rubber wheels of the gurney electrically isolate the gurney, the EMT's foot creates a new electrical pathway, and the EMT will get shocked.

Street Smart

Many defibrillators use a technology called "biphasic defibrillation," which allows use of a lower overall energy setting while still providing effective energy to the heart muscle. The EMT should be familiar with the machine and technology used by his agency.

SKILL 29-1 *Operation of an Automated External Defibrillator*

PURPOSE: To perform an external defibrillation, when indicated, on a patient in cardiac arrest.

STANDARD PRECAUTIONS:

☑ Automated external defibrillator
☑ Personal protective clothing

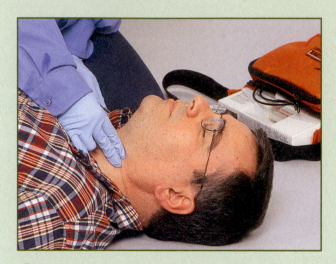

1 The EMT must confirm that the patient is in cardiac arrest.

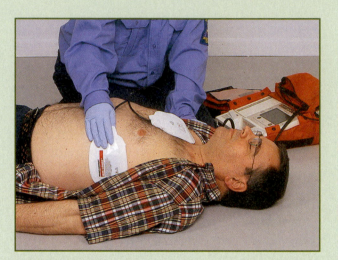

2 The EMT applies the electrode pads to the anterior chest wall, one to the apex of the heart at the lower left rib cage and the other to the right sternal border below the clavicle.

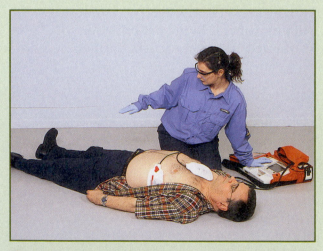

3 The EMT then turns the power on the AED while calling *"all clear."* The EMT must ensure that no one is touching the patient.

(continues)

SKILL 29-1 *(continued)*

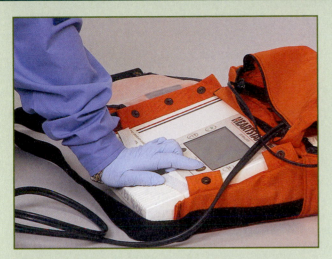

4 The EMT then presses the *analyze* button and presses the *shock* button, as advised. Again, the EMT must ensure that no one is touching the patient.

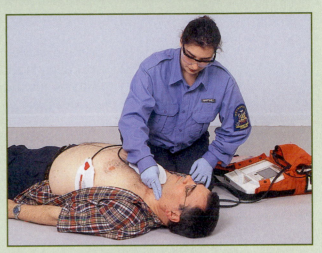

5 After the series of shocks has been performed, the EMT must check for the presence or absence of a pulse. If the pulse is absent, then CPR must be continued for another minute. If the patient's pulse returns, then the EMT checks for breathing. If the patient's pulse does not return, then another round of shocks may be indicated.

The AED electrode pad is placed in about the same location as the pacemaker. If a pacemaker is located under the skin, as indicated by a bulge about the size of a silver dollar, then the AED pads should be moved slightly to the left and down several inches toward the feet so that the electrode is not over the pacemaker.

If the AED electrode is placed immediately over the pacemaker, the AED may sense the pacer's impulse, seen as a spike on the ECG, and think the heart is beating regularly. Even more important, if the AED functions correctly, detects the ventricular fibrillation, and a defibrillation is delivered, the pacer will absorb some of the defibrillation energy and may not work properly afterward.

Automatic Implantable Cardioverter/Defibrillator

Using state-of-the-art microelectronics and more powerful microprocessors, physicians and biomedical engineers have created an AED that can be placed within the body. The **automatic implantable cardioverter/defibrillator (AICD)** is used for patients who are at risk for developing recurrent ventricular tachycardia or fibrillation.

Often the patient's family will tell the EMT that the patient has an AICD. Many patients also carry an instruction card in their wallet or purse.

Similar to a pacemaker, the AICD has a generator/defibrillator and a set of wires that leads to the heart. When the AICD senses an *event*, such as ventricular fibrillation, it signals the defibrillator, which in turn shocks the heart.

Because the AICD is internal and the wires are attached directly to the heart, it takes very little energy to defibrillate the heart, 5–15 joules. The energy is so low, and the shock so small, that if the AICD

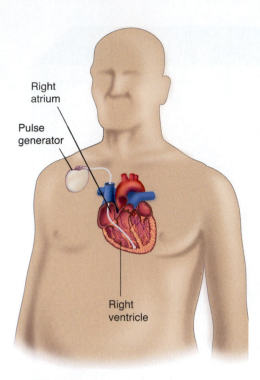

Right
atrium

Pulse
generator

Right
ventricle

FIGURE 29-17 An automatic
implantable cardioverter/defibrillator is an
internal AED.

should function, or fire, while the EMT is doing CPR, he may feel a mild tingling in the arms. This is *not* dangerous to the EMT yet can be diminished by use of gloves, which act as an insulator.

The most common type of AICD looks very similar to an artificial pacemaker and is typically located in the same location under the right clavicle (Figure 29-17). When an AICD is detected, the AED electrode pads should be moved slightly to the left of normal and several inches toward the feet, in the same placement as used for a patient with a pacemaker.

Medication Patches

The use of transdermal patches has become increasingly popular. These self-adhesive patches contain medication that is slowly absorbed through the skin of the patient. Patches are an easy and convenient way of administering a medication that must have a steady level in the bloodstream. Alternatively, the patient would have to take a pill several times a day.

Examples of transdermal patches include nitroglycerin patches, used for cardiac patients; nicotine patches, used for cigarette cessation programs; and hormone replacement patches, used in cancer prevention or treatment.

These transdermal patches often have an aluminum backing or the drug's paste medium is *reactive* to the defibrillation. Consequently, when the patient is shocked, the patch either ignites, making a popping sound, or heats up, burning the patient.

Patches are generally worn on the upper chest, on the upper back, or on the shoulders. Before operating the AED, the EMT must *completely* expose the patient's chest wall and look for patches.

Gloves should always be worn when removing a patch. Lift the corner of the patch by the tab and pull. The patch should come off easily. If medication is still visible on the patient's skin, use a 4-by-4 pad and wipe it off.

Hypothermia

Hypothermia is a condition in which the body temperature drops below 95°F (normal body temperature is 98.6°F). When the body temperature drops even further, to 90°F, the heart becomes quite irritable and the patient is at risk for ventricular fibrillation.

Examples of patients who could suffer hypothermia include winter hikers, persons immersed in cold water for a long time, and homeless persons. Whenever a patient has been outdoors for a prolonged period, consider the possibility of hypothermia.

The cold heart is resistant to attempts at defibrillation. Most medical protocols and the American Heart Association's Advanced Cardiac Life Support (ACLS) course advocate delivering one set of stacked shocks only. If the heart does not respond to these initial attempts, continue CPR and immediately transport the patient to the most appropriate emergency facility.

Transport

The patient in cardiac arrest, or having been reversed from cardiac arrest, is a critically ill patient. Transport should be accomplished quickly, and the patient should be brought to the closest appropriate hospital. Local protocols often govern the destination of particular patients on the basis of hospital capability.

ALS should always be requested early in the resuscitation of a cardiac arrest victim. ALS providers can offer additional medications and other procedures to the patient. If no ALS provider has arrived on the scene by the time the patient is packaged and ready to go, an intercept should be attempted while en route to a hospital.

Postarrest Care

After the first set of shocks, and every set afterward, the EMT should perform a *reverse CPR check*. Start by checking the carotid pulse. If a pulse is detected, then the EMT should proceed to checking for breathing.

It is common that for several minutes after a successful defibrillation, and cardiac arrest reversal, the patient will need manual ventilation, using a bag-valve-mask or similar device.

If the patient is breathing adequately, then place the patient on a high-concentration oxygen mask and proceed to check the patient's level of consciousness.

If the patient remains unconscious and has no evidence of trauma, turn the patient over onto her side in the recovery position. The recovery position facilitates drainage of secretions from the mouth and decreases the risk of aspiration. The electrodes should be left in place so that defibrillation may be quickly performed if cardiac arrest should recur.

Ongoing Assessment

During transport, the patient should be closely monitored. The ongoing assessment should involve continuous monitoring of the breathing and pulse. Recurrence of cardiac arrest is not uncommon. The sooner it is discovered, the more likely the EMT will be successful in reversing it again.

Should pulse and breathing be lost, the patient should again be placed on her back; everyone should be clear of the patient; and the AED should be allowed to analyze the rhythm.

Field Termination

There are some circumstances in which resuscitative efforts will not be indicated. Circumstances in which death is obviously irreversible are discussed in Chapter 3 and should be reviewed.

In some areas, ALS personnel may have a protocol to terminate resuscitative efforts once they have become futile. Termination is often done with direct contact with a physician.

Despite the death of the patient, it is important for the EMT to offer support to the family or friends who are present. Family on scene will need support when the decision is made that the patient is dead.

After death has been declared, the EMT must remember to show respect for the deceased. Speak to the family, calling the patient by his or her common name. Use direct language, including the word *dead*. Do *not* use terms such as "gone to a better place," as these leave room for misinterpretation.

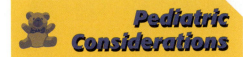

Pediatric Considerations

It is recommended that patients who weigh less than 25 kilograms (kg) or are under 9 years of age be defibrillated with a machine that is specifically designed for use on children. Typically a smaller amount of electricity is used and the machine might be programmed to respond to electrical patterns more commonly seen in pediatric patients.

While these pediatric-capable defibrillators are intuitively preferred, recommendations based upon the available literature conclude that an adult AED may be used on children older than 1 year of age if that is the only machine at hand. Nonetheless, services that respond to a large number of pediatric patients might consider maintaining an AED that is specifically recommended for this age group.

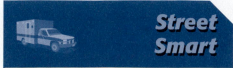

Street Smart

It is often useful to the family to have one person on the crew explain everything that is going on with their loved one from the very beginning of the resuscitation. It is not difficult for an EMT to tell the family that their loved one's heart is not beating and that she is not breathing, but what they need to hear is that you are trying to get the heart restarted and are providing breaths for the patient.

These explanations may help the family come to terms with the fact that everything is being done, and may also help them accept the death, if that is the outcome.

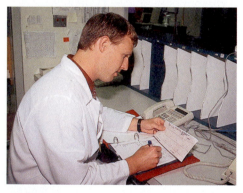

FIGURE 29-18 Medical control will want to review the Patient Care Report whenever an AED is used by EMTs.

This is not the time for morbid humor but a time for reverence. Though humorous situations do sometimes occur at death, leave the laughter until later.

Be prepared for the family's reactions to death. Any reaction is possible, from denial to anger and rage to bargaining. These normal behaviors represent either some way of fleeing the message or fighting the messenger. Do not take any behaviors personally.

Senior EMTs or clergy, or both, should be on hand, if possible, to deal with grieving family members. Any death notification is a time for high emotions and can lead to surprising reactions.

POSTCALL

After a cardiac arrest call, the EMT needs to document all actions accurately on the Patient Care Report (PCR). If CPR was not initiated, the rationale for no CPR must be explained. If CPR and the AED were used, then all care surrounding the event must be documented. A readout of the AED's memory or a copy of the tape should be attached to the PCR.

This documentation is generally reviewed by the quality improvement committee. A physician is often a part of this committee when cardiac arrest calls are reviewed (Figure 29-18). The committee will review the call for adherence to protocols as well as for comparison with EMS standards. Nationally, EMS strives to have CPR begin within 4 minutes, and defibrillation within 8 minutes.

All supplies used during cardiac arrest resuscitation should be replenished immediately. Supplies typically used include defibrillation electrode pads (with cables) and the cassette tape or module. The batteries should be rotated out of service, for recharging, and replaced with fresh batteries. Use of a checklist can make this process easier.

Competency Assurance

Many EMTs do not have an opportunity to use an AED regularly. However, EMTs are expected to be proficient with the use of an AED at all times. Therefore, it is important that EMTs practice AED use regularly. A semiannual refresher course in the use of an AED is a minimum expectation for many EMTs.

Physician oversight is a very important component to any defibrillation program. The involvement of a physician in the refresher courses as well as call reviews can help improve the medical care given by the EMT. Physicians are also involved in protocol development regarding the use of AEDs and resuscitation situations. The EMT should be familiar with all relevant protocols in his area.

Debriefing

A cardiac arrest can be one of the most stressful calls to which an EMT will respond. In some cases, the EMT may know the patient or the patient's family. This personal involvement creates some special stress for the EMT.

Whenever a patient dies, an EMT will reflect on the care that was given. Concerns about errors that may have been made and questions about personal competency surface. It is important that the EMT explore these questions and resolve them.

A postcall debriefing may help the EMT work through the problems and, more important, improves performance for the next call.

CONCLUSION

The advent of AED technology has improved the chances of survival from prehospital cardiac arrest. An EMT, armed with an AED, can provide definitive care in this critical situation. Combining assessment, AED, and CPR, the EMT can contribute to the successful resuscitation of a victim of cardiac arrest.

TEST YOUR KNOWLEDGE

1. List, in order, the steps of assessment for a patient in cardiac arrest.
2. Why is early defibrillation important?
3. What are the indications for the AED?
4. Which ECG rhythms are "shockable" and which are "nonshockable"?
5. What is the difference between a fully automatic and a semiautomatic defibrillator?
6. List several safety considerations for the AED.
7. List several special conditions when the AED may have limited use.
8. What is the importance of ALS to the care of the cardiac arrest patient?
9. What is the function of the physician in AED practice?
10. What is a debriefing useful for?

INTERNET RESOURCES

For additional resources on cardiac arrest and defibrillation, check out these Web sites:

- American Heart Association, http://www.americanheart.org
- HeartCenterOnline, http://www.heartcenteronline.com
- National Center for Early Defibrillation, http://www.early-defib.org

FURTHER STUDY

The critical moment. (1997). *Journal of Emergency Medical Services, 22*(1), supplement.
Newman, M. (1998). The chain of survival revisited. *Journal of Emergency Medical Services, 23*(5), 46–52.

CHAPTER 30

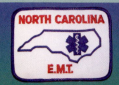

Altered Mental Status

KEY TERMS

AEIOU TIPS
altered mental state
Alzheimer's disease
anticonvulsant
aura
clonic phase
diabetes mellitus
diabetic coma
diabetic ketoacidosis (DKA)
diet-controlled diabetes
epilepsy
generalized seizure
gestational diabetes
grand mal seizure
hyperglycemia
insulin-dependent diabetes
insulin shock
keto-acid
Kussmaul's respiration
non-insulin-dependent diabetes
partial seizure
petit mal seizure
postictal phase
seizure
status epilepticus
tonic phase

OBJECTIVES

Upon completion of this chapter, the reader should be able to:

1. Define the terms *awake* and *oriented*.
2. Define the term *altered mental state*.
3. List several causes of an altered mental state.
4. Describe the general underlying conditions that create altered mental status.
5. Describe how insulin works.
6. Describe the treatment of diabetes.
7. Describe the signs and symptoms of hypoglycemia.
8. Define the term *seizure*.
9. Differentiate between a generalized and a partial seizure.
10. Describe the care of the seizing patient.
11. Describe the care of the postictal patient.
12. Describe the most common causes of seizures.

OVERVIEW

A patient may act confused or disoriented or may "just not be acting right" for many reasons. Concerned family members or citizens may recognize that the patient is in need of immediate medical attention and call emergency medical services (EMS).

Often people are frightened by the person and call the police. The police, in turn, call EMS when the medical emergency is recognized. In both of these cases, the patient is experiencing a change in behavior that may be due to illness or disease, in other words, an **altered mental state**.

Several potentially dangerous medical conditions can create altered mental states. It is important for an emergency medical technician (EMT) to understand these conditions and to be able to assess the patient for them.

More important, the EMT must quickly treat the patient before the condition worsens. In some of these conditions, the failure of the EMT to quickly assess and intervene may cause the patient to suffer permanent disability or die.

MENTAL STATES

EMTs may encounter many patients who, for some unknown reason, are experiencing an altered mental state. An altered mental state is easiest to define when it is compared with the definition of a normal mental state.

A person who is awake, alert, and appropriately interactive with the environment has a normal mental state. A normal mental state requires that the person have an adequate supply of blood, carrying oxygen and sugar (glucose), circulating in the brain.

The awake, alert patient who is ill or injured will usually cooperate with the care that is being given by answering simple questions. The awake, alert patient will also follow instructions, sometimes described as following commands.

Normally, a person is oriented. An oriented person has the ability to comprehend who he is, where he is, and generally what time it is. In other words, the patient is oriented to person (self), place (where he is), and time (what time it is).

✳ *Strange Behavior*

"Officer, I was stopped and I thought he started up, so I started up, then he suddenly stopped again and I slammed into him," Darryl related as he shifted through the glove compartment looking for the car's registration. "I immediately got out of my car and asked him if he was all right and he mumbled something crazy."

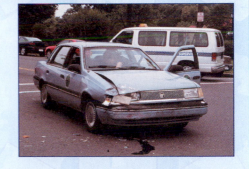

"Sir, I'm not a police officer, and I don't need to see your registration. I'm an EMT with the quick response team," Andy replied.

"Whatever man, I'm telling you he's not right," Darryl countered. "He's acting weird, man."

"We'll check him out, sir. Please remain seated in your car until we can get back to you," Andy instructed.

As Andy approached the car, he started to survey the vehicle for damage. Clearly it was a minor fender bender with minimal rear-end damage. "Sir, are you all right?" Andy called out. The driver, an elderly male, looked up at him and said, "What happened? How come the fire department's here?"

Andy couldn't help but notice the smell of cigarettes and stale urine. On the floorboard of the car were several empty beer cans. As Andy continued to survey the scene, he listened to the driver. His speech was slurred, as though he was drunk, and he repeated his questions over and over again.

- What are the probable causes for this patient's altered mental state?
- What important medical history should an EMT obtain in this case?
- What are the immediate treatment priorities?

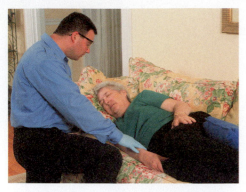

FIGURE 30-1   The determination of the level of consciousness is made at the beginning of the initial assessment.

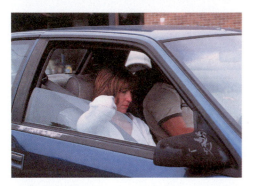

FIGURE 30-2   A patient's orientation is always relative to the surroundings that she is in.

TABLE 30-1

Some Treatable Causes of Altered Mental Status

Problem	Effect
Congestive heart failure	Hypoxia
Diabetes	Hypoglycemia
Gross external hemorrhage	Hypoperfusion
Internal bleeding	Hypoperfusion
Lung disease (e.g., emphysema)	Hypoxia
Oxygen-poor environment (confined space)	Hypoxia
Partial foreign body airway obstruction	Hypoxia
Smoke inhalation	Hypoxia

EMTs determine a patient's mental status at the beginning of the initial assessment, using the AVPU scale (Figure 30-1). Review Chapter 13 for further details about AVPU assessment. If the patient is awake and oriented to person, place, and time, then he is alert and considered to be in a normal mental state.

Altered Mental Status

Any time a patient is confused or disoriented about person, place, or time, he has an altered mental state. The patient who is indifferent, apathetic, and generally detached from his surroundings is also experiencing an altered mental state.

Examples of statements, made by a patient, that would lead an EMT to think the patient is disoriented and, therefore, has an altered mental state follow.

- "Where am I?"
- "What just happened?"

A failure to remember what just happened is called *amnesia*. Amnesia can be due to a head injury.

After a motor vehicle collision (MVC), most people are concerned about themselves (Am I hurt?), the other driver (Is he hurt?), and damage to the car (Figure 30-2). A driver who appears to be uninterested in his own injuries should be assumed to have an altered mental status.

CAUSES OF ALTERED MENTAL STATUS

There are many reasons why a patient would have an altered mental state. Some are due to chronic health conditions. For example, elderly patients with Alzheimer's disease are often confused. **Alzheimer's disease** is a progressive, irreversible deterioration of intellectual function. Chapter 41 discusses this condition in more detail.

However, many altered mental states are due to acute changes within the body that are the result of disease or trauma. These acute and potentially reversible changes can lead to serious long-term complications or even death, if left untreated.

These acute changes usually involve the loss of either sufficient oxygen or sugar in the brain. Table 30-1 lists some potentially reversible causes of an altered mental state. The EMT is trained to identify and treat these causes of altered mental status.

The EMT should never assume that a patient who is not awake, alert, and oriented is normal. Erring on the side of caution, the EMT should always treat every patient as if the patient has a potentially reversible cause for his altered mental status.

A mnemonic to help an EMT remember some of the more common causes of altered mental status is **AEIOU TIPS**. Table 30-2 provides some relatively common conditions an EMT will encounter that could produce an altered mental status. The table explains each letter in the mnemonic, although some providers differ on the meaning of each letter.

TABLE 30-2

Conditions That Lead to an Altered Mental Status		
Letter	**Condition**	**Contributing Factor**
A	Alcohol	Effects of ethanol or any other form of alcohol (Chapter 35)
E	Epilepsy	Seizures (Chapter 30)
I	Insulin	Too much insulin results in low glucose levels in the blood (Chapter 30)
O	Oxygen deprivation or drug overdose	Insufficient oxygen can result in brain hypoxia (Chapter 8); overdose on certain types of medications can result in poor brain perfusion (Chapter 35)
U	Uremia	Kidney failure results in buildup of toxins in the bloodstream (uncommon)
T	Trauma	Injuries to the head (Chapter 21)
I	Infection	Any overwhelming infection or any infection involving the brain (Chapter 30)
P	Psychiatric disorder/Poisoning	Behavioral disorders (Chapter 32) or poison (Chapter 36)
S	Stroke	Causes a lack of blood supply to a portion of the brain (Chapter 31)

Each of the conditions listed can lead to potentially life-threatening complications. The first four represent the most common patient presentations an EMT might encounter.

DIABETES MELLITUS

The brain uses glucose and oxygen to create energy. Without an abundant supply of both, the brain will malfunction. The outward signs are confusion, combativeness, lethargy, and even coma.

Sugar (glucose) is obtained from the food we eat in a process called digestion. However, it is not enough to simply eat large quantities of food. Somehow the glucose has to get to the cells of the brain, where it can be used for fuel.

Glucose is transported to the brain in the blood. Once it is in the brain, it must be *carried* into the brain's cells, where it can be used for energy. The carrier for glucose into the brain's cells is a hormone called insulin (Figure 30-3). Without insulin, the glucose remains in the blood and cannot be used by the cells.

Insulin is produced in a gland called the pancreas, which is located under the liver. For reasons yet unknown, the pancreas of some people slows or even stops working. The result is a disease called **diabetes mellitus**. There are several variations to this disease.

Insulin-Dependent Diabetes

In cases in which the pancreas no longer produces insulin, the patient must take insulin supplements. Insulin is given as an injection.

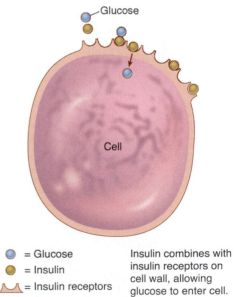

Glucose

Cell

🔵 = Glucose
🟡 = Insulin
⋀⋀ = Insulin receptors

Insulin combines with insulin receptors on cell wall, allowing glucose to enter cell.

FIGURE 30-3   Insulin is the carrier of sugar from the blood into the cells.

Sugar Sickness

"Police unit twelve and Ambulance three. Meet a party, Yellowstone rest area, Interstate 85. Possible EMS."

As Claire slowly pulled the ambulance into the rest area, she noticed a new-model car with the passenger-side door wide open and a woman attending a man sitting in the front seat.

Turning off her emergency lights to prevent drawing undue attention to the situation, Claire listened to Charlie, the highway patrolman, who was first on scene.

"Claire, the woman says that it's her husband. Something about his sugar sickness acting up again," Charlie started to say when suddenly the woman cried out, "Can someone help him before he passes out!" The woman appeared to be struggling with her husband.

- What is the nature of this emergency?
- What actions should the EMT take immediately?
- Would the actions be different if the patient were unconscious?

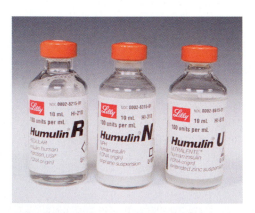

FIGURE 30-4 Insulin comes in short-acting and long-acting varieties.

Without these insulin supplements, the glucose the patient eats cannot get to the brain's cells. The result is an increase in the blood glucose levels and a brain that is starved for fuel. Frequently this type of diabetes occurs in children. For this reason, it was once called juvenile diabetes. The more descriptive term **insulin-dependent diabetes** is now more commonly used.

Supplemental Insulin

Insulin was first obtained from the pancreas of pigs and cows (pork or beef insulin) and was used by physicians to treat diabetic patients. Human insulin used today is artificially created by genetic engineering. This human insulin has fewer side effects than did the pork and beef insulin.

Regular insulin is a short-acting insulin. *Longer-acting* insulin, called NPH or Lente, sustains the patient's blood sugar at even levels throughout the day. Many patients with diabetes mix these two types of insulin, depending on the time of day (Figure 30-4).

Insulin is taken in correlation with regular meals. Because glucose levels in the bloodstream rise after a meal, more insulin has to be available at mealtimes to help utilize this fuel.

Non-Insulin-Dependent Diabetes

In some other cases, the pancreas does not produce enough insulin for the amount of glucose that is in the bloodstream. The pancreas can be stimulated to produce more insulin by medications called *oral hypoglycemic agents*. Patients with this condition do not require insulin and are referred to as having **non-insulin-dependent diabetes**. Without these oral medications, these patients may also have rising blood glucose levels. Because there is still some insulin production, however, in this case the brain is not completely starved for fuels. The small amount of insulin that is present carries some glucose into the brain's cells. Patients who require supplemental insulin may use intermittent subcutaneous injections throughout the day. Other patients may have a continuous infusion of insulin through an insulin pump.

Table 30-3 lists common diabetic medications, including oral hypo-glycemic agents.

Other Forms of Diabetes

Some diabetic patients do not require any medications to keep their blood glucose under control as long as they carefully regulate their intake of sugars. By controlling their dietary intake of sugars, these patients with **diet-controlled diabetes** can avoid the need to take medications.

When a woman becomes pregnant, her body's need for insulin increases. If her pancreas is unable to supply the insulin her body demands, high blood glucose levels result (Figure 30-5). When her pregnancy is over, her insulin demands drop back to former levels. This type of pregnancy-induced diabetes is called **gestational diabetes**.

Signs and Symptoms

When the pancreas stops creating sufficient insulin, the blood sugar starts to build up. A high blood sugar level, called **hyperglycemia**, has several effects on the patient.

First, the patient's kidneys try to rid the body of the excess sugar. When the kidney starts to excrete sugar, or *spill sugar*, the sweetened urine also removes water as well. The increased volume of urine created is called *polyuria*. This can quickly lead to dehydration.

With a loss of so much water through urine, the body starts to crave more water and the patient starts to drink water excessively, a condition called *polydipsia*.

In the interim, the cells of the body, including the brain cells, have gone without glucose. These cells continue to send messages for more glucose, and the patient starts to eat larger amounts of food. This condition is called *polyphagia*. Despite the fact that the patient is eating large amounts of food, the sugar is not getting into the cells, and the patient starts to lose weight. Table 30-4 summarizes the signs of the onset of diabetes.

Acute Diabetic Problems

Even the most attentive diabetic patient will sometimes find himself having a problem regulating his glucose levels. The EMT will often be called to help manage the diabetic patient when the glucose level has gone to either extreme.

Hyperglycemia

The development of hyperglycemia, seen in untreated or under-treated diabetes, is a prolonged event, taking from 12 hours to as much as several days to create any significant problem. When glucose cannot be used for fuel, because of an inability to get it into the cells, the body must find a fuel source elsewhere. This alternative fuel source comes in the form of fats. Fats can be broken down to form energy and waste products. This form of energy is much less efficient

TABLE 30-3

Some Common Diabetic Medications	
Injected insulin	Humulin
	Novolin
	Iletin
	Lantus
Oral hypoglycemic agents	Diabinese
	Glucotrol
	Micronase
	DiaBeta
	Glynase
	Orinase

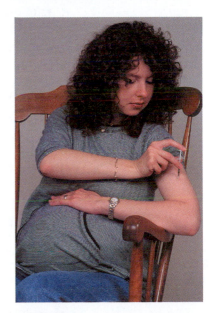

FIGURE 30-5 A pregnant woman can develop diabetes during her pregnancy.

TABLE 30-4

Signs of Onset of Diabetes Mellitus
Excessive thirst
Frequent urination of large amounts
Excreting sugar into urine
Sudden unexplained weight loss
Constant hunger

than the standard glucose breakdown and cannot support normal body functions for long.

When sugar is used, or metabolized, by a cell, the by-products are water and carbon dioxide. Water and carbon dioxide are eliminated by the kidneys or the lungs. When fats are metabolized, an organic acid called a **keto-acid** (or ketone) is created. These keto-acids are the by-products of ineffective metabolism. A diabetic patient who has changed to fat metabolism is at risk of developing a condition called **diabetic ketoacidosis (DKA)**.

DKA is a condition characterized by hyperglycemia and a buildup of keto-acids in the blood. Keto-acids are toxic to the body. In addition, the high blood sugar has resulted in excessive urination (polyuria) and loss of significant water and electrolyte stores. DKA occurs only in patients who are dependent upon insulin supplements and only when they have not taken sufficient amounts of the hormone. This condition is potentially life threatening if not recognized and treated immediately.

Signs and Symptoms of Diabetic Ketoacidosis

Keto-acids, or ketones, are partially eliminated in the urine, like sugar. Ketones are also exhaled on our breath, like carbon dioxide. Ketone-laden breath is sweet-smelling like Juicy Fruit gum. However, this is an ineffective process and not all the ketones are eliminated.

As the ketones build up, and the acid level in the blood increases, the patient starts to breathe faster and deeper, in an effort to *blow off* the excess acid. This very deep, almost sighing, breathing is called **Kussmaul's respiration** (Figure 30-6) and is characteristic of diabetic ketoacidosis.

Because of the dramatic fluid level changes that occur in the body, the patient may experience other symptoms. Many patients complain of stomachaches and cramps, followed by vomiting. Most will experience weakness and *malaise* (a sluggishness or lethargy that is associated with sickness).

Unchecked, the combination of dehydration, acidosis, and lack of glucose inside of the brain's cells leads to mental confusion and delirium. Without any medical intervention, diabetic ketoacidosis can lead to coma and even death. An unconscious diabetic patient, who is hyperglycemic, is said to be in a **diabetic coma**.

Management of DKA

Aside from assessing and managing the airway, breathing, and circulation (ABC), there is very little an EMT can do for this high-priority patient in the field. Patients with DKA and any patient with an altered mental status should be given high-flow oxygen. Rapid transport to the emergency department is the best treatment. Whenever possible, an advanced life support (ALS) intercept should be arranged while en route.

Hyperosmolar Hyperglycemic Non-ketonic Coma

A form of diabetes, often seen in obese or elderly patients, occurs as the pancreas fails to produce sufficient insulin for the body's needs.

Normal breathing

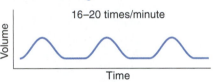

Kussmaul's respiration

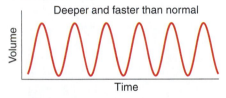

FIGURE 30-6 Kussmaul's respiration is deep, sighing breaths.

While these patients may supplement their insulin needs with insulin injections, there are times when insulin demands fall below insulin supply. At those times these patients' blood sugar starts to rise to dangerously high levels. However, unlike patients who are not producing any insulin, these patients do not metabolize fats and therefore do not produce keto-acids, causing a syndrome called hyperosmolar hyperglycemic non-ketonic coma (HHNK).

The symptoms of the patient who is hyperglycemic and in diabetic ketoacidosis and the patient who is hyperglycemic and in HHNK are the same, with the notable exception of Kussmaul's respiration and ketones on the breath; ketones smell like Juicy Fruit gum on the breath.

In both cases the patient may experience an altered mental state and may lapse into coma. When faced with these diabetic emergencies the EMT should provide oxygen and transport the patient immediately.

Hypoglycemia

DKA or HHNK as a result of high blood sugar is dangerous, but its onset is gradual, generally allowing the patient time to seek medical attention. The opposite condition of a low blood sugar, called hypoglycemia, occurs very suddenly, usually within an hour, and can quickly lead to brain damage and even death. Hypoglycemia is a true medical emergency.

Insulin allows blood glucose to go into cells, where it is used for fuel. When the glucose goes into the cells, the blood glucose level falls. Diabetic patients time their insulin injections around meals. The insulin should "peak" just after the meal.

If the insulin peaks at the wrong time, then the insulin will lower the blood glucose to dangerously low levels. There are numerous reasons why the amount of insulin injected would not match the blood glucose.

If the patient eats a meal later than expected, then the insulin would peak prematurely. If the patient fails to eat a meal, the insulin still works and the blood sugar will drop to dangerously low levels.

Signs and Symptoms of Hypoglycemia

When the blood glucose level falls, the body reacts. Adrenaline is excreted into the blood. Adrenaline helps to stimulate the release of stored sugar. Adrenaline also stimulates the heart to beat faster. Adrenaline can make the patient shaky, sweaty, and agitated. Because these body reactions are similar to the reactions that are seen in shock, severe hypoglycemia is sometimes called **insulin shock**.

The lack of glucose to the brain results in its malfunction. Confusion, agitation, and combativeness are commonly seen in hypoglycemia. Without more blood glucose, the patient will progress from confusion to unconsciousness. Often when the blood glucose gets dangerously low, the patient will have a seizure. Without any treatment, the brain starts to suffer damage and the patient may die.

Management of the Hypoglycemic Unconscious Patient

When a patient with diabetes collapses into unconsciousness, family or bystanders may call EMS. The first-arriving EMT is usually told that

Street Smart

Despite all the explanations offered about diabetic emergencies, it is sometimes difficult for an EMT to distinguish hypoglycemia from hyperglycemia in the field. It is usually safe to assume that the blood sugar is low if the patient is a confused diabetic. If the patient is unconscious, treat and transport the patient immediately.

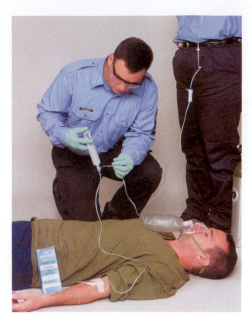

FIGURE 30-7 Advance life support personnel can rapidly reverse hypoglycemia with sugar (dextrose) via an IV.

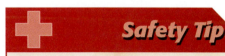

Safety Tip

The patient who is hypoglycemic often appears to the layperson to be intoxicated. The patient's speech is slurred, his walking gait is uneven (drunken staggers), and he appears confused. Never assume that a diabetic is "just drunk." The chance of surviving untreated hypoglycemia is poor. Treat the possibility of hypoglycemia first.

the patient is a diabetic. An EMT should also look for a MedicAlert® patient directive or other similar medical alert identification as part of her assessment. Medical identification or MedicAlert patient directives provide critical information on patient history, especially when the patient is unconscious. Thus, the MedicAlert patient directives speak for the patient when the patient is unable to speak for himself.

If an unconscious patient is thought to be diabetic, the EMT should assume that the patient could be hypoglycemic. An initial assessment should be performed, with time taken to open, assess, suction, and secure the airway. High-concentration oxygen should be given via either a bag-valve-mask or a partial non-rebreather mask, as appropriate.

The EMT should not delay the transportation of the patient and should proceed to package the patient immediately. Minutes count, and the patient should be taken to the closest ALS provider, whether that is the emergency department or interception with an ALS unit. Glucose administered through an intravenous (IV) will rapidly reverse the hypoglycemia and can be lifesaving (Figure 30-7).

Management of the Hypoglycemic Conscious Patient

If the patient is conscious, proceed with the initial assessment. Is the patient combative or confused? If the patient is altered in mental status and a diabetic, suspect hypoglycemia. Be sure that the patient is able to maintain his own airway. That will be very important shortly. Administer high-concentration oxygen via facemask. The patient's body is under stress and will need the supplemental oxygen.

The SAMPLE history (see Table 10-5) will provide the details that will confirm that the patient is experiencing a hypoglycemic episode. If the confusion occurred suddenly, consider hypoglycemia. If the change in mental status occurred after missing a meal or after strenuous exercise, consider hypoglycemia.

Check for medications that the patient might be taking. Insulin is usually stored in the refrigerator. The insulin vial is very small, about the same size as a bottle of nitroglycerin. Syringes may be evident as well as sharps containers for used syringes.

The type of diabetes the patient has will help the EMT to look for either insulin or an oral hypoglycemic agent. Many other medications interact with or interfere with the action of these medications. If the patient just started a new medication or recently changed medications (or doses), the change could have affected the patient's blood sugar level. Find and record all medications that the patient is taking.

The physical examination of the hypoglycemic patient should reveal signs similar to those of the patient in shock. The patient's skin will be cool and moist. The heart will be racing, or tachycardiac. However, unlike the blood pressure in hemorrhagic shock, the blood pressure of the hypoglycemic patient will initially be somewhat elevated. (No fluid has been lost to cause the blood pressure to drop.)

Glucose Administration   If the patient is maintaining his own airway, the patient should be placed on high-concentration oxygen. The EMT should then administer oral glucose. Further details regarding this medication and its administration should now be reviewed in Chapter 26.

Street Smart

Hypoglycemia affects brain function. That is why the patient may appear intoxicated when, in fact, he is hypoglycemic. Similarly, sometimes hypoglycemia will appear to look like a stroke (Chapter 31).

Most EMTs would think that the elderly patient who is weak on one side, has slurred speech, and lapses into unconsciousness has had a stroke. However, hypoglycemia can have similar impacts on the brain.

An EMT should treat any altered mental status in a diabetic patient, regardless of age, as if it were hypoglycemia.

Safety Tip

Caution is advised when looking for insulin. Insulin is an injected medication, implying that a needle was used. These insulin syringes are small, about the same size as a tuberculin syringe used for tuberculosis (TB) testing.

Sharps containers, the storage space for used needles and syringes, may be too expensive for a patient who is on a fixed income. Some diabetics resort to using empty coffee cans or empty plastic milk jugs in an effort to save money. Although these containers are safe alternatives, they are usually not well marked. Be alert and always keep safety in mind.

TABLE 30-5

Hyperglycemia (Diabetic Coma) versus Hypoglycemia (Insulin Shock)		
	Hyperglycemia	**Hypoglycemia**
Onset	Gradual (12–48 hours)	Sudden (<1 hour)
Level of consciousness	Confused, combative	Confused, combative
Heart rate	Tachycardia	Tachycardia
Skin	Warm and dry	Cool and moist
Pupils	Normal	Dilated
Blood pressure	Normal	Slightly elevated
Respiration	Deep (Kussmaul's)	Rapid and shallow

Oral glucose should never be administered to a patient who cannot control his airway. An unconscious patient cannot control his airway. Aspiration of glucose is potentially dangerous. Because the danger of aspiration is always present, if the patient should suddenly become unconscious, the EMT should always have a suction device ready at the patient's side to suction out any remaining material. Table 30-5 summarizes the differences between hypoglycemia and hyperglycemia.

Fingerstick Glucose Testing

Diabetic patients often test their blood glucose at home using special machines. Some EMTs have also started testing the blood glucose of patients with altered mental status while in the field. This simple procedure, outlined below, is quick and provides the EMT with a qualitative measure of the patient's blood glucose. However, the EMT should never delay administering oral glucose to a conscious patient who has an altered mental status and a history of diabetes.

Medication Notes

Generic name: Oral glucose
Trade name: Insta-Glucose, and others
Indications: Suspected low blood glucose
Contraindications: Patients who cannot control their own airway and cannot swallow their own secretions should *not* be given oral medications.
Dose: One tube, or one container
Route: Oral only

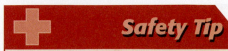

Safety Tip

If the patient is a known diabetic and is combative, stand back. The EMT is under no obligation to tackle a combative patient. On the other hand, the EMT cannot sit back and wait for the patient to become unconscious.

Quickly obtain assistance, usually from a law enforcement officer, to restrain the patient. A specific plan should be ready for these types of emergencies. Review Chapter 32 for more details on how to handle a combative patient.

When it is safe, quickly proceed with administering the oral glucose. Any delay and the patient may lapse into unconsciousness and lose his ability to protect his airway.

If the opportunity does not present itself, then the EMT should immediately transport the patient to either the emergency department or an ALS unit, whichever is closest.

Time is of the essence. Quick thinking and action on the part of the EMT can prevent a bad situation from getting worse.

There are many commercially available home use blood glucose testing machines, called glucometers. All have one common feature, that is, they require a blood sample for analysis. How that sample is obtained and tested is widely variant. Each manufacturer has guidelines for the proper operation of its model of glucometer.

While glucometers are very dependable and rarely need adjustment, it is common practice to test their accuracy regularly, at least once weekly, with a premixed sugar solution of specific strength called a reagent.

After the EMT's introduction and assessment, a determination is made to test the patient's blood glucose. Common indications for testing blood glucose include patients with an altered mental status, for example, confusion or combativeness, after ingestion of unknown poisons (toxins), after a convulsion, or any diabetic patient with a medical emergency.

Next the EMT should explain to the patient the reason why a blood sample is being taken. This can be done while assembling the necessary equipment such as a lancet (a skin puncture device), alcohol-soaked pads, personal protective equipment (PPE) such as gloves, a sterile gauze pad, and a self-adhesive bandage.

After donning gloves, the EMT should select a site, often a fingertip of the nondominant hand, avoiding areas with burns, rashes, or scars. Next the EMT should prepare the site by cleansing it with the alcohol-soaked pad, allowing time for the alcohol to dry. It is important to allow the alcohol to dry on the skin so that it will not mix with the blood and alter the blood sample. Massaging or warming the selected site will increase blood flow and increase the chances of first time success.

The EMT should then grasp the patient's finger with her nondominant hand, placing her thumb at the base of the patient's nail bed and wrap her fingers around the side of the finger. This permits the best leverage for obtaining a blood sample. The EMT should then remove the cover from the lancet, or follow the manufacturer's instructions, and firmly, and with authority, press the lancet against the skin. Any hesitancy may cause the patient unnecessary discomfort. The object of this procedure is to produce a swift, deep puncture.

From the wound, the EMT should squeeze a single large, round droplet of blood and wipe it off on the gauze pad. The EMT should then squeeze a second droplet of blood by milking the finger with her fingers. The squeezing action (milking) should be gentle; vigorous milking dilutes the sample.

This sample is then placed on the glucometer test strip; some glucometers draw the sample into a sensor using capillary action. The glucometer should then proceed with a countdown to the reading, usually about 15–30 seconds.

While awaiting the results of the blood glucose test, the EMT should apply a sterile gauze pad to the fingertip and ask the patient to apply direct pressure to the site. Once the glucometer provides a reading, it should be recorded and appropriate action should be taken according to the reading.

It is the EMT's responsibility to properly discard the lancet into an approved sharps container and to discard all bloody dressings into an appropriate container. Any blood spilt should be quickly wiped up with an absorbent dressing and the area wiped down with a hypochlorite solution such as 1:10 bleach in water.

After approximately 5 minutes, the EMT should confirm that the bleeding has stopped. If the bleeding continues, then more direct pressure is required. If the bleeding has stopped, then a self-adhesive bandage may be applied.

SEIZURE DISORDERS

As was described in Chapter 5, the brain is a group of specialized cells that interact to convey messages to and from every part of the body. The brain controls all activities within the body through these complex interactions. If part of the brain becomes irritated, it can create confusing messages. This event can result in confusion, unconsciousness, or repeated involuntary muscle contractions known as a **seizure**. The events in the brain that result in a seizure can be thought of as a sort of short circuit of the brain's electrical system.

Seizures can indicate a potentially life-threatening problem, which may need prompt medical attention. The EMT should take the necessary steps to stabilize the patient in the field, then transport as soon as possible.

Some seizures are not necessarily life threatening. A patient with a history of seizures may even refuse to be transported to the hospital.

The EMT's responsibility is clear in both cases. The EMT should try to protect the patient from further harm and encourage the patient to accept transportation for further medical evaluation.

The EMT should remember that there are a variety of reasons why a patient might have a seizure, and most cannot be treated in the field. The most appropriate prehospital care for a patient who has had a seizure is transportation to the hospital for further medical evaluation.

✳ *Seizure*

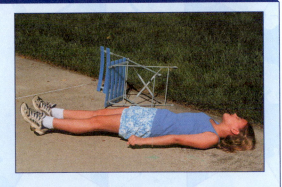

"9-1-1, what is your emergency?" Darlene, an emergency communications specialist, asked the caller as she noted that the caller was using one of the new cell phones that gave her his exact location by coordinates. "We are in the park, near the swings. This girl, she fell down."

"Is she conscious?" asked Darlene in a calm voice.

"She's shaking and jerking and stuff," replied the caller.

"Please stay on the phone, it's a free call. I am dispatching the park police to your location now."

- What is the likely nature of this emergency?
- What are the assessment priorities for this patient?
- What are the treatment priorities for this patient?
- What special concerns should the EMT have for this patient?

TABLE 30-6
Causes of Seizures
Alcohol withdrawal
Brain tumor
Eclampsia (toxemia of pregnancy)
Fever (common in children)
Hypoglycemia
Hypoxia
Infectious disease (e.g., food poisoning)
Metabolic disorders (e.g., endocrine disease)
Poisons (e.g., camphor, cyanide, strychnine)

Causes of Seizures

The most common reason that a person would have a seizure is epilepsy. **Epilepsy** is a condition characterized by repetitive seizures of a similar nature. Although seizures can sometimes be traced to a specific area of the brain, the cause of epilepsy is often unclear.

Isolated seizures, or seizures that have defined causes, are not due to epilepsy. Certain toxins, or poisons, can build up in the blood and cause the patient to have a seizure. Hypoxia and hypoglycemia can cause a patient to have a seizure. Table 30-6 lists some of the more common causes of seizures.

Types of Seizures

Seizures affect the brain's ability to function. Think of the brain as a large circuit board, with electrical pathways, that operates a machine, called the body. If a bucket of water is poured over a circuit board, as the water advances, the circuit board starts to short-circuit, and eventually the entire circuit stops working.

When the brain's "electrical circuits" malfunction, owing to a short circuit in the brain, the patient experiences a seizure (Figure 30-8). If the malfunction is isolated to a small portion of the brain, a **partial seizure** results. This type of seizure may affect the speech or the motor function of a portion of the body.

If the seizure affects the entire brain, the patient will experience a dramatic set of events involving the whole body. These total body seizures are called **generalized seizures**.

Phases of a Generalized Seizure

The source of a seizure is called the *origin*. If the origin is in the visual center, the patient may see a flash of color. If the origin is in the olfactory area, the patient may sense a strange smell. These sensations serve as a

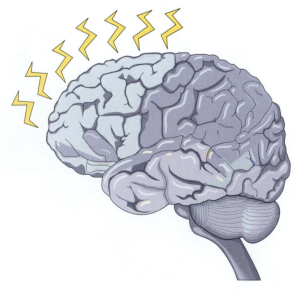

Partial seizure

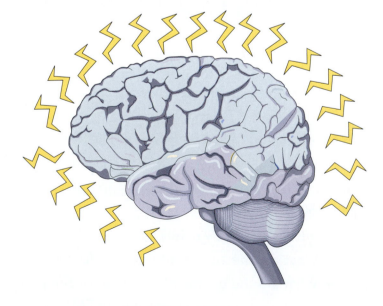

Generalized seizure

FIGURE 30-8   Chaotic firing all over the brain results in a generalized seizure.

warning sign at the onset of a seizure. This phenomenon is referred to as an **aura**. Auras are usually very brief. The patient typically does not have time to react, to sit down, for example, before the next phase.

After the aura passes, the patient loses consciousness. As the irregular electrical activity moves throughout the entire brain, the patient collapses to the ground.

Tonic-Clonic Phase

Next, the entire body stiffens in the **tonic phase**. The forceful contraction of all the muscles of the body, in the tonic phase, lasts for about 30 seconds. During this time, the back arches and the extremities straighten.

The sudden contraction of the diaphragm may cause air to be forcefully exhaled against a partially closed voice box. A high-pitched sound can be produced that sounds like a scream and has been referred to as the "epileptic cry." Any sputum in the airway may be forcefully expelled as well. This expulsion results in "foamy" sputum erupting from the mouth.

During the tonic phase, the diaphragm and the chest wall muscles remain contracted and the patient stops breathing. If the tonic phase, is prolonged, the patient may become hypoxic and cyanotic.

As the muscles become exhausted, the body relaxes momentarily, only to contract again. This intermittent contraction and relaxation of the muscles is called the **clonic phase**. During this phase, the patient may unintentionally empty his bladder.

The intermittent contraction and relaxation of muscles results in the patient's body thrashing around, striking any nearby objects, and can result in serious injury.

Postictal Phase

Most seizures last for only about 3–5 minutes. During that time, the muscles have been working extremely hard. Not surprisingly, the patient feels completely exhausted once the seizure ends (Figure 30-9). This phase is called the **postictal phase**. (Postictal translates as "after the blow.") This phase will usually gradually resolve and the patient will become more awake and oriented but will likely be tired from the event.

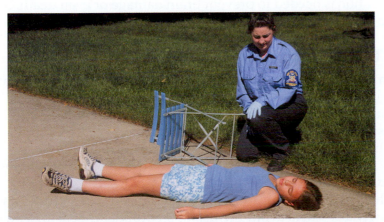

FIGURE 30-9 The period of time immediately after the tonic-clonic phase is called the postictal phase.

Street Smart

The public, in the past, labeled a partial seizure as a **petit mal**. Similarly, the term **grand mal** was applied to a generalized seizure. These two imprecise lay terms are still widely used today.

Some people describe the patient who is having a seizure as "throwing a fit" or having a "convulsion." The terms *fit* and *convulsion* are also old terms for a seizure.

Cultural Considerations

Many patients with epilepsy are referred to as "epileptics." The use of a diagnosis to describe a person is demeaning and reduces that person to being thought of only as a "disease." These people are patients with epilepsy and should be referred to, correctly, by their name and not by a label.

Street Smart

In the past, some thought that the patient in a seizure had been taken by "evil spirits." The scream and the violent shaking were attributed to the soul's resisting the evil spirits. Even today, people will refer to a seizure episode as an "attack."

Safety Tip

Another myth that accounted for epilepsy was the disease theory. It was theorized that the epilepsy patient was diseased with *rabies*. Epilepsy is not caused by rabies.

However, a patient with a serious infection of the brain, called *meningitis*, can experience a seizure. The EMT should take Standard Precautions when caring for a seizure patient. If the patient is feverish, the EMT should wear a mask as well as gloves.

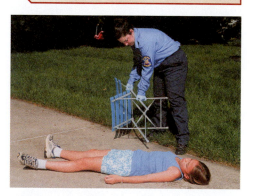

FIGURE 30-10   Protect the seizing patient from injury.

Street Smart

In the past, well-meaning people would force a spoon between the teeth of a seizing patient to prevent the patient from biting his tongue. Although this precaution may have prevented the patient from biting his tongue, more often it resulted in broken teeth.

The Epilepsy Foundation of America does not advocate the use of bite blocks when a patient experiences a seizure. The idea is that it is less expensive and less involved to suture a laceration to the tongue than it is to repair broken teeth.

Management of the Patient with a Seizure

Field treatment of a patient with a seizure disorder is dependent on which phase of the seizure the patient is experiencing. Typically, an EMT arrives to find the patient postical, after the tonic-clonic phase, and can assist the patient with recovery.

Repeated seizures do occur. The EMT must always be prepared to protect the patient in case of another seizure.

The Actively Seizing Patient

Witnessing a seizure can be frightening. The EMT should calmly proceed with protecting the patient during the seizure. First, do not attempt to restrain the patient. Instead, remove any objects the patient may inadvertently strike (Figure 30-10). If possible, remove or loosen any tight clothing that may create a strangulation hazard.

If possible, turn the patient's head to the side to allow drainage of saliva. Remember, do not restrain the patient's head. Restraining the patient's head may create whiplash-like muscle injury.

Do *not* force anything into the mouth of the seizing patient. If the patient *had* an oral airway in place, leave it. Never force an oral airway, a bite block, or other device between the teeth of a seizing patient. To do so may result in broken teeth, which may then obstruct the airway.

High-flow oxygen should be administered via a non-rebreather mask. If the patient is not breathing adequately, the EMT may need to assist ventilations with a bag-valve-mask device. Constant attention should be paid to the airway and breathing status of the seizure patient until he is able to manage on his own.

Carefully observe the patient during the seizure. Note the time of onset and the duration of the seizure. Note which body parts were involved as well as the presence of any cyanosis. Be prepared to support the patient immediately after all muscle activity stops.

Status Epilepticus

If the patient continues to convulse, without interruption, or the patient has a series of seizures, without regaining consciousness, the patient is in a condition called **status epilepticus**.

Status epilepticus is a medical emergency. Rapid advanced-level intervention is needed to prevent brain damage or even death. Status epilepticus is therefore a high-priority situation.

The Postictal Patient

When the patient is postictal, the EMT should be sure that the patient has an adequate airway. If the patient has bitten his tongue while seizing, there may be blood in the airway. The blood should be suctioned out using a Yankauer suction tip.

If the airway is clear, consider rolling the patient onto his left side, in the recovery position. This position allows the patient's secretions to naturally drain from the mouth and nose.

If the patient is responsive only to painful stimuli, consider an oral airway. Many EMTs avoid the use of an oropharyngeal airway, concerned that it will stimulate vomiting. In those cases, a nasopharyngeal airway may be used.

The patient should be given high-concentration oxygen. Although the patient's color may have returned, the body just endured an exhausting physical exercise. Oxygen helps the patient to recover.

If the patient's breathing is shallow, it is appropriate to assist the patient's breathing, for a moment, with a bag-valve-mask device. Remember, although epilepsy is the most common cause of seizures, there are other causes also. These other causes can produce respiratory depression or arrest.

Usually, there is no serious bleeding unless injury occurred during the seizure. Proceed with obtaining a set of vital signs. Remember that the vital signs obtained are going to be more consistent with those of an athlete who just ran a 100-yard dash than with those of a sleeping patient.

Once the ABCs have been addressed, the EMT should perform a rapid head-to-toe assessment utilizing DCAP-BTLS (see Table 14-3) to assess for the possibility of any injuries that may have occurred during the seizure. Note whether the patient has been incontinent of urine (involuntary bladder emptying).

Anticonvulsants

After being diagnosed with recurrent seizures, the patient will be placed on medication. The frequency and severity of seizures can be controlled by medications called **anticonvulsants**. These medications, if taken as directed, are sometimes effective in preventing further seizures. More than half of patients on anticonvulsants will remain seizure free. Table 30-7 lists some anticonvulsants.

CONCLUSION

There are many causes for alterations in mental status. Because diabetic emergencies and seizures are commonly seen by the EMT, having a basic understanding of these conditions will help her to manage the situation more effectively. No matter the cause of an altered mental status, the EMT's initial priorities are to assess and manage the ABCs.

In general, quick, effective, and professional behavior on the part of the EMT can prevent a change in the patient's mental status from becoming deadly. Accurate assessment of the situation, coupled with good decision making about treatment and transportation priorities, results in better patient outcomes.

TEST YOUR KNOWLEDGE

1. What does it mean to say that the patient is awake and alert?
2. What is meant when it is said that a patient has an altered mental state?
3. What are some general causes of an altered mental state?
4. What are the general underlying conditions that can create an altered mental state?
5. What is insulin, and how does it affect metabolism?

Street Smart

There are many advantages to using a nasopharyngeal airway for a postictal patient. One, if the patient should seize again, an airway is in place and the patient can be ventilated if needed. Two, as the patient becomes more conscious, he will not be stimulated to vomit. Last, as the patient becomes more responsive, he will attempt to remove the nasopharyngeal airway from his nose. This attempt signals the EMT that the patient is improving.

Safety Tip

The EMT should take Standard Precautions to prevent possible contamination by body fluids. Minimally, gloves should be worn.

Cultural Considerations

Be sensitive to the patient's right to privacy. Some patients, after having had a seizure, are embarrassed because the seizure occurred in public. In simple-to-understand terms, tell the patient who you are and that he may have just seized. Then tell the patient what you are going to do.

The EMT should cover the patient, if possible. Consider moving the patient to a more private location or the back of the ambulance before proceeding with detailed assessments.

TABLE 30-7

Commonly Prescribed Anticonvulsants

Generic Name	Trade Name
carbamazepine	Tegretol
clonazepam	Klonopin
ethosuximide	Zarontin
phenobarbital	Luminal
phenytoin	Dilantin
valproic acid	Depakote

6. What is the treatment for diabetes?
7. What occurs if diabetes is left untreated?
8. What is a generalized seizure?
9. What is the difference between a generalized and a partial seizure?
10. How does an EMT care for an actively seizing patient?
11. How does an EMT care for a postictal patient?
12. What are some of the common causes of seizures?

INTERNET RESOURCES

For additional information on diabetes, visit these Web sites:

- American Diabetes Association, http://www.diabetes.org
- Children with Diabetes, http://www.childrenwithdiabetes.com
- National Institute of Diabetes and Digestive and Kidney Diseases, http://www.niddk.nih.gov
- WebMD, http://www.diabetes.com

For additional information related to epilepsy and seizure disorders, visit these Web sites:

- American Epilepsy Society, http://www.aesnet.org
- Epilepsy Foundation, http://www.epilepsyfoundation.org
- Epilepsy Project, http://www.epilepsy.com

FURTHER STUDY

Cobaugh, D. (1999). Inhalant abuse. *Journal of Emergency Medical Services, 24*(10), 66–69.

Goss, J. (1999). Clinical clues to illicit drug use. *Journal of Emergency Medical Services, 24*(3), 110–118.

LeDuc, T. (1997). Alcoholism: America's pervasive disease. *Journal of Emergency Medical Services, 22*(5), 76–79.

Meade, D., & Fending, D. (1996). PCP. *Emergency Medical Services, 25*(6), 29–34.

Murphy, P. (1995). Brain storm. *Journal of Emergency Medical Services, 20*(11), 58–60.

Murphy, P., & Alfaro, S. (1999). Meningitis. *Journal of Emergency Medical Services, 24*(5), 74–79.

Nicholl, J. (1999). Prehospital management of the seizure patient. *Emergency Medical Services, 28*(5), 71–79.

CHAPTER 31

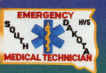

Stroke

KEY TERMS

cerebrovascular accident (CVA)

Cincinnati Prehospital Stroke Scale

dysarthria

embolus

expressive aphasia

facial droop

hemorrhagic stroke

infarct

ischemia

ischemic stroke

penumbra

pronator drift

receptive aphasia

stroke

thrombus

transient ischemic attack (TIA)

OBJECTIVES

Upon completion of this chapter, the reader should be able to:

1. Describe the pathophysiology of ischemic stroke.
2. Describe the pathophysiology of hemorrhagic stroke.
3. Discuss the typical signs and symptoms seen in a stroke.
4. Identify several conditions that might mimic stroke symptoms.
5. Demonstrate the appropriate assessment techniques for a patient with signs and symptoms of stroke.
6. Describe the appropriate management of the patient suffering from a stroke.
7. Discuss the time-dependent nature of this condition.

OVERVIEW

As the third leading cause of death and the leading cause of disability in the United States today, stroke is a problem that an emergency medical technician (EMT) is very likely to encounter in clinical practice. Early identification of the possibility of stroke as a diagnosis and appropriate decision making on the part of the EMT can have a significant impact on the morbidity and mortality associated with this condition.

PATHOPHYSIOLOGY

A **stroke** is injury to brain tissue that occurs as a result of disruption of blood flow to part of the brain. This disruption can occur in one of two general ways. A stroke is also called a **cerebrovascular accident (CVA)**.

Stroke is the third leading cause of death in the United States and is the number one leading cause of disability. Because a stroke results in irreversible brain damage, the patient loses a part of her body function. This often results in lifelong disability and necessitates long-term

Possible Stroke

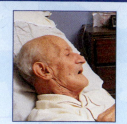

Carla entered the apartment first. She was led down the hall to the master bedroom where an elderly man was lying in bed. "Good morning, sir. My name is Carla, and I am an EMT. What seems to be the problem today?" Carla inquired. "Well," the patient tried to say, "I feel very weak and I can't seem to move my left arm." His speech was somewhat slurred and difficult to understand.

Carla proceeded to obtain further history while her partner, Ruscan, started to assess the patient and check his vital signs. "160 over 120," reported Ruscan. "I wonder what his baseline pressure is?"

Carla turned to the patient's daughter and asked, "When did all this start?" The daughter explained that the patient's weakness started during breakfast. With the help of a neighbor, she was able to get him back to bed, maybe an hour ago. When he did not get better, she called 9-1-1.

"Let's get him packaged," Carla ordered Ruscan while she put the oxygen mask in place, "and get him to the Stroke Center at Memorial."

- What are the signs and symptoms of a stroke?
- What are risk factors for a stroke?
- What should an EMT do to treat the patient who is possibly suffering from a stroke?

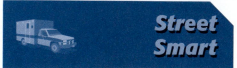

Street Smart

The lay public sometimes refers to a stroke as a "brain attack" because of its similarity in physiology to a "heart attack," the lay term for a myocardial infarction. Both conditions involve death of tissue due to lack of adequate blood flow to the area.

care. Early recognition and diagnosis of stroke can lead to earlier treatment and the potential for a better outcome.

While 70% of stroke victims regain functional independence, 30% are permanently disabled. Furthermore, 20% of stroke survivors continue to require institutional care 3 months after the event. Despite the profound way that stroke affects so many people, there is general misunderstanding about the condition. It is often thought that once a person has a stroke, nothing can be done in treatment. On the contrary, over the last decade, advances in treatment are resulting in improvements in recovery of many patients with stroke.

The treatment of stroke is a very time-dependent issue. The longer an area of brain is without oxygen, the more damage is done. Many therapies for stroke are only effective when utilized very early on in the event. This means that public education regarding stroke symptom recognition and how to access emergency services rapidly is paramount if we are to have a chance to impact this disease process. Secondly, the EMT must be able to quickly recognize the symptoms and signs of stroke and be knowledgeable regarding the services available in his region to treat this incredibly time-sensitive condition. It is important that patient care protocols address the management of stroke as a true medical emergency.

Types of Stroke

Brain cells are dependent upon continuous flow of oxygenated blood in order to function normally. Anything that interrupts the normal flow of blood will cause malfunction of the cells that depend upon it. The causes of stroke can be easily divided into two main categories: ischemic and hemorrhagic.

Ischemic Stroke

Ischemia is the injury of tissue that occurs as a result of blockage of the vessel that normally supplies that tissue with blood. The vast majority of strokes, about 85%, are ischemic in nature. Most **ischemic strokes** occur as a result of chronic narrowing of vessels by atherosclerosis followed by the gradual accumulation of platelets and other blood components, called a **thrombus**, eventually resulting in a complete blockage of the vessel. This process is similar to what is seen in the coronary vessels described in Chapter 28. Figure 31-1 illustrates the anatomy of a thrombus.

Blood flow may also be interrupted when a blood clot that is formed elsewhere in the body travels through the bloodstream and gets lodged in one of the vessels supplying the brain. This type of traveling debris is called an **embolus** and also interrupts blood flow to the tissue beyond where it is lodged. Figure 31-2 illustrates this concept.

Another less common mechanism whereby the brain is deprived of oxygenated blood is during periods of severe shock when the blood pressure falls so low that flow to the brain is not maintained. In this case, the entire brain is without oxygen and severe brain injury may result.

Regardless of the cause of the interruption in blood flow, the brain cells that are deprived of oxygenated blood will die within a very short period of time. A group of cells that have died as a result of prolonged lack of oxygen are referred to as an **infarct**. When cells die, they release chemicals that may cause injury to the surrounding cells. The area of brain tissue that surrounds an infarct is called the **penumbra**. The penumbra is a group of brain cells that are injured yet have the chance of recovery if appropriate treatment is begun rapidly. Figure 31-3 depicts this concept.

Transient Ischemic Attack

Occasionally, a patient may have decreased blood flow to an area of the brain that is only temporary. When this occurs and the symptoms resolve completely in under 24 hours, the term **transient ischemic attack (TIA)** applies. A TIA is usually associated with a thrombus that the body is able to resolve on its own. Patients who have a TIA are at a high risk of having a stroke in the near future. In fact, certain patients have as high as a 25% risk of stroke in the first year after a TIA, the highest incidence being in the first month.

Patients who call emergency medical services (EMS) for stroke symptoms that resolve spontaneously must still be transported for immediate evaluation. A physician may be able to help the patient modify her risk factors and use medications to try and prevent a further event.

Hemorrhagic Stroke

The second category of stroke is known as **hemorrhagic stroke**. This category accounts for less than 15% of strokes. In hemorrhagic stroke there is a rupture of one of the cerebral vessels. This may occur as a result of chronic high blood pressure causing a weakening of the vessel, or as a result of an abnormality such as an aneurysm in the blood vessel. In either case, rupture of a vessel in the brain will decrease

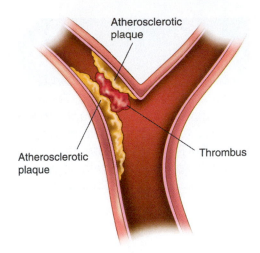

FIGURE 31-1 Platelets and other blood factors can adhere to the irregular surface of a plaque, resulting in a thrombus.

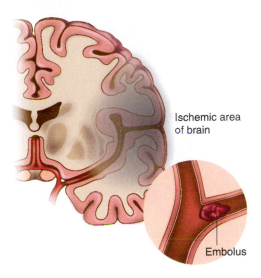

FIGURE 31-2 An embolus can lodge in a cerebral vessel, resulting in ischemia to the brain tissue supplied by that vessel.

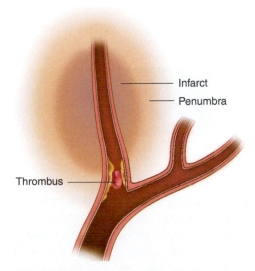

FIGURE 31-3 The penumbra is a potentially salvageable area of brain tissue.

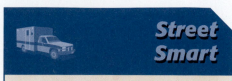

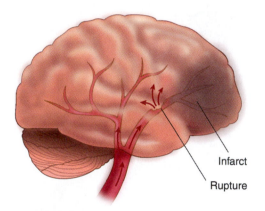

FIGURE 31-4 In hemorrhagic stroke, the rupture of a blood vessel results in decreased blood flow to an area of brain tissue.

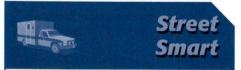

blood flow to the brain tissue supplied by that vessel, resulting in an area of infarct. Figure 31-4 shows this pictorially.

In addition to the decrease in blood flow to the area supplied by that vessel, the blood that leaks out of the vessel can cause injury to the surrounding brain tissue in several ways. Blood itself is irritating to brain cells and can cause injury when it leaks outside the vessel. Additionally, when a significant amount of blood accumulates, it can compress surrounding brain tissue, also resulting in injury. In this case, intracranial pressure may become elevated, in much the same way it does in a patient with a traumatic hemorrhage in the brain. Increased intracranial pressure is discussed in detail in Chapter 21.

Risk Factors

Factors that put a person at risk for a stroke include anything that can result in vessel occlusion or vessel weakening and rupture. People with known vascular disease, such as patients with coronary artery disease or hypertension, are at risk. Diabetes over a long period of time can result in vascular abnormalities. Irregular heart rhythms can cause blood clots that can block vessels. Any cause of very high blood pressure, such as cocaine use or uncontrolled hypertension, can result in stroke. Anyone who has previously suffered a stroke is at risk of experiencing another.

Signs and Symptoms

The signs and symptoms that are present in a patient experiencing a stroke will depend upon the area of the brain that is affected. The most common cerebral vessel affected by a stroke is the middle cerebral artery. In this case, the patient will present with weakness and/or numbness in the face and arm on one side. Often the leg on the same side is involved to some extent as well. Speech may be difficult to understand, called **dysarthria**, if the muscles in the mouth that normally allow clear speech are affected.

Other symptoms that people suffering from a stroke may complain of are listed in Table 31-1. Many of these symptoms are very nonspecific. The EMT must maintain a high index of suspicion when treating patients who may be at risk for stroke.

Although their presentation is sometimes similar to those suffering from an ischemic stroke, patients suffering from a hemorrhagic stroke often present with a headache and signs of increased intracranial pressure.

If the symptoms of stroke are discovered early in the course of the event and the diagnosis is made quickly, therapies may be instituted to reduce the possibility of long-term disability. The symptoms present at the onset of a stroke do not necessarily remain throughout the stroke. If treatment is initiated early enough, some brain tissue may be salvaged and some function may return. The EMT plays an important role in recognizing this condition rapidly.

Assessment

During the assessment of a patient with symptoms and signs of stroke, the EMT should assess for immediate life threats, as with any other critically ill patient. Additionally, an accurate history of the events preceding the call for EMS will be crucial, as management decisions are made in the hospital. A focused neurologic examination will provide the EMT with information that will allow for decisions to be made regarding management, both by the EMT and by the hospital staff.

Initial Assessment

Certain patients having a stroke may have problems that present an immediate threat to the patency of the airway, adequacy of breathing, or circulatory status. Immediately after ensuring the safety of the scene, the EMT should perform an initial assessment and immediately address any potential life-threatening issues at that point. Chapter 13 details the initial assessment that should be performed on every patient.

Focused History

If the patient is awake and able to answer questions, the EMT should perform a focused history that includes the history of present illness and questions regarding past medical history, allergies, or medications taken. If the patient is not able to provide the history, the EMT should obtain relevant historical information from family or others who are present. Particular attention should be paid to determining the exact time of onset of the current symptoms. The management of stroke is very time sensitive. Certain therapies are only employed if they can be initiated within a very narrow window of 3 hours from symptom onset. Other therapies have a slightly wider window of opportunity. However, in any case, it is imperative that the time of onset of the symptoms be identified as accurately as possible. Chapter 16 discusses the focused history and physical exam of the medical patient.

Focused Physical Examination

The focused physical examination should include a brief neurologic examination. The neurologic examination should include five pieces of information.

The patient's mental status should be described. The level of consciousness on the AVPU scale (see Chapter 13) is helpful, as is describing the patient's orientation to person, place, and time. If the patient is awake and able to answer questions, the EMT can ask her for her name, where she is, and what time of day it is. These questions can be repeated as needed by other providers to assess for changes in mental status.

An examination of the patient's pupils is appropriate during the first examination and during each reassessment (Figure 31-5). Their shape and response to light should be assessed. Normally, pupils are round, of equal size, and respond by constricting when exposed to a light source. Any irregular shape, size difference from one side to another, or abnormal response to light may be a sign of possible brain injury.

The patient should be asked to perform several tasks as part of the remainder of the neurologic examination. First, the EMT should ask the patient to raise the arms straight out in front of her with palms facing up. Then the patient should be instructed to close the eyes and

TABLE 31-1
Symptoms Associated with Stroke
Generalized or focal weakness
Paralysis on one side of the body
Paresthesias on one side of the body
Difficulty in speaking
Headache
Vomiting
Visual changes
Dizziness

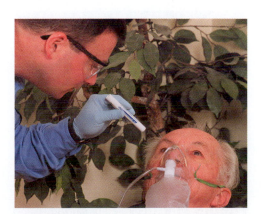

FIGURE 31-5 Examining the pupils for size and reactivity to light should be a routine part of every assessment.

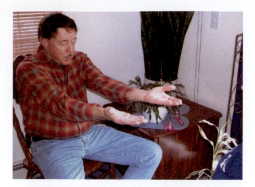

FIGURE 31-6 The presence of pronator drift indicates arm weakness, sometimes due to a stroke.

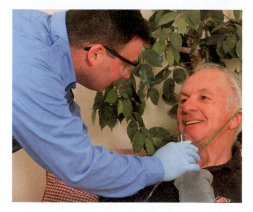

FIGURE 31-7 Asking the patient to smile can help to demonstrate weakness of the facial muscles on one side of the face.

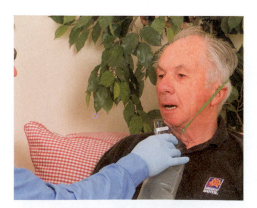

FIGURE 31-8 Garbled or slurred speech can result from weakness of the muscles in the mouth and throat, sometimes associated with stroke.

attempt to keep the arms still for 10 seconds (Figure 31-6). If one arm drifts, it indicates weakness on that side and should be carefully noted. This weakness is called **pronator drift** and is a useful way to test for arm weakness.

Next, the patient should be asked to smile and show the teeth (Figure 31-7). Normally, both sides of the face should move equally, and the smile should be equal on both sides. If one side of the face does not move as well, it is called a **facial droop** and indicates facial muscle weakness. This test can be performed easily by the EMT.

Lastly, the EMT should note the clarity of the patient's speech (Figure 31-8). If speech seems garbled, slurred, or inappropriate, that should be noted. Garbled speech is called **dysarthria** and can be indicative of a stroke.

Depending upon the area of the brain that is affected, the patient's speech may be affected in a different way. Expressive aphasia is one such condition. If a patient is speaking with inappropriate words, but forming them clearly, she is said to have **expressive aphasia**. This is often frustrating to the patient. In the most extreme case, the patient will be unable to speak at all. **Receptive aphasia** exists when the patient seems to not understand words that are spoken to her. This condition is sometimes difficult to differentiate from uncooperative behavior related to a change in mental status. Each of these speech alterations indicates injury to the area of the brain that controls the patient's speech.

A focused neurologic exam such as this can be rapidly accomplished by the EMT. The combination of assessment of arm drift, facial droop, and speech is known as the **Cincinnati Prehospital Stroke Scale** and has been found to be easily completed by any level of provider, from EMT to physician. Additionally, it is an accurate predictor of the diagnosis of acute stroke and can be utilized to make decisions regarding the patient's management. Table 31-2 summarizes the Cincinnati Prehospital Stroke Scale.

There are other well-known standardized stroke scales that are specifically designed to be utilized in the prehospital environment for the assessment of the patient with an acute stroke. Two such scales are the 3-item Los Angeles Motor Scale and the 15-item shortened National Institutes of Health Stroke Scale. The EMT should become

TABLE 31-2

The Cincinnati Prehospital Stroke Scale		
	Normal	**Abnormal**
Arm drift	Both arms move equally or not at all.	One arm drifts compared to the other.
Facial droop	Both sides of the face move equally.	One side of the face does not move at all.
Speech	Patient uses correct words without slurring.	Patient uses inappropriate words, slurs, or is mute.

familiar with whatever standardized assessment is recognized in his area of practice.

Some types of strokes affect a part of the brain that does not cause abnormality on any of these tests. Therefore, the EMT should consider stroke not only in patients who have such abnormalities but also in any person who has suspicious symptoms.

Baseline Vital Signs

As with every patient the EMT encounters, the patient suffering from a stroke will need careful assessment. Baseline vital signs are a part of that assessment. It is not unusual for the blood pressure to be elevated in some types of stroke. The EMT should take careful note of any vital sign abnormalities and report them to hospital staff.

Management

We know that every minute during a stroke, brain cells are being damaged and time is of the essence to try and limit permanent injury of the brain. While the treatment of a stroke is a true emergency, the prehospital management of stroke is somewhat limited. The job of the EMT is to recognize the symptoms and provide expedient transport to a hospital capable of managing the condition.

The hospital management of the patient will center on making the diagnosis and ruling out other causes of the symptoms, then in providing definitive therapy to reestablish blood flow to the affected area of the brain when this is possible. In the case of a hemorrhagic stroke, the treatment will focus on controlling the blood pressure and limiting further injury.

In the case of ischemic stroke, intravenous medications may be given to break up the clot and allow blood to flow again to the affected area of the brain. In highly specialized centers, these thrombolytic medications may be administered directly into the artery affected by a specially trained physician. Additionally, similar to what is done in cardiac angioplasty, tiny tools can sometimes be utilized inside the vessel to assist in the reestablishment of blood flow. These procedures, while only available at certain centers, might offer fewer side effects and a more direct means of reestablishing blood flow to the injured brain.

Hospitals that are able to offer advanced therapies to stroke victims at all times are referred to as stroke centers. Timeliness of transport is of key importance, as these therapies may only be utilized if the patient presents to the hospital within a very short window of time. The EMT should be familiar with the capabilities of hospitals in his region and should follow protocols, carefully regarding where stroke patients should be transported.

During transport the EMT will continually assess the patient and take steps to prevent worsening injury, if possible. Such steps include appropriate management of the airway, breathing, and circulation (ABCs). If the patient is not able to effectively maintain her own airway, the EMT should take the appropriate action. Chapter 7 discusses the techniques used for airway maintenance.

Increased intracranial pressure may result in an abnormal breathing pattern. If the patient is not breathing effectively, the EMT must assist her as described in Chapter 8.

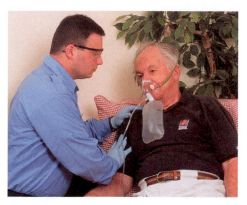

FIGURE 31-9 The patient suffering from a stroke may be profoundly weak on one side and may need help to keep from falling.

Stroke is a condition in which part of the brain is not receiving enough oxygen; therefore, high-flow oxygen should be provided to every patient with a possible stroke.

During a stroke, the brain senses lack of blood flow to the affected area. In compensation, the blood pressure may elevate in an attempt to provide blood flow to the involved area. This may result in very elevated blood pressures. Occasionally, a stroke may result from or cause low blood pressure. If this is the case, the EMT should take steps to support the blood pressure as described in Chapter 9.

In the nonhypotensive patient, keeping the head of the bed elevated to at least 30 degrees may help to decrease intracranial pressure by allowing venous drainage of blood out of the head more easily. This upright position is recommended unless management of the airway and breathing precludes it.

Differential Diagnoses

A focused neurological examination should be done for any patient suspected of having suffered a stroke. An abnormal finding on any of these tests may indicate a stroke, although other conditions can cause some of them. Table 31-3 lists some of those which should be considered.

The EMT may not be able to differentiate between stroke and many of these other conditions; however, the treatment an EMT can offer is very much the same for each. Management of the ABCs with timely transport to the appropriate hospital is indicated in each case.

Transport

As soon as the possibility of stroke is recognized, the EMT should take steps to initiate transport by the most expedient means to the most

TABLE 31-3

Other Diagnoses to Consider in the Presence of Strokelike Symptoms	
Hypoglycemia	Low blood sugar
Bell's palsy	An inflammatory condition of the nerve controlling the muscles of one side of the face
Traumatic brain injury	Injury to the brain from trauma
Seizure	Localized paralysis may remain after a seizure for hours to days
Migraine	Complicated migraines may result in neurologic abnormalities that resolve upon resolution of the migraine
Drug toxicity	Toxic levels of some medications (e.g., Lithium, Dilantin, Tegretol) may cause neurologic abnormality

appropriate hospital. Advanced life support should be requested to intercept if indicated in local protocols. In some areas of the country, stroke patients are specifically triaged to hospitals that have specialized stroke teams and capabilities to provide advanced therapies very quickly. In some cases, if the most appropriate hospital is a significant distance from the patient, a helicopter might be the most expedient means of transport. The EMT should become familiar with protocols in his area.

Early notification of the destination hospital is very important in the case of a stroke patient. Such advanced notification allows the hospital to mobilize necessary resources and prepare to manage this patient in the most expeditious manner.

Ongoing Assessment

The importance of repeated, ongoing assessments in the stroke patient cannot be overstated. Any changes in the patient's vital signs, mental status, pupils, or focused neurologic examination are of importance to the treating team at the hospital and should be noted carefully.

? Ask the Doc

The National Association of EMS Physicians and the Air Medical Physicians Association each have position statements that support the rapid transport of stroke patients to hospitals having specialized capabilities to manage these conditions.

CONCLUSION

Stroke affects more than 700,000 people in the United States each year. As a true medical emergency, stroke is a condition that an EMT must be very familiar with. Protection of the patient from further injury during expedient transport to an appropriate facility will be the cornerstone of the prehospital management of this condition.

TEST YOUR KNOWLEDGE

1. What are the anatomic changes seen in an ischemic stroke?
2. What are the anatomic changes seen in a hemorrhagic stroke?
3. What are the typical signs and symptoms seen in a stroke?
4. Name several conditions that might mimic stroke symptoms.
5. Describe the appropriate assessment techniques for a patient with signs and symptoms of stroke.
6. List the management priorities for the patient suffering from a stroke.
7. Why is the management of a stroke so time sensitive?

INTERNET RESOURCES

For additional information on stroke, visit these Web sites:
- American Heart Association, http://www.americanheart.org
- American Stroke Association, http://www.strokeassociation.org
- Brain Attack Coalition, http://www.stroke-site.org
- Internet Stroke Center, http://www.strokecenter.org
- National Stroke Association, http://www.stroke.org

FURTHER STUDY

Air Medical Physician Association. (2004, April 13). Appropriateness of medical transport and access to care in acute stroke syndromes: Position statement of the Air Medical Physician Association. Salt Lake City, UT: Author.

Gerard, D., & Maniscalco, P. (2000). Brain attack: New perspectives on stroke. *Emergency Medical Services, 29*(1), 51–55.

Kothari, R. U., Pancioli, A., Liu, T., Brott, T., & Broderick, J. (1999, April). Cincinnati Prehospital Stroke Scale: Reproducibility and validity. *Annals of Emergency Medicine, 33*(4), 373–378.

Llanes, J. N., Kidwell, C. S., Starkman, S., et al. (2004, January–March). The Los Angeles Motor Scale (LAMS): A new measure to characterize stroke severity in the field. *Prehospital Emergency Care, 8*(1), 46–50.

Tirschwell, D. L., Longstreth, W. T., Jr., Becker, K. J., et al. (2002, December). Shortening the NIH Stroke Scale for use in the prehospital setting. *Stroke, 33*(12), 2801–2806.

CHAPTER 32

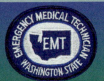

Abnormal Behavior

KEY TERMS

addiction

anxiety disorder

auditory hallucination

behavioral emergency

bipolar disorder

command hallucination

delirium

delirium tremens (DTs)

dementia

dependency

depression

excited delirium

hallucination

hobble restraint

medically necessary restraint

mental illness

organic disorder

positional asphyxia

psychiatry

show of force

substance abuse

suicide

tactile hallucination

takedown

visual hallucination

withdrawal symptoms

OBJECTIVES

Upon completion of this chapter, the reader should be able to:

1. Define what constitutes a behavioral emergency.
2. Describe several functional reasons for a behavioral emergency.
3. Describe several mental illnesses that could result in a behavioral emergency.
4. List several signs and symptoms of severe or clinical depression.
5. List several symptoms, or features, of psychotic behavior.
6. Describe how substance abuse withdrawal can lead to a behavioral emergency.
7. List signs and symptoms of a behavioral emergency.
8. Describe several concerns an EMT should have about scene safety on the scene of a behavioral emergency.
9. Describe the general approach to a call involving a behavioral emergency.
10. Describe how a person might be verbally persuaded to accept medical care.
11. Describe how a person would be safely restrained.
12. Discuss the medical–legal issues surrounding restraint by EMTs.
13. Describe the dangers, for the patient as well as the crew, during a patient restraint.
14. List unacceptable restraint devices and techniques for patient restraint.
15. Describe the important elements in an ongoing assessment of the medically restrained patient.

OVERVIEW

Mental illness is any disorder that affects the mind and is exhibited in a person's behavior. Although mental illness, and **psychiatry**, which is the study of mental illness, is a complex topic, emergency medical services (EMS) can be called for some very simple reasons.

Aggressive Behavior

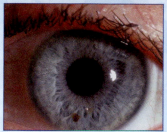

Tom regularly checked on his father every other day just to make sure he was all right and that he had everything he needed. Smitty, Tom's father, was a widower, and since his wife had died 5 years ago he was prone to "hitting the bottle."

Today Tom just had a feeling something wasn't right. The front door was open and the window was broken. Approaching carefully, he could see the old man sitting in his overstuffed chair. He had a crazy look in his eyes.

Calling out to Smitty, Tom asked, "Hey, are you all right?" That's when the old man got out of his chair and charged at Tom. Tom, being younger and quicker, easily ducked the old man's fist and headed straight to his truck. Calling 9-1-1 he told them, "Smitty's out of his head. Better send the sheriff up here."

- What signs and symptoms of a potential behavioral emergency are present in this case?
- What are some of the potential causes of this abnormal behavior?
- What are the EMT's first priorities?

Typically, EMS is called whenever the patient's behavior is seen as dangerous to himself or others or when the patient's behavior is socially unacceptable. Therefore, emergency medical technicians (EMTs) are less interested in the specific diagnosis of mental illness than in understanding the types of behaviors that would generate a call for EMS.

This chapter discusses mental illness within the context of the accompanying abnormal behavior. This chapter further discusses how an EMT should respond to those behaviors.

BEHAVIORAL EMERGENCY

A **behavioral emergency** can be defined as any situation in which the patient exhibits a behavior that is unacceptable, dangerous, or intolerable to the person, the family, or the community. Attempted suicide is an extreme example of a behavioral emergency. A subtle example of a behavioral emergency is the clinical depression that may have led up to the suicide attempt.

Often, a behavioral emergency is brought to the attention of authorities, such as police, because of the violent nature of the behavior. This is not always the case. Concerned persons who call on the public, such as letter carriers or drivers for Meals on Wheels, may call EMS if they find a client acting in a manner that is not typical for the client and is potentially unsafe (Figure 32-1). Family members, close friends, and interested bystanders will call 9-1-1 when a person is "not acting right."

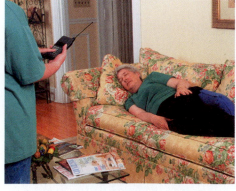

FIGURE 32-1 Concerned citizens and family members call EMS to report a behavioral emergency.

Organic Disorders

Abnormal behaviors have been attributed to people who are "not thinking right." This is a simplistic definition, but it does point to the core of the matter. Abnormal behavior is the result of a malfunction in the brain.

The brain can malfunction for a variety of reasons. For example, the brain fails without adequate oxygen and glucose. Any disease or physical condition that causes the brain to malfunction is an **organic disorder**. Table 32-1 is a list of organic disorders. It is important for an EMT to understand, evaluate, and treat any organic disorder.

Hypoxia-induced abnormal behavior is a common organic disorder an EMT can treat readily through oxygen administration (Chapter 8). Hypoglycemia is another organic disorder an EMT can treat quickly, using oral glucose (Chapter 30).

The key is that the EMT must have a suspicion that the patient's abnormal behavior may be due to a medical, or organic, cause, not to a psychiatric cause. If the EMT is wrong, then no harm has come to the patient. If she is right, the EMT may have prevented brain injury and possibly even death.

Dangerous Assumptions

Some people, when witnessing abnormal behavior, dismiss the patient's illness as "just plain crazy." If an EMT dismisses a patient in this manner, she may be missing a life-threatening condition.

As a medical professional, the EMT must first safeguard the patient's life. With this concept in mind, an EMT must evaluate and treat any serious medical conditions that could create abnormal behavior.

The mnemonic AEIOU TIPS, discussed in Chapter 30, is helpful for understanding possible organic causes of altered mental states.

Mental Disorders

Any disorder that impairs the brain's function, the way the brain thinks, without a firm physical (organic) cause is considered a mental illness. The outward evidence of mental illness is usually bizarre or irrational behavior.

Substance abuse, depression, and psychosis are examples of common mental illnesses; they are discussed in detail later in this chapter. An EMT might encounter a patient suffering from any one of these disorders. The focus of the EMT is not to diagnosis the illness, but rather to deal effectively with the potentially dangerous behavior that is being exhibited by the patient.

Signs and Symptoms

Although each behavioral disorder is characterized by its own specific signs and symptoms, those that will most often result in an emergency call for the EMT are listed in Table 32-2.

Scene Size-Up

The initial dispatch information should alert the EMT to the potential for violence on scene. Radio reports of "shots fired," "suicide attempted," and the like should warn the EMT of the potential for personal injury and an unsafe scene.

TABLE 32-1
Some Organic Disorders That Cause Abnormal Behavior
Hypoxia
Hypoglycemia
Hypoperfusion
Head injury
Drug overdose
Excessive cold
Excessive heat

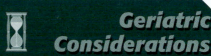

Geriatric Considerations

Patients over the age of 65 are at risk for the "three Ds": depression, dementia, and delirium. The EMT should attempt to differentiate between dementia and delirium. Depression is discussed later in the chapter.

Dementia is a gradual loss of cognitive (thinking) function. A common cause of dementia in the elderly is Alzheimer's disease. Alzheimer's disease is a progressive neurological disease that is associated with a gradual loss of intellectual function.

Delirium, on the other hand, is a sudden erratic change in behavior. A delirious patient may be frightened, disoriented, incoherent, and combative. Delirium may be the result of a stroke, infection, fever, or accidental overdose of medications (review AEIOU TIPS). A sudden change in mental state, such as confusion and bizarre behavior, requires immediate medical assessment in the emergency department.

TABLE 32-2

Signs and Symptoms of a Behavioral Emergency

Mental confusion

Extreme agitation

Inappropriate anger

Weeping and crying

Violence

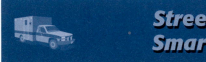

Street Smart

Some EMS calls are also crime scenes. Attention should be paid to the details on scene. Take extreme care to avoid destroying footprints, tire tracks, or broken glass.

Do not touch or move suspected weapons. Call police immediately for assistance, and consider retreating from the scene until they arrive. Always wear gloves whenever handling any object on scene.

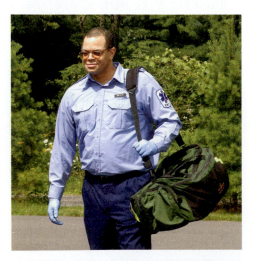

FIGURE 32-2 Equipment should be carried in a manner that will allow the EMT to make a quick getaway if a patient becomes violent.

Occasionally, the street address is known to EMS. There may have been previous EMS calls at the same location for injuries secondary to fighting, for example. Many communications centers have a location's call history on computer.

Never enter an unsafe scene. If the scene involved weapons, the EMT should place, or stage, the ambulance far enough back to be out of sight and out of the line of fire. Turn off any warning lights that might alert those on scene of your presence. Stay in the vehicle until the scene is declared safe by police.

As the EMT approaches the scene, she should perform a visual sweep of the scene, looking for telltale signs of violence, such as broken glass, blood on the ground, empty alcohol containers, and spent gun shell casings.

Scene Safety

An EMT should take several important safety measures whenever she is entering a scene. Never enter a potentially violent scene alone. Always have a police officer clear the scene first. Then proceed into the scene, with a partner or a police officer. Using the "buddy system" improves the EMT's chances of remaining safe.

Whenever an EMT is approaching a potentially violent scene, she should be thinking about escape. The EMT should look for nearby objects that will provide cover (protection from bullets) and may provide concealment.

Carry all portable gear over one shoulder only or in one hand by the straps (Figure 32-2). Never sling portable gear over both shoulders. A violent patient could grab the portable gear bag and use it to drag the EMT off her feet.

If it is necessary to make a hasty retreat, slip the bag off the shoulder and onto the ground in the path of any pursuers.

Have a portable radio immediately available for emergency use. Observe radio silence when approaching the patient. Extraneous radio chatter may be both distracting and alarming to the patient.

At night, only the first EMT should have a flashlight. All personnel should walk in a single file to decrease their target profile. The first EMT should hold the flashlight out to the side of the body, again, to decrease the target profile.

If it is a street call, and a crowd has assembled, study the crowd carefully. The mood of the crowd, heard in the tone and words of the bystanders, should key the EMT to the potential for further violence.

If it is a house call, stand to the side of the door and knock loudly. Do not depend on doorbells. Call out loudly. Use terms like "ambulance" or "rescue squad." Pick terms that any patient will understand. If possible, leave doors open to provide a ready escape route.

The EMT, or her partner, should always make sure that the path to the exit or doorway is open and clear of obstacles. If a hasty retreat is necessary, the EMT should carefully back out of the situation. The EMT should never turn her back on the potential assailant until she is clear of the doorway or a considerable distance away.

Finally, the EMT should stand a safe distance from the patient; over an arm's length away is usually sufficient. Never stand too close to the patient. The patient may feel threatened and respond violently.

Furthermore, an EMT should never sit or kneel in front of a seated patient. Instead, the EMT should crouch down while still on the balls of the feet. From this crouched position, the EMT will be able to quickly respond to threats by springing up and retreating to safety (Figure 32-3).

Objects around the patient that could be used as weapons should be removed if possible. Alternatively, the patient can be lured away from them. The EMT should always be alert and prepared for potential violence.

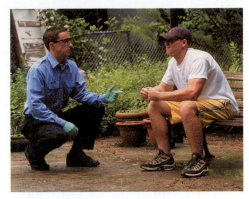

FIGURE 32-3 Never kneel or sit in front of a patient. Instead, crouch in front of the patient at least an arm's length away.

Assessment

The general approach to assessing a potentially violent patient is to "stop, look, and listen." Observe the patient carefully. Angry patients often stand bolt upright, legs spread slightly apart, ready for a fight. Other signs of potential violence include clenched fists, hands stiffly forced into the pocket, or arms folded tightly across the chest.

Look into the patient's eyes. The saying goes that "the eyes are the windows to the soul." Many times the EMT can tell whether the patient is angry, frightened, or confused just by looking into the eyes.

The eyes also often signal when a patient is going to make a sudden move, for example, when reaching for a weapon. Maintain good eye contact. Good eye contact communicates the EMT's confidence to the patient.

The initial assessment can be done at a safe distance. The patient who is awake, on his feet, and exhibiting potentially violent behavior likely has a patent airway, adequate respirations, and no gross circulatory problem. The EMT should not attempt close physical assessment if it is felt to be dangerous.

History and Focused Physical Examination

As the EMT gathers the history, she is listening to the patient's voice. An angry patient will use angry words and profanity. The patient's speech may be pressured, trying to get a complete thought out in just one breath.

Signs of agitation include rapid pacing, rigid posture (Figure 32-4), and quick irregular movements. Rapid darting eye movements, like those of a trapped animal looking for an escape, may indicate the patient's panic.

If it is safe to do so, a history of the present illness and SAMPLE history (see Table 10-5) can be obtained from family members if the patient is unable or unwilling to provide them himself. The focused physical examination may be limited for safety reasons, but if she is able to, the EMT should assess the patient from head to toe for signs of obvious injury. Vital signs should be measured when it is safe to do so, and should be repeated as often as necessary.

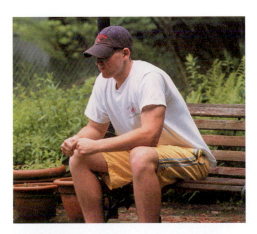

FIGURE 32-4 Body language often says what the patient is feeling.

Management

Regardless of the situation, the EMT must maintain a calm and professional manner. As a matter of practice, only one EMT should talk to the patient, if possible. This approach allows the EMT–patient relationship to be developed. Hopefully, the patient will begin to trust the EMT and then agree to care and transport.

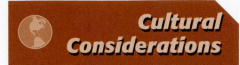

Cultural Considerations

Some patients may consider direct eye contact as a challenge or an affront. Staring contests, as these behaviors are called, are counterproductive to the task at hand.

The intent is to calm the patient and to get the patient to trust the EMT. If the patient appears to be offended by direct eye contact, then the EMT should avoid it.

The EMT should identify herself clearly and tell the patient what her intentions are. The EMT should speak in a calm, reassuring manner, directing the conversation to the patient. Good eye contact with the patient helps improve patient rapport, in most cases.

Verbal Persuasion

One of the EMT's goals is to defuse the angry situation and convince the patient to cooperate with care. The key to achieving that goal is good, effective communication. Effective communication with an angry, agitated, or confused patient first requires that the EMT speak slowly and clearly. The EMT should state her name and purpose plainly to the patient. If the patient does not understand what is being said, repeat the message until he does understand.

The EMT should ask the patient about his concerns. If the patient asks a question, answer the question honestly. Patients will sense when an EMT is lying.

If the patient wants to talk about his hallucinations, reassure the patient that the hallucinations are temporary. Hallucinations can be very frightening to the patient. Remind the patient that you are there to help and protect him.

Seek the patient's cooperation. Encourage the patient to "speak up." Talking about emotions and feelings starts the therapeutic process. For an EMT to be effective, she need only be a good listener.

If the patient is refusing transportation and he needs medical attention, be firm and reject his refusal. Explain to the patient, in simple terms, that his refusal is unacceptable and that he must go to the hospital.

If the patient remains uncooperative, explain to the patient the consequences of failing to go to the hospital. Some patients may feel threatened and lash out unexpectedly. The EMT should be prepared to withdraw in case of a physical attack.

Even when the patient is visibly shaken, stay calm. The patient may direct hurtful comments toward the EMT. Remember that the patient is ill, and the comments said are said under duress. An EMT always maintains a professional attitude, never taking comments personally, remembering that the patient is suffering from an illness that alters his thought processes.

Physical Restraint

There comes a point, in a behavioral emergency, when it is clear that verbal persuasion is not going to be effective. The patient will display signs of **excited delirium**.

The patient in an excited delirium will demonstrate hyperactive irrational behavior. Often, excited delirium is the result of drug intoxication or mental illness, such as schizophrenia. The patient is frequently described as being *out of control*.

Unchecked, the patient will become increasingly agitated and will become violent. Therefore, the patient who is experiencing excited delirium is clearly in danger of harming others or himself.

When a patient is out of control and is a clear danger to himself or others, then a decision has to be made to restrain the patient for his own protection. The decision to restrain a patient should be made only after all other means of persuasion have been exhausted. Family members may be helpful in convincing the patient to cooperate.

Medical Necessity

A patient may be restrained against his will for a legitimate medical necessity. The government provides physicians limited authority, usually under the mental health law, to restrain a person when the patient is a danger to himself or others.

When a restraint is performed for this reason, it is called a **medically necessary restraint**. A medically necessary restraint is ordered by a doctor and done only for the safety of the patient or others.

It is apparent that restraint is a treatment, but it is different from most treatments in that the patient is not permitted to refuse it. To refuse a treatment, the patient must be competent. It is assumed that any person who is thinking of harming himself or others is irrational and therefore incompetent. If the patient is incompetent, then the patient cannot refuse treatment.

Medically necessary restraint differs from police custody. Police officers are afforded wider authority to stop, detain, and, if necessary, restrain citizens—in other words place them in custody—for the purposes of law enforcement. Medically necessary restraint is a treatment ordered for a patient who is incompetent to make his own decision.

In some jurisdictions, the law allows police to take protective custody of certain incompetent individuals. (Review Chapter 2 on medical responsibilities for a discussion on competency and permission.) The idea of protective custody follows logically. If the patient is incompetent, then he cannot refuse treatment. In this case, the patient is restrained by police until EMS arrives.

An EMT is permitted to use only reasonable force to restrain a patient. Reasonable force might be defined as the strength it would take to overpower the patient and no more. In other words, it is the minimum force needed to confine a patient without undue risk of injury to either the patient or the EMT.

The objective of the restraint is to protect the patient from himself, not to harm him. Use of more force than is necessary to restrain the patient might be called excessive force.

If excessive force is used, or if the patient should not have been restrained in the first place, then the patient has been denied his civil rights. In those cases, the patient or patient's family may elect to start legal action against the EMT. Criminal charges for assault could also be filed against the EMT for use of excessive force.

The EMT's best protection when determining when to use restraint is to follow local protocols and carefully document the need for such restraint.

Restraint Procedure

At some point in the patient assessment, it may become apparent that the patient will not cooperate with the plan of care. The patient may be clearly demonstrating that he intends to harm himself or others. A physician (through protocols) or, more commonly, a law enforcement officer makes the decision to restrain the patient and have him brought to the emergency department. When these conditions have been met, then the patient must be restrained using a **takedown** procedure.

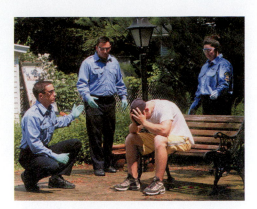

FIGURE 32-5 A show of force is sometimes all that is necessary to obtain a patient's cooperation.

A takedown is the planned orderly restraint of a patient for a medical purpose. Before the takedown is actually performed, there must be a strategy on how to proceed with the takedown. This preplanning helps ensure the safety of all providers involved and, more important, the safety of the patient.

To control the patient's extremities is to control the patient. Most takedown procedures involve obtaining and maintaining control of the extremities.

While the first EMT is attempting to verbally persuade the patient to cooperate with the treatment plan (talking the patient down), another EMT should be establishing a safe strategy for the takedown.

First, always ensure that there are enough crew members, usually a minimum of four people, for a safe restraint. If there are not enough to effect a safe takedown, the group should withdraw until reinforcements arrive.

Each crew member must be assigned a role for the takedown. Typically, one person is assigned the role of team leader. Each member of the team will be assigned a specific job, often maintaining control of a body part. The team leader will signal the team when to move, quickly, to restrain the patient. The signal, usually a verbal cue such as "OK" or a hand gesture, tells all team members to proceed to restrain the patient's limbs.

With a strategy in place, the team moves into position. The EMT negotiating with the patient should signal the team to move forward at the right moment (Figure 32-5). When the team leader moves the team forward, what she has effectively done is to say that the discussion has failed.

At this time, the EMT talking with the patient should make one last effort to convince the patient to agree to care by pointing out the large number of people behind him. The patient, seeing a large number of determined individuals, called a **show of force**, may see the intelligence in cooperating and quietly comply with the first EMT's request. If the show of force fails, then, on cue, the team should move forward quickly to surround and take the patient down.

Having the stretcher near is convenient. Then the patient can be positioned on the stretcher. At other times, flexible stretchers are used. The next section discusses alternative restraint techniques.

Total Body Restraint

The most effective restraint would totally encapsulate the patient, preventing the patient from moving yet allowing the patient to be carried. A blanket, flexible stretcher, or similar apparatus is an effective total body restraint device.

If a flexible stretcher is used, the patient must first be placed on the stretcher. Once the patient is on the stretcher, the bedroll is opened and wrapped around the patient. The sheet is snugly wrapped around the patient, while the patient's arms are down along his sides. Next the blankets are crossed over the patient, opposite the direction of the sheet.

Layering linen over the patient while folding the linen in opposite directions is called the *papoose* technique (Figure 32-6). Papoose is very effective for children or for weak or elderly patients.

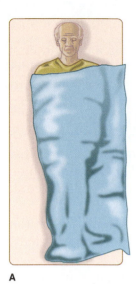
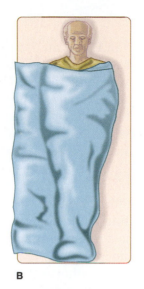
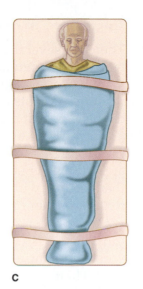

A   B   C

FIGURE 32-6 The papoose is an effective restraint technique for small or elderly patients.

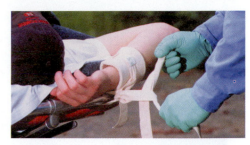

FIGURE 32-7 Secure one arm over the patient's head.

Finally, the stretcher straps are secured at the shoulders, hips, and thighs. Additional 9-foot straps placed around the entire apparatus can help secure the patient.

The EMT should take care to continually monitor the respiratory status of the restrained patient, as overly tight restraints can restrict breathing.

Extremity Restraint

After the team has completed the takedown and the patient's limbs are being physically restrained, the patient must be moved to a transportation device, such as the stretcher.

If the gurney wheels are lockable, then lock them. If they are not, the EMT must remember to place a foot under a wheel to act as a chock. Nothing is more difficult than trying to restrain a squirming patient on a moving gurney.

The patient is lifted by all four extremities and placed, faceup, onto the stretcher. Placing the patient faceup is important to prevent respiratory compromise in the prone position. It also allows the EMT to monitor the patient's airway, breathing, and circulation (ABCs).

Secure one arm above the patient's head, at the crossbar at the head of the gurney. Place the other hand, preferably the nondominant hand, down at the patient's side. By having his arms placed in opposing directions, the patient cannot get leverage and use the large abdominal muscles to sit up (Figure 32-7).

Place the gurney's strap under the patient's armpits. Keep the strap high and tight. Another strap should be placed immediately above the patient's knees. Again, with the knees held down, the patient is prevented from using the large thigh muscles for force. If the legs are strapped at or below the knees, then the patient can squirm out from under the strap.

Finally, if necessary, restrain the ankles. First, secure the two ankles, one to the other. Then secure the ankles to the gurney. Often this last step, securing the ankles to the gurney, is unnecessary and makes the move to the hospital gurney more difficult.

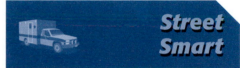

Street Smart

The use of a **hobble restraint** is not acceptable in EMS. A hobble restraint, also known as "hog-tying," places a patient on his stomach with his wrists and ankles tied together behind him.

When an exhausted patient is placed facedown, after a vigorous physical confrontation, he may not have the strength to lift his chest and breathe deeply. The result is the patient slowly suffocates and eventually could go into respiratory arrest. There are reports of people having died because they were placed in hobble restraint. Death from being restrained in this situation is called **positional asphyxia**.

Many police departments now ban the use of hobble restraints. If the patient is found "hobbled," immediately roll the patient onto his side to allow him the chance to breathe deeply.

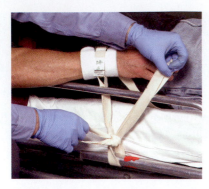

FIGURE 32-8 A restraint looped over the patient's wrist with a half-hitch is an effective restraint device.

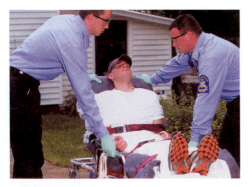

FIGURE 32-9 A chest restraint allows the patient to remain seated.

Restraint Devices

There are several devices an EMT can use to restrain a patient. First, there are triangular bandages. Cravats, triangular bandages folded lengthwise, are strong and versatile. EMTs often use cravats for restraint. Cravats fold into small packets about the size of the palm of the hand and fit easily into a uniform pocket, out of sight.

Cravats also apply the force of the restraint across a broad swath, preventing the restraint from cutting into the patient's flesh. When applied to a wrist or an ankle, the cravat is looped *twice* over the limb, then secured with a half-hitch. The *tails* of the cravat are then secured to the stretcher railing (Figure 32-8).

Strong roller gauze (Kling or Kerlix) can be used as well. Caution must be exercised because a roller bandage can cut into the patient's wrists, creating a soft tissue injury.

Psychiatric hospitals use a leather restraint device, a commercially manufactured restraint device that consists of a loop of leather with a locking device on a strap that is applied to each wrist. The top wrist loops are then secured to a waist belt or to the rails of the stretcher. Like the wrist restraints, in an ankle restraint a leather loop goes around the ankle. Ankle restraints are usually secured to the stretcher by a belt wrapped around the foot of the stretcher.

Although leather restraints are more expensive than other devices, they can be fixed on the patient quickly. Leather restraints have the added advantage of being padded. Padding prevents friction burns to the wrist and ankles as the patient struggles.

In nursing homes, elderly patients who are prone to falling or wandering off are restrained with a chest harness. A chest harness is vest-like and goes over the patient's head in a T-shirt fashion. Some chest harnesses have panels made of cotton; others have panels made of nylon mesh. Both varieties of chest harnesses are strong and durable.

The chest harness has fabric belts sewn into the vest. These belts can be fastened behind the patient's back, out of reach, to keep the patient in the chair.

A chest harness is a very effective means of restraining a patient while still allowing him to sit upright (Figure 32-9). Certain elderly patients, those with heart failure, for example, cannot tolerate lying flat for extended periods without feeling short of breath. Furthermore, the chest harness allows the EMT access to the patient's arms for purposes of taking blood pressures.

Safety Tip

If the patient is spitting at people, the EMT should be sure to wear eye protection as well as a mask. Placing a mask on the patient may be effective, but a determined patient will manage to get the mask off and spit at the EMT. Be proactive, and protect yourself by shielding your eyes.

Street Smart

When securing a patient to a stretcher, be sure to secure the limbs to a nonmovable rail. If the limbs are secured to lower bars in the carriage and the stretcher is quickly raised to the high position, then the patient's pinned arms will be injured, and possibly even broken.

As a matter of practice, all restrained patients should be transported on a stretcher in the low position. This practice prevents a squirming patient from overturning the stretcher.

Safety

If a situation deteriorates and safety is compromised, the team should withdraw. Police are trained in effective restraint techniques. In those cases, the police should be encouraged to restrain the patient.

Once the patient has been restrained, then the EMT, at her earliest convenience, should replace the police restraints (handcuffs, ties) with medical restraints. Often patients become exhausted after a vigorous restraint and are easier to manage.

If the patient must remain in handcuffs, then the police officer should accompany the patient to the hospital.

Transport

Once the patient has been safely secured to the stretcher and is in the back of the ambulance, the EMT should transport the patient to the closest appropriate hospital. Every EMT should be familiar with the capabilities of each nearby institution. Some emergency departments have a separate psychiatric facility, which may be appropriate for a patient with an acute mental illness. The EMT should always follow local protocols regarding transport of the psychiatric patient.

Ongoing Assessment

Whenever a patient is restrained, it is imperative that the EMT maintain a constant vigil. The EMT has eliminated the patient's ability to care for himself. The patient is completely dependent on the EMT for safety. This is no small matter. It is frightening to the patient and places the burden of the patient's safety entirely on the EMT.

The EMT should check pulses, movement, and sensation in the extremities at least every 10 minutes (Figure 32-10). The patient's ABCs should be reassessed at least every 5 minutes.

Documentation

A restraint call involves a great deal of documentation. The EMT must document the patient's condition. It is important to document the efforts that were made to avoid using the restraint before it was decided that the restraint had to be used. If medical control was contacted for orders to restrain, that contact must be documented. If a police officer ordered restraint, in some jurisdictions, then the officer's name, badge number, and agency should be noted.

Safety Tip

The safest place to sit when transporting a restrained patient is at the head of the patient. If the patient should get an arm out of the restraint, he cannot generate a great amount of force to strike the EMT. The arm muscles are weaker when extended overhead.

Being at the patient's head affords the EMT the opportunity to reassure the patient, while monitoring the airway and level of consciousness.

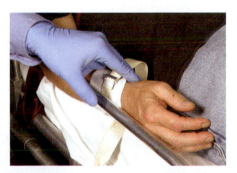

FIGURE 32-10   Distal pulses should be checked every 5–10 minutes.

Street Smart

A patient who is restrained is in a compromised position. He or she cannot defend against unwanted attacks and thus feels very vulnerable. The patient may perceive activities, such as performing a detailed physical examination, as sexual in nature.

Avoid allegations of sexual misconduct by either putting an EMT of the same sex in the patient compartment or, at least, leaving the compartment door open between the driver and the EMT. Many agencies require the EMT to call in the mileage at the start of the trip and at the end of the trip as well.

Safety Tip

The EMT should never allow a patient to talk him into releasing restraints once they have been applied. If it was deemed necessary to place the restraint, then it should remain in place until arrival at the receiving facility. It is unsafe for a sole EMT to attempt to rerestrain a previously violent patient in the back of a moving ambulance.

The method of restraint must be noted. The ongoing assessment of the patient must clearly indicate the EMT's attention to the ABCs as well as to the extremities.

PSYCHIATRIC DISORDERS

Although there are a number of psychiatric disorders, they all have some features in common. First, the patient may completely lose touch with reality or at least have distorted perceptions of reality. The patient may no longer be able to interact appropriately with the environment and does not see the world as others do. The difficulty lies in the fact that the patient's distorted perceptions of reality can eventually result in a complete loss of touch with reality.

Overall, many psychotic patients suffer from some impairment of their ability to conduct their activities of daily living (ADLs). ADLs are the human routines that sustain the person, including eating, sleeping, working, and having hobbies. When the ADLs are neglected, the patient either becomes unhealthy or becomes a danger to himself.

These patients are truly in need of prompt medical attention. Medications and psychiatric intervention can help these patients regain a grasp on reality and a chance to return to normalcy.

Depression

Depression is a condition in which sadness and despair predominate the moods of a person. These feelings become overwhelming and can lead to neglect of family, friends, and self. Depression is seen in many people, to some extent, under certain almost predictable circum-

Attempted Suicide

The woman caller on the phone was frantic: "Please hurry, I think my son may be trying to kill himself."

"Ma'am, where is your son now? Does he have any weapons?" asked the communications specialist.

As emergency units were being dispatched, the caller gave the whole story. Her son had recently completed his junior year of high school and didn't do as well as he had hoped. In fact, he would probably have to repeat the year. Coping also with the fact that his father had recently died, her son had become increasingly more withdrawn and solitary.

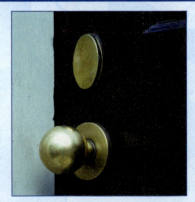

Today, however, he seemed rather upbeat for a change and went up to his room to listen to his music. That was at two o'clock. At five o'clock she called up to him to come down for dinner. When she got no answer, she went and knocked on his door. When he failed to answer her calls, she tried the door, only to find that it was locked from the inside. Frightened, she called the emergency number for help.

- What are the clinical signs and symptoms evident in this case?
- What would be the EMT's priorities on this scene?
- How should an EMT respond to a despondent patient?

stances. For example, after a severe life disappointment, a person usually goes through a period of depression. This situational depression resolves itself, usually with support from friends and family, and the person returns to normalcy.

Clinical depression occurs in about one-third of the U.S. population, at least once in their lives. Extreme emotional trauma, such as the death of a spouse, can lead to clinical depression. Table 32-3 lists some common causes of depression.

Signs and Symptoms

If the depression is severe or the patient does not have sufficient support mechanisms, the depression can lead to abnormal behavior. The patient will experience mental apathy, or melancholy. As the patient becomes increasingly depressed and despondent and starts to neglect his ADLs, *clinical depression* may ensue. This condition is present when the mental condition results in physical problems such as changes in appetite, weight gain or loss, sleeping difficulties, and illness. Table 32-4 lists signs and symptoms of clinical depression.

Assessment

When called to the scene of a depressed patient, the EMT should take careful note of her surroundings. Any description of the living conditions and any evidence of an overdose, drug use, or other means of self-harm are important to pass on to hospital personnel.

Management

In the care of the depressed patient, it is important for the EMT to be supportive. Regardless of the reason for the depression, the EMT cannot begin to understand exactly what the patient is going through. Simply to be there and to offer medical help and a hand to hold will be appreciated.

The person with severe depression is often unable to make decisions easily or quickly. Any decisions that must be made, such as which hospital to go to or which shoes to put on before transport, may need significant coaxing by the EMT. A supportive, yet decisive manner is most useful.

Safety Tip

Note that all of the causes of depression listed in Table 32-3 are common life stresses. During the course of a lifetime, most individuals develop coping mechanisms to deal with these stresses. If the individual becomes overwhelmed by these stresses, or has insufficient coping mechanisms to deal with them, the individual may become victim to depression.

EMTs encounter these stresses frequently. Both sympathy and empathy for these patients add to the stress that the EMT feels, possibly leading the EMT into depression. It is important that EMTs know how to cope with stress successfully. Chapter 4 provides some insight into commonly encountered stress in EMS and how to cope with it.

TABLE 32-3

Causes of Depression

Death of child
Loss of job
Death of spouse
Divorce
Financial catastrophe
Terminal illness

TABLE 32-4

Signs and Symptoms of Clinical Depression

Loss of appetite
Loss of weight
Overeating
Insomnia (sleeplessness)
Hypersomnia (sleeps all day)
Decreased libido (loss of sex drive)
Feelings of worthlessness, helplessness, or hopelessness
Excessive guilt
Recurrent thoughts of death
Suicidal ideation
Frequent crying
Emotional lability (mood swings)

TABLE 32-5

Methods of Suicide

Gunshot
Hanging
Drowning
Poisoning
Lacerating arteries (slashing)
Burning
Jumping from a height
Intentional overdose
Inhalation of toxic gases
Intentional motor vehicle collision

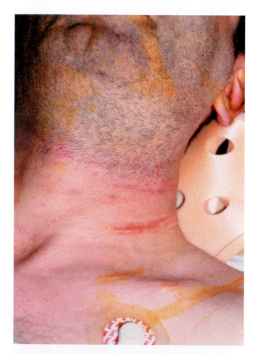

FIGURE 32-11 Suicide is the final result of depression in many cases. Note the rope marks on the neck of this man who attempted suicide. (Courtesy of Wayne Triner, DO, Albany Medical Center, Albany, NY.)

Suicide

When a patient voluntarily takes his own life, he has committed **suicide**. Suicide is a national health problem. Every year, about 25,000 Americans attempt suicide. That is one suicide attempt every 90 seconds.

Although EMTs do not perform suicide risk assessments, it is valuable for an EMT to know the risk factors of suicide so that she can have a "heads-up" attitude about suicide.

Depression is the leading risk factor for suicide. Depressed elderly males who are either divorced or widowed are at greatest risk of committing suicide. There is also an increased incidence of suicide around the holidays, when families traditionally gather. The patient remembers and misses loved ones. These feelings can lead to worsening depression and suicide. Similarly, there is an increased incidence of suicide around anniversaries and birthdays.

More females attempt suicide, but more males actually kill themselves. Any attempt at suicide is a cry for help (Figure 32-11). Although 80% of people who attempt suicide will do so repeatedly, every suicide attempt should be taken seriously. Eventually, the person will successfully kill himself if appropriate help is not obtained. Table 32-5 lists some common mechanisms encountered during an attempted suicide.

Signs and Symptoms

When assessing the potential suicidal patient, the EMT should look carefully for signs of self-inflicted injury or of illness secondary to poisoning or overdose. The specific signs and symptoms present will be related to the method of suicide that the patient attempted.

Street Smart

Many questions are raised when a dead body is discovered. The police have an interest in determining whether the person died because of suicide or murder. EMS has an interest in determining whether the patient is dead or is in need of medical treatment.

EMS and police, working together, can accomplish both missions without compromising either. Only one EMT need enter a scene to confirm the patient's condition. Carefully noting what she touches and where she steps, and trying to preserve evidence, the EMT should approach the patient.

Once the EMT is at the patient's side, the EMT should determine whether resuscitation is possible. (Review Chapter 3 for determination of death.) If it is not, then the EMT should carefully withdraw. If the patient is in cardiac arrest and cardiopulmonary resuscitation (CPR) is needed, the EMT should consider dragging the patient, using an emergency move, to another area.

In the meantime, other EMS personnel should stand by, or stage, in an adjacent area. When the patient is brought out, then CPR may be started.

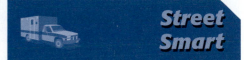

Management

In caring for the person who is suspected of being suicidal, the EMT should be direct in her questioning. It is important that she be clear whether the patient intended to harm himself or not. If there is any physical evidence of an attempt to self-harm, or if a bystander claims that the patient threatened to harm himself, the EMT should assume that the patient is a potential danger to himself. This patient must be transported to an emergency department for evaluation by a physician regardless of his desires. The EMT should treat whatever injuries she finds in a focused physical exam.

Bipolar Disorder

Manic-depressive disorder, or **bipolar disorder**, is a type of mental illness characterized by extremes of emotion ranging from total elation to deep depression.

Signs and Symptoms

One day the patient may feel all-powerful, euphoric, and full of energy. The patient can also become extremely agitated and irritable. On other days, the patient is depressed, withdrawn, and feels worthless. The patient will have all the signs and symptoms of clinical depression.

Management

The drug lithium is often prescribed to control the manic phase of the disorder. Along with lithium, an antidepressant medication may also be prescribed. Although certain medications can control the extreme emotional swings, the patient must be compliant with his medications to get the desired effect. Table 32-6 lists common antidepressants.

TABLE 32-6

Common Antidepressants	
Generic Name	**Trade Name**
Amitriptyline	Elavil
Amoxapine	Asendin
Bupropion	Wellbutrin
Doxepin	Sinequan
Fluoxetine	Prozac
Imipramine	Tofranil
Nortriptyline	Pamelor
Sertraline	Zoloft

Mentally Ill

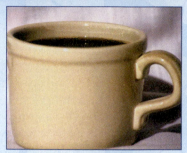

"Meet the officer, front of the coffee shop, Madison at Lark," was all the information that Maggie was given. She knew the spot. Just down the road from the psychiatric center and across from the park, it was a favorite gathering place.

Maggie pulled up next to the curb and got out. She immediately recognized Bret, the beat cop, and Mr. Gibbons, who liked to be called "Michael the archangel."

Today, it seems that Michael had tangled with a customer from the doughnut shop. The customer, frightened, had insisted that the cashier call the police for that "strange man out there." Although Michael was indeed loud, cursing, and shaking his fist skyward, he was not acting any differently than normal—that was, until Bret had asked him to quiet down and move along.

When Michael had refused, stating he had his orders from God, Bret had called for EMS. "Maggie, take him back in, and get him tuned up again," Bret ordered.

- What signs and symptoms of a psychiatric disorder are evident?
- What past medical history might be important?
- What would be the EMT's treatment priorities in this case?

The patient with bipolar disorder who seems to be out of touch with reality or in any danger of causing harm to himself or others must be transported safely to the emergency department.

Schizophrenia

Schizophrenia is a poorly understood mental disease that may be due to a neurochemical imbalance. Schizophrenia is defined by its several distinguishing elements or psychotic features.

Signs and Symptoms

In general, the schizophrenic patient is *out of touch* with reality. The patient imagines a fantasy world and lives out his life in that fantasy. Part of that fantasy may involve **hallucinations**. Hallucinations are sensations or perceptions that have no basis in reality.

For example, some patients with hallucinations may feel as if bugs are crawling on their skin. These hallucinations are called **tactile hallucinations**. In reality, there are no bugs on the patient's skin.

Other hallucinations may be **visual hallucinations**. Seeing snakes all around is an example of a visual hallucination. Finally, the patient may have an **auditory hallucination**. Hearing voices is an example of an auditory hallucination.

Management

The EMT should ask the psychotic patient, "Are you hearing voices?" Certain auditory hallucinations are called **command hallucinations**. The voices in a command hallucination are telling the patient what to do.

If the patient answers yes, continue to probe. Ask the patient what the voices are saying. Do not act surprised if the patient answers something to the effect of, "The voices say you are the devil and I should kill you." Remember that the patient is out of touch with reality. The patient does not see the EMT as someone who will help him, but rather as someone who may harm him.

Command hallucinations can be very compelling, and therefore powerful, to the patient. The patient may act violently toward the EMT. The EMT should always be prepared for a tactical retreat. Continually reassure the patient that he has control and the hallucination will pass. Encourage the patient to keep you informed of what the voices are saying. Table 32-7 lists other common psychotic features.

Patients with schizophrenia are often prescribed medications to try to calm their symptoms and help them live normal lives. These medications are called *antipsychotics*, some of which are listed in Table 32-8.

Anxiety Disorder

Anxiety is a normal response to stress. Anxiety becomes abnormal when the response is exaggerated or inappropriate to the situation. Abnormal anxieties, or **anxiety disorders**, collectively represent the largest group of mental illnesses in the United States.

The causes of anxiety disorders are varied. Table 32-9 provides a partial listing of causes of anxiety disorders. Regardless of the cause, the results are the same—exaggerated or inappropriate anxiety.

Signs and Symptoms

The patient suffering from an anxiety disorder will have symptoms of anxiety when exposed to the stimulus that he is afraid of. Sometimes the stimulus is a tangible thing, such as a bee; other times, it is not as readily found, as in the case of panic attacks. Table 32-10 lists some of the more common signs and symptoms found in the patient suffering from an anxiety disorder.

TABLE 32-7

Psychotic Features

Feature	Definition
Delusions of grandeur	False belief that the person is something he is not
Hallucinations	False perceptions having no basis in reality
Muted catatonia	Inability to speak or respond
Paranoia	Persistent persecutory delusions
Persecution complex	Belief that everyone is intent on harming the patient
Somatic illness	Complaint of illness with no physical evidence

TABLE 32-8

Common Antipsychotic Medications

Generic Name	Trade Name
Chlorpromazine	Thorazine
Clozapine	Clozaril
Fluphenazine	Prolixin
Haloperidol	Haldol
Mesoridazine	Serentil
Perphenazine	Trilafon
Thioridazine	Mellaril
Thiothixene	Navane

TABLE 32-9

Anxiety Disorders

Feature	Definition
Obsessive-compulsive disorder (OCD)	Irresistible urge to do an act repeatedly (ritualistic behavior)
Panic disorder	State of extreme uncontrollable fear; also called panic attack
Phobia	Intense and irrational fear of something (there are 700 described phobias)
Post-traumatic stress disorder (PTSD)	Maladaptive response seen after a psychologically distressing event

TABLE 32-10

Signs and Symptoms of an Anxiety Disorder

Anxiety

Diaphoresis

Dilated pupils

Fear

Hyperventilation

Palpitations

Shortness of breath

Sweatiness

Tachycardia

Tremulousness

Substance Abuse

The misuse of a drug or other substance, in order to alter the person's perception or mood, is called **substance abuse**. Substance abuse, including alcoholism, is a significant health problem in America. Substance abuse can lead to a number of chronic debilitating diseases that cost Americans almost a trillion dollars a year in health care and related costs.

Substance abuse often leads to abnormal behavior. The EMT is expected to be able to deal with the patient while the patient is under the influence of any mind-altering substance (Figure 32-12).

Often people will use illicit (illegal) drugs to alter their mood or mental state. Most illicit drugs create a heightened sense of well-being, or euphoria, called *getting high*. Often these drugs are impure. Numerous materials—including baking soda, talcum powder, and rat poison—are used to dilute, or *cut*, these drugs, in order to sell more drugs. Many of these substances are toxic. For this, and other reasons, any patient who is suspected of substance abuse should be seen in the emergency department. Table 32-11 lists some commonly abused street drugs.

As a patient repeatedly consumes certain drugs, his body will start to need that drug. This physical need for a drug is called an **addiction**. Not all drugs are physically addicting. Over time, patients may

FIGURE 32-12 Substance abuse, including drug abuse, can lead to behavioral emergencies.

Withdrawal

The war monument was a favorite hangout for the local street alcoholics and a frequent place for EMS calls. Tonight was no different. Joel was usually unkempt, but he normally was not disagreeable. Joel was what people call a "nice drunk."

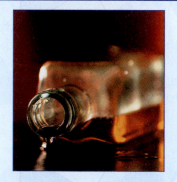

(Courtesy of PhotoDisc.)

Today, he was arguing with everybody and telling them all, "I can kick it. I don't need no help from nobody." But he confided in a friend that he did need some help, and that's how EMS appeared at the old war monument.

Approaching the scene, careful not to step on the wine bottles strewn about the ground, EMTs Campion and Hilts knelt down and asked Joel what was wrong. Joel reluctantly spoke up and said, "I've got the shakes, man. Can you help me out?"

- What signs and symptoms of substance abuse are evident?
- What past medical history might be important?
- What would be the EMTs' treatment priorities in this case?

TABLE 32-11

Commonly Abused Drugs			
Name	**Street Names**	**Source**	**Effect**
Amphetamines	Uppers, speed	Manufactured	Stimulant
Caffeine		Coffee, chocolate	Stimulant
Cocaine	Coke, crack	Coca plant	Euphoria
Hashish	Tar	Resin of cannabis	Euphoria
Heroin	H, smack, horse	Opium plant	Euphoria
Inhalants	Huffing, bagging	Lighter fluid, gas	Euphoria
Lysergic acid diethylamide (LSD)	Acid	Chemistry lab	Euphoria
Marijuana	Pot, grass, weed	Cannabis plant	Euphoria
Nicotine		Cigarettes, tobacco	Stimulant
Sedatives	Downers, barbs	Manufactured	Sedative

develop a craving for a drug. Called **dependency**, this craving is largely psychological. The combination of dependency and addiction helps to explain why drugs are so widely abused.

Overdose

When too much of a substance is ingested, inhaled, or injected into the body, the substance becomes toxic to the body. A toxin, or poison, interferes with the body's metabolism. Too much of a toxin will eventually kill the patient. Any intoxication is, by definition, an overdose of the drug.

Drug Withdrawal

Withholding a drug from an addicted patient can have many unpleasant physical and psychological effects, called **withdrawal symptoms**. Withdrawal symptoms vary widely according to the type of drug, the patient's length of addiction, and the drug's effect on the body.

A program of gradual drug withdrawal, under medical supervision, is called detoxification. A detoxification program minimizes the impact of withdrawal symptoms while ridding the body of the unwanted drug.

Withdrawal from any drug without medical supervision can be very dangerous. Sudden withdrawal from heroin, for example, can lead to sweating, tremors, diarrhea, vomiting, and cramps in the stomach and legs. Unexpected withdrawal from other drugs can lead to sudden cardiac death.

Alcohol Withdrawal

Alcoholic patients are both psychologically dependent upon and physically addicted to alcohol. Chronic alcoholism causes damage to every organ system, but especially to the liver and the heart. Common physical problems associated with chronic alcoholism are heart disease, hypertension, cirrhosis of the liver, pancreatitis (inflammation of the pancreas), and gastrointestinal problems. Alcoholic patients also suffer from depression (alcohol is a depressant), insomnia, impotence, and amnesia (blackouts).

Signs and Symptoms   For all these reasons, alcoholic patients may try to stop drinking. Within 24 hours, the patient may start to experience acute alcohol withdrawal symptoms. The symptoms of alcohol withdrawal include marked tremors (shaking), sweating, weakness, nausea, vomiting, and diarrhea. In addition, the EMT may find that the patient is tachycardiac and hypertensive.

Sudden alcohol withdrawal can lead to **delirium tremens (DTs)**. Delirium tremens is a state of mental confusion, anxiety attacks, and hyperexcitability, frequently with visual hallucinations.

Some patients may be quiet and paranoid, possibly fearful of the snakes or monsters that are frequently hallucinated. Others may be excited, trembling, or talking or yelling incoherently.

Management   Without immediate medical treatment, the patient having the DTs may experience seizures, status epilepticus, and possible cardiac arrest. The EMT should provide supportive care, including oxygen administration; close observation of the airway, breathing, and circulation; a darkened room; and quiet transportation. Any patient who is going through the DTs must be evaluated in the emergency department immediately.

CONCLUSION

Behavioral emergencies present a unique challenge to the EMT. The EMT must maintain her professional dignity, often in the face of personal attack. The EMT must attempt to assess and treat any medical conditions that may be causing the abnormal behavior. Finally, the EMT must maintain safety for both herself and her patient.

The single most important principle an EMT must keep in mind is that this is a patient, a person in need of medical attention. This patient needs her help and her compassion, despite appearances to the contrary.

TEST YOUR KNOWLEDGE

1. What is a behavioral emergency?
2. What are several reasons that a patient might have a behavioral emergency?
3. What mental illnesses could cause the patient to have a behavioral emergency?
4. What are the signs and symptoms of severe depression?

5. What is a psychotic feature?
6. What are several drugs of abuse that can lead to behavioral emergencies?
7. What are some of the behaviors an EMT can practice to protect himself on scene?
8. What does it mean when it is said that the patient was restrained out of a medical necessity?
9. What is a show of force?
10. How would a patient be restrained to a stretcher?
11. How often does an EMT check a restrained patient?

INTERNET RESOURCES

For additional information on mental illness, visit these Web sites:

- NAMI, http://www.nami.org
- National Resource Center on Homelessness and Mental Illness, http://www.nrchmi.samhsa.gov
- Rethink, http://www.rethink.org

For additional information on drug abuse, visit these Web sites:

- National Institute on Drug Abuse, http://www.nida.nih.gov
- National Youth Anti-Drug Media Campaign, http://www.theantidrug.com

For additional information related to suicide, visit these Web sites:

- American Association of Suicidology, http://www.suicidology.org
- American Foundation for Suicide Prevention, http://www.afsp.org
- Suicide Awareness Voices of Education, http://www.save.org

FURTHER STUDY

Abdon-Beckman, D. (1997). An awkward position: Restraints and sudden death. *Journal of Emergency Medical Services, 22*(3), 88.

Ball, R. (1998). Waiting to exhale—Treatment of hyperventilation. *Journal of Emergency Medical Services, 23*(1), 62–69.

Doyle, T., & Vissers, R. (1999). An EMS approach to psychiatric emergencies. *Emergency Medical Services, 28*(6), 87–88.

Goss, J. (1997). Somatoform disorders. *Journal of Emergency Medical Services, 22*(12), 58–64.

LeDuc, T. (1997). Depression. *Journal of Emergency Medical Services, 22*(11), 84–88.

CHAPTER 33

Abdominal Pain

KEY TERMS

abdominal aortic aneurysm (AAA)

acute coronary syndrome (ACS)

appendicitis

bowel obstruction

cholecystitis

diverticulitis

ectopic pregnancy

esophageal varices

gastroenteritis

hematochezia

hemetemesis

melena

pancreatitis

pyelonephritis

renal stone

ulcer

OBJECTIVES

Upon completion of this chapter, the reader should be able to:

1. Identify the organs that lie within each quadrant of the abdomen.
2. Describe the more common diseases affecting abdominal organs that may cause abdominal pain.
3. Identify two extra-abdominal conditions that can cause a complaint of abdominal pain.
4. Discuss the assessment techniques used during the management of the responsive patient complaining of abdominal pain.
5. Discuss the assessment techniques used during the management of the unresponsive patient who may have complained of abdominal pain.
6. Describe the management priorities for a patient with abdominal pain.

OVERVIEW

Abdominal pain is the most common complaint of patients visiting emergency departments, accounting for 57 of every 1,000 adult visits in the United States. Accordingly, abdominal pain is a common reason for a call to emergency medical services (EMS). While the etiology of the pain does not usually impact the emergency management provided by an emergency medical technician (EMT), it is useful for pre-hospital providers to understand the potential for serious illness when a patient complains of abdominal pain. This chapter describes the more common nontraumatic conditions that cause abdominal pain and outlines the appropriate management techniques to be utilized by the EMT.

ANATOMY REVIEW

Prior to a detailed discussion of the management of patients with abdominal pain, it is wise to briefly review the relevant anatomy that was introduced in Chapter 5. The abdomen is defined as the space

My Belly Hurts

Mr. Jones feebly attempted a smile when he saw the EMT enter the room. Sarah, an EMT on duty with the Keene Volunteer Rescue Squad, approached the elderly man and noted his pale, sweaty skin and saw that he was leaning significantly in the chair he was sitting in. After performing an initial assessment and administering oxygen, Sarah listened to Mr. Jones explain that he had been experiencing a tearing pain in the center of his abdomen that radiated toward his back for approximately one hour. When he became dizzy and nearly passed out he decided to call EMS.

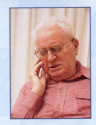

- What are the priorities in caring for Mr. Jones?
- Should he be managed as a low-priority or high-priority patient?
- What should the medical assessment focus on?

bordered superiorly by the muscular diaphragm, posteriorly by the retroperitoneum, anteriorly and laterally by the abdominal wall musculature, and inferiorly by the bony pelvis. This is illustrated in Figure 33-1.

There are several organ systems contained within the abdomen. The digestive organs of the gastrointestinal tract include the stomach, small and large intestines, liver, gallbladder, and pancreas. These organs are responsible for a number of things, most notably perhaps is digestion of nutrients that are ingested.

The genitourinary system, comprised of the kidneys, ureters, and bladder excrete bodily wastes and maintain a fluid and electrolyte balance within the body. Additionally, while the male genitals are largely located outside the borders of the abdomen, both male and female genital organs serve important functions in hormone regulation and can lead to abdominal pain when disease occurs.

The spleen and blood vessels that are located in the abdomen are part of the hematologic system and are involved in the flow of blood through the body. Figure 33-2 illustrates the location of each of these organs within the abdomen.

When discussing abdominal anatomy, it is useful to use the commonly known topographic descriptions noted in Figure 33-3. While this is not the only means of describing abdominal anatomy, it is likely the most commonly utilized in the prehospital setting.

CAUSES OF ABDOMINAL PAIN

While there are many disease processes that can cause a patient to have abdominal pain, the specific etiology may not be obvious to the EMT. The focused history and physical exam may lend clues to the underlying problem, but the EMT will often not have sufficient information to exclude the presence of a serious illness. For this reason, the patient with abdominal pain should be treated aggressively by the EMT, assuming the presence of a significant disease process. Because of this potential, advanced life support (ALS) involvement is often indicated in the prehospital management of the patient with abdominal pain. Local protocols govern this practice.

Abdominal wall musculature (lateral and anterior borders)

Diaphragm (superior border)

Pelvic floor (inferior border)

FIGURE 33-1   The abdomen has defined borders.

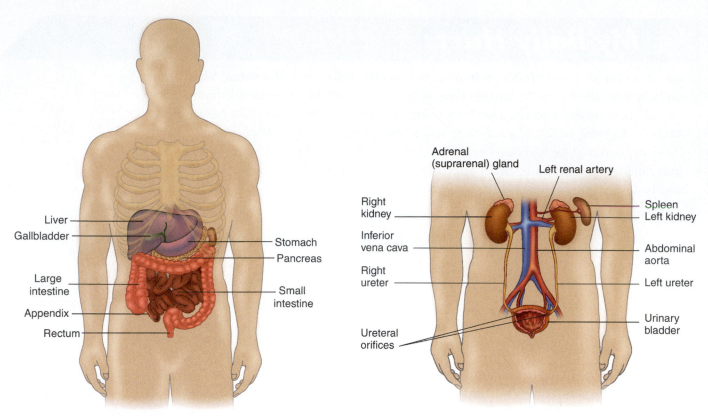

FIGURE 33-2 Several organ systems are found within the abdomen.

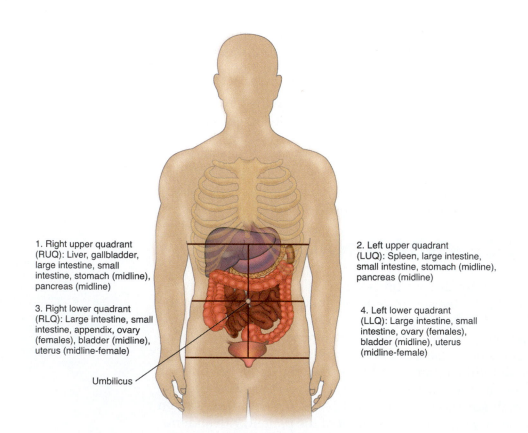

1. Right upper quadrant (RUQ): Liver, gallbladder, large intestine, small intestine, stomach (midline), pancreas (midline)

2. Left upper quadrant (LUQ): Spleen, large intestine, small intestine, stomach (midline), pancreas (midline)

3. Right lower quadrant (RLQ): Large intestine, small intestine, appendix, ovary (females), bladder (midline), uterus (midline-female)

4. Left lower quadrant (LLQ): Large intestine, small intestine, ovary (females), bladder (midline), uterus (midline-female)

FIGURE 33-3 Abdominal topography can be described in four quadrants.

The EMT should treat the patient with abdominal pain for the potential of serious illness and appropriately manage shock and other obvious threats to life found during the initial assessment. The determination of a diagnosis is not necessary in order to provide these basic treatments; however, it is useful for the EMT to have a basic knowledge of the specific conditions that can cause abdominal pain.

Gastrointestinal

The gastrointestinal system is comprised of the organs involved in digestion of foods. This system begins at the mouth and includes all of the organs pictured in Figure 33-4.

Disease in any part of the gastrointestinal system can cause abdominal pain. Alteration of the function of this system can result in serious imbalances in the body's fluid and electrolyte balance as well as in the stores of glucose. Some of the more common disease processes originating in this system are described next.

Peptic Ulcer Disease

The stomach is normally responsible for producing acid that is effective in breaking down foods for digestion. These acids are powerful and have the potential to cause injury to the lining of the stomach as well, if protective mechanisms are not in place. When these protective mechanisms are not functional, the result can be irritation of the stomach lining or even erosion through the entire wall of the stomach

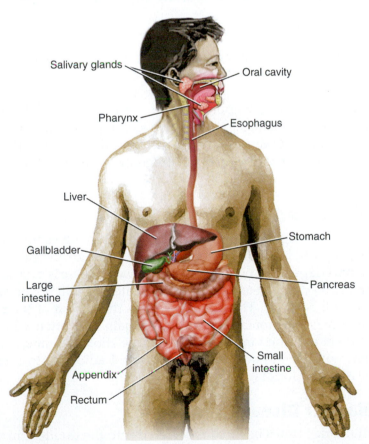

FIGURE 33-4 The gastrointestinal sytem includes all organs involved in the digestion of food.

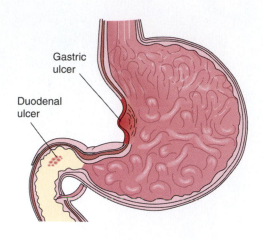

Gastric
ulcer

Duodenal
ulcer

FIGURE 33-5 Peptic ulcer disease can cause gastric or duodenal ulcers.

(Figure 33-5). Such erosion is referred to as a gastric **ulcer**. Ulcers occur commonly in the first part of the duodenum as well. If an ulcer involves a blood vessel, serious bleeding can occur. The patient with an ulcer may have abdominal pain located in the middle of the upper abdomen, often referred to as the epigastrium. If the ulcer involves a blood vessel the patient may vomit blood, called **hemetemesis**.

Additionally, blood that passes through the gastrointestinal tract will undergo some digestion, resulting in black-colored, tarry stools. This type of stool is characteristic of bleeding in the upper gastrointestinal tract and is called **melena**. Significant blood loss can occur as a result of a bleeding ulcer. The EMT should be aware of the potential for hemorrhagic shock. Definitive treatment involves reduction of acids and enhancement of protective mechanisms within the stomach. In severe cases surgery may be required to repair perforations of the stomach.

Esophageal Varices

There are veins that run through the distal esophagus that can, in certain disease states, become distended and rupture, resulting in massive uncontrolled bleeding. These distended veins are called **esophageal varices** and are most commonly seen in patients with severe liver disease. A patient with ruptured esophageal varices will present with repeated episodes of hemetemesis and likely signs of shock. This patient may or may not complain of pain. The mortality associated with such an event is 50% even with treatment. Hospital treatment involves halting the bleeding and replacing the lost blood.

Gastroenteritis

Usually a viral irritation of the stomach and intestines, **gastroenteritis** is a condition that results in vomiting, diarrhea, and, often, abdominal pain and fever. If vomiting and diarrhea are profuse, gastroenteritis can lead to significant dehydration and hypovolemic shock. Definitive goals in management involve slowing the fluid losses and ensuring adequate hydration. While the condition is most often self-limiting, in its most severe form, gastroenteritis can result in significant morbidity and mortality.

Bowel Obstruction

Normal functioning of the gastrointestinal tract involves the passage of solids, liquids, and gases from one end through the other. This movement is dependent on a clear passageway. If there is a narrowing or complete blockage at any point, these materials will not be able to pass and will back up. This backup causes distension of the bowel and sometimes the stomach, resulting in pain and often vomiting. Such a **bowel obstruction** can have multiple etiologies, and curative treatment will depend on the specific cause. Radiologic testing will often be required for diagnosis.

Gallbladder Disease

The gallbladder stores bile that is secreted into the duodenum when needed to assist in absorption of fatty foods. Occasionally, solid material can accumulate in the gallbladder, forming gallstones. These gall-

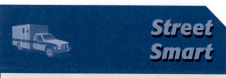

Street Smart

Blood that collects in the stomach can undergo some digestion over time. When vomiting occurs the black/brown appearance of this blood is often referred to as "coffee grounds." This is in contrast to bright red emesis, which is due to fresh bleeding. In either case blood loss may be significant.

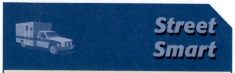

Street Smart

The patient with bleeding from esophageal varices may have such massive hemetemesis that her ability to maintain her own airway may be in jeopardy. The EMT should be prepared to intervene if needed.

stones can cause a blockage of bile flow (Figure 33-6), resulting in distension of the gallbladder and pain. This distention can lead to inflammation and infection of the wall of the gallbladder. This condition is called **cholecystitis** and results in fever, right upper abdominal pain, and often vomiting. Backup of bile can result in excess accumulation of its components in the bloodstream, resulting in a yellow color to the skin, called jaundice. Jaundice is commonly seen in gallbladder disease. Decompression or surgical removal of the gallbladder is sometimes indicated.

Appendicitis

The appendix is a narrow appendage at the junction of the small and large intestines, often located in the right lower quadrant of the abdomen. In 6% of the American population, the appendix becomes obstructed with some solid material, distends, and may rupture (Figure 33-7). This condition is called **appendicitis** and presents most often with right lower abdominal pain. Other associated symptoms may include poor appetite, nausea, and fever. Surgical removal of the appendix is necessary.

Diverticulitis

Many people have small outpouchings of the large bowel called diverticuli. They are most commonly found in the descending colon located in the left side of the abdomen, although they can be found throughout the large intestine. If one of these diverticuli becomes obstructed, it can distend, become inflamed, and perforate similar to the process described in appendicitis (Figure 33-8). When diverticuli become diseased, the resulting condition is called **diverticulitis**. Patients with diverticulitis complain of abdominal pain and may notice red blood in their stool. Passage of bright red blood from the rectum is known as **hematochezia** and is usually indicative of a disease process in the lower gastrointestinal tract. Diverticulitis may require surgery in severe cases.

Pancreatitis

One of the jobs of the pancreas is to secrete enzymes into the duodenum that aid in digestion. If the ducts that contain these digestive enzymes become blocked, they can become distended and result in inflammation of the organ. Inflammation of the pancreas is called **pancreatitis** and often results in severe upper abdominal pain and vomiting. Patients with pancreatitis can become quite ill and may require prolonged hospitalization.

Genitourinary

While there are many disease processes that involve the genitourinary tract, we discuss the more common acute conditions that might result in a call for EMS assistance.

Renal Stones

As blood flows through the kidneys, salts and water are filtered out into the ureters as urine. Sometimes there can be particulate material

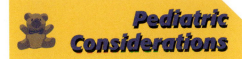

Pediatric Considerations

Children are much more sensitive than adults to fluid losses. A small child who has gastroenteritis may quickly develop life-threatening hypovolemic shock.

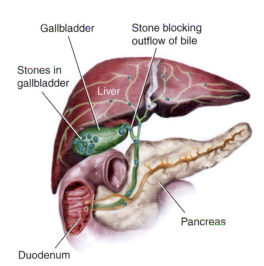

FIGURE 33-6 Gallstones can block the outflow of bile from the gallbladder.

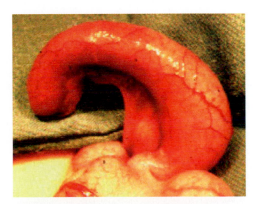

FIGURE 33-7 Definitive treatment for appendicitis is surgical removal of the inflamed appendix. (Courtesy of the Division of Pediatric Surgery, Brown Medical School, Providence, RI.)

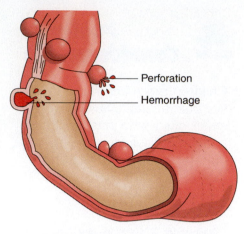

FIGURE 33-8 Diverticuli can perforate or cause internal bleeding.

that crystallizes in the urine, resulting in a formed piece of solid material referred to as a stone. These **renal stones** can become lodged in the ureter during attempted passage to the bladder. Severe flank pain is often experienced by the patient who has a renal stone that has become lodged in a ureter. Classically, the pain radiates along the anatomy of the genitourinary system, that is, from the flank to the groin. Vomiting is also common, and pain medications are crucial to the management of this condition. While renal stones are not immediately life threatening, the pain can often be quite severe and rapid transport is most appreciated by affected patients.

Pyelonephritis

Infection of the urinary tract can involve the bladder alone, or may ascend through the ureters into the kidneys, resulting in **pyelonephritis**. The kidneys are extremely well vascularized and when bacteria are allowed to infiltrate these organs, the risk of the infection spreading into the bloodstream is high.

Patients who have infections involving the kidneys may have pain over one or both flanks, vomiting, and high fever. This type of severe infection can result in significant morbidity and mortality if not rapidly treated with appropriate antibiotics. Patients with pyelonephritis may require hospitalization for intravenous antibiotic therapy.

Ectopic Pregnancy

In a small percentage of pregnancies, implantation occurs outside the uterus. This is called an **ectopic pregnancy**. The most common place for an ectopic pregnancy to occur is in a fallopian tube (Figure 33-9).

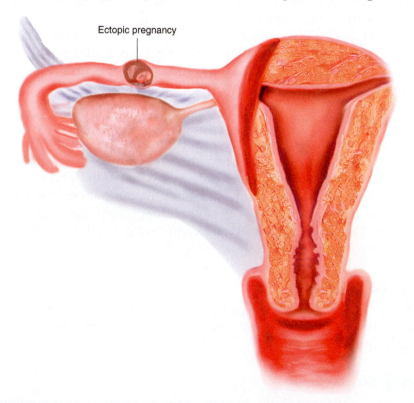

FIGURE 33-9 An ectopic pregnancy will rapidly outgrow the confines of the fallopian tube.

As you might imagine, as the pregnancy advances, the fallopian tube would not be large enough to accommodate its occupant. Sometime between 6 and 12 weeks (often before some women realize they are pregnant) the fallopian tube becomes quite distended and is in danger of rupturing. If this should happen the results would be catastrophic bleeding. For this reason, ectopic pregnancy is the second leading cause of maternal mortality in the United States. Early symptoms of this condition might be lower abdominal pain with or without vaginal bleeding in a woman of childbearing age. The woman may or may not realize she is pregnant so it is important for the EMT to consider the possibility of this life-threatening condition in any woman of childbearing age who complains of lower abdominal pain. Careful evaluation by a physician and sometimes surgical intervention is required. Ectopic pregnancy is further discussed in Chapter 36.

Vascular

There are several large blood vessels that pass through the abdominal cavity. Disease within these vessels can result in abdominal pain, or, in some cases, what patients perceive as back pain since the aorta and vena cava lie rather posteriorly in the retroperitoneal space.

Abdominal Aortic Aneurysm

The abdominal aorta carries blood at arterial pressures out of the chest and to the abdominal organs and lower extremities. As a person ages, the structure of the arteries may change. In some cases, the walls of the vessels may become weakened, allowing a ballooning out to occur. This balloonlike widening of a weakened artery is called an aneurysm. When this occurs in the section of the aorta passing through the abdomen, it is called an **abdominal aortic aneurysm (AAA)**. If the wall of the aneurysm becomes stretched thin enough, it may leak or rupture. This leads to massive bleeding and death if not rapidly repaired. Even with immediate surgical treatment, many patients who suffer from a rupture of an aortic aneurysm will die. Typical symptoms of an AAA might include abdominal or back pain. If there has been any blood loss, evidence of shock may be noted. Syncope is not uncommon as the presenting complaint with a ruptured AAA due to the rapid loss of blood and resultant profound shock.

Extra-Abdominal

There are some conditions that can commonly cause the patient to feel abdominal pain when the pathology is not in the abdomen at all. These are referred to as extra-abdominal sources of abdominal pain. The reason for this is complex but has to do with shared sensory nerves between the diseased organ and the abdomen. The more common serious conditions that mimic an abdominal emergency are discussed next.

Acute Coronary Syndrome

Women and patients who suffer from diabetes are at higher risk than other populations to have atypical symptoms of an **acute coronary syndrome (ACS)**. These patients may not describe the chest pain and

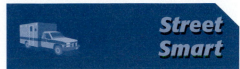

Street Smart

In some cases, a pulsatile mass may be felt or seen on abdominal exam, corresponding to a large aneurysm. The importance of gentle abdominal examination and gentle handling of the patient in this case cannot be overstated. Unnecessary force put on an already weakened vessel can lead to rupture. If a pulsatile mass is noted in the abdomen, no further palpation should occur at the hands of the EMT.

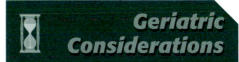

Geriatric Considerations

While an AAA may occur at any age, the majority of patients who require treatment for this condition are over the age of 60. The EMT should keep this life-threatening diagnosis in mind when caring for patients in this age group with complaints of abdominal pain.

Safety Tip

The EMT must always remember to take precautions and don the personal protective equipment that is appropriate to the situation. A patient with coughing may have a respiratory infection that may be transmitted through respiratory secretions. Consideration of a mask would be appropriate in this case.

shortness of breath that are commonly associated with a heart problem. In fact, abdominal complaints are not uncommon as symptoms of ACS in these patients and others as well. Yet another potential life-threatening diagnosis presenting with abdominal pain, the EMT must consider ACS when a patient has risk factors for such. Appropriate management for this potential is crucial to decrease morbidity and mortality associated with this condition, discussed in detail in Chapter 28.

Pneumonia

Fairly common in children and occasionally in adults, pneumonia can cause abdominal pain. Typically, the patient with pneumonia has some symptoms consistent with this respiratory infection, such as cough, fever, or difficulty breathing. While the EMT may have been called for a patient with abdominal pain, if upon assessment the patient appears to be short of breath, appropriate action must be taken as outlined in Chapter 27.

ASSESSMENT

The assessment of the patient complaining of abdominal pain will follow the principles of those for the medical patient detailed in Chapter 16. As always, the first task is to perform a scene size-up and ensure the safety of the situation for the EMT and his team.

Initial Assessment

The initial assessment is always completed next and must include the EMT's general impression as he initially views the patient. It is important to take note of the environment as well as the appearance of the patient as the EMT approaches. The findings of the initial assessment will guide the remainder of the assessment. If the patient is responsive, the airway, breathing, and circulation are assessed and any immediate life threats are addressed appropriately.

Because many of the disease states that can cause abdominal pain can be a threat to life, the EMT must assume that possibility and manage the patient as a high priority. The airway should be addressed as needed and any necessary breathing assistance should be provided. Even when the patient is not having trouble breathing, supplemental oxygen should be applied in patients with abdominal pain, given the potential for shock. The patient's circulatory status should be assessed and managed as appropriate, with the Trendelenburg position utilized for signs of hypoperfusion.

Focused History

When the patient is able to provide the history of the present illness, the EMT should listen carefully to the events leading up to the call for EMS. An acronym that is sometimes used to guide the gathering of such details is OPQRST. Chapter 16 discusses this in detail and should be reviewed.

Additionally, questions about the patient's past medical history following the SAMPLE (see Table 10-5) format should be asked. If the patient is unable to provide this information, friends, family members, or bystanders should be briefly questioned.

In the unresponsive patient, this historical information will be obtained only after the EMT performs a rapid medical assessment as detailed in Chapter 16. If staffing permits, while the EMT performs this assessment, another member of the team can obtain important details from people nearby the patient.

Focused Physical Exam

In the responsive patient, a focused physical exam should be completed after the history has been taken. In a patient with a complaint of abdominal pain, the EMT should pay careful attention to the assessment of the abdomen. This assessment should include visual inspection and palpation.

Palpation of the abdomen should be done gently, beginning in an area farthest from the noted site of pain. The EMT should press down in each of the four quadrants of the abdomen. He should note the patient's response to pressure in each area. Tensing of muscles over an area of pain is called guarding and is worthy of note. Sometimes, the entire abdomen will feel tense, or rigid, when the intra-abdominal process is generalized. This finding of abdominal rigidity is also important to note. Any obvious masses felt during this examination should be documented carefully. It is important that one person only perform the abdominal palpation when possible. Repeated palpation of the abdomen in a patient complaining of abdominal pain is unnecessary and uncomfortable for the patient.

In the unresponsive patient, the EMT should perform a head-to-toe assessment as detailed in Chapter 16, looking for any signs that might point to the reason for unresponsiveness. If it is known that the patient complained of abdominal pain prior to losing consciousness, careful attention should be paid to the abdominal exam during this rapid medical assessment.

Vital Signs

The initial and repeated measurement of respirations, pulse, and blood pressure can provide important information regarding the state of a patient's health. This should be done immediately after the rapid medical assessment in the unresponsive patient and may be accomplished after the focused physical exam in the responsive patient.

As discussed in this chapter, abdominal pain can be a symptom that represents any one of a number of disease states that can lead to shock and hypoperfusion. Careful attention to the vital signs will be paramount as the EMT assesses the patient for signs of shock. The measurement of orthostatic vital signs in the awake patient may be appropriate to assess for signs of hypovolemia. This measurement of blood pressure and heart rate in a supine and standing position is discussed in Chapter 9.

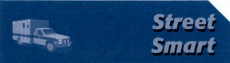

Street Smart

When a patient complains of abdominal pain, it is important to ask her to indicate with her own hand exactly where she notes the pain. This allows the examiner to avoid the painful area early on in the assessment. Immediately pressing on a painful area during an assessment may cause the patient such upset that the remainder of the assessment may be unreliable or difficult to complete.

MANAGEMENT

It is important to remember that there are many potential causes of abdominal pain and that as many as 50% may go undiagnosed. Regardless of the cause, the principles of early management are the same in all cases. Some patients with abdominal pain may be profoundly ill upon presentation to EMS, others may be early in the course of their illness, and yet others may have a non–life-threatening cause for their pain. In any case, the EMT is responsible to thoroughly assess the patient and assume the potential for serious disease. Management of the airway, breathing, and circulation will be appropriate for any patient with abdominal pain during transport to definitive care.

TRANSPORT

Transport should be initiated as soon as it is possible during the previously described phases of assessment. It is important to maintain the patients in whatever position they find most comfortable during movement and ambulance transport. Often in patients with abdominal pain, drawing the knees up toward the abdomen can be of comfort and should be allowed. The mode of transport and destination facility will be determined based on the patient presentation and local protocols.

In most patients with abdominal pain, ALS assistance would be of potential benefit, although transport should not be delayed. An intercept during transport would be appropriate, although the EMT should take note of local protocols regarding this issue. Additionally, early notification of the receiving facility will ensure that it is adequately prepared for the arrival of a potentially ill patient.

Ongoing Assessment

As with any patient, it is important to continually observe for changes in assessment findings. As described in Chapter 17, the key parts of the assessment should be repeated during the transport and any changes noted carefully and passed on to the receiving staff at the hospital.

CONCLUSION

The EMT will have multiple occasions to care for patients with the complaint of abdominal pain. Some patients will be overtly ill with clear evidence of shock upon presentation. Others may not show physical evidence of hypoperfusion or have abnormal physical findings upon the initial examination. All patients with abdominal pain, no matter their initial presentation, have the potential for serious morbidity and mortality. The EMT must realize this and structure his management priorities around it.

TEST YOUR KNOWLEDGE

1. Name the organs that lie within the following abdominal quadrants.

   a. Right upper quadrant

   b. Left upper quadrant

   c. Right lower quadrant

   d. Left lower quadrant

2. What are some of the more common diseases affecting abdominal organs that may cause abdominal pain?

3. Name two extra-abdominal conditions that can cause a complaint of abdominal pain.

4. What type of assessment would be appropriate for these two types of patients?

   a. The responsive patient complaining of abdominal pain

   b. The unresponsive patient who may have complained of abdominal pain

5. What are the management priorities for a patient with abdominal pain?

INTERNET RESOURCES

There are many Internet resources that can be accessed to review the different etiologies for abdominal pain. Search the Internet for specific conditions or try these sites.

- MedicineNet, http://www.medicinenet.com
- MedlinePlus, http://www.nlm.nih.gov/medlineplus

FURTHER STUDY

Beebe, R., Scott, A., & Fong, E. (2002). *Functional anatomy for emergency medical services*. Clifton Park, NY: Thomson Delmar Learning.

CHAPTER 34

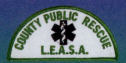

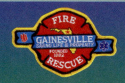

Environmental Emergencies

KEY TERMS

active rewarming

acute mountain sickness

afterdrop

air embolism

black widow spider

Boyle's law

brown recluse spider

chilblains

conduction

convection

coral snake

decompression sickness

evaporation

frostbite

frostnip

heat cramps

heat exhaustion

heat stroke

high-altitude cerebral
edema (HACE)

high-altitude pulmonary
edema (HAPE)

hyperbaric chamber

near-drowning

nitrogen narcosis

passive rewarming

pit viper

(continues)

OBJECTIVES

Upon completion of this chapter, the reader should be able to:

1. Describe the various mechanisms by which the body loses heat.
2. Describe the various mechanisms by which the body generates heat.
3. Identify local cold injuries and describe the proper treatment for these conditions.
4. List signs and symptoms of generalized hypothermia.
5. Describe the emergency medical care of the patient with generalized hypothermia.
6. List signs and symptoms of heat exhaustion and heat stroke and differentiate between the two.
7. Describe the emergency medical care of the patient with heat exhaustion and heat stroke.
8. Identify the complications of near-drowning.
9. Describe the emergency medical care of the near-drowning victim.
10. Identify signs and symptoms of diving-related emergencies.
11. Describe the emergency medical care of diving-related emergencies.
12. Identify signs and symptoms of altitude emergencies.
13. Describe the emergency medical care of altitude emergencies.
14. Identify the priorities in caring for the victim of a lightning strike.
15. Describe the emergency medical care of a victim of a bite or a sting.

OVERVIEW

The emergency medical technician (EMT) will be called to care for patients who have been exposed to various environmental dangers. It is important that prehospital providers recognize when environmental factors, such as heat or cold exposure, cause a medical emergency.

The principles of emergency medical care for the patient suffering from heat or cold exposure are dependent upon the EMT's recognizing the problem.

In addition to simple exposure to the elements, many outdoor activities may create other emergencies that the EMT must be familiar with. Water and altitude emergencies, lightning strikes, bites, and stings will be reviewed so that the EMT may be better prepared to recognize and deal with problems related to these environmental issues.

TEMPERATURE REGULATION

The human body functions within a very narrow range of temperature. If the body temperature is allowed to go outside of this narrow range, organ systems may malfunction.

A part of the brain called the hypothalamus is largely involved in temperature regulation. This centrally located part of the brain controls the body's set point, which can be thought of as the ideal temperature that the body wants to settle at for a particular time. For the most part, that temperature is within one degree of normal body temperature. Normal body temperature is 98.6°F, or 37°C.

The body is constantly faced with things that cause heat loss. On the other hand, many normal body activities generate heat that may need to be released. **Thermoregulation** can be thought of as an attempt to balance the amount of heat lost and heat gained in order to maintain a constant body temperature.

Heat Loss

Because the body generates heat with nearly every metabolic activity, there is a need to get rid of excess heat. There are four general ways that heat can be removed from the body: radiation, convection, conduction, and evaporation.

Radiation

Radiation accounts for about 60% of the heat lost from the body at normal room temperatures. It is defined as the transfer of heat from the warm body into the cooler environment just by the fact that a temperature gradient exists. Warmth will leave the body and move into the cooler surrounding environment. Radiation is seen when a person who feels very hot steps into an air-conditioned room and suddenly feels cooler. The excess heat is being dispersed into the cooler environment. Figure 34-1 illustrates this means of heat loss. Of course, when the ambient temperature rises, less heat will be dispersed in this manner.

Convection

Air currents passing by a warm surface will pick up heat and transfer it away from that surface. This means of heat loss can be important to people out of doors and is called **convection**. This can be illustrated by thinking of a person who feels very hot, then stands in front of a fan and feels cooler. The excess heat is moved away from the person

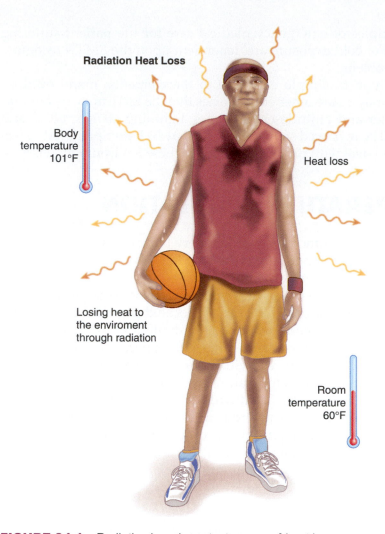

Radiation Heat Loss

Body temperature 101°F

Heat loss

Losing heat to the enviroment through radiation

Room temperature 60°F

FIGURE 34-1 Radiation is an important means of heat loss.

by the cooler currents of air moving past. Figure 34-2 depicts the concept of heat loss by convection.

Conduction

If a warm object is in direct contact with a cooler object, heat will be transferred to the cooler object. This **conduction** of heat happens regularly when injured patients are left lying on the cold ground. It is important that EMTs be aware of this means of heat loss in order to prevent excess heat loss from occurring in their patients. Conduction is illustrated in Figure 34-3.

Evaporation

Another major means of heat loss in warm environments is **evaporation**. This involves the transfer of heat into body fluids such as sweat, which then dissipates as it evaporates. Evaporation accounts for about 30% of the body's normal heat loss. If the humidity in the environment is high, the moisture on the body's surface will not evaporate; therefore, no heat loss occurs in this manner.

A large part of the heat lost by evaporation is via the moisture in the respiratory tract. During ventilation, the movement of air into and out

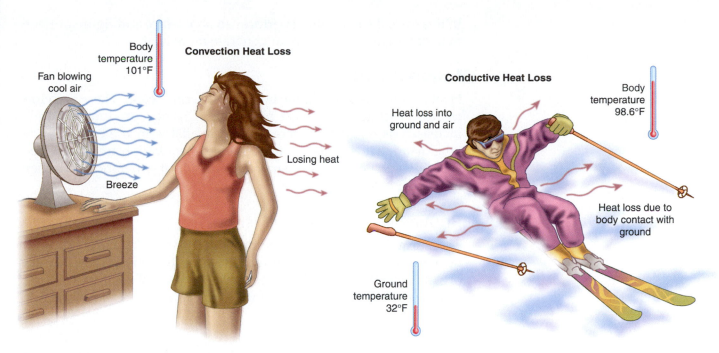

FIGURE 34-2   Convection is a mechanism that allows for heat loss.

FIGURE 34-3   Conductive heat loss is a means of heat dispersal.

of the lungs allows significant loss of moisture, and therefore of heat. Figure 34-4 illustrates evaporative heat loss from surface perspiration and from the respiratory tract.

Maximizing Heat Loss

Understanding the four major means of losing heat from the body, you can imagine several ways that the body can maximize their use. In particularly warm environments, sweating usually occurs. The skin may become flushed, and the rate of breathing and the heart rate will likely increase. All of these are reactions that the body has to maximize heat loss by these different mechanisms.

Sweating and increasing the respiratory rate increase heat loss by evaporation. The flushed skin is a result of superficial vasodilation, which brings more of the blood up toward the surface, where it may come into closer contact with the cooler environment for additional loss of heat. Increasing the heart rate will increase the number of times the blood passes close to the surface of the body, where it can dissipate some excess heat.

Heat Gain

Having discussed the body's mechanisms for getting rid of excess heat, we must also understand how the body gains heat. Heat gain can be a desired increase in temperature to make up for heat loss somewhere else, or it can be an undesirable increase and the heat gained must then be dissipated in some way.

As already mentioned, the normal metabolism of the body produces heat. In particularly cold environments, the amount of heat lost may be greater than the amount generated with normal metabolism.

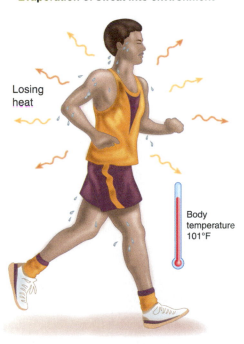

FIGURE 34-4   Humans utilize evaporation to disperse excess heat from the body.

In this case, the body must perform an about-face and figure out how to maintain its temperature or generate more heat.

Internal Sources

Heat is generated inside the body by several means. These activities create a baseline level of heat generation. This heat production may be increased as needed to increase heat available in the body. On the other hand, if these internal means of heat generation are diminished, the body will not have its usual amount of heat generation, and there may be a net loss in heat.

Routine Cellular Metabolism

The normal functioning of the body generates a certain amount of heat via metabolism. The minute-to-minute activity of cells and organs generates heat. Increased activity would create more heat. Decreased activity would generate less heat.

Muscle Contraction

The other major internal means of heat generation comes from contraction of muscles. As individual muscles contract, heat is produced. Heat generation by muscle contraction explains the rise in body temperature noted after heavy exercise or seizure activity. Both involve plenty of muscle contraction.

The body may also create extra muscle contraction when a rise in temperature is desired. These extra muscle contractions are seen as shivering. Shivering is a very effective means of increasing heat generation and creating a net rise in heat gain and therefore a rise in body temperature.

External Sources

Body heat can also be gained from external sources. Just as heat can be lost into a cooler environment, heat can be gained from a warmer environment. In extremely hot environments, such as in a sauna or very hot weather, the body will gain heat if the ambient temperature is higher than the body temperature.

Preservation of Body Heat

Just as the body has means of maximizing heat loss by vasodilation, sweating, and increased respiratory rate and cardiac output, heat gain can also be maximized in an attempt to preserve body temperature in a cold environment.

Vasoconstriction will draw warm blood away from the surface of the skin to prevent heat loss to a cooler environment. *Piloerection* is a term that simply refers to hair standing up, essentially goosebumps. This primitive reflex is an attempt to maintain body heat.

Shivering in a cold environment will increase the body's production of heat. Stimulation of the sympathetic nervous system will result in an elevated heart rate and will increase the body's metabolic rate, causing a greater amount of internal heat production.

Recognition of these signs of heat preservation may enable the EMT to more quickly identify a patient suffering from an environmental medical emergency.

Individual Factors

There are individual factors that may impair a person's ability to maintain body temperature within the ideal range.

Extremes of Age

Persons at extremes of age may be unable to protect themselves from extremes of heat or cold. This inability may be a result of physiologic issues, or these patients may simply not be able to remove themselves from the hot or cold environment or may not be capable of taking proper precautions, such as wearing protective clothing for the temperature. The EMT should be extra vigilant for temperature-related problems in infants and elderly patients.

Medical Conditions

In addition to extremes of age, any person who has chronic medical problems is likely to be at risk of having impaired thermoregulatory ability. Conditions such as diabetes, cardiac disease, thyroid disease, and many other chronic disease states put a patient at higher risk of suffering a heat- or cold-related illness due to an impaired ability to adequately balance heat loss and heat gain.

Acute medical problems such as shock, head injury, burns, generalized infections, injuries to the spinal cord, or hypoglycemia can also impair a patient's thermoregulatory ability. The EMT must therefore be attentive to maintaining body temperature in patients with problems such as these.

Drugs

Certain medications can decrease the body's ability to maintain an appropriate body temperature. Any medication that affects the sympathetic or parasympathetic nervous system or the metabolic rate has a chance of altering the patient's thermoregulatory ability.

EMTs should be aware that patients who are taking multiple medications are at high risk of being unable to adequately protect themselves from extremes of temperature by thermoregulation.

COLD EXPOSURE

Prolonged exposure to a cold environment can result in a wide spectrum of injuries and illnesses. The EMT must be familiar with the management of local cold injuries as well as systemic cold illness.

Local Cold Injuries

The spectrum of cold illness starts at a local level. Skin injury and musculoskeletal injury as a result of cold exposure are very common and can be easily recognized and managed by the EMT.

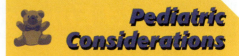

Pediatric Considerations

Infants and young children are small and have a large body surface area relative to body mass or volume because they have a smaller muscle mass and less body fat. In addition, infants cannot shiver. Instead, they have a specialized adipose tissue, called brown fat, that is stimulated by cold to produce heat.

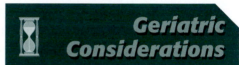

Geriatric Considerations

Elderly patients and patients with chronic medical illnesses also are at increased risk of suffering cold emergencies. They may lose their ability to sense cold and to take appropriate protective measures. The ability to increase heat production and to conserve heat may be altered by their age or by medical conditions.

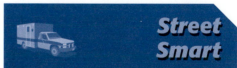

Street Smart

Most acutely ill patients will have trouble maintaining body temperature. It is therefore an important part of the management of the critically ill patient to prevent heat loss. Heat loss can easily be prevented by removing any wet clothing, moving the patient off any cold surface quickly, and covering the patient with a blanket as soon as the necessary assessment and treatment have been done.

Cold Emergency

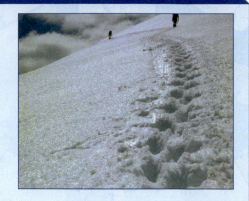

On a cold December morning around Christmas, emergency medical services (EMS) is called to meet the local forest ranger. Ranger Pete reports that he is caring for a hunter who was brought out of the woods by his friends because "he was acting drunk." The hunting buddies swore that they hadn't been drinking, so Pete, sensing something might be amiss, called EMS to check the hunter out.

The patient's buddies report that he had been with them all morning standing on watch waiting for deer. Then he suddenly got up, slowly walked a few feet from his stand, and sat down in the middle of a snowbank. He then started taking off his winter coat. When he answered their questions about what he was doing, they noticed he had notably slurred speech. His only complaint was pain in his feet and tingling in his hands.

Using a CB radio, they had contacted Ranger Pete and told him that they would meet him at the end of the old logging road just north of the river fork. They complained that they had had a difficult time getting their buddy out of the woods because he was becoming increasingly uncooperative.

- What could be wrong with this hunter?
- What are the priorities in management of this condition?
- What signs and symptoms should the EMT attempt to assess?
- What are the short- and long-term consequences of this condition?

Chilblains

Chronic exposure of skin to cool, windy, damp weather can result in painful inflamed skin lesions called **chilblains**. These patchy skin lesions are often swollen and red to bluish and cause significant itching and burning. In longer-term exposures, the skin may blister or ulcerate. Symptoms of chilblains may develop up to 12 hours after the exposure.

The area of skin that was affected will often be hypersensitive to cold after this injury, resulting in discomfort and increased chance of future cold injury. Women are particularly susceptible to this injury. The face and hands are the most commonly affected areas because they are often left exposed to the cool, damp wind.

Trench Foot

Prolonged exposure of skin to cool, wet conditions can result in a condition called **trench foot**. Trench foot refers specifically to the injury seen after wearing wet footgear or being immersed in water for a prolonged period of time. The classic patient suffering from trench foot is a soldier who has spent a prolonged period of time standing in a trench full of water.

The injured extremity will initially be cold, pale, and swollen and will have diminished sensation and circulation. After it is rewarmed, the area will become increasingly swollen, red, warm, and painful.

This stage will often last from 4 to 10 days. The patient is often left with some sensory deficit and local hypersensitivity to the cold.

Frostnip

When unprotected skin is exposed to freezing temperatures, local injury can occur that is very similar to that seen in thermal burns. The mildest form of this local cold injury is called **frostnip**. Affected skin will be blanched and numb but will be easily rewarmed, and the tissue will have no permanent damage.

Frostbite

Actual tissue damage that has occurred as a result of exposure to freezing and below-freezing temperatures is called **frostbite**. If the surface of the skin and superficial subcutaneous tissues are affected, the tissue will appear white with blisters (Figure 34-5). Tissue affected by superficial frostbite will feel soft and pliant and will flush as it is rewarmed. This type of injury is often quite painful as rewarming occurs.

When the tissue damage has extended deeper into the tendons, muscles, and nerves, the part will be cold and hard with a classic woodlike feel to it. Tissues affected by deep frostbite will be pale or mottled and will not regain circulation after rewarming. It is common for digits to become necrotic and be sloughed off (Figure 34-6).

Management of Local Cold Injuries

The management for all local cold injuries is very similar. The priorities in management include removing the patient from the cold or wet environment, removing any cold and wet articles of clothing, and rewarming the injured part.

Rewarming should involve immersion into warm water for up to 30 minutes. The less severe the injury, the less time it will take to warm it up. The EMT should attempt rewarming only if she is confident that she will be able to protect the patient from further cold injury and avoid refreezing of the injured tissue.

If circumstances prevent immediate rewarming or if refreezing is a possibility, then the affected extremity should not be rewarmed. Instead, the area should be carefully bandaged and splinted to prevent further injury during transport.

Gentle handling of the injured tissue is important to prevent any further damage. After rewarming, the part should be carefully bandaged and splinted to avoid any rough movement. When the EMT is bandaging cold-injured skin, it is important not to allow contact with other skin. Gauze padding should be placed between fingers or toes to prevent the injured tissue from sticking to the opposing skin.

Finally, the patient suffering from a local cold injury should be evaluated in the hospital for evidence of any other injuries or effects from the exposure.

General Hypothermia

When net heat loss is greater than net heat gain, body temperature will fall, resulting in a condition called hypothermia. Hypothermia can be defined as a core body temperature of less than 95°F. The severity

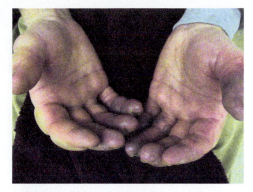

FIGURE 34-5 Superficial frostbite can be quite painful. (Courtesy of Kevin Reilly, MD, Albany Medical Center, Albany, NY.)

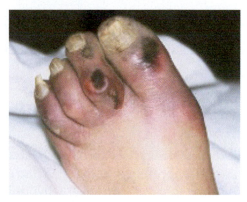

FIGURE 34-6 Deep frostbite results in permanent damage to tissue. (Courtesy of Deborah Funk, MD, Albany Medical Center, Albany, NY.)

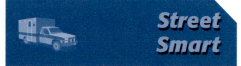

Street Smart

When rewarming the injured area, the EMT should use clean water that is warm but not too hot to touch. Generally, water that is around 104°F is adequate. If the water is too hot for the EMT to immerse her hand in, then it should be allowed to cool before immersing the patient's injured extremity in it!

Dry heat should never be used because it can cause further tissue damage.

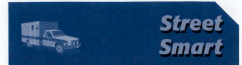

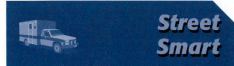

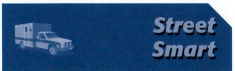

of hypothermia ranges from mild illness, when the temperature is just under 95°F, to severe hypothermia, when the body temperature is below 86°F.

Symptoms of hypothermia are related to failure of organ systems. The severity of the symptoms of this cold-related illness is directly related to the temperature. The colder the body temperature, the more dramatic the signs and symptoms. Decreasing mental status and motor function are well correlated with the increasing degree of hypothermia.

Signs and Symptoms

Some of the first signs seen in the hypothermic patient are poor coordination, memory disturbances, reduced sensation, mood changes, dizziness, and difficulty with speech. Patients suffering from early hypothermia may not realize that they are having a problem. Judgment is usually impaired, and often the hypothermic patient will begin taking off clothing, despite the cold weather. This is sometimes referred to as paradoxical undressing.

The mildly hypothermic patient will show signs of the body's attempts to maintain a normal temperature and decrease heat loss. Vasoconstriction results in pale, cool skin. Heart rate and respiratory rate are often increased. Shivering is common as the body attempts to generate additional heat.

As the body temperature falls, the above signs become more pronounced. Muscles and joints become stiff, and below 86°F shivering no longer occurs. At these low body temperatures, organ systems do not function well at all. Breathing will slow or even cease; pupils will no longer react; heart rate will slow; and blood pressure will fall. Eventually, if treatment is not provided immediately, the heart will stop completely and the patient will die.

Management

Management cannot start without recognition. The EMT should be sure to assess the skin temperature of every patient and determine whether the environment could have caused a low body temperature, given the patient's current health state. If mild hypothermia is clearly evident, the EMT must first remove the patient from the cold environment if possible. The patient should not be allowed to walk or exert himself and must be handled very gently.

The next priority in caring for the hypothermic patient is to prevent any further heat loss by removing any cold, wet clothing and covering the patient in warm blankets. Oxygen should be administered and should be warmed and humidified if possible.

Treatment that is geared toward preventing any further body heat loss is called **passive rewarming**. Actions taken to actually try to increase body temperature are considered **active rewarming**.

Active rewarming by the EMT consists of placing heat packs or hot-water bottles in the groin, axillary, and cervical regions (corresponding to areas where major vessels come close to the surface) and increasing the heat inside the ambulance (Figure 34-7). Medical control may sometimes give specific instructions to give the patient warm, high-calorie liquids by mouth. The EMT is to give liquids only if specifically instructed to do so by medical control and only if the patient is awake and able to hold the cup and drink the liquid himself. The EMT should never administer anything by mouth to a patient who has a decreased level of consciousness. Every EMT should be familiar with her local protocols regarding rewarming the hypothermic patient.

If a patient is hypothermic but is awake and responding appropriately, the EMT should institute both passive and active rewarming measures. If the patient has a decreased level of consciousness, only passive rewarming should be attempted. External active rewarming in severe hypothermia can actually cause a drop in the core body temperature. This phenomenon is referred to as **afterdrop**.

Afterdrop results when peripheral vasodilation occurs and the cold blood from the surface and extremities is shunted into the core of the body, causing a drop in core body temperature. In severe hypothermia, it is better not to attempt to actively rewarm the patient but to simply prevent further heat loss, transport the patient, and support vital signs as necessary. Other, more invasive, techniques of active rewarming can be started at the hospital, so the EMT should not delay transport of the hypothermic patient.

The profoundly hypothermic heart is very irritable and can easily go into ventricular fibrillation. At cold temperatures, defibrillation may not be effective. The EMT should always be very gentle when handling the hypothermic patient to try to prevent the onset of ventricular fibrillation as a result of rough handling. When a patient is found in cardiac arrest, the EMT should follow her usual protocols for CPR and defibrillation and should contact medical control as soon as possible (see Chapter 29 for more details).

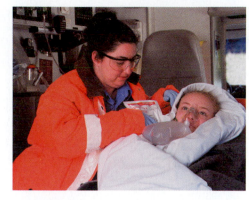

FIGURE 34-7   The EMT will likely treat patients suffering from hypothermia during cold weather.

Prevention Among Emergency Workers

As prehospital providers, EMTs will often practice in environments that do not have a controlled temperature. Many emergencies require the EMT to work outside for prolonged periods, even in very cold or very hot weather.

It is important that the EMT take steps to protect herself and her crew from adverse events related to extremes of temperature. Proper clothing for the weather is essential to working in the outdoor setting.

Several layers of clothing that can be taken off or put back on depending on the working environment are ideal for the prehospital health care worker. Gloves, hat, and face and ear protection are just as important as the heavy winter coat that keeps the body warm. Serious cold injury can occur very rapidly and affects many outdoor workers every winter. Figure 34-8 shows an EMT dressed appropriately for working outdoors on a cold winter day.

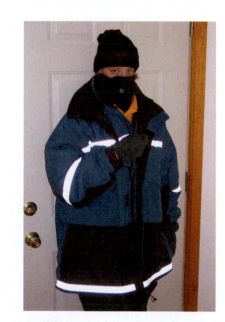

FIGURE 34-8   Proper dress can help prevent hypothermia in cold environments.

HEAT EXPOSURE

When overall heat gain is greater than heat loss, the body temperature will rise. This condition is called hyperthermia. Exposure to a hot environment does not always cause hyperthermia. Prolonged exposure to heat may result in a range of problems.

Heat Cramps

One of the body's responses to a hot environment is perspiration. The perspiration will evaporate, and heat will be lost. Perspiration is made up of water and salts. In very hot environments, more than a liter of sweat can be lost each hour. A person can become quickly dehydrated and have significant electrolyte (salt) abnormalities.

When muscles become dehydrated and are deprived of certain electrolytes, they may spasm. These painful, involuntary spasms of muscles are called **heat cramps**. Heat cramps most often occur in the calf, thigh, or shoulder muscles and usually affect people who are not used to the heat.

Management

Heat cramps are very uncomfortable but cause no permanent damage. A patient suffering from this condition should be removed from the hot environment and allowed to gently massage the painful area. Oral rehydration with water or an electrolyte solution will often result in complete recovery. Popular sport drinks are often given along with water for rehydration in a hot environment.

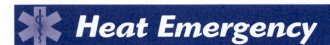

Heat Emergency

The local Miracle Marathon draws hundreds of runners from all over the region. Some runners train for months in preparation for this race; others are pure amateurs.

Today, race day, is an oppressively hot summer day with temperatures running in the 90s, and the humidity almost as high.

Race officials have provided aid stations at 1-mile intervals along the route as well as a small field hospital at the finish line in anticipation of the large number of athletes who might become ill or injured.

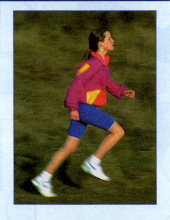

EMTs Hsiung and Weatherby volunteered for duty and have been assigned to the treatment sector of the field hospital. As soon as they arrive, patients start to be brought in.

"This runner went down at the halfway point," yells the race volunteer over the din inside the tent, "and we brought her here in the back of the pickup."

The patient is disoriented, thrashing about, and grossly diaphoretic. Her pulse seems to be racing as well. The physician in charge orders the EMTs to assess the patient and start basic life support treatment, then report their findings.

- What could be wrong with this runner?
- What are the priorities in management of this patient?
- What signs and symptoms should the EMTs look for to determine whether the patient is suffering from heat exhaustion or heat stroke?
- What will be the short- and long-term consequences of this patient's condition?

Heat Exhaustion

As do cold-related illnesses, heat-related illnesses involve a spectrum of disorders that may begin as mild and without treatment may progress to a life-threatening condition. Some people who are exposed to heat compensate very effectively; others have minor consequences such as heat cramps. Some patients are not able to compensate for the excess heat and suffer a generalized heat-related illness.

The mildest form of generalized heat-related illness is called **heat exhaustion**. This syndrome is characterized by symptoms such as dizziness, malaise, muscle aches, headache, fatigue, nausea, vomiting, and light-headedness. Often the patient suffering from heat exhaustion will have lost a great deal of fluid in sweat and may appear quite dehydrated or even have signs and symptoms of compensated shock.

The patient may have a normal or slightly elevated body temperature and elevated heart and respiratory rates and may have pale, clammy skin. The mental status in heat exhaustion is always normal. If the patient has an altered mental status, then he has a much more serious condition.

Management

Patients suffering from heat exhaustion should immediately be removed from the hot environment, and any excess clothing should be taken off. Because these patients are dehydrated, rehydration is a mainstay of therapy. Oral rehydration with water and electrolyte solutions is possible if the patient is not nauseated or vomiting. Sometimes intravenous hydration is necessary and must be provided by advanced-level providers or by hospital staff.

Patients suffering from heat exhaustion will usually fully recover after adequate hydration, although this illness may aggravate other underlying medical conditions such as diabetes or heart disease. The EMT should be alert for such complicating factors in caring for these patients.

The EMT will encounter many situations in which heat exhaustion is very common, one of which is standing by at the scene of a fire. Firefighters wear heavy, restrictive protective clothing. Even when the weather is not hot, the firefighter will often be exposed to extremely hot temperatures while fighting a fire.

It is crucial that appropriate rehabilitation be provided for the firefighters on a regular basis in order to enable them to cool off and rehydrate themselves (Figure 34-9). The EMT will often be responsible for this type of "rehab station" and must be able to properly care for the firefighters and recognize the signs of a serious heat illness.

Many areas have a recommended protocol for managing patients in such a situation. Other situations in which frequent assessments of persons involved in strenuous physical activity in a hot environment might be necessary include marathons and outdoor concerts or other events. The EMT should be familiar with local protocol for such situations. An example of such a protocol is seen in Table 34-1.

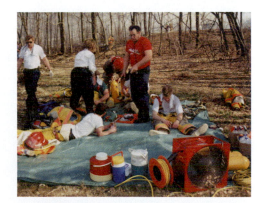

FIGURE 34-9 EMTs may be responsible for maintaining rehabilitation at the scene of a fire. (Courtesy of David J. Reimer Sr.)

Heat Stroke

A life-threatening form of heat illness is present when the heat-exposed patient is found to have an altered mental status. Altered

TABLE 34-1

Emergency Incident Rehabilitation

The following guidelines are intended for use at events where fluid loss is a concern for participants or spectators. These guidelines may also be used at fire scenes to treat firefighters.

The use of this protocol assumes that the person has no significant complaint. If a person arrives at the rehab area complaining of chest pain or shortness of breath or has an altered mental status, keep the patient NPO (nothing by mouth) and follow the protocol appropriate to the patient's complaint.

At fire scenes, the "rehab area" should be located near the self-contained breathing apparatus (SCBA) bottle-changing, triage, or staging area.

1. When the person arrives in the rehab area for the first time:
   A. Encourage the person to drink at least 8 ounces of fluid.
   B. An EMT should do a visual evaluation (the look test) for signs of heat exhaustion or fatigue.
   C. If vital signs are not within the criteria listed below, protective gear should be removed, and the person should rest for at least 15 minutes and be given continued oral rehydration.
   D. If vital signs return to criteria limits, the person can be released to return to duty.
   E. If vital signs are still beyond the limits, continue rehab for another 15 minutes and determine whether further intervention may be needed.
   F. If after 30 minutes the vital signs are still beyond the limits, advanced life support (ALS) transport to the hospital should be initiated.

2. When a person arrives in the rehab area a second time:
   A. Protective gear and constrictive clothing should be removed, and the person given at least 8 ounces of fluid to drink.
   B. An EMT should do a visual evaluation for signs of heat exhaustion and fatigue.
   C. If vital signs are not within criteria limits, further hydration should be provided and the person should rest for 15 minutes.
   D. Continue procedure 1F as above.

3. Vital signs criteria:
   A. Blood pressure: systolic <150 mm Hg or diastolic <100 mm Hg
   B. Respirations: <24 per minute
   C. Pulse: <110 per minute (An irregular pulse mandates ALS intervention, electrocardiogram (EKG) monitoring, and removal from active duty or the event.)

4. Other considerations:
   A. Names and vital signs for each patient should be recorded on a log sheet for the incident.
   B. A full patient care report (PCR) should be written on any transported person.
   C. Electrolyte solutions are encouraged.
   D. More aggressive treatment should be used during extremes of temperature.
   E. Consider carbon monoxide poisoning during prolonged exposure to smoke.
   F. Other agency procedures may be used in place of these guidelines as appropriate.

If any questions exist regarding the treatment of a patient according to this protocol, contact Medical Control for advice.

(Adapted from 2000 REMO ALS Treatment Protocols, New York, Hudson-Mohawk Region. Courtesy of the Regional Emergency Medical Organization, Albany, NY.)

mental status indicates brain malfunction. This condition is called **heat stroke**. The patient suffering from heat stroke may have been exposed to very high temperatures for a short period of time or may have been exposed to moderate temperatures for a prolonged period of time. Alternatively, exposure to moderate temperatures combined with intense exertion and internal heat generation will have the same result.

For heat stroke to occur, the overall heat gain must greatly exceed heat loss and the body temperature must rise considerably. Temperatures exceeding 106°F are not uncommon in this condition.

The EMT must be able to recognize the signs of heat stroke and rapidly initiate therapy because more than 70% of patients with heat stroke will die if the body temperature is not lowered within 2 hours.

The signs of heat stroke include hot skin, with or without associated sweating; elevated body temperature; and altered mental status with a history of heat exposure. The progression of the disease may include seizures, coma, and eventually death.

Management

Removal of the patient from the hot environment and aggressive cooling measures should be initiated as soon as heat stroke is suspected. The EMT should carefully monitor the airway, breathing, and circulation and be prepared to support them if necessary. Oxygen should be administered as for any patient with an altered mental status.

The most effective means of cooling victims of heat stroke is to completely undress them, then spray them with tepid water, and allow fans to blow over the body. Alternatively, ice packs can be placed in the groin, armpit, and neck regions.

The EMT should initiate transport as soon as possible. An advanced life support (ALS) intercept should be requested, and transport to the closest hospital, in accordance with local protocols, should be initiated.

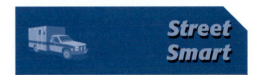

Street Smart

Ice-cold water should not be used to cool victims of heat stroke. The icy water may induce shivering, which would result in an increase in body temperature—exactly the opposite outcome of the goal of therapy.

Prevention Among Emergency Workers

EMTs often work in hot environments. It is vitally important that they realize they are susceptible to heat-related illnesses! Proper clothing and adequate hydration with frequent breaks from intense heat or exertion are important to keep the rescuers healthy.

WATER-RELATED EMERGENCIES

Nearly 8,000 people die each year in the United States as a result of drowning. More than 40% of these drowning deaths are children. EMTs should consider participating in community events that teach water safety in an effort to prevent these devastating incidents.

Near-Drowning

The term *drowning* refers to submersion in water that results in death within 24 hours. If death does not occur in this time period, the term used to describe the event is **near-drowning**.

Although near-drowning by definition does not cause death, it is nonetheless a devastating event. If the brain is left without oxygen for

Possible Drowning

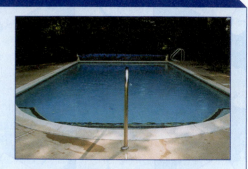

The first-arriving police unit arrived at the private residence of Ms. Roberta Freeman within minutes. She had called 9-1-1 and reported that her 2-year-old had wandered away. She was frantic at the door, screaming over and over, "My baby, my baby, where's my baby!"

Officer Lee calmly asked the mother to look upstairs in the house and under the beds and he would start to look outside. As Ms. Freeman stepped inside the doorway, Officer Lee made his way around to the backyard.

He immediately noticed an in-ground pool and remembered that small children are often attracted to pools. As soon as he entered the backyard, his worst fear was confirmed. Lying facedown in the shallow end of the pool was Justin.

He quickly entered the pool and carried Justin to the deck. Then, using his radio, he called in "Infant submerged, unknown downtime."

- What is the definition of near-drowning?
- What are the priorities in management of this child?
- Does the temperature of the water make a difference in long-term outcome?
- What are the short- and long-term consequences of this condition?

a period of time, severe neurologic injury will result. It is the job of the EMT to quickly evaluate and provide emergency medical care to victims of near-drowning. Early rescue and resuscitation will improve the prognosis of the near-drowning victim.

Series of Events

The series of events occurring in a drowning incident is somewhat variable, although the final result is always hypoxia. Upon submersion, victims may hold their breath, causing blood oxygen levels to fall and carbon dioxide levels to rise. They are eventually forced to take a breath by the rising carbon dioxide levels in the blood.

Upon inhalation, water entering the airway will cause laryngospasm and bronchospasm. Often, this airway spasm will prevent any further water from entering the lungs. Water also is swallowed, often in large amounts, resulting in stomach distension.

As blood oxygen levels continue to fall, the heart rate will slow. As the heart rate slows, the blood pressure will fall. If rescue does not occur at this point, the victim will suffer a cardiopulmonary arrest.

The speed with which rescue occurs will often determine how likely resuscitation is to be successful.

Cold Water

When submersion occurs in cold water, the resulting hypothermia seems to have a protective effect upon the patient's organs. The reason is unclear. Survival of cold-water drowning victims has been recorded after even 40 minutes of submersion. The EMT should keep this fact in mind when resuscitating patients who have been submerged in cold water for any length of time.

Management

The first priority of management of the near-drowning victim is to remove the patient from the water. The EMT should be sure not to place herself or her team in danger of harm during this rescue. Only persons trained in water rescue should venture into water after a submerged victim.

A good rule of rescue to remember when dealing with water rescues is "reach, throw, row, then go." This is to remind the rescuer to try as many techniques as possible to help the victim that do not involve going into the water. Figures 34-10 through 34-13 depict this series of rescue techniques. The EMT who is likely to encounter water emergencies frequently in her job should consider further training in water rescue. A rescuer who is not trained in water rescue who enters the water has a good chance of becoming a victim herself. She will have served no purpose other than to distract further rescue efforts from the initial victim as rescuers attempt to rescue the EMT.

When rescuing a victim from the water, the EMT should consider the possibility of spinal injury. If there is any likelihood that spinal injury exists, as might happen in a dive into a shallow pool or onto rocks, careful attention to spinal immobilization must be a priority.

Upon removal of the victim from the water, the EMT should perform an initial assessment and treat any cardiac or respiratory compromise. There is no need to attempt to remove water from the patient's lungs, although vomiting is common as water returns from the stomach after having been swallowed. The EMT should have suction readily available.

All near-drowning victims should be transported to a hospital. Delayed respiratory difficulty can occur as a result of exposure of the airways to water. Near-drowning victims who are awake upon rescue from the water generally have a good prognosis if proper treatment is provided.

Diving Emergencies

Although diving emergencies certainly are not common throughout the country, many EMTs will be called upon to care for patients who have been scuba diving and are suffering complications. It is important for the EMT to understand a few basic points about diving emergencies.

Boyle's Law

A quick lesson in physics can improve an EMT's understanding of diving emergencies. One concept is all that is necessary to understand why divers get into trouble. **Boyle's law** describes that the volume of a gas varies inversely with the surrounding pressure. This concept is more easily understood with examples.

Consider a bag of air that is put under 25 feet of water. Pressure is exerted upon that bag of air by the water. The pressure will compress the air into a smaller volume, allowing it to fit into a smaller bag.

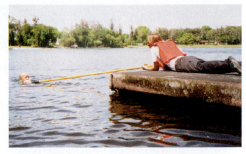

FIGURE 34-10 In any attempt to rescue a patient from a body of water, the first technique used is to reach out while maintaining a secure hold on a stable object.

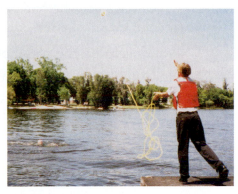

FIGURE 34-11 If the EMT is unable to reach a victim in the water, the next step is to throw a rescue rope or flotation device for the patient to hold onto.

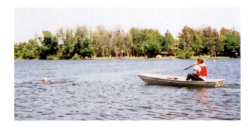

FIGURE 34-12 If the rescuer has been unable to reach the victim by reaching or throwing, he should use an appropriate watercraft to reach the patient if he is trained to do so.

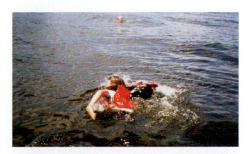

FIGURE 34-13 Only if all other methods have failed or are not available should a rescuer enter the water to go after a water bound victim, and only if he is properly trained to do so.

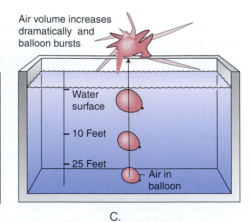

Scuba Accident

EMTs Lorento and Alfonso were enjoying their first day on beach patrol. Both EMTs had requested a transfer from South-Central to Beach Patrol for a change of pace and a little relaxation.

Their first call of the day was at a local beach resort where scuba diving lessons are offered to tourists. The divemaster had called EMS for a woman who claimed she was unable to walk after surfacing from a dive.

As Lorento started his initial assessment of the patient, Alfonso questioned the divemaster about the events preceding the call. They discovered that she was a novice diver who had dived to a moderate depth and immediately upon surfacing from her dive was unable to support herself or control her legs.

- What might be the cause of the patient's symptoms?
- How should the EMTs treat her?
- What considerations in transport are relevant to this condition?

Take that small bag of air from under the 25 feet of water and bring it back up to the surface. As the pressure around it is removed, the air will expand back to its original volume. If left in the small bag, it may pop the bag as it expands. Figure 34-14 depicts this concept.

This concept of Boyle's law explains diving-related emergencies. This section will discuss the most commonly seen diving emergencies related to pressure problems that the EMT should be familiar with.

Descent

Divers can have complications upon descent due to the compression of air in enclosed body spaces. These types of problems are appropriately called "squeeze"-related problems.

Squeeze

As you might expect, the term *squeeze* refers to the compression of a volume of air in an enclosed space as the diver goes farther down

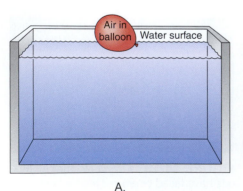

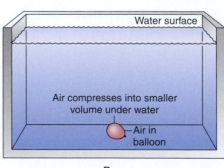

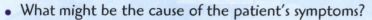

FIGURE 34-14 A. Air takes up a defined volume of space at sea level. B. The same amount of air is compressed into a smaller volume when under 25 feet of water. C. As air is brought from a depth back to sea level, the amount of space it takes up will increase.

under water and the pressure of the surrounding water increases. There is often a pocket of air in a diver's ears and sinuses that can be compressed with the increase in pressure during a dive.

Divers often employ a technique of breathing that equalizes the pressures in these spaces as they descend in the water. If the pressures are not equalized, the air enclosed in these spaces will be "squeezed," causing pain and even damage to the area. The eardrum may even perforate with the increased pressure.

Symptoms of ear squeeze or sinus squeeze are pain during descent that often will force the diver to ascend immediately. If squeeze occurs, the diver should not be permitted to dive again until he has been examined by a physician at a hospital. EMTs should facilitate this exam by transporting the patient to the hospital for evaluation.

Management

Management of ear and sinus squeeze is generally limited to pain medicines prescribed by a physician. The EMT should advise the patient not to dive and to be examined by a physician to determine the extent of any injury. If the eardrum ruptures in this manner, permanent hearing loss may result.

Ascent

Just as divers can have problems with compression of air in enclosed spaces on the way down, they can have problems with expansion of air on the way up. Some of these ascent-related emergencies can actually be life threatening and therefore are important for the EMT to understand.

Decompression Sickness

A commonly known diving injury occurs during a rapid ascent as the pressure upon the diver decreases. The gases that were used for breathing during the dive are compressed and can become trapped in tissues in that form. If the diver ascends too rapidly to allow proper decompression of these gases, they can expand, forming bubbles. These bubbles can become stuck in joint spaces and in various tissues such as muscles, lung tissue, the brain, or the spinal cord. This condition is known as **decompression sickness**. This condition can occur if the patient takes an airplane flight within 24 hours of a dive—such as returning home from vacation.

Symptoms often do not occur for 1–6 hours after the dive has been completed and consist of pain in the areas listed above. The most common complaint is severe aching joint pain, although neurologic problems such as paralysis can occur as can respiratory problems if the lungs are involved. The classic joint pain is likely the origin of the term *the bends*.

Pulmonary Overpressurization Syndrome

Another emergency of ascent is related to expanding air within the lungs as pressure decreases and the volume of air proportionally increases. A diver should always ascend slowly and exhale constantly during this time to allow the excess volume of air to escape.

If an ascent is too rapid or if the diver does not exhale, the volume of air in the lungs increases and can actually cause the tiny alveoli in the lungs to rupture. This so-called **pulmonary overpressurization syndrome (POPS)** will result in immediate symptoms of chest pain and difficulty breathing. Figure 34-15 illustrates this process.

Air Embolism

If a diver has sustained alveolar rupture during POPS, the air may actually rupture into a pulmonary blood vessel. Air that enters the bloodstream can travel wherever that blood vessel goes. The air bub-

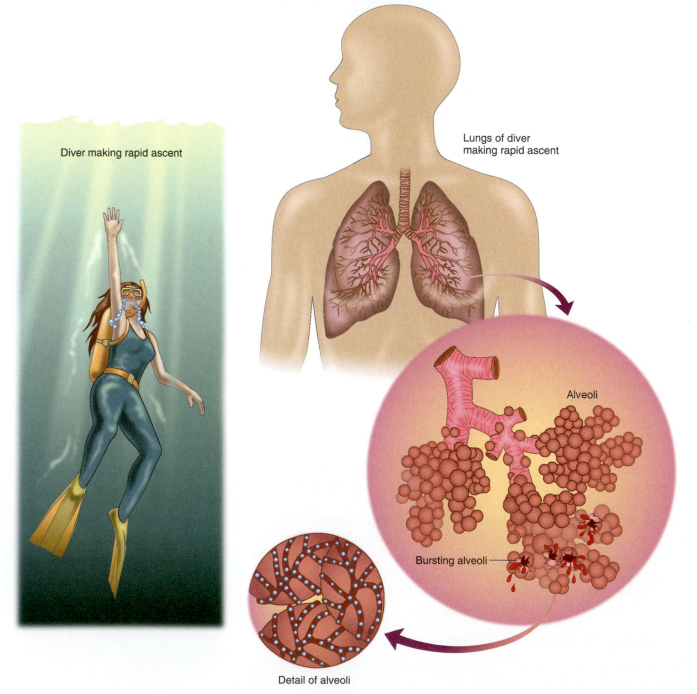

Diver making rapid ascent

Lungs of diver making rapid ascent

Alveoli

Bursting alveoli

Detail of alveoli

FIGURE 34-15   Expanding air can rupture a lung if not allowed to properly escape during ascent from a dive. Air can rupture into a pulmonary blood vessel during ascent from a dive.

ble will become lodged in a small vessel and cause an inflammatory reaction that will result in a rapidly forming blood clot. Air that is traveling through the bloodstream is called an **air embolism**.

Since the vessels most commonly affected by this condition are the pulmonary capillaries, the air bubbles will follow the pulmonary vessels into the left heart. From there, they will then be sent to any organ in the body along the arterial system. The bubbles will travel in the arteries until they reach a small vessel that they cannot pass through. The resulting blood clot will occlude blood flow and cause severe pain, ischemia, and infarction of the tissue.

The symptoms of this air embolism are evident immediately upon ascent and may consist of severe pain, paralysis, or even unconsciousness or strokelike symptoms, depending upon the location of the embolism.

Management

The management of all emergencies of ascent involves support of the airway, breathing, and circulation as appropriate. In addition, 100% oxygen should be administered to all patients who have symptoms of ascent emergencies. The patient should be placed in a supine position and transported immediately to a hospital for treatment.

Definitive treatment of these types of emergencies involves placing the patient in a specialized type of device called a **hyperbaric chamber**. These hyperbaric chambers create a simulated dive and allow recompression of air. Only specialized hospitals have hyperbaric chambers. The EMT who works in an area where scuba diving is common should be familiar with his surrounding hospitals and know where the closest chamber is located.

Nitrogen Narcosis

One additional diving-related emergency the EMT should be familiar with is **nitrogen narcosis**. Sometimes called "rapture of the deep," this illness is a reversible condition caused by the anesthetic effect of nitrogen at high partial pressure. Nitrogen is one of the gases that is in a diver's air bottle.

The patient suffering from nitrogen narcosis will appear as though he is intoxicated during the dive. The incidence increases with the depth of the dive and completely resolves with ascent.

Management

It would be uncommon for the EMT to see residual signs of nitrogen narcosis after the diver has surfaced. If signs of intoxication or other mental status changes are present after a dive, air embolism to the brain or other, non-dive-related, medical illnesses should be suspected.

ALTITUDE EMERGENCIES

At high elevations, the partial pressure of oxygen is less than that at sea level, essentially creating a hypoxic environment. It makes sense, then, that altitude-related emergencies are related to hypoxia.

People who live at high altitudes have grown accustomed to, or acclimated to, the lower oxygen levels. Those who are not acclimated to this environment can become ill.

Altitude-related emergencies are a spectrum of illnesses that begin with a mild disease called acute mountain sickness and progress to a life-threatening emergency known as high-altitude pulmonary edema. The EMT who practices in an area that services high altitudes should be familiar with these illnesses.

Acute Mountain Sickness

Persons who are not acclimated to a high altitude can suffer from **acute mountain sickness (AMS)**. It is usually seen during a rapid ascent above 2,000 meters, or 6,600 feet, above sea level.

Symptoms of AMS begin with light-headedness and mild breathlessness. After a period of around 6 hours, other symptoms may occur such as headache, nausea, weakness, and fatigue. These symptoms will progress to severe headache, vomiting, and weakness if treatment is not provided.

High-Altitude Cerebral Edema

If left untreated, AMS can progress and may result in cerebral edema. This condition is called **high-altitude cerebral edema (HACE)**. Altered mental status, trouble walking, decreasing level of consciousness, and focal neurologic weakness can all be symptoms of this extreme progression of mountain sickness.

High-Altitude Pulmonary Edema

The most lethal complication of mountain sickness is **high-altitude pulmonary edema (HAPE)**. Early symptoms of this very serious condition include dry cough and dyspnea on exertion.

✳ *Altitude Emergency*

The alert tones went out. "Southern Tier Blue Team, assemble at Black Mountain trailhead. All team members prepare for a possible backcountry rescue."

EMTs Yates and Butts had just completed their wilderness EMT course and were prepared for this first mission. The patient was a young woman who was visiting the high country for the first time. She was complaining of a headache, a nonproductive cough, and severe shortness of breath. Her shortness of breath had started right after she had arrived from Miami and had become progressively worse. Initially, the trouble breathing occurred only when she exerted herself, but now it had become so severe that she could not tolerate lying flat.

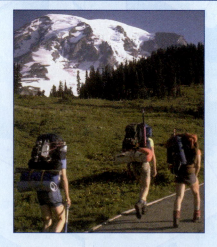

- What could be wrong with this young woman?
- What are the priorities in emergency medical care of this condition?
- What are the potential consequences of not treating this type of illness?

If the condition is allowed to progress, the patient will become weak and will have dyspnea even while at rest. Crackles will be clearly heard in the lungs as fluid builds up in the alveoli. Without treatment, this condition may become fatal.

Management

The management of any of the altitude-related emergencies involves oxygen and descent. Mild mountain sickness may be treated with oxygen and special medications to help the body more rapidly acclimate to the altitude. More severe symptoms of AMS or of HACE or HAPE should be taken very seriously, and descent should be initiated immediately while oxygen is administered to the patient.

LIGHTNING STRIKES

Each year there are 300 fatalities and 1,500 injuries in the United States related to lightning strikes. Most deaths are due to immediate cardiac arrest. Among survivors, 75% sustain some sort of significant permanent disability or complication.

A direct lightning strike involves the instantaneous delivery of 100 million volts that usually rapidly pass over the victim's body. People who are not directly struck by lightning can still be injured as a result of a side splash of current from the initial impact site. Lightning injuries can be separated into minor and severe injuries.

Minor Injuries

Minor injuries from a lightning strike result in a stunned patient. Confusion, amnesia, and short-term memory difficulties are common. Other common symptoms may include headache, muscle pain, numbness, and temporary visual or auditory problems. Most patients

✳ *Lightning Strike*

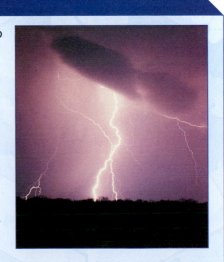

"Rescue nine, Ambulance nine-five-two, and Engine twenty-one respond to the municipal golf course, at the 13th hole, for a possible lightning strike."

Emergency crews arrive at the 13th hole to find a man in cardiac arrest with CPR being performed by a caddie. Three other patients are lying about the hole. The three other patients have various complaints, but all appear to be minor.

"At first we just tingled. Then all of a sudden, swish, boom, and crash," remarks one golfer. "I looked over and poor Harry was down and the caddie was doing CPR. I used my cell phone to call EMS."

The thunderstorm continues as the captain calls for backup to assist in caring for the multiple victims.

- What are the priorities in management of these patients?
- How is the triage concept different in a lightning strike than in any other situation?
- What are some of the consequences of a lightning strike?

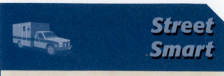

with minor lightning injuries gradually improve and do not generally have long-term problems.

Common findings after lightning strikes are that more than 50% of people struck have ruptured eardrums. Superficial skin burns are fairly common although not often serious.

In addition to the electrical injury, blunt trauma is common as a result of the force from the strike or secondary to a fall afterward. The EMT should be alert for possible traumatic injury such as broken bones and an injured spine. It is always a wise idea to assume the presence of traumatic injury and immobilize the patient to prevent any worsening of injuries.

Severe Injuries

In severely injured people, the electricity produces a sudden direct current (DC) countershock that results in a halt in all cardiac electrical activity, and cardiac arrest results. After a few minutes, the heart may spontaneously resume its electrical activity. The lungs, on the other hand, may still be stunned as a result of the high-voltage shock and may not allow breathing to begin again. Persistent respiratory arrest will result in hypoxia. Hypoxia to the irritated heart may result in ventricular fibrillation. The state in which the severely injured patient is found depends on the timing of the rescuer arrival.

Early in this sequence of cardiac arrest, good airway and ventilatory management will likely result in a reversal of cardiac arrest and a favorable outcome. The longer the heart goes without oxygen, the less likely resuscitation is to be successful.

Even without causing cardiac arrest, a lightning strike results in a loss of consciousness in more than 70% of victims. Permanent neurologic injury to the brain or spinal cord may result.

Management

The first priority in the management of the victim or victims of a lightning strike is scene safety. The EMT must be sure that it is safe to allow her crew to approach the victims. It may be necessary to enlist the assistance of the fire department if there is still a risk of electrical injury in the vicinity owing to downed power lines or other damage caused by the storm.

The next important consideration is to decide who should be treated first if there are multiple victims. In the case of lightning strikes, the principles of triage are reversed. People who are not in cardiac arrest upon the arrival of the rescuers will likely survive, and the people in cardiac arrest will likely be easily reversed. If personnel are limited, it may be reasonable to expend the limited resources in attempting to resuscitate the cardiac arrest victim. Chapter 44 will discuss the usual methods of triage.

Understanding the physiology of lightning injuries, the EMT should provide support for the airway, breathing, and circulation as needed and immobilize patients who may have suffered a blunt traumatic injury.

All victims of lightning strikes should be evaluated at the hospital because some of the consequences of a lightning strike can be delayed hours to days.

BITES AND STINGS

The EMT may get called to treat victims of envenomations from a variety of sources. Although bite and sting emergencies are not common, it is useful for the prehospital provider to be familiar with the most serious varieties she may be called to treat.

Snakes

The only venomous snakes native to the United States are rattlesnakes, copperheads, and water moccasins (all pit vipers) and coral snakes. Although there are nearly 8,000 reported venomous snake bites each year, the reported mortality rates are low. Despite the low number of deaths due to snake bites, the EMT who practices in an area where these snakes are found is likely to be called to treat a victim of a bite. It is therefore important for her to recognize the venomous nature of the snake and be knowledgeable about the effects of the bite and the appropriate prehospital treatment.

The degree of poisoning after a bite may range from a completely dry bite (25% of bites) to a severe envenomation, with symptoms evident immediately after the strike. The symptoms seen with each type of snake bite vary slightly, so they will be covered individually.

Pit Vipers

A **pit viper** can be recognized by its two movable fangs and the depression (pit) that is seen in front of each eye (Figure 34-16A). The typical pit viper bite will have two fang marks with local pain and swelling (Figure 34-16B).

In more severe envenomations, the patient will also develop more extensive edema and systemic symptoms such as nausea and signs such as tachycardia. In very severe envenomations, the patient will appear acutely ill, with hypotension, tachycardia, altered mental status, respiratory distress, and spontaneous bleeding.

Coral Snake

"Red on yellow, kill a fellow; red on black, venom lack." This rhyme can be recalled when identifying a true **coral snake**. These venomous reptiles can be recognized by their brightly colored body with red and yellow bands directly opposed in addition to black bands (Figure 34-17).

The bite of the eastern coral snake is toxic and causes neurologic decompensation in its victims. Tremor, salivation, respiratory paralysis, seizures, and other neurologic problems can occur after a significant bite.

Management

Every patient who is bitten by a snake should be evaluated in the hospital. The patient should be kept calm. The bitten extremity should be immobilized and kept below the level of the heart.

If the patient has any symptoms other than local pain and swelling, oxygen should be administered and the EMT should consider an ALS intercept. Transport should not be delayed in an attempt to find or identify the snake.

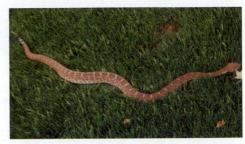

A.

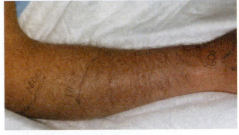

B.

FIGURE 34-16 A. A pit viper can be recognized by the sunken pit in front of each eye. B. The bite produces local pain and swelling. (Courtesy of Sean Bush, MD, Loma Linda Medical Center, Loma Linda, CA.)

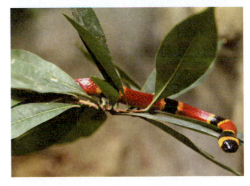

FIGURE 34-17 Despite its beautiful coloring, the coral snake is quite venomous. (Courtesy of PhotoDisc.)

Safety Tip

In the past, it was taught to cut the snake bite and attempt to suck out the venom. This treatment is no longer practiced and is not appropriate prehospital management because it tends to cause more tissue damage than the bite itself and places the EMT at risk.

Spider Bite

Camping in the high country of the Sierras had always been a dream of Matt's, and when he had an opportunity to take a group of Scouts into the wildlands, he jumped on it.

The first day was mighty grueling, and Matt slept like a log that night. The next morning Matt rolled out of bed, slipped his feet into his boots, thinking he was ready for the trail ahead, and suddenly felt a sharp pain on the bottom of his left foot.

He violently threw the boot off his foot and yelled out, "Ouch! Something just bit me!" Examining his foot, Matt noted that it had started to swell, and he was wondering how he was going to hike the 20 miles back out if he needed to.

- What is the likely source of the pain and swelling?
- What would be the immediate treatment?
- Are all bites treated the same?

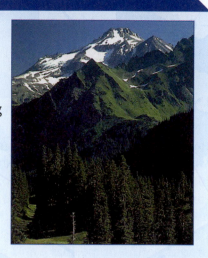

Street Smart

The EMT should obtain a description of the snake but should never attempt to capture the snake in order to identify it. It is useful for the hospital staff to know the species of snake that bit the patient, but not at the expense of the EMT's safety! Most areas will have an animal control officer who can come and capture or identify the snake.

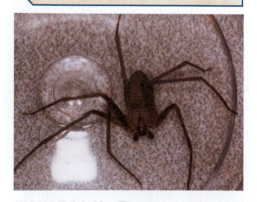

FIGURE 34-18 The venomous brown recluse spider is found most commonly in the southern and western United States. (Courtesy of Sean Bush, MD, Loma Linda Medical Center, Loma Linda, CA.)

Spiders

Most spider bites are harmless. There are two species of spider whose bites may result in some long-term consequences. The brown recluse and black widow spiders are the offending arachnids.

Brown Recluse Spider

Most commonly found in the southern and western United States, the **brown recluse spider** is about 1/4 to 3/4 inch long (6–20 mm). Its brown body has a violin-shaped mark on the back (Figure 34-18). The bite of the brown recluse results in a mildly red lesion that can develop severe pain, a blister, and bluish discoloration (Figure 34-19).

The severe form of the spider bite may become necrotic and result in large areas of skin and tissue being damaged. A rare systemic reaction to this envenomation may occur 1–2 days after the bite and may result in death.

Black Widow Spider

The female **black widow spider** is a jet-black spider, around 1 inch (25 mm) long, and has a red hourglass mark on the abdomen (Figure 34-20). The male is much smaller and harmless. This spider is found throughout the United States in crevices, woodpiles, stables, and garbage piles. More frequent encounters are reported in the warmer months.

The black widow spider bite is initially painful, and within 1 hour the patient may have redness, swelling, and generalized painful muscle cramping. This severe muscular pain can last for several days and may result in muscle weakness that lasts for weeks to months. Although less common, other serious complications of the black widow spider bite include severe hypertension, respiratory failure, shock, and coma.

Management

The emergency treatment of these spider bites is merely supportive: bandaging of the site and transport of the patient to the hospital where specific medications may be administered for the more serious symptoms. Although most spider bites will not result in serious symptoms, some can be fatal and all patients encountered by the EMT should be transported to the hospital for complete evaluation.

Scorpions

Scorpions are most frequently encountered in the southwestern United States and very rarely cause fatal injury in adults (Figure 34-21). A scorpion sting usually results in a slightly reddened area and causes a stinging or burning feeling. Occasionally, local tissue damage can occur.

Severe reactions more often occur in children and can consist of hypertension or hypotension, heart arrhythmias, throat spasms, muscle twitching, abdominal pain, and respiratory trouble.

Management

Most scorpion stings will require only pain medication; however, patients with severe reactions can decompensate very quickly. Patients who were stung by a scorpion and call EMS should be transported to the hospital for further evaluation.

Patients whose sting is limited to localized symptoms can be transported without any specific treatment. Patients who have any evidence of symptoms in addition to local stinging and pain should be placed on oxygen, and an ALS intercept should be considered. The EMT should carefully monitor the airway, breathing, and circulation during transport of these patients.

Marine Animals

The variety of injuries the EMT may see as a result of encounters with marine animals will certainly vary depending upon her area of practice. These injuries may vary from a shark bite to a jellyfish sting, and each is treated differently. Some marine injuries can be extremely painful and are potentially fatal.

Management

The EMT who regularly cares for patients exposed to such marine animals should seek out further specific training to help recognize and treat such injuries. In general, the EMT should assess the patient as she would any other patient and support the vital signs as appropriate.

CONCLUSION

The EMT will encounter many patients who have been exposed to a variety of environmental factors. Many of these may cause a life-threatening problem. It is the responsibility of the EMT to be familiar with those environmental emergencies that are universally common, such as those covered in detail in this chapter.

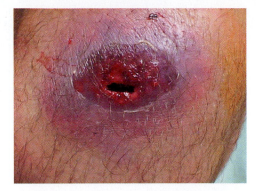

FIGURE 34-19 A characteristic wound from a brown recluse spider. (Courtesy of Deborah Funk, MD, Albany Medical Center, Albany, NY.)

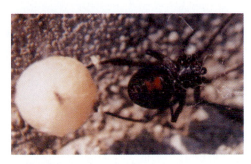

FIGURE 34-20 The black widow spider has been found throughout the United States in crevices, woodpiles, stables, and garbage piles. (Courtesy of Sean Bush, MD, Loma Linda Medical Center, Loma Linda, CA.)

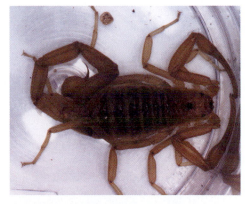

FIGURE 34-21 Scorpion bites rarely cause significant illness. (Courtesy of Sean Bush, MD, Loma Linda Medical Center, Loma Linda, CA.)

Further training is encouraged for those EMTs who will routinely be exposed to patients who suffer from other specific types of environmental injuries or illnesses.

TEST YOUR KNOWLEDGE

1. What are the various mechanisms by which the body loses heat?
2. What are the various mechanisms by which the body generates heat?
3. What are the local cold injuries, and what is the proper treatment for these conditions?
4. What are the signs and symptoms of generalized hypothermia?
5. What is the appropriate emergency medical care of the patient with generalized hypothermia?
6. What are signs and symptoms of heat exhaustion and heat stroke?
7. What is the emergency medical care of the patient with heat exhaustion or heat stroke?
8. What are the complications of near-drowning?
9. What is the emergency medical care of the near-drowning victim?
10. What are signs and symptoms of diving-related emergencies?
11. What is the emergency medical care of diving-related emergencies?
12. What are signs and symptoms of altitude emergencies?
13. What is the emergency medical care of altitude emergencies?
14. What are the priorities in caring for the victim of a lightning strike?
15. What is the emergency medical care of a victim of a bite or a sting?

INTERNET RESOURCES

The following Web sites contain additional information related to the content in this chapter. Search by the topics covered in the chapter for even more information. Share helpful Web sites with your colleagues.

- Divers Alert Network, http://www.diversalertnetwork.org
- Diving Medicine Online, http://scuba-doc.com
- Hyperbaric Medicine Unit of Aberdeen Royal Infirmary, Scotland, http://www.hyperchamber.com
- Hypothermia.org, http://www.hypothermia.org
- Outdoor Places, http://www.outdoorplaces.com
- Survive Outdoors, http://www.surviveoutdoors.com

FURTHER STUDY

Gurr, D., & Brown, T. (1998). Zapped. *Journal of Emergency Medical Services, 23*(12), 66–69.

Margolis, G. (1998). Immersion hypothermia. *Journal of Emergency Medical Services, 23*(9), 66–70.

Schulmerich, S. (1999). When nature turns up the heat. *RN, 62*(8), 35–39.

Stewart, C. (2000). When lightning strikes. *Emergency Medical Services, 29*(3), 57–59.

CHAPTER 35

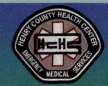
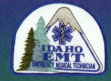
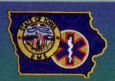

Poisoning and Allergic Reactions

KEY TERMS

allergen
allergic reaction
overdose
Poison Control Center
poisoning

OBJECTIVES

Upon completion of this chapter, the reader should be able to:

1. List various ways that poisons can enter the body.
2. Describe signs and symptoms associated with different types of poisonings.
3. Discuss the emergency medical care of the patient who has been poisoned.
4. Discuss the special considerations required in the emergency medical care of the intentional overdose patient.
5. Identify the potential airway issues in the poisoned patient.
6. Discuss the indications and contraindications for activated charcoal in the poisoned patient.
7. Recognize the need for medical control and advanced life support in the poisoned patient.
8. Recognize the patient experiencing an allergic reaction.
9. Describe the emergency medical care of the patient with an allergic reaction.
10. Differentiate between a simple allergic reaction and anaphylaxis.
11. Describe the implications of anaphylaxis in regard to airway management.
12. State the indications and contraindications for the epinephrine auto-injector.
13. Identify the importance of medical control and advanced life support in the care of the patient with anaphylaxis.

OVERVIEW

The term *poison* has been used for hundreds of years to describe a deadly substance. Exposure to such substances can cause predictable or unpredictable reactions. When a person is exposed to a substance and becomes ill as a result, it is referred to as **poisoning**. When that exposure is deliberate, the term **overdose** is sometimes used. If a generally harmless substance causes an unexpected activation of the person's immune system, it is called an **allergic reaction**.

It is important that the emergency medical technician (EMT) be familiar with these concepts and understand the priorities in the management of poisoned patients and patients suffering from allergic reactions.

POISONING

Thousands of children are poisoned each year as they explore their environments. Many adults become ill each year as a result of poisoning as well. Some poisonings are unintentional; others are deliberate.

People can become ill after exposure to harmful substances via several routes. Although the general concepts are similar, each mechanism has unique differences in management.

General Assessment

As with all emergency situations, it is important that the EMT evaluate the scene for safety before approaching the patient. Some poisons, if still present on the scene, can be harmful to emergency providers. Appropriately trained hazardous materials technicians should be called to assist if it is thought that the substance involved makes the scene unsafe. Scene safety is discussed further in Chapter 44.

Once safely removed from any danger, poisoned patients all require a thorough assessment and history to be done by the EMT. If the patient does not have any acutely life-threatening issues, the EMT should carefully look for specific evidence of illness related to the poisoning.

The history obtained should include specific information regarding the poisoning as well as the usual SAMPLE (see Table 10-5) history and relevant medical history.

Specific History

If the exact name of the substance that the patient was exposed to is available, the EMT should carefully record it and relay it to hospital personnel. If the container or a sample of the substance is available and can safely be collected, the EMT should consider bringing it to the hospital for identification.

The exact time of exposure to the poison should be determined. Some remedies are useful only during a certain time frame. If the exposure was more than a single event, the EMT should determine over how long a period of time the patient was exposed to the substance. If the amount of the substance that was involved is measurable, the EMT should record the amount as well.

The EMT should determine and document whether anyone provided any type of treatment for the patient before the EMT's arrival. Often, the family of a poisoned person will call the **Poison Control Center** hot line. Personnel trained to recommend treatments for specific poisonings staff this hot line. There are Poison Control Centers all over the United States. It is a useful resource for laypersons and medical personnel as well. Some emergency medical services (EMS) systems recommend that EMTs call Poison Control for advice in

Safety Tip

Substances that could be harmful to the EMT or hospital staff should not be collected. A description of the container or the name if available would be sufficient information to relay to hospital staff.

Street Smart

If the poison involved is a medication, the number of missing pills can be estimated by counting those remaining in the bottle. The total number of pills dispensed in the bottle is noted on the prescription label. It is always best to bring the bottle and the remaining medication to the hospital. Hospital staff can confirm the identity of the drug and calculate the number missing.

managing a poisoned patient. The EMT should follow local protocols regarding whom to contact.

Many decisions regarding treatment of the poisoned patient involve calculations based upon the patient's weight. If possible, the EMT should determine what the patient weighs. Parents often know what their child weighs and can relate that information if asked.

General Management

Although every situation is unique and each toxic substance creates its own problems that need individualized care, there are some general management principles that the EMT can use when caring for all poisoned patients.

Scene Safety

As repeatedly stressed, the priorities in management of the patient who has been potentially poisoned begin with safety of the emergency team. The EMT should be sure that the scene is safe for his team to enter.

Life-Threatening Problems

The EMT should use his general impression and initial assessment to identify and treat any immediately life-threatening problems. It is not uncommon for a poisoned patient to develop airway, breathing, or circulatory compromise. The EMT should follow the principles of supporting these systems as previously learned.

Specific management techniques should be utilized as appropriate for the situation and as directed by medical control.

Medical Direction

After addressing any immediate life threats, the EMT should consult with medical control regarding further management. Some systems have set up protocols to be used as off-line medical control in this circumstance. The EMT should be familiar with local protocols and follow them carefully.

Other systems require on-line consultation with a physician or that physician's designee. That designee may be the Poison Control Center in the case of the poisoned patient. Again, the EMT should follow local protocol.

Transport

Once immediate life threats have been addressed, the EMT should collect any remaining pills, containers, or labels that can identify the potential poison and transport the patient to the most appropriate medical facility. In some cases, identification of the substance will be crucial in providing appropriate in-hospital care (Figure 35-1).

Ongoing Assessment

The EMT should realize that the poisoned patient has the potential to decompensate very quickly. Even if the patient appears well upon first assessment, the poison may not have yet absorbed fully into the

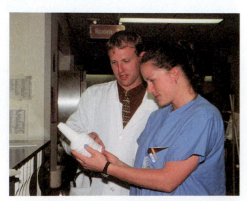

FIGURE 35-1 Some therapies for poisoned patients are dependent upon accurate identification of the substance involved.

Accidental Poisoning

An elderly woman meets EMS at the door and ushers the two EMTs into her living room. She explains that she called the emergency number after she found her 4-year-old grandson playing with her heart pills.

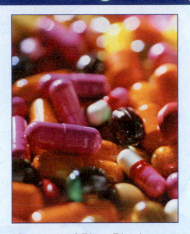

(Courtesy of PhotoDisc.)

The grandmother explains, "But I only left him for a moment." While EMT Rodriguez attempts to calm the visibly distraught grandmother, EMT Ruoff notes that the child is happily playing on the floor and wonders just how much trouble those pills can cause.

- What signs and symptoms should the EMT look for in this child?
- What are the management priorities in the patient after the suspected ingestion of a poison?

bloodstream. Once this has absorbed, the patient may rapidly decompensate. Consequently, the EMT must continually reassess the poisoned patient for hints of such decompensation. Table 35-1 lists some signs of decompensation in the poisoned patient.

Certain poisons cause characteristic changes in the patient's vital signs. The EMT should carefully monitor the patient's heart and respiratory rates, blood pressure, skin color and temperature, and pulse oximetry.

ALS Intercept

If the patient's condition exceeds the EMT's abilities, an advanced life support (ALS) intercept should be considered. Medical control may be helpful in deciding when this is necessary.

Transport should be accomplished in a timely fashion, and the EMT should continually reassess the patient and be prepared for possible decompensation.

If any further decontamination is needed, notification of the destination facility is critically important so that it may make appropriate arrangements.

INGESTED POISONS

Perhaps the most common route of poisoning is by oral ingestion. Children often will put just about anything into their mouth. If allowed to have access to a potentially harmful substance, a child may unintentionally poison herself.

A different situation may exist in adults. Certainly the possibility of unintentional poisoning exists, but the rates of deliberate poisoning

TABLE 35-1

Signs of Decompensation— Poisoning

Decreasing mental status

Increasing heart rate

Seizure

Decreasing respiratory rate

Respiratory arrest

Hypotension

Cardiac arrest

increase in adulthood. Care of these patients involves some different considerations.

Intentional Ingestions

When a person deliberately ingests a substance that she believes to be harmful, it is referred to as an overdose. Often the patient is suffering from severe depression and is attempting to harm or even kill herself.

In this situation, it is the duty of the EMT to treat the patient and prevent any further harm. A patient who has attempted or threatened to harm herself should be transported to an appropriate hospital for medical and psychiatric treatment. This person should not be given the option to refuse further treatment, even if she does not appear to acutely need medical care. The care of the patient who may be a danger to herself is covered in detail in Chapter 32.

Signs and Symptoms

Ingested poisons can cause myriad physical findings and symptoms (Figure 35-2). The earliest are often related to the gastrointestinal tract, as this is the part of the body first contacted by the substance. The airway can also be affected if the poison injures the mouth and throat.

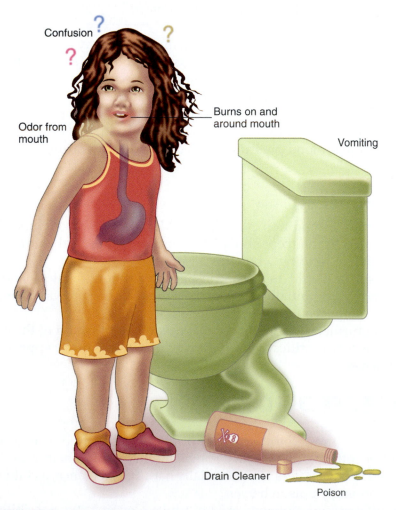

Confusion

Odor from mouth

Burns on and around mouth

Vomiting

Drain Cleaner

Poison

FIGURE 35-2 Ingested poisons can cause injury to the mouth and throat and will absorb into the stomach vessels and be distributed throughout the body.

The EMT should look for these specific signs and symptoms when evaluating the patient who has ingested a poison. Table 35-2 lists these signs and symptoms.

Management

A general impression and initial assessment will identify any potential airway, breathing, or circulatory problems. These issues must be addressed immediately upon their recognition.

Potential life-threatening problems in the patient who ingested a poison may include loss of airway patency because of mouth and throat burns if the substance ingested was a caustic substance. The patency of the airway may be in jeopardy also if the patient is unconscious as a result of the effects of the ingested poison.

Any pills or harmful material that remain in the patient's mouth should be removed. If the patient is conscious, she should be asked to spit into a basin. Often a suction catheter can be used to remove any material from the unconscious person's mouth. Certain ingested substances can rapidly cause heart or brain malfunction, resulting in shock, seizures, or decreased level of consciousness. If faced with a patient with evidence of hypoperfusion, the EMT should treat her as outlined in Chapter 9. Seizures and altered mental status can be managed according to the priorities discussed in Chapter 30.

Activated Charcoal

The ideal way to manage a potentially harmful oral ingestion is to prevent some or all absorption of the poison. Activated charcoal can prevent absorption of certain ingested substances if administered within 1–2 hours of ingestion.

This suspension of charcoal in a liquid binds to some poisons, preventing them from being absorbed. It should be given only to patients who have ingested a noncaustic substance and who are awake and able to drink the liquid without potential for airway compromise.

Activated charcoal should never be administered to a patient with an altered mental status or who has ingested a caustic substance. The EMT should follow local protocol for specific recommendations.

INHALED POISONS

The priority of emergency personnel responding to the scene of a potential poisoning by inhalation must be their own safety. If the dispatch information is suspicious for an airborne poison, personnel trained to operate in such an environment should immediately be called to assist. The EMT should take the time to survey the scene for any potential airborne poison and should not enter a scene that is considered to be potentially dangerous.

Signs and Symptoms

After inhaling a poison, a patient will likely have complaints surrounding the respiratory system (Figure 35-3). Depending on the nature of the substance, however, the signs and symptoms may be

TABLE 35-2

Signs and Symptoms of Ingestion Poisoning

Nausea
Vomiting
Diarrhea
Altered mental status
Abdominal pain
Chemical burns around the mouth
Breath odor of chemical
Difficulty breathing

Street Smart

Certain poisons can create a characteristic odor to the breath. During the assessment of the airway, the EMT should note any odors on the patient's breath.

Medication Notes

Generic name: Activated charcoal
Trade name: Actidose, Super-Char, and more
Indications: Recent ingestion of poison
Contraindications: Patients who cannot control their own airway and swallow their own secretions or who have been given ipecac should *not* be given oral medications.
Dose: 1 g/kg body weight (50–100 g for typical adult)
Route: Oral

✳ *Inhalation Poisoning*

"I couldn't get the sink clean, so I mixed the green stuff with the bleach," explained the dishwasher. The initial call was for an odor or gas in a local restaurant.

When EMS arrived, people were streaming out of the building, coughing and acting as if they were choking. Several more complained of trouble breathing.

While the paramedic was establishing EMS command and calling for more resources, EMT Butler proceeded to corral the patrons into one area so they could all be treated.

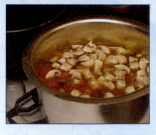

(Courtesy of Morguefile.)

- What are the immediate priorities for responding emergency personnel?
- What are the priorities in the emergency medical care of these patients?
- What are signs and symptoms characteristic of inhaled poisons?

quite extensive. Table 35-3 lists common signs and symptoms seen in the patient who has inhaled poison.

Management

Once properly trained providers have removed the patient from the potentially harmful area, the EMT can safely assess and treat the patient.

The general impression and initial assessment will allow the EMT to identify and treat any potentially life-threatening conditions immediately. Oxygen should always be administered to the patient who appears to have inhaled a potentially harmful substance.

TABLE 35-3

Common Signs and Symptoms of Inhalation Poisoning
Difficulty breathing
Chest pain
Cough
Hoarseness
Dizziness
Headache
Confusion
Seizures
Altered mental status

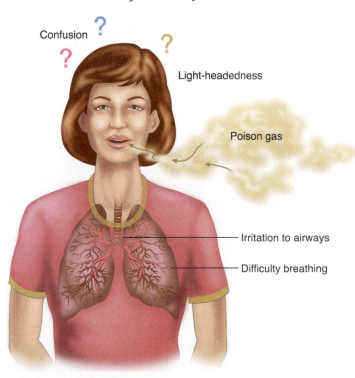

FIGURE 35-3 Inhaled poisons can cause irritation and injury to the upper and lower airways and may impede effective oxygenation.

INJECTED POISONS

Although uncommon, another type of poisoning involves the injection of a harmful substance. Intentional injection of a substance known to be harmful falls under the category of overdose, as discussed earlier.

Sometimes a patient will not know of the toxic nature of the substance and therefore the poisoning is unintentional. Another unintentional source of toxic injection is from creatures such as snakes, spiders, or scorpions. The management of these venomous injections is discussed in Chapter 34.

Signs and Symptoms

The signs and symptoms associated with an injected poison depend significantly on the specific poison (Figure 35-4). Some commonly seen signs and symptoms that the EMT should look for are listed in Table 35-4.

Management

In keeping with the high priority of safety in the management of any patient, the EMT should be aware of the sharp nature of the injecting device and should take care to ensure proper disposal of any contaminated sharps.

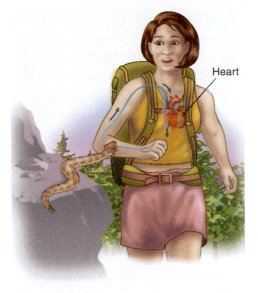

FIGURE 35-4 An injected poison will directly enter the bloodstream and be distributed around the body. Local blood vessel irritation is often seen.

✳ *Overdose*

"I don't feel well," complained Marty, a pale, thin young man, probably in his early 20s. He was found on the front stoop of a known crack house, and police were standing by as the crew started their work.

"Marty, can you tell me what you were doing?" asks Lt. McGreevy.

"Doing, doing," Marty spits out. "I've been doing whatever I can score, that's what I've been doing."

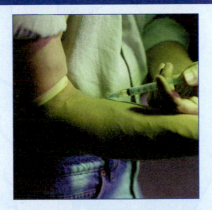

(Courtesy of PhotoDisc.)

The track marks on the inside of his forearms were prominent, with long, angry–looking streaks running up into his armpit.

"He told me," he continued, "that it was some fine horse. But I think he lied to me."

- What are the priorities in management of the patient with an injected poison?

- What are some signs and symptoms commonly seen in patients who have been poisoned in this manner?

TABLE 35-4

Signs and Symptoms of Injection Poisoning
Pain at injection site
Weakness
Dizziness
Chills
Fever
Nausea
Vomiting

TABLE 35-5

Signs and Symptoms of Absorption Poisoning

Liquid or powder on skin

Burns

Itching

Irritation to skin

Redness to area of exposure

Difficulty breathing

The patient should be removed from any potential danger. If any systemic signs and symptoms are present, the EMT should encourage the patient to lie quietly, with the affected part (the body part that suffered the bite, sting, or injection) lower than the heart. This position will decrease the flow of toxin toward the heart. Oxygen should be administered, and the patient should be transported as appropriate.

ABSORBED POISONS

Certain types of substances have the ability to be absorbed through intact skin. Others can cause injury to the skin upon contact.

Signs and Symptoms

The patient who is exposed to an absorbable poison will have symptoms that are specific to that agent but will often exhibit signs and symptoms such as those listed in Table 35-5 and shown in Figure 35-5.

Management

The principles of scene safety cannot be stressed enough in the case of absorbed poisons. Often, the offending agent is still in contact with

Hydrochloric acid

Irritation of skin

FIGURE 35-5 Some substances can be absorbed directly through the skin into surface blood vessels; others cause injury to the skin itself.

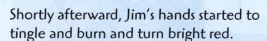

✳ *Absorbed Poison*

Jim was moving several barrels of cleaning chemicals from the warehouse to the storeroom, as he had been instructed to, when a couple of them tipped over, spilling their contents all over the floor.

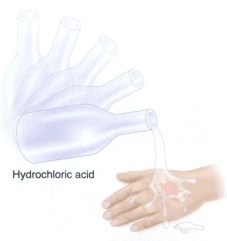

Hoping to avoid embarrassment, Jim thought he could quickly mop up the chemicals with a couple of rags. So he set about to do just that, using his bare hands.

Shortly afterward, Jim's hands started to tingle and burn and turn bright red. Alarmed, Jim reported to the company's infirmary immediately. There, he was cared for by an industrial nurse, Mary-Beth, who was assisted by EMT Baker.

Jim tried to explain what had happened and concluded his story with the statement, "I've burned my hands." Realizing the importance of his hands to a laborer like Jim, EMT Baker activated the company's emergency battalion and requested the ambulance.

- What are the priorities in the management of the patient who has been exposed to a topical poison?

- What signs and symptoms might be seen in such a situation?

the patient, presenting a significant danger to the unprepared EMT. Only emergency providers with training specific to this situation should attempt to enter the scene. These providers will appropriately decontaminate the patient and bring her to a safe area where the EMT can then provide the appropriate medical treatment.

If the exposure is limited and the substance easily recognized and dealt with, the EMT may choose to initiate decontamination according to local protocols. The appropriate initial care for any potentially harmful substance on the skin is to remove the substance by first brushing away any solid material. This step should be followed by extensive flushing with copious amounts of clean water. All clothing around the site should be removed before flushing. This decontamination should be done on scene.

If the patient's eyes were exposed to the substance, they should be irrigated thoroughly with clean water for at least 20 minutes. Contact lenses should be removed promptly. Care should be taken not to contaminate the unaffected eye by directing the irrigation from the middle of the face toward the affected eye as illustrated in Figure 35-6.

Care should be taken to properly collect and dispose of any contaminated runoff from the irrigation or flushing of a contaminated patient.

ALLERGIC REACTIONS

An allergic reaction occurs when the body is exposed to a particular substance that the immune system is particularly sensitive to. The immune system is the part of the body that responds to foreign materials such as viruses and bacteria and fights against them to prevent illness.

Occasionally a person's immune system may be particularly sensitive to a material that may be otherwise thought of as harmless. Every person's immune system responds to substances differently. A substance that causes an exaggerated immune system response resulting in an allergic reaction is called an **allergen**. Some common allergens are listed in Table 35-6.

Anaphylaxis

The actual effects on the body of an activation of the immune system can range from a local irritation at the site of the exposure to a life-threatening

Street Smart

Large-scale flushing may be impractical in the back of a moving ambulance; therefore, any flushing should be accomplished on scene. The only exception would be if the patient's condition warranted immediate transport or if only eyes were involved. The irrigation of eyes involves a more controlled flow of water and can be more easily accomplished in the rear of an ambulance.

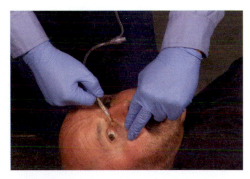

FIGURE 35-6 When the EMT is irrigating a contaminated eye, it is important to avoid cross-contaminating the uninvolved eye.

Street Smart

There are many different ways to effectively provide eye irrigation. If one eye is involved, intravenous (IV) tubing can be hooked up to normal saline and used to irrigate the eye. Alternatively, if these supplies are not available, oxygen tubing can be pushed through the punctured cap of a plastic bottle of normal saline with the same effect.

If both eyes are involved, a nasal cannula attached to IV saline may be placed over the bridge of the nose, allowing even flow to both eyes simultaneously.

TABLE 35-6

Common Allergens
Insect stings (bees, wasps, etc.)
Foods (nuts, seafood, peanuts, etc.)
Plants
Medications

Allergic Reaction

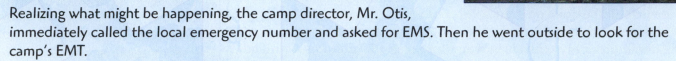

"What luck!" thought 17-year-old camp counselor-in-training Cathie. "First I pull latrine duty, then I get stung by a bee!"

Cathie proceeded directly to the camp office to report that she had been stung. By the time she got there, she was covered with raised red bumps and was itchy all over.

She was surprised when she heard her own voice, as she said, "I've been stung." Her speech was thick, and her tongue felt swollen.

Realizing what might be happening, the camp director, Mr. Otis, immediately called the local emergency number and asked for EMS. Then he went outside to look for the camp's EMT.

- What is an allergic reaction?
- What differentiates an allergic reaction from life-threatening anaphylaxis?
- What are the management priorities for a simple allergic reaction?

reaction called anaphylaxis (see Chapter 9). Anaphylaxis is a serious form of allergic reaction that may result in shock and even death.

Pathophysiology

The body's reaction to an extreme immune response involves several body systems, and substances are released from different cells throughout the body. These substances cause the signs and symptoms that are classically seen with an allergic reaction. Figure 35-7 illustrates the physical findings seen in an allergic reaction.

Skin

One of the most common signs of an allergic reaction is a rash. The rash associated with an acute allergic reaction is a characteristic pattern of raised reddened areas of skin called hives, or urticaria. The hives are actually created by tiny patches of dilated blood vessels with localized swelling caused by the chemicals released when triggered by the immune system. Figure 35-8 illustrates the pathophysiology behind hives.

Hives can be localized to just the area of exposure, as is seen in a bee sting. If the allergy is to an ingestion, such as peanuts, the hives may be more generalized. Hives tend to be very itchy, and the patient will want to scratch all over.

A mild allergic reaction may be limited to hives. Although this condition is very uncomfortable, isolated urticaria is not life threatening. The patient with hives, however, should be assessed for the presence of other signs of a severe allergic reaction.

Respiratory

In addition to causing localized inflammation of the skin, the immune response can cause inflammation and edema in the upper airway and lungs.

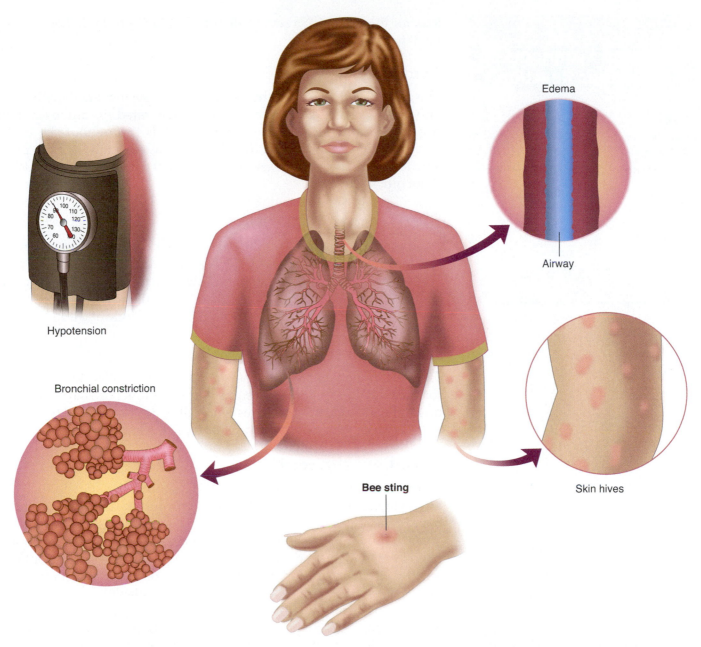

FIGURE 35-7 A severe allergic reaction involves several body systems.

Edema

Airway

Hypotension

Bronchial constriction

Bee sting

Skin hives

Swelling of the face, lips, and tongue is an ominous sign of a severe allergic reaction. If allowed to progress, the swelling can continue and completely occlude the patient's airway, making breathing impossible.

Signs of significant swelling in the airway are a hoarse voice, indicating swelling of the vocal cords, or an inspiratory upper airway sound called stridor. These signs indicate a dangerously narrowed upper airway.

Inflammation in the lower airways and lungs will result in constriction of the bronchioles. As the space for airflow is narrowed, the patient will begin to feel short of breath. The sound of the air rushing through the narrowed airways is called wheezing and can be heard upon auscultation of the chest.

These signs of airway and respiratory compromise may became very obvious but may initially be quite subtle. The EMT must specifically

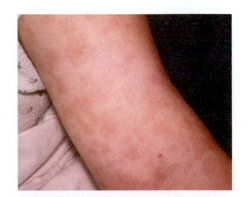

FIGURE 35-8 Hives are often the result of allergic reactions such as this reaction to penicillin. (Courtesy of the Centers for Disease Control Public Health Image Library.)

TABLE 35-7

Signs and Symptoms of an Allergic Reaction

Mild Allergic Reaction	Severe Allergic Reaction (Anaphylaxis)
Skin	
Warmth	Warmth
Redness	Redness
Hives	Hives
Itching	Itching
Localized swelling	Swelling
Respiratory	
No signs or symptoms	Throat tightness
	Shortness of breath
	Cough
	Wheezing
	Stridor
	Hoarseness
	Tachypnea
Cardiovascular	
No signs or symptoms	Tachycardia
	Hypotension
	Dizziness
	Other signs and symptoms of a hypo-perfused state
Other	
Itchy, watery eyes	Itchy, watery eyes
Headache	Headache
Runny nose	Sense of impending doom
	Runny nose

look for these signs of a severe allergic reaction in order to begin treatment immediately.

Cardiovascular

The generalized effects on the cardiovascular system are usually seen only with a severe reaction. This exaggerated immune system response results in dilation of blood vessels throughout the body. Such generalized dilation of blood vessels causes a fall in blood pressure and a sharp rise in heart rate. These will result in hypoperfusion if not quickly treated.

Signs and Symptoms

It is important to realize that the patient suffering from an allergic reaction may initially have signs of only a mild reaction but can progress to severe anaphylaxis in a matter of minutes. The typical allergic reaction begins within 30 minutes of exposure to the allergen. Table 35-7 lists the most common signs and symptoms of an allergic reaction.

Assessment

The key in management of the patient with an allergic reaction is for the EMT to recognize the signs and symptoms of anaphylaxis. A mild allergic reaction requires very little treatment by the EMT. Anaphylaxis will result in death if not quickly and properly treated.

Initial Assessment

During the initial assessment, the EMT should specifically look for any evidence of airway swelling and respiratory or cardiovascular compromise.

High-flow oxygen should be administered and, if signs of hypoperfusion are evident, the patient should be placed in a Trendelenburg position, kept warm, and immediately transported to the closest hospital, with an ALS unit called to intercept if available.

If the patient's breathing is inadequate, ventilations should be assisted with 100% oxygen. If the patient suffers a cardiac arrest, the EMT should institute appropriate supportive measures and rapidly transport.

The ongoing assessment should be repeated frequently because patients suffering from an allergic reaction can quickly worsen and require additional treatments.

History and Focused Physical Examination

A history and focused physical exam can provide crucial information to the EMT. Table 35-8 lists some important historical questions the EMT should ask of the patient with evidence of an allergic reaction.

Management

The patient with a severe allergic reaction will decompensate quickly without rapid treatment. The EMT should initiate treatment as appropriate through the initial assessment, including oxygen and ventilatory assistance if needed.

Some patients who have experienced previous anaphylactic reactions are prescribed a lifesaving medicine, epinephrine, by their physician. The EMT may assist the patient to use this medication with approval from medical control.

Epinephrine

Epinephrine is an injectable medication that dilates the bronchioles and constricts the blood vessels. These effects are useful in the patient suffering from an anaphylactic reaction.

Along with these useful effects, epinephrine has many unwanted and potentially harmful side effects. Therefore, the EMT must be thoroughly familiar with its indications and should consider its use only for a patient who has been prescribed it by a physician, unless local protocols allow differently.

Clear indications for use of epinephrine include those signs and symptoms listed in Table 35-9. Epinephrine is not indicated for use in a mild allergic reaction without evidence of airway, breathing, or circulatory compromise. Further details regarding this medication can be found in Chapter 26.

Transport

The patient suffering from an allergic reaction should be transported to the closest appropriate hospital. If any evidence of a severe reaction is present, an ALS intercept should be called for if available. ALS providers carry additional medications that may be useful in the management of the anaphylactic reaction.

Frequent reassessments during transport are critical so that any decompensation can be quickly recognized and appropriately dealt with. Table 35-10 lists signs of patient decompensation.

If these signs of deterioration become evident, the EMT should contact medical control for advice on further management. High-flow oxygen with ventilatory support if necessary, proper Trendelenburg positioning, and heat maintenance are indicated for the patient with evidence of hypoperfusion.

If the patient continues to decompensate, the EMT should be prepared to initiate basic cardiac life support measures to include

TABLE 35-8

Questions Related to Allergic Reactions

Is there a previous history of allergic reaction?

How severe was the previous reaction?

What was the patient exposed to?

What were the nature and timing of the exposure?

What symptoms are evident?

Has there been any progression of the symptoms?

Has your doctor prescribed medication for you to use in this situation?

What interventions have been attempted?

Street Smart

Some states allow nonphysicians to carry and administer epinephrine in the case of a severe allergic reaction. The EMT should be familiar with local regulations and obtain the relevant training if he is expected to utilize this medication without a physician's prescription.

Medication Notes

Generic name: Epinephrine
Trade name: EpiPen
Indications: Life-threatening allergic reaction
Contraindications: None in the presence of an indication
Dose: 0.3–0.5 mg for adults
0.15–0.3 mg for children
Route: Intramuscular

TABLE 35-9

Indications for Use of Epinephrine

Airway	Throat tightness
	Hoarseness
	Stridor
Breathing	Shortness of breath
	Wheezing
	Dyspnea
Circulation	Hypotension

TABLE 35-10

Signs of Decompensation— Allergic Reaction

Decreasing mental status

Increased difficulty breathing

Decreasing blood pressure

cardiopulmonary resuscitation (CPR) and automated external defibrillator (AED).

In most cases, with appropriate therapy, the patient with an allergic reaction will improve quickly. If the patient does not improve, the EMT should continue to administer high-flow oxygen and monitor the patient for deterioration as discussed previously.

All patients suffering from an allergic reaction should be transported to the hospital for further treatment and observation.

CONCLUSION

The body reacts to different substances in different ways. Some reactions can be predicted on the basis of the type of exposure, but some are quite unpredictable.

Exposures can be to substances known to be harmful or to harmful amounts of otherwise unharmful substances. These poisonings can result in severe illness. Exposure to a substance that causes an allergic reaction can also cause very severe illness.

No matter the nature of the exposure, the EMT must be familiar with the concepts of assessment and management of these patients.

TEST YOUR KNOWLEDGE

1. List various ways that poisons can enter the body.
2. Describe signs and symptoms associated with different types of poisonings.
3. Discuss the emergency medical care of the patient who has been poisoned.
4. Discuss the special considerations required in the emergency medical care of the intentional overdose patient.
5. Identify the potential airway issues in the poisoned patient.
6. Discuss the indications and contraindications for activated charcoal in the poisoned patient.
7. Discuss the need for medical control and advanced life support in the poisoned patient.
8. Describe the patient experiencing an allergic reaction.
9. Describe the emergency medical care of the patient with an allergic reaction.
10. Differentiate between a simple allergic reaction and anaphylaxis.
11. Describe the implications of anaphylaxis in regard to airway management.
12. State the indications and contraindications for the epinephrine auto-injector.
13. Identify the role of medical control and advanced life support in the care of the patient with anaphylaxis.

INTERNET RESOURCES

The following Web sites provide additional information on allergies and poisoning. Search the Internet using the types of poisons and allergic reactions discussed in this chapter for additional information. Share your results with your colleagues.

*   American Academy of Allergy, Asthma, and Immunology, http://www.aaaai.org
*   American Association of Poison Control Centers, http://www.aapcc.org
*   Asthma and Allergy Foundation of America, http://www.aafa.org
*   Food Allergy and Anaphylaxis Network, http://wwwfoodallergy.org

FURTHER STUDY

Fortenberry, J. E., Laine, J., & Shalit, M. (1995). Use of epinephrine for anaphylaxis by emergency medical technicians in a wilderness setting. *Annals of Emergency Medicine, 25*(6), 785–787.

Haynes, B. E., & Pritting, J. (1999). A rural emergency medical technician with selected advanced skills. *Prehospital Emergency Care, 3*(4), 343–346.

Hellman, M. (1996). Pediatric poisonings. *Emergency Medical Services, 25*(6), 21–29.

Hunt, D. (1997). Curse of the black scorpion. *Emergency Medical Services, 26*(10), 37–44.

Marciano, S. (1997). Mammalian animal bites. *Emergency Medical Services, 26*(10), 50–55.

Phillips, K. (1997). Nicotine poisoning. *Emergency Medical Services, 26*(9), 38–40.

Shepard, S. (1996). Plant exposures. *Emergency Medical Services, 25*(6), 39–40.

EMS *in Action*

It was 4 A.M. when my phone rang. I hoped it was the ambulance corps and not an emergency in the family, and it was. The dispatcher at the volunteer agency asked if I could make a connection with an ambulance that was on a maternity call five miles from my home. The crew consisted of a driver with no training and a new EMT, John, who was 20 years old and looking for help. He thought the birth was imminent. I advised the dispatcher to let John know I would be en route and to load the patient and meet me on scene or at the interstate entrance. I got dressed and headed for the scene, arriving just as he was loading the patient in the ambulance. She was having contractions and did not want to move very fast.

John had asked an EMT on rescue to assist him until I arrived. I got into the ambulance to find the expecting mother in full, hard labor. (This was her second child.) She was not crowning yet, so we proceeded to the hospital. About four blocks later she said she was having severe pressure pains. On examining her, she was crowning. We pulled over to the side of the road to deliver. I asked John to open the OB kit. He was very nervous, and when he opened it, it spilled onto the stretcher. I moved all the contents to the bench and prepared the mother with his help. He didn't want to deliver the baby but just watch, as he had never done this before.

There was a complication when the head delivered. The sac was not broken, so I ruptured it, the head delivered, and the cord was wrapped around the neck. I removed the cord, and the delivery proceeded without any further complications. John was in awe throughout the delivery. He breathed a sigh of relief when it was over. We cared for the baby, cleaned the mother up, and started for the hospital again.

There is nothing more rewarding than delivering a baby. John gained enough confidence in this delivery to deliver another a few weeks later. Two seasoned EMTs were on crew with him. He stepped up and advised his partners that he would take charge. When it was over, they asked him how he handled it so calmly. He just said, "Oh, it was nothing."

J. Penny Shutts, CIC, AEMT, NREMT-B
Instructor and Advanced Provider
Sandy Creek, New York

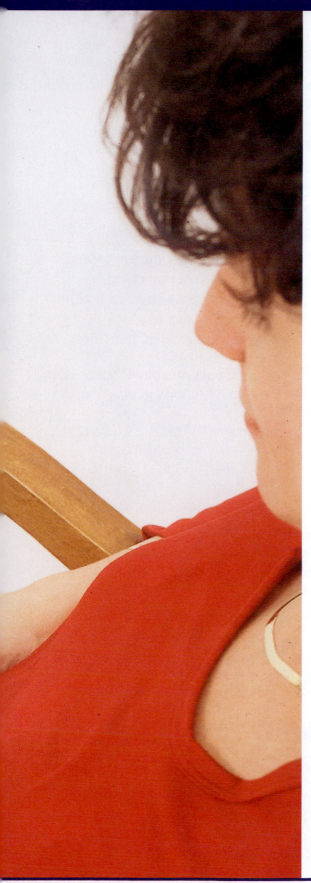

Maternal Health Emergencies

Although childbirth heralds the start of a new life, it also can be the harbinger of disaster if something goes wrong. The EMT's role in childbirth is usually one of an assistant, while the mother will naturally birth the baby.

However, the EMT must constantly assess both mother and child for signs of distress and be prepared to support the mother throughout the pregnancy as well as the childbirth.

This section reviews the special problems with pregnancy and the special role of the EMT as birth assistant.

CHAPTER 36

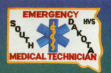

Prenatal Problems

KEY TERMS

abortion

cervix

childbirth

eclampsia

ectopic pregnancy

fallopian tube

fetus

fundus

miscarriage

ovary

ovulation

ovum

placenta

placenta previa

placental abruption

quickening

sexual assault

spontaneous abortion

supine hypotensive
   syndrome

uterus

OBJECTIVES

Upon completion of this chapter, the reader should be able to:

1. Identify the components of the female reproductive system.
2. Explain how the body changes during pregnancy.
3. Describe the care of the pregnant patient with abdominal pain.
4. Explain how to care for a victim of a sexual assault.
5. Review the risk factors that contribute to complications of pregnancy.
6. Describe the care of the pregnant patient with vaginal bleeding.
7. Explain the care of the woman who is suffering from pre-eclampsia and eclampsia.
8. Explain what protective mechanisms the fetus has against blunt trauma.

OVERVIEW

Pregnancy can be a truly wonderful time in a woman's life. It can be a dangerous time in her life as well. In the late nineteenth and early twentieth centuries, many women died during pregnancy due to complications of childbirth. Although that does not happen as often today, some of the same risks still exist.

An emergency medical technician (EMT) may be called to the scene of a woman who is having a complication of pregnancy. At those scenes, the EMT has not one life but two lives to consider. An EMT's prompt attention to life-threatening complications can help to ensure the survival of both mother and child in many cases.

ANATOMY REVIEW

The **uterus**, also called the womb, is a muscular chamber that holds the products of conception until birth. The nonpregnant uterus looks like an inverted bottle and is located inside the pelvis. The superior portion of the uterus, or the bottom of the bottle, is called the **fundus**. At the inferior portion of the uterus, or the neck of the bottle, is the **cervix**. The cervix is a ring of muscle that closes the uterus to the outside world. Through this small muscular opening, a baby is carried, or

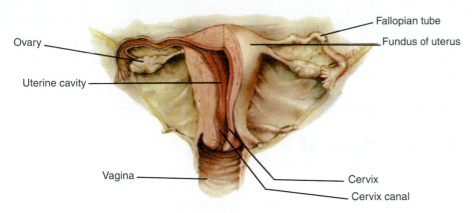

Ovary

Uterine cavity

Fallopian tube

Fundus of uterus

Vagina

Cervix

Cervix canal

FIGURE 36-1 The female reproductive system.

born, into the vagina. The baby then travels down the vagina, or birth canal, in a process called **childbirth**. The anatomy of the female reproductive system is illustrated in Figure 36-1. Further review can be found in Chapter 5.

CONCEPTION AND PREGNANCY

Attached to either side of the uterus are two tubes, called **fallopian tubes**. The fallopian tubes lead to the **ovaries**. The ovary is the source for a woman's lifetime supply of eggs. When an egg is released from an ovary, during a process called **ovulation**, it travels down the thin-walled fallopian tubes. (The fallopian tube has the same diameter as the lead of a pencil.) Once inside the fallopian tube, if sperm is present, fertilization of the egg may take place. The fertilized egg, now called an **ovum**, then travels into the uterus where, under normal circumstances, it will implant into the uterine wall on the uterine lining (Figure 36-2). Once the ovum is implanted in the uterine wall, it begins to grow and becomes first an embryo, and then a **fetus**.

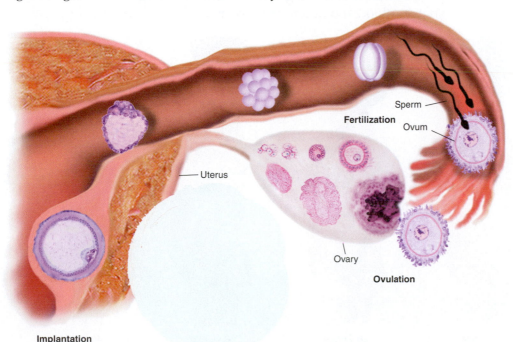

Sperm

Fertilization

Ovum

Uterus

Ovary

Ovulation

Implantation

FIGURE 36-2 The fertilized egg becomes an ovum and is implanted in the uterine wall.

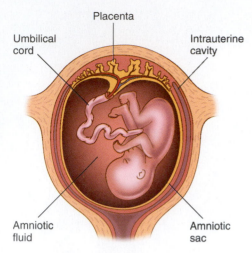

FIGURE 36-3 The anatomy of a pregnant uterus.

Early in the fetus's development, a bridge is created from mother to infant called the **placenta**. The lay term for placenta is the afterbirth. The placenta is important to the developing fetus. The placenta carries oxygen and nutrients from the mother to the fetus (Figure 36-3). Without a placenta firmly attached to the uterine wall, the fetus is at risk for hypoperfusion and hypoxia.

The Changes of Pregnancy

Pregnancy begins when the fertilized ovum implants in the uterine wall and continues for 37–40 weeks. The 9-month pregnancy is divided into three time periods, or trimesters. The first trimester is when implantation occurs and organs first start to appear in the fetus. The second trimester is a period of rapid growth and development for the fetus. During the third and last trimester, the fetus completes development.

Following fertilization, in the first trimester, powerful hormones are released that have a dramatic impact on the woman's body, preparing it for the rest of the pregnancy. Blood flow is increased to the uterus in anticipation of the demands of the placenta and the needs of the fetus. The blood volume in the body increases about 30%–35%. Because of this, more blood must be lost before the pregnant patient shows signs of hypoperfusion. The increased blood volume also leads to an increased heart rate, on average 10–15 beats per minute. However, the baseline blood pressure normally drops approximately 10–15 mm Hg during pregnancy. The changes in vital signs during pregnancy are illustrated in Figure 36-4.

As the uterus expands, it presses against the mother's diaphragm and makes breathing more difficult. The mother starts to breathe more rapidly and to take more shallow breaths. On average, the mother gains between 2 and 3 pounds of weight for every month of pregnancy. This weight gain represents the weight of additional fluid, such as blood and amniotic fluid, as well as the weight of the baby.

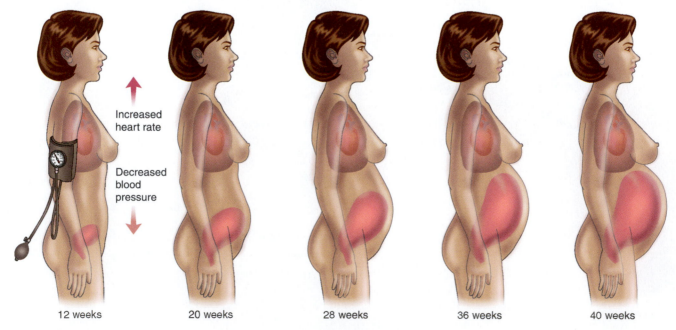

FIGURE 36-4 Breathing, heart rate, and blood pressure all change in pregnancy.

Abdominal Pain

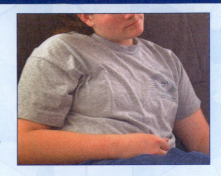

"Mom, I'm going to stay home! I don't feel so well," Erin yelled down the stairs. "OK, honey, but you'll miss your senior picture. Call me at the office if you get worse," her mother yelled back as she went out the front door.

Her mother had been at work less than an hour when the phone rang. "Mom, I really hurt," Erin cried. Her mother said, "Look, I'm coming home, and I'll call the ambulance as soon as I hang up." Mrs. Ward then called the local emergency number and explained to the operator how to locate the house, where to find the emergency key to get into the house, and that she would be home in about 30 minutes.

"Hello! It's Officer McCall, Cherry Valley Police. Hello!" cried out the police officer as he entered the house. "In here!" Erin replied. Led by Officer McCall, the ambulance crew walked toward the low sounds of sobbing and into the living room. The girl was curled in fetal position on the sofa, with the phone on the floor, and obviously had been crying. "My belly hurts, it really hurts!" she said.

- Based on the patient presentation, what medical conditions might an EMT suspect?
- What are the assessment priorities for this patient?
- What are the management priorities for this patient?
- How could this patient deteriorate?

ABDOMINAL PAIN IN WOMEN OF CHILDBEARING AGE

There are many different reasons for a woman to have abdominal pain. Some are related to pregnancy; most are not. Abdominal pain due to a complication of pregnancy, however, can be life threatening. Because a woman may not know she is pregnant early on, any sexually active woman of childbearing age with lower quadrant abdominal pain is treated as though she were pregnant. The childbearing years start when a female has her first menses at menarche. Some women start their menses as early as 8 or 9 years of age, although 11 is the average age of menarche for women in the United States. Menses, the root of the word "menstruation," is the periodic discharge of blood and tissue from the uterus through the vagina, commonly called a woman's period. Until menopause, the end of a woman's fertility, menstruation occurs approximately every 28 days when a woman is not pregnant. Menarche, represented by a woman's first menses, is the beginning of a woman's period of fertility.

Ectopic Pregnancy

Immediately after intercourse, the fertilized ovum is supposed to travel down the fallopian tubes and enter the uterus. For one reason or another, the ovum may fail to descend into the uterus, and a pregnancy may develop outside of the uterus. A pregnancy that develops outside of the uterus is called an **ectopic pregnancy** (Figure 36-5).

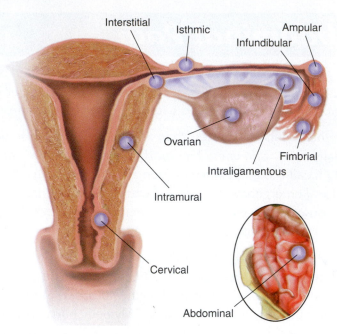

FIGURE 36-5 An ectopic pregnancy can occur at many sites outside the uterus.

In some cases, the ectopic pregnancy develops in the fallopian tube. The fallopian tubes are very thin, and the developing ovum eventually ruptures the fallopian tube. The rupture of a fallopian tube from an ectopic pregnancy can cause significant internal bleeding. Unchecked, the bleeding can eventually lead to shock, and even death. A woman is at greatest risk for a ruptured ectopic pregnancy between her 6th and 12th week of pregnancy.

Assessment

The symptoms of an ectopic pregnancy include lower abdominal pain and possibly even scant vaginal bleeding. The abdominal pain may be described as crampy or achy. If internal bleeding is significant, the patient may have symptoms consistent with hypoperfusion such as dizziness, thirst, and anxiety.

The signs of an ectopic pregnancy are similar to the signs of any severe hemorrhage. Tachycardia, tachypnea, pallor, and other signs of hypoperfusion will be present. Hypotension is a grave indication of severe internal bleeding. Lower abdominal tenderness to palpation is also usually found.

Management

The focus of prehospital care of the pregnant woman who may have an ectopic pregnancy is to treat the hypoperfusion. The EMT should always provide high-concentration oxygen, regardless of pulse oximetry readings. While the mother may be well oxygenated, the developing fetus may be hypoxic, and there is no method by which an EMT can measure the fetus's oxygenation. The EMT also should place the patient in the modified Trendelenburg position to improve circulation to the uterus. Finally, the EMT should cover the mother with a blanket to preserve body warmth for both mother and child.

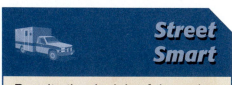

Street Smart

Despite the denials of the patient or the results of home pregnancy tests, an EMT should always consider the possibility of pregnancy in a woman of childbearing age with a complaint of lower abdominal pain. Accordingly, the EMT must err on the side of caution and treat every female of childbearing age who has a complaint of lower abdominal pain as if she may have an ectopic pregnancy.

Transportation

If the patient presents with clear signs of hypoperfusion, she should be transported immediately. An advanced life support (ALS) intercept should be arranged if possible so that intravenous (IV) lines can be established. It is important to transport the mother to an appropriate facility that is capable of dealing with hemorrhage and can provide blood if the need should arise.

SEXUAL ASSAULT

EMTs treat all cases of violent sexual attack as **sexual assault**. A sexual assault can be a rape, sodomy, or even unwanted sexual touching. Sexual assault can occur to both men and women. A sexual assault is a psychological, as well as a physical, trauma to a person. Often sexual assault is not about sex but about one human being controlling or dominating another human being. This form of power struggle results in violence and trauma.

Assessment

The first priority in any trauma is to care for the patient's physical well-being. If life-threatening injuries are present, the EMT should complete an initial assessment and treat the injuries. However, the EMT should be sensitive to the psychological trauma that has occurred as well. If it is possible, a same-sex EMT should care for the patient. The EMT should respect the patient's requests for privacy, up to and including the patient's right to refuse a physical examination (Figure 36-6).

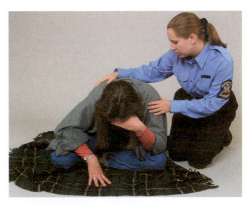

FIGURE 36-6 Active listening and a caring attitude help the sexual assault victim.

✴ *Rape*

Officer Gould was making her usual rounds on campus when her radio crackled and a message came across the air. The dispatcher announced, "Units in the vicinity of the soccer field, acknowledge and respond to the south end for a panic alarm activation."

Officer Gould, who was near the soccer field, responded to the dispatcher with "on scene," as the first-arriving unit. As she looked around, she saw a young woman, maybe in her late teens, standing behind a tree. "Probably a freshman," Gould thought as she approached the woman.

As she moved closer, Gould could see that the young woman was partially clothed and that she was valiantly trying to hold up the remains of her shirt to cover her chest. The words that the young woman spoke cut through the cold night air like a knife. "I've been raped," the woman told the officer.

- Based on the patient presentation, what injuries might an EMT suspect?
- What are the assessment priorities for this patient?
- What are the management priorities for this patient?
- How could this patient deteriorate?

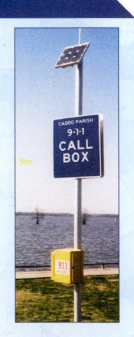

It is not appropriate for an EMT to ask the patient to recount the assault. An insensitive EMT who barrages the patient with questions about the assault can cause feelings of fear, anxiety, guilt, and indignity in the patient. Instead, the EMT should listen carefully to the patient's complaints, focusing on the physical injuries that may have occurred. The EMT should never take a patient's refusal to talk personally.

An EMT should never perform a genital assessment of a sexual assault patient unless significant trauma or severe bleeding is present. If that is the case, the EMT should focus on treating the injury, then cover the patient's body. Trauma from a sexual assault usually consists of lacerations, bruising, and associated bleeding. The bleeding typically can be controlled by bulky dressings.

Management

Although rape is a criminal matter, the law does not require the patient to report the crime. Some patients, for a variety of valid reasons, decide not to pursue criminal charges at the time. The EMT must respect the patient's wishes. The responsibility of the EMT is to treat the patient. If the patient does wish to press criminal charges, the EMT should contact a law enforcement officer (LEO) for assistance. Detectives with special training in sex crimes often investigate sexual assault cases.

The EMT is not responsible for collecting evidence; however, the EMT who removes clothing or personal effects from the patient when an LEO is not present should place these articles in a plain brown paper bag. The paper bag should then be folded and taped shut, and initialed by the EMT. The bag should be kept by the EMT until it can be personally handed over to an LEO.

The patient should be discouraged from bathing, douching, voiding, or hand washing immediately after the assault. Law enforcement officers may want an opportunity to collect evidence from the victim's body. A sexual assault "evidence kit" is usually available for this purpose.

A special case is the sexual assault of a minor. In some states, sexual assault of a minor must be reported as child abuse. The EMT should know the local and state laws regarding the reporting of child abuse.

In a case of alleged sexual assault or rape, the EMT's documentation may be very useful in the prosecution of the attacker. It is important that the EMT completely and accurately document the patient's physical condition. The patient care report will likely be reviewed by lawyers and may even be used in a court of law in testimony. Therefore, it is important that the EMT keep her descriptions of the patient's condition simple and in terms that a layperson, like a juror, would understand. It is also important that the EMT try to document any statements made by the patient, in the patient's own words if possible, regarding the assault or rape on the patient care report. The EMT should be especially careful to keep the documentation impartial and objective.

Transportation

All victims of sexual assault and rape should be encouraged to be evaluated at a hospital in a timely manner. Medical care always takes precedence over police reporting. The LEO can always follow the patient to the hospital to get a report.

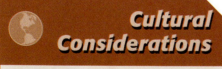

Cultural Considerations

EMTs make many decisions, on behalf of their patients, without a conscious thought. A sexual assault may leave a person with a sense of powerlessness and loss of control. Whenever possible, the EMT should involve the patient in decision making. Even making simple decisions can help patients feel as though they are regaining control of their life and body.

In some cases, patients request care only in the field and do not want to be taken to the hospital. In those cases, the EMT should respect the patient's wishes and offer the patient the opportunity to call emergency medical services (EMS) again if she should change her mind.

COMPLICATIONS EARLY IN PREGNANCY

Prenatal care can help to reduce the risk of complications of pregnancy and to ensure the delivery of a healthy baby. Unfortunately, not every woman knows that she is pregnant in the first trimester, when some of the risks are greatest.

Women who smoke tobacco products or who drink alcohol are at greater risk of prenatal complications. Women who suffer from diabetes before pregnancy experience more complications of childbirth. Some women develop diabetes during pregnancy because of the pregnancy. This type of diabetes is called gestational diabetes and may spontaneously resolve with the completion of the pregnancy. Other women, who decide to become pregnant later in their reproductive lives, are also at greater risk for the complications of pregnancy.

Bleeding During Early Pregnancy

Occasionally, a woman experiences light bleeding early in her pregnancy. Many of these pregnancies will be normal; however, it is impossible to know what the bleeding means without examination by a physician.

Excessive Bleeding

The EMT team and the sheriff's deputy were met at the door by a middle-aged woman who reeked of cigarette smoke. "It's my daughter, she's in the bathroom." With those words, the woman turned around, sat down in her chair, and continued to watch the soap opera on television.

Walking in single file down the narrow hallway, the team came to a closed bathroom door. From behind the closed door came a muffled, "I'll be right there." In about a minute, the door opened and a teenaged girl motioned Shelley, one of the EMTs, inside, and indicated that the men should stay out.

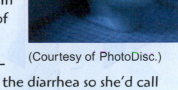

(Courtesy of PhotoDisc.)

"Look," the girl started, "I'm pregnant, but my Momma don't know. I'm bleeding down there," indicating her crotch. "More than usual. I told Momma I had the diarrhea so she'd call EMS." While listening to the girl's story, Shelley peered into the toilet. It was full of blood.

- Based on the patient presentation, what medical conditions might an EMT suspect?
- What are the assessment priorities for this patient?
- What are the management priorities for this patient?
- How could this patient deteriorate?

Spontaneous Abortion

Many pregnancies are not completed, or carried for the full term. A pregnancy may end prematurely for a variety of reasons. The termination of a pregnancy before a fetus reaches the stage of viability, at about 20 weeks, is termed an **abortion**.

If the embryo is imperfect or conditions are not right, the woman may lose the pregnancy very early in the pregnancy. The woman may experience what is called a **spontaneous abortion**. A spontaneous abortion, also called a **miscarriage**, occurs in 1 out of every 200 pregnancies.

Usually a spontaneous abortion occurs in the first 6–12 weeks of pregnancy. A woman who is unaware that she is pregnant may spontaneously abort the pregnancy without her knowledge. The only change that she might note is that her menstrual flow, her period, is heavier than normal. Today, home pregnancy tests can determine that a woman is pregnant within the first 2 weeks. A woman who knows she is pregnant may interpret any bleeding as a spontaneous abortion, or miscarriage.

A spontaneous abortion may be accompanied by abdominal pain. It is difficult to differentiate between a spontaneous abortion and an ectopic pregnancy without an ultrasound. Because an ectopic pregnancy is potentially life threatening and a spontaneous abortion usually is not, the EMT should treat for the worst possibility. Any woman of childbearing age with lower abdominal pain should be assumed to be having an ectopic pregnancy and treated accordingly.

Assessment of the Pregnant Woman

The assessment of a pregnant woman should begin the same way as for any other patient, with a scene size-up and initial assessment. Any life-threatening problems found in the initial assessment should be addressed at that time. The focused history and physical examination of the pregnant woman who is responsive should be based upon her presenting complaint. Additional factors that are important to obtain as part of a pregnant woman's history, regardless of her complaint, are how far along she is in her pregnancy; whether she has had prenatal care; whether she has had any complications with the pregnancy; and how many times she has been pregnant before this pregnancy. This information, along with the usual SAMPLE history (see Table 10-5) and a history of the present illness, will be useful in the care of the patient.

When measuring vital signs, the EMT should remember the expected slight elevation in heart rate and respiratory rate and drop in blood pressure that are found toward the end of pregnancy. The remainder of this chapter covers other specific assessment techniques and the management of conditions related to pregnancy.

Signs and Symptoms

The EMT should ask the patient whether there is any pain or cramping associated with the bleeding. If the answer is yes, the EMT should ask when the pain began and have the patient characterize it. The EMT should also ask when the bleeding started. A rough estimate of blood loss can be determined by asking for a pad count. A pad count

---

Street Smart

Any pregnancy is a highly emotional event. Emotional support for the patient is very important. Pregnancy is a very private condition, and the EMT should be kind and considerate of the patient's rights to privacy.

The EMT also must ask the patient sensitive questions about the pregnancy as a part of the history gathering during the assessment. If possible, a female EMT should attend the patient while these questions are being asked because this may make the patient more comfortable.

Cultural Considerations

Some cultures, for example, Arab-Americans, prefer that a woman attend a woman who is pregnant. The patient, or the patient's family, may not be pleased to know that a male is asking personal questions or examining the patient. The EMT should be sensitive to these cultural differences in her community and be prepared to respond to them appropriately.

is the number of sanitary napkins, or tampons, that the woman has used since the bleeding began.

The other physical signs found in the woman who may be miscarrying are the same signs and symptoms of hypoperfusion from hemorrhage. The EMT should assess the patient for signs of pallor, tachycardia, and tachypnea.

Management

Care of the patient who is having, or may have had, a spontaneous abortion is largely supportive. The EMT should complete an initial assessment and gather the SAMPLE history. High-concentration oxygen should be administered and the patient prepared for immediate transportation. Occasionally, a patient may show the EMT a sanitary pad. The EMT should note the color and consistency of the blood on the pad; it is not necessary for an EMT to ask to see a sanitary pad; it is enough that the patient said she is bleeding. The EMT should try to save any blood clots or tissue that may be found (Figure 36-7). Any plastic cup with a lid is an acceptable container for this material, which should be given to hospital staff so they may examine it.

COMPLICATIONS OF PREGNANCY

Once a woman has passed the sixth month of her pregnancy and entered the last trimester, the chances of successfully completing the pregnancy are greatly increased. By the third trimester, the infant may survive if it is born at this early date. Some risks to the mother, however, still exist. The EMT should recognize the risks involved with complications in the third trimester and transport the mother and child immediately to an appropriate facility.

Bleeding Late in Pregnancy

Any vaginal bleeding during pregnancy should be considered serious. Vaginal bleeding can be life threatening to both the mother and the fetus. Any vaginal bleeding during pregnancy should be evaluated by a medical provider as soon as possible. Sudden vaginal bleeding, especially in the third trimester of pregnancy, may indicate that there is a problem with the placenta.

Placental Abruption

Vaginal bleeding may indicate that the placenta has prematurely detached from the uterine wall, a condition that is called **placental abruption**. Placental abruption results in a decreased blood flow to the fetus and significant blood loss for the mother. This condition most commonly follows some kind of trauma. Even minor falls can be the inciting factor for an abruption; therefore, every woman in her third trimester of pregnancy who suffers even a minor injury should be evaluated at the hospital in a timely fashion.

The woman with a placental abruption (Figure 36-8) may complain of abdominal pain followed by vaginal bleeding. Vaginal bleeding may not be present if the bleeding is contained behind the placental barrier and does not leak out of the uterus through the cervical opening.

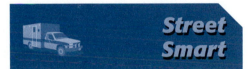

FIGURE 36-7 Blood clots and tissue should be collected and delivered to the emergency department.

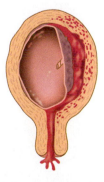

FIGURE 36-8 A detached placenta is called a placental abruption.

Vaginal Bleeding

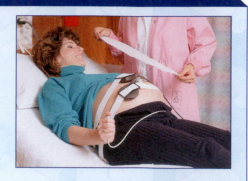

"Dr. Fitz's office," the receptionist announced. "Did someone there call EMS, ma'am?" asked EMT Waite. "Yes, please come in," replied the receptionist. "Down to the end of the hall, last door on the left. The nurse will meet you there."

Pulling the stretcher behind them, the two EMTs went down the narrow hall to the last door on the left and knocked on the door. "Come in," shouted a voice from within. The EMTs were then led to the cramped examining room, where they met their obviously pregnant patient.

"Hello," EMT Waite said to the patient. Immediately the nurse provided a long patient history that included 28 weeks of pregnancy and heavy, painless vaginal bleeding for the past 2 hours.

The last remark was like a slap in the face for the EMTs. Heavy, painless vaginal bleeding for 2 hours! The two EMTs immediately leapt into action.

- Based on the patient presentation, what medical conditions might an EMT suspect?
- What are the assessment priorities for this patient?
- What are the management priorities for this patient?
- How could this patient deteriorate?

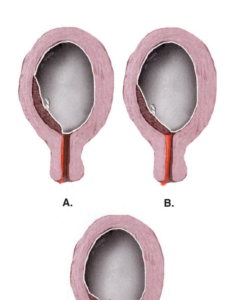

A.   **B.**

C.

FIGURE 36-9 A misplaced placenta is called placenta previa.

Placenta Previa

Another situation that may result in third trimester vaginal bleeding occurs when the placenta is placed abnormally low in the uterus and the placenta has grown over the opening of the uterus, or the cervix (Figure 36-9). This condition, which is known as a **placenta previa**, results in significant vaginal bleeding without any associated pain and can rapidly result in hemorrhagic shock for the mother and lack of blood flow to the fetus. Placenta previa occurs about once in every 200 pregnancies, and usually in first-time mothers.

Toxemia of Pregnancy

During her pregnancy, a woman may develop a condition called toxemia of pregnancy. Toxemia of pregnancy literally means the "poisoned pregnancy." If let untreated, toxemia of pregnancy can lead to coma and death. The cause of toxemia is not known, but the condition occurs more commonly in women during their first pregnancy. Women who are very young, less than 17 years, or older, more than 35 years, are also at greater risk of developing toxemia. Toxemia of pregnancy is more commonly called **eclampsia** today. Eclampsia can be divided into two stages: pre-eclampsia and eclampsia.

Pre-eclampsia

A woman with pre-eclampsia may experience a variety of symptoms, including mild to severe hypertension and edema of the face and hands. Some patients with pre-eclampsia complain of severe headaches and visual disturbances.

The woman with pre-eclampsia should be transported quietly to the hospital with oxygen in place. Bright lights and loud sirens may induce a seizure and should be used only if the mother is unconscious. ALS intercept and medical direction should be obtained as indicated by local protocol.

Eclampsia

The hallmark that separates eclampsia from pre-eclampsia is a seizure. The seizure indicates severe brain irritation. If the eclampsia is not treated, the patient will lapse into a coma. The EMT should initiate rapid transportation to the closest ALS unit or hospital while managing the airway, breathing, and circulation (ABCs) of mother and child. Eclamptic seizures can be treated with intravenous medications; therefore, the EMT must transport the patient immediately.

Management

An EMT should *not* perform either internal or external vaginal examination of a pregnant woman in the field unless she is anticipating an imminent delivery of the infant. The EMT can study the signs of an imminent birth in Chapter 37.

The EMT need not distinguish between the conditions causing bleeding in the third trimester. Instead, the EMT should consider the patient to be having a complication of pregnancy and should transport her immediately.

The bleeding can be profuse and life threatening to both mother and fetus. The mother should be assessed and reassessed for signs of hypoperfusion. It is assumed that if the mother is hypoperfused, then the fetus is in distress. The mother should be transported on her left side in the modified Trendelenburg position; she also should be kept warm with a blanket and be given continuous high-concentration oxygen provided via a non-rebreather facemask.

BLUNT ABDOMINAL TRAUMA

The developing fetus has a number of protections from outside forces. In the early stages of pregnancy, the pelvis provides a bony shield against blunt and penetrating trauma. As the fetus develops and enlarges, outgrowing the confines of the pelvis, amniotic fluid is produced in larger and larger quantities. The amniotic fluid surrounds the fetus and acts as a shock absorber. As much as 500–1,000 cc of this almost-clear fluid can be found in the amniotic sac within the uterus, surrounding the fetus as a protective cushion.

At about the 12th week of pregnancy, the uterus expands outside the protective confines of the pelvis. In the third trimester, the pregnant uterus markedly protrudes past the rest of the body's silhouette and, thus, becomes more prone to injury.

In severe cases of blunt trauma, the force can be so great that the uterus actually ruptures. This rupture is more common in women who previously had a cesarean section because of the weakened uterine wall. A uterine rupture can quickly lead to serious life-threatening internal hemorrhage.

Spousal Abuse

As the EMTs parked the ambulance, they could see a police officer leading a man away from the house in handcuffs. Puzzled by what they were seeing, EMT Nabinger approached the police supervisor, Sgt. McNally, and inquired, "What's going on? We got a call for a woman who had fallen."

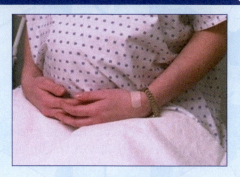

"More like pushed, down a flight of stairs," Sgt. McNally replied. "She's over there, in the patrol car. Look, I've got to take a statement, so do you mind if I listen in while you guys get your history?"

"It's entirely up to her," Nabinger told McNally, "but as far as I'm concerned, you're welcome to come." As McNally turned to wave down a passing patrol car with red lights flashing, he added, "Oh, by the way, she's 6 months pregnant. I'll be with you guys in a minute."

"Six months pregnant," Nabinger thought. He felt his stomach begin to knot.

- Based on the patient presentation, what injuries might an EMT suspect?
- What are the assessment priorities for this patient?
- What are the management priorities for this patient?
- How could this patient deteriorate?

Assessment

The assessment of the pregnant patient who has experienced a blunt trauma is no different than that of any other patient except that the EMT must remember she is treating not one patient, but two. The second patient, the fetus, is much more sensitive to changes in blood volume. Therefore, the EMT must have a heightened awareness and a higher index of suspicion that bleeding may be occurring internally.

Scene Size-Up

The mechanism of injury is the key to understanding why a pregnant woman who has sustained a blunt trauma may be bleeding internally. A variety of mechanisms, from assaults to vehicular collisions, can cause blunt trauma, and the severity of the trauma is a function of the force involved. How fast was the vehicle moving? How many stairs did she fall down? The EMT must ask these and other questions as she approaches the scene and does her scene size-up.

Falls

The additional weight of the infant shifts the woman's center of gravity forward. This change makes a pregnant woman prone to falling forward. This condition, a forward center of gravity and a resultant tendency to fall, makes the uterus prone to injury from blunt trauma. Injury to the uterus can occur from some very common mechanisms of injury. For example, the expectant mother may trip on a curb she cannot see and fall forward, striking her abdomen and suffering blunt trauma.

It is important that the EMT document not only the fall but also the height from which the patient fell, as well as the type of surface on which the patient landed. The EMT also needs to perform a standard assessment for head and spine injury.

Intentional Trauma

Some women, including those who are pregnant, are victims of domestic violence. Spouses and fathers of unexpected babies may be angry about the pregnancy. The pregnant abdomen then becomes the target of the attack. Pregnant women have been shot in the abdomen, pushed down a flight of stairs, and punched or kicked in the abdomen. The attackers may intend to cause a miscarriage as well as punish the woman for the pregnancy.

Motor Vehicle Collisions

Pregnancy doubles the chance of injury in a motor vehicle collision. As the body is thrown forward, the bulging abdomen becomes the area of first contact. Both mother and child can be adversely impacted. Restraint devices, like seat belts and padded steering wheels, can help to lessen the blow. Yet, some women fail to wear their seat belt properly. Saying that the seat belts are "uncomfortable," they wear the seat belts higher on the abdomen, and not across the pelvis where the seat belt is supposed to be (Figure 36-10). Some expectant mothers think that wearing a seat belt will actually increase the chance of injury to their unborn baby. Research has shown that seat belts, a lap belt with a shoulder restraint, actually decrease the rates of maternal mortality and uterine injury. EMTs should encourage all pregnant women to wear their seat belts when driving.

Assessment

After the scene size-up and consideration of the mechanism of injury, the EMT should proceed with the initial assessment. The treatment priorities for a pregnant patient are the same as those for a nonpregnant patient. The EMT should secure the airway, assess and assist respiration, control bleeding, and rapidly transport high-priority cases.

The EMT also should ask the mother whether she felt a gush of fluid from her vagina. If she did, then her membranes may have ruptured. Fluid leaking from the vagina may be amniotic fluid, or it may be blood. The presence of blood should lead the EMT to suspect either placental abruption or possibly a ruptured uterus. In both cases, the patient needs rapid transportation to the closest appropriate facility.

At or before the 20th week of pregnancy, a mother may feel fetal movement, called **quickening**. The EMT should ask the mother whether she can feel her baby move. The fetus is usually more active after trauma. However, a still baby may just be a quiet baby. The EMT should not alarm the mother by making any rash statements about the baby being injured because the baby is not moving.

The EMT should carefully palpate the pregnant woman's abdomen to assess for tenderness (Figure 36-11). A pregnant uterus normally feels firm and should be nontender. The abdomen should be examined for signs of trauma. Reddened areas, abrasions, contusions, and

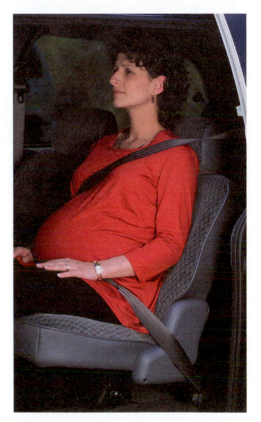

FIGURE 36-10 A properly worn seat belt can decrease injuries sustained by a pregnant woman in a motor vehicle collision.

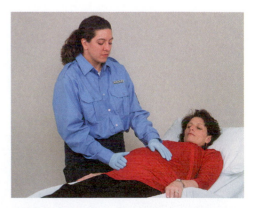

FIGURE 36-11 The EMT should feel for point tenderness as well as fetal movement.

point tenderness may indicate the place where the force struck the abdomen.

It is difficult to assess fetal heart sounds in the field, so the EMT should not spend time trying to ascertain whether these sounds are present. Instead, the EMT should advise the hospital about the situation so that a fetal heart monitor will be ready when the patient arrives.

The EMT should ask the mother whether she is feeling any cramps or labor pains, and should ask her to make a comparison between her present level of discomfort and that caused by her worst menstrual cramps. Usually labor pains are worse than the patient's worst menstrual cramps.

The EMT should ask the mother whether she was wearing her seat belt at the time of the accident and should examine the car for air bag deployment. If the air bag has been deployed, the EMT should look at the steering wheel under the air bag for deformity.

Management

When trying to manage the pregnant patient who has suffered a traumatic injury, the EMT is faced with not one, but two, patients. How does the EMT manage both? While the concept of caring for two seriously injured patients may be daunting, the EMT need only concentrate her skills on the mother. The infant's survival is tied to the mother's survival. Simply stated, "Save the mother to save the baby."

The EMT should concentrate on the ABCs. High-concentration oxygen is always appropriate. Even if the mother is well oxygenated, the fetus may not be because of vasoconstriction and shunting. As with any other injured patient, the pregnant trauma patient should have spinal immobilization if appropriate. Oxygen should be administered if it is indicated by the injury. Any pregnant woman with abdominal pain after trauma should receive high-flow oxygen.

Hypoperfusion in Pregnancy

When the body loses blood, vasoconstriction of selected organs occurs, shifting or shunting blood to more vital organs. The skin is usually the first organ to shunt blood, followed by muscles, gut, kidneys, heart, lungs, and lastly, brain. The pecking order of hypoperfusion is different during pregnancy. When the pregnant body loses blood, the placenta is the first organ to vasoconstrict, shunting blood away from the fetus to the mother's vital organs.

It is difficult for an EMT to assess fetal distress. However, an EMT can assess the mother and indirectly infer the fetal condition. When the mother's skin is pale and clammy, that would imply that the placenta is vasoconstricted and the fetus is in distress.

Because of the changes of pregnancy, the traditional signs of hypoperfusion may not be as reliable. A pregnant woman's resting heart rate is naturally higher than usual, and her resting blood pressure is slightly lower than usual. These findings should not be mistaken as signs of hypoperfusion and impending shock. The EMT should remember that the increased blood volume, about 35% more blood volume than normal, will allow for more blood loss before a significant drop in blood pressure occurs. The EMT should take repeated vital signs during an ongoing assessment and report any changes immediately.

Transportation

The patient should be transported to the closest appropriate facility. When the EMT considers transportation destinations, she should consider the fetal-monitoring capabilities of the hospitals. The EMT should follow local triage protocols regarding destination hospitals.

Typically, a trauma patient is immobilized to a backboard supine to protect the spine. A pregnant trauma patient should also be immobilized to the backboard; however, the weight of the uterus, when the mother lies flat, compresses the vena cava and stops blood from returning from the lower extremities to the heart. Immediately the patient's heart receives about 30% less blood return than is normal. The patient's blood pressure will drop suddenly, and the patient may even lose consciousness. The sudden loss of blood pressure when a pregnant woman lies flat is called **supine hypotensive syndrome**.

Supine hypotensive syndrome happens more commonly in the third trimester and is easily treated. Once the patient has been immobilized, head and body, to the backboard, the backboard is tilted onto the left side at about a 15-degree angle. A bedroll or rolled blanket placed under the backboard works well to maintain this position (Figure 36-12). If tilting the backboard is not possible, an EMT can take two hands and manually shift the uterus to the left side, off the vena cava. After either technique is utilized, the blood pressure should immediately return.

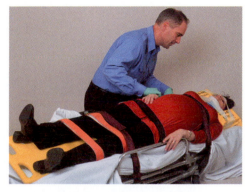

FIGURE 36-12 Tilting the backboard as little as 15 degrees can prevent supine hypotensive syndrome.

CONCLUSION

The changes of pregnancy present many challenges to the EMT who is trying to manage the complications that can occur during a pregnancy. By providing competent, professional prehospital care, however, the EMT can be part of helping to bring a new life into the world.

TEST YOUR KNOWLEDGE

1. What are the components of the female reproductive system?
2. What changes occur in the body of a pregnant woman?
3. What are several factors that increase a woman's risk of a complication during pregnancy?
4. What special considerations should be given to a sexual assault victim?
5. What are the signs of placenta previa?
6. What mechanisms protect the fetus from blunt trauma?
7. How would an EMT treat pre-eclampsia?

INTERNET RESOURCES

For additional information related to pregnancy, visit these Web sites:

- Childbirth.org, http://www.childbirth.org
- Ectopic Pregnancy Trust, http://www.ectopic.org
- Pregnancy.org, http://www.pregnancy.org

Information related to rape and sexual assault can be found at these Web sites:

- Hope for Healing, http://www.hopeforhealing.org
- Rape, Abuse and Incest National Network, http://www.rainn.org

FURTHER STUDY

Cascio, A., & Polk, D. (1997). Trauma in the pregnant patient. *Journal of Emergency Medical Services, 22*(8), 90–97.

Gregoire, A. (1997). When the trauma patient is pregnant. *RN, 60*(2), 44–50.

Mattera, C. (1999). Obstetrical complications. *Journal of Emergency Medical Services, 24*(3), 124–128.

Phillips, K. (1996). Teen abortion. *Emergency Medical Services, 25*(5), 41–43.

CHAPTER 37

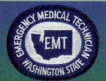

Emergency Childbirth

KEY TERMS

amniotic sac

bloody show

Braxton Hicks contractions

breech presentation

cardinal movements of labor

cervical dilation

cesarean section

crowning

effacement

first stage of labor

gravidity

labor

meconium

molding

multiparous

parity

premature delivery

primiparous

prolapsed umbilical cord

second stage of labor

third stage of labor

OBJECTIVES

Upon completion of this chapter, the reader should be able to:

1. Describe the normal female anatomy during pregnancy.
2. Describe the components of the three stages of labor.
3. Identify signs and symptoms of impending delivery.
4. Recognize the importance of a brief predelivery history.
5. Describe how to assist with a normal delivery in the field.
6. Identify the presentation and the prehospital management of a prolapsed umbilical cord.
7. Describe how to manage a breech or a limb presentation.
8. Describe special considerations with the passage of meconium-stained amniotic fluid.
9. Identify special considerations associated with multiple gestations or premature delivery.
10. Describe the proper care of the mother postdelivery.

OVERVIEW

Even though pregnancy is a common condition, childbirth rarely occurs in the field. Most women prefer to deliver their infants within a hospital or other health care facility. Some women, however, do choose to deliver their infants at home, with or without professional assistance. The emergency medical technician (EMT) may be called to assist with such a delivery in the case of complications. Also, sometimes a woman progresses through labor so quickly that she has no time for the trip to the hospital. In these situations, the EMT is called upon to assist with rapid transport and, if necessary, to facilitate the delivery.

Because EMTs do not frequently encounter an emergency involving childbirth, they should review the basic principles of childbirth often. Such review and continuing education are important with this and any other conditions the EMT may infrequently encounter.

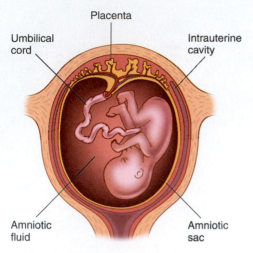

FIGURE 37-1 Amniotic fluid surrounds the fetus, providing a physiologic cushion.

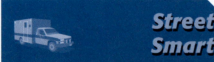

Street Smart

Random contractions that occur in the third trimester that are not associated with cervical effacement and dilation are not true contractions. They are termed **Braxton Hicks contractions** or "false labor." Although EMTs are not expected to distinguish false labor from actual labor, these contractions are typically shorter and less intense than true contractions. Braxton Hicks contractions do not result in delivery of an infant.

ANATOMY REVIEW

A review of relevant anatomy aids in a discussion of the process of childbirth. As a pregnancy progresses, the uterus enlarges in the abdomen, pushing other structures aside. Inside the uterus, the fetus grows and develops over the course of the pregnancy.

The fetus receives all necessary nutrients via the placenta, which is firmly adhered to the uterine wall. The umbilical cord is the connection between the placenta and the fetus.

The fetal-placental unit is surrounded by a membrane, called the **amniotic sac**. This sac encloses the growing fetus and the amniotic fluid that serves as a protective cushion. Figure 37-1 illustrates this anatomy.

As the pregnancy nears its conclusion, the lower uterine segment, or cervix, begins to thin out. This thinning of the cervix is referred to as **effacement**. As the fetal head descends into the pelvis, it slowly stretches the cervix open. This progressive opening of the thinned cervix is called **cervical dilation**. This process can be seen in Figure 37-2.

NORMAL CHILDBIRTH

In most circumstances, childbirth is accomplished without complications. However, the EMT needs to be familiar with the normal progression of childbirth in order to assist in delivery if needed.

Stages of Labor

The term **labor** refers to the process by which the uterus expels the products of conception, namely, the fetus and placenta. For purposes of discussion and management, this process can be divided into three separate stages. The EMT must be able to recognize which stage of labor an expectant mother is in, as this may alter management decisions.

Stage One

Toward the end of pregnancy, as the fetal head moves down into the pelvis, the cervix thins and begins to dilate. When this occurs, a collection of mucus is expelled from the cervix. This expulsion of a small amount of bloody mucus is known as a **bloody show**. The bloody show does not indicate labor has begun; it is merely a sign of cervical thinning.

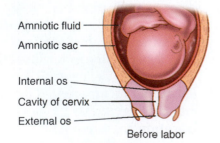 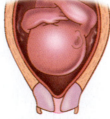 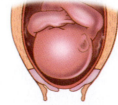 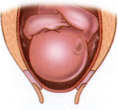

Before labor Early effacement Complete effacement Complete dilation

FIGURE 37-2 As the fetal head descends, the cervix thins and opens to allow the baby to pass through.

When a pregnancy reaches its full term, usually around 40 weeks, the uterus begins to contract. The contractions become increasingly frequent and intense as the uterine muscle attempts to force the baby out.

The organized uterine contractions push the fetal head down into the pelvis, causing further effacement and dilation of the cervix. For the fetus to exit the uterus, the cervix must be completely effaced and dilated to 10 centimeters. This process of cervical effacement and dilation is known as the **first stage of labor** and takes anywhere from a few to upward of 30 hours. Usually, women who have had children before progress through this stage more rapidly.

At some point during the first stage of labor, the amniotic sac usually ruptures, resulting in expulsion of amniotic fluid. Normally amniotic fluid is fairly clear. Any odor or color to the fluid should be noted, as it may impact later management.

Occasionally, the amniotic sac does not rupture spontaneously during this stage of labor. In such cases, the EMT will have to actually open the sac as the infant's head delivers. The sac can be opened easily by pinching the membrane and twisting or pulling it away from the infant's presenting part.

Stage Two

After the cervix is completely dilated, the **second stage of labor** begins. During this stage, more coordinated uterine contractions force the fetal head through the uterine opening and into the vaginal canal.

As the fetal head descends and pushes against the rectum, the mother may have an intense feeling of the need to move her bowels. This feeling is followed by increasing vaginal pressure as the infant continues his descent.

Impending delivery is evident as the fetal head becomes visible at the perineum. The fetal head pushes through the vagina and forms a bulge at the vaginal opening, stretching the perineum. This appearance of the fetal head at the vaginal opening is called **crowning**.

Crowning is initially evident during forceful uterine contractions. As the head is pushed farther into the birth canal, the infant's head bulges at the perineum even between contractions. A few more coordinated contractions usually facilitate delivery of the infant.

At this point, with the onset of each contraction, the mother is encouraged to inhale, hold her breath, and bear down steadily for as long as she can. This pushing helps to bring the baby through the birth canal.

As the space for the infant to come through is relatively small, the infant makes a series of natural movements upon descent through the birth canal. These movements are known as the **cardinal movements of labor** and are pictured in Figure 37-3. The EMT who is familiar with these movements can assist an infant through these maneuvers during an emergency delivery in order to bring the infant through the easiest path to the outside world.

The second stage of labor ends upon delivery of the infant. This stage of labor lasts an average of 30–60 minutes, although it can occur very quickly. The EMT must be able to recognize the woman who is in this stage of labor so that the EMT can prepare for an emergency delivery.

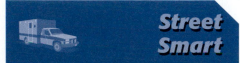

Street Smart

A woman who has had children previously is referred to as **multiparous**, whereas a woman who is in her first pregnancy is called **primiparous**. Multiparous women usually progress much more quickly through labor than primiparous women.

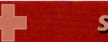

Safety Tip

Despite an overwhelming urge to do so, the EMT should not allow the mother in this stage of labor to go to the bathroom. Delivery of an infant into a toilet is not ideal and can cause injury to both mother and infant.

Street Smart

Many couples learn a method of controlled breathing that can help facilitate effective pushing during contractions. One such method is called Lamaze. The mother's partner acts as her coach. If the parents have practiced such a technique, they should be encouraged to use it.

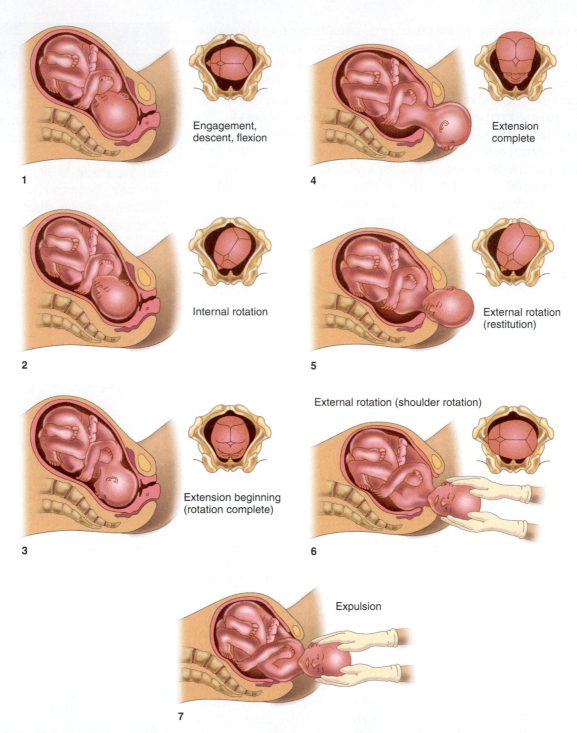

1   Engagement, descent, flexion

2   Internal rotation

3   Extension beginning (rotation complete)

4   Extension complete

5   External rotation (restitution)

6   External rotation (shoulder rotation)

7   Expulsion

FIGURE 37-3   The infant makes a series of natural movements to maneuver his way out through a narrow birth canal.

Stage Three

After delivery of the infant, the uterus rapidly decreases in size. With the change in shape of the uterus, the placenta separates from the inner uterine wall and is expelled through the vagina. This usually happens within 30 minutes of delivery of the infant. The delivery of the placenta is the **third stage of labor**. Transport usually can be accomplished safely during this stage of labor.

Placental delivery is often accompanied by a gush of blood, as the placenta is a very vascular organ. Anywhere from 250 to 500 cc of blood loss is expected. The increase in maternal vascular volume helps the mother's body compensate for this loss.

The placenta should be delivered into a bucket, bag, or other container so that it can be taken to the hospital with the patient. The obstetrician will examine the placenta to make certain that it has been entirely expelled. In rare cases, a piece remains inside the uterus and may continue to bleed or become infected. A physician who finds that a piece of placenta is missing may need to check the patient for retained placental tissue inside the uterus.

Safety Tip

Childbirth always involves splashing blood and body fluids. The EMT should use proper personal protective equipment, including, at a minimum, gloves, goggles, and a gown.

 # Delivery

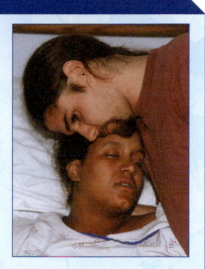

"This has got to be the biggest snowstorm on record," said Mike as he stirred his coffee and looked out the window. The words had barely left Mike's lips when the call went out. "Woman in labor, contractions less than 4 minutes apart. 200 Ponderosa."

Fortunately, a county snowplow was standing by for just such an emergency. The snowplow quickly swung onto the ambulance ramp and cleared a wide path, then proceeded, at about 20 miles per hour, toward 200 Ponderosa. The ambulance followed it.

After what seemed like forever, the ambulance finally arrived. Grabbing the obstetrics kit as well as the first-in bag, Mike went to the door and knocked. He was met at the door by a middle-aged man who ushered the crew into a second-floor bedroom.

Sitting up in a knees-to-chest position was a woman in her mid-30s who was panting. Around the bed were three other children, all playing and seemingly oblivious to their mother's situation.

"Hi, my name is Mike, and don't worry," Mike said. "Hi, my name is Dawn," the patient replied, "and this isn't what I had planned. The nurse-midwife was supposed to be here by now." Mike was quick to reply, "It's understandable, the snow is about 3 feet high now. Tell me, how do you feel?"

Dawn stopped panting, looked at Mike, and said, "I feel like pushing!"

- What are the signs of impending delivery?
- What should be included in the assessment of a woman in labor?
- What equipment should the EMT prepare if he thinks childbirth is imminent?
- What should the EMT do if the umbilical cord presents first?
- What should the EMT do if the infant's buttocks present first?
- What would the EMT do if the amniotic fluid were green-tinged?
- What would the EMT do if the patient said, "I'm having twins"?
- What would the EMT do if the mother was delivering ahead of schedule?
- What should the EMT do for the mother after the delivery?
- What should the EMT do for the infant after the delivery?

EMERGENCY CHILDBIRTH

Although some people believe the ideal place for delivery of an infant is in the presence of a physician or other similarly trained personnel, the EMT may be faced occasionally with a mother who delivers before safe transport can be accomplished. The EMT must recognize this situation when it happens and be prepared to facilitate a controlled delivery in the field.

When an EMT is called to care for a woman in labor, the best course of action is to rapidly evaluate the patient and begin transport expediently. Delivery by an obstetrician in a hospital is always a better prospect than delivery by an EMT on the living room floor or in the back of the ambulance.

If the EMT believes that delivery is imminent, he should prepare for delivery in the field. Whether delivery is done right where the mother is found or in the back of the ambulance is dependent upon how quickly the delivery progresses. Table 37-1 lists some signs of impending delivery.

History

Despite the rapid progression of a delivery, the EMT should attempt to ask the patient a few relevant historical questions. The answers to these questions may have a large impact on the management of the upcoming delivery.

The due date is an important piece of information for the EMT. If a delivery is occurring more than 4 weeks before the due date, it is considered to be premature. The EMT must be aware of some special considerations when delivering a premature infant. This topic is covered in more detail later in this chapter.

Any known complications with the pregnancy should be elicited. If the mother has had no prenatal care or doctor's attention prior to the delivery, it is unlikely that she will be aware of any problems. On the other hand, the mother who has been under a doctor's care during the course of the pregnancy may be able to provide the EMT with valuable information. The presence of twins, for example, is certainly a relevant factor that the EMT should know about prior to the actual delivery so that appropriate preparations can be made for two infants, rather than one.

If the amniotic sac has already ruptured, the color of the amniotic fluid should be noted. The presence of a green tinge is indicative of meconium and will have implications for the immediate care of the infant upon delivery. This topic is discussed in more detail later in the chapter.

If the time is available, the EMT may initiate a more detailed focused history during transport. The EMT should question the mother about the timing of her contractions. Knowing when they started, how much time is between them, and how long each one lasts will give the EMT an idea of how far the labor has progressed. The longer the contractions last and the closer together they become, the closer the patient is to delivery.

Past pregnancy history can be detailed with the total number of pregnancies, including the current one, being noted. In addition, the

TABLE 37-1

Signs of Impending Delivery

Crowning

Feeling of need to move bowels

Increasing vaginal pressure

Increased need to push

number of live children born should be determined. These numbers can be expressed by a commonly used convention: the total number of pregnancies is referred to as **gravidity**, and the number of live children born is referred to as the **parity**.

The initials "G" and "P" are often used to represent the gravidity and the parity. A woman who is pregnant with her first child is G1P0 because she is with her first pregnancy and has yet to deliver a child. A woman who is in her third pregnancy and has delivered two previous live infants is G3P2.

These numbers can be broken down further and detailed, but for the purposes of an initial history, the EMT should report the gravidity and parity as described.

Assessment

The usual initial assessment and measurement of vital signs should be performed, as they would be on any patient. The focused physical assessment of the expectant mother should be based upon her complaint. If she is complaining of contractions or describes rupture of her membranes, the EMT should briefly examine the perineum for signs of crowning or any abnormality.

When performing an examination of the perineum, the EMT should make every attempt to respect the mother's privacy by doing the examination in a private area and keeping the mother covered as much as possible. A sheet draped over the mother's lower body will provide some privacy, although the examining EMT obviously needs to look beneath the sheet. The best position to facilitate the examination is with the mother lying on her back with her heels drawn up toward her buttocks and her knees allowed to fall to the sides.

The EMT should visually inspect the perineum during and between contractions. Any evidence of bulging or of obvious crowning should be noted. The presence of amniotic fluid should be noted, along with its color. Anything protruding from the vaginal opening should be noted.

The EMT has no need to touch any part of the mother's genitalia and should never perform an internal vaginal examination to determine the position of the fetal head. The EMT should also perform this visual inspection of the perineum with another health care professional present in order to avoid any allegations of inappropriate behavior.

When this examination has been completed, if imminent delivery is not expected, the mother may be prepared for transport. Supplies should be readily available during transport to facilitate delivery and care of an infant if needed.

This examination should be repeated only if the patient's symptoms change and the EMT suspects that an examination might reveal a change. For example, if the contractions have become more frequent and the mother feels an urge to move her bowels, the perineum should be reassessed.

Preparation for Delivery

If the EMT suspects delivery is likely to occur soon, he should prepare quickly for it. The first and most important thing to do is to apply

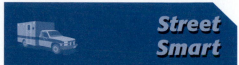

Street Smart

Some mothers prefer to deliver their babies at home. This plan may have been discussed and organized in conjunction with the mother's health care provider. A physician may attend a home delivery, but more often, a specially trained health care provider, called a midwife, is present. Midwives receive training specifically to facilitate home deliveries if that is the wish of the parents. These providers may call emergency medical services (EMS) if they encounter any unforeseen complications during the delivery process.

appropriate personal protective equipment. Childbirth can be quite messy, so the EMT should apply gloves, face and eye protection, and a gown.

The remaining supplies needed to facilitate a delivery are nicely packaged in commercially available kits. The contents of such a kit are listed in Table 37-2 and shown in Figure 37-4.

An EMT who plans to facilitate a delivery should consider contacting medical control. Many regional protocols require a medical control decision to attempt a delivery on the scene. It is helpful to have the medical control physician on the telephone or radio during the delivery to help with any unforeseen complications.

At least two EMTs should facilitate a delivery. One EMT can tend to the mother, while the second can care for the newly born infant.

Creating a calm and controlled atmosphere is the best way to accomplish an emergency delivery in a controlled manner. A controlled delivery is healthier for both the mother and the infant. Uncontrolled expulsion of the infant can result in severe tears to the mother's perineum and in injuries to the baby.

Normal Delivery

Since EMTs infrequently deliver babies, they will find it helpful to review this skill in a step-by-step manner. Skill 37-1 presents the steps involved in an emergency delivery. Most deliveries are completed without any difficulty, but the EMT should know about potential complications and how to manage them. Complicating circumstances are dealt with later in the chapter.

TABLE 37-2

Contents of a Typical Obstetrics Kit	
Supply	**Use**
Surgical scissors	To cut the umbilical cord
Clamps	To clamp the umbilical cord
Bulb suction	To suction the infant's mouth and nose
Towels	To dry and warm the infant, to drape over the mother's perineum
Gauze sponges	To apply pressure to the perineum
Gloves	To protect the EMT's hands
Baby blanket	To wrap the infant
Sanitary napkins	To place over the vagina after delivery of the placenta
Plastic bag	To contain the placenta after delivery

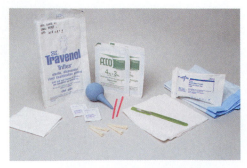

FIGURE 37-4 The EMT should be familiar with the contents of an OB (obstetrics) kit.

SKILL 37-1 *Emergency Delivery*

PURPOSE: To assist the mother in the natural delivery of a newborn infant.

STANDARD PRECAUTIONS:

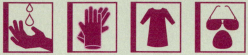

- ☑ Surgical scissors or cord clamps
- ☑ Bulb suction device
- ☑ Towels
- ☑ Gauze sponges
- ☑ Baby blanket
- ☑ Sanitary napkins
- ☑ Plastic bag or bucket
- ☑ Personal protective equipment

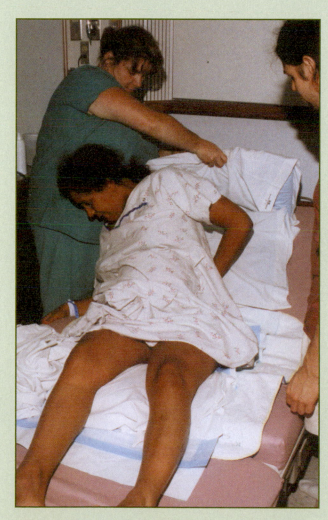

1 The EMT should position the mother supine with knees drawn up and spread apart, and can assist the mother by helping her to elevate her buttocks on a pillow or blankets.

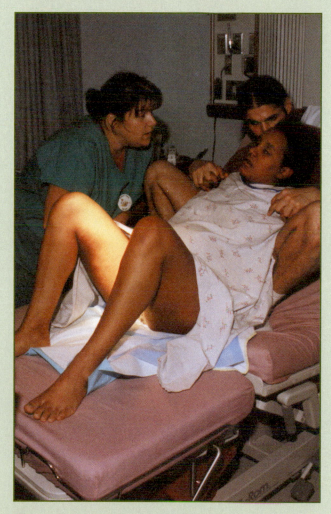

2 The EMT should create a clean area around the vaginal opening with clean towels or paper barriers.

(continues)

SKILL 37-1 *(continued)*

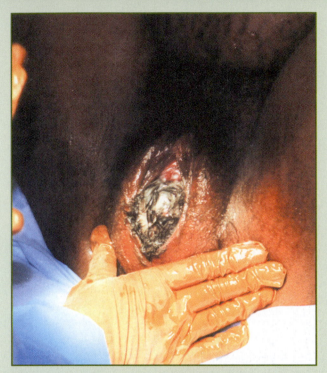

3 As the infant's head appears during crowning, the EMT should place her fingers gently on the skull and exert very gentle pressure to prevent explosive delivery.

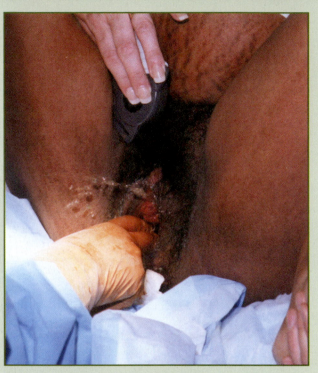

4 If the amniotic sac has not broken, the EMT should use her thumb and forefinger, or a clamp, to puncture the sac and push it away from the infant's head and face.

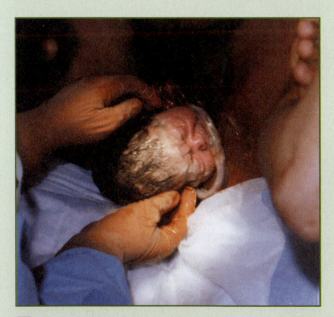

5 As the infant's head is delivered, the EMT should determine whether the umbilical cord is around the neck and, if it is, slip it over the infant's head or shoulder. If it is not possible to slip the cord, the EMT should clamp the cord in two places, cut the cord between the clamps, and unwrap the cord from the infant's neck.

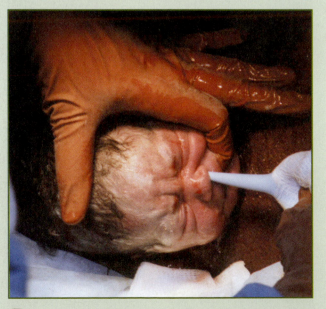

6 After the infant's head is born, the EMT supports the head and suctions the newborn's mouth and then the nose several times with the bulb suction device.

(continues)

SKILL 37-1 *(continued)*

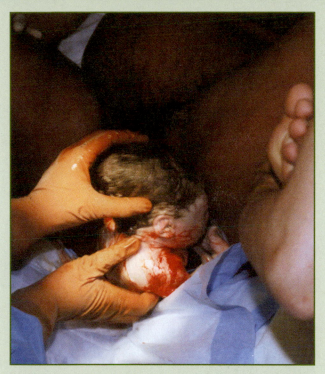

7 As the torso and full body are born, the EMT supports the infant with both hands. As the feet are born, the EMT should grasp them firmly.

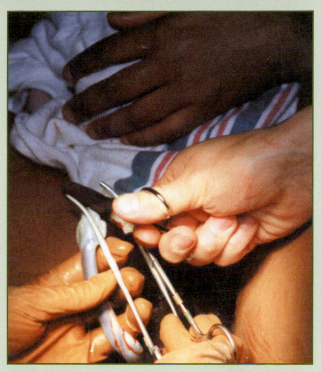

8 After pulsations cease in the umbilical cord, the EMT should clamp the cord in two places, with the closest clamp about 4 fingers' width away from the infant, and then cut the cord between the clamps.

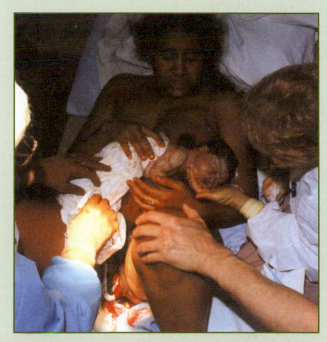

9 Then the EMT should gently dry the infant with towels and wrap the infant in a warm blanket. The infant should be placed on its side, preferably with the head slightly lower than the trunk.

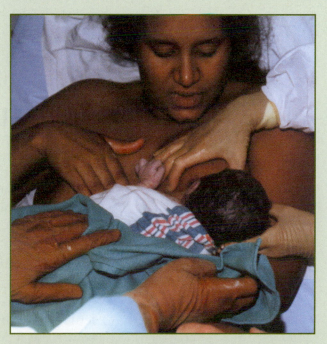

10 Another EMT should monitor the infant and complete initial care of the newborn.

(continues)

SKILL 37-1 *(continued)*

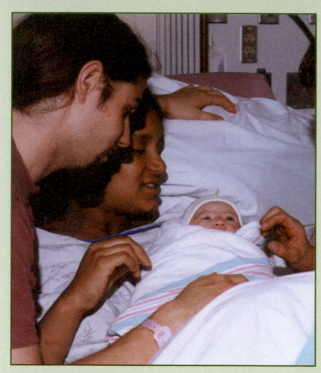

11 The EMT should place a sterile sanitary napkin between the mother's legs and have her close her legs. The EMT should also comfort the mother and monitor vital signs.

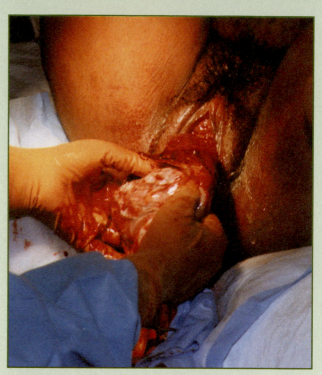

12 While preparing the mother and infant for transport, the EMT should watch for delivery of the placenta. When the placenta is delivered, the EMT wraps the placenta in a towel, places it in a plastic bag or container, and transports it to the hospital with the mother.

SPECIAL DELIVERY SCENARIOS

Unfortunately, every delivery does not go as smoothly as planned. The presence of complications during childbirth can be dangerous to both mother and infant. The EMT should be familiar with the more common special delivery situations and be prepared to manage them appropriately.

Prolapsed Umbilical Cord

Occasionally, during the fetal movement down into the birth canal, the umbilical cord becomes lodged between the birth canal and the fetus's head. In this case, the umbilical cord may exit the birth canal before the fetal head. This condition is called **prolapsed umbilical cord** and is depicted in Figure 37-5.

A prolapsed umbilical cord results in the fetal head compressing the blood supply that passes through the cord as the fetus descends in the canal. This condition can be life threatening to the infant and, therefore, must be quickly recognized and managed by the EMT.

Signs and Symptoms

The mother with a prolapsed umbilical cord often presents with contractions like any other laboring mother. Sometimes she will be aware of something coming out of her vagina. Upon initial perineal examination, the EMT will see the silvery-white umbilical cord coming from the vaginal opening.

Because the umbilical cord carries the blood flow to the infant, it normally pulsates with the beat of the mother's heart. If the cord is not pulsating, it is probably being compressed inside the birth canal and all blood flow to the infant has been cut off.

Management

Management by the EMT of a mother with a prolapsed umbilical cord begins with the discovery of the condition upon visual perineal examination. The mother should be immediately placed on 100% oxygen and put into a head-down or buttocks-raised position to allow gravity to lessen pressure in the birth canal.

The EMT should insert a sterile gloved hand into the vagina and push the fetal presenting part (usually the head) away from the cord. If blood flow is reestablished, pulsations of the cord should be visible. This technique is demonstrated in Figure 37-6.

The mother should be rapidly transported in the head-down, buttocks-up position with the EMT constantly maintaining pressure on the infant's head to keep it from compressing the umbilical cord. Medical control should be contacted as soon as possible during transport.

Breech Presentation

The majority of infants are delivered head first, but occasionally the fetus fails to rotate into a head-down position prior to the onset of labor. When the fetal buttocks or lower extremities are low in the uterus at the time of labor, these parts exit the birth canal first.

The fetal part that is first visible at the perineum is called the presenting part. When the presenting part is the fetal buttocks or lower extremities, it is called a **breech presentation**.

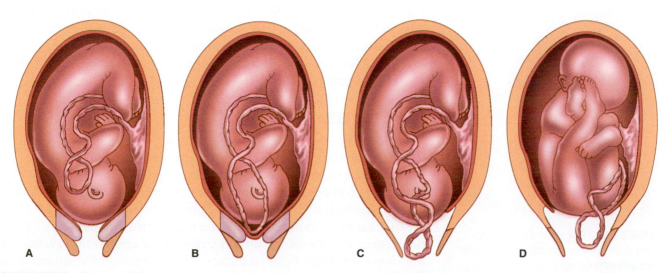

A   B   C   D

FIGURE 37-5   If the umbilical cord precedes the infant's head, the head will compress the cord as it descends into the birth canal.

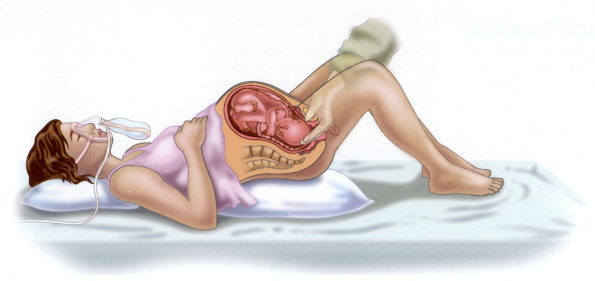

FIGURE 37-6 The EMT can help to prevent complete compression of the umbilical cord and the vessels within it by holding the infant's head away from it during contractions.

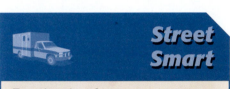

Street Smart

Rarely, the fetus may present with one limb, usually a foot, protruding from the birth canal. This condition is unlikely to result in an easy delivery, and the patient should be treated just as for a breech presentation with rapid transport to the closest appropriate hospital.

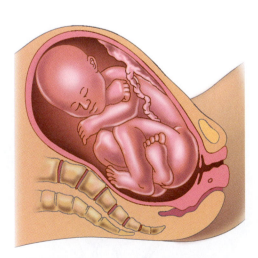

FIGURE 37-7 Because the breech newborn is at greater risk for injury during delivery, physicians often choose to perform a cesarean section.

The breech newborn is at greater risk for injury during delivery. A prolapsed umbilical cord is seen more often with a breech presentation also. Recognition of this condition by the EMT is imperative so that appropriate management may be initiated. Figure 37-7 illustrates this difficult position of the infant.

Because the position of the baby is not ideal, delivery can be complicated and dangerous. Often obstetricians choose to perform a surgical delivery through the abdomen, called a **cesarean section**, to avoid injury to the infant during a vaginal delivery.

Signs and Symptoms

The mother who has a fetus in the breech position experiences labor like any other mother. As the fetus descends in the birth canal, the buttocks or legs become visible at the perineum, rather than the head.

Management

Once the breech presentation has been recognized, the EMT should place the mother on 100% oxygen and position her head down with her pelvis elevated. This position may help to slow delivery. Transport should be initiated immediately to the closest appropriate hospital. Medical control should be established while en route according to local protocols.

Meconium

During the normal course of labor, the amniotic sac breaks, allowing the amniotic fluid to be expelled from the vagina. This fluid is normally clear and watery. Occasionally, however, the fluid has a green tinge. This color is due to the presence of meconium in the fluid.

Meconium is the term for newborn feces. The very mature fetus or the distressed fetus may expel some meconium into the amniotic fluid. Because he is completely bathed in this fluid upon delivery, the infant may have amniotic fluid in his mouth and nose. If the infant were to breathe in, or aspirate, the meconium, it would be potentially harmful.

Aspiration of meconium into the lungs can result in serious infection and injury to the newborn's lung tissue. Recognition of the presence of meconium is crucial so that appropriate steps may be taken to prevent its aspiration by the infant.

Signs and Symptoms

When an EMT is evaluating a mother in labor, he should always question her regarding the color of the amniotic fluid upon rupture of her membranes. The EMT also should note the color of any fluid present during his initial perineal examination.

The thicker the meconium is in the fluid, the more hazardous it is to the newborn. Very thin, watery, yet slightly green-tinged fluid is not as big a risk as fluid as thick as pea soup. Regardless of the viscosity of the fluid, the EMT must take special measures during delivery to prevent injury to the infant's lungs.

Management

Upon recognition of the presence of meconium, the EMT should immediately make preparations for its management. Transport should be initiated so that the newborn may be cared for by advanced medical personnel as soon as possible. The delivery should be allowed to progress in as controlled a manner as possible.

As soon as the infant's head has been delivered, the EMT should ask the mother to stop pushing. It is often helpful to ask her to concentrate on her breathing in order to overcome the urge to push the baby out completely. The infant's nose and mouth must be suctioned several times to remove any meconium present. Once this has been accomplished, the EMT should encourage the mother to continue to push and deliver the infant.

Upon delivery, the infant should not be immediately stimulated, but should be placed on a firm surface where the EMT can again suction the infant's mouth and nose. The infant should then be assessed and resuscitated as appropriate. Involving advanced life support (ALS) providers in the care of the newborn with meconium aspiration is often helpful.

Multiple Gestation

One in 90 pregnancies in the United States results in twin births. A twin birth is the delivery of two infants during one pregnancy. Complications of pregnancy and delivery are increased with multiple gestations.

Compared to a single-infant pregnancy, which delivers at 40 weeks, twins tend to deliver at an average of 37 weeks, triplets at 33 weeks, and quadruplets at 29 weeks. Earlier delivery means that the infants have less time in utero for development. The special considerations associated with premature deliveries are discussed later.

Signs and Symptoms

The mother who is carrying more than one fetus often knows this and can share the information if specifically asked. A mother who has not had prenatal care may not realize that she is carrying more than one fetus. The EMT should specifically question the mother regarding this issue prior to delivery.

If this history is not obtained or not known, the EMT will become aware of the presence of more than one infant when the uterus does not decrease in size significantly after delivery of one infant. Often the second infant is not in a head-first position.

Management

Because the risk of complications is increased in delivery of multiple gestations, the mother laboring with multiple gestations should be transported immediately in hopes that delivery can occur at the hospital. When caring for the mother, the EMT should prepare multiple delivery kits. A twin delivery will require two complete delivery kits and two complete infant resuscitation setups. Additional trained providers should be available if delivery is to occur in the field.

Premature Delivery

Most normal pregnancies end at an average of 40 weeks. This length of a pregnancy is necessary to allow complete development of the fetal organs. One of the last organ systems to mature is the pulmonary system. Infants who are born prematurely can be underdeveloped with incompletely matured lungs. The earlier the delivery, the more likely it is that complications will occur.

A delivery that occurs prior to 36 weeks of gestation is considered to be a **premature delivery** and ideally would not be attempted in the field. The premature infant is very prone to injury during delivery and may require extensive resuscitation that is available only at the hospital.

Signs and Symptoms

When caring for the woman in labor, the EMT should always determine the gestational age or the due date of the pregnancy. If the due date is more than 4 weeks away or the estimated gestational age is less than 36 weeks, the labor is premature.

Management

If a mother presents in labor prior to 36 weeks of gestation, the EMT should initiate transport as soon as possible. The destination hospital should be notified, and medical control should be established if recommended by local protocol.

If delivery is imminent, the EMT should prepare for it. A smaller infant usually is delivered much more quickly than a full-term baby. Care should be taken to cover the premature newborn to prevent loss of body heat. The premature infant is at great risk of developing hypothermia.

Any necessary resuscitation should be performed unless the small size of the very premature newborn makes this resuscitation physically impossible. Infants born prior to 24 weeks generally do not survive due to inadequately matured organ systems.

POSTDELIVERY CARE

After delivery is completed, the EMT should transport the mother and the infant to the hospital in a timely fashion. If she is able, and the infant is healthy, the mother should be allowed to hold the infant. The EMT should frequently reassess the flow of vaginal bleeding. Excessive bleeding is defined as greater than 500 cc or if the mother exhibits signs or symptoms of hypoperfusion.

Mother

After the placenta is delivered, the uterus normally contracts and bleeding slows. If the uterus does not contract, it may continue to bleed heavily. If excessive bleeding occurs, the EMT can attempt to cause contraction of the uterus.

Uterine contraction can be stimulated by firm uterine massage. The EMT should place his hand on the lower abdomen just above the pubis and firmly knead the area. The massage may be uncomfortable for the patient but will help to slow the bleeding. Figure 37-8 demonstrates this technique. Uterine massage should continue until the bleeding stops.

If excessive bleeding has occurred, the EMT should treat the mother for shock by applying high-flow oxygen and placing her supine or in a Trendelenburg position. The EMT should perform ongoing assessments frequently and arrange for an ALS intercept if possible.

Infant

The initial resuscitation of the newborn is centered on an initial assessment of activity, color, breathing, pulse, and tone. It is helpful to have a second EMT care for the infant. If the newborn is sick and requires active resuscitation, the infant may need to be transported in a separate ambulance so that adequate room is available for care. The care of the newborn is considered in the next chapter.

CONCLUSION

Childbirth is a common process, yet the EMT does not often encounter a delivery in the field. Most deliveries will be uncomplicated and the EMT will merely facilitate the process. However, complications during childbirth can be devastating for both the mother and the baby.

The EMT should be familiar with normal labor and delivery and also must be able to recognize and appropriately manage patients with complicated deliveries or special delivery considerations. Because EMTs do not handle deliveries often, they should review the procedures frequently.

TEST YOUR KNOWLEDGE

1. What changes take place in female anatomy during pregnancy?
2. What are the components of the three stages of labor?

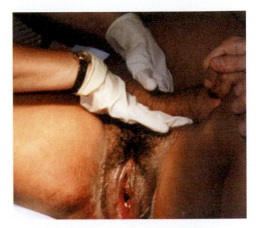
FIGURE 37-8 Firm massage of the empty uterus helps to stimulate uterine contraction.

Street Smart

The EMT should not be alarmed at the cone shape of the infant's head. The infant's cranial bones are not yet fused and can easily move around to facilitate passage through the narrow birth canal. This process is called **molding** and is nearly always seen in infants delivered vaginally. The shape of the infant's head will return to normal within several days.

3. What are signs and symptoms of impending delivery?

4. What is the importance of a brief predelivery history?

5. How can an EMT assist with a normal delivery in the field?

6. What is the proper care of the mother postdelivery?

7. What is the presentation and the prehospital management of a prolapsed umbilical cord?

8. How should the EMT manage a breech or a limb presentation?

9. What are some special considerations associated with multiple gestations or premature delivery?

10. What are the special considerations with the passage of meconium-stained amniotic fluid?

INTERNET RESOURCES

Visit these Web sites for additional information on childbirth and complications of childbirth:

- Breech Babies.com, http://www.breechbabies.com
- Center for the Study of Multiple Births, http://www.multiplebirth.com
- Childbirth Solutions, http://www.childbirthsolutions.com
- Childbirth.org, http://www.childbirth.org

FURTHER STUDY

Mattera, C. (1998). Emergency childbirth. *Journal of Emergency Medical Services, 23*(7), 60–69.

EMS in Action

Tavoris Allen, Jay Tsultim, and Ryan English were on their way down Interstate 75 to their evening paramedic class at Manatee Technical Institute (MTI) in Bradenton, Florida. It was just before 6 P.M., and they were running late. It was their habit to put their stethoscopes around their necks when they got in the car to travel to class. They wanted to be prepared for training when they walked through the classroom door. This evening, however, they would have to be prepared for more than class.

The trip was routine by now, four nights a week plus clinicals. It was a rigorous schedule on top of their day jobs. Allen had already worked his day as a firefighter EMT with Hillsborough County Fire Rescue. Tsultim, a Web designer, and English, in service with the U.S. Coast Guard, were also firefighter EMT volunteers for Hillsborough. They made the daily commute to class a bit easier by carpooling.

As they approached the Ellenton exit, traffic dramatically slowed. They were about to take the exit to avoid the traffic jam ahead when a man ran across the road calling for help. Then they saw the accident. A sedan and a pickup had collided. As the three EMTs went into rescue mode, they quickly assessed the scene to identify the most critical need. At first they thought it would be the man crouched in a fetal-like position, but he was conscious, though dazed. Then they heard a woman scream, "My baby! My baby!"

They turned to where the newborn lay looking lifeless, behind the mangled sedan. An early arriver was trying to administer chest compressions, but the newborn, now purple in color, was not getting enough air. He was in cardiac distress with agonal breathing. He had regurgitated and had probably suffered the trauma of head injury. The newborn was in very bad shape.

(*continues on page 809*)

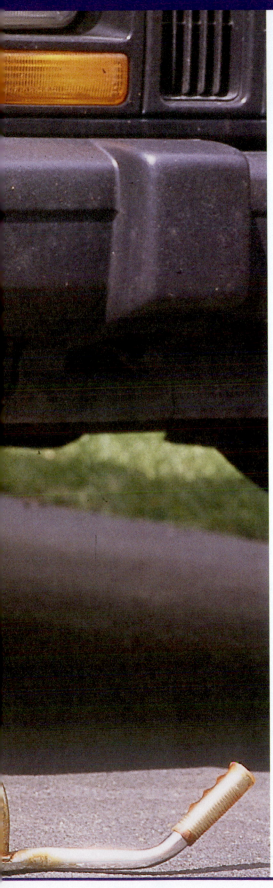

Childhood Emergencies

Children represent so much to most of us. They represent the dreams and hopes of our future, and for this reason, when a child is sick both parent and child are affected emotionally. Furthermore, children present special challenges to the EMT because children are, after all, not just little adults.

Finally, an EMT feels more pressure to succeed with a child's care than with an adult's and feels more of a sense of failure if she does not. All of these factors add up to create more stress for the EMT.

By understanding the special developmental considerations of children as well as the importance of parenting to the child's total care, the EMT may feel less anxiety about caring for a child.

CHAPTER 38

Newborn Care

KEY TERMS

acrocyanosis
Apgar
fontanels
molding
neonate
vernix caseosa

OBJECTIVES

Upon completion of this chapter, the reader should be able to:

1. Demonstrate how to obtain an Apgar score on a newborn.
2. Discuss the implications of the Apgar score for the newborn.
3. Identify the treatment priorities for a newborn.
4. Describe the care of a newborn with respiratory distress.
5. Demonstrate a focused physical examination for a newborn.
6. Identify which pregnancies may have complications.
7. Demonstrate the resuscitation of a newborn in cardiac or respiratory arrest.

OVERVIEW

Although most deliveries are without complications, in the first hour of life, a newborn is at high risk for a number of potentially fatal problems. An emergency medical technician (EMT) may be caring for the newborn and mother during that first hour. The EMT can successfully meet the challenge by integrating a few new concepts into existing knowledge of prehospital emergency care.

THE NEWBORN

Immediately after a prehospital delivery, the EMT is faced with caring for two patients. Ideally, one EMT is assigned to care for the mother, while another takes responsibility for the care of the newborn.

A newborn, up to 1 month of age, is called a **neonate**. Immediately after birth may be the most stressful period in life for a neonate. The newborn must quickly adjust to life outside the womb or he will not survive.

The EMT's role is to support the newborn struggling to meet the demands of life. The EMT is primarily interested in preventing complications, such as hypothermia, and alerting the hospital of any difficulties.

INITIAL ASSESSMENT OF THE NEWBORN

The **Apgar** score was developed in 1952, by Dr. Virginia Apgar, as a standard tool for measuring the health of a newborn. Since then, many health care professionals involved in the care of neonates have utilized this tool.

The Apgar score measures heart rate, respiration, muscle tone, response to stimuli, and color. The Apgar score is based on the newborn's condition at 1 minute after birth and 5 minutes after birth. Table 38-1 details the point assignments associated with this well-known scoring system.

The EMT should integrate the Apgar scoring tool into her initial assessment of the newborn. The initial assessment of a newborn starts with an assessment of level of consciousness. While a newborn is not expected to interact with the environment, he should be awake and active.

First, the EMT should try to straighten the legs (Figure 38-1). If the newborn is active and kicking, the newborn is awarded 2 points. If the newborn slowly/weakly flexes the legs back into the fetal position, 1 point is awarded. If no motion is detected, no points are given.

Proceeding to the airway, the EMT should take the bulb syringe and suction the nostrils (Figure 38-2). If the newborn coughs or sneezes, a strong protective reflex, the EMT awards 2 points. If the newborn merely grimaces, the EMT awards only 1 point. If the newborn does not react to this noxious stimulus, no points are awarded.

Next, the EMT assesses the newborn's breathing. The strong cry of a newborn is an excellent indication of good respiratory effort

TABLE 38-1

Apgar Score

A = Appearance
  2—Completely pink
  1—Cyanotic extremities
  0—Central cyanosis

P = Pulse
  2—Greater than 100 bpm
  1—Less than 100 bpm
  0—No pulse

G = Grimace
  2—Cough or sneeze
  1—Grimace
  0—Unresponsive

A = Activity
  2—Active
  1—Flexion
  0—No motion

R = Respiration
  2—Good respiration, strong cry
  1—Slow or irregular respiration, weak cry
  0—Apneic

 ## Assessing the Newborn

"Wow, this is really cool!" thought Jose as he wiped the newborn with a dry towel. Jose had just seen a live birth for the first time. The baby was perfect. She had tiny hands, a little blue, but perfect. And the fingernails are so small, Jose thought. She had a hearty wail that indicated she was moving good air, and she was just kicking, kicking, kicking. So much life in this little one, he thought to himself.

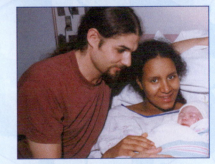

Returning to reality, Jose told himself, "Back to work, time for an Apgar score to see how this little one is doing." Looking at the laminated card that he had taken out of the birth kit, he called out, "The Apgar is 9!"

- What is the importance of obtaining an infant Apgar score?
- What signs would the EMT observe that might indicate the newborn is having difficulty adjusting to life?
- What actions would the EMT take to try to support the newborn who is having difficulty?
- What would be the EMT's response to the mother of a newborn with a birth defect when the mother asks, "Is my baby all right?"

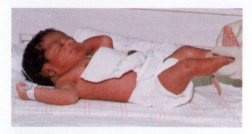

FIGURE 38-1 An active, kicking newborn is awarded 2 points on the Apgar score.

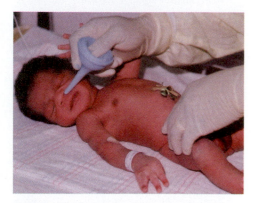

FIGURE 38-2 If the newborn sneezes when his nostrils are suctioned, he is awarded 2 points on the Apgar score.

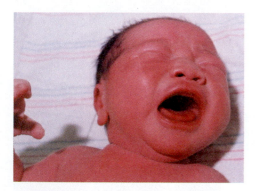

FIGURE 38-3 The newborn with a strong cry is awarded 2 points on the Apgar score.

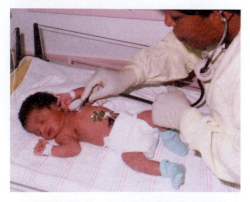

FIGURE 38-4 A newborn with a heart rate greater than 100 beats per minute is awarded 2 points on the Apgar score.

(Figure 38-3). A strong cry is awarded 2 points. If the newborn's breathing is shallow or irregular, only 1 point is awarded. If the newborn is apneic, no points are awarded.

Circulation is assessed using both pulses and color. The EMT may attempt to obtain a brachial pulse in the newborn's upper arm. If the brachial pulse is difficult to palpate, then the EMT should count the apical pulse (Figure 38-4). The EMT puts her stethoscope over the newborn's heart and then counts an apical pulse. An apical pulse is counted by listening to the heartbeat at the apex, or bottom, of the heart.

Immediately after childbirth, it is sometimes possible to gently grasp the umbilical cord and feel the pulsation of the heart. A pulse may be also counted in this manner.

A newborn's heart rate should be very fast, greater than 100 beats per minute. If the pulse rate is greater than 100 beats per minute, two points are awarded. If the pulse rate is less than 100 beats per minute, 1 point is awarded. If no pulse is present, no points are awarded.

Another indicator of good circulation is capillary bed perfusion. A hearty circulation will flush the capillary beds of the hands and feet, making them appear pink. If the palms of the hands or the soles of the feet are pink, 2 points are awarded (Figure 38-5). If cyanosis, a bluish or gray pallor, is present in the feet and hands, 1 point is awarded. If the newborn is centrally cyanotic, as well as peripherally cyanotic, no points are awarded. A bluish or gray pallor to the chest is called central cyanosis.

The newborn's level of consciousness, airway, breathing, and circulation (ABCs) are all assessed using the Apgar tool. Each should be awarded points, and the infant assigned a total Apgar score.

Most newborns lose at least one point in color/appearance in the initial 1-minute assessment. **Acrocyanosis**, cyanosis of the extremities, may be normal in the newborn within the first hour after birth.

An Apgar score of 7 to 10 points usually indicates that the newborn is having no difficulty adjusting to life outside the womb. A score between 4 and 6 points indicates that the newborn is moderately depressed. Several actions the EMT can take to stimulate a moderately depressed newborn are discussed later in this chapter.

A score of 3 or less indicates a high-priority newborn that will require vigorous resuscitation in the field and probable admission to a neonatal intensive care unit. Despite vigorous resuscitation, newborns with a 1- and 5-minute Apgar score of 3 or less have a 50% chance of survival.

Management of the Newborn

The first priority of management of a newborn, as with any other patient, is maintaining the airway. Newborns are obligatory nose breathers. When at rest, a newborn will naturally choose to breathe through the nose. This is an important protective function of the body.

The nose not only heats and humidifies the air that is inhaled but also filters the air, trapping bacteria in mucus. In the first 30 minutes to an hour after birth, the newborn produces large amounts of mucus.

The EMT must keep the newborn's nostrils clear of mucus. A bulb syringe is convenient for this purpose. First, the newborn should be placed head down to facilitate drainage. Picking up the syringe, the EMT should compress the bulb to express the air within the bulb. Keeping the bulb compressed, the EMT should place the tip of the syringe gently into the nostril. Once the tip is within the nostril, the bulb is released and the mucus is suctioned into the bulb. The bulb is emptied onto a 4 × 4, and the process repeated with the other nostril.

If the mucus is thick and tenacious, a flexible French suction catheter may have to be used. A great deal of caution must be observed, as the suction can injure tender tissues within the nostrils. The suction should be set at the lowest setting on the suction machine. The tip of the French catheter should be gently inserted no more than one-half inch into the nostril. Low-pressure suction should be applied, as the catheter is withdrawn, for no more than 10 seconds. The process should be repeated for the other nostril.

If the newborn's respirations are still depressed or irregular, oxygen should be gently administered. Oxygen tubing, connected to an oxygen regulator turned to 4 liters per minute, is held about 1 inch away from the newborn's mouth and nose. If the infant does not immediately improve, or "pink up," from this blow-by oxygen, the liter flow can be increased.

After about 30 seconds to a minute, the newborn should be reassessed. If the newborn still has poor respiratory effort, or is bradycardic (heart rate less than 100), the newborn's respiration must be assisted with a bag-valve-mask (BVM) and high-concentration oxygen.

Indications that an infant may be experiencing respiratory distress include seesaw respirations, marked chest retractions, and audible grunting. Seesaw respiration is the result of an exaggerated paradoxical movement of the chest and the abdomen as the infant uses abdominal muscles to assist the weak diaphragm to breathe.

As the diaphragm tries to draw in more air, the skin between the ribs is also drawn in, causing the skin to retract. This sign of respiratory distress is called intercostal retractions. With intercostal retractions, the outline of each rib becomes more prominent. When the newborn is in serious distress, sternal retraction also may be observed (Figure 38-6).

Respiratory failure is more commonly seen in the premature newborn and the newborn with congenital heart defects. Eventually, these newborns may go into respiratory arrest.

If the newborn shows signs of respiratory distress or failure, the EMT should transport the newborn immediately. In some cases, it may be appropriate to delay the mother's transportation in order to rapidly transport the newborn.

If the mother permits, a newborn who is healthy should be put to the mother's breast (Figure 38-7). It is a good sign if the newborn appears interested in suckling, as this indicates that the newborn is stabilizing and is ready to take nourishment.

Breast-feeding is also good for the mother. Stimulation of the nipple in turn stimulates hormones that increase uterine contractions. As the uterus contracts, the placenta is delivered and bleeding slowed.

A newborn is very prone to hypothermia. The EMT can take several steps to ward off heat loss and hypothermia. A great deal of heat is lost via the evaporation of the amniotic fluid that once bathed the infant. To prevent this heat loss, the newborn should be immediately dried with a clean towel.

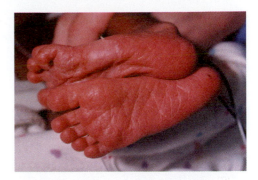

FIGURE 38-5 If the soles of the feet and the palms of the hands are pink, the newborn is awarded 2 points on the Apgar score.

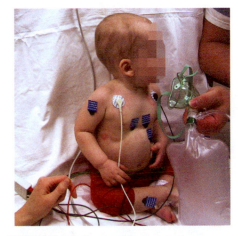

FIGURE 38-6 An infant must be watched carefully for signs of respiratory distress.

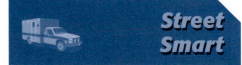

Street Smart

The new mother may be concerned about oxygen being administered to her new baby because she may have heard that oxygen can affect an infant's vision. Oxygen toxicity leading to visual impairment occurs only after prolonged exposure to high concentrations of oxygen, so concerns about vision should not affect the EMT's decision to use this lifesaving drug. The EMT should explain to the new mother that the lowest concentration of oxygen that is effective is being used, and only for a very short amount of time.

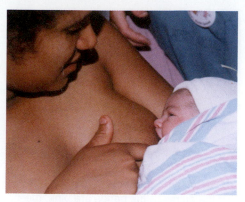

FIGURE 38-7 Breast-feeding helps the mother's uterus contract and return to normal.

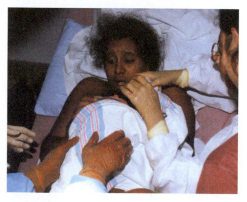

FIGURE 38-8 Placing the newborn against the mother's body will help to maintain body temperature.

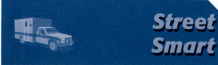

Street Smart

The newborn radiates a great deal of heat into the atmosphere from the large head. To reduce this type of heat loss, a cap or bonnet should be placed on the neonate. Additionally, to prevent further heat loss, the newborn should be swaddled in a warmed cotton blanket.

The newborn should not be placed on a table or other solid surface for assessment, as the heat loss from conduction, contact on a cold surface, can lead to hypothermia. Initially, the newborn should be placed on a blanket while being assessed. When the EMT is done with the assessment, the newborn should be placed on a surface close to body temperature, such as in the mother's arms (Figure 38-8).

FOCUSED ASSESSMENT OF THE NEONATE

After completing the newborn's initial assessment and assigning an Apgar score, the EMT should perform a thorough detailed physical examination, looking for normal characteristics and noting any abnormalities.

General Appearance

The newborn is typically found in a fetal position, with the knees flexed and the chin resting on the chest. Premature newborns and hypoxic newborns take a more relaxed posture, with legs and arms extended.

The newborn's skin should be red and flushed when he is crying. The hands and feet may be cyanotic. Hypothermia may increase the degree of acrocyanosis that is seen. Cyanosis may be transient, lasting only seconds, as the lungs are exercised and eventually begin to function properly all the time.

The EMT may notice a white, cheesy substance on the newborn's skin. This substance is called **vernix caseosa**. It is thought to help protect the newborn from heat loss. The EMT need not remove it immediately.

At first glance, the newborn's head may appear to be misshapen. A misshapen head after a vaginal delivery is a natural finding; it results from a process called **molding** that involves compression of the newborn's skull during delivery. The head will return to its normal shape in approximately 1–2 days.

The EMT should observe for the soft spots, or **fontanels**. The fontanels are the junction of the bones of the skull. Eventually, the fontanels close as the newborn matures. Usually there are only two fontanels that can be seen, one anterior and one posterior. Crying, coughing, and lying down may cause the newborn's fontanels to bulge temporarily. If a fontanel is depressed, the child may be dehydrated.

Light-skinned newborns usually have dark blue eyes, while dark-skinned newborns have brown eyes. The newborn's eyes commonly appear to lack focus, scanning back and forth. The EMT may also notice some blood in the sclera; this is a result of the newborn's compression during delivery and is not significant.

As was previously mentioned, the nose may create a large amount of mucus and needs to be suctioned frequently. Nasal flaring is a sign of air hunger. The EMT should further assess the newborn to determine whether further treatment is necessary.

The newborn's chest should be assessed for signs of respiratory distress. The respiratory findings should be reported to a physician.

The umbilical cord should be carefully inspected. Immediately after birth, the umbilical cord should appear bluish-white. Any odor or drainage should be reported.

Finally, the EMT should assess the extremities for movement. Almost every new mother wants to know whether the newborn has 10 fingers and 10 toes. The EMT should check the fingernail beds for capillary refill. Persistent cyanosis may indicate either hypoxia or hypothermia.

Birth Trauma

Birth trauma is usually associated with a difficult delivery. Babies with above average weight commonly suffer some birth trauma. The EMT may notice that the newborn is not moving the arms symmetrically. This could indicate that the clavicle has been fractured. The EMT need not splint the clavicle but should simply handle the newborn gently and report any deformity or loss of motion to the physician.

Birth Defects

One of the first questions an EMT may have to answer from a mother is, "Is my baby all right?" If the answer is no, the mother has to immediately deal with the loss of the "perfect baby."

Mothers sometimes react angrily, crying "why me?" Other mothers go into denial. The EMT must be prepared for these possibilities in order to deal with her own emotions and still help the mother to cope with hers.

Usually a physician is responsible for explaining the circumstances to the new parents; however, in the case of emergency medical services (EMS), that may not be possible. If the mother asks the EMT whether her baby is all right, it is probably best to briefly explain to the mother what has been found, in simple terms that she can understand.

Parents attach a great deal of meaning to the behaviors and facial expressions of caregivers. The EMT must remain professional and non-judgmental at this time. The EMT should present the newborn as something precious and emphasize the well-formed portions of the body.

The EMT should defer any questions about the deformity to the physician, and yet try to be open, caring, and honest.

NEWBORN RESUSCITATION

When a newborn is in cardiopulmonary arrest, the EMT must react quickly. Otherwise, the newborn may suffer permanent brain damage and possibly even death. Fortunately, the EMT can fall back on some basic procedures that should be familiar. These basic procedures will be effective in the majority of cases. The EMT need only modify these procedures somewhat, according to the size of the newborn. See Figure 38-9.

Not all newborns breathe spontaneously at birth; some need assistance. The EMT can identify early those newborns who are more likely to need resuscitation by taking an accurate history. Newborns

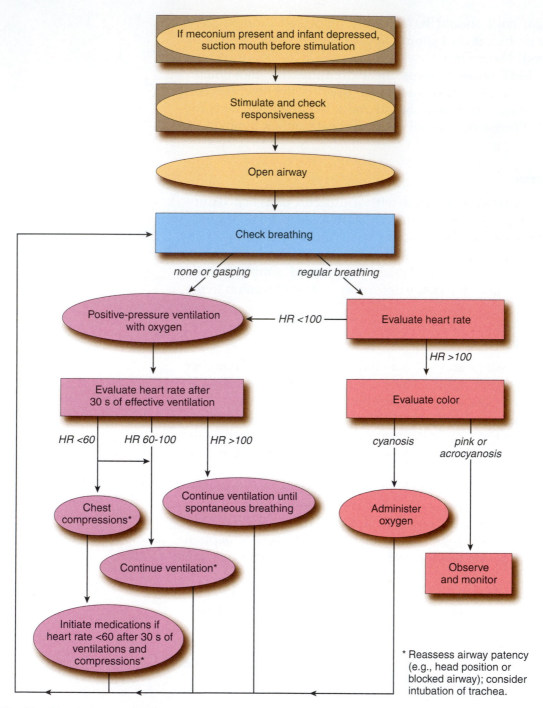

FIGURE 38-9 Algorithm for advanced life support of the newborn. (Reprinted courtesy of the American Academy of Pediatrics.)

of high-risk pregnancies, listed in Table 38-2, are the most likely newborns to require some assistance.

A newborn depressed from hypoxia will be bradycardiac and may even be pulseless. To reverse this condition, the EMT need only reverse the hypoxia in the majority of cases. Therefore, the EMT should focus her attentions on the newborn's breathing.

Some newborns need only a little encouragement to breathe better. Slapping the newborn on the buttocks or flicking the newborn's heels is a waste of precious time. Instead, the EMT should lay the newborn

✳ *Infant in Distress*

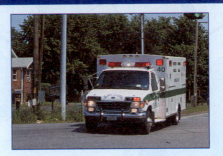

"Infant not breathing at 34 Indian River Boulevard." As this announcement came over the loudspeaker, for a moment, it seemed like nobody was breathing. You could have heard a pin drop. Then a flurry of activity began as people ran to the ambulance bays.

The infant alarm people had called the fire department and left a message that an "apnea" monitor had been installed at 34 Indian River Boulevard for a "high-risk infant."

As the ambulance proceeded down Liberty Street, the wail of the siren blocked out everything. Daphne sat on the bench, looking at the action wall and thinking to herself, "OK, be calm. What am I going to need? What am I going to do?"

The ride seemed to take an eternity.

- Which infants are at "high risk" for cardiac arrest?
- What are the treatment priorities?
- When does an EMT start compressions?
- What does it mean when an infant has green goop in his mouth immediately following childbirth?

TABLE 38-2

High-Risk Pregnancy

Premature delivery
Multiple births
Prolapsed umbilical cord
Severe maternal bleeding
Meconium aspiration

Street Smart

In some cases, a newborn is not born alive. Newborns can be *stillborn* for a number of reasons. Prolonged compression of the umbilical cord or hypotension of mother or child are just a couple of reasons that a newborn can be stillborn.

Whatever the explanation, the newborn will be unresponsive, apneic, and pulseless. The EMT should begin resuscitation, regardless of how bleak the outlook. While the effort may appear to be fruitless, the mother and the EMT need to know that all that could have been done for the newborn was attempted. When the mother and child arrive at the hospital, professional counselors will be available to help the family cope with the loss.

---

on his back and vigorously dry the newborn, in a circular motion, with a clean towel (Figure 38-10). This is often all it takes to stimulate the newborn to breathe.

If this is unsuccessful, the EMT must proceed to the ABCs. The cornerstone of newborn resuscitation is attention to airway and breathing. In fact, 80% of apneic newborns can be resuscitated with basic management of the airway and breathing alone.

The EMT should open the newborn's airway, using a modified jaw thrust. Care should be observed to ensure the head is not tilted back. Overextension of the newborn's neck can actually close off the airway. The newborn's head should be in a neutral position. Often padding is needed under the newborn's back to keep the head in a neutral position.

The nostrils and the mouth should be suctioned clear of mucus, blood, and other fluids. Suctioning should not last longer than 10 seconds.

A newborn has a very large tongue compared to that of an adult. In most cases, an oral airway pushes the tongue backward and creates an airway obstruction, but usually an oral airway is not needed.

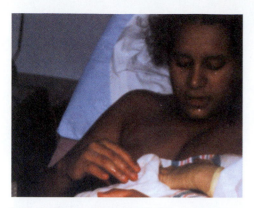

FIGURE 38-10 Stimulation, such as a back rub, is often all that is needed to help a newborn breathe better.

If the newborn remains bradycardiac (less than 100 bpm) or pulseless, the EMT must proceed to positive pressure ventilation. It is important that the EMT carefully observe ventilation technique. Overly aggressive ventilation can lead to hyperinflation of the lungs and stomach. A distended stomach reduces lung expansion and risks regurgitation. An overinflated lung can burst, creating a pneumothorax.

Ventilation should continue at a rate of between 40 and 60 breaths a minute or a breath every second. The volume of each breath should be only enough to see the chest rise.

If the heart rate remains below 60 beats per minute despite positive pressure ventilation, then cardiac compressions should be started. For cardiopulmonary resuscitation (CPR) to be effective, the spine must be supported during compressions. A newborn's chest usually can be encircled by the EMT's hands. The EMT's interlocked fingers on the newborn's back provide a platform for compressions. The EMT's two thumbs can then compress the chest.

If the newborn is small or premature, the EMT may have to overlap her thumbs before beginning compressions. If the newborn is large, which is often the case with newborns of diabetic mothers, or if the EMT's hands are compromising chest expansion, then two fingers should be placed on the chest over the midsternum. Compression should be about one-half to two-thirds of an inch deep and be maintained at a rate of 120 times a minute.

Two EMTs can perform effective ventilation and compression provided they work together. One EMT is at the head of the patient delivering ventilation, one every fifth compression, and the other EMT continues to deliver chest compressions. Figure 38-11 shows the inverted pyramid developed by the American Heart Association as a guideline for neonatal resuscitation.

Street Smart

The use of narcotics can cause respiratory depression in the user. In the case of a pregnant woman, the effects carry over to the unborn child. If the mother is suspected of having used a narcotic before delivery, the newborn should be transported immediately. An advanced life support (ALS) unit should be contacted to intercept with the ambulance. Positive pressure ventilation should be continued until ALS personnel can establish intravenous access and administer the narcotic antidote, Narcan (naloxone).

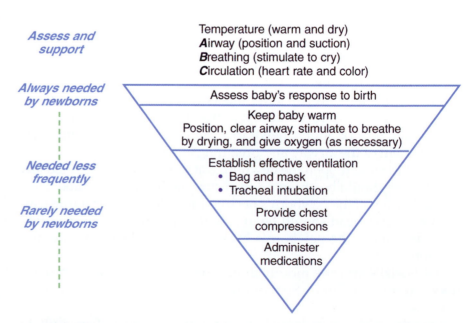

FIGURE 38-11 The resuscitation triangle starts with the basics and ends with the advanced life support procedures. (Reproduced with permission, *PALS Provider Manual*, © 2002, American Heart Association.)

Meconium Aspiration

Meconium is the first feces of a newborn. It is made up of bile and mucus and has a greenish color to it. Meconium may pass into the amniotic sac during delivery if the newborn is distressed.

Aspiration of meconium by a newborn can cause difficulty in the newborn's ability to breathe. If the EMT observes meconium, she should proceed with the newborn's resuscitation, as previously described, and transport the newborn immediately. The EMT should give more attention to clearing the airway with suction and should consider providing supplemental oxygen as needed. If possible, ALS providers should be intercepted.

EMS in Action

(continued from page 798)

Without a word to each other, the MTI classmates went into action to save the baby's life. None of them had ever rescued an infant so young—12 days old—but the team was focused on one objective: to sustain the tiny infant's life. Every second counted. An infant has only 6 to 12 minutes without oxygen before cardiac arrest and death can occur.

Instinct, training, experience, and teamwork came together as the three executed the cardiopulmonary resuscitation (CPR) procedures. With such a small child, it was important to stay especially calm and carry out the procedures with kid gloves. Too much force in breaths or compression could do further harm.

Tsultim rolled up a towel to raise the infant's shoulders to align the airway and began breaths, while English counted the brachial pulse. It was 52—too low. English began compressions as Tsultim held the head and cervical spine and used the mouth-to-cheek technique for breaths, keeping the rescue team to as few in number as possible around the tiny child. While English and Tsultim administered CPR, Allen put his stethoscope to work monitoring lung sounds and making sure the brachial pulse was sustained.

The three continued CPR for what seemed like forever, but in reality was about 5 minutes, when the ambulance arrived. Allen lifted the infant as Tsultim held his head in line with his body, carrying him inside the ambulance onto a stretcher. They placed a BVM with oxygen on the baby, but lost the brachial pulse. They continued compression while the ambulance medic administered endotracheal intubation, suction, and intraosseous infusion.

As the EMTs applied the leads and watched the heart rate and beat, the brachial pulse returned. The infant's color began to improve. Allen, Tsultim, and English had kept the baby alive. Their job was done and the ambulance sped the infant to the hospital.

MTI's modest rescuers figured it was all in a day's work, made it to class late, and proceeded with their night's lab practicing IVs in the back of a moving ambulance. But, as MTI's east campus administrator, Priscilla Haflich, put it, "We're very proud of our heroes. They exemplify our mission to produce the best in skilled health care professionals."

The three got an extra A+ for that evening's session: The infant is enjoying a healthy recovery and a second chance at life.

Priscilla Haflich, BA, MA, MEd, EdD
East Campus Administrator, Manatee Technical Institute
Bradenton, Florida

CONCLUSION

By applying a new understanding about newborns to previous knowledge of prehospital emergency care, the EMT is able to competently manage the newborn.

TEST YOUR KNOWLEDGE

1. What are the signs of a newborn in respiratory distress?
2. How is an Apgar score obtained?
3. What are the elements of the Apgar score?
4. What are the implications of the Apgar score?
5. What unique features does an EMT look for in the focused physical examination of the newborn?
6. What are "high-risk" pregnancies?
7. What are the steps of resuscitation of a newborn?
8. At what rate should the EMT do CPR compressions on a newborn?

INTERNET RESOURCES

Additional information and resources related to neonatal resuscitation can be found at these Web sites:

- American Heart Association, http://www.americanheart.org
- Neonatal Resuscitation Program, American Academy of Pediatrics, http://www.aap.org (Click on the link for Neonatal Resuscitation Program.)
- Neonatal Resuscitation Program, Manitoba, Canada, http://www.nrp.mb.ca

FURTHER STUDY

Hamilton, S. (1999). Prehospital newborn resuscitation. *Emergency Medical Services, 28*(5), 39–45.

Suslowitz, B. (1998). The empty crib. *Journal of Emergency Medical Services, 23*(3), 86–88.

CHAPTER 39

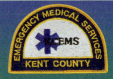

Pediatric Medical Emergencies

KEY TERMS

abdominal thrusts

asthma

back blows

chest thrusts

croup

debriefing

epiglottitis

febrile seizure

intercostal retraction

meningitis

sternal retraction

sudden infant death
   syndrome (SIDS)

OBJECTIVES

Upon completion of this chapter, the reader should be able to:

1. Identify the developmental considerations for infants, toddlers, preschool children, school-age children, and adolescents.

2. Recall the differences in anatomy and physiology of the infant, child, and adult patient and describe how they affect emergency care.

3. Describe some general techniques that are useful in taking a history and performing a physical examination on a pediatric patient.

4. Describe the typical response to illness of the infant or child.

5. Describe several causes of pediatric airway emergencies and the emergency management of them.

6. Describe several causes of pediatric respiratory emergencies and the emergency management of them.

7. Identify the signs and symptoms of hypoperfusion in the infant and child.

8. State the most common causes of cardiac arrest in infants and children and how they impact emergency management of this condition.

9. Describe several causes of pediatric altered mental status and the emergency management of them.

10. Recognize the need for EMT debriefing following a difficult pediatric transport.

OVERVIEW

Caring for ill or injured children can be a stressful situation for an emergency medical technician (EMT). Care of children is based upon the age of the child. Children of different ages are susceptible to different types of illnesses. Familiarity with general techniques of pediatric assessment and with the common illnesses in each age group can help the EMT to feel more comfortable when faced with an ill or injured child.

NORMAL CHILDHOOD DEVELOPMENT

Although every child is not the same, there are some well-known developmental characteristics that are similar in children of the same age. It is important for an EMT to understand some of these characteristics. Understanding these similarities, as well as the differences, will impact the way an EMT cares for a pediatric patient.

Newborn

Although it is somewhat uncommon for the EMT to be called to care for a newborn, or neonate (0 to 1 month of age), it is important for him to be familiar with the expected normal findings. Even though it does not seem that a neonate interacts much with its environment, these tiny babies have very well-developed senses of smell and hearing. Early in life, they tend to recognize the smell of their mother and the sound of her voice.

It may be useful for the EMT to allow the newborn's mother to hold the newborn during the assessment and care, as much as possible given the newborn's condition. This may calm the newborn and allow a more accurate examination. When the neonate is quiet, the EMT can do the parts of the examination that require quiet, such as listening to lungs, counting respiratory rate, observing the work of breathing, and noting skin color. These are things that can be difficult to determine in the screaming newborn.

It is in this first month of life that many congenital illnesses are discovered. A congenital illness is an illness that the child is born with. The signs and symptoms of the illness may not have been evident immediately at birth, but may begin to show up as the child grows and develops.

Common illnesses that may develop during this time in life are jaundice, vomiting, respiratory distress, and fever. Some of these illnesses are discussed in the previous chapter; others are discussed later in this chapter.

Young Infant

The young infant, aged 1 to 5 months, is growing rapidly. Babies usually double their birth weight during this time period. The visual acuity of the young infant is improving, and she begins to follow objects with her eyes. Curiosity and amazement are predominant findings in infants as they observe their environments. Typically, nonsensical verbalizations begin in this time period.

Common illnesses and injuries seen in this age range, which are discussed more throughout this and the next chapter, include sudden infant death syndrome, vomiting, diarrhea, meningitis, child abuse, and accidents. Examination techniques for this age group are similar to those used with the neonate. These infants are becoming curious and will definitely watch all movement around them intently. Slow movements and gentle handling are the keys to the successful assessment of the young infant.

Safety Tip

If a newborn is to be transported, it is important that she be adequately and safely secured in the ambulance. It is recommended that any newborn be transported in an approved infant car seat appropriately strapped into the ambulance stretcher or bench unit. If the ambulance does not have an appropriately sized car seat for the neonate, the parents likely will.

When examining an infant of any age, the EMT should remember that they are at increased risk for hypothermia. The EMT should keep the infant covered as much as possible and try to warm the hands and stethoscope prior to coming into contact with the infant. Much of the initial examination can be done without even touching the infant. Observing the infant's mental status (alertness), airway patency, respiratory rate, and skin color is easily done without actually touching the infant.

Older Infant

The older infant, from 6 to 12 months of age, is becoming more active and is likely to be standing and walking. This increased mobility will lead to an increased risk of injury during exploration. Infants in this age group sometimes do not like being around strangers. The stress they feel in this situation is referred to as *stranger anxiety*. The EMT can help to alleviate this anxiety by gaining the parent's confidence first, and allowing the infant to remain as close to the parent as possible.

Common presenting problems in this age group are febrile seizures, vomiting, diarrhea, dehydration, bronchiolitis, motor vehicle collisions, croup, child abuse, poisonous ingestion, and falls.

Toddler

The 1- to 3-year age group is often called the toddlers. At this age, children are constantly moving around. They often are becoming increasingly independent. Despite their apparent desire for independent play and need to do things for themselves, toddlers often do not like to be separated from their parents. They should be allowed to remain close to a parent whenever possible during emergency care.

This increase in mobility and perception of independence can lead to more accidents. The most common emergencies seen in this age group are motor vehicle accidents, vomiting, diarrhea, febrile seizures, ingestions, falls, child abuse, croup, meningitis, and ingestion of foreign bodies.

When examining the toddler, it is important to remember that the child will need much encouragement and reassurance. The child may believe her illness or injury is a punishment and is often afraid of the possibility of pain. Something as simple as a blood pressure cuff must be demonstrated before it is applied to the fearful toddler.

The toe-to-head approach for an assessment is very useful in this age group. Involving the child in the examination with constant reassurance is also helpful. Making a game out of the exam is often a good way to gain the child's cooperation.

Preschool

As the child gets older and enters the preschool age (3 to 5 years), motor development continues. These children are starting to play more sophisticated games. They are often very attached to parents and personal belongings. A teddy bear will go a long way in gaining the confidence of this child.

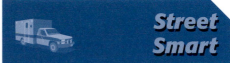

Street Smart

A useful examination technique for a toddler is to begin the assessment at the feet. This is less threatening to the child than beginning an assessment at the head.

If the child appears acutely ill on the first general impression, the priority will be to complete the initial assessment. A very sick child often does not care about the EMT's examination technique. This fact alone should alert the EMT that the child is sick. Whenever an EMT assesses a child, skill and confidence are important in order to gain the confidence of the parents.

It is very important to provide simple and honest explanations to the preschool child for every part of any examination. This will help to alleviate some of the fear of the unknown and fear of pain that the child may be experiencing. Making the examination a game is also useful in this age group.

Common presenting problems in the preschool age group include croup, asthma, ingestions, motor vehicle collisions, burns, child abuse, foreign body ingestions, drownings, epiglottitis, febrile seizures, and meningitis.

School-Age

The school-age child (6 to 12 years old) has a brain that is now 90% of the adult weight. These children are also physically growing quickly and are very active. The combination of rapid growth and high levels of activity can result in clumsiness and an increase in injuries. In a child this age, it is important to take the history directly from the child, confirming only important information with an adult. The child will have more confidence and respect for the EMT if it is clear that she is being listened to and taken seriously.

During the assessment, it is often helpful for the EMT to share his findings and to provide reassurance. Protection of modesty during an examination is also important at this age. The child should be moved out of her group of friends so she can feel free to express her feelings and pain without fear of embarrassment. Fear of permanent injury or disfigurement is a very real concern to these children. Common occurrences in this age group are drowning, motor vehicle collisions, bike accidents, fractures, falls, sports injuries, child abuse, and burns.

Adolescent

From the ages of 12 to 15 years, the adolescent is undergoing various degrees of growth and development. The teenager places a great deal of importance on body image and can be temporarily devastated by what seems to the EMT to be a minor illness or injury.

In the teen years, peers become more important in the child's life, and the child becomes much more independent. Risk-taking behavior is common in this age group. Drug- and alcohol-related emergencies are increasingly common in the teen years. Despite their apparent lack of concern for injury, adolescents are often afraid of permanent disfigurement once they have sustained an injury. Other common emergencies in this age group are mononucleosis, asthma, motor vehicle collisions, sports injuries, suicide gestures, sexual abuse, and pregnancy.

GENERAL CONSIDERATIONS

When caring for infants and children, the EMT must first remember that these patients are not small adults. They are people with many age-specific differences about their bodies and age-related illnesses of which an EMT must be aware.

The EMT may face a significant challenge when called to care for a pediatric patient. The child may not be able to provide an account of

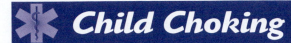

Child Choking

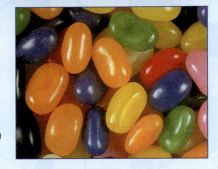

The 9-1-1 communicator picked up the phone to hear a man yelling, "He is choking!" Calmly, she proceeded to give the distraught parent step-by-step instructions while she turned the address over to another communicator. As ambulances were speeding to the address, the communicator explained each step.

By following carefully scripted instructions, the communicator was able to talk the man through the appropriate maneuvers to remove the jelly bean from his son's airway. By the time the EMTs arrived at the house, she could hear the child crying loudly in the background. The communicator told the parent, "Sir, the ambulance is there; you're in good hands. Let them do their job, and, sir, good luck."

- What makes a child's airway different from an adult's?
- How can the EMT differentiate between a partial and a complete airway obstruction?
- What should be done for the child with a complete airway obstruction from a foreign body?
- What are the potential causes of pediatric airway obstruction?
- What should be done after the airway has been cleared?

the illness or injury as well as an adult. The child also does not have as much experience with illness or injury. In addition, the EMT may not have a lot of experience caring for children.

When treating a pediatric patient, the EMT also has to care for the child's parents. With experience, the EMT will learn that in many situations, the care he provides to the parent through careful explanation and compassionate support will be instrumental in successful management of the child's illness. Many times, if the EMT can keep the parents calm and gain their confidence, he will be much more successful in obtaining a history and performing a physical examination on the child (Figure 39-1).

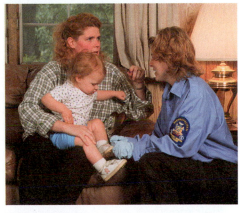

FIGURE 39-1   Many times when an EMT is called to care for a child, she must also care for the parent by providing reassurance.

Initial Approach

As the EMT initially approaches the pediatric patient, he should immediately lower himself to the child's eye level. If the child is seated, the EMT should kneel beside the child, rather than stand and tower over him. This simple act puts the child more at ease and gives the parent the sense that the EMT is comfortable with the situation.

It is helpful for the EMT to introduce himself to the child as well as to the parent. Identifying his position and his reason for being there is also useful.

Gathering a History

When gathering a history regarding a child's illness, the EMT needs to alter his technique based upon the child's age. If the child is old enough to respond to any sort of question, the EMT should question the child in a friendly manner. If the child is too young or too ill to speak, the parent will be the primary source of information. If the original questions are asked of the child, the parent should be asked for confirmation. Often the parent will add details that are useful to the EMT. However, the EMT must remember to ask the child the questions first.

Performing a Physical Examination

When assessing an infant or child, the most important part of the examination is sometimes gained by careful observation. Observing the child's interaction with the environment, the comfort with which she speaks and breathes, and how she holds and moves her body will tell the EMT how sick the child may be. The child who is talking a mile a minute and running back and forth in a room is not likely to be in danger of losing her airway or requiring ventilatory support.

Simple observation can tell the EMT a lot about his patient, and because it involves no touching or hurting, the child will not mind that it is being done. After allowing the child to become accustomed to his presence, the EMT should initiate the necessary physical examination. There are different examination techniques that can be used for each age group, based upon the child's expected response or level of interaction. However, some general points about the examination of the infant or child will be helpful to the EMT.

The EMT should always try to gain the child's confidence before attempting to physically touch the child. The EMT should be honest about examination requirements and should move slowly and gently. If it is possible, allowing the child some control during the examination may help the child to feel more in control of the entire situation and, for that reason, less afraid. For example, asking the child which body part should be examined next or what she thinks will be found there can give the child a sense of control and lessen her fear.

The EMT who is trying to gain the child's acceptance so that physical examination may be performed should consider placing simple assessment tools, like a stethoscope, within reach of the child so that the child is not afraid of the equipment. Similarly, using the equipment on mom or dad before using it to assess the child may help lessen the child's anxiety (e.g., listening to dad's lungs first).

Any part of the examination that is expected to cause pain should be done last. If a painful, swollen, deformed extremity is manipulated before any other examination is done, the child will not be likely to allow the EMT to perform any further examination without a fight.

It is helpful for the EMT to remember the normal physical findings for each age group. Infants and children have ranges for normal vital signs that differ from those of the normal adult. Table 39-1 lists the normal pediatric vital signs by age. The EMT should be familiar with these ranges and may want to carry a card or other reference that lists these important numbers.

COMMON PEDIATRIC ILLNESSES

Although children can suffer from illnesses that are common to adults, there are some unique differences about how a child presents with the same illness. There are also some illnesses that are classically found only in children. It is useful for the EMT to be familiar with the clinical presentation of an illness for a child.

Street Smart

In the past, well-meaning emergency care providers would take an examination glove and blow it up into a balloon. This practice should be discouraged. Children, seeing adults making balloons from gloves, may be led to believe that gloves are toys and inadvertently pick up and place a contaminated glove in their mouth.

TABLE 39-1

Normal Pediatric Vital Signs by Age

Age	Respiratory Rate	Heart Rate	Systolic BP
Newborn	30–60	100–160	50–70
1–6 weeks	30–60	100–160	70–95
6 months	25–40	90–120	80–100
1 year	20–30	90–120	80–100
3 years	20–30	80–120	80–110
6 years	18–25	70–110	80–100
10 years	15–20	60–90	90–120

AIRWAY PROBLEMS

Children have relatively small airways when compared to those of an adult. The child's smaller upper airway can become more easily blocked by secretions or foreign bodies. For this reason, airway problems are more common in children than in adults.

Foreign Body Obstruction

The curious nature of a child often results in her getting into places that a parent may have never imagined. Younger children, especially, tend to put every new object in the mouth for a taste test. This investigative nature can and does often lead to airway obstructions by foreign bodies.

A typical story would be of a child playing with some small object. The child suddenly becomes quiet, with or without associated coughing. A parent who discovers the child immediately may realize what has happened. If the parent does not find the child until after the airway has been occluded for a few minutes, the parent will likely find the child unconscious.

The progression of events in an airway obstruction in a child is for the object to be inhaled into the airway. When the inhaled object reaches an airway that is too small to get through, it becomes lodged and blocks any further airflow in or out. If this airway is a very proximal airway, such as the trachea, the child will not be able to breathe in or out at all. After a short period of time without oxygen, the blood will become low in oxygen, causing the brain to malfunction, and the child becomes unconscious. If the condition is not remedied quickly, the heart will begin to slow as a result of the low oxygen levels and will eventually stop. This progression of events from airway obstruction to cardiac arrest can happen in as little as a couple of minutes.

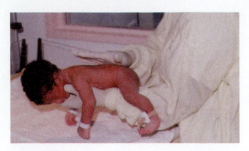

FIGURE 39-2 Back blows alternating with chest thrusts is the appropriate treatment for a foreign body airway obstruction in an infant.

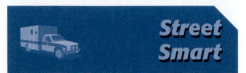

Street Smart

Remember that the infant's airway is very narrow and flexible. The proper position for opening the airway is neutral. If the head is hyperextended, the airway can be kinked like a straw and occluded. Careful attention should be paid to the position of an infant's airway.

The child's head should be placed in the neutral-plus position. This is neutral plus a little extension. This is the ideal position for opening the airway of a child to avoid excessive hyperextension and inadvertent airway occlusion.

Neck flexion may be avoided by placing a small towel or other material for padding under the child's torso, lifting the body even with the relatively larger head.

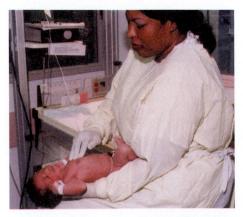

FIGURE 39-3 The positioning for chest thrusts on an infant is one finger width below the nipple line.

Incomplete Obstruction

If an airway obstruction is not complete, evidenced by the ability of the child to cry, speak, or cough, the EMT should encourage the child to cough. Oxygen should be applied, and the EMT should calmly but quickly initiate transport. As long as the child is still able to verbalize and move enough air to keep her chest rising and her skin a well-oxygenated pink color, the EMT should take no action other than to initiate transport. If at any point the obstruction becomes complete, it should be managed as described in the following text.

Assessment

The initial assessment of the child with a foreign body in the airway often reveals the source of the problem. If the object has completely occluded the airway, the child will likely be unconscious by the time emergency medical services (EMS) arrives. The initial management involves opening the airway and checking for breathing. When no breathing is noted, two breaths are given. In the case of a complete airway obstruction, the EMT will be unable to get a breath into the child. Just as the child was unable to breathe spontaneously because of the obstruction, air cannot be forced through by the EMT.

The next step is to reposition the child's airway. The pediatric patient has a relatively large tongue that can create an airway obstruction. With a slightly different airway position, the rescue breath may be effective. If still no effective ventilations are provided, the EMT should assume a complete airway obstruction and proceed with foreign body airway obstruction procedures.

Management

The appropriate management of a complete airway obstruction depends on the child's age. The following section is an overview of the procedures for relieving an obstructed airway. The EMT should refer to either the American Red Cross or the American Heart Association manual for complete details.

Infant

The infant under 1 year of age can be lifted into the EMT's arms, turned face downward, with the head lower than the chest. In this position, the EMT firmly strikes the infant between the shoulder blades five times. Figure 39-2 demonstrates this technique.

These five **back blows** are then followed by turning the child over to a faceup position, where **chest thrusts** can be performed. These chest thrusts involve placing two fingers one finger width below the nipple line and thrusting inward one-half to three-fourths of an inch as shown in Figure 39-3. The combination of these two maneuvers will hopefully generate enough intrathoracic pressure to result in the foreign body being expelled.

If the infant remains conscious, the cycle should continue with back blows being followed by chest thrusts until the object is expelled or the infant becomes unconscious.

If the infant is unconscious, after five back blows and five chest thrusts have been completed, the EMT should look into the infant's mouth to see whether the foreign body is visible, as illustrated in Figure 39-4. If it is, it should be removed with the EMT's little finger. If no foreign body is visible, the EMT should avoid a blind finger sweep, as this may push an unseen object farther into the infant's throat.

At this point, the EMT should attempt once again to ventilate the infant. This series of steps should be continued until the infant can be successfully ventilated. When ventilation is successful, two breaths should be given and the infant's pulse checked.

Child

In a child aged older than 1 year, an airway obstruction is managed in a manner similar to the way it is in the adult patient with a few important differences.

Once the complete obstruction has been recognized, the EMT should initiate **abdominal thrusts**. In the unconscious child, that involves placing the child supine and placing the heel of one hand in the epigastric region of the child's abdomen. The other hand should be placed behind the first, and together the hands should be thrusted upward and inward in an attempt to increase the pressure in the chest and expel the obstructing foreign body. Each thrust should be an individual attempt to force the object out. This should be repeated five times.

After five abdominal thrusts, the EMT should go to the head of the child and again open the airway and look inside. If an object is seen, it should be removed using a small finger. If no object is seen, the EMT should not place a finger in the child's mouth, as that can cause injury or force any object farther in. Ventilation should again be attempted. If it is not possible and the foreign body remains, the EMT should repeat the procedure, beginning with five more abdominal thrusts.

Once the foreign body has been removed and an effective ventilation has been delivered, the EMT should give two full breaths and perform a pulse and breathing check. The conscious child with a complete airway obstruction should be managed as an adult would be, with abdominal thrusts being performed from a position behind the child (Figure 39-5). These thrusts are continued until the object is expelled or the child loses consciousness.

Transportation

If the ventilation is unsuccessful, the EMT should immediately prepare for transport. Advanced life support (ALS) personnel can be helpful in these circumstances. ALS personnel have advanced airway skills and equipment and may be able to use this equipment, such as magill forceps, to remove the foreign body.

If the ventilation is successful and the apparent source of the obstruction recovered, the child should still be transported to the emergency department for evaluation. Trauma to the soft tissues of the throat can lead to swelling and more airway difficulty.

TROUBLE BREATHING

The single most common medical emergency for a child is trouble breathing. Small airways can become narrowed and occluded for a

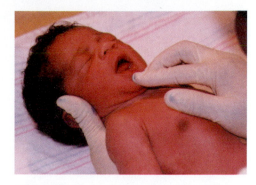

FIGURE 39-4 When treating the infant with a foreign body airway obstruction, the EMT should never reach into the airway with his fingers unless the object is actually seen.

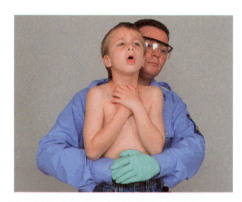

FIGURE 39-5 A child who is choking but conscious should have the Heimlich maneuver performed upon him to relieve the upper airway obstruction.

number of reasons. Regardless of the cause, the result is the same, breathing difficulties. Several common childhood illnesses that can lead to breathing difficulties are discussed here.

Croup

One illness that can result in airway narrowing and trouble breathing in a child is croup. **Croup** is a viral illness that causes swelling of the upper airways, specifically the larynx, the trachea, and the bronchi. This infection is most commonly seen in the fall and winter. It often begins with usual upper respiratory infection symptoms such as cough, runny nose, and sore throat, and then progresses to troubled breathing. Croup commonly lasts several days and is *not* usually associated with a very high fever, although a low-grade fever is possible. Children ages 6 months to 4 years are typically affected by this illness.

Epiglottitis

Another condition that affects a child's airway is a bacterial infection of the epiglottis, called **epiglottitis**. Epiglottitis is far less common than croup, but it is more likely to cause life-threatening airway obstruction. Because this condition is most commonly caused by a bacteria, children are routinely vaccinated against the bacteria that causes it. Children who have not been vaccinated are at increased risk of epiglottitis.

Epiglottitis involves an inflammation of the epiglottis, the floppy piece of tissue that covers the tracheal opening during swallowing. The normal epiglottis serves a protective purpose by covering the tracheal opening into the lungs and preventing aspiration when swallowing occurs; but when the epiglottis becomes swollen and inflamed, it can cover the tracheal opening, block the airway, and create an airway obstruction.

Assessment

Croup is characterized by a harsh-sounding cough that has been likened to a seal barking. This harsh sound is created by a forceful expelling of air through a swollen and irritated airway. If the swelling is severe, the child can develop inspiratory stridor. Symptoms of croup usually are worse at night than during the day.

The child with epiglottitis will present with the sudden onset of a high fever and brassy cough. A sore throat is a common complaint, and the child often breathes shallowly with obvious dyspnea, stridor, and an inability to handle secretions, visibly drooling in some cases.

Management

The most severe cases of epiglottitis can result in a complete airway obstruction. In this case, the foreign body removal techniques will not be effective. The EMT has to do his best to ventilate the child with a bag-valve-mask and quickly transport the child to the closest appropriate hospital.

Complete airway obstruction happens very rarely with croup. Management of the patient with croup involves calm transport to the hospital with delivery of humidified oxygen. Humidification of the inspired air often helps air to pass more easily through the child's narrowed airway.

Transportation

During transport, the child with respiratory distress should be allowed to sit in whatever position is most comfortable for the child. The parent should be allowed to sit close to the child to help calm the child. Blow-by oxygen may be helpful, as long as it does not agitate the child. When agitated, the child with croup often experiences an increase in symptoms, and a child with epiglottitis can develop a complete airway obstruction.

Some EMTs are taught to use a nebulizer system for administration of certain inhaled medications. Several milliliters of sterile saline may be placed in a nebulizer and with oxygen applied may be held near the child's mouth and nose. If the child tolerates this technique, the resulting mist of saline and oxygen can create the necessary humidification to ease the child's work of breathing somewhat.

The EMT should never attempt to visualize the oropharynx of any child who has symptoms that sound even remotely like epiglottitis. Any pharyngeal manipulation can result in a complete airway obstruction. If a complete airway obstruction does occur, despite the EMT's careful avoidance of the airway, the EMT should ventilate the child with a bag-valve-mask and transport the child quickly to the closest hospital. Advanced life support may be helpful but should be intercepted while en route to the hospital.

PEDIATRIC ASTHMA

Asthma is a very common disease state that involves reversible spasm of the smaller airways in the chest. In addition, there is a component of inflammation that serves to further narrow the airways. Asthma is a very common disease in children. Some children actually outgrow the disease as they grow older. Asthma is also commonly seen in adults and is addressed in Chapter 27. Asthma can be caused by many factors as outlined in Table 39-2.

Respiratory Infections

Although asthma is certainly a common disease in children, it does not account for all episodes of respiratory distress in children. Probably one of the most common causes of respiratory difficulty in children is an upper respiratory infection. Infections of the upper respiratory tract, such as a simple cold, can cause enough inflammation and secretions in the child's airway to cause difficulty breathing. Clearing of the secretions often helps to ease the child's breathing.

Assessment

Asthma is characterized by periods in which the child is well and periods in which the child is in bronchospasm. The bronchospasm is often brought on by a recognized trigger, such as those listed in Table 39-2.

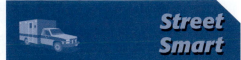

TABLE 39-2

Common Triggers of Asthma
Cold
Exercise
Animal dander
Dust
Smoke and other airborne irritants
Respiratory infections

✳ *Asthma Attack*

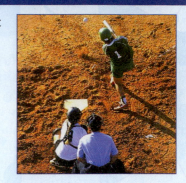

"You're out!" yelled the umpire as the boy slid into home plate. "All that effort for nothing," thought Jose, as he watched from the bleachers. Jose had been standing by at the Little League game for an hour when one of the coaches brought one of his players over to be "checked out."

The 8-year-old boy was complaining that he was having trouble breathing. The boy stated that he had a history of asthma but does not like to use his puffer because it makes him "nervous." Jose started his initial assessment, noting that an anxious father was jogging toward them.

- What is asthma?
- What can trigger an asthma attack?
- What are the signs and symptoms of asthma?
- What is the treatment for asthma?

TABLE 39-3

Signs of Respiratory Difficulty in a Child

Increased respiratory rate

Shallow respirations

Intercostal retractions

Accessory muscle use

Nasal flaring

Sternal retractions

Noisy respirations

FIGURE 39-6   The child in respiratory distress often has intercostal retractions that are visible to the EMT if he looks for them.

This bronchospasm causes the child to feel short of breath. Severe bronchospasm can sometimes generate a cough as well. If the EMT places his stethoscope on the patient's chest, under the clavicles, he will hear the characteristic wheezing sound of asthma.

The child suffering from an asthma flare-up, or exacerbation, often describes her chest as feeling "tight." This is because the airways are in spasm and it is difficult to breathe air in and out through such narrowed passages. A cough is sometimes a predominant feature of this condition. Signs of respiratory difficulty in a child are listed in Table 39-3.

These signs of increased respiratory difficulty are evidence of the increased work the child is putting into getting air into and out of the chest. Increasing the rate of breathing brings in more air, and usually the volume of each breath is less than the volume of a normal breath.

The use of thoracic muscles to help the diaphragm in creating an effective breath is evidenced by visualization of the outline of each rib with each breath. This obvious retraction of the skin between each rib is called **intercostal retraction** and is a fairly reliable sign of respiratory distress in a child (Figure 39-6). In more severe cases, the sternum is actually pulled inward with all of the effort to breathe. This is called **sternal retraction** and is a sign of severe respiratory distress in a child.

When a child is trying to increase the amount of air she pulls into her lungs, often the mouth is open and the nares flare widely to allow for more air entry. It takes a lot of energy to breathe when all of the airways are narrowed to near-collapse.

The child who is in respiratory distress for a protracted period of time may become physically exhausted. When the child is no longer able to maintain the extra work of breathing, the child will experience a respiratory failure. Signs of respiratory failure are listed in Table 39-4.

Management

The signs of respiratory failure, listed in Table 39-4, may indicate that the child is in need of immediate ventilatory support. The EMT must recognize these signs and provide such support or the child will

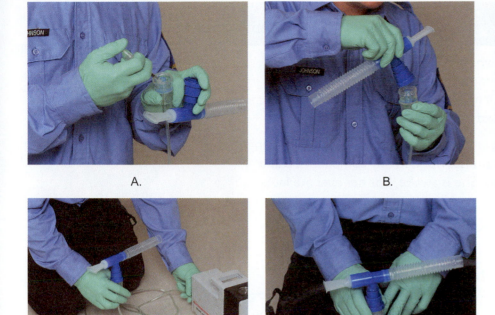

A.

B.

C.

D.

FIGURE 39-7 The prescribed liquid medication is placed into the nebulizer and either the compressed air or oxygen turned on to 8 liters per minute (lpm).

TABLE 39-4
Signs of Respiratory Failure in a Child
Cyanosis
Altered mental status
Abdominal breathing
Decreasing respiratory rate
Bradycardia

progress to cardiac arrest. Methods for ventilation are described in Chapter 8.

The child suffering from asthma often has bronchodilating medication prescribed by her physician. The EMT can assist a child with the metered dose inhaler just as he assists the adult patient with an inhaler. Chapter 26 describes the use of the metered dose inhaler. The EMT should refer to local protocols before assisting a child with a metered dose inhaler.

Very small children who cannot cooperate with the administration of a metered dose inhaler can be given the same medication via a special apparatus called a nebulizer. Parents are often prescribed a small air compressor that blows air into a small medication-filled chamber. This creates an aerosol that may then be inhaled by the small child. Figure 39-7 illustrates the use of such a device. The EMT should follow local protocols regarding medication administration.

HYPOPERFUSION

There are several causes of hypoperfusion in the pediatric patient. One of the most common causes of hypoperfusion is a large fluid loss resulting in hypovolemia. The blood volume of a child is much smaller than that of an adult, and therefore a child cannot afford to lose much fluid before experiencing hypovolemia and hypoperfusion. Common causes of pediatric fluid loss include dehydration and blood loss from trauma.

Vomiting and diarrhea from common viral illnesses can cause massive fluid losses in a child. If a child is not given enough to drink

Street Smart

Some pediatric bag-valve-mask devices come with an additional valve called a "pop-off" valve. These pop-off valves are designed to release pressure when the lungs become full. Sometimes these valves prematurely release because of back-pressure from a collapsed airway or a kinked trachea. For this reason, the EMT should disable the pop-off valve and pay close attention to airway position as well as lung inflation to ensure that the child is receiving adequate ventilatory volumes.

✳ *Ill Child*

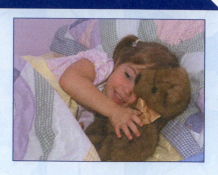

Dana, the EMT-in-charge, is led down the hall to the bedroom. Charity, the girl's mother, says, "She's not acting right. She sleeps all the time, and she isn't keeping anything down." Dana finds out that the mother called the pediatrician's office, who directed her to call 9-1-1.

The child has had diarrhea for the past three days and just started vomiting this morning. Other than that, the girl has not had any complaints. Dana finds a pale, listless child lying in bed. She is awake, but her eyes are lackluster and her lips are cracked.

- Can vomiting and diarrhea lead to hypoperfusion?
- What are the signs of hypoperfusion?
- What should the EMT do to treat the hypoperfusion?

Street Smart

Capillary refill is very dependable as a sign of hypoperfusion in children. A child with poor capillary refill, that is, longer than 2 seconds, should be treated aggressively and transported immediately.

to replenish the fluid lost, the child will become dehydrated. Dehydration from nausea and vomiting can quickly lead to hypoperfusion and hypovolemia in small children.

Assessment

It is important that the EMT recognize signs of hypoperfusion in the pediatric patient. A child is generally able to compensate for volume loss fairly well by increasing the heart rate and shunting blood away from the skin and abdominal organs. These compensatory mechanisms lead to tachycardia, pale skin, delayed capillary refill, and nausea. Decreased urine output from poor kidney perfusion is evidenced by a decrease in the number of wet diapers.

If the volume loss continues or the child is not treated, compensation will fail and the heart will no longer be able to adequately perfuse the brain, resulting in an altered mental status. The child who does not recognize her parents or who does not act appropriately should be considered to be very sick indeed.

The last evidence of decompensation in the pediatric shock patient is a fall in blood pressure. When the heart is no longer able to generate enough forward pressure to allow a normal blood pressure, the blood pressure falls. A falling blood pressure in a child is a very bad sign. The heart then begins to fail, resulting in a slower heart rate. Unless treated quickly, this child will die.

Management

The EMT must recognize the early signs of hypoperfusion so that he can initiate proper treatment and begin transport of the child to the most appropriate facility. Waiting for a falling blood pressure and hypotension before diagnosing hypoperfusion is a mistake.

CARDIAC ARREST

The most common cause of cardiac arrest in children is respiratory arrest. Children do not often have a cardiac event that leads to cardiac

EMS in Action

My story has to do with a cardiac arrest of a 9-year-old boy on the school grounds. It was a typical spring day when my unit got dispatched delta on a fall at the elementary school.

My paramedic partner and I responded within seconds of the tap out. The school was only about four blocks away, so it took less than a minute to arrive. On our arrival we were shocked to see a playground teacher and a bystander doing CPR on the boy. My partner instructed me to grab the life pack, med box, and airway kit as he called back to dispatch and informed them that we had a code 99 in progress and to send for fire responds as well as the other medic unit.

When I reached the patient, he was pulseless and apneic. I bared his chest and applied the AED pads; no shock was advised. The other units were now starting to arrive and we began CPR and set up for a field intubation. My partner dropped in the tube and we started a line and pushed every drug we could at this kid. Tension was really starting to build at this time, and we knew we had to go. We were able to start pacing the patient but he was a PEA rhythm. We loaded the patient after being on scene for about 15 minutes (but it seemed longer than that). The drive to the hospital was about 28 minutes. On the way we got pulses back and then lost them again. But we never gave up, because no one in EMS likes to lose.

We continued CPR for another 45 minutes in the ER. I am sad to say that despite all efforts by field EMS and the hospital staff, we were not able to revive him. This is without a doubt the hardest call I have ever run in my short career as an EMT. You think to yourself that school is supposed to be a safe place for kids, and not a place where they will get hurt or, even worse, die. This call was the one that almost made me quit and pursue other options. I know that I am not the only one who has felt this way. When I say that no one in EMS likes to lose, I think that we are type-A people who are competitive and try harder and longer even when there is no hope left. I felt a major defeat that day.

One reason I am still pursuing my paramedic certification is the help I got from senior medics such as my partner and other medics in the company. I learned that not everyone can be saved and that as hard as we try, we cannot control everything. If I can pass one thing on that I learned from this experience, it is to talk about it. Talk to anyone who will listen, do not dwell on it alone because it will tear you apart. Even writing this story a month and half later still helps. I will never forget that day, but I have moved on and hope to be in paramedic school soon.

Scott Thompson, EMT-IV Tech
North County EMS
Yacolt, Washington

arrest. More often what happens is the child goes into respiratory failure that leads to profound hypoxia. In turn, profound hypoxia leads to cardiac failure and the cardiac arrest.

Therefore, an EMT's priority in pediatric cardiac arrest is to provide good ventilation with 100% oxygen, along with cardiac compressions. The importance of good ventilation in the pediatric patient cannot be overemphasized. Often, treatment of the respiratory arrest will lead to a reversal of the cardiac arrest.

SIDS

The sudden, unexplained death of an infant in the first year of life is known as **sudden infant death syndrome (SIDS).** This somewhat mysterious syndrome occurs at a rate of 2 in 1,000 live births and is the leading cause of death in children 1 week to 1 year of age. The peak incidence is from 2 to 4 months of age and usually occurs during the infant's sleep. Males are more commonly affected than females. The winter months also seem to account for more cases of SIDS than other times of the year.

Although it is not known exactly what the cause of death is in these otherwise healthy infants, several risk factors have been associated with its occurrence. Infants of mothers of low socioeconomic groups are at increased risk, as well as infants of low birth weight.

An EMT may be called to the scene of a family who is unable to wake their infant from a nap. If the child is found to be in cardiac arrest, the EMT should initiate resuscitative efforts and transport the infant to the closest appropriate hospital. Emotional support must be provided to the parents as well. The EMT must avoid making any comments that might suggest blame to the parents. The cause of death in SIDS is unknown, and parents often blame themselves.

During the resuscitation, it is probably helpful for the EMT to explain to the parents each intervention. Explaining that the infant is not breathing, that the heart is not beating, and that those things are being supported during transport will inform the parents about what is being done for their child. If the resuscitation is not successful, the parents will have seen firsthand the work that went into trying to save their infant.

Because the death of an infant is such a difficult situation to deal with, both for the parents and for the providers, an extra provider may need to be present to help support the parents while the primary EMT cares for the infant.

ALTERED MENTAL STATUS

There are several causes of an altered mental status in a child. The EMT must first focus on the child's airway, breathing, and circulation. If the EMT finds that all of these are normal, he must investigate other possible causes. This section discusses the most common causes of an altered mental status in the pediatric patient.

Seizures

Many children suffer a seizure at some time in their childhood. Probably the most common type of seizure seen in children is called a **febrile seizure**. This type of seizure is caused by a rapid increase in body temperature. Usually associated with some type of infection, this fever causes the brain to short-circuit, in a way, resulting in a seizure.

A febrile seizure usually does not last more than a few minutes, although rarely it does last much longer. The child has a brief period of lethargy and confusion followed by a return to a more normal mental state, just as is seen after a nonfebrile seizure.

A child who has had a febrile seizure is at higher risk of having future such events whenever the child experiences a high fever, but the child is not at increased risk for chronic seizures like epilepsy.

When the EMT is called to treat a child who has had a seizure, if the child feels very hot to touch, the EMT should perform his usual initial assessment and manage the airway and breathing as appropriate.

Childhood Seizure

The 14-year-old babysitter met EMS at the door. "Thank goodness you guys got here so fast!" she blurted out. "He's in here. I've called his mother. I didn't know what to do. This is my first job. Did I do the right thing?" "Miss, slow down, relax," George responded as he carried his pediatric bag into the living room.

On the couch, a small boy, maybe 3 years old, was lying on his side covered with a blanket. He was talking gibberish and responded slowly when the babysitter, Irene, called his name. Irene explained that the boy had not been feeling well, and he had been running a fever. Suddenly, the boy had gone into convulsions, which prompted her to call 9-1-1.

Irene could not offer much history, except that she was sure that the boy had never seized before and now he was not acting right. Just then, the boy's mother came running into the room, and Irene exclaimed, "He was shaking all over!"

- What are some causes of altered mental status in a child?
- What is a febrile seizure?
- What should the EMT do for the child who may have had a seizure?
- Are there potential causes other than seizure for the altered mental status?
- What questions should the EMT ask the mother?

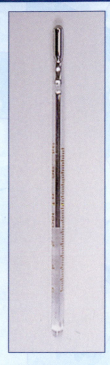

(Courtesy of PhotoDisc.)

Usually manual repositioning of the airway and some simple suctioning solve any airway issues after a seizure. The application of 100% oxygen by mask is usually appropriate.

The history of an infection or fever is usually obtained. The child should be undressed from any bulky clothing, and moistened washcloths or towels should be wiped over the child's body to moisten the child's skin. A fan should then be applied to the child so that evaporation may allow a decrease in body temperature.

Diabetes

Diabetes is a condition of altered glucose utilization that can affect children as well as adults. Chapter 30 deals with this condition in detail. The EMT should realize that the child who has a history of diabetes and who has an altered mental status may be suffering from low blood sugar, or hypoglycemia.

If the child is able to maintain her own airway and swallow on command, the EMT may give the child some sugar by mouth. If the child is unconscious or cannot effectively handle airway secretions, nothing should be placed in the mouth, and transport should be initiated immediately. An ALS intercept should be requested.

Behavioral

Although not very common, children can suffer from behavioral disorders that result in abnormal behavior. If there is a known history of such a disorder, the EMT should consider it. In the absence of a

Street Smart

Rapid cooling of the feverish child using cold, wet towels can induce hypothermia. Gentle cooling with moist hand towels is in order. Often all that is needed is disrobing the child and letting the heat dissipate naturally. The EMT, or parent, should never use rubbing alcohol to cool a child.

history of a similar reaction because of a behavioral disorder, the EMT should assume that any abnormal behavior is the result of a medical illness and should treat the child as a medical emergency.

Poisoning

Because of their inquisitive nature, children are at high risk of being poisoned. Children who can get into household cleaners, cosmetic products, and medications may become poisoned. The first indication of such a poisoning may be an altered mental status. Earlier signs of poisoning may include the presence of a spilled bottle of some chemical or medication, smells on the child's breath, discoloration of the mouth or lips, and vomitus with pill fragments or a chemical smell.

If a poisoning is suspected, the EMT should maintain the child's airway and breathing, and then follow local protocol. Some regions advocate calling a Poison Control Center, while others require the EMT to contact local medical control first. Regardless of protocol, the child who is poisoned is in need of rapid transport to an appropriate hospital.

It may be useful to the hospital staff if the EMT brings any potential containers so that the poison may be more rapidly identified and appropriate treatment started.

Infections

Because children play in close contact with many other children, they are susceptible to contracting many infectious diseases that are spread by casual contact. Some common infectious diseases spread from child to child include colds, the flu, gastroenteritis (stomach bug), strep throat, mononucleosis (a viral infection), and chickenpox.

Many of the illnesses spread among children are not life threatening. **Meningitis**, on the other hand, is an infectious disease that can be caused by a virus or a bacteria and is transmitted by coughing and sneezing. It is an infection of the lining surrounding the brain and spinal cord, and it can be very serious, especially when it is caused by particular types of bacteria. A child with meningitis may have a fever, headache, stiff neck, rash, and altered mental status. A child with meningitis may have a seizure. A child with these symptoms should be considered to have a potentially serious illness and should be transported to the hospital immediately.

Assessment

The focus of assessment for any child with an altered mental status remains on the airway, breathing, and circulation. Treating a child's troubled breathing, for example, improves the child's mental status.

Every child is different. If the EMT is unsure about whether the child's mental status is normal, he should ask the parent or caregiver. The parent will be able to ascertain whether the child has returned to baseline.

Management

A number of minor treatments can be offered by the EMT in the instances described earlier. The most common treatment, however, is

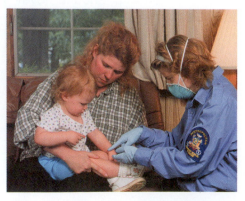

FIGURE 39-8 It is a good policy for the EMT to isolate herself from any potentially infectious respiratory secretions.

simply caring support of the child and family and transportation to the hospital.

STRESS IN CARING FOR CHILDREN

The EMT should recognize that caring for sick and injured children can be quite stressful, not only for the EMT, but for the child, the parents, and other health care providers as well.

Child

An ill or injured child is often forced to endure examination by a complete stranger who is sometimes dressed in a scary uniform. This may happen without the benefit of having a parent nearby. The illness itself is frightening to the child, and the fact that a stranger is doing strange things to her is even scarier.

The EMT should realize the potential for such fear and do everything in his power to reduce the child's anxiety. Knowing the normal stages of development and the needs of a child of a particular age group can be helpful. Probably the best way the EMT can put a child at ease is by being honest and calm, and by allowing a parent to be nearby if the parent is also able to be calm.

The EMT should never lie to a child if he expects that child to trust him or another provider. If a procedure will hurt, the EMT should tell the child that it will hurt and also how long it will hurt and what will happen when it is over.

Family

The family of a sick child is under a great deal of stress. The EMT must not only care for the sick child, but must make time to care for the anxious parents as well. Keeping the parents informed and allowing them to participate when that is appropriate will help to reassure them. If the parents are calm, the chances of keeping the child calm are increased.

Occasionally, a parent will be unable to be calm and quiet. If attempts to put the parent at ease are unsuccessful, the best plan of action is to separate the child from the parent. A parent who is hysterical only worsens the anxiety of the child. The EMT might have better luck with the child alone in this case. If a parent is separated from the child, a separate provider should be assigned to the parent and should continue trying to calm and support the parent.

Provider

Perhaps because EMTs do not care for children often, caring for a sick child is nearly always stressful for the EMT. It is important to realize in advance that feelings of fear and anxiety when faced with an ill child are normal. These feelings must be put aside at the time of the incident so that appropriate care may be given.

Later, after the call, the EMT should take a moment to allow his feelings to surface. Talking about the situation with coworkers is often helpful. This type of informal **debriefing** after a stressful call is necessary to prevent a buildup of such feelings of stress and anxiety.

CONCLUSION

Caring for an ill child is often an anxiety-producing event for the EMT. Knowledge of normal child development and the common illnesses affecting the pediatric population can help the EMT to feel more at ease with the situation.

TEST YOUR KNOWLEDGE

1. What are some general techniques that are useful in taking a history and performing a physical examination on a pediatric patient?

2. What are some developmental considerations for infants, toddlers, preschool children, school-age children, and adolescents?

3. What are the differences in anatomy and physiology of the infant, child, and adult patient and how do they affect emergency care?

4. What is the typical response to illness of the infant or child?

5. What are several causes of pediatric airway emergencies and how are they managed?

6. What are several causes of pediatric respiratory emergencies and how are they managed?

7. What are the signs and symptoms of hypoperfusion in the infant and child?

8. What are the most common causes of cardiac arrest in infants and children and how do they impact emergency management?

9. What are several causes of pediatric altered mental status and how are they managed?

10. Why does an EMT need to debrief following a difficult pediatric transport?

INTERNET RESOURCES

For further research and information related to the development of children, visit these Web sites:

- Child Development Institute, http://www.cdipage.com
- Foundation for Child Development, http://www.ffcd.org
- National Association For Child Development, http://www.nacd.org
- NCAST-AVENUW, University of Washington, http://www.ncast.org
- Society for Research in Child Development, http://www.srcd.org

These Web sites provide information related to asthma:

- American Academy of Allergy, Asthma and Immunology, http://www.aaaai.org
- Asthma and Allergy Foundation of America, http://www.aafa.org
- U.S. Environmental Protection Agency, http://www.noattacks.org

Learn more about sudden infant death syndrome by visiting these Web sites:

- American SIDS Institute, http://www.sids.org
- National SIDS/Infant Death Resource Center, http://www.sidscenter.org
- Sudden Infant Death Syndrome Network, http://sids-network.org

FURTHER STUDY

Ball, R. (1999). Seize the moment—Assessment and management of febrile seizures. *Journal of Emergency Medical Services, 24*(3), 78.

Deschamp, C., & Sneed, R. (1997). EMS for children with special healthcare needs. *Emergency Medical Services, 26*(11), 57–62.

Ojanen-Thomas, D. (1996). Assessing children—It's different. *RN, 59*(4), 38–45.

Perkin, R. M., & van Stralen, D. (1999). My child can't breathe. *Journal of Emergency Medical Services, 24*(9), 42–48.

Perkin, R. M., & van Stralen, D. (2000). Pediatric passages. *Journal of Emergency Medical Services, 25*(3), 50–58.

Raidow, S. (1998). Meeting the emotional needs of the pediatric patient. *Emergency Medical Services, 27*(4), 28.

Shaner, K., & Bechtal, N. (1997). Bridging the gap. *Emergency Medical Services, 26*(3), 46–50.

Werfel, P. (1998). The gentle art of pediatric assessment. *Journal of Emergency Medical Services, 23*(3), 58–64.

CHAPTER 40

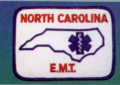

Pediatric Trauma Emergencies

KEY TERMS

central venous catheter
cerebrospinal fluid shunt
child abuse
feeding tube
mandated reporter
mechanical ventilator
tracheostomy
tracheostomy tube

OBJECTIVES

Upon completion of this chapter, the reader should be able to:

1. Recognize trauma as the leading cause of pediatric mortality.
2. Explain how pediatric anatomy alters patient assessment.
3. Explain how pediatric anatomy relates to chest trauma.
4. Explain how pediatric anatomy relates to abdominal trauma.
5. Explain how pediatric anatomy relates to head injuries.
6. Discuss the causes of pediatric spinal trauma.
7. Explain the treatment of pediatric spinal trauma.
8. Explain how pediatric anatomy relates to bone injury.
9. Identify pediatric trauma cases that are high priority.
10. Discuss pediatric burn care.
11. Define and recognize examples of child abuse.
12. Discuss the emergency care of the child with special needs.

OVERVIEW

Pediatric trauma is the number one killer of children over 1 year of age. In fact, trauma accounts for more pediatric deaths in the United States than all other causes of pediatric death combined.

Pediatric trauma death is largely preventable. The majority of these deaths occur in motor vehicle collisions in which, if proper restraints were worn, the number of fatalities would be less.

When a collision does not end with a fatality, it often results in an injury that causes permanent disability or disfigurement. For a child, this lifelong affliction impacts the child's development, both mentally and physically.

Perhaps one of the most anxiety-producing emergencies for an emergency medical technician (EMT) is pediatric trauma. Fortunately, an EMT does not need to learn a new set of skills. For the majority of pediatric trauma cases, the EMT need only integrate a few new facts into an already developed skill set. With practice, an EMT can become as comfortable with pediatric trauma care as with adult trauma care.

PEDIATRIC TRAUMA ASSESSMENT

The maxim "children are not small adults" is particularly applicable to pediatric trauma care. Children have significant anatomic and psychological differences compared to adults. These differences make children more prone to certain injuries. The EMT must consider these differences when assessing a child.

Anatomic Differences

The anatomic differences between a child and an adult are directly related to the child's physical development. As a child matures, the body changes to adultlike proportions. During that period of growth, the child can be categorized into several groups; frequently, groups are based on age.

Nevertheless, the EMT should remember that every child is an individual and should treat every child individually. There are large 12-year-olds who should be treated as adolescents, and there are small teenagers who may have to be treated like children.

Some anatomic differences are common among children of all age groups and diminish as the child gets older. These differences should be taken into account when an EMT is assessing and treating a child.

For instance, a child's head is proportionally larger than an adult's head, which makes the child more "top heavy" and more prone to head injuries. A child also has a higher ratio of body surface area to

Interstate Car Accident

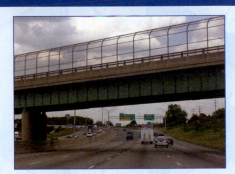

The siren screamed as the pumper raced through the streets. The report was, "Child hit by a car on Highway 66." An engine, an ambulance, and a paramedic-rescue had all been dispatched to the scene.

Emotions were running high when the crew left the station. Just four days before, the crew had worked a pediatric arrest caused by a fall from a third-story window. The child did not survive.

Now they were faced with another pediatric trauma, and this one was on the interstate. Cars would be speeding along the highway at speeds of more than 70 miles per hour. "Where the heck was the mother?" Mario thought angrily. "Why wasn't she watching the kid?"

Refocusing his thoughts, Mario, the EMT on the engine, started to consider his priorities once he was on the scene. "C-spine first," he reminded himself.

- What are the typical causes of pediatric trauma?
- What are the anatomic differences between a child and an adult?
- What are the indications for transporting a child to a trauma center?
- How would an EMT manage a chest injury? An abdominal injury? A spinal cord injury? A long bone fracture?
- How should an EMT respond to child abuse?

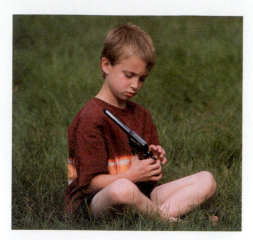

FIGURE 40-1 Children do not understand the consequences of their actions.

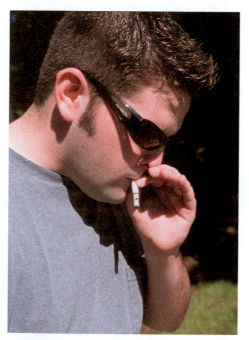

FIGURE 40-2 Adolescents are likely to experience problems from their experimentation.

mass, which means a child has more skin per pound of body weight. Therefore, a child loses heat faster and is more prone to hypothermia than an adult under similar circumstances.

Mechanism of Injury

Why is death from trauma more prevalent in children? The answer stems, in part, from the nature of a child. Each age range, from toddlers to adolescents, has unique psychological characteristics that put children at risk for different types of trauma.

Small children are curious. A child learns a great deal about the world by exploring it. A toddler will put small objects into the mouth to taste them and, therefore, is at risk for foreign body airway obstruction.

School-age children will play with implements of daily living, such as matches, in which case the result may be burn trauma. Sometimes children sense that something, like a gun, is forbidden and test the boundaries of adult tolerance (Figure 40-1). These children do not understand that serious injury or even death can result from mishandling a weapon.

In general, a child is less likely than an adult to understand that certain acts can result in serious injury. A child does not understand that running into the road to get a ball can have disastrous results.

Adolescents, on the other hand, understand these risks and choose to take them. Adolescent risk-taking behavior, such as drinking and driving, all too often results in death or serious injury. Adolescents are still curious, but in different ways than toddlers. An adolescent is more willing to experiment, such as by using illicit drugs (Figure 40-2). Table 40-1 relates types of trauma to the age of the child.

Initial Assessment

Some say that 90% of a pediatric assessment can be made from the door. This statement certainly can be applied to pediatric trauma assessment. Chapters 12 through 17 discuss the phases of assessment

TABLE 40-1

Pediatric Trauma by Age Category		
Age Category	**Types of Trauma**	**Examples**
Toddlers	Blunt trauma	Motor vehicle collision
	Drowning	Pool and bucket
	Burn trauma	Scalding
	Poisoning	Household cleaners/pills
School-age	Blunt trauma	Motor vehicle collision
	Falls	Bicycle
	Burn trauma	Intentional fires
Adolescents	Blunt trauma	Motor vehicle collision
	Penetrating trauma	Suicide/homicide
	Poisoning	Overdose

in detail and should be reviewed prior to this discussion of special considerations during pediatric trauma assessment.

General Impression

As the EMT approaches the child, she should stop, just for a moment, and form a general impression of the child. Immediately the EMT should try to ascertain the degree of the child's distress. Is the child in no apparent distress, in severe distress, or somewhere in between? An EMT does not need a great deal of experience with sick children to make this decision; she need only compare the way the sick child is acting with how a normal child acts.

Mental Status

A normal child is active, almost constantly moving. A sick child is often inactive, keeping unusually still. A normal child's eyes are bright, attentive, and constantly scanning the environment (Figure 40-3). A sick child's eyes are dull and lackluster. The sick child appears self-absorbed and disinterested in his environment.

When a child is hurt, he usually wants the comfort of his parents. He may cry, kick, and exhibit other attention-getting behavior. The EMT should determine whether the child is showing these age-appropriate behaviors. If the child appears distracted by an injury or, worse, disinterested in his parents' attention, the child probably has significant injuries.

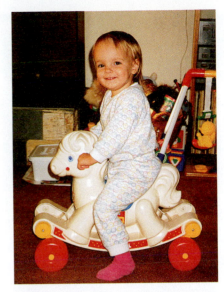

FIGURE 40-3 A normal child is awake and alert, active and interactive with her environment. (Courtesy of the Williams and Light Family.)

Airway

In general, a child's airway is smaller and more prone to obstruction than an adult's airway. A blockage can be life threatening in many cases. An EMT should carefully assess a child's airway and take pains to keep it clear.

Normally, a child breathes through his nose. Infants are natural, or obligatory, nose breathers. When a child is breathing through his open mouth, the child either is in pain or has "air hunger."

Breathing

The muscles in a young child's chest wall are not well developed. To breathe deeply, the child uses his abdominal muscles to help the diaphragm muscle. When the child is breathing fast and deep, a kind of seesaw breathing motion is seen.

A child's sternum is very soft, still largely made of cartilage. With a very deep inhalation, the negative pressure created by the diaphragm literally sucks in the sternum, which is called sternal retraction.

Similar to sternal retraction, intercostal retractions draw in the skin between the ribs with every deep breath. These signs—mouth breathing, sternal and intercostal retractions, and seesaw respiration—are all signs of a child having severe difficulty breathing. Chapter 39 contains more information on pediatric medical emergencies.

Circulation

Even a small amount of blood loss can be significant to a child. Comparatively, a child's blood volume is much smaller than an

TABLE 40-2

Pediatric Transport Criteria

Trauma triage—Child should be transported to a level one pediatric trauma center.*

Vital signs
  Signs of severe hypoperfusion
  Sustained tachycardia
  Bradycardia
  Hypotension

Presenting injury
  Uncontrolled airway**
  Severe difficulty with breathing
  Uncontrollable bleeding
  Paralysis or paresthesia
  Open fracture
  Penetrating trauma
  Head injury
  Severe facial trauma

Mechanism of injury
  Pedestrian struck at speed greater than 20 mph
  Dragged by a motor vehicle
  Fall three times or greater than child's height
  Unrestrained passenger in a rollover
  Ejected from motor vehicle
  Restrained passenger in high-speed crash (>50 mph)
  Passenger where another passenger died

* If a level one trauma center is within a reasonable distance. The EMT should always follow local protocols.
** The child should be taken to the closest available hospital, preferably a trauma center.

adult's. Loss of as little as 12 ounces (350 cc), or the amount in a soda can, can be life threatening.

Focused Trauma History and Physical Examination

Chapter 14 discusses trauma assessment in detail. The specific techniques used in assessing children of different ages should also be reviewed in Chapter 39. The priorities in the pediatric trauma assessment, as with adult assessments, are based upon the injuries found in the initial assessment and upon the mechanism of injury. Table 40-2 lists injuries and mechanisms of injury that are considered high priority in a child. These criteria can be used to triage a pediatric patient to the most appropriate hospital, according to local protocols.

BLUNT TRAUMA

Anybody struck by a motor vehicle has the potential for being seriously injured. A car weighing as much as a ton can transfer a great deal of energy and create very significant injuries. The injuries a child may sustain, if struck by a motor vehicle, are a function of the height of the child and the height of the car.

When a sports car strikes a teenager, the direct trauma from the bumper can cause lower leg injuries. When the teen is thrown, chest and head injuries also can occur. If a truck strikes a school-age child, the direct injury may cause immediate head injuries.

In most cases of accidents with motor vehicles and pedestrians, some blunt trauma occurs. Blunt trauma can result in internal bleeding, hypoperfusion, and shock.

Sometimes assessing injuries from blunt trauma in a child is difficult. There may be outward signs of deformity, contusions, abrasions, and burns; but sometimes these signs are initially quite subtle. If the EMT relates size and age of the child to the specific mechanism of injury, she can predict the area of injury and may be better able to discover these subtle signs.

Hypoperfusion

A child's body has a wonderful capacity to compensate for blood loss. Shunting blood to the vital core organs, the child is able to mobilize lifesaving stores of blood from the skin and abdominal organs.

Outwardly, the child will become very pale and diaphoretic. The child's capillary refill will become increasingly prolonged, beyond the normal 2 seconds. The child may even complain of nausea.

During this time, the heart continues to pump adequate amounts of blood to the vital organs, keeping them alive. The child's body is able to compensate in this manner up to a certain point.

There comes a point, however, when a significant volume of blood is lost and the child rapidly decompensates. The child's peripheral pulses become weaker, as the body shifts, or shunts, blood from the extremities to the vital organs.

The EMT can feel the result of this shunting of blood by comparing radial pulses and carotid pulses (Figure 40-4). In the presence of hypoperfusion and shunting, the radial will feel weaker than the carotid. This comparison of pulses will confirm that the child is shunting blood to the vital organs and may be in danger of decompensating.

As the bleeding continues, the child's capillary refill times increase and the child begins to become less responsive (Figure 40-5). These signs—weaker peripheral pulses, delayed capillary refill, and lethargy—and the other signs of hypoperfusion, in the face of trauma, are indications that the child has likely lost a significant amount of blood.

A loss of consciousness and a slow, or bradycardiac, heart rate may be signs of imminent cardiac arrest. Any child who is unconscious or bradycardiac is a high priority.

Management

The principles of management of hypoperfusion are similar whether the patient is an adult or a child. The EMT must realize, however, that the signs of hypoperfusion in a child are not as obvious as those in an adult, and the child may decompensate quickly.

Ensuring adequacy of oxygenation and circulation is the basic goal in the management of the pediatric patient suffering from hypoperfusion. Chapter 10 discusses hypoperfusion and its management in more detail.

Chest Injury

A child's rib cage has a large amount of soft cartilage that makes it very flexible. When a blunt force is applied, the rib cage will bend inward, then spring back to its original position.

An unsuspecting EMT might never question the possibility of a severe underlying injury unless she understood that a child's ribs are very flexible. When an EMT observes an abrasion or a contusion on a child's chest, she should consider what internal organs may have been injured.

It takes a great deal of force to break a child's ribs. Severe internal injury is usually associated with a pediatric rib fracture.

Management

The management of pediatric chest injuries is similar to that described in Chapter 23. Oxygenation, ventilation when needed, and stabilization of obvious chest injuries should be accomplished during the initial assessment.

The EMT must keep in mind that fewer signs of external trauma will be evident in the small child, despite potential serious internal injuries. Evidence of difficulty breathing or circulatory compromise in the child, along with an appropriate mechanism of injury, should prompt the EMT to suspect chest injury.

Abdominal Injury

Unlike those of an adult, a child's liver and spleen are only partially protected by the rib cage. That leaves these solid, blood-filled organs more susceptible to injury. Blunt trauma to the child's abdomen may tear, or lacerate, a child's liver or spleen.

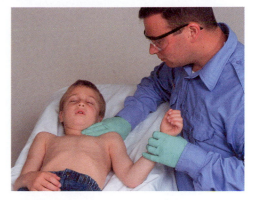

FIGURE 40-4 Pulse differences between central and peripheral pulses may indicate hypoperfusion.

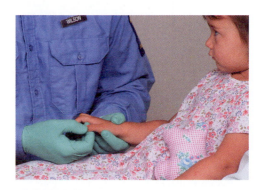

FIGURE 40-5 Capillary refill is a dependable indicator of perfusion in children.

An EMT should have a high index of suspicion that if a child was struck in the abdomen and has signs of hypoperfusion, then the child may have internal bleeding from abdominal injuries.

Management

A child with signs of abdominal injury, such as tenderness or bruising, should be carefully monitored for signs of hypoperfusion and shock. The principles discussed in Chapter 23 should be reviewed. A child with potential intra-abdominal injuries should be transported, if possible, to a hospital that is capable of managing pediatric surgical emergencies.

Head Injury

The signs and symptoms of a pediatric head injury are similar to those of an adult's head injury. Loss of consciousness, headaches, and blurred vision are all examples of signs of head injury. Chapter 21 should be reviewed for further signs and symptoms.

Children are more likely to experience nausea and to subsequently vomit from a head injury than an adult. Nausea and vomiting is so common with a pediatric head injury that an EMT should suspect a head injury in a traumatized child who has nausea or vomits.

The EMT must be prepared to turn a head-injured child quickly onto his side and suction the airway clear if the child should vomit while supine on the long backboard. For this reason, a suction device should always be ready for use.

An EMT may witness a child experience a seizure after a trauma. These post-traumatic seizures may be caused by a head injury. The first concern when the child seizes is to maintain the airway without compromising the child's spine. The child should be protected from further injury during the seizure. Remember that a postictal period of decreased level of consciousness is common after a seizure. The EMT should continue to support the child's airway and breathing as needed during this period.

Management

The management of the child with a head injury is also based upon adequacy of oxygenation, ventilation, and circulation. The injured brain is dependent upon receiving an adequate supply of oxygenated blood. Chapter 21 reviews the details of management of head injuries.

Spinal Injury

In any deceleration injury, such as a fall or a motor vehicle collision, there is potential for neck injury. Children are perhaps at greater risk for this type of injury given their relatively larger and heavier heads. The large head is thrown forward in the incident, forcibly flexing or extending the neck. This mechanism can result in injury to the spine. Chapter 22 discusses spine injuries in detail. Table 40-3 summarizes mechanisms of injury related to spinal trauma.

Management

Management of any spinal injury always begins with moving the spine into neutral alignment and maintaining manual stabilization of

TABLE 40-3

Causes of Pediatric Spinal Trauma by Classification

Motor vehicles
    Motor vehicle collisions
    Motor vehicle versus pedestrian
    Motorcycles—on and off road
    All-terrain vehicles
    Snowmobiles

Sports
    Swimming/diving
    Football
    Rock climbing
    Downhill skiing/snowboarding

Crime
    Gunshot wounds
    Knife wounds
    Blunt trauma—assault

the head and neck. The EMT may need to take anterior stabilization when a child is in a car seat. The EMT should not cover the child's ears; loss of hearing can be frightening to a child.

If the EMT can get above and behind the car seat, manual stabilization can be held from above, as demonstrated in Figure 40-6. The EMT needs to explain to the child what is going to happen before it happens in order to reduce the child's apprehension and improve the child's cooperation.

An initial assessment of the child should be performed, including oxygen administration as indicated. If the child is high priority, he should be removed from the car seat quickly.

Car seats are not designed as pediatric immobilization devices. The EMT must either modify the car seat or remove the child from the car seat. Reasons to remove a child from a car seat include ease of access to the child. It is difficult to manage an airway, suction a child, or even splint an injured extremity while the child is still in the car seat.

There are several advantages to leaving a child in a car seat. One reason is that the child may be more comfortable and cooperative if he is left in the familiar surroundings of his car seat. Another reason is convenience; it is more convenient to move a child from the motor vehicle to the ambulance gurney if the child is in a car seat. If a child can be reasonably immobilized in the car seat, he may be left in it with padding as necessary to immobilize the head, neck, and spine in alignment. If this is not possible, the child must be removed and immobilized in a pediatric immobilization device.

A cervical collar should be applied as soon as practical. There are a variety of pediatric cervical collars available on the market, and children come in a variety of sizes. The EMT should carefully match the right size collar to the patient (Figure 40-7).

In some cases, especially in the case of infants, it is difficult to find a properly fitting cervical collar. In those cases, a rolled towel can be placed around the neck, in the form of a horseshoe collar, and then secured at the chest. Figure 40-8 demonstrates the use of a towel as a cervical immobilization device.

Throughout the process of applying a cervical collar and afterward, the EMT must maintain continuous manual stabilization.

Immobilization in Car Seat

While maintaining manual stabilization, the EMT should consider whether it is necessary to pad behind the child's thorax. When a child is flat, his large head can lift his cervical spine out of alignment. It may be necessary to pad behind the child's thorax to move the cervical spine back into alignment.

If it is necessary to pad the thorax, the EMT will have to first release the restraint straps and/or lift the front guard from the child. The EMT would then gently slide either a folded blanket, towel, or foam pad into place behind the child (Figure 40-9).

The child is properly immobilized, and in neutral spinal alignment, when the opening of the ear is directly over the middle of the shoulder. The EMT should then resecure the restraint straps or replace the front guard, immobilizing the torso before proceeding to immobilizing the head.

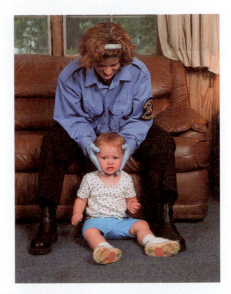

FIGURE 40-6 Manual stabilization may be held from a superior position.

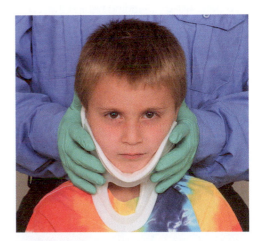

FIGURE 40-7 Pediatric cervical immobilization collars must fit the patient.

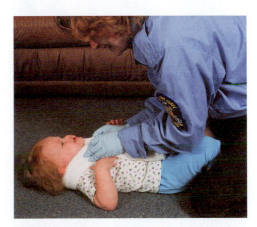

FIGURE 40-8 A cervical immobilization device may be improvised from a rolled towel.

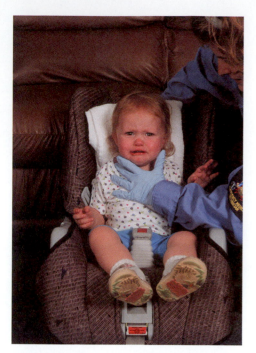

FIGURE 40-9 Padding behind the thorax helps to maintain neutral cervical spine alignment.

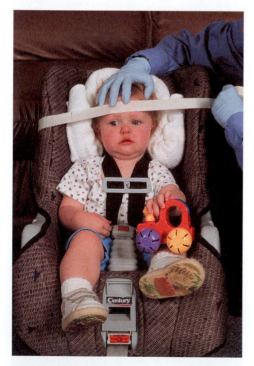

FIGURE 40-10 Rolled towels may be used as head blocks and the entire assembly taped into place.

The head may be immobilized in the car seat by placing two rolled towels on each side of the child's head. The head and towels can then be secured by placing a length of tape around the car seat, as demonstrated in Figure 40-10. Sandbags are *not* acceptable for use as head blocks. If the child must be turned suddenly, to clear the airway, for example, the sandbags would act like a counterweight to the body, forcing the neck out of alignment.

The child, immobilized securely in the car seat, should be placed on and fastened to the ambulance gurney. When the gurney is secured in the ambulance, the EMT should sit where the child can see her without turning his head.

Removing a Child from a Car Seat

Sometimes it is necessary to quickly remove a child from a car seat, for example, if the child is in respiratory and/or cardiac arrest or has an uncontrolled airway. Using a shortboard, several EMTs can quickly remove a child from a car seat. There are also commercial pediatric immobilization devices available. If using such a device, the EMT should follow the manufacturer's recommendations regarding proper use.

If a short backboard is to be used, one EMT must first maintain manual stabilization of the spine. Another EMT then places a short backboard at the head of the car seat. It may be necessary to place a mat or block under the short backboard to make it level with the lip of the car seat. Another EMT removes, or cuts, the restraint straps on the car seat and then quickly applies the properly sized cervical immobilization device.

Slowly tilting the seat backward, while maintaining manual stabilization of the head and spine, the EMTs should center the top of the car seat with the bottom of the short backboard.

The EMT at the head maintains stabilization while the other EMT grasps the child under the arms and slightly lifts and slides him, along his long axis, onto the short backboard. It may be necessary to lift the child onto a thorax pad placed on top of the short backboard.

Once the child is on the short backboard, his torso should be immobilized to the board. The spaces between the straps and the child may need to be padded. Straps should be placed under the arms, at the top of the chest, as well as across the hips. The restraint straps should not severely restrict the child's breathing.

Bony Injury

A child's bones are somewhat flexible and seldom break. It takes a great deal of force to create a fracture of the bone of a child. An EMT should have a high index of suspicion that there may be other more significant injuries if she observes what appears to be a fracture.

Management

Any painful, swollen deformity needs to be immobilized and then evaluated by a physician. However, the EMT should not be distracted by painful bony injuries and ignore more life-threatening injuries.

BURNS

The mere thought of a child with severe burns makes the most experienced EMT anxious. By applying the basic principles of adult burn care, reviewed in Chapter 24, and modifying them to accommodate the pediatric patient, the EMT can feel better about patient care and help improve the patient's outcome.

Children become burn victims for a variety of reasons. A child playing with matches may unwittingly start a house fire. A toddler exploring his world may unintentionally pull a pot of hot water off the stove. A burn may also be a result of child abuse; an adult may inflict a burn upon a child.

Management

The EMT is immediately concerned about maintaining an open airway. Inhalation of smoke and superheated air can cause upper airway swelling. The pediatric airway is narrow. A small amount of swelling, or edema, can completely close off the airway in a matter of minutes.

The EMT should listen for the sounds of stridor, a low-pitched inspiratory sound created in the throat as air rushes through a narrowed airway. The EMT should then look into the mouth for evidence of burn injury. A reddened throat, soot on the tongue, and singed nose hairs are all signs of burn injury to the airway.

Toxins, such as carbon monoxide, may have been inhaled by the child. Carbon monoxide interferes with oxygen absorption and can lead to hypoxia. High-concentration oxygen should be administered via a pediatric mask as soon as possible for every burn victim.

The percent of body surface area burned should be estimated. The percentage of body surface area for each part of the body differs in a child and an adult. A special pediatric chart must be used to properly estimate burn area. Chapter 24 on burns contains this chart.

Children have a relatively large surface area compared to weight ratio, making them more prone to hypothermia. Hypothermia is a major concern for the pediatric burn patient. An EMT must be cautious that the use of local irrigation does not create hypothermia, further complicating the patient's situation. Chapter 24 should be reviewed for further specific details of burn care.

CHILD ABUSE

Whenever the pattern of injury does not match the reported mechanism of injury, an EMT must consider the possibility of child abuse. Between 500,000 and 4 million children are abused each year in the United States, and some of these children present for emergency medical care.

Child abuse is an emotional, physical, or sexual injury inflicted upon a child by a parent or another person who is entrusted with the care of the child. Injury from child abuse arises from an act, such as a beating, or from a parent's failure to act properly. A parent's failure to act is called neglect.

EMS in Action

Often in EMS we are faced with the questions of why, what, and when. Our patients answer these questions when we interview them during an assessment. What may not be as frequent are the situations that prompt *us* to face those same questions during our shift.

I remember the day well, July 17, another warm sultry day in St. Louis. Working the second shift based out of a city hospital, we could look forward to a busy evening. My unit was given an assignment of a 345, or urgent shooting, on the city's south side. Communications also indicated this may be a psychological case, as they stated the victims were children. My partner and I looked at each other and instantly knew this call was real. Pulling up to the address, the street was empty. It was as if time had stopped, everything was quiet. The police had arrived and we followed them into the apartment. We found three children ranging in age from 24 months to 7 years all mortally injured with gunshot wounds to the head. Everything seemed to take on a surreal quality; my partner calling for additional units, contacting the pediatric hospitals to give reports, directing first responder help. IVs were placed, victims were intubated and ventilated, additional units arrived and assisted with transportation.

I remember thinking, what will my student think of this call? Why did this have to occur? When will these sad feelings about young lives extinguished leave? Some of these questions I have answers for. I can review the technical aspect of this assignment and see that everything worked well; our treatments successful. We were able to obtain IVs, to intubate, and to transport. Successful technical skills do not always influence outcomes, such as in this case. I also see how everyone involved came together to protect and shelter each other: police, nurses, and EMS.

This day became something different to each of us. I chose to incorporate it into what I call heartbeats, that split second when everything changes and you know you will never be the same. I choose to do something positive with these heartbeats, even if it is to just remember. Remember to take care of yourself and your partner. Remember to care for your equipment. Remember to seek new learning opportunities. Every moment, in everything you do, you make a difference in other people's lives. In that difference lies their healing and your power. Always remember that.

Charlene Jansen, EMT-P
EMS Program Coordinator
St. Louis Community College

If an EMT observes several injuries in various stages of healing, she should suspect child abuse (Figure 40-11). If an EMT responds to the same address repeatedly for injuries that are inconsistent with the mechanism of injury, she should suspect child abuse.

An EMT may be the only witness to the caregiver taking a child to several different emergency departments to avoid suspicion of child abuse. The EMT should report her observations to a physician.

If a child's recall of the events that caused the injury is substantially different from the caregiver's story, the EMT should suspect child abuse. If the child appears fearful of a parent or caregiver, the EMT should suspect child abuse.

It is not the EMT's place to approach a parent or caregiver with such suspicions. The EMT's first and immediate concern is to care for the child. After completing the call, the EMT should report her suspicions to the emergency department physician.

In some states, the EMT is required by law to report suspicions of child abuse; such an EMT is a **mandated reporter**. In most states, an EMT is not required to report suspected child abuse but may decide to report it to a mandated reporter. Physicians and registered nurses are typical mandated reporters. These health care professionals will make sure that the child is safe, that the suspicions are investigated, and that help is provided to both the child and the parent.

CHILDREN WITH SPECIAL NEEDS

In the course of the EMT's practice, she will likely encounter a child who has some sort of disability, including physical or mental limitations. Some of these children with disabilities are dependent upon advanced technology for survival. The EMT should be familiar with some of the more common tools used to help these children live comfortably.

When assessing a child who has such special health care needs, the EMT must realize that her own idea of a normal baseline for mental status or vital signs may not be that child's baseline. The EMT should realize that many of the children who rely on different technological tools have vital signs outside the normal range for their age. The parents or caregivers usually have a clear understanding of what is normal and abnormal for the child. The EMT should rely upon the information provided by the caregiver.

The techniques used for assessment and management of the airway, breathing, and circulation are often the same as those used for other children, except in certain circumstances where technological equipment alters the management.

Tracheostomies

A **tracheostomy** is an opening in the front of the neck that has been surgically created to allow for the placement of a rigid tube, called a **tracheostomy tube**. This rigid tube is placed for many different reasons, all of which center around a need for an artificial airway to maintain adequate oxygenation and ventilation. Figure 40-12 shows an illustration of a child with a tracheostomy tube in place.

Management

The child with a tracheostomy may encounter problems related to his tracheostomy tube. Frequent secretions can cause obstruction and difficulty breathing. The EMT can use a small French suction catheter to clear out the tracheostomy tube to help the child breathe more easily.

If oxygen delivery is necessary, the oxygen mask should be directed toward the tracheostomy. If ventilations are necessary, the EMT can accomplish this by attaching a bag-valve-mask directly to the tracheostomy tube (most will fit; others may require an adapter that the parents will often have) and ventilating as usual. Alternatively, the EMT can ventilate the patient with a mask over the mouth and nose while sealing the tracheostomy site with a finger (Figure 40-13).

If an EMT is having difficulty managing a child with a tracheostomy, she should arrange for an advanced life support (ALS) intercept while beginning transport to the closest appropriate hospital.

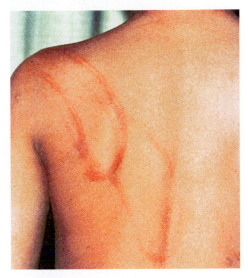

FIGURE 40-11 Bruising in specific patterns such as the loop of a strap often is an indicator of child abuse. (Courtesy of Emergency Medical Services for Children, NERA, Torrance, CA.)

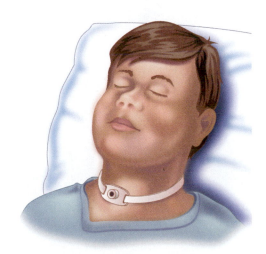

FIGURE 40-12 A tracheostomy tube creates an open airway for a child who may have difficulty maintaining one on his own.

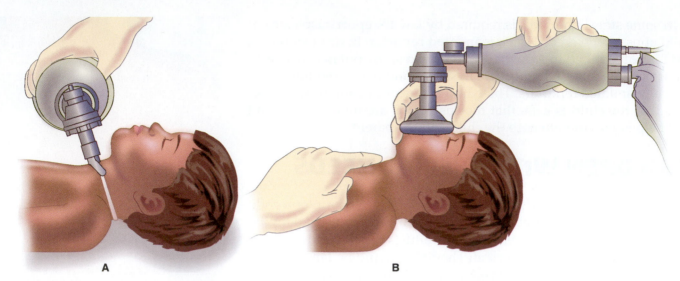

A   **B**

FIGURE 40-13   A. The child with a tracheostomy tube can be ventilated by attaching the bag-valve-mask directly to the tracheostomy tube. B. The child with a tracheostomy may also be ventilated by sealing the tracheostomy with a finger and providing mask ventilation over the mouth and nose.

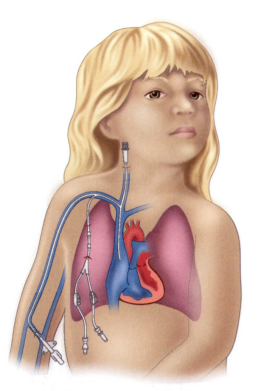

FIGURE 40-14   Central venous catheters are used to administer intravenous medications or to withdraw blood samples from the venous system.

Mechanical Ventilators

Some children who have problems breathing adequately on their own are dependent on machines to do the breathing for them. These machines are called **mechanical ventilators** and can be very small and portable.

Management

The parent or caregiver will know how to operate the child's ventilator, and the EMT should not attempt to manipulate it. If the child is having respiratory difficulty while on the ventilator, the EMT may disconnect the child's tracheostomy tube from the ventilator tubing, suction the tube as necessary, and use a bag-valve-mask to assist the child's ventilations. The parent can be asked to shut off the ventilator so that it does not alarm. The EMT who is providing ventilation to a child should arrange to intercept with an ALS provider.

If the child who is dependent upon a mechanical ventilator requires transport for another reason, the parent may choose to bring the ventilator if it is portable. The EMT should assist the parent in this situation. Alternatively, the EMT can use a bag-valve-mask to provide ventilation for the child during the transport. Any questions regarding the management of the child on a ventilator should be directed to an on-line medical control physician.

Central Venous Catheters

Children who require frequent intravenous medications or frequent blood sampling often have a **central venous catheter** in place. This is an intravenous catheter that is placed in one of the large vessels, often in the upper arm or the upper chest (Figure 40-14). This catheter may be used by trained personnel to administer medications or withdraw blood.

Management

Because the EMT does not administer intravenous (IV) medications or draw blood samples, she will likely have no need to use these catheters. Care should be taken when caring for a child with a central venous catheter to keep the site clean.

If there is bleeding from the catheter, the EMT should kink the tubing and then find a clamp to use to close off the tubing so as to not allow further bleeding. If the bleeding is from the site of entry, direct pressure with a sterile dressing may be applied while the child is being transported to the closest appropriate hospital.

Feeding Tubes

Feeding tubes are soft, flexible tubes that are placed into the stomach, either through the nose or through the anterior abdominal wall. These tubes are used to provide liquid nutrition to children who are otherwise unable to obtain nutrition. The tube placed through the nose is called a nasogastric tube, while the tube that is surgically placed through the anterior abdominal wall is called a gastrostomy tube (Figure 40-15).

Management

Rarely will a feeding tube contribute to an emergency situation, but an ambulance may be called to transport a child who has such a tube. The EMT should take care to keep the site of the tube clean and avoid any pulling of the tube. Occasionally the child will need transport to the hospital if a feeding tube has been accidentally removed. The EMT should never attempt to replace the tube, but should bring the tube with the child to the emergency department where a physician can manage the problem.

Cerebrospinal Fluid (CSF) Shunts

A **cerebrospinal fluid shunt** is a special catheter that is used to drain excess CSF off the brain and into the abdomen, where it can be easily absorbed. There are several conditions that do not allow adequate drainage of CSF from the brain and that require this therapy. These shunts, also called ventriculo-peritoneal (VP) shunts, are under the skin and extend from the ventricles of the brain down the side of the neck and chest wall and into the peritoneal cavity (Figure 40-16).

An EMT may be called to care for a child who is suffering from a complication of his primary disease or as a result of the shunt itself. Infection is a common reason for emergency evaluation. Fever in a child with a shunt must be evaluated immediately. Infection of the shunt can result in brain infection.

Failure of the shunt to work also may result in a rise in intracranial pressure if CSF is unable to adequately drain. This condition is evidenced by vomiting, altered mental status, seizures, or cardiorespiratory compromise.

Management

The EMT should treat the child with a CSF shunt for the presenting problem as indicated. Airway, breathing, and circulation management is done in the same manner as for any other child. The child with possible shunt failure or infection should be evaluated immediately by a physician.

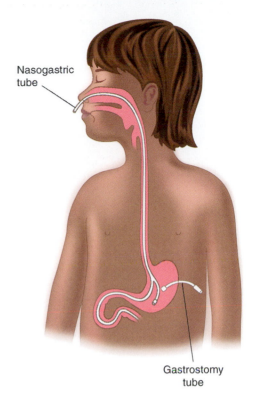

FIGURE 40-15 Nasogastric and gastrostomy tubes can be used to supply nutrition to a child who cannot eat by mouth.

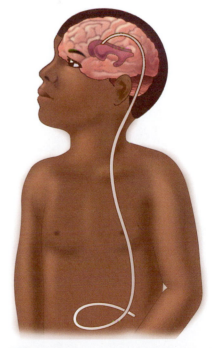

FIGURE 40-16 A cerebrospinal shunt allows drainage of CSF from the brain into the peritoneal cavity.

CONCLUSION

Pediatric trauma care is challenging for an EMT. The added emotional component makes the EMT's job that much harder. However, if an EMT remembers her basic care principles and modifies them to accommodate the pediatric patient, she can render competent pediatric emergency care.

TEST YOUR KNOWLEDGE

1. What is the leading cause of pediatric mortality?
2. How does pediatric anatomy alter an EMT's patient assessment?
3. How does pediatric anatomy relate to chest trauma?
4. How does pediatric anatomy relate to abdominal trauma?
5. How does pediatric anatomy relate to head injuries?
6. What are some causes of pediatric spinal trauma?
7. What is the treatment for pediatric spinal trauma?
8. How does pediatric anatomy relate to bone injury?
9. What pediatric trauma cases are considered high priority?
10. How would an EMT care for a pediatric burn patient?
11. What is child abuse?
12. What are some examples of child abuse?
13. Name some of the technological devices upon which a child with special health care needs may be dependent.

INTERNET RESOURCES

These Web sites offer additional information on pediatric trauma and child abuse:

*   Child Abuse Prevention Network, http://child-abuse.com
*   Childabuse.org, http://www.childabuse.org
*   Prevent Child Abuse America, http://www.preventchildabuse.org

FURTHER STUDY

Ladebauche, P. (1997). Childhood trauma: When to suspect abuse. *RN, 60*(9), 38–40.

Liebesfeld, M. (1997). When love hurts. *Emergency Medical Services, 26*(3), 29–39.

Quirk, P., & Adelson, P. (1997). Shaken-baby syndrome and the EMS provider. *Emergency Medical Services, 27*(9), 32–38.

Santamaria, J. (1999). September–October. Pediatric diving injuries for the pre-hospital care provider. *NAEMT News,* 10–14.

Ventura, M. (1997). Airbag safety alert. *RN, 60*(4), 43.

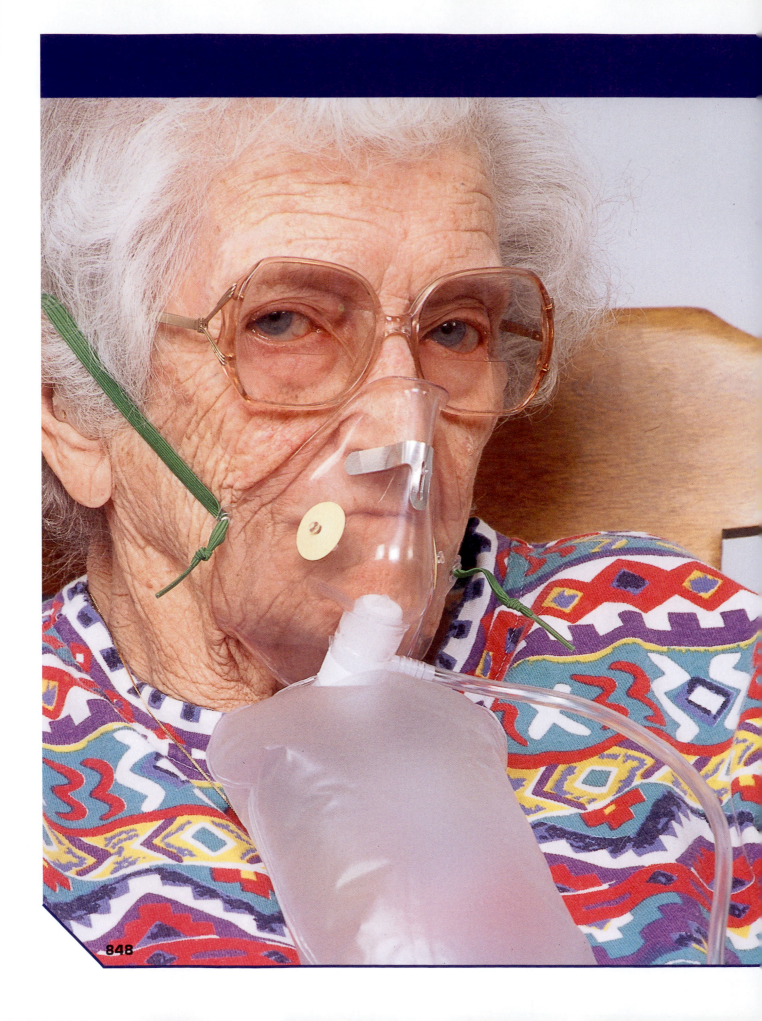

Geriatric Emergencies

In a phrase, America is graying. That means to say that Americans, as a people, are getting older, on average, and this fact represents a special challenge to the EMT.

An EMT must understand the changes that occur with aging and the particular health problems that accompany those changes. This section helps the EMT understand those changes and thus manage the problems that occur because of those changes.

EMS in Action

I was working on my first ambulance job out of EMT school doing BLS transports in Oakland, California. My partner and I were dispatched to a nursing home for a patient who was experiencing shortness of breath. Upon arrival, I found an 85-year-old female in bed and struggling to breathe. She wore a nasal cannula that was providing 3 lpm of oxygen. A sign above her bed identified that she had COPD. The nurse confirmed the COPD and told me that the patient used oxygen 24 hours a day and may have also been suffering from pneumonia. This poor woman was fighting for every breath and beginning to show signs of hypoxia. I decided to move her to a non-rebreather mask at 15 lpm of oxygen. In the time it took us to transfer her to the gurney she was improving. Her color was returning, her respirations were easier, and she had begun to calm considerably.

We moved her to the ambulance and I climbed into the back with her. I immediately moved the non-rebreather mask tubing from the portable tank to the rig's onboard oxygen system and turned the regulator valve until the needle rested on 15 lpm and I could hear the airflow. As my partner navigated the ambulance out of the parking lot and toward the emergency room, I began the detailed physical exam. My patient was actually in very good condition other than the COPD and whatever her current respiratory problem was.

(continues on page 865)

CHAPTER 41

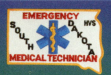

Geriatric Medical Emergencies

KEY TERMS

arthritis

delirium

dementia

elder abuse

osteoporosis

polypharmacy

silent myocardial infarction

OBJECTIVES

Upon completion of this chapter, the reader should be able to:

1. Identify the neurologic changes characteristic of aging.
2. Identify the cardiovascular changes characteristic of aging.
3. Identify the respiratory changes characteristic of aging.
4. Identify the gastrointestinal changes characteristic of aging.
5. Identify the genitourinary changes characteristic of aging.
6. Identify the musculoskeletal changes characteristic of aging.
7. Identify the integumentary changes characteristic of aging.
8. Describe the problems that can occur with polypharmacy.
9. Define the term *dementia*.

OVERVIEW

Today, advances in medicine, sanitation, hygiene, and control of infectious disease have led to an increase in the life expectancy in the United States to more than 75 years. Our concept of what age constitutes "old age" has significantly changed. As the body ages, there are characteristic changes that leave us susceptible to particular disease processes.

Geriatrics is the study of the diseases of elderly adults. This chapter discusses those diseases most relevant to the emergency medical technician (EMT).

THE AGING OF SOCIETY

People aged 85 and older are the fastest growing age group in the United States. The U.S. Census Bureau estimates doubling of the size of the older-than-85 group by the year 2025. Chronological age does not determine a person's state of health. Every person ages differently.

Elderly people as a group have more health problems than younger people do. Studies have shown that geriatric patients utilize emergency medical services (EMS) three to four times more frequently and require more advanced life support care than younger adults do. Emergency department (ED) usage shows similar trends with patients over the age of 65 accounting for 15% of visits while this age group makes up only 12% of the population. Furthermore this group accounts for 43% of all hospital admissions and 48% of intensive care admissions from the ED. The more complicated nature of an elderly person's medical problems often requires more time and resources to manage effectively.

It is certainly relevant for the EMT to be familiar with the normal changes associated with aging and the disease processes most commonly found in the elderly.

PHYSIOLOGIC CHANGES ASSOCIATED WITH AGING

From the moment we are born, our bodies start to age. This aging process is inevitable. Some changes, such as hair loss or graying, may be obvious, but others may be more subtle until they lead to a problem. This section discusses some of the more subtle changes that occur in each organ system as a body ages.

Varied Complaints

"A-2, respond priority two, the Rockenstire residence, 2401 North Main Street. Elderly woman, complains of a fever," the speaker boomed.

The crew, Ivan and Caitlyn, were greeted by an elderly woman, probably in her late 70s, who ushered them through the doorway and into her living room. "Would you like some tea?" was her first response. "No, thank you, ma'am," said Ivan. "Why did you call EMS today, ma'am?"

Mrs. Rockenstire proceeded to list about half a dozen complaints, including trouble breathing when she walked to the mailbox, a sore hip from a fall several days ago, and a general allover ache she thought was from her arthritis.

"Mrs. Rockenstire, what specifically is bothering you today, something that you want checked out at the hospital?" implored Caitlyn as she sought the one answer to the question that would mean the patient needed medical attention.

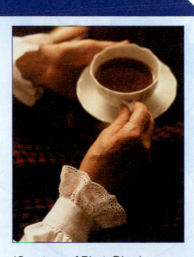

(Courtesy of PhotoDisc.)

- What physiologic changes are common as a person ages?
- How does this affect a person's health?
- How might this impact the EMT's care?

Neurologic

Some of the changes in the neurologic system may be more obvious as a person ages. Visual acuity notably decreases, as evidenced by the need for glasses as one gets older. The senses of hearing, taste, and smell also become less acute.

These changes may seem like a mere inconvenience, but they can have devastating effects in some cases. Poor vision can lead to an increased risk of falls and subsequent injuries. Loss of hearing and sense of smell can take away the ability to recognize warning signals such as smoke alarms or the smell of smoke or gas.

Many times, the progressive decline in these sensory abilities is not noticed by the person, but by family members. Glasses and hearing aids may help to reduce the effects of this aging process. The EMT should make an effort to bring any such physical aids with the patient to the hospital. This will facilitate patient comfort and communication in the hospital. Of course, care should be taken not to misplace these often costly devices.

When caring for an elderly patient, the EMT should determine whether any sensory deficits are prominent. If so, he should be sure to accommodate the problem. On the other hand, the EMT should also not assume that every elderly person is hard of hearing or cannot see. Each patient should be individually assessed and treated.

If a hearing deficit is present, the patient is sometimes described as *hard of hearing*. Several techniques may be used that improve effective communication between the EMT and the patient who is hard of hearing. These techniques are listed in Table 41-1. Be sure to mention to the hospital staff that the patient has a hearing deficit. If the patient has hearing aids, allow her to put them in so that communication is made easier.

Cardiovascular

As vessels age, their elasticity decreases, resulting in stiffening. This stiffening can result in higher blood pressures. In addition, the buildup of fatty deposits throughout life accumulates to decrease the size of the inner lumen of the vessel.

These changes in the vessels lead to a decreased ability to change the amount of blood flow to a particular area based on need. The person's tolerance of exercise decreases. As the heart continues to pump against these stiffening vessels, it becomes less and less efficient as a pump, further decreasing the individual's exercise ability.

These changes in the cardiovascular system put the elderly person at increased risk of a heart attack or heart failure. The incidence of these two conditions increases with increasing age. These conditions are discussed in Chapters 27 and 28.

Respiratory

Decreasing elasticity in the chest wall and lung tissue also results in decreased lung volumes. The alveoli and the cilia that clear the lungs of unwanted particles also become less efficient.

This results in increased risk for infection in the lungs and a decreased ability to compensate for it. Elderly patients with respira-

---

TABLE 41-1

Communication Techniques for Patients with Hearing Deficits

Directly face the patient when speaking.

Be sure the patient is looking at you when speaking.

Speak slowly and clearly.

Stand close to the patient when speaking, and speak in a loud, yet clear tone of voice. Yelling is not necessary.

Street Smart

When communicating with the person who is hard of hearing, the EMT can place a stethoscope in the patient s ears and speak into the head. This may allow some magnification of the sound for the patient and may improve her ability to hear.

tory infections such as pneumonia can become very ill very quickly. Chapter 27 reviews the common respiratory diseases.

Gastrointestinal

One of the most obvious findings in old age is the loss of teeth. While this may seem merely an inconvenience, it does limit the food a person can eat, which can potentially lead to malnutrition.

Decreased motility of the gastrointestinal system results in less efficient absorption of nutrients and problems with elimination. Constipation is a very common problem among the elderly.

Genitourinary

A loss of bladder tone and a decrease in the bladder's capacity can result in embarrassing incontinence and also increase the risk for urinary tract infection.

Progressive decreasing blood flow to the kidneys results in a decline in kidney function. This can result in difficulty maintaining an appropriate fluid and electrolyte balance, as this is primarily regulated by the kidney. Dehydration is very common in the elderly.

Many medications are eliminated by the kidney. If the kidney function is decreased, medications may not be eliminated as quickly as expected. If medication doses are not appropriately decreased, this can lead to a buildup in the body. This buildup can have harmful effects on the patient.

Musculoskeletal

A progressive loss in the calcium content of the bones, called **osteoporosis**, occurs more commonly in women than in men as they age. This loss of calcium leaves the bones weaker and at increased risk of breaking. Sometimes even minor trauma can result in bone fractures in an older patient.

A decrease in the flexibility of joints, together with an inflammation within those joints, called **arthritis**, can lead to decreased mobility of the patient.

Integumentary

Integumentary refers to the skin and the structures immediately underlying it. A loss of subcutaneous fat and water content leaves an elderly person's skin dry and wrinkled. It is at increased risk of tearing and does not heal as quickly as younger skin. Care should be taken during movement and transport to avoid damage to an elderly patient's sensitive skin.

The loss in the fatty layer under the skin leaves the elderly person much more susceptible to hypothermia in the cold. Elderly people are unable to insulate themselves as well as younger persons. In addition, the decrease in water content and declining function of the sweat glands leave the elderly patient unable to effectively dissipate heat, leading to heat-related illnesses as well.

Finally, as the body ages, the hair loses color, becoming gray or white. Hair also does not grow as quickly and becomes less prevalent on the body. Figure 41-2 summarizes the physiologic changes that occur as the body ages.

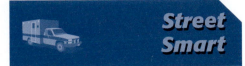

Street Smart

Falls are quite common in elderly patients. EMS may be called when an elderly patient has fallen and is unable to get up (Figure 41-1). When evaluating these patients, the EMT must remember that even a minor fall can result in broken bones. Before assisting the patient to her feet, a thorough assessment should be performed to ensure that no bones are painful, swollen, or deformed. The management of bony injuries is discussed in Chapter 25.

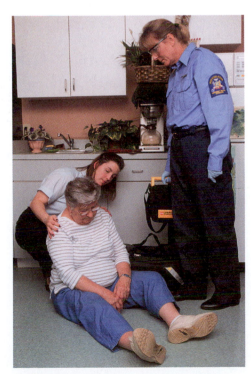

FIGURE 41-1 Falls are common among the elderly. A detailed assessment should be performed to ensure no bones have been broken.

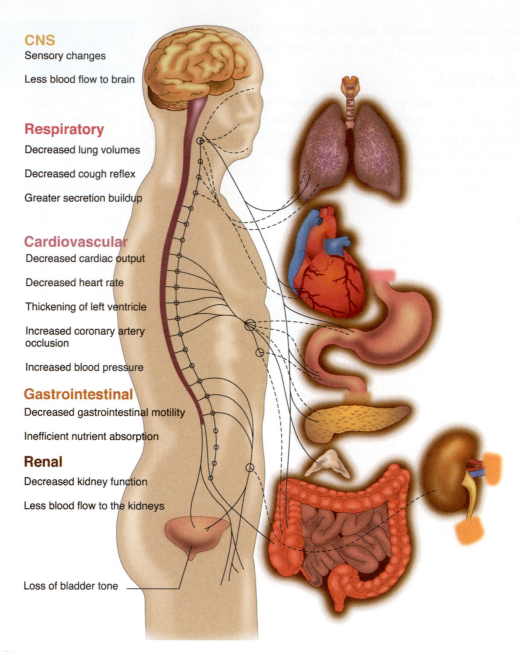

CNS

Sensory changes

Less blood flow to brain

Respiratory

Decreased lung volumes

Decreased cough reflex

Greater secretion buildup

Cardiovascular

Decreased cardiac output

Decreased heart rate

Thickening of left ventricle

Increased coronary artery occlusion

Increased blood pressure

Gastrointestinal

Decreased gastrointestinal motility

Inefficient nutrient absorption

Renal

Decreased kidney function

Less blood flow to the kidneys

Loss of bladder tone

FIGURE 41-2   There are changes in nearly every organ system that become evident as a person ages.

ASSESSMENT OF THE ELDERLY PATIENT

Although the steps in assessing the elderly patient are the same as those used to assess any other patient, there are some special considerations in the assessment of this population.

Scene Size-Up

When going into a patient's home, an EMT has a unique opportunity that the hospital staff will not have. The EMT is able to observe the patient's living conditions. As people age, they sometimes find it increasingly difficult to do the things that they once were able to do without difficulty, such as cook, clean, or shop for necessities. If the patient does not have family or friends who help her perform these duties, she may find them impossible to complete. The result may be a home that is not in an ideal livable condition for an elderly person.

The EMT should take time to look around the room he is in and note the general condition of the home. When looking for the patient's medications, the EMT may have occasion to enter the kitchen. He should take a moment to look around and see how well the kitchen appears to be stocked. The general appearance of the home should give the EMT an idea of the patient's ability to care for herself.

If the EMT is concerned about the patient's ability to adequately care for herself, he should ask the patient whether any help is available to her. Many older patients have family, friends, or visiting health care personnel who help them manage. If the EMT finds that a patient seems unable to care for herself adequately based on the condition of the home, he should notify the receiving hospital personnel. Hospital personnel can involve a social work team to determine whether the patient needs further assistance.

Initial Assessment

The principles of the initial assessment remain the same no matter what the age of the patient. Assessing mental status and ensuring an adequate airway, breathing, and circulation are the priorities in elderly patients as well as younger patients. Chapter 13 reviews these principles in detail.

Focused History and Physical Examination

Based on whether the patient is suffering from a medical or traumatic problem, the EMT will follow the assessments that are detailed in Chapters 13 to 16.

It must be realized that obtaining a history from an elderly patient may have challenges. Communications difficulties may contribute and the complexity of the problem may be difficult to communicate in an efficient manner. The EMT should make the effort to obtain an accurate and thorough history when the patient's condition and time permits. It is not uncommon for family, friends, or others to have significant contributions to the history of the patient's illness or injury. If these people do not accompany the patient to the hospital, the EMT is the only person who is able to obtain such information. It is crucial that any such information obtained is well documented and relayed to receiving staff.

Transport

During transport of the elderly patient, the EMT should remember the changes in the body that occur in this age group and protect the patient from further harm. Careful transferring will avoid further injury to fragile skin or bones. Adequate protection from excessive heat or cold is important to prevent hyperthermia or hypothermia.

Ongoing Assessment

As reviewed in Chapter 17, the ongoing assessment should be performed during transport to find any changes that may be occurring during this time.

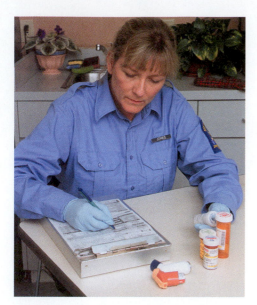

FIGURE 41-3 Many elderly adults are prescribed multiple medications; during history taking, the EMT should note the medications used.

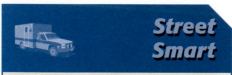

It is a good practice to gather all the patients medications into a container and bring them along to the hospital for review by the receiving staff. However, the EMT must realize that these medications are often quite costly. Special care should be taken to ensure that these items do not get misplaced.

GENERAL MEDICAL CONSIDERATIONS IN THE ELDERLY

The EMT will frequently be called to care for an elderly patient. It is important to be familiar with some of the general considerations that may affect the health of these patients.

Medication Use by the Elderly

As adults get older, they are more likely to have medical problems. Medications are usually prescribed to help the person deal with these problems. If more than one illness is present, more than one medication will probably be prescribed (Figure 41-3). The average elderly American takes more than four prescription drugs and two or more over-the-counter drugs.

The use of multiple medications by a single patient is known as **polypharmacy**. Polypharmacy, while sometimes necessary to treat multiple disease processes, increases the risk of medication side effects. If one medication has two possible side effects and another medication has another two possible side effects, that leaves the patient with four possible side effects. The elderly patient's body responds to medications in different ways.

In addition, the more medications that are prescribed, the more difficult it becomes to remember when to take each one. Medication compliance decreases with every drug that is added to the list that is prescribed. The use of multiple medications can be fraught with complications.

Each of these factors leads to up to one third of elderly persons developing adverse effects to medications. Furthermore, they are at least twice as likely to have undesirable side effects of medications as younger adults. In fact, 1 in 20 hospital admissions among the elderly is thought to be due to adverse reactions to medications.

It is important that the EMT carefully document each of the patient's medications and pass that information on to the receiving staff at the hospital. A complete knowledge of the patient's medication history may help the physician to appropriately manage the patient.

Susceptibility to Disease

The physiologic changes associated with aging leave the elderly person at increased risk for multiple illnesses and injuries. Table 41-2 lists some medical problems that become more prevalent in the elderly.

Altered Presentation of Disease

Along with the increase in incidence of illness, the elderly patient presents health care workers with a challenge. Because of the changes associated with normal aging, they may not present with the typical complaints of an illness. Disease states are more often discovered in advanced stages in elderly patients because their presence may not have been obvious earlier.

An example is a heart attack. Perhaps because of alterations in nerve stimulation, an elderly patient who is suffering from a myocardial infarction may not experience chest pain. The patient's perception of any discomfort may be greatly altered. The symptoms in the elderly patient may be atypical or absent altogether. The occurrence of a heart attack without the presence of the classic pattern of chest pain is called a **silent myocardial infarction**. A silent myocardial infarction is more likely to occur in an elderly patient.

The index of suspicion for serious disease in the elderly patient has to be even higher than it is with a younger patient because of elderly patients' altered presentation patterns.

Mistreatment of the Elderly

In other countries, elderly people are considered to be wise and are given a position of respect. The young routinely care for their parents and elderly relatives until they die. In the United States, the philosophy of caring for the elderly is a little different.

Many families choose to place elderly relatives in a facility where they can receive care from trained staff. The industry of adult homes, nursing homes, and skilled care facilities is growing daily as our society makes arrangements to care for its elderly. Nevertheless, many elderly people do still live on their own, receiving assistance from special programs for meals, transport, and daytime activities.

Their dependence on others for help places the elderly person at risk for mistreatment. Mistreatment of an elderly person is known as **elder abuse** and is unfortunately very prevalent in the United States today. General estimates of elderly abuse in this country suggest that it may affect 10% of the elderly population. With more than 1 million victims reported annually, yet gross underreporting is assumed, EMTs must be aware of the possibility of this problem in the patients for which they care.

Elder abuse can consist of physical or psychological abuse as well as neglect or exploitation. The elderly person who is living with family is often at greatest risk, although patients in nursing homes have been victims as well.

Just as in other forms of abuse, the EMT is often the first health care provider to become aware of the possibility of abuse. Any suspicions the EMT has based on what is seen in the home should be communicated to hospital staff so that further investigation can take place.

COMMON ILLNESSES IN THE ELDERLY

Although any illness can occur at nearly any age, there are some illnesses that occur more commonly or require unique considerations in an elderly population.

Altered Mental Status

Elderly patients may develop an altered mental status that is subtle and only recognized by family members or may have a dramatic disturbance in their level of consciousness, prompting a call to EMS. The causes of an altered mental state in an elderly patient are many and

TABLE 41-2

Prevalent Medical Conditions in the Elderly

Hypertension

Heart attack

Heart failure

Kidney disease

Complications of diabetes

Stroke

Dementia

Falls

Infections

Fractures

often multifactorial. Many issues inherent to the elderly make assessment of this condition difficult at best. There are several disease states that cause an altered mental status that are worthy of review here.

Dementia

A common illness seen in the elderly is dementia. **Dementia** is a syndrome that is characterized by a progressive decline in intellectual function that usually leads to deterioration of occupational, social, and interpersonal functions. The incidence of dementia increases with age, with as many as 50% of people over age 85 having some degree of dementia.

Difficulties with memory are often the first symptoms or signs of dementia. The onset of this disease process is usually quite subtle. A gradual progression over a period of years is characteristic of this syndrome. Often the patient does not even notice the symptoms. Many times this illness goes unrecognized for a significant period of time. It may become apparent during a period of stress, when the symptoms of the dementia may be acutely worsened. Any medical or psychological stress can temporarily worsen the condition.

Loss of memory may lead to the EMT encountering the patient who has wandered away from home and does not remember where she lives. The patient with dementia may not even recall her own name.

There are many different causes of dementia, some of which are reversible. The most common cause of dementia in the United States is Alzheimer's disease.

✳ *Disorientation*

"Ma'am, you can't shop here dressed like that," the store manager pleaded with the elderly woman, then turned to address the EMT. "Thank goodness you're here, Officer."

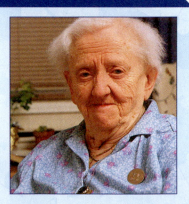

"Sir, I'm an EMT, not a police officer," Mario said. Then he asked, "What's going on here?" "I need more cat food!" Mario turned in the direction of the voice. In front of him stood an elderly woman, probably in her mid-80s, dressed in a nightgown and slippers. "Ma'am, how did you get here? There's 3 feet of snow outside, and it's still coming down!" The words had scarcely left his lips when he realized that the patient was not paying attention.

Just then Mario heard someone yelling, "Mother, Mother!" He saw a middle-aged woman rushing toward them. "I'm sorry, Officer, sometimes Mother gets confused and wanders off. I'll take her home immediately." Mario waved his hand to stop her. "Please, let me check her out," Mario said to the daughter. "She's been outside in the freezing cold. I want to make sure she's all right."

- What is the difference between delirium and dementia?
- What are some of the causes of dementia?
- How should the EMT treat the patient with dementia?

Alzheimer's Disease

Alzheimer's disease is responsible for 60% of cases of dementia in the United States. The incidence of this condition increases sharply with age. The cause of the disease is unknown, but it has been found to be somewhat genetic in nature, although with variable expressions. Some people who have been diagnosed with Alzheimer's disease are hardly symptomatic, while others are completely nonfunctional, relying on others for all of their activities of daily living.

The clinical expression of this disease is with dementia of varying degrees. There are very subtle changes found in the brain tissue of patients who suffer from this disease. Not much is known about the etiology of the disease; therefore, treatments are largely experimental.

Delirium

Delirium can be defined as an acute change in mental status occurring secondary to a potentially reversible medical condition. While delirium can exist in conjunction with dementia, it is important to realize the acute nature of the process in this case. Elderly patients are at high risk for delirium during the course of even minor illnesses due to physical sensitivity to illness and to medications prescribed for those illnesses. Medications are the most common reversible cause of delirium, even when they are used appropriately.

Rather than a disease process on its own, delirium can be thought of as a marker for another disease. Often the underlying disease is one that may pose a serious threat to life, such as myocardial infarction, stroke, pneumonia, gastrointestinal bleeding, overwhelming infection, traumatic brain injury, or pulmonary embolus. Classic symptoms and signs of these conditions may be absent in the elderly patient, the only sign of illness being the acute confusional state.

Because patients suffering from delirium may not be able to provide an adequate history, EMTs may not have the historical clues to guide their management of such conditions. For this reason, the elderly patient with an acutely altered mental status should be treated as if a potential life threat existed.

When possible, the EMT should attempt to obtain a history from family, friends, caregivers, or other personnel who might be able to provide clues to the patient's current condition. Of key importance is a description of the patient's baseline mental status and how the current presentation differs. Additionally, symptoms of recent illness or any medication changes, whether over the counter or prescription, should be elicited.

Trauma

In the over 65 population, trauma is the fifth leading cause of death. This population accounts for 20% of all trauma patients and nearly 30% of fatalities. Injuries that might be easily survived by a younger adult may often be fatal in an elderly person. Furthermore, those who survive their injury will often require long-term care. The EMT should be aware of the high morbidity and mortality associated with even seemingly minor trauma in this patient population and take care to

Safety Tip

The patient with an altered mental status may be agitated and could pose a threat to the safety of herself or the EMT. Physical restraint may be required to protect the patient and the EMS team. If this is felt to be necessary, care should be taken to avoid injuring the patient, remembering that the elderly patient is more sensitive to minor trauma. Chapter 32 addresses the process of restraint in more detail.

provide expedient transport to a facility capable of managing geriatric trauma. When assessing the elderly trauma victim, the EMT must also remember that the physiologic changes associated with aging result in subtle visible physical findings, even when significant disease is present. For example, the elderly patient can lose a significant amount of blood before showing any signs of shock. Rapid decompensation, once a critical threshold is reached, is classic. The EMT must look carefully for those subtle signs, such as confusion, and treat aggressively to prevent further decompensation. Regional trauma protocols often have special considerations for elderly patients, often mandated treatment at a trauma center after a significant mechanism of injury even when no physical abnormalities are noted. While an EMT will not be in a position to diagnose specific injuries in any definitive way, it is worthwhile to review the unique factors associated with specific injuries in the geriatric population.

Falls

Falls account for the most significant injuries in the elderly, although motor vehicle accidents, pedestrian accidents, violent assault, and burns contribute to the numbers of injured elderly adults as well.

Falls occur in nearly one third of adults over age 65 who live independently, and at an even higher rate in institutionalized adults. One in 10 falls results in an injury that requires emergency department care. The frequency of falls and severity of injuries sustained increases with each decade of life.

There are many reasons for falls in the elderly, and these can be separated into several categories. It is useful for the EMT to consider these factors as he obtains a history and observes the patient's home environment. The first category is environmental objects that contribute to a fall. This includes things in the patient's environment that cause a trip, slip, or fall. Poor lighting, lack of handrails, loose floor coverings, and unstable furniture are a few examples of how environmental issues can lead to a fall.

Physiologic factors can also lead to a trip, slip, or fall. Degenerating vision, poor balance, decreasing strength, and slower reaction times are among the physiologic changes associated with aging that frequently contribute to falls. It is obvious that physiologic factors can add to environmental objects and create a fall. If the EMT notes things in the patient's home environment that seem a likely contributing factor to a fall, he should report this to hospital staff. It may be useful for a social worker to visit the patient's home and assess the safety of the environment in order to prevent further injury.

The last category of factors leading to falls in the elderly are pathologic processes that result in the patient falling down. Acute neurologic conditions, cardiac conditions, and other potentially serious disease processes can lead to a loss of consciousness and a fall. In obtaining a history, it is important for the EMT to question the patient regarding symptoms preceding the fall such as palpitations or dizziness. Additionally, witnesses to the incident should be questioned about any noted loss of consciousness, seizure activity, or other obvious sign of illness.

Head Injuries

Traumatic brain injury is a leading cause of trauma death in the elderly population. In the elderly patient, a Glasgow Coma Scale of 8 or less is associated with a mortality of greater than 90%. Subdural hematomas are seen with three times the frequency as seen in a younger population. This is due largely to the normal shrinkage of brain tissue within the skull, known as atrophy, resulting in more movement of the brain with sudden movements of the head. Violent movement of the brain within the skull can lead to tearing of veins and subsequent bleeding into the subdural space.

The addition of medications that are meant to thin the blood and prevent clotting can worsen this condition. Elderly patients are more often prescribed such medications. Even minor head trauma can lead to a significant injury. Often the bleeding is slow in nature and results in a delay in the onset of any symptoms. Subtle symptoms such as confusion or headache may occur several days to weeks after an injury. The EMT should ask specifically regarding any injury in the weeks preceding the current problem. Chapter 21 reviews the management of the patient with a head injury in detail.

Chest and Abdomen

Aging, brittle bones are more susceptible to fracture. An elderly patient may sustain a fractured rib with a mechanism as benign as a strong cough or sneeze. A careful physical exam may reveal point tenderness over a fracture site or even crepitus as a result of bone ends rubbing together. Rib fractures may be associated with significant internal organ injury.

Mortality from intra-abdominal injury can exceed four times that seen in younger patients. Additionally, the physical exam of the elderly adult's abdomen may be falsely reassuring due to the altered response to peritoneal irritation. The classic rigid, tender abdomen may not be present despite significant intra-abdominal injuries. Chapter 23 discusses the assessment and management techniques utilized in the case of chest and abdominal injury.

Spine

Many elderly adults have chronic degenerative changes in their spines that result in pain. After sustaining trauma, it may be difficult to determine whether any pain in the neck or back is due to previous disease or to new injury. It is best for the EMT to assume the presence of a new injury and take precautions to prevent further injury by providing spinal immobilization in any case where significant trauma exists or even in the case of minor trauma with neck or back pain. Chapter 22 discusses spine injuries in detail.

Extremities

Fractures to extremities can occur with minor trauma or even with no noted trauma at all in the elderly population. Bones are more susceptible to injury due to the normal aging process, and the presence of abnormality in a bone causing a spontaneous fracture is more common in this population. The EMT should be vigilant to the possibility of a fractured bone even when a history of trauma is not clear. Any extremity pain should be suspicious and treated as a possible fracture as described in Chapter 35.

Acute Myocardial Infarction (AMI)

It may be obvious that as people get older, their risk of cardiovascular disease increases. In fact, more than half of myocardial infarctions happen in elderly persons. What is not always obvious, however, is their presentation of the disease. Elderly patients very often do not have the classic symptom complex expected with an AMI as described in Chapter 28. The presence of atypical or no apparent symptoms can lead to a delay in presentation and treatment. Perhaps for this reason and due to multiple coexisting medical conditions, the elderly patient has double the risk of dying from a heart attack as someone younger. AMI is the leading cause of death in the over 65 population, accounting for two thirds of deaths in this age group.

The EMT should be vigilant to consider the possibility of AMI in elderly patients who have complaints such as shortness of breath, nausea, dizziness, weakness, and sweating even without the presence of chest pain. Proper treatment and transport decisions as discussed in Chapter 28 can have an impact on the outcome of the elderly patient with an AMI.

Abdominal Pain

The complaint of abdominal pain in a patient over the age of 65 is much more likely to result in hospital admission, need for surgery, and significant morbidity and mortality than in any other age group. The EMT should take note of the likelihood of a serious condition existing when abdominal pain is the complaint in the elderly patient. This is true even in the absence of classic physical findings. The elderly patient may not exhibit guarding or rigidity due to relatively thin abdominal musculature and other anatomic changes associated with aging. Chapter 33 discusses specific causes of abdominal pain and the treatment of each.

Infection

For a multitude of reasons elderly patients are more susceptible to infection, and as with many other disease processes in this age group, will often present atypically. Many elderly patients with severe infections do not even have a fever. The presenting complaint may be as nonspecific as a poor appetite, feeling tired, or confusion. Respiratory infections, urinary tract infections, intra-abdominal infections, and soft tissue infections are the most common sources for serious infection in the elderly population. Many times, an elderly patient with a particular infectious problem will require hospitalization when a similar disease in a younger person would be easily treated at home.

Stroke

While it was discussed in Chapter 31 that stroke can occur in any age group, it cannot be denied that advancing age is a significant risk factor, and the majority of strokes do occur in an elderly population.

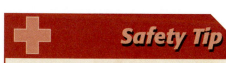

Safety Tip

Nearly 30% of newly diagnosed cases of tuberculosis are found in patients over 65 years of age. Tuberculosis is an infectious disease that is transmitted by respiratory droplets and is many times difficult to treat. Recalling the atypical presentation of infection in the elderly, the EMT should have a low threshold for donning appropriate personal protective equipment if treating an elderly patient with a cough, fever, or other concerning symptoms.

Elderly patients may delay accessing EMS and often have higher rates of death and significant disability after a stroke. The EMT may be able to impact these statistics through early recognition and expedient transport to an appropriate hospital.

Depression

Many elderly patients suffer from some degree of depression. In one study of nonhospitalized patients, nearly a third had some symptoms of mild depression, with 6% classified as severe. Not unexpectedly, the rates are higher among hospitalized patients. Depression in the elderly can present to the EMT in several ways. In some cases, the patient can become confused as a result of the depression. The EMT may be called for an altered mental status. Alternatively, the patient may not be able to care properly for herself due to her depressed state and this may result in a call for EMS. At the extreme, EMS may be activated for a suicide attempt. The suicide risk is highest among elderly men. While the depressed mood of the patient may be very obvious to the EMT, there is often a coexisting medical condition that results in a need for EMS.

Alcohol Abuse

Abuse of alcohol is exceedingly common in the elderly population in the United States. It is estimated that more than 2.5 million elderly people abuse alcohol. In this age range, women seem to be affected more than men. Chronic alcohol use can lead to a number of serious medical problems, especially in an elderly person. Gastrointestinal bleeding, injury from falls, and other trauma can be related to the abuse of alcohol. More details regarding the presentation and management of alcohol abuse can be found in Chapter 32.

Undernutrition

For a multitude of reasons, nearly one fifth of elderly patients presenting to emergency departments in the United States are undernourished. It is thought that depression, lack of money, lack of transportation for shopping, inability to manage cooking, and problems with chewing and swallowing all contribute to this important issue. Undernutrition can lead to immune compromise and resultant infections. Additionally, worsening of chronic medical conditions can be seen. If an EMT identifies any of these problems in an elderly patient, it would be appropriate to report such concerns to the receiving staff at the hospital so that appropriate referrals can be made to assist the patient with her nutritional needs.

CONCLUSION

The aging of our society makes it necessary for the EMT to become familiar with the normal changes associated with aging as well as the common illnesses encountered in this age group. The EMT's rapid recognition of the potential for serious illness or injury can lead to greatly improved outcomes for elderly patients.

TEST YOUR KNOWLEDGE

1. What are the neurologic changes characteristic of aging?
2. What are the cardiovascular changes characteristic of aging?
3. What are the respiratory changes characteristic of aging?
4. What are the gastrointestinal changes characteristic of aging?
5. What are the genitourinary changes characteristic of aging?
6. What are the musculoskeletal changes characteristic of aging?
7. What are the integumentary changes characteristic of aging?
8. Describe the problems that can occur with polypharmacy.
9. Define the term *dementia*.

INTERNET RESOURCES

For more information related to issues common to the geriatric population, visit these Web sites:

- AARP, http://www.aarp.org
- American Geriatrics Society, http://www.americangeriatrics.org
- *Geriatric Times Magazine*, http://www.geriatrictimes.com

FURTHER STUDY

Andresen, G. (1998). As America ages: Assessing the older patient. *RN, 61*(3), 46–56.

Andresen, G. (1998). Dx dementia. *RN, 61*(6), 26–30.

Ball, R. (1997). Geriatric assessment: The patient over 65. *Journal of Emergency Medical Services, 22*(3), 96–100.

Dickinson, E. T., Verdile, V. P., Kostyun, C. T., et al. (1996, February). Geriatric use of EMS. *Annals of Emergency Medicine, 27*(2), 199–203.

Keller, V., & Baker, L. (2000). Communicate with care. *RN, 63*(1), 32–33.

Morris, M. R. (1998). Elder abuse: What the law requires. *RN, 61*(8), 52–53.

Nixon, R. G. (2003, February). Geriatrics and their meds: Problems and perils. *Emergency Medicine Service, 32*(2), 35–38, 40–42.

Sanders, A. B. (1996). *Emergency care of the elder person.* St. Louis, MO: Beverly Cracom Publications.

Werfel, P. (1998). Geriatric assessment and specialized pathology. *Journal of Emergency Medical Services, 23*(11), 63–71.

EMS in Action

(continued from page 849)

Since I was new and needed the practice, I completed ongoing assessments on my patients every 5 minutes regardless of their condition. A few miles into the transport I noticed that my patient was taking a downturn. Her respirations took more and more effort, she was losing color, and her mental status was definitely decreasing. My heart started pounding and I replayed my training over in my head. She was already in the Fowler's position. There were no kinks in the oxygen tubing. What was I supposed to do? My patient had a do not resuscitate order and, as my partner pulled into the hospital parking lot, I sat back trembling and thought that I was about to watch a patient die for the first time.

I then noticed the onboard oxygen regulator needle sitting impotently on 0 lpm. I knew our main oxygen tank was full; I had checked the gauge myself at the start of the shift! I cranked the valve one way and then the other. Nothing. I ripped the tubing off the tree and reattached it to the portable tank, setting it to 15 lpm. The oxygen was flowing again and by the time we got the patient through the ER doors, she had stabilized again.

After sheepishly explaining to the ER doctor that I had almost killed the patient by not checking the basics, I returned solemnly to the ambulance to try and figure out what had gone wrong. The main oxygen tank was still full, but the main valve was closed. The previous crew had shut off everything at the end of their shift. When I attached the non-rebreather mask and opened the regulator, it had bled the line. There had been enough oxygen for me to see the needle go to 15 lpm and that was it. Although having a crew shut off the main valve to the onboard oxygen tank is uncommon, I now always check it at the beginning of each shift. Sometimes twice.

Brian Bricker, NREMT
EMS Instructor
Bricker Professional Education, Inc.
Norman, Oklahoma

CHAPTER 42

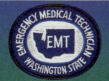

Advance Directives

KEY TERMS

advance directive

do not resuscitate order
(DNR)

health care proxy

hospice

living wills

out-of-hospital DNR

Patient Self-Determination
Act

power of attorney (POA)

standard comfort measures

terminal

OBJECTIVES

Upon completion of this chapter, the reader should be able to:

1. Describe an advance directive.
2. Differentiate the different types of advance directives.
3. Explain how the Patient Self-Determination Act affected EMS.
4. Distinguish comfort measures from resuscitation.
5. Discuss treatment decisions in the field when:
   a. A patient does not have an advance directive
   b. The patient's advance directive is insufficient per local protocols

OVERVIEW

Advances in medicine have created opportunities for people to live longer and more productive lives. Advances in medicine have also made it possible to delay the inevitable, death. As medicine and society struggle with this life or death contradiction, patients have tried to assert their right to make the decisions about their own lives, to decide when they want to be allowed to die.

Those decisions, which before were made in the hospital, are increasingly being made by and for patients who are out of the hospital and in the community. Emergency medical services (EMS) is increasingly confronted with the issue. This chapter discusses the situation in which an emergency medical technician (EMT) is faced with an order to not start cardiopulmonary resuscitation (CPR) on a patient in cardiac arrest.

ADVANCE DIRECTIVES

When an EMT is confronted with a terminally ill patient, she may also be confronted with a potential role conflict. First, the EMT may see herself in the role of lifesaver—a person who would make a valiant effort to save another human's life regardless of how futile that effort may be. However, the EMT may also be faced with a patient who is asking her to not fulfill her role as a lifesaver. Instead, the patient may be asking the EMT to fulfill her role as a compassionate caregiver, a person who understands the patient's pain and suffering and would do nothing to prolong it. The patient may even ask the EMT *not* to start CPR if he should die.

This conflict is not unique to EMTs. Physicians and nurses—in fact, all health care professionals—have had to grapple with this life or death decision. Should they start CPR on a terminally ill patient when they suspect it may cause needless pain or, worse, is contrary to the patient's wishes?

Advances in medicine have made it possible to substantially prolong life. However, the question that always arises is, "at what cost to that person's quality of life?" Some patients have decided they do not want heroic efforts made to save their lives. They state that they have lived long enough and do not want to live life suffering. Other elderly patients are concerned that if they survive after resuscitation, they will become a burden on their families.

These patients have used a variety of methods to make their wishes known before they die and to prevent the interference of health care providers in what is seen as a natural act, the act of dying. Collectively these efforts to express patients' wishes before they become incapacitated are called **advance directives**.

This chapter does not attempt to answer the moral and ethical questions surrounding decisions regarding advance directives or to definitively answer the complex legal questions that surround the

✦ A Natural Death

"9-1-1, what is your emergency?" Taking a deep breath, the patient's daughter, Ruby, started to explain. "I think my father is dead. Could you please send someone over here to check on him?"

The patient, an elderly man lying in bed, is pulseless. The man's wife, Doreen, is standing next to him. She keeps asking that nothing be done and that he be left alone to "die in peace; that's what he would have wanted."

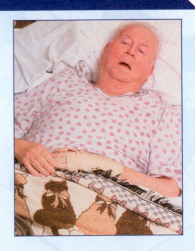

Ruby tells the EMT that her father was gasping for breath and she got scared, so she called 9-1-1. Her father has had a long history of Alzheimer's disease and heart failure, and the doctors have told Ruby that nothing more can be done for him.

Looking down at the elderly man, a man who had obviously fought his disease for a long time, the EMT notes that the patient looks oddly at peace.

- Is the EMT obligated to start CPR?
- Is there any order or directive that could have an impact in this case?
- Would medical control help in this situation?

issue. The intent of this chapter is to provide an EMT with a basic foundation for understanding advance directives and their impact on the practice of an EMT.

General Principles of Consent and Refusal

The foundation of every advance directive is the fundamental principle that every patient has a right to control his own body. Control means the patient must consent before a health care professional may begin any treatment. Logically, if the patient can consent, the patient can refuse treatment as well. It is an established fact in American jurisprudence that a patient may refuse treatment, even if the foreseeable outcome will be death.

What if the patient becomes unconscious and is unable to consent or refuse? The legal principle of implied consent assumes that the patient could have changed his mind at the last moment and wanted treatment. In other words, the dying patient might have wanted to be resuscitated but was unable to express his wish. Therefore, it is common practice to start resuscitation of the unconscious patient, based on the principle of implied consent.

Patients Impacted by Advance Directives

Advance directives are not restricted for use only by the elderly. Persons with profound disabilities may, for legitimate reasons, decide not to have extraordinary measures taken to prolong their lives, despite the fact that technology is available to prolong that life.

An EMT should never think that a person who is physically disabled has a decreased mental capacity. The two are not directly related. Similarly, patients with incurable diseases also may decide to stop or restrict treatment that they view as a futile delay of the inevitable.

Finally, the treatment of a disease that has afflicted a patient may reach the limits of modern technology. Medicine cannot offer these patients any more hope. These patients are at the end of their disease; in other words, their condition is **terminal**.

Types of Advance Directives

Many instruments, some that are legal documents and others that are medical orders, have been used to prevent someone from being resuscitated. The single unique characteristic of these advance directives is that they enable health care professionals to follow a patient's expressed wishes after his death.

Living Wills

Living wills may represent one of the oldest forms of advance directive. **Living wills** are documents that specifically address the wishes of the patient in regard to resuscitation. The instructions in a living will are meant to be followed by the patient's physician and other health care providers if the patient is unable to express these instructions for himself.

In most cases, living wills are created by the patient with the assistance of a lawyer, and without input from a physician. An example of

---

Pediatric Considerations

Discussions of consent and refusal assume that the patient has the legal capacity to consent, by virtue of age and competency, and to make decisions. In the case of children and others who are legally incompetent, it is the responsibility of the family, physician, and courts to make that determination. If a decision, an advance directive, is made in this fashion, it is legally binding on all health care providers who care for that patient.

a living will can be found in Figure 42-1. A patient's living will is witnessed by adults and signed by the patient in the same manner as other wills. However, a living will does not designate or rely on an agent to enforce it. (An agent is usually a family member or friend entrusted with making decisions on behalf of the patient.) Rather, a living will assumes that the physician or health care provider will

Declaration

Declaration made this _____ day of _____ (month, year).

I, _____, being of sound mind, willfully and voluntarily make known my desire that my dying shall not be artificially prolonged under the circumstances set forth below and do hereby declare:

If at any time I should either have a terminal and irreversible incurable injury, disease, or illness or be in continual profound comatose state with no reasonable chance of recovery, certified by two physicians who have personally examined me, one of whom shall be my attending physician, and the physicians have determined that my death will occur whether or not life-sustaining procedures are utilized and where the application of life-sustaining procedures would serve only to prolong artificially the dying process, I direct that such procedures be withheld or withdrawn and that I be permitted to die naturally with only the administration of medication or the performance of any medical procedure deemed necessary to provide me with comfort care.

In the absence of my ability to give directions regarding the use of such life-sustaining procedures, it is my intention that this declaration shall be honored by my family and physician(s) as the final expression of my legal right to refuse medical or surgical treatment and accept the consequences from such refusal.

I understand the full import of this declaration and I am emotionally and mentally competent to make this declaration.

Signed:_____

City, Parish, and State of Residence_____

The declarant has been personally known to me and I believe him or her to be of sound mind.

Witness:_____

Witness:_____

FIGURE 42-1   The living will was one of the first advance directives. (Courtesy of the Louisiana Hospital Association, Baton Rouge, LA.)

accept the living will as being the patient's last request and will abide by that decision.

Therefore, there is an implicit understanding within a living will that a physician will comply with the patient's final wishes. But a living will is not legally binding; and on occasion, especially during emergencies, the patient is treated by an emergency physician or other health care provider who is not the patient's primary or attending physician. This person may not know the circumstances surrounding the decision to create the living will and may not agree with the patient's decision. In addition, some physicians believe that a patient, who is not a physician, is not capable of making a wise medical decision alone and that, therefore, living wills should not be recognized as a matter of principle.

Durable Power of Attorney

A **power of attorney (POA)** allows a designated person to make decisions on behalf of another who is unable to make decisions. This decision-making authority is usually restricted to business or personal matters. Seldom is a durable power of attorney used to make medical decisions. Typically, a patient assumes that a physician will make the best decision on his behalf and that a POA is not necessary.

Ordinarily, a power of attorney expires when the patient expires. The unique quality of a durable power of attorney—health care (DPOA-HC) is that it outlasts the patient. A durable power of attorney allows a patient to designate an agent, frequently a spouse or offspring, to make life-and-death decisions for him in the event he cannot make those decisions himself. A sample durable power of attorney can be found in Figure 42-2.

Like a living will, a durable power of attorney is a legal document, and not a medical document. Because this document is prepared without advice or recommendations from a medical professional, some physicians prefer to make the decisions they consider to be best for the patient regardless of the presence of such a document. Occasionally, when a physician disagrees with the family and proceeds with treatments despite the family's protest, conflicts erupt between family members and physicians.

Do Not Resuscitate Orders

In some cases, the judgment of the physician attending the patient is that, in his medical opinion, any efforts at resuscitation will be futile. Such a physician can write a medical order to be followed by all health care providers to prevent further life-preserving therapies, up to and including CPR.

This medical order will state that if the patient's heart and/or breathing should stop, no attempt should be made to revive the patient. This order to not resuscitate a patient is called a **do not resuscitate order (DNR)** (Figure 42-3).

A DNR order is usually written after the physician has spoken to the patient and family and all have agreed that resuscitation will not be in the patient's best interests.

Part I. Durable Power of Attorney for Health Care

- If you do NOT wish to name an agent to make health care decisions for you, write your initials in the box | Initials

This form has been prepared to comply with the "Durable Power of Attorney for Health Care Act" of Missouri.

1. Selection of agent. I appoint:
Name:_____
Address:_____

> It is suggested that only one Agent be named. However, if more than one Agent is named, anyone may act individually unless you specify otherwise.

Telephone:_____
as my Agent.

2. Alternate Agents. Only an Agent named by me may act under this Durable Power of Attorney. If my Agent resigns or is not able or available to make health care decisions for me, or if an Agent named by me is divorced from me or is my spouse and legally separated from me, I appoint the person(s) named below (in the order named if more than one):

First Alternate Agent
Name:_____
Address:_____
_____
Telephone:_____

Second Alternate Agent
Name:_____
Address:_____
_____
Telephone:_____

> This is a Durable Power of Attorney, and the authority of my Agent shall not terminate if I become disabled or incapacitated.

Part I. Durable Power of Attorney for Health Care (Continued)

3. Effective date and durability. This Durable Power of Attorney is effective when two physicians decide and certify that I am incapacitated and unable to make and communicate a health care decision.

- If you want ONE physician, instead of TWO, to decide whether you are incapacitated, write your initials in the box to the right. | Initials

4. Agent's powers. I grant to my Agent full authority to:

A. Give consent to, prohibit, or withdraw any type of health care, medical care, treatment, or procedure, even if my death may result;

- If you wish to AUTHORIZE your Agent to direct a health care provider to withhold or withdraw artificially supplied nutrition and hydration (including tube feeding of food and water), write your initials in the box to the right. | Initials

- If you DO NOT WISH TO AUTHORIZE your Agent to direct a health care provider to withhold or withdraw artificially supplied nutrition and hydration (including tube feeding of food and water), write your initials in the box to the right. | Initials

B. Make all necessary arrangements for health care services on my behalf, and to hire and fire medical personnel responsible for my care;

C. Move me into or out of any health care facility (even if against medical advice) to obtain compliance with the decisions of my Agent; and

D. Take any other action necessary to do what I authorize here, including (but not limited to) granting any waiver or release from liability required by any health care provider, and taking any legal action at the expense of my estate to enforce this Durable Power of Attorney.

5. Agent's Financial Liability and Compensation. My Agent acting under this Durable Power of Attorney will incur no personal financial liability. My Agent shall not be entitled to compensation for services performed under this Durable Power of Attorney, but my Agent shall be entitled to reimbursement for all reasonable expenses incurred as a result of carrying out any provision hereof.

Part II. Health Care Directive

- If you DO NOT WISH to make a health care directive, write your initials in the box to the right, and go to Part III. | Initials

I make this HEALTH CARE DIRECTIVE ("Directive") to exercise my right to determine the course of my health care and to provide clear and convincing proof of my wishes and instructions about my treatment.

If I am persistently unconscious or there is no reasonable expectation of my recovery from a seriously incapacitating or terminal illness or condition, I direct that all of the life-prolonging procedures which I have initialed below be withheld or withdrawn.

I want the following life-prolonging procedures to be withheld or withdrawn:

- artificially supplied nutrition and hydration (including tube feeding of food and water) . . . . | Initials
- surgery or other invasive procedures. . . . . | Initials
- heart-lung resuscitation (CPR) . . . . | Initials
- antibiotic. . . . . | Initials
- dialysis. . . . . | Initials
- mechanical ventilator (respirator). . . . . | Initials
- chemotherapy. . . . . | Initials
- radiation therapy. . . . . | Initials
- all other "life-prolonging" medical or surgical procedures that are merely intended to keep me alive without reasonable hope of improving my condition or curing my illness or injury. . . . . | Initials

However, if my physician believes that any life-prolonging procedure may lead to significant recovery, I direct my physician to try the treatment for a reasonable period of time. If it does not improve my condition, I direct the treatment be withdrawn even if it shortens my life. I also direct that I be given medical treatment to relieve pain or to provide comfort, even if such treatment might shorten my life, suppress my appetite or my breathing, or be habit forming.

IF I HAVE NOT DESIGNATED AN AGENT IN THE DURABLE POWER OF ATTORNEY, THIS DOCUMENT IS MEANT TO BE IN FULL FORCE AND EFFECT AS MY HEALTH CARE DIRECTIVE.

Part III. General Provisions Included in the Directive and Durable Power of Attorney

YOU MUST SIGN THIS DOCUMENT IN THE PRESENCE OF TWO WITNESSES. IN WITNESS WHEREOF, I have executed this document this_____day of _____, year____.

_____
Signature
Print name _____
Address _____

The person who signed this document is of sound mind and voluntarily signed this document in our presence. Each of the undersigned witnesses is at least eighteen years of age.

Signature_____   Signature_____
Print name _____   Print name _____
Address _____   Address _____

> ONLY REQUIRED FOR PART I — DURABLE POWER OF ATTORNEY

STATE OF MISSOURI   )
) as
_____OF_____   )

On this_____day of_____, year_____, before me personally appeared to me known to be the person described in and who executed the foregoing instrument and acknowledged that he/she executed the same as his/her free act and deed.

IN WITNESS WHEREOF, I have hereunto set my hand and affixed my official seal in the County of _____, State of Missouri, the day and year first above written.

_____
Notary Public

My Commision Expires:_____

FIGURE 42-2 The durable power of attorney gives legal authority to someone to make health care decisions after death. (Reprinted with permission of the Missouri Bar.)

DNR DOCUMENTATION FORM 1
CONSENT FOR DNR ORDER BY ADULT PATIENT WITH CAPACITY

PATIENT IDENTIFICATION PLATE

The patient's consent to a DNR order must be obtained at or about the time the order is issued. The patient's consent may be either oral or written.

ORAL CONSENT must be given in the presence of a physician and another witness.

Physician's Statement
I have provided the patient with information about his or her diagnosis and prognosis, the reasonably foreseeable risks and benefits of CPR, the range of available resuscitation measures, and the consequences of a DNR order. The patient has expressed the decision to consent to a DNR order orally in my presence.

_____   _____
Physician Signature   Date

Witness's Statement
The patient has expressed the decision to consent to a DNR order orally in my presence.

_____   _____
Witness Signature   Date

_____
Print name

ALTERNATIVELY, WRITTEN CONSENT may be given and signed by the patient and two adult witnesses. If written consent is obtained, a copy must be placed in the chart.

After consent is obtained, the DNR order is to be issued by the attending physician and entered on the physician's order sheet.

If the attending physician objects to a DNR order, he or she must either:
— transfer the patient to another attending physician, or
— notify the medical director that dispute mediation is required

REMINDER: The DNR order must be reviewed by the attending physician at least **every three days** to determine if the order is still appropriate in light of the patient's condition. A notation must be made in the chart to reflect that review. It is **not** necessary to repeat the consent process when the order is reviewed.

FIGURE 42-3 A do not resuscitate order is a physician's order to not revive the dying patient.

The Patient Self-Determination Act

In 1991, the United States Congress sought to enact a body of law that would protect the rights of the patient as well as provide some direction to physicians on how to react to patient requests for advance directives. That law was the **Patient Self-Determination Act** of 1991.

The Patient Self-Determination Act is binding on any institution or organization that accepts Medicare or uses federal funding. It was specifically directed toward the population of patients that was already in health care institutions.

Health Care Proxy

The Patient Self-Determination Act also created a new entity, the **health care proxy**. The health care proxy is a person who is appointed by the patient to make decisions on behalf of the patient. The health care proxy is similar to a DPOA-HC, except that an attorney need not be involved in the process.

The health care proxy can make broad decisions, for instance, about resuscitation, for the patient. The health care proxy can also make specific decisions, for example, regarding tube feedings or machine ventilation. A sample health care proxy can be found in Figure 42-4. In some states, the decision of a health care proxy is not binding on an EMT in the out-of-hospital environment. The exception may be when an EMT is transferring a patient from one health care facility to another. The EMT should follow local protocols regarding health care proxies, DNR orders, and interfacility transfers.

Out-of-Hospital DNR Orders

In some circumstances, a patient who is not in a health care institution may wish to not be resuscitated. The patient may have been discharged for home care, for example, yet still desire the protection a health care proxy or a DNR order offers from unwanted intrusions into his private life by well-meaning EMTs. Physicians, as well as EMS authorities, have sought a way to provide such patients the same rights out of the hospital as they would have within the hospital.

The **out-of-hospital DNR** provides that means and is used in some states to give direction to EMTs faced with a dying patient. The out-of-hospital DNR is a binding medical order issued by the physician attending the patient that prevents the EMT from starting lifesaving measures such as CPR.

An out-of-hospital DNR should be written either on the physician's letterhead or on a preapproved DNR form (Figure 42-5). It should be clearly written, leaving no room for ambiguity. A statement such as "no heroics" can be meaningless. A statement like "no CPR or defibrillation" leaves little doubt about the patient's or the physician's wishes.

Frequently, a standard legal form is used that EMTs can quickly identify as a legitimate medical order. In some states, a specified state form must be used.

Problems with Out-of-Hospital DNRs

Problems have arisen in the field with out-of-hospital DNRs. In an emergency, family members may be confused and forget where the

Advance Directive

Part A

APPOINTMENT OF HEALTH CARE AGENT

(Optional Form)

(Cross through if you do not want to appoint a health care agent to make health care decisions for you. If you do want to appoint an agent, cross through any items in the form that you do not want to apply.)

1. I, _____, residing at
   _____
   _____ appoint the following individual as my agent to make health care decisions for me _____
   _____
   _____ (full name, address, and telephone number)
   Optional: If this agent is unavailable or is unable or unwilling to act as my agent, then I appoint the following person to act in this capacity _____
   _____
   _____ (full name, address, and telephone number)

2. My agent has full power and authority to make health care decisions for me, including the power to:
   a. Request, receive, and review any information, oral or written, regarding my physical or mental health, including, but not limited to, medical and hospital records, and consent to disclosure of this information;
   b. Employ and discharge my health care providers;
   c. Authorize my admission to or discharge from (including transfer to another facility) any hospital, hospice, nursing home, adult home, or other medical care facility; and
   d. Consent to the provision, withholding, or withdrawal of health care, including, in appropriate circumstances, life-sustaining procedures.

3. The authority of my agent is subject to the following provisions and limitations:
   _____
   _____
   _____
   _____
   _____

4. My agent's authority becomes operative (initial the option that applies):
   _____ When my attending physician and a second physician determine that I am incapable of making an informed decision regarding my health care;
   or
   _____ When this document is signed.

5. My agent is to make health care decisions for me based on the health care instructions I give in this document and on my wishes as otherwise known to my agent. If my wishes are unknown or

FIGURE 42-4 A health care proxy was created by the federal Patient Self-Determination Act of 1991.

unclear, my agent is to make health care decisions for me in accordance with my best interest, to be determined by my agent after considering the benefits, burdens, and risks that might result from a given treatment or course of treatment, or from the withholding or withdrawal of a treatment or course of treatment.

6. My agent shall not be liable for the costs of care based solely on this authorization.

By signing below, I indicate that I am emotionally and mentally competent to make this appointment of a health care agent and that I understand its purpose and effect.

_____   _____

   Date   Signature of Declarant

(Signature of Declarant) The declarant signed or acknowledged signing this appointment of a health care agent in my presence and based upon my personal observation appears to be a competent individual.

_____   _____

   Signature of Witness 1   Signature of Witness 2

FIGURE 42-4   (continued)

DNR is located. In some cases, family members may not be present to produce the document at the time the patient expires.

To help with this problem, some states are using DNR bracelets or necklaces. These bracelets minimally have imprinted on them the patient's name and the words "Do Not Resuscitate." EMTs should review the local medical protocols before accepting a DNR bracelet or necklace as a directive to be followed.

Resuscitation Decision Making

An out-of-hospital DNR is effective only if it is accepted by medical control and meets all the criteria that have been established by medical control. The medical directors in some communities have chosen not to allow an EMT to accept an out-of-hospital DNR. Although this decision may seem to eliminate the issue of out-of-hospital DNRs, in reality, the problem is often not that simple.

Family members may become very agitated if CPR is started and may feel that they have the right to decide the patient's treatment. The EMT should try to explain to the family that the EMT is under medical orders to start CPR. If the family becomes hostile, the EMT should either move the patient to the ambulance quickly or make a tactful retreat and call for law enforcement officers.

**State of New York
Department of Health**

**Nonhospital Order Not to Resuscitate
(DNR Order)**

Person's Name_____

Date of Birth ___/___/___

Do not resuscitate the person named above.

Physician's Signature _____

Print Name _____

License number _____

Date ___/___/___

It is the responsibility of the physician to determine, at least every 90 days, whether this order continues to be appropriate, and to indicate this by a note in the person's medical chart. The issuance of a
new form is **NOT** required, and under the law this order should be considered valid unless it is known
that it has been revoked. This order remains valid and must be followed, even if it has not been
reviewed within the 90 day period.

FIGURE 42-5 Some EMS systems use a special out-of-hospital DNR form.
(Reprinted with permission of the New York State Department of Health.)

If an out-of-hospital DNR is accepted by medical control, it must
meet a few basic conditions before an EMT can accept it as legitimate.
An out-of-hospital DNR should clearly state the name of the patient
and the limitations for his care. For example, the out-of-hospital DNR
may state that no external chest compressions may be done or that the
EMT may not assist ventilation. Some out-of-hospital DNRs are effective only for a specified period of time. State law may stipulate that an
out-of-hospital DNR is effective for only 30 or 60 days. The EMT must
know the local protocols regarding DNRs.

Some opponents of out-of-hospital DNRs argue that an EMT has to
be a "street lawyer" to be able to react correctly when confronted with
a pile of "legal papers" and a dying patient whose treatment decisions
are in question.

When in doubt and without further guidance, if an EMT is unsure
of how to proceed, the EMT should always err in favor of helping the
patient through the emergency. If EMS was called, it can be assumed
that an emergency existed and that the patient would have wanted
resuscitation under the principle of implied consent; therefore, routine patient care is in order. The EMT should then immediately contact medical control for further instructions on how to continue or
discontinue treatment.

STANDARD COMFORT MEASURES

Despite having a valid DNR order, a patient's family may decide to call EMS for a variety of other good reasons. The family may be unsure of how to react to the situation, such as the patient's choking, so they call EMS. Alternatively, the patient may be extremely uncomfortable, and the family may think that EMS can provide pain medication. For all these reasons and more, EMS is called to the home of a patient with a DNR.

A DNR means that an EMT should not start CPR on a pulseless patient. A DNR does not mean that the EMT should not provide care for the patient who is not in cardiac arrest. Supportive care designed to ease the patient's suffering is called **standard comfort measures**. Examples of standard comfort measures include suctioning the patient's airway clear of secretions and the administration of oxygen if the patient's breathing is labored.

Ventilating the nonbreathing patient, however, is not a standard comfort measure. It is a part of resuscitation. An EMT should consult with her medical director, before the call, about what procedures fall under standard comfort measures and what procedures are considered resuscitation.

Hospice

An EMT may encounter hospice staff while on the scene of a terminally ill patient. **Hospice** programs provide supportive care to dying patients and their families both in special hospice centers and at home. A hospice nurse may call EMS to help transfer a patient to a hospice center or for assistance with patient care in a crisis.

Hospice nurses provide care that is outlined in a predetermined set of medical orders. These medical orders may differ from those of an EMT. These differences may lead to conflicts on the scene. The EMT should meet with hospice staff in their community to discuss these differences beforehand in order to prevent conflict and ensure a seamless provision of care between patient care providers. If a hospice nurse is on scene and there is a question regarding treatment, the EMT should contact medical control for direction.

CONCLUSION

At first glance, advance directives can appear very confusing. EMTs have felt like they are in the unenviable position of having to make snap decisions about life and death. For this reason, it is important that an EMT know her local medical protocols regarding out-of-hospital DNRs. Moreover, whenever an EMT is in doubt, the EMT should contact medical control for advice and direction.

The core issue with an out-of-hospital advance directive often revolves around performing CPR or not performing CPR. In some cases, it may not be in the patient's best interest to have CPR performed. The EMT who does not perform CPR may, in appropriate circumstances, be providing the best care for the patient.

TEST YOUR KNOWLEDGE

1. What is an advance directive?
2. What are the types of advance directives?
3. What is a comfort measure as opposed to a resuscitation treatment?
4. What should an EMT do if a terminal patient does not have an advance directive?
5. What should an EMT do if the advance directive is incomplete?

INTERNET RESOURCES

Search the Web using the following key terms for additional information related to this chapter:

- Advance directives
- Living wills
- Do not resuscitate orders
- Health care proxy

FURTHER STUDY

Heckerson, E. (1997). Termination of field resuscitation. *Emergency Medical Services, 26*(8), 51–56.

EMS in Action

Just because it's a bright, sunny day, don't think that bad things cannot happen. On October 7, 2003, at 1445 hours, my station received a call to a westbound entrance gate for the Ohio Turnpike, which passes through my town. The initial call was for a rolled-over tractor-trailer that had struck the tollbooth and gate. Luckily, we thought, the State of Ohio had recently gone to unmanned tollbooths due to previous accidents at this location, so our main concern was for the driver of the truck and any hazardous items that may have been released from the crash. The initial response was my paramedic engine company with three personnel and a paramedic unit staffed by an EMT–Basic and two paramedics.

On arrival I sized-up the scene for hazards and saw a tractor-trailer flipped over on the driver's side halfway through the gate to the turnpike. As I dismounted my apparatus, I was stunned to see a small car smashed under the trailer. The car was now approximately 18 inches high and looked as though it had been in a car compactor such as those you would see in a junkyard. Even more disconcerting were the cries of a passenger in the car, "Get me out of here!"

The truck driver had apparently tried to avoid an accident by swerving into another lane of the toll gate. Excessive speed was a factor according to the Ohio Highway Patrol. As the driver swung the semi into another lane, he ran out of space entering the gate, and the truck rode up onto the concrete barrier between the lanes. Then the truck flopped over onto the car and its two passengers. The truck was fully loaded with frozen food.

Quickly, my crew and I formulated a plan for rescue. A medical helicopter from Metro-Health Medical Center in Cleveland was requested, since that hospital provides Level 1 trauma care to our area. I ordered a protective hose line to be pulled and on standby in case we needed to suppress any fires. We then set about cribbing and stabilizing the trailer so that it would not move or shift while we tried to remove the patients from the car.

While all of this was being done, one of the paramedics began assessing the passenger we had heard crying. She was talking and breathing OK. She stated that she was 40 years old and did not think she was bleeding anywhere, but her back and neck hurt from her being pushed down across the front seat. She was alert and knew what had happened and what was going on. This proved that her ABCs, as well as her level of consciousness, were intact. The passenger calmly stated that she knew that the driver of the car was deceased.

(*continues on page 911*)

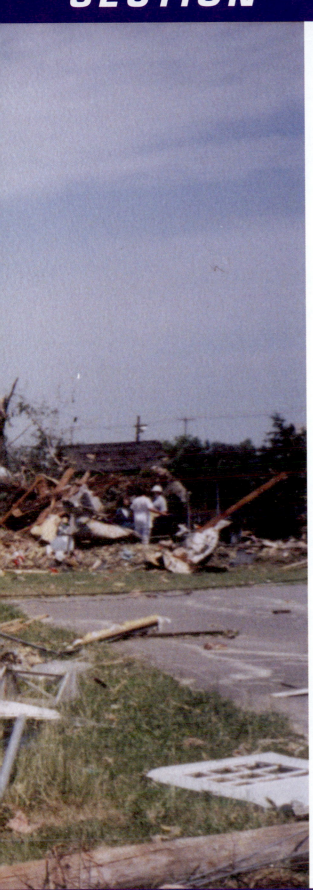

EMS Operations

One of the more exciting, and more stressful, times in an EMT's career is when he is faced with a special situation, such as a hazardous materials spill or multiple patients.

These emergencies can occur during times of natural disaster or during the calm of night. Whenever they do occur, the EMT must be prepared to respond to the emergency quickly and appropriately.

This section on EMS operations details the actions that an EMT should take at the scene of a special situation as well as how the EMT should respond to the everyday emergency.

CHAPTER 43

Emergency Vehicle Operations

KEY TERMS

approach path

controlled intersection

covering the brake

due regard

emergency ambulance

emergency ambulance
  service vehicle (EASV)

emergency services vehicle
  (ESV)

emergency vehicle operator
  (EVO)

Emergency Vehicle
  Operators Course
  (EVOC)

flashback

four-second rule

hot-load

landing zone (LZ)

LZ officer

panic stop

right-of-way

rotor wash

sharps container

shoreline

siren mode

spotter

surrounding area

(continues)

OBJECTIVES

Upon completion of this chapter, the reader should be able to:

1. Explain the importance of adequate preparation prior to an emergency call.
2. Describe personnel considerations in daily EMS operations.
3. Describe equipment considerations in daily EMS operations.
4. List the phases of an emergency call and the important considerations in each phase.
5. Explain the emergency vehicle operator's considerations during an emergency response.
6. Describe proper emergency vehicle positioning at the scene.
7. List the two general indications for air medical transport from an emergency scene.
8. Describe the factors that go into landing zone preparation.
9. Discuss the importance of safety when operating around a helicopter.
10. List activities that should be completed on the emergency crew's return to the station.

OVERVIEW

In addition to the vast amount of medical knowledge that the new emergency medical technician (EMT) will accumulate, he also must learn the basics of emergency medical services (EMS) operations. This chapter discusses vehicle and equipment readiness as well as emergency response and the transportation of the sick and injured to definitive care.

READINESS

The best way to do a job well is to be well prepared to do the job. The EMT will have a hard time caring for a patient who is ill or injured if his vehicle will not run, his equipment is defective, or needed medical supplies are missing. Before the alert is sounded and the pager tones go out, the EMT must check both his medical supplies and equipment completely, as well as ensure the readiness of his emergency vehicle for emergency operation.

Emergency Vehicle Classifications

Wherever someone gets hurt or is ill and calls for help, EMS must be able to respond to the scene, regardless of the location of the scene. EMS responds in a wide variety of environments, and frequently each environment requires a specialized vehicle. Table 43-1 lists just a few specialized vehicles used by EMTs to respond to the scene of a medical emergency.

Every call for EMS has two components: the emergency response phase that brings both medical personnel and equipment to the scene and the transportation phase in which the patient is taken to the emergency department. Police cruisers and fire apparatus are two examples of an **emergency services vehicle (ESV)** typically used to quickly

Shift Change

It is eight o'clock in the morning and shift change time at the 13th Street station. The oncoming EMTs put on the coffee and head for the equipment bay to begin their daily equipment check. Tru, the new EMT on crew, says, "I hear that these new turbo diesels can really fly!" To which her partner Barney replies, "We aren't going to test that theory today. The roads are wet from last night, and the temperature is supposed to stay around 30 degrees. Too much chance of icing up."

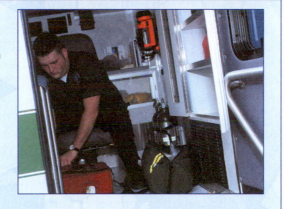

Tru looks a little dejected when Barney says, "Look, why don't you ride in the back today, and I'll drive." Picking up the vehicle checklist, Barney starts to perform a routine vehicle inspection while Tru inspects the equipment in the rear of the ambulance.

- What is necessary preparation for duty as an EMT?
- Why is it necessary to perform an equipment check at the beginning of every shift?
- Why is it necessary to perform a vehicle inspection at the beginning of every shift?

TABLE 43-1

EMS Vehicles

Condition	Vehicle
1. Snow and ice	Ice rescue platforms and sleds
	Snowmobiles
	Snow tractors
2. Off road	Dirt bikes
	Four-wheel all-terrain vehicles
	Four-wheel trucks
3. Water	Airboats
	Aluminum boats
	Deep submergence rescue vehicles
	Hovercraft
	Personal watercraft
4. Mass gatherings	Bicycles
	Buses
	Motorcycles
	Motorized carts
5. Remote wilderness	Fixed-wing aircraft
	Helicopters

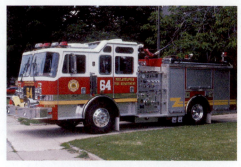

A.

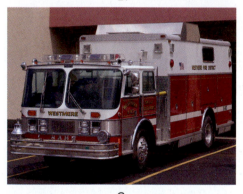

B.

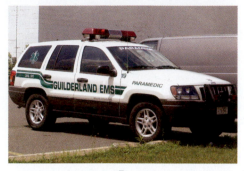

C.

FIGURE 43-1 Many types of vehicles are used for emergency response. (B. and C. are courtesy of David J. Reimer Sr.)

get equipment and trained personnel to the scene, but not capable of transporting the patient to definitive care. Figure 43-1 shows examples of these vehicles.

Emergency ambulances are designed for both emergency response and patient transportation. There are several different types of ambulances, each with its own distinctive features and advantages.

The van style type II ambulances are often preferred by urban EMS systems because they are easier to handle on narrow city streets. Modular type III ambulances are preferred by paramedic systems for the roominess of the patient compartment.

Many fire-based EMS systems prefer the truck style type I ambulances because of their additional compartment space and load-carrying capacity. Figure 43-2 shows examples of two types of ambulances commonly used in the United States.

Medical Supplies

To care for an ill or injured person, the EMT needs certain basic medical supplies and equipment. The specific medical equipment that is required onboard an ambulance is often regulated by state or local agencies. This equipment can be divided into equipment needed on scene and equipment that will be needed during transport.

Portable Medical Supplies

Once EMS has arrived on scene, the medical supplies must be carried to the patient's side. Typically, these medical supplies are carried in either durable hard plastic cases or flexible cloth bags. The supply kits are known by a variety of names—for example, jump kits, first-in bags, and first-aid boxes.

All of these portable medical kits must minimally contain the medical supplies needed for immediate lifesaving treatments. An **emergency ambulance service vehicle (EASV)** should minimally carry the equipment that is dictated by state or regional medical authorities. These legally mandated minimal stocking regulations exist to protect the public and often come with substantial penalties or fines for noncompliance. Table 43-2 shows a typical equipment list for a portable medical kit.

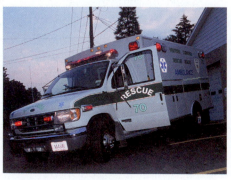

A.

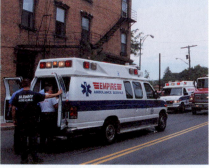

B.

FIGURE 43-2 Several types of ambulances are commonly used in the United States.

TABLE 43-2

Portable Medical Kit

Portable hand lantern
- ❑ Working bright
- ❑ Charging light on

Portable electric suction unit
- ❑ Operational >300 mm Hg
- ❑ Yankauer suction
- ❑ Suction tubing

Portable AED unit
- ❑ Automated external defibrillator
- ❑ Defibrillation pads
- ❑ Scissors
- ❑ Hand towel
- ❑ Spare battery

Medical supply bag

Center compartment

Airway/breathing equipment
- ❑ Hand-powered suction unit (backup)
- ❑ Oropharyngeal airways (variety)
- ❑ Nasopharyngeal airways (variety)
- ❑ K-Y Jelly packets
- ❑ Bag-valve-mask (BVM) with tubing

- ❑ BVM assembly
- ❑ BVM masks (variety)
- ❑ Non-rebreather mask
- ❑ Pediatric mask
- ❑ Nasal cannula
- ❑ Petroleum gauze
- ❑ Portable oxygen (minimum 500 psi)
- ❑ Pulse oximeter with probe (optional)

Infection control pocket
- ❑ Goggles
- ❑ Gloves in baggie
- ❑ Red bags—small
- ❑ Waterless hand cleaner

Vital signs equipment
- ❑ Stethoscope
- ❑ Scissors
- ❑ Blood pressure cuff—adult

Side compartment—front

Tape bag
- ❑ 1-inch tape
- ❑ 2-inch tape
- ❑ 3-inch tape

Bandages bag
- ❑ Military compress
- ❑ 2-inch roller bandage (two-headed)
- ❑ 3-inch roller bandage (one-headed)
- ❑ Triangular bandages/ cravats

Dressings bag
- ❑ 4 × 4 gauze
- ❑ 5 × 9 gauze
- ❑ Burn sheet (1)
- ❑ Trauma/universal dressing

Miscellaneous
- ❑ Ice pack
- ❑ Glucose
- ❑ Ring cutter
- ❑ Seat-belt cutter

Side compartment—back
- ❑ Cervical collar—no neck/XS
- ❑ Cervical collar—short
- ❑ Cervical collar—regular
- ❑ Cervical collar—tall
- ❑ Cervical collar—pediatric
- ❑ Cervical collar—universal

Emergency Ambulance Supplies

A well-stocked emergency ambulance is a minimal expectation of the public. Every EMT should know where each piece of equipment is in his ambulance. During an emergency, there is no time to refer to a checklist or search through compartments. Further guidance on minimal emergency ambulance supplies is provided by the American College of Emergency Physicians in its position paper titled "Guidelines for Ambulance Equipment."

All the supplies and equipment in an EASV should be securely fastened or stored within a compartment. In the event of a collision, unsecured equipment can become a projectile, injuring the patient or the crew. A simple seat-belt style restraining belt will secure a 10-pound automated external defibrillator (AED), for example, and prevent it from becoming a danger to the crew. Many newer ambulances have rolling or sliding doors that allow easy access to equipment within the compartment while preventing the equipment from shifting during a crash. Table 43-3 lists the general medical supplies that might be required to be onboard an ambulance.

TABLE 43-3

Onboard Patient Care Equipment

Action wall—interior
- ☐ Bag-valve-mask with tubing
- ☐ Suction onboard/test at 300 mm Hg
- ☐ Yankauer tip and tubing
- ☐ Goggles
- ☐ Oxygen regulator—wall
- ☐ Onboard oxygen—500 psi minimum
- ☐ Latex gloves—small/ medium/large/extra large
- ☐ Nonlatex gloves—small/ medium/large/extra large
- ☐ Penlight

Vital signs supplies
- ☐ Blood pressure cuff—adult
- ☐ Blood pressure cuff—large adult
- ☐ Blood pressure cuff—pediatric
- ☐ Stethoscope/bell and diaphragm
- ☐ Spare tips and diaphragm
- ☐ Trauma scissors

Airway supplies
- ☐ Suction tubing
- ☐ Suction canisters
- ☐ Yankauer tips
- ☐ Water for suction—500 cc
- ☐ Cups for sterile water
- ☐ Nasopharyngeal airways (2 each) size 30, 32, 36, French
- ☐ Oropharngeal airways (2 each) size 04, 06, 08
- ☐ Emesis basins

Breathing supplies
- ☐ Adult bag-valve-mask with tubing
- ☐ Facemask—small adult

- ☐ Facemask—adult
- ☐ Facemask—large adult
- ☐ Flow-restricted oxygen-powered ventilation device
- ☐ Pediatric bag-valve-mask
- ☐ Pediatric mask
- ☐ Spare oxygen regulator
- ☐ Spare oxygen rings/tips
- ☐ Non-rebreather masks
- ☐ Nasal cannula
- ☐ Pediatric oxygen masks
- ☐ Pediatric nasal cannula
- ☐ Oxygen humidifier

Circulation supplies

Sterile dressings
- ☐ 2 × 2 dressings
- ☐ 4 × 4 dressings
- ☐ 5 × 9 dressings
- ☐ Ace bandages

Clean bandages
- ☐ Gauze dressings
- ☐ Gauze roller 2-inch
- ☐ Gauze roller 4-inch
- ☐ Gauze roller 6-inch
- ☐ Kerlix roller 6-inch
- ☐ Tape 1-inch
- ☐ Tape 2-inch
- ☐ Tape 3-inch
- ☐ Military compress
- ☐ Binder bandage

Major wound dressing
- ☐ Trauma/universal dressing
- ☐ Aluminum foil—nonsterile
- ☐ Sterile water—1,000 cc
- ☐ Tape 4-inch

Burn care
- ☐ Sterile water for irrigation
- ☐ Sterile sheets
- ☐ Sterile facemasks
- ☐ Prefabricated wet dressings

Fracture management
- ☐ Trauma scissors
- ☐ Sports "shark" cutting tool
- ☐ Cravats
- ☐ Ice packs
- ☐ Tape 1-inch
- ☐ Tape 2-inch
- ☐ Tape 3-inch

Splints
- ☐ Prefabricated arm short splint
- ☐ Prefabricated leg short splint
- ☐ Prefabricated leg long splint
- ☐ Ladder splint
- ☐ Padded board splint—short
- ☐ Padded board splint—medium
- ☐ Padded board splint—long
- ☐ Unipolar traction splint
- ☐ Bipolar traction splint
- ☐ Pediatric traction splint

Hazardous materials supplies
- ☐ Nitrile gloves
- ☐ Nitrile booties
- ☐ Duct tape
- ☐ Tyvek one-piece suit
- ☐ Goggles
- ☐ Dust mask
- ☐ Disposable stethoscope
- ☐ Disposable blankets

(continues)

TABLE 43-3 (continued)

Childbirth supplies	☐ Nitrile gloves—small, medium, large	☐ Portable stretcher
☐ Sterile obstetrics (OB) kit	☐ Spill kits	☐ Extrication collars
☐ Silver swaddler		☐ Straps
☐ Sterile sheets	**Patient comfort supplies**	☐ Short backboard
☐ Sterile aprons—cloth	☐ Bedroll (blanket and sheet)	☐ Flexible spinal immobilization device
☐ Goggles	☐ Pillow	
☐ Large sealable bags for placenta	☐ Blanket	☐ Head immobilization device
	☐ Sheets	☐ Rescue basket
	☐ Pillowcases	☐ Webbing
Infection control supplies	☐ Towels	
☐ HEPA/N95 masks—small	☐ Face towels	**Advanced life support (ALS) supplies**
☐ HEPA/N95 masks—medium	☐ Bedpan—fracture	☐ Electrocardiogram (ECG) electrodes
☐ HEPA/N95 masks—large	☐ Toilet paper	
☐ Dust mist mask	☐ Urinal	☐ IV solution—1,000 cc saline solution
☐ Goggles	☐ Paper chux	
☐ Red bags—small		☐ IV solution—250 cc saline solution
☐ Clear garbage bags—small	**Patient carrying devices**	
☐ Red bags—extra large	☐ Long backboards	☐ Microdrip IV tubing
☐ Spray bottles (empty)	☐ Stairchair	☐ Macrodrip IV tubing
☐ Bleach (small bottle)	☐ Flexible stretcher	☐ Extension tubing
		☐ Pressure bag

Nonmedical Supplies

In addition to actual equipment used to care for patients and appropriate training in caring for patients, the EMT should have access to appropriate equipment that will allow him to safely get to the patient, care for her, and get her to an appropriate facility. Table 43-4 lists recommended rescue equipment to have on hand.

Safety Equipment

Proper preparation and familiarity with safety equipment are essential to prevent the EMT from becoming ill or getting injured (Figure 43-3).

Street Smart

For years EMS relied on the standard wooden backboard for spinal immobilization. Many of these backboards are still in service today. However, concerns about potentially infectious materials permeating the surface of these boards have forced many services to replace them with new plastic-type backboards.

If a wooden backboard is still in service, the EMT should ensure that the surface is intact, a waterproof finish covers the surface completely, and the ends are not splintered. Worn or damaged backboards cannot be easily decontaminated and should be replaced.

Safety Tip

With the increasing use of advanced life support personnel, many EASVs are equipped with a **sharps container**, an impervious container for disposing of needles and the like. An EMT should be very careful when replacing these sharps containers to prevent an accidental needle stick and subsequent blood-borne pathogen exposure. Emptying small sharps containers into large sharps containers is not a recommended practice. Overfilling of the sharps containers is a common cause of needle-stick incidents.

TABLE 43-4

Rescue Equipment for Ambulance

Incident management
- ❏ Triage tags with pencils
- ❏ EMS command vest
- ❏ Triage vest
- ❏ Staging vest
- ❏ Transportation vest
- ❏ Treatment vest
- ❏ Clipboards
- ❏ Multiple casualty incident (MCI) plan

Rapid vehicle rescue
- ❏ Step-blocks
- ❏ Cribbing
- ❏ Toolbox
  - ❏ Phillips screwdriver

- ❏ Standard screwdriver
- ❏ Mallet
- ❏ Claw hammer
- ❏ Hacksaw with blades
- ❏ Oil can
- ❏ Can of oil
- ❏ Bolt cutters
- ❏ Gloves—leather
- ❏ Goggles
- ❏ Vise grips
- ❏ Lineman's pliers
- ❏ Channel pliers
- ❏ Duct tape
- ❏ Orange surveyor's tape
- ❏ Window punch
- ❏ Razor

- ❏ Cold chisel
- ❏ Linoleum cutter
- ❏ Contact paper
- ❏ Tarp—blue
- ❏ Disposable blankets

Shore-based water/ice rescue
- ❏ Rope in a bag
- ❏ Personal flotation device (PFD)
- ❏ Whistles
- ❏ 200 feet of nylon rope
- ❏ Carabiners
- ❏ Loops of webbing
- ❏ Basket stretcher
- ❏ 30 feet of webbing

Personal protective equipment is discussed in detail in Chapter 6. Other safety equipment that may be necessary includes protective helmets, coats, and gloves. Additional equipment, such as fire extinguishers, flares, traffic cones, and reflective safety vests, is also useful and may be required by local or state regulation.

Maps

Regardless of how well an **emergency vehicle operator (EVO)** knows an area, it is always wise to have local maps readily available in the emergency ambulance service vehicle. Knowing the quickest way to get to a patient and to get the patient to a hospital is important. A quick look at a map before starting the response will confirm the appropriate route (Figure 43-4).

The term *ambulance driver*, as used in the past, failed to fully explain the role of an EMT or other designated individual who was part of the EMS team. The term *emergency vehicle operator* more fully encompasses the EMT's many responsibilities, which include driving the ambulance, helping to establish scene safety, assisting with the patient's packaging and transportation, and decontaminating the emergency vehicle. Furthermore, the term *ambulance driver* is based on the assumption that the EMT will always be operating an ambulance. The various vehicles listed in Table 43-1 demonstrate the large variety of emergency vehicles an EMT might be called on to operate.

Protocols/Procedures Manual

Most EMTs operate under a set of protocols. These protocols and any relevant standard operating procedures are often in writing. These

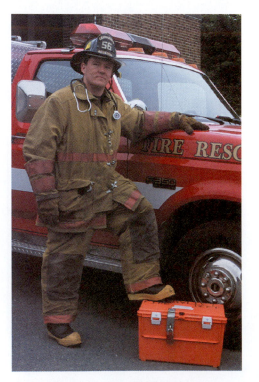

FIGURE 43-3   The EMT should use whatever safety equipment that is appropriate for the specific emergency situation.

documents should be in a place that is readily available to the EMT. For example, the recommended procedure for what to do if the ambulance is involved in an accident should be in the vehicle, where the EVO can reference it at the time it is needed. Treatment protocols can be referenced if needed while providing patient care.

Communications Devices

As discussed in Chapter 18, emergency personnel need to be in constant communication with their emergency communications center. Communication is usually done by radio. Most vehicles have a mobile radio mounted in them, and portable radios are often used by the providers outside the vehicle (Figure 43-5). The EMT should be familiar with the operation of all communications devices prior to responding to any emergency call.

Cellular or wireless telephones are often used by emergency personnel in place of or in addition to radios. If a portable telephone is to be used, the EMT should know where it is located, how it is charged, and how it is operated. Keeping a list of commonly needed telephone numbers with the telephone is useful.

DAILY PREPARATION

There are a number of things the EMT should make a part of his daily work routine. These routines help to ensure the EMT is prepared to provide EMS.

Personnel

The personnel expected to respond to emergency calls should not only be properly trained, but they should also be well rested, as well as physically and mentally prepared for an emergency operation. The work environment should be such that it allows for these qualities. Chapter 4 discusses this type of work environment in more detail.

Staffing for ambulances is often guided by local regulation. Usually at least one EMT is required to be in the patient compartment. Two trained providers are preferred, especially with high-priority patients who may need multiple interventions performed simultaneously.

Equipment Preparedness

At the start of his daily duties or at the beginning of his tour of duty, the EMT should carefully check all the equipment he may need to use during the shift. He should check to be sure that all the required items are where they belong and are functioning appropriately. Any equipment that requires an electrical charge should be tested to ensure that it is charged. Any battery-operated equipment should be tested to ensure a full charge on the batteries. Oxygen tanks should be tested and filled as needed.

Everything should be clean and in working order. If anything is not functioning properly, the EMT should take steps to fix the problem prior to his receiving an emergency call.

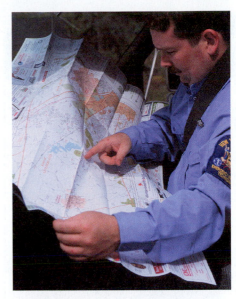

FIGURE 43-4 The EVO should take a few moments to confirm the location of the incident and the appropriate route to take.

✚ Safety Tip

The EVO of an emergency vehicle should always look at a map prior to starting to drive. He should never try to read a map as he drives the vehicle. Driving an emergency vehicle requires the undivided attention of the EVO. The person riding in the passenger seat can read the map book if needed.

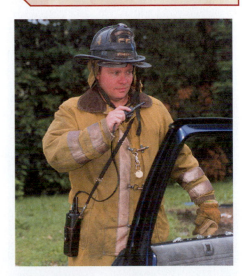

FIGURE 43-5 The EMT must be familiar with the use of different types of communication devices.

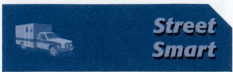

Every emergency ambulance service vehicle should have a backup communications system. This planned redundancy is critical to ensure that EMS will be ready and available in time of disaster. It is not unusual for downed trees to block microwave links or for radio towers to be struck by lightning, both of which can cause communication problems, especially if a service depends on cellular telephone technology. Past experience demonstrates that during times of natural disaster and public emergencies, a large number of cell-phone calls by concerned civilians can quickly tax and then overwhelm the available cellular system.

TABLE 43-5

Inspection of Emergency Ambulance Service Vehicle

Safety check

- ❑ Tires (soft or flat?)
- ❑ Leaks under vehicle
- ❑ Front radio mic
- ❑ Turn signals
- ❑ Reverse lights
- ❑ Headlights high/low
- ❑ Light bar front
- ❑ Light bar rear
- ❑ Red corner flashers
- ❑ Scene light left
- ❑ Scene light right
- ❑ Siren wail
- ❑ Compartment lights
- ❑ Portable radio

(continues)

Equipment Failure

Every EMS service should have a policy and a procedure for reporting defective equipment. Reporting defective equipment ensures that patient care will not be compromised while permitting corrective action to be taken by the service. The United States Food and Drug Administration (USFDA) may require an EMT to report any medical equipment failures under its mandatory medical device reporting regulations as well (Figure 43-6).

Vehicle Preparedness

The EVO should carefully check the EASV at the start of his shift and follow a mechanical checklist to ensure that the vehicle is sound and fully operational. Table 43-5 lists items that should be inspected in the EASV at the start of every shift. Properly checking the EASV at the start of a shift will uncover potentially dangerous mechanical problems. These issues should be properly dealt with prior to taking any emergency calls.

NEW YORK STATE DEPARTMENT OF HEALTH
Emergency Medical Service Program

Equipment Failure Report

S A M P L E   F O R M

Date Problem Reported: Month Day Year

Type of Failure
- ❑ Vehicle — Vehicle #   Mileage
- ❑ Vehicle's Radio — Vehicle #
- ❑ Portable Radio — I.D. #
- ❑ On-board Equipment — Type

Vehicle/Equipment Failure Discovered   (Check only one box in this section)
- ❑ While completing ambulance daily/shift inspection
- ❑ Enroute to a call or hospital
- ❑ On scene of a call
- ❑ Other (describe) _____

Was patient on board?   ❑ Yes   ❑ No

Time Crew Affected

Time failure discovered:	
Time failure reported:	
Time taken out of service:	
Time put back in service:	
Total out of service time:	

Did the crew go back into service with:
❑ Same equipment   ❑ Different equipment

Was anyone injured by the failure?   ❑ Yes   ❑ No

If yes, report all accidents to the supervisor.

Description of Problem: _____

Impression of Problem Cause: _____

DOH-2502 (11/88) p. 1 of 2

Reporting Crew Member's Signature

FIGURE 43-6 An EMT should report and fill out an equipment failure report as needed. (Reprinted with permission of New York State Department of Health.)

Mechanic's Report on Vehicle Failure/Supervisor's Report on Equipment Failure

Description of problem and/or part(s) found defective: _____

_____
_____
_____

Description of repairs/replacement solving problem: _____

_____
_____

☐ Internal repair   ☐ Outside vendor repair

Name _____ | Date repairs completed: / /

_____ Mechanic's Signature   _____ Ambulance Supervisor's Signature

Comments: _____
_____
_____
_____
_____

Once actions are completed on this report, it should be filed in either the individual vehicle's maintenance file, the communications equipment repairs file, or the equipment repair file.

DOH-2502 (11/88) p. 2 of 2

FIGURE 43-6 (continued)

RESPONSE

During a call, the EMT can think about several different phases of emergency operation. Each phase has specific considerations that must be acknowledged by every member of the crew.

Alarm and Alert

The crew must be notified of the call for EMS in some fashion. Usually the crew is notified by the communications center via radio, pager, or telephone. The communications specialist at the center is notified of the need for medical assistance either directly by the patient or through another dispatch center. Many systems provide communications specialists with special emergency medical dispatch (EMD) training so that they will know how to obtain critical patient information for responding EMS units.

Street Smart

Every EASV should be part of a preventive maintenance (PM) program. A PM helps to reduce the incidence of mechanical breakdown in the field and costly repairs, as well as prolongs the service life of the vehicle. The adage "an ounce of prevention is worth a pound of cure" is true as it relates to the EASV.

En Route

As the emergency call is dispatched, Marc checks the wall map to be sure he is thinking of the most appropriate route to the scene. Nigel unplugs the ambulance, opens the bay door, and starts to climb into the driver's seat. "Not yet, Nigel, you can drive after the course. Until then, it's still me," barks Marc. "Back into your seat!"

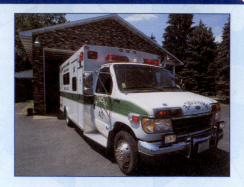

With seat belt fastened, Nigel picks up the radio and advises the communications center that "Rescue 2 is en route." The center responds, "A rollover with possible entrapment." Nigel asks, "What do you think we'll find when we get there, Marc?"

- What are the responsibilities of each crew member prior to and during an emergency response?
- What are some of the EVO's considerations during an emergency response and on arrival at the scene?
- What do your local traffic laws require of emergency vehicles during an emergency response?

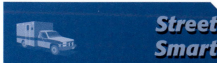

Street Smart

Although it goes without saying that the EVO should not be intoxicated on alcohol or illicit drugs when driving, other substances also can impair the EVO's condition. Many prescription and over-the-counter medications can lead to drowsiness and slowed reactions. Nasal decongestants and cough remedies contain substances that can dull the EVO's senses. The label of any medication should be read carefully for such warnings. If a medication is necessary, the EVO should consider requesting reassignment rather than put the crew and the patient or himself at risk.

Initial Information

Initially, the communications specialist provides the EMT with the information necessary to find the patient and to consider what equipment he will be likely to need to care for the patient. This information should include the nature of the call, the location of the patient, the presence of more than one patient, and any special problems such as limited access. Additionally, the communications specialist should have the name, location, and telephone number of the caller so that if any further information is needed, the caller can be called back.

Departure

Once the nature and location of the call have been given, the EVO should look up the location of the incident on a map and decide on the most appropriate route to take. Also, the EVO should ensure that any **shorelines**, electrical power sources from the building to the ambulance, have been removed and that the crew members are wearing safety belts. Only after these things have been done should the vehicle be put into drive gear.

Driving

Many times the priority of a response, based on preapproved guidelines, is assigned by the communications specialist. A high-priority call, sometimes called a priority one response or a Delta response, is likely to require a response with red lights and sirens being used. Lower-priority calls should be responded to at normal speed while observing usual vehicle and traffic laws.

Emergency Vehicle Operator

Although anybody with a driver's license can drive an ambulance in most states in the United States, possession of a driver's license should not be the minimum standard. The person who is entrusted with the lives of the patient and the crew should be appropriately trained to drive an emergency vehicle. Many states mandate that the EVO attend an approved **Emergency Vehicle Operators Course (EVOC)**.

The EVO should be physically and mentally prepared for emergency responses. He should be capable of performing calmly under stress. Tolerance of other motorists and a positive attitude about his abilities as an EVO are essential. There is no place for *road rage* behind the wheel of an emergency vehicle.

The EVO also should be given time to become familiar with the characteristics of the vehicle he is to be driving. He should not drive an emergency vehicle for the first time with lights and siren on in bad weather conditions to respond to an emergency. The EVO should drive the emergency vehicle under normal operating conditions and on dry roads on several occasions before driving it to an emergency.

Driving Safety

Safe driving is an essential part of every emergency response. With the amount of time the EMT will spend in a moving vehicle during the course of his job, he cannot afford to practice unsafe driving habits. Safe habits that begin early in an EMT's career will serve him well throughout his career.

The EVO should always adjust the driver's seat as well as the mirrors when he enters the vehicle. The mirrors are particularly important in an ambulance. The interior driver's mirror is useful for observing the patient's compartment. With one less mirror, the EVO is dependent on the two outside mirrors. The EVO should be aware that the passenger-side mirror, the one the EVO must depend on as he makes his way through stopped traffic, often has a very limited view.

The EVO must be properly restrained in the vehicle with a seat belt while the vehicle is in motion. The use of seat belts protects vehicle occupants from serious injury in many motor vehicle crashes. Since 1987, the National Fire Protection Association (NFPA) has advocated the use of seat belts for all fire department vehicles, including fire department ambulances. The EVO also must remain attentive to all his surroundings. He should maintain a safe following distance and avoid situations that could result in his vehicle being blocked in.

Warning Devices

Bells, whistles, lights, and sirens do not give the EVO the **right-of-way** on the road. The right-of-way, a legal right for passage ahead of someone else, must be given by other drivers on the road. Even when the right-of-way is given to the EVO, he must exercise **due regard** for other drivers on the road, practicing good judgment and not endangering other motorists needlessly.

Failure to exercise due regard for other motorists may result in collisions, injuries, and legal complications, including criminal charges. While the Good Samaritan law can provide the EMT with some protection while the EMT is rendering medical care, the EVO does not have any similar protection and must accept full responsibility for his actions.

To improve safety and to alert other drivers, elaborate markings, flashing lights, and sirens have been created. None of these improvements, however, can replace good judgment when the EVO is driving.

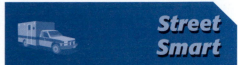

Street Smart

The EMT and the EVO should make a regular practice of wearing seat belts regardless of whether they are responding to an emergency or just driving to the store. All of the occupants in an ambulance are highly visible to the public, and the public notices whether the EMT and the EVO are wearing their seat belts. An EMT, as a health care professional, should set the example and wear his seat belt whenever he is in "mobile service."

Safety Tip

The vehicle's headlights should be on whenever the vehicle is in motion. Studies have shown that even during daylight hours, the use of headlights can reduce the chances of a collision by more than 15%. The headlights permit other drivers to recognize the ambulance sooner as another vehicle in motion.

Markings Almost 30 years ago, the U.S. federal government attempted to standardize ambulance markings for a number of reasons. One reason was that if ambulances were similar in appearance, the public could more readily identify them on the road. Subsequently, the federal government advanced what has become the standard for ambulance construction, the Federal Specification for the Star-of-Life Ambulance (KKK-A-1822E). The original federal specifications called for all ambulances to be white and to have a broad Omaha Orange stripe around the entire ambulance.

White is believed to be the most visible color to other motorists. However, the EVO should be aware that white blends in more easily with snow, fog, smoke, and haze. Therefore, the EVO must be more vigilant of other drivers in such conditions.

Many EMS systems initially adopted the standard orange stripe but eventually abandoned it in favor of more distinctive coloring. This decision involves no potential harm in view of the fact that the National Research Council has reported that there was no special research to support the choice of Omaha Orange.

Most ambulances also display the word *ambulance* and the blue star of life prominently on all sides of the ambulance. To enhance recognition of the ambulance in the rearview mirror, the word *ambulance* is spelled backward and in capital letters, ƎƆИA⅃U8MA, on the hood of the ambulance.

Many ambulances have a highly reflective tape placed around the entire vehicle to enhance visibility at night. The EVO should remember that this reflective tape is visible only when light strikes it directly. Therefore, reflective tape does not add any special protection when the ambulance crosses an intersection at an angle to the headlights of other vehicles.

Emergency Warning Lights There is no standardization of the color of emergency warning lights across the United States. Many states have chosen red lights, the original emergency color recognized by a majority of the public as meaning emergency. Others have chosen blue lights, believing that blue light is more visible, particularly at night when the danger to emergency workers is greatest. Finally, other states and EMS systems have put white light into the combination of emergency warning lights that are displayed.

Studies have shown that white light is highly visible during both day and night operations. Many emergency service providers have equipped emergency ambulance service vehicles with alternating headlights, also referred to as **wig-wags**.

Recently, the Federal Specification for the Star-of-Life Ambulance added one yellow light, midship and rear facing. Research has shown that a yellow light can be seen for a great distance. Yellow is now identified as the standard "warning" color; it warns motorists of an impending danger ahead. To prevent or reduce the number of rear-end mishaps at motor vehicle collisions, a blinking yellow light has been added.

Three types of emergency lights, sealed beam, LED, and strobe, are used on emergency vehicles. Each type has its advantages. The long, steady flash of a sealed beam allows drivers visual reaction time to identify the light and determine its location. The bright flash of the strobe allows the light to be seen for great distances but has the drawback of **flashback** during snow or rainstorms. Flashback occurs when the bright light of a strobe bounces off the rain or snow and back into the EVO's eyes. The newest emergency warning lights are light-emitting diodes (LED). The LED, a small semiconductor device that emits light when charged with electricity, does not tend to fail when hit, and it is visible over greater distances than standard emergency lighting. As an added bonus the LED has a greater useful life, 100 times greater, than an incandescent bulb and uses 80–90% less energy than an incandescent bulb. LED studies performed at the Lighting Research Center of the Rensselaer Polytechnic Institute, New York, have demonstrated the utility of LED in many applications, including emergency vehicle lighting. Current experience with LED emergency lights for emergency vehicles suggests that, in the future, the LED may be the primary emergency light system.

Light Patterns   The number of light pattern configurations rivals the number of light combinations. However, there are a few constants in every light pattern. At least one forward-facing flashing light is placed in the grill of the ambulance. This light permits drivers who are immediately in front of an ambulance and unable to see the lights on the roof to recognize that an emergency vehicle is behind them.

When on the scene of a road call at night, the emergency ambulance needs to have its outline illuminated so that other drivers can discern its location in the dark. This is usually accomplished by placing a flashing light in each corner of the roof.

Finally, most emergency ambulances have additional scene lights affixed to the ambulance compartment. Some of these scene lights help to illuminate the scene, and the rear-facing scene lights illuminate the crew as they load the patient into the ambulance.

Emergency warning lights have long been recognized as important to the on-scene safety of emergency personnel. Yet despite the ever-increasing variety and patterns of emergency warning lights on emergency vehicles, a number of firefighters, law enforcement officers, and emergency medical technicians are killed every year while on American highways by other motorists. Twenty-five percent of all firefighter fatalities are the result of crashes with other vehicles while either responding to or returning from an emergency.

In an effort to reduce the number of emergency vehicle-related fatalities in the United States, the United States Fire Academy (USFA), together with the United States Department of Transportation (USDOT) and the Society of Automotive Engineers (SAE) have established the Fire Service Emergency Vehicle Safety Initiative. Part of that initiative is to study the effect and effectiveness of emergency lights, including incandescent lights, strobe lights, LED lights, light patterns, and light colors. The results of these studies will be forwarded to the NFPA, a national fire consensus group whose recommendations are widely accepted by the fire and EMS communities.

Audible Warning Devices   The earliest emergency vehicles used a bell that rang loudly to announce the vehicle's presence and provide

Street Smart

The use of lights and sirens on a limited-access highway is highly questionable. The time saved by going over the posted speed limit is often insignificant and not worthwhile when compared to the risks of high-speed driving. Some states and highway authorities forbid the use of lights and sirens by emergency vehicles on superhighways.

a warning of danger. Modern electronic sirens are a far cry from the distant ancestor, yet they accomplish essentially the same task. Most emergency ambulances in the United States have two basic **siren modes**. These siren modes are characteristic patterns of sound designed to alert other motorists.

The first siren mode is the **wail**. The wail is a long unwinding of the sound after it reaches a peak. This monotonous up-and-down sound travels well over long distances and is almost universally perceived by drivers as an emergency alert. The other sound, called a **yelp**, is a short staccato sound that almost chirps at other motorists. The yelp is more effective than the wail within shorter distances and around obstacles.

Some newer electronic sirens have other tone patterns besides the traditional wail siren and the yelp siren. One of those new sirens, the hi-lo siren, is frequently added to the collection of sirens. The hi-lo is the primary siren sound for emergency vehicles in Europe and has been gaining in popularity in the United States. The hi-lo takes advantage of a wider spectrum of sound across the audible frequencies. It is a sound that more readily overcomes environmental noises, has better penetration of enclosed vehicles, and has a rapid cycling time. Better penetration allows more rapid identification of the sound—alerting—and the rapid cycling of the siren allows drivers to better locate the source of the sound, a result of comparing the tonality of two sounds and establishing their location and movement, called Doppler shift.

However, there is some controversy about the hi-lo siren. The more traditional siren mode, the wail, created by the Q mechanical siren, a trademark of the Federal Signal Company, has been in existence for 50 years, and American drivers have been conditioned to associate that sound with an emergency vehicle. Some EMS authorities believe that the unfamiliar hi-lo siren would not alert drivers to the presence of an emergency vehicle as quickly as the traditional wail siren sound.

There are times when this difference may be used to an advantage for the EVO. If one emergency vehicle unavoidably must follow another emergency vehicle, from a safe distance, the presence of another siren sound, hi-lo, for example, may alert motorists that once one emergency vehicle has passed, another emergency vehicle is approaching.

In the past, sirens were mounted on the roof with the lights, which meant that the driver had to listen to this almost deafening noise for prolonged periods. Today, almost all sirens are mounted ahead of the driver in the grill, where the sound is less deafening.

Although technology has improved sirens, it has not improved their effectiveness. Soundproofing built into new cars can reduce outside noise interference, including sirens, by as much as 40%. The volume of high-powered car radios and speakers also can mask outside sounds. These factors, combined with the fact that there are more hearing-impaired drivers on the road today, create a dangerous driving environment for the EVO.

Drivers who do not hear and recognize the siren until the last moment may react suddenly and unpredictably when they finally hear the siren. The EVO must drive defensively to avoid collisions with these drivers. Methods of defensive driving are discussed later in this chapter.

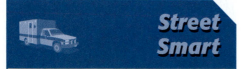

Street Smart

New ambulances also are sound-proofed, thereby preventing the EVO from hearing other emergency vehicles as well. Therefore, it is a good driving practice to operate the ambulance with the driver's-side window rolled down a few inches, regardless of the weather. This affords the EVO a better opportunity to hear other emergency vehicles and to respond appropriately. It also helps to prevent driver fatigue due to carbon monoxide poisoning as a result of a rusted or faulty exhaust system.

Some emergency ambulances come with either mechanical or electronic airhorns. While these devices can be very effective for alerting motorists ahead of the impending arrival of an emergency ambulance into an intersection, the sound can be very irritating as well. The EVO should never use the airhorn to "punish" another motorist for failing to bear right and give up the right-of-way.

Most siren systems also contain a public address (PA) system. This system is very useful in times of disaster when public notification of evacuation, for example, is needed. The PA system is seldom used when the ambulance is in emergency response mode. However, when an emergency ambulance is entrapped by other vehicles in a gridlock, the EVO can use the PA system to give directions to the other drivers. This is effective only if the other drivers understand. Therefore, the EVO should very slowly and clearly describe any vehicle about which he is giving directions, for example, "The gray car with Florida license plates, please move to the shoulder of the road." The EVO should not be surprised if drivers do not immediately react. The PA system is seldom used, and drivers are often confused about the "voice" they hear.

Priority Response

Red lights and sirens should be used with caution, if used at all. In the past, most emergency vehicles routinely used red lights and sirens as warning devices for every response and for every patient transport to the hospital. This is no longer the case.

The use of red lights and sirens tremendously increases the risk of collision and subsequent personal injury. The EVO and the EMT must always question the use of red lights and sirens before proceeding on an EMS call. Advances in the field of prehospital medical treatment as well as the widespread use of emergency medical dispatch have made these red lights and siren responses unnecessary in many cases.

Furthermore, in many jurisdictions there is no immunity from liability for driving with red lights and sirens. The burden of the safe operation of the emergency vehicle lies with the EVO. In fact, the largest percentage of lawsuits against EMTs are directly related to the operation of the emergency vehicle.

Laws and Regulations Every state has laws and regulations governing the use of emergency warning devices and the operation of emergency vehicles. The EVO should be familiar with local laws and regulations related to each of the issues listed in Table 43-6.

Driving Conditions

Every EVO should adjust his driving to the conditions of the road. Any changes in weather or road conditions should be noted and dealt with appropriately.

Adverse Weather Driving in poor road conditions is a way of life for the EVO and EMT. When others will not drive, the EMT and all other emergency services providers have no choice. When an emergency arises, EMS must make a reasonable effort to respond regardless of the conditions. However, the EVO and the EMT can maximize the chance of success by thinking ahead and being proactive instead of reactive to the driving conditions.

Street Smart

The mere sound of a siren causes our adrenaline to rise, and we become anxious. This response may not be beneficial to a patient, particularly a cardiac patient. Many EMS systems transport their conscious chest pain patients without lights or siren. If the siren is used, the EVO should first alert the patient and the patient's family that he is going to be using it. This warning can help to reduce the anxiety that the siren creates.

TABLE 43-6

Motor Vehicle Laws Pertaining to Ambulance Operation

Vehicle parking or standing

Procedures at red lights, stop signs, and intersections

Regulations regarding speed limits

Direction of flow or specified turns

Emergency or disaster routes

Use of audible warning devices

Use of visual warning devices

School buses

When an ambulance stops for a flashing red light of a school bus, the EVO should wait for the school bus to turn off the flashing lights prior to attempting to pass it. This will decrease the chance of misunderstood hand signals and minimize the chance of inadvertently striking a child.

When approaching an intersection, most EVOs switch from the wail siren mode to the yelp siren mode. However, some less-experienced EVOs rapidly switch between different siren modes, assuming that this makes the emergency vehicle more noticeable. This assumption demonstrates a fundamental misunderstanding of siren operation.

For a siren to be effective, the listener/driver must first hear it, identify from which direction the sound is coming, and visually confirm the source—in this case, an ambulance. Rapidly changing sounds do not permit the listener/driver to identify the direction of the sound and only serve to confuse and frustrate the listener/driver. Changing the siren mode at about 100 feet from the intersection and then leaving it in one single mode for at least 60 seconds is the most effective method.

For example, when heavy snowfall and drifting conditions make roads almost impassable, the assistance of a county snowplow, to lead the way, can be invaluable. Similarly, the EMT should monitor both highway department radio traffic as well as National Weather Service reports for information about flash floods and road closings.

If compelled to drive in these conditions, the EVO must exercise extreme caution. For example, the speed should be reduced, and the vehicle should be driven in a lower gear if needed. Asking communications to recontact the residence and advise the patient of the delay is helpful, since the EVO and EMT are less inclined to take risky actions if the patient knows they are being delayed by the weather.

Heavy Traffic   Heavy traffic is a fact of life for many EMTs operating in suburban and urban systems. Drivers on the way to or from work may not be willing to grant the emergency ambulance the right-of-way. Other drivers may attempt dangerous maneuvers like the squeeze play. The squeeze play occurs when a driver on the right of the ambulance tries to move in front of the ambulance, around another car, and then back into the traffic. This maneuver can result in a rear-end collision for the ambulance.

The EVO should avoid weaving in and out of traffic in order to make progress. Instead, the ambulance should remain in the outside passing lane and wait for the traffic to yield the right-of-way.

Whenever the EVO is negotiating the ambulance through heavy traffic, he should consider **covering the brake**. By putting one foot over but not on the brake, the driver effectively cuts down his reaction time for emergency braking and may prevent a collision.

Controlled Intersections   **Controlled intersections**, intersections with traffic signal devices, are the most common place for a crash involving an emergency vehicle. Other motorists may not hear or see the approach of the emergency vehicle in time to stop. Extreme care must always be used when passing through intersections. When going against the red traffic light, the emergency vehicle should come

Inexperienced EVOs and EMTs think that using the lights and siren during bad weather will improve their response times. Research, however, has shown that EVOs drive the ambulance 15 miles per hour faster when the lights and siren are used than when they are driving without lights and siren. This increased speed may be inadvisable during poor weather and even poorer driving conditions. It is often better to arrive safely a few minutes later than not to arrive at all.

to a near-complete stop (Figure 43-7). The EVO should try to make eye contact with each of the drivers in the other vehicles before proceeding through the intersection cautiously.

Many driving authorities advocate that the driver look right, then left, and then right again before proceeding. This routine encourages the EVO to always scan the intersection for dangerous situations.

When multiple emergency vehicles are traveling the same route, the EVOs must use extreme care. The presence of more than one emergency vehicle can be confusing to motorists and is extremely dangerous. Once one emergency vehicle passes, the motorist may not realize that another is coming and might not appropriately yield to it.

Because of the associated danger, multiple emergency vehicles that must travel the same route should maintain a wide following distance and should be extremely attentive to surrounding traffic. Multiple vehicles on the same route, however, should be avoided when at all possible.

Braking   The EVO should always consider the impact that braking will have on the patient. If the patient has a broken leg, for example, a sudden unexpected stop can violently force the bone ends together, causing more injury and significant pain. Therefore, the EVO should anticipate stops and start to slow as he approaches the stopping place. For example, when the EVO sees a prolonged or stale green light, he can anticipate that it will change to a red light in just a moment.

The first action in slowing an ambulance is to take the right foot off the accelerator. This allows the engine to slow the vehicle. Then the EVO should gently start to depress the brake pedal. A quick jab at the brake pedal will cause the ambulance to lurch forward and potentially cause more injury to the patient.

To avoid **panic stops**—fast, unexpected braking—the EVO should maintain a safe traveling distance that allows the EVO time to react if the situation should suddenly change. The **four-second rule** is often recommended by expert drivers and Emergency Vehicle Operators Course instructors. To follow the four-second rule, the EVO need only pick an object, like a sign on the side of the road, and count the time between when the vehicle in front of him passes it and when he passes it. The total elapsed time should be greater than 4 seconds.

Often new EVOs have a difficult time estimating the distance that it will take to stop the ambulance. Part of the reason is because their normal driving and braking experience is with a standard automobile. The emergency ambulance is actually as heavy as a light truck (about 10,000 pounds) and, thus, takes more time to stop and covers more distance in the interim. Table 43-7 shows the braking distance of a light truck at various speeds. Note that as the speed increases, the braking distance increases at a much greater rate.

In the past, ambulance drivers were taught to "pump the brakes." Pumping the brakes has been a questionable practice for some time. The theory states that a steadily applied brake will heat up to about 700 degrees and then fail or "lock up." Hypothetically, the pumping action of the driver allows the brakes time to cool and, thus, grip better.

New brakes are made of composite materials that resist overheating, and most ambulances have antilock braking systems (ABS) that automatically pump the brakes for the driver. Therefore, the EVO

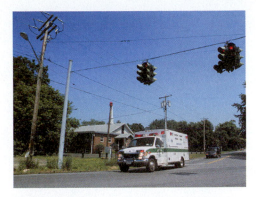

FIGURE 43-7   A complete stop at a red light gives the EVO time to be sure that all other vehicles in the intersection know of his intention to drive through it.

Safety Tip

The use of police escorts should be discouraged because of the danger that is created when multiple emergency vehicles pass motorists. The motorist, hearing a siren and seeing one emergency vehicle pass, may think the right-of-way is clear and proceed back onto the roadway and into the path of the second emergency vehicle. In reality, little time is saved by using an escort, and the risk greatly outweighs the benefit.

Street Smart

Every EMS system should have a policy and procedure for collisions involving the ambulance. Unfortunately, ambulance collisions are a reality in EMS. The EMT involved in an ambulance collision must ensure that arrangements are being made to dispatch another EMS unit to the EMS call.

TABLE 43-7

Braking Distance—Light Truck (10,000 pounds)

Speed (mph)	Reaction Time (ft)		Braking (ft)		Total Distance (ft)
10	11	+	7	=	18
20	22	+	30	=	52
30	33	+	67	=	100
40	44	+	125	=	169
50	55	+	225	=	280
60	66	+	360	=	426

needs to know that he must apply the brakes in a steady and forceful fashion, and the ambulance will do the rest.

Sometimes, panic stops are unavoidable. Panic stops occur when something, such as a dog or a child running after a ball from between two parked cars, suddenly and unpredictably moves in front of the ambulance. If the EVO remembers, he should simultaneously warn the occupants to brace for impact while applying the brake. This warning may give an EMT who is standing in the patient compartment time to sit down.

Whenever the ambulance comes to a complete stop, the EVO should be able to see the rear wheel of the vehicle in front of him. In this position, if the ambulance needs to pull out to respond to a call or the vehicle in front should stall, there is room to evade the vehicle ahead and proceed. Many EMS systems encourage their EVOs to drive in the outside or passing lane at all times. Then if the ambulance needs to "light up" to respond to a call, it does not need to wait for traffic to clear in front of it before it can respond.

Crew During an emergency response, the crew should remain quiet so as not to distract the EVO. The crew should be constantly on the lookout for potential dangers and should immediately, but calmly, relay them to the EVO if found. The crew should remain restrained in their seats until the vehicle has come to a complete stop and the EVO has indicated that it is safe to unbuckle seat belts and exit the vehicle.

ARRIVAL

On arrival at the scene, EVOs have much to do aside from actual patient care. The EVO must always think about the positioning of the vehicle, placement of lights, possible destinations, and routes to those destinations.

Emergency Lights

When arriving at a residence for a house call, the EVO should consider turning off or reducing the number of flashing lights. Flashing

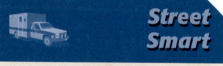

Street Smart

It is the complacent EVO who gets into a crash with the ambulance. Failure on the part of an EVO to anticipate, recognize, and respond appropriately to the dangers of the road is what leads to ambulance collisions. This assertion is supported by the well-established fact that the majority of ambulance collisions occur on clear days with good visibility. This fact should be a sobering thought for an EMT.

lights in residential neighborhoods tend to attract children, adding to the danger present when operating an emergency vehicle.

When the ambulance arrives at the scene of a roadside call, the EVO should consider shutting down his headlights to prevent them from blinding oncoming traffic. Furthermore, on the scene of a motor vehicle collision, the large number of flashing lights from the large number of emergency vehicles serves only to confuse the other drivers in traffic. Therefore, the EVO should consider leaving only the corner flashers lighted on the ambulance to illuminate its position for other drivers.

Positioning

The emergency vehicle should always be positioned in a place that is safe for the emergency crew. It should always be uphill and upwind from any potential hazards. Generally, staying 100 feet from any wreckage is a good idea at a motor vehicle crash.

When arriving on the scene of a traffic accident, if no police or other units have arrived yet, the ambulance should park 100 feet in front of the wreckage and leave all emergency warning lights on (Figure 43-8). The headlights should be shut down, unless they are needed to illuminate the scene, to avoid the blinding of oncoming traffic. This protective positioning serves to block the crew and the patients from passing traffic. It is important to remember to set the parking brake.

If other units have arrived and taken up the protective position, the ambulance should proceed approximately 100 feet past the wreckage (Figure 43-9). This positioning will leave the vehicle free for easy egress from the scene when it becomes necessary.

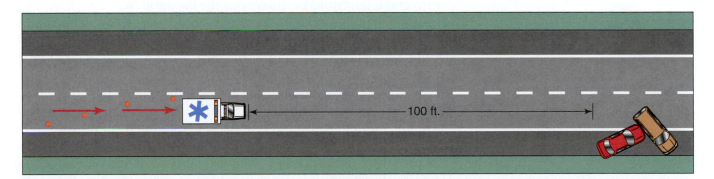

FIGURE 43-8 The first vehicle to arrive at a motor vehicle crash should be used to shield the accident scene from passing traffic.

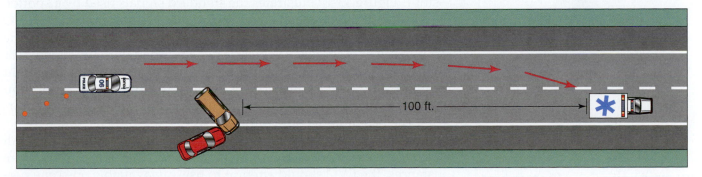

FIGURE 43-9 If the scene is already shielded on arrival, the ambulance should be positioned just beyond the accident scene to allow for an easy exit.

On the scene of an incident at which multiple emergency vehicles are arriving, the EVO is wise to stay with the ambulance at all times. He can then move the ambulance if necessary to prevent it from becoming blocked in. A path of exit must always be available for the ambulance so that it may leave expediently once a patient is loaded. A more extensive discussion of vehicle positioning and scene safety considerations is contained in Chapter 12.

Backing and Parking

A large percentage of ambulance collisions involve the rear passenger section, the portion of the ambulance that cannot be seen by the EVO. Emergency vehicles have unintentionally backed over and injured or killed civilians and fellow emergency service providers. By following a few simple rules, the EVO can avoid a backing collision.

First, backing the ambulance or any emergency vehicle should be avoided whenever possible. Careful consideration of the scene location and the probable direction of travel to the hospital by the EVO will help him decide the best approach to the scene in order to avoid having to back up.

Whenever backing is unavoidable, a **spotter** should be used. A spotter is a person who observes the ambulance as it is in reverse and directs the EVO to avoid obstacles. Note the use of the phrase *avoid obstacles*; every time an ambulance is backing up, there are obstacles and potential collisions. A spotter extends the EVO's perception of right, left, and rear space.

The spotter should be clearly visible in the EVO's mirrors, standing about 10–15 feet to the left rear of the ambulance. Spotters should *never* be allowed to ride either the tailboard or running boards. One bump and a fall could be disastrous for the spotter.

With the spotter in sight, the EVO should start to move the ambulance slowly in reverse, with one foot covering the brake. The EVO should always keep the spotter in sight. If the EVO loses sight of the spotter, he should stop immediately.

The spotter should signal the driver which direction the vehicle should turn, using standard signals. To direct the ambulance straight back, the spotter would put one hand above his head and wave the ambulance back. To direct the ambulance to turn in one direction or another, the spotter should point with both hands in the direction of travel. To direct the ambulance to come to a complete stop, the spotter would cross his arms and clench his fists while simultaneously yelling "stop." Figure 43-10 illustrates the standard signals used by a spotter.

Backing in the dark can be more difficult. When possible, the EVO should utilize the rear scene lights to illuminate the spotter. If the ambulance or emergency vehicle is not equipped with functional rear scene lights, the spotter should utilize two flashlights. A flashlight with a traffic wand attached can be very useful. Under no circumstances should the spotter point the flashlight at the ambulance mirrors. The bright light could blind the EVO.

In certain situations, the ambulance is staffed with only an EVO. All other personnel are actively engaged with rescue. In those rare instances, the EVO should attempt to use any available on-scene personnel. If this is not possible, the EVO should stop the ambulance,

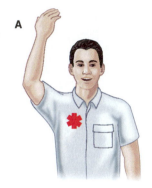

A

Straight back

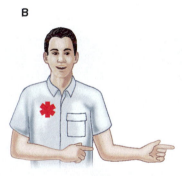

B

Turn

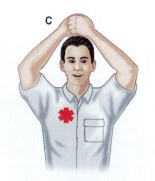

C

Stop

FIGURE 43-10 Only a few basic hand signals are needed by the spotter.

proceed to the rear, and perform a complete survey of the area behind the ambulance.

Whenever the ambulance is parked, the emergency brake should be engaged as a precaution. At every EMS call, sooner or later, an EMT and the patient will be behind the ambulance. Therefore, it is only prudent to maximize the crew's safety and engage the emergency brake.

Scene Size-Up

On arrival at the scene, the EVO should advise the communications specialist that he has arrived. It is important to keep the communications specialist up to date on locations and activities. The first-arriving crew should immediately perform a scene size-up and relay key information back to dispatch.

Appropriate personal protective equipment should be put on prior to any emergency personnel entering any scene. The safety of the scene must be immediately assessed. Any dangers to incoming crews should be quickly reported. The safety of the vehicle positioning should again be confirmed.

The mechanism of injury or nature of illness should be quickly apparent during this initial scene survey. If there are multiple patients, the initial crew should immediately assess the need for additional resources and advise the communications specialist, and then begin appropriate triage. Mass casualty incidents are discussed in detail in Chapter 44.

The information relayed to the communications specialist after the initial scene survey should include a confirmation of the nature of the incident; an estimated number of patients; and the need for further resources such as police, fire, or air support, and the priority of their responses.

On-Scene Actions

Calm management and organization is key to the management of any emergency scene. Whether there is 1 patient or 100 patients, calm operation in an organized fashion facilitates appropriate care and timely transportation of the patient(s).

On-Scene Stabilization

On every scene, the EMT has the responsibility to adequately assess every patient in a timely fashion. This assessment should follow previously outlined guidelines and should end with a determination of priority. Any necessary stabilization should be done, and plans for transport should be made as soon as is practical.

Often the EVO is responsible for preparing stretchers, stairchairs, and other means of conveyance for the EMT. This team approach often reduces the time involved prior to transportation of the patient.

Transportation

Once appropriate stabilization techniques have been utilized, the patient should be prepared for transfer. The principles of patient movement are discussed in Chapter 11. The transfer should be made as expediently as the patient's condition requires.

Helicopter Transport

The EMT will likely have occasion to call for air medical assistance at some point in his career. Helicopter transport has a significant role in prehospital emergency care for both trauma and medical patients. The EMT should be familiar with the capabilities of the air medical agencies that service his area and should know how and when to contact them.

Utilization   There are two general indications for utilizing a helicopter to transport a patient to a hospital. The first indication is if the patient's condition is high priority and very rapid transport to a particular hospital will be beneficial.

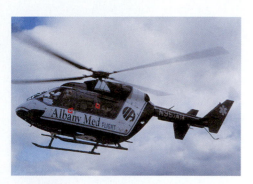

FIGURE 43-11   Air medical service can provide important, even lifesaving, skills and training at the scene of any emergency.

Helicopters travel at speeds much faster than ambulances, and they do not have to follow roads. They can proceed, literally, in the line of sight from point A to point B (Figure 43-11). Therefore, they can get to places faster than a ground vehicle.

Many regions have specific protocols governing the utilization of air medical services. These protocols often describe high-priority patients who are a significant distance from the most appropriate hospital as being appropriate for helicopter transport. The EMT should be familiar with the local helicopter utilization protocols.

The next indication for helicopter transport is dependent on the composition of the helicopter crew. If the crew can perform interventions that the patient needs quickly and the ground crew is unable to perform them, it may be appropriate to call for air medical assistance.

Some helicopter services carry medications that are not carried by ground providers. Sometimes helicopter crews have advanced skills or are trained in specialized rescue techniques. The EMT should be familiar with the capabilities of local air medical agencies.

When requesting a helicopter response, certain basic information is needed. The exact location of the incident, nature of such incident, and number of patients and their specific injuries is often required on initial dispatch. Many regions have policies to request the helicopter to stand by if it seems that it may be needed, but all of the information has not yet been obtained.

For example, a report of a very serious accident with multiple injured patients in an area that is a significant distance from any trauma center may merit notification of air medical support. In this case, the helicopter can be put on standby so that the crew is ready to respond in a short period of time if they are actually needed. Once EMS crews arrive on the scene and actually evaluate the situation, they can request the aircraft to respond if needed or allow it to return to service.

Landing Zone   If a helicopter is requested, the ground personnel must find a safe place for it to land. This area is usually referred to as a landing zone. A **landing zone (LZ)** is an area intended for the purpose of landing and taking off in the helicopter. One person who is familiar with the requirements of an LZ should take charge of its preparation. This person is referred to as the **LZ officer** and is the only person who should be in communication with the aircraft as it approaches.

When choosing an appropriate LZ, there are several things to consider. First, it should be located as close to the actual scene of the incident as possible while still being safe. Often, in the case of a car accident, the LZ can be in a field adjacent to the road or even in the road itself if traffic can be stopped. If a suitable area is not available close by, a more remote LZ may be chosen. In that case, the ground personnel should make arrangements to either bring the patient to the LZ or bring the helicopter crew to the patient.

Landing zones must be a certain size and have certain safety features. Most medical helicopters require a **touchdown area** of between 75 feet square and 100 feet square. The preference is 100 feet square, since that is large enough for both day and night operations, as well as for landing the larger aircraft that the military routinely uses.

The touchdown area is the actual site where the aircraft will land. It should be fairly level and free of any obstacles such as trees, signs, posts, or markers. If the area is unpaved, shrubs, brush, grass, weeds, and so forth should not be higher than 24 inches. Any slope should not be more than 5–10 degrees.

The area above and around the touchdown area is called the **surrounding area** and should be free of any obstacles in which the helicopter could get tangled. When evaluating the surrounding area, the LZ officer should take note of any trees, poles, towers, signs, or wires that are in the surrounding area (Figure 43-12). These should be reported to the pilot of the helicopter as LZ hazards when the helicopter approaches the scene. The specific locations of such hazards must be made clear because sometimes it is difficult to see hazards such as wires from the air.

Additional information that is useful for incoming pilots includes a report of the wind direction and intensity and the condition of the

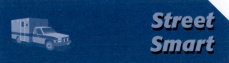

Street Smart

How does an EMT know if the slope is greater than 10 degrees? One method of determining slope is called the WALT method. The acronym WALT stands for "walk and look triangle."

First, the EMT puts a traffic cone or other marker midzone. Then he walks a distance of six times his height, or about 35 feet or 12 normal strides. The EMT then turns and looks at the landing zone. The EMT's line of sight should be even with or just a little higher than the traffic cone. If it is, the LZ is considered acceptable. The EMT should then go back and remove the traffic cone.

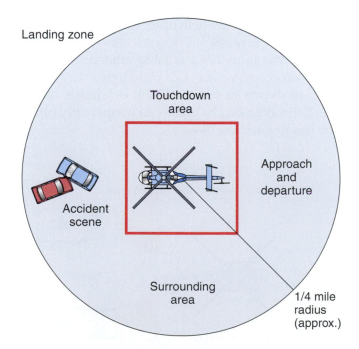

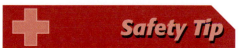

Safety Tip

A significant cause of helicopter crashes is **wire strikes**. When a helicopter's rotor spins around and makes contact with a wire, the rotor usually shatters and the aircraft plummets earthward.

It is imperative that the LZ officer make the location of any wires clear to the pilot. Using the directions of the compass, the LZ officer should call out the wire locations, for example, "Poles with wires in the northwest corner." The LZ officer should avoid the use of "left" or "right," as these terms are confusing to the pilot.

FIGURE 43-12 The LZ officer should choose a touchdown area that has an obstacle-free surrounding area and approach path.

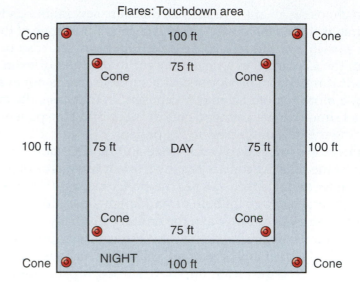

FIGURE 43-13 The marking of an LZ should be clear to the pilot from the air.

touchdown area. For example, if there are moderate winds out of the southwest and the ground surface is muddy, the pilot should be made aware of these conditions when he is given the initial information about the LZ hazards.

Approach Although a helicopter is capable of taking off and landing straight up and down, having a clear path for a more favorable approach angle is preferable. The **approach path** should be free of towers, poles, wires, trees, and so forth.

Because of the confusing nature of many accident scenes, it is often helpful to clearly mark the intended touchdown area with cones, flares, or other secured markers at its four corners (Figure 43-13). Any markers that are used should be carefully secured, since the wind created by the rotor blades as the helicopter lands can be quite forceful. This wind is called **rotor wash**.

If appropriate markers are not available, emergency vehicles can be used on two or four corners of the LZ. Headlights may be used to illuminate the LZ as shown in Figure 43-14, but lights must never be directed at the helicopter. Bright lights can temporarily blind the pilot, making a safe landing impossible.

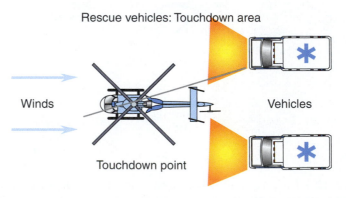

FIGURE 43-14 Emergency vehicle headlights can be used to mark a landing zone.

Landing Zone Safety As the touchdown area is prepared, the LZ officer must be sure to secure any loose debris, clothing, hats, or anything else that may blow around as the helicopter lands. A loose piece of debris can be blown into the rotor blades of the helicopter and cause significant damage, which may render the aircraft useless.

As the aircraft is approaching the touchdown area, any nearby personnel should wear goggles or face visors to protect their eyes from blowing debris. Alternatively, they should turn their backs to the winds created by the helicopter's rotor until the helicopter has landed and shut down.

If the accident is near the LZ, the patient and any exposed crew members should be appropriately protected from blowing debris during the final approach of the aircraft. Doors and windows to nearby vehicles should be kept closed, and any nearby traffic should be held if it has any potential for coming into contact with the aircraft in the LZ area.

Because it is certainly exciting to watch, rescues that involve helicopters often draw a crowd of onlookers. These people should be kept at a distance of at least 200 feet from the touchdown area for their own safety.

As the aircraft approaches the touchdown area, the LZ officer should continue to observe its descent from a safe distance of at least 100 feet. Nobody should be within 100 feet of the touchdown area until it is safe to approach. The pilot of the aircraft will indicate when it is safe to approach the aircraft. If an unsafe situation develops during the final approach, the LZ officer should immediately and calmly contact the pilot with the information.

LZ Hand Signals The LZ officer really needs to know only two hand signals to communicate with the pilot. While facing the pilot at the edge of the LZ, the LZ officer simply stands with his arms outstretched, indicating that the aircraft's approach is safe. The LZ officer should not be concentrating on how the aircraft is descending but should be looking around the aircraft for dangers.

If a wire strike suddenly seems possible, an individual runs out to meet the helicopter, or another danger under or around the helicopter arises, the LZ officer should signal to the pilot of the immediate danger, using a vigorous crossing and uncrossing of his arms over his head. This **wave-off** will cause the pilot to quickly abort the landing.

Touchdown Operations around the helicopter while it is on the ground also have several rules. In general, nobody should ever approach the aircraft while it is running unless he is signaled to do so by the pilot. This includes the LZ officer as well. The pilot will usually direct the appropriate movement about the aircraft. If an EMT is signaled that he may approach the aircraft, he should always approach from the front, the twelve o'clock position, within clear view of the pilot. Personnel should never approach a helicopter from the rear, the six o'clock position. The danger zones around the aircraft are illustrated in Figure 43-15. On the rear of the aircraft tail is a tail rotor that spins very fast. It spins so fast that it is nearly invisible. The tail rotor is very dangerous. If an EMT is hit by a spinning tail rotor, he would be very seriously injured and possibly even killed.

Safety Tip

Many EMS agencies require that a pumper be at standby whenever a helicopter lands. If that is the case, then the pumper should be staged to the side of the LZ, away from the approach path. The firefighters should stand by in full turnout gear with a charged line standing behind the pumper.

The pumper will act as a barrier from flying debris and a heat shield until the firefighters can make their attack. For fire suppression, rapid deployment of foam is best.

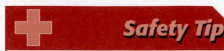

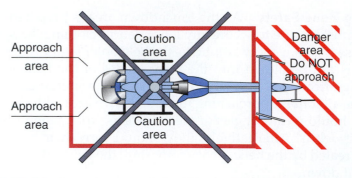

FIGURE 43-15 Ground personnel should be familiar with the danger zones around a helicopter.

The height of the main rotor blades may require that approaching personnel duck down to avoid being struck by them. For this reason, it is good practice for an EMT to wear a safety helmet whenever he is around an aircraft. If approaching a helicopter on a slope, the EMT should approach from the downhill side to avoid being struck by the main rotor blades on the uphill side. See Figure 43-16 for an illustration of this concept.

Most helicopter crews will come to the patient, away from the aircraft, to quickly assess the patient. Any necessary treatment will be initiated, and then movement of the patient to the aircraft will be directed by the pilot and helicopter crew.

When carrying the patient to the waiting aircraft, the EMT should stay close to the patient's side, semicrouched, and walk at a deliberate pace. The EMT should never run to the helicopter. The EMT should never carry anything, including IV fluids, over his head as he approaches the aircraft.

Liftoff Once the patient has been safely loaded, all ground personnel should leave the landing zone in the direction indicated by the pilot or helicopter crew and should remain at least 200 feet away from the aircraft while it prepares to lift off. A great deal of rotor wash will again be generated as the aircraft lifts off. Again, no bright lights or flashes should be aimed at the aircraft during this time, as they could create a vision problem for the pilot.

Although general safety issues surrounding operation around helicopters are similar between agencies, ground EMS personnel should routinely practice and train with their local helicopter agencies so that safe operation around the aircraft becomes second nature.

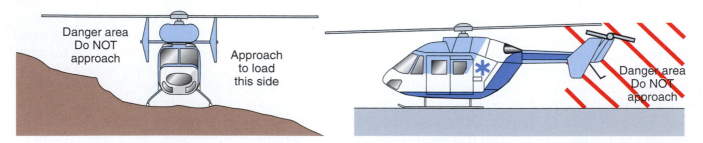

FIGURE 43-16 When approaching a helicopter that has landed on a slope, always approach from the downhill side to avoid injury. Never approach the aircraft from behind.

Ambulance Transport

Typically, the patient is transported to the hospital in an ambulance. The decision whether to use lights and sirens is dictated by the patient's condition. Thus, the EMT must make the decision and inform the EVO. It is important that the EMT and the EVO understand the reason for the decision. When a patient is potentially unstable, the EVO should be made aware that it may be necessary to "step up" the response to lights and sirens if the patient's condition should deteriorate.

Transport to Facility   Once the patient and the crew have been safely secured in the ambulance, the EVO should notify the communications specialist of the intended destination and the time of departure from the scene. Just as with the response to the scene, the EVO should plan the route prior to beginning the drive.

Most transports to a hospital are done without red lights and siren. The crew should weigh the risks associated with using these warning devices against the benefit of a potentially quicker transport time. If red lights and sirens are used at all in this phase of response, they should be used only for high-priority patients. Extreme care should be used during this high-risk transport.

Often a family member wants to travel with the patient to the hospital. This may be appropriate if the family member is calm and can offer some support to the patient on arrival at the hospital or can provide hospital staff with useful information. The family member generally should ride in the front passenger seat of the ambulance, using a seat belt.

A family member who is hysterical and might create a distraction to the crew or the EVO during transport should not be allowed to ride in the ambulance. Instead, the crew should enlist the assistance of the police or a supervisor in transporting the distraught family member to the hospital.

As soon as possible during transport, the EMT in charge should contact the receiving facility and give them a brief verbal report. This report should include information that will help the receiving staff to properly prepare for the patient. This radio report is described in Chapter 19.

Arrival at Facility

Immediately upon arrival at the hospital, the EVO should notify the communications specialist. The ambulance should be safely positioned at the ambulance entrance. Often this requires backing up. It is always wise for an EVO to request a person to step out of the ambulance to watch the vehicle back up. This is insurance against unseen obstacles behind the ambulance. An emergency department entrance is a busy place. There is always a risk of inadvertently striking a person or another vehicle.

Once the vehicle is adequately parked, the EVO should assist the medical crew in taking the patient out of the ambulance and into the emergency department.

Transfer of Care

The patient should be transferred to the stretcher that is designated by the triage staff at the emergency department. This should be done

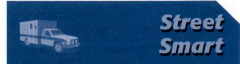

Street Smart

The landing team should remain assembled for about 5 minutes after liftoff. If an in-flight emergency should occur, the aircraft may need to return quickly to a secured landing zone.

Street Smart

Occasionally, family members want to follow the ambulance to the hospital in a private vehicle. If the EVO is expecting to use the emergency warning lights and siren, he should advise the family *not* to follow him. A private vehicle following an ambulance through intersections is, at best, breaking the law and, at worst, risking a serious collision in the intersections.

Pediatric Considerations

It may be appropriate to allow parents of children being transported to ride in the back with their child. This may provide a more comfortable atmosphere for the child. The emergency crew should make this decision on a case-by-case basis.

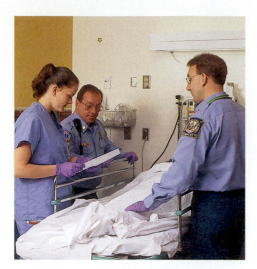

FIGURE 43-17 When transferring patient care to hospital staff, the EMT should give a complete verbal report to the accepting nurse and/or physician.

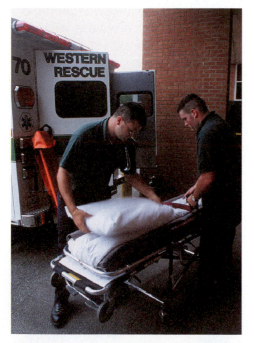

FIGURE 43-18 When restocking the ambulance after a call, the EMT should clean the stretcher of any visible contamination and make it up with clean linen.

following principles of safe lifting and patient transfer discussed in Chapter 11. Once the patient is safely on the hospital stretcher, she should be made comfortable. Any oxygen should be transferred to the hospital's oxygen supply. Any IV lines should be hung appropriately on IV poles or hangers.

Prior to leaving the bedside, the prehospital crew should raise the bedside rails on the stretcher to prevent the patient from accidentally falling. A complete verbal report should be given to an appropriate staff member, usually a nurse, prior to leaving the patient's side (Figure 43-17). Any personal or other items belonging to the patient should be given to the receiving staff.

Charting

The written chart should be completed as soon as possible after patient care has been transferred to the hospital staff. Usually a written report with the details of the incident must be placed in the patient's hospital records before the EMT returns to service. The report enables hospital staff to refer to the Patient Care Report if any questions regarding prehospital care are asked. More information on documentation is contained in Chapter 20.

Cleaning

The crew should turn its attention to cleaning and decontaminating the ambulance before returning to service. Specifics about decontamination and routine vehicle cleaning are contained in Chapter 6.

Restocking

The next order of business is to restock the ambulance in preparation for the next call. Some hospitals provide replacement items for equipment used, such as oxygen masks and IV supplies. Additionally, some hospitals may exchange clean for dirty linen. The linen on the stretcher should always be replaced with clean linen (Figure 43-18).

Return to Station

Once the necessary paperwork, cleaning, and restocking have been accomplished, the crew should return to the station to finish preparations for the next call. On their departure from the hospital, dispatch should be notified. When the vehicle has been completely cleaned and restocked, the crew should notify dispatch that the ambulance is in-service, which means the crew is ready to take another call.

Restock and Refuel

Certain restock items, such as backboards and oxygen tanks, may not be available at the hospital. These items should be restocked as soon as possible on return to the station. Additionally, the vehicle should be refueled as needed. The fuel tank of an emergency vehicle should be maintained above one-half full at all times to ensure adequate fuel for prolonged emergency operations.

Reports

On return to the station, any further paperwork should be completed. It is always wise to complete any documentation that is relevant to the call as soon as possible after completion of the call. It is generally easier to recall specifics soon after the event than days later. Furthermore, events documented at the time of the event ring more true in a court of law than facts remembered days or even weeks later and may affect whether a document can even be received into evidence in court.

Debriefing

Regardless of the nature of the event, it is a good idea for the crew to discuss the call. A brief discussion of any problems or concerns can be helpful in preventing similar incidents or problems on future calls. Concerns from any crew member should be addressed, and the crew should ask themselves, "Could we have done anything differently?"

The postcall debriefing following each call should become routine. It allows issues to come to the surface quickly, rather than be hidden away until the problems are much larger.

CONCLUSION

The well-trained EMT not only will be an effective caregiver but also will understand the safety issues surrounding operation of emergency vehicles. Specifics of ground and air medical operations should be a part of any EMT training program.

 EMS in Action

(continued from page 880)

The passenger-side door was cut off the car and the patient was immobilized on a long board with a cervical collar, head-blocks, and multiple straps. Her breath sounds were assessed as clear in all fields, and a detailed assessment showed no significant injuries to the patient. Oxygen and an IV were established before she was flown to Metro-Health Medical Center, where she was evaluated and released that evening. She was extremely fortunate that as the trailer rolled over and crushed the roof of the car, she was pushed down across the front seat.

After the passenger was extricated and care transferred to the flight crew, one of my crewmen crawled into the car and confirmed the status of the driver. Unfortunately, she was not as lucky as her friend. The truck driver was also treated at the scene for minor cuts and was taken into custody by the Ohio Highway Patrol. A heavy-duty tow truck pulled the flattened car from under the trailer. It was not until 1830 hours that the toll gate reopened.

The lesson here is that a scene may not always be what you are expecting it to be, and even when that scene looks awful, the condition of the patient may surprise you as well. My entire crew returned with no injuries to themselves because we worked smartly, and as a team. We ensured safety first before rescue or intervention. With what we were facing that day, my entire crew believes that this call was nothing less than a success.

Greg Laborie, NREMT-P, EMSI
North Ridgeville Fire Department
North Ridgeville, Ohio

TEST YOUR KNOWLEDGE

1. Explain the importance of adequate preparation prior to an emergency call.
2. Describe personnel considerations in daily EMS operations.
3. Describe equipment considerations in daily EMS operations.
4. List the phases of an emergency call and the important considerations in each phase.
5. Explain the EVO's considerations during an emergency response.
6. Describe proper emergency vehicle positioning at the scene.
7. List activities that should be completed on the emergency crew's return to the station.
8. List the two general indications for air medical transport from an emergency scene.
9. Describe the factors that go into landing zone preparation.
10. Discuss the importance of safety when operating around a helicopter.

INTERNET RESOURCES

Additional resources related to this chapter can be found at these Web sites:

- Ambulance.com, http://www.ambulance.com
- Emergency Vehicle Owners and Operators Association, http://www.evooa.org
- Road Safety International, http://www.roadsafety.com

Search using key terms related to this chapter to find additional information on operations of the emergency vehicle.

FURTHER STUDY

Anderson, R. (1998). Touchdown! Establishing a helicopter landing zone. *EMS Rescue Technology, 1*(2), 64–66.

Burns, L. (1999). So you want to drive an ambulance? *Emergency Medical Services, 28*(11), 53–59.

Meade, D., & Dernocoeur, K. (1998). Street smarts: Principles of vehicle placement. *Emergency Medical Services, 27*(11), 34–36.

Spivak, M. (1998). Learning to drive . . . All over again. *Emergency Medical Services, 27*(11), 41–43.

U.S. General Services Administration. (2002, June). *Federal specification for the star-of-life ambulance.* Washington, DC: U.S. General Services Administration. Retrieved September 27, 2004, from http://www.ntea.com/Downloads/AMD_KKK-A-1822E.pdf.

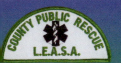

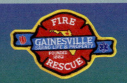

CHAPTER 44

Public Safety Incident Management

KEY TERMS

briefing

chain of command

Chemical Transportation Emergency Center (CHEMTREC)

cold zone

command post

decontamination corridor

Emergency Response Guidebook (ERG)

emergency response team

field hospital

first responder awareness level

guides

hazardous material

hot zone

incident commander (IC)

Incident Management System (IMS)

limited victim incident (LVI)

Material Safety Data Sheet (MSDS)

medical group supervisor

morgue

multiple casualty incident (MCI)

(continues)

OBJECTIVES

Upon completion of this chapter, the reader should be able to:

1. Recognize the presence of hazardous materials.
2. Discuss the role of an EMT on the scene of a hazardous materials incident.
3. Explain how to use the *Emergency Response Guidebook*.
4. Classify what areas would be in the hot zone, cold zone, and warm zone.
5. Explain the different hazardous materials identification systems in use for fixed facilities and transportation.
6. Explain the initial role of an EMT on the scene of a multiple casualty incident.
7. Describe the Public Safety Incident Management System.
8. Explain the concept of chain of command.
9. Describe the roles of the following officers:
   Safety
   Research
   Public information
   Staging
   Triage
   Treatment
   Transportation
10. Describe the START Triage System.

OVERVIEW

A response to a scene with multiple patients or unknown chemical exposure may be a very stressful scene for the responding emergency medical technician (EMT). These scenes can often be confusing and chaotic. It is the EMT's responsibility to assist with establishing order in these situations. How these scenes are managed in the first few minutes often dictates the overall outcome of the entire incident. This chapter acquaints the EMT with how to act safely and effectively in those first few minutes.

SAFETY AND HAZARDOUS MATERIALS

Every EMT is responsible for the safety of herself and the crew. An EMT's ability to be safe is dependent on an ability to identify dangerous situations. Some situations are clearly dangerous, yet many dangerous situations are not realized until it is too late. To prevent these unfortunate circumstances, the EMT must be trained to become "aware" of the telltale signs in the environment that warn of a dangerous substance.

A **hazardous material** can be defined as any substance that can cause injury or death to an exposed person. A hazardous material spill would, therefore, represent a dangerous situation for an EMT and the public. It is important an EMT learn to identify spilled hazardous materials. Identifying a hazardous material affords an EMT the chance to avoid a potential exposure and subsequent injury.

Federal Regulation

The federal Hazardous Waste Operations and Emergency Response (HAZWOPER) regulation requires that EMTs and all other emergency

✴ *Tanker Rollover*

Traffic was at a standstill, and we were crawling along the shoulder of the road. The fog was so thick you could barely see a hand in front of your face.

The initial dispatch information was for a "possible injury accident near exit 24." As we approached the exit, the fog suddenly changed colors from white to brown, and the air smelled like rotten eggs.

We immediately stopped and started to back up. Grabbing the binoculars, I looked ahead. There it was, a tank trailer on its side. It appeared to be on fire. Brown–black smoke was billowing from its underside.

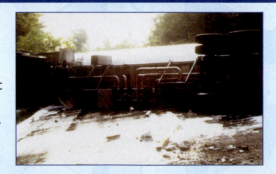

(Courtesy of Craig Leroy, Troy Fire Department, Troy, NY.)

- What are the indications that this is a hazardous materials incident?
- What other signs should the EMT look for?
- What would be the EMT's initial priorities?
- If this was a building, what signs would the EMT look for?
- Would the EMT's priorities change?

responders be trained regarding hazardous materials. Specifically, section 29 of the *Code of Federal Regulations* (CFR), subsection 1910.120, requires that training be provided to "those likely to witness or discover a hazardous substance release and who have been trained to initiate the emergency response sequence by notifying the proper authorities of the release." (EPA 40 CFR 311 covers federal and local government employees.)

Those parties likely to discover a hazardous substance release are generally referred to as first responders. The term *first responders* does not refer to the level of medical training, but instead refers to who would arrive on the scene of such an incident first.

In many situations, the EMT may be a first responder. Therefore, an EMT must be trained to identify hazardous materials and notify proper authorities. This training is called the **first responder awareness level**. It should be noted that while an EMT is expected to be able to identify a potential hazardous material incident, she is not expected to take any action to stop the incident. The responsibility of an EMT trained at the first responder awareness level is strictly to identify the hazardous situation and retreat until properly trained personnel arrive.

When an EMT identifies a potential hazardous materials incident, other, more specially trained responders will be called to render the situation safe. The next responders, the **operations level responders**, are expected to act and minimize the spread of the spill as well as prevent further injuries. The actions of these operations level responders are primarily defensive. By establishing a perimeter and remaining at the periphery, these responders are primarily protected by distance.

Eventually, specially trained hazardous material technicians and specialists, usually part of an **emergency response team**, will arrive to rescue contaminated patients as well as control, confine, contain, and decontaminate the area. The EMT is the first link in the hazardous materials response and plays an important part in every hazardous materials response. Early identification of a spill and prompt notification of the proper authorities by an EMT improves the chances of a more favorable outcome.

Assessment

The assessment of the patient with a potential hazardous materials exposure starts by making sure the EMT is not the next patient. To do this, the EMT must proceed carefully and methodically through the steps of a patient assessment with a constant eye on personal safety.

Scene Size-Up

Whenever an EMT is approaching a scene, she should slow down and maybe even stop to assess the scene for obvious hazards. The EMT should try to look at the whole scene, not just the narrow setting surrounding the incident. The use of binoculars can improve an EMT's ability to observe the whole scene without getting dangerously close (Figure 44-1).

Smoke may indicate there is fire. Fire markedly increases the number of dangers present, including explosion as well as toxic vapors.

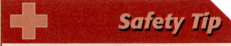

Safety Tip

Many hazardous materials, also known as hazmats, are routinely used in manufacturing processes as well as transported across the country. Every EMT is advised to obtain hazardous materials awareness training. This training should comply with all pertinent Occupational Safety and Health Administration (OSHA) regulations regarding the detection and response to hazardous materials.

These hazardous materials awareness courses typically take approximately 4–8 hours to complete. At the completion of the course, the EMT should expect to be able to identify hazardous materials and understand how to properly respond to a hazardous materials incident.

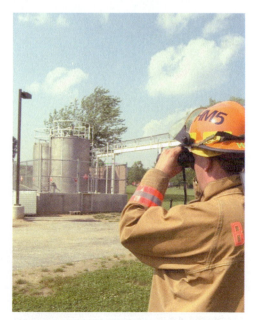

FIGURE 44-1 Using binoculars, the EMT should try to get the global picture.

Typically, smoke rises in the air. Spilled chemicals may release toxic vapors that tend to stay closer to the ground. In fact, more than 80% of toxic vapors are heavier than air. To protect herself and her crew, the EMT should stage the ambulance far away from any smoke or vapors. She should also place the ambulance upwind and uphill of the vapors. These actions will decrease the chance of an accidental exposure.

The EMT should then assess the risk, preferably using binoculars to see the entire scene. There are a numbers of signs or clues to the presence of possible hazardous materials on scene.

The initial actions of the EMT on the scene of a potential hazardous materials spill is critical to the long-term impact of the event. To help the EMT remember which actions to take, the mnemonic **SIN** can be helpful.

The *S* in SIN stands for safety. First and foremost the EMT must be concerned about her safety. Staging the ambulance uphill and upwind, and at a safe distance, from the incident is the EMT's first priority.

Once the EMT is now in a safe area, in an area called the cold zone as illustrated in Figure 44-11, the EMT should turn her attention to the *I* in SIN. The *I* stands for isolation, meaning establishing a perimeter around the incident. The next section deals with hazardous material identification and the use of the *Emergency Response Guidebook* to establish an isolation zone and the borders of the perimeter.

Last, the EMT should deny entry into the area until qualified personnel are on scene. Denying entry, that is, No entry, is the *N* in SIN and indicates the importance of establishing public safety.

Hazmat Identification

Hazardous materials are transported every day by plane, boat, truck, and train. In some circumstances, the type and shape of the transporting vehicle give the EMT an idea of what type of hazardous materials may be involved. For example, when a train car derails and a tanker car is breached, it is probable that a large amount of fluid will be spilled.

Similarly, the name of the carrier may provide some clue to the cargo it contains. For example, a tanker truck marked "North Country Oil Company" is likely to be carrying petroleum products (Figure 44-2).

The shape of the container on the vehicle may also provide valuable additional information. Round containers with rounded ends are likely to be carrying materials such as gases or liquids, which may be under pressure. Any material under pressure is an explosive hazard.

Hazardous Materials Placards The United States Department of Transportation (USDOT) has adopted the United Nations (UN) standard for identifying a hazardous material using **placards**. A placard is a system of symbols placed on three sides of a container indicating the vehicle is carrying a certain class of hazardous materials. For an example of a placard for an explosive, see Figure 44-3.

Placards are usually $10^3/_4$-inch diamonds that are colored and numbered. Each placard will have unique colors, symbols, and numbers to identify the class of the materials. The colors may also indicate the danger present. For example, an all-orange placard also indicates

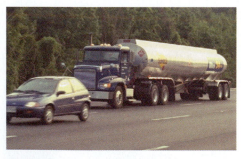

FIGURE 44-2 The name of the carrier may be a clue to the cargo.

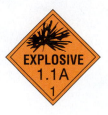

FIGURE 44-3 A placard indicates that hazardous materials may be aboard.

a danger of explosion. The placard in Figure 44-3 has both the orange color as well as the symbol for an explosive.

The symbol is also intended to provide a broad warning. A skull and crossbones, for example, indicates that the material is poisonous. A test tube with a liquid dripping onto a dissolving hand is indicative of a corrosive substance (Figure 44-4).

Perhaps more important than the colors and symbols are the numbers. These numbers symbolize that a specific substance belongs to a certain classification of hazardous materials. When several different potentially hazardous materials are being carried, the primary hazard will be identified. While a placard number may not precisely identify the material, it does tell the EMT to what general class the most hazardous material belongs. This, in turn, can provide the EMT with some basic information on how to respond in the worst-case scenario.

Fixed Facility Hazardous Materials

Hazardous materials incidents can occur in situations other than in transit. Spills at a manufacturing plant or fires may create a hazardous materials incident. When an EMT arrives at any scene, she should stop, look, and listen for signs of danger. The location of the call, for example, a chemical storage facility, may alert her to the possibility of a hazardous materials incident. The nature of the plant, for example, a petroleum distillation operation, may also alert her to the type of hazardous materials.

Using binoculars, the EMT may observe large numbers of people exiting the building. She may also observe clouds of smoke or the fog of a vapor. Instead of the UN placard system, the EMT might observe a diamond-shaped warning sign with four more diamonds inside. This is the National Fire Protection Association's **(NFPA) 704 symbol** (Figure 44-5). The NFPA recommends safety practices to the industry but cannot enforce these practices. The NFPA is an advisory group, not a law enforcement organization. Therefore, in some instances, a community may not have adopted the standard.

In many instances, local communities have adopted the NFPA recommendations and made them into legal ordinances under the fire or building codes. In those cases, the EMT will observe the diamond-shaped NFPA 704 symbol. Each diamond within the diamond represents a certain type of hazard. The red diamond represents the fire potential. An EMT would be interested in the blue diamond that represents health risk. At the bottom of the diamond is a white diamond. Special hazards, such as radioactive material, may be indicated by a spinning propeller (Figure 44-6).

Inside each of the diamonds is a number from 0 to 4. This number represents the nature of the most dangerous hazardous material within the facility. For example, a 4 in the health hazard would indicate a material that is "too dangerous to health to expose workers." According to the NFPA standards, the number 4 in the blue diamond represents a health hazard in which, "A few whiffs of the material could cause death."

Preplans and MSDS In many cases where there is a high life hazard, public safety officials may have already planned for the potential

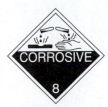

FIGURE 44-4 Symbols may also provide a clue to the nature of the cargo. A dripping test tube indicates a corrosive.

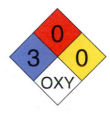

FIGURE 44-5 The NFPA 704 symbols are placed on fixed storage facilities.

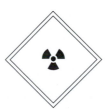

FIGURE 44-6 Symbols within the white diamond warn of special dangers.

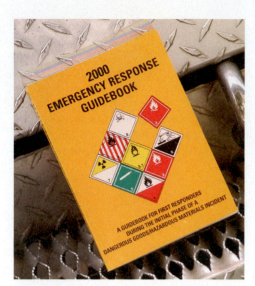

FIGURE 44-7 The *Emergency Response Guidebook* (ERG) is a valuable tool containing much-needed safety information.

of a disaster. This preplan often includes information about the substance as well as a general plan of approach. The health and safety information is often listed on a **Material Safety Data Sheet (MSDS)** that must be maintained by law at every site where dangerous or hazardous chemicals are stored. The EMT should ask to see the MSDS if it is available.

Incident Response Plan

Federal regulations (29 CFR 1910.120) require that every community have a plan of response for hazardous materials incidents. In many cases, emergency medical services (EMS) and other public safety agencies have adopted the Incident Management System.

Initial Actions

Once an EMT has identified a placard number, the EMT would refer to the *Emergency Response Guidebook* **(ERG)** (Figure 44-7). The ERG provides responders with instructions and information on how to handle the first 30 minutes of a hazardous materials spill, also known as hazmat.

First, the placard numbers are cross-referenced in the yellow section of the ERG. Using the number, the EMT can find a reference in the ERG directing her to the **guides** in the orange section. These guides provide the EMT with instructions for evacuation distance, perimeter boundaries, and potential hazards. Every emergency vehicle should have an ERG readily available.

Small containers and quantities of hazardous materials may not be marked by the DOT UN placard. However, the contents of these small containers will be listed on **shipping papers**. Shipping papers accompany any hazardous material while it is in transit. Also called a bill of lading, shipping papers contain the chemical name of the materials, as well as the UN designation (Figure 44-8). These shipping papers may be found in the map pocket of a truck door or in the possession of the driver or pilot of the vehicle.

The shipping papers will also list a description of the material as well as immediate health hazards and the fire/explosion risk. The shipping papers must also list a telephone number to call for technical assistance. Many trucking companies use the services of **Chemical Transportation Emergency Center (CHEMTREC)**, at 800-424-9300, for 24-hour technical assistance in the event of a chemical spill.

The EMT may also open the ERG to the blue section and, using the chemical name, find the cross-reference to the guide. Turning to the guide in the orange section, the EMT will find fundamental emergency response information. Figure 44-9 contains instructions for using ERG found on the inside cover of the book.

Evacuation Distances In some cases, the hazardous material is so dangerous that an evacuation of all civilians in the vicinity must take place immediately. When an EMT comes across a highlighted entry in either the yellow section, UN placard numbers, or in the blue section, the chemical names, she should immediately refer to the guide in the green section for evacuation information.

```
┌─────────────────────────────────────────┐
│                                           │
│   SHIPPING PAPER                          │
│ ─────────────────────────────────────    │
│     PAPER 1 OF 1                          │
│ ─────────────────────────────────────    │
│    TO:    Wafers R Us                     │
│           88 Valley Street                │
│           Silicon Junction, CA            │
│ ─────────────────────────────────────    │
│    FROM: Essex Corporation                │
│          5775 Dawson Avenue               │
│          Coleta, CA 93117                 │
│ ─────────────────────────────────────    │
│    QT     HM                              │
│    DESCRIPTION 1 Cyl                      │
│    WEIGHT         25 lbs                   │
│ ─────────────────────────────────────    │
│    RQ     Phosgene, 2.3, UN1076,          │
│           Poison, Inhalation              │
│           Hazard, Zone CA                 │
│ ─────────────────────────────────────    │
│   This is to certify that the above named materials are │
│   properly classified, described, packaged, marked and │
│   labeled, and are in proper condition for transportation │
│   according to the applicable regulations of the │
│   Department of Transportation. │
│ ─────────────────────────────────────    │
│   Shipper:       Essex Corp               │
│   Carrier:       Knuckle Bros.            │
│   Per:           Shultz                   │
│   Per:                                    │
│   Date:          6/27/00                  │
│   Date:                                   │
│ ─────────────────────────────────────    │
│   SPECIAL INSTRUCTIONS                    │
│             24 Hr. Emergency Contact      │
│             Ed Shultz, 1-800-555-555      │
│                                           │
└─────────────────────────────────────────┘
```

FIGURE 44-8   Shipping papers also list the contents of a shipment.

The green section of the ERG contains readily available information about isolation and evacuation distances for both day and night operations (Figure 44-10).

Perimeters Once a hazardous material has been identified, a perimeter must be established to prevent further contamination of civilians and emergency responders. The immediate vicinity of the hazardous material spill considered contaminated and a risk to rescue personnel is called the **hot zone**. Emergency services personnel, including EMS, are not allowed under any circumstances to enter the hot zone without special protective equipment.

The outermost perimeter beyond which it is considered safest for all emergency services providers is called the **cold zone**. EMS usually stages and sets up an aid station in the cold zone at the perimeter's

RESIST RUSHING IN !
APPROACH INCIDENT FROM UPWIND
STAY CLEAR OF ALL SPILLS, VAPORS, FUMES AND SMOKE

HOW TO USE THIS GUIDEBOOK DURING AN INCIDENT INVOLVING DANGEROUS GOODS

O N E **IDENTIFY THE MATERIAL** BY FINDING ANY **ONE** OF THE FOLLOWING:

THE 4-DIGIT ID NUMBER ON A PLACARD OR ORANGE PANEL

THE 4-DIGIT ID NUMBER (after UN/NA) ON A SHIPPING DOCUMENT OR PACKAGE

THE NAME OF THE MATERIAL ON A SHIPPING DOCUMENT, PLACARD OR PACKAGE

IF AN **ID NUMBER** OR THE **NAME OF THE MATERIAL** CANNOT BE FOUND, SKIP TO THE NOTE BELOW.

T W O **LOOK UP THE MATERIAL'S 3-DIGIT GUIDE NUMBER** IN EITHER:

THE ID NUMBER INDEX..(the yellow-bordered pages of the guidebook)

THE NAME OF MATERIAL INDEX..(the blue-bordered pages of the guidebook)

If the guide number is supplemented with the letter "P", it indicates that the material may undergo violent polymerization if subjected to heat or contamination.

If the index entry is highlighted, **LOOK FOR THE ID NUMBER AND NAME OF THE MATERIAL** IN THE TABLE OF INITIAL ISOLATION AND PROTECTIVE ACTION DISTANCES (the green-bordered pages). If necessary, **BEGIN PROTECTIVE ACTIONS IMMEDIATELY** (see the section on Protective Actions).

USE THE FOLLOWING GUIDES FOR ALL EXPLOSIVES:

DIVISION 1.1 (EXPLOSIVES A) - GUIDE 112
DIVISION 1.2 (EXPLOSIVES A & B) - GUIDE 112
DIVISION 1.3 (EXPLOSIVES B) - GUIDE 112
DIVISION 1.4 (EXPLOSIVES C) - GUIDE 114
DIVISION 1.5 (BLASTING AGENTS) - GUIDE 112
DIVISION 1.6 - GUIDE 112

THREE **TURN TO THE NUMBERED GUIDE** (the orange-bordered pages) **AND READ CAREFULLY.**

NOTE **IF A NUMBERED GUIDE CANNOT BE OBTAINED BY FOLLOWING THE ABOVE STEPS**, AND A PLACARD CAN BE SEEN, LOCATE THE PLACARD IN THE TABLE OF PLACARDS, THEN GO TO THE 3-DIGIT GUIDE SHOWN NEXT TO THE SAMPLE PLACARD.

IF A REFERENCE TO A GUIDE CANNOT BE FOUND AND THIS INCIDENT IS BELIEVED TO INVOLVE DANGEROUS GOODS, TURN TO **GUIDE 111** NOW, AND USE IT UNTIL ADDITIONAL INFORMATION BECOMES AVAILABLE. If the shipping document lists an emergency response telephone number, call that number. If the shipping document is not available, or no emergency response telephone number is listed, IMMEDIATELY CALL the appropriate **emergency response agency listed on the inside back cover of this guidebook.** Provide as much information as possible, such as the name of the carrier (trucking company or railroad) and vehicle number.

FIGURE 44-9 The inside cover of the *Emergency Response Guidebook* (ERG) provides information on how to use the book.

edge. EMTs in this zone should not be at any risk of contamination. Figure 44-11 illustrates these zones.

Management

Before treatment can begin, the victim must be cleansed and decontaminated. This process of decontamination can be lengthy. In the interim before the arrival of the first patient, the EMT should try to ascertain exactly what the contaminants are and then contact medical control for instructions on how to treat the patient.

TABLE OF INITIAL ISOLATION AND PROTECTIVE ACTION DISTANCES

ID No.	NAME OF MATERIAL	SMALL SPILLS (From a small package or small leak from a large package)				LARGE SPILLS (From a large package or from many small packages)			
		First ISOLATE in all Directions		Then PROTECT persons Downwind during-		First ISOLATE in all Directions		Then PROTECT persons Downwind during-	
		Meters (Feet)		DAY Kilometers (Miles)	NIGHT Kilometers (Miles)	Meters (Feet)		DAY Kilometers (Miles)	NIGHT Kilometers (Miles)
2420	Hexafluoroacetone	60 m	(200 ft)	0.3 km (0.2 mi)	1.0 km (0.6 mi)	215 m	(700 ft)	0.8 km (0.5 mi)	3.5 km (2.2 mi)
2421	Nitrogen trioxide	60 m	(200 ft)	0.2 km (0.1 mi)	0.5 km (0.3 mi)	155 m	(500 ft)	0.5 km (0.3 mi)	1.6 km (1.0 mi)
2438	Trimethylacetyl chlonde	60 m	(200 ft)	0.2 km (0.1 mi)	0.5 km (0.3 mi)	155 m	(500 ft)	0.5 km (0.3 mi)	1.9 km (1.2 mi)
2442	Trichloroacetyl chloride	60 m	(200 ft)	0.3 km (0.2 mi)	1.0 km (0.6 mi)	215 m	(700 ft)	0.8 km (0.5 mi)	3.4 km (2.1 mi)
2474	Thiophosgene	95 m	(300 ft)	0.3 km (0.2 mi)	1.1 km (0.7 mi)	215 m	(700 ft)	1.0 km (0.6 mi)	4.2 km (2.6 mi)
2477	Methyl isothiocyanate	60 m	(200 ft)	0.2 km (0.1 mi)	0.6 km (0.4 mi)	185 m	(600 ft)	0.6 km (0.4 mi)	2.4 km (1.5 mi)
2480	Methyl isocyanate	125 m	(400 ft)	0.5 km (0.3 mi)	2.3 km (1.4 mi)	305 m	(1000 ft)	1.9 km (1.2 mi)	8.2 km (5.1 mi)
2481	Ethyl isocyanate	185 m	(600 ft)	1.3 km (0.8 mi)	6.1 km (3.8 mi)	520 m	(1700 ft)	5.0 km (3.1 mi)	11.0+ km (7.0+ mi)
2482	n-Propyl isocyanate	155 m	(500 ft)	1.3 km (0.8 mi)	5.8 km (3.6 mi)	490 m	(1600 ft)	4.7 km (2.9 mi)	11.0+ km (7.0+ mi)
2483	Isopropyl isocyanate	155 m	(500 ft)	1.3 km (0.8 mi)	5.8 km (3.6 mi)	490 m	(1600 ft)	4.7 km (2.9 mi)	11.0+ km (7.0+ mi)
2484	tert-Butyl isocyanate	155 m	(500 ft)	1.1 km (0.7 mi)	5.3 km (3.3 mi)	460 m	(1500 ft)	4.3 km (2.7 mi)	11.0+ km (7.0+ mi)
2485	n-Butyl isocyanate	155 m	(500 ft)	1.1 km (0.7 mi)	5.3 km (3.3 mi)	460 m	(1500 ft)	4.3 km (2.7 mi)	11.0+ km (7.0+ mi)
2486	Isobutyl isocyanate	155 m	(500 ft)	1.1 km (0.7 mi)	5.3 km (3.3 mi)	460 m	(1500 ft)	4.3 km (2.7 mi)	11.0+ km (7.0+ mi)
2487	Phenyl isocyanate	155 m	(500 ft)	1.1 km (0.7 mi)	4.8 km (3.0 mi)	460 m	(1500 ft)	4.0 km (2.5 mi)	11.0+ km (7.0+ mi)
2488	Cyclohexyl isocyanate	155 m	(500 ft)	1.0 km (0.6 mi)	4.7 km (2.9 mi)	460 m	(1500 ft)	3.9 km (2.4 mi)	11.0+ km (7.0+ mi)
2495	Iodine pentafluoride	DANGEROUS: When spilled in water, see list at the end of this table.							
2521	Diketene, inhibited	60 m	(200 ft)	0.2 km (0.1 mi)	0.6 km (0.4 mi)	155 m	(500 ft)	0.5 km (0.3 mi)	2.3 km (1.4 mi)
2534	Methylchlorosilane	60 m	(200 ft)	0.2 km (0.1 mi)	0.8 km (0.5 mi)	185 m	(600 ft)	0.6 km (0.4 mi)	2.9 km (1.8 mi)

FIGURE 44-10 The green section of the *Emergency Response Guidebook* (ERG) provides minimum evacuation distances.

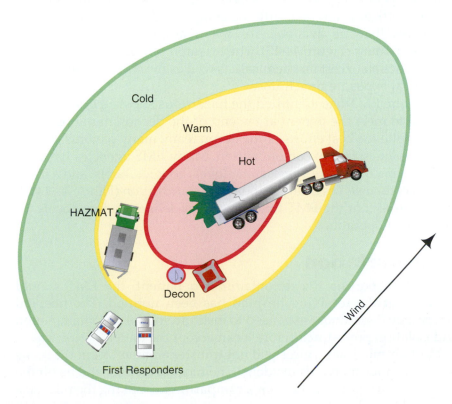

FIGURE 44-11 The area within the hot zone is contaminated.

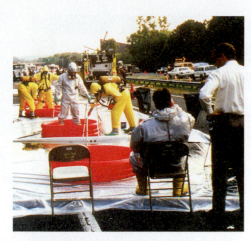

FIGURE 44-12 EMS usually awaits the arrival of patients at the end of the decontamination corridor in the cold zone. (Courtesy of the Baltimore County Fire Department.)

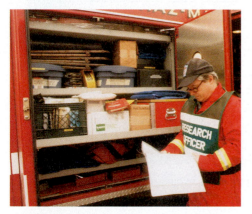

FIGURE 44-13 The great number of chemicals may require that a specialist, a research officer, be available to the incident commander.

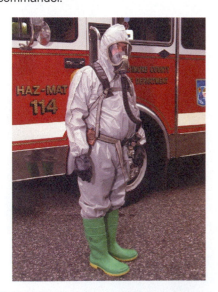

FIGURE 44-14 An EMT should wear appropriate personal protective equipment to prevent secondary contamination.

Decontamination

Specially trained responders from an emergency response team, wearing proper protective equipment, will enter and rescue patients. These patients are then carried or moved into a **decontamination corridor** (Figure 44-12). The decontamination corridor bridges the hot zone and the cold zone in an area called the warm zone. The decontamination corridor is the area where the hazardous materials are cleaned off the rescuers and patients.

The usual method of decontamination involves dilution of the substance with large amounts of water, and perhaps, chemical degradation. The decontamination, or decon, area is usually clearly marked with cones and barrier tape. There is an entrance abutting the hot zone and an exit near the cold zone. EMTs who will be transporting the patient for further medical evaluation would be at standby, at the exit in the cold zone.

Treatment

The care of a chemically exposed patient is the same as the care for a poisoned patient. First, the offending substance has to be identified. In many cases, this is more difficult than one might anticipate. There are more than 100,000 known hazardous chemicals used by industry. Many chemicals have very similar spellings. It is critically important that the EMT obtain the correct spelling of the chemical.

General first aid information to treat the chemically exposed patient is provided in the ERG, but this is often insufficient for protracted medical operations. In those cases, other resources, including poison control, must be contacted for further instructions. Many hazmat emergency response teams have a special **research officer**. The research officer is familiar with the computer databases and printed references that are available for the treatment of the chemically exposed patient (Figure 44-13). The research officer understands the mode of action of certain chemicals as well as the chemical effects and the critical exposure time frames.

Once the EMT has identified the hazardous substance, she would prepare to meet the patient at the end of the decontamination corridor. Despite the best efforts of the decon team, many patients still are not completely free of contamination. Many EMS agencies have the EMTs wear a one-piece Tyvek suit, gloves, goggles, boots, and a mask to protect themselves from secondary contamination (Figure 44-14). It is important that the EMT follow local guidelines and protocols for this type of operation.

Transportation

Before transporting the decontaminated patient, the EMT should ensure that the receiving hospital has been notified. The hospital emergency department may need to institute special decontamination and isolation procedures before it can accept the patient.

Most air medical services will not transfer a patient from the scene of a hazardous materials incident. Chemicals that may still be on the patient can off-gas into the pilot's compartment, making the pilot sick and unable to fly.

Ongoing Assessment

The complex chemical interactions that can occur make it difficult to treat the poisoned hazmat patient. The EMT should maintain a constant vigil over the patient and treat the patient as a high-priority patient.

MULTIPLE PATIENT ENCOUNTER

When an EMT arrives on a scene where there are many patients, she might think that she has to act differently. She may become confused, even overwhelmed, by the sheer number of patients. Yet, the patient care approach for a hundred patients is the same as the patient care approach for one patient.

Someone has to be the leader to direct the activities of others on arrival and throughout the call. In some systems, this may be a crew chief or a lieutenant. In a major incident, it would be the incident commander.

A crew chief is responsible for the safety of the crew and the patient. In a major incident, this would be the safety officer. (The responsibilities of the various officers are described later in this chapter.)

The ambulance has to be positioned in anticipation of transporting the patient to the hospital. Typically, the emergency vehicle operator

✦ *School Bus Accident*

A truck loaded with topsoil was making its way down Route 7, lumbering along at a leisurely 30 miles per hour when it approached Cornish Hill. Easing the truck into low gear, the driver had already started the descent when he realized that he had lost his brakes.

Concerned about what was ahead, the trucker frantically sounded his airhorn and tried to downshift. Glancing ahead, his heart stopped. Crosswise in the middle of the road was a school bus. There was no way to avoid the crash. He just braced for impact.

Sitting on the opposite corner was Officer Lee, sipping his coffee and just observing the intersection. He suddenly realized what was going to happen. Dropping his coffee in his lap, he picked up the radio and shouted, "School bus accident, corner of Route 7 and Cornish Hill." He then bounded from the patrol car to the carnage that was before him.

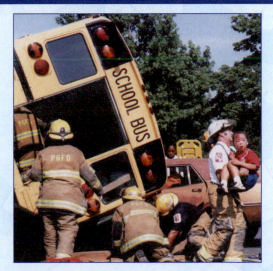

(Courtesy of Craig Smith.)

- What is the responsibility of the first-arriving emergency responder to the scene of a major incident?
- What are the advantages of the Incident Management System?
- What are the various officers in the EMS sector?
- What are the roles and duties of these officers?
- How does a major incident compare to a typical EMS call?

(EVO) prepares the ambulance for the arrival of the patient. In a major incident, this would be the staging officer.

Someone has to go to the patient and assess the patient, decide whether the patient is high or low priority, and then communicate that decision to the crew. Often this is the EMT attendant. In a major incident, this would be the triage officer.

Someone has to treat the patient. This, again, is usually the EMT attendant or a team of EMTs and/or first responders. In a major incident, this would be the treatment officer.

Finally, someone has to notify the communications center, as well as the hospital, that the patient is being transported to the hospital. The EVO would normally perform these tasks. In a major incident, these tasks would be performed by the transportation officer.

On a routine call for EMS, each member of the crew assumes many roles in the course of providing patient care. When the number of patients increases, the roles must be distributed to other supporting personnel.

Yet, the tasks and objectives remain essentially the same. An EMT, with the assistance of supporting personnel, has a duty to provide emergency medical care to sick and injured patients.

An EMT must remember that the tasks that need to be accomplished for many patients are the same as the tasks that need to be completed for one patient. The EMT must then delegate those responsibilities to others.

THE MULTIPLE CASUALTY INCIDENT

A **multiple casualty incident (MCI)** can be defined as "more patients than EMTs." In some systems, as few as three patients constitutes an MCI. Some EMS systems make a distinction between a smaller and a larger number of patients, calling a smaller number of patients a **limited victim incident (LVI)** and a larger number of patients an MCI. This distinction is useful for assigning roles and responsibilities. The responsibilities do not change, just the number of people performing them.

For example, at a collision between a school bus and a passenger car, where there are only minor injuries, it may only be necessary to establish a triage and treatment center. In other cases, where there are sufficient ambulances immediately available, it may not be necessary to establish a treatment area. These examples of an LVI can often be dealt with by establishing just the EMS sector described later in this chapter.

Public Safety Incident Management System

At a major incident, there may be many other problems, beyond just providing patient care. A public safety incident may be the result of criminal activity. Whenever there is a crime, law enforcement will become involved. Some of these public safety emergencies are spawned by fire or spilled hazardous chemicals. Fire suppression and hazard mitigation is the responsibility of the fire service.

Some public safety emergencies, such as floods, are protracted events, going on for weeks and even months. Public safety personnel would have to be fed, housed, and periodically relieved during these incidents.

The only way to deal with the complexities of these scenes is to develop a management approach that is flexible as well as expandable. This management system includes the leadership of all three emergency services at the local, state, and federal levels, as well as allows for industry participation.

The complexity of the problem of managing a large-scale incident came to a pinnacle after a series of tragic wildfires in California in the fall of 1970. The fragmented and disjointed efforts by the large number of public services (police, fire, and EMS) present resulted in less-than-satisfactory results.

Public safety leaders, supported by work from the original FIREscope project, advanced the concept of the Incident Command System (ICS). Over the years, the ICS has evolved into the present Public Safety Incident Management System.

The **Incident Management System (IMS)** is a system of organization and administration that involves all emergency service providers and provides for a calculated response to the typical challenges faced at a large-scale event. The IMS focuses on the three critical tasks of incident management, namely, command, control, and communications. Table 44-1 highlights the characteristics of the IMS.

Incident Command

The Incident Management System requires that there be an **incident commander (IC)** for every incident. The IC is in command and has overall responsibility for the entire incident.

There are two forms of incident command: singular and unified. Each form has its place in the management of a public safety incident. In a smaller incident involving just one agency, it makes sense that the head of the service, for example, the police chief, would be the incident commander.

In larger incidents or multijurisdictional incidents, several service leaders may share joint command. The advantages of a joint "unified" command are several. For example, when resources are limited, services can share assets.

There may be a fire chief, police chief, and EMS chief in the **command post**. The command post is a centralized location, often off site, where the heads of public safety agencies gather and regulate on-scene operations (Figure 44-15). Each chief is responsible for her own service, but all share the responsibility for incident management.

Often the leadership within a unified command rotates according to the incident needs. For example, in a house fire, initially fire suppression is the first priority. Naturally, the fire service takes prominence at this time. As victims are rescued, EMS may take dominance. Finally, after the fire is extinguished, the police arson investigators may have priority.

Chain of Command

The IC must delegate her responsibilities to others and still remain in control of the incident. In other words, others are assigned roles and

---

TABLE 44-1

Characteristics of the Incident Management System

1. **Agency autonomy:** Each emergency service must still be able to operate under its command structure.

2. **Effective span of control:** Supervisors must effectively oversee the individuals assigned to them.

3. **Modular organization:** As the incident expands in either size or length of time, the system must be able to accommodate the change.

4. **Common terminology:** Organizational positions and tasks must have commonly recognized titles.

5. **Common action plan:** Officers discuss approaches so as to not to be at cross-purposes.

6. **Management by objective:** Objectives must be clearly stated and achievable.

7. **Functional clarity:** Each group must understand its specific purpose.

8. **Integrated communications:** A means by which all emergency services officers can communicate with one another.

9. **Comprehensive resource management:** The ability of commanders and officers to share and save resources.

10. **Shared support:** Utilization of common support staff by all emergency services, such as a public information officer.

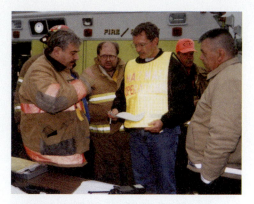

FIGURE 44-15 The incident commander establishes an incident command post. (Courtesy of David J. Reimer Sr.)

duties, but each reports to a supervisor, who ultimately reports to the incident commander. This reporting mechanism is called the **chain of command**.

The chain of command ensures that the IC and others in the chain of command have the best information about current conditions. The chain of command also permits the IC to stand back and look at the larger perspective. An IC cannot be giving detailed instructions for every activity, micromanaging, and still be able to comprehend the complexity of a large event.

The chain of command assumes delegation of authority. The IC delegates authority to others, who in turn assign tasks and duties. Borrowing from business management principles, a manager cannot supervise more than six or eight subordinates at one time. Limited supervisory responsibility is called span of control. By limiting span of control, the IC ensures the best supervision of personnel. Figure 44-16 illustrates the hierarchy of the chain of command.

Command Personnel

There are often several officers attached to the incident commander. These officers are charged with certain functional duties that are common to all services and all incidents.

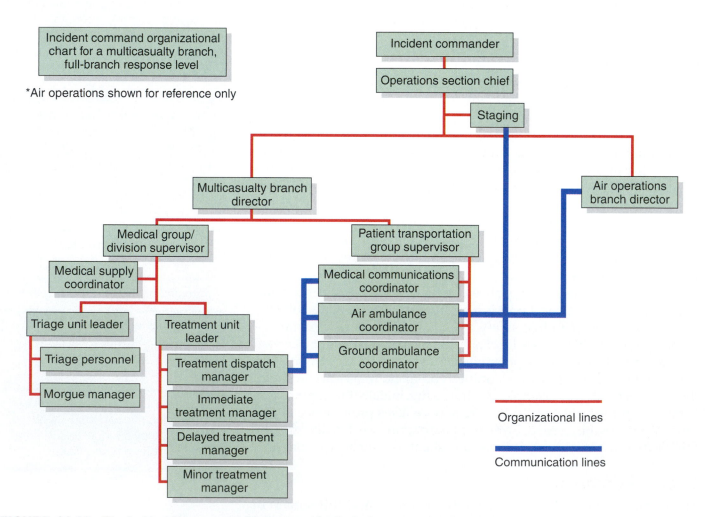

FIGURE 44-16 The Incident Management System provides for both command and control.

Safety Officer The **safety officer (SO)** is designated by the incident commander and is responsible for the safety of all personnel. The SO should be a trained person who understands the common hazards seen at an incident, as well as techniques to mitigate those hazards.

The SO should understand all applicable safety codes, including the Occupational Safety and Health Administration (OSHA) regulations and the National Fire Protection Association (NFPA) recommendations.

The SO has special emergency authority and can countermand any order given, including an order by the IC. The SO exercises that authority to stop unsafe actions and protect the lives of personnel on scene (Figure 44-17).

If the IC does not assign an SO, the IC retains the responsibility and the liability for the safety of all personnel on the scene.

Public Information Officer

A public safety incident is a newsworthy event in most communities. Agents for the media will appear on almost any scene and ask for information about the incident. It is the responsibility of the incident commander to respond to these requests.

The IC may decide to assign a **public information officer (PIO)** to meet with the media and report the state of affairs at the incident (Figure 44-18). In larger systems, the media will start to identify the PIO and seek her out.

The IC may also decide to request that the highest elected official act as the PIO. Again, these highly visible officials remove attention from the IC and allow her to return her attention to her duties.

Role of the EMT in Incident Management

The EMT is not expected to fully understand the complexities of the entire Public Safety Incident Management System. The objective of every EMT is to understand when to activate the IMS and how to participate in the IMS as a provider.

The following section details the steps involved in activating and participating in EMS operations.

EMS OPERATIONS SECTOR

From an EMS perspective, there are five tasks in a public safety emergency. The first task is to take control of the situation, in other words, to take command. The second task is to assemble needed resources and personnel. The third task is to locate and sort the patients according to the severity of their injuries. The fourth task is to render needed medical care according to that severity. The fifth task is to transport patients for further medical evaluation as soon as possible. The IMS utilizes a group of EMS officers within the operations sector who are charged with each of these tasks.

Medical Group Supervisor

The first officer has overall responsibility for EMS operations, as well as interfacing with other emergency services commanders. When an

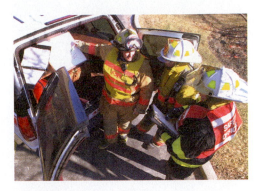
FIGURE 44-17 The safety officer reports directly to the incident commander and has responsibility for the safety of all personnel.

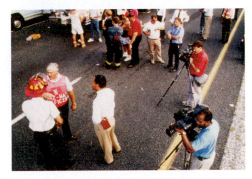
FIGURE 44-18 The public information officer interfaces with the media and the press. (Courtesy of the Baltimore County Fire Department.)

Street Smart

The very nature of most public safety incidents creates a great deal of stress in providers. When the incident is over, it is very common for special critical incident stress debriefing (CISD) teams to meet with providers. However, these CISD sessions occur after the fact, after the damage has been done. In some systems, there is a special **trauma intervention program (TIP)**. TIP teams operate in the field during an incident, identifying providers who are at risk and attempting to remove or reduce the stress on those individuals. These TIP teams operate freely throughout the arena with the permission of the IC.

EMT is in charge of the first-arriving unit, she should establish her authority as the person in charge of EMS. The EMT would assume the title of **medical group supervisor** until she is relieved by another, higher-ranking EMS officer.

The next task is to establish a command post. Some systems use a flag or even a traffic cone to denote the command post, while others have command vehicles such as a paramedic supervisor's car. Establishing a command post helps direct other responding chief officers to a central location. In many cases, a simple over-the-air declaration is all that is needed, for example, "Medcom, this is unit 24 establishing EMS command at the corner of Madison and Lark."

If a command post already exists, for example, the fire chief has established a command post, then the medical group supervisor should link up with the fire chief and create a unified command post.

After determining the nature of the incident, and perhaps the potential number of casualties, the IC should make a declaration. A declaration, often called the first-in report, communicates the problem present and the resources that may be needed to resolve the problem. An example of a first-in report might be: "Unit 24 reporting a school bus struck by a dump truck, possible 40 victims, smoke showing. EMS command is declaring an MCI and will be going to Plan B. Please send heavy rescue." Table 44-2 summarizes the elements needed in a declaration.

If a large number of resources is needed, a preplanned disaster response system may have to be activated. By declaring a "Plan B," as in the preceding example, the EMT knows which police, fire, and other EMS units will be dispatched to her location.

Some EMS systems have created **tactical command sheets**. These tactical command sheets provide specific instructions for how to proceed with managing a specific incident (Figure 44-19). While these tactical command sheets can be very useful, they are only a tool. The EMT must evaluate each scene individually and consider what resources may be needed.

TABLE 44-2

Elements of the First-In Report

1. Incident location—with cross street if available	5. What is the initial victim estimate?
2. Type and cause of incident— as much as known	6. What are the probable injuries?
3. Is the incident open, with victims accessible, or closed, victims inaccessible and need rescue?	7. What is the best access to the scene for other responders?
	8. Where should staging be located?
4. Is the incident contained, the cause ceased or continuing, the danger persistent?	9. What additional resources are needed?
	10. What preplan is being utilized?

GUILDERLAND EMS Incident Tactical Work Sheet

Call Location_____ Medical Command Location_____

_____Establish unified command with Fire & Police · _____Put on EMS Command bib _____Advise inbound units where to stage
_____Designate Triage Officer   _____Advise crews to stay with units until given instructions
_____Advise units to switch radios to 7.15.(Level 2 & Level 3) **LEVEL 1, RESCUES & SIGNAL 30's STAY ON GEMS CHANNEL.**

Level 1 3-6 Patients	Level 2 7 - 15 Patients	Level 3 16 + Patients	Rehab & Rescues	Signal 30 (Major Fires)
_____ Declare MCI _____ EMS All Call _____ Request other units _____ Cover Town ALS _____ Cover Town BLS _____ Roll Call Hospitals	_____ Declare MCI _____ EMS All Call _____ Request other units _____ Cover Town ALS _____ Cover Town BLS _____ Roll Call Hospitals _____ Call in EMS Coordintor _____ Call in Medical Director _____ Medical Supply _____ Transport Officer _____ Treatment Officer _____ Staging Officer _____ Field Com.	_____ Declare MCI _____ EMS All Call _____ Request other units _____ Cover Town ALS _____ Cover Town BLS _____ Roll Call Hospitals _____ Call in EMS Coordintor _____ Call in Medical Director _____ Medical Supply _____ Transport Officer _____ Treatment Officer _____ Staging Officer _____ Field Com.	_____ Assess # and Types of Units Needed. (With Fire Command) _____ Establish Perimeter _____ Designate Triage Area _____ Designate Rehab Area _____ Second BLS Unit ? _____ Second ALS Unit ? _____ Medical Supply ?	_____ Establish Perimeter _____ Designate Triage Area _____ Designate Rehab Area _____ Call in EMS Coordinator _____ Call in Medical Director _____ Second BLS Unit ? _____ Second ALS Unit ? _____ Medical Supply ? _____ Transport Officer ? _____ Treatment Officer ? _____ Staging Officer ?
3 - 5 Ambulances Needed	6 - 10 Ambulances Needed	11 + Ambulances Needed		

Hospital Roll Call	AMCH	ST. PETERS	MEMORIAL	VA	ELLIS	ST. CLARES	ST. MARYS	SAMARITAIN
CAN TAKE								
# PT. SENT								

NUMBER OF PATIENTS BY PRIORITY

1 (RED)	2 (YELLOW)	3 (GREEN)	0 (BLACK)	TOTAL

RESPONDING UNITS			
GUILDERLAND	M15_____ M18_____ M19_____ M30_____ R1_____ R5_____ R40_____ R50_____ R60_____ MED. SUPPLY_____ EMS20_____ EMS5_____ EMS10_____	BETHLEHAM ONESQUETHAW RAVENA ROTTERDAM	5181_____ 5182_____ 2585_____ 2687_____ 2689_____ A10_____ A30_____
COLONIE	621_____ 622_____ 631_____ 632_____ 641_____ 642_____ 651_____ 652_____ 653_____		A40_____ A32_____
ALBANY COUNTY VOORHEESVILLE HELDERBURG DELMAR	M1_____ M2_____ M3_____ 5680_____ 5685_____ 5384_____ 5386_____ 5388_____ 0981_____	DUANSBURG MOHAWK CAPITAL DISTRICT	

FIGURE 44-19 Tactical command sheets provide the EMT with a standardized approach that must be customized for each incident. (Reprinted with permission of Guilderland Emergency Medical Services, Guilderland, NY.)

Transfer of Command

To prevent any interruptions in operations and to decrease the likelihood of miscommunication, whenever another person such as an EMT or a high-ranking official assumes EMS command, she will need a **briefing**. A briefing is usually performed one on one, as one EMS commander provides the most up-to-date information about the current state of affairs (Figure 44-20). Any tactical command sheets that were used are reviewed, as well as any status boards. A transfer of command and the responsibility of command is not completed until the new commander accepts the report. Often this acceptance of command is acknowledged over the air, for example, "Medcom, supervisor fifteen is assuming EMS command." The duties of the EMS commander are summarized in Table 44-3.

Staging Officer

Without clear instructions, incoming units will proceed directly to the scene. Within minutes the scene may be a mass of emergency vehicles, each interfering with the other. To prevent this chaos, a **staging area** is usually established.

A staging area is an off-scene location where personnel and vehicles assemble and await assignment. A typical staging area is a parking

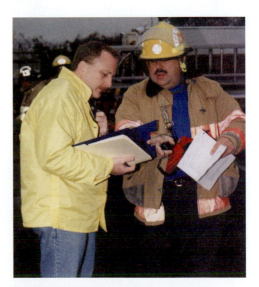

FIGURE 44-20 EMS command is transferred only after a complete situational briefing. (Courtesy of David J. Reimer Sr.)

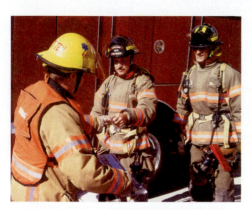

FIGURE 44-21 The staging officer assembles needed vehicles, personnel, and equipment.

TABLE 44-3

Medical Group Supervisor	
Duties	9. Authorizes release of information
1. Assesses the situation	10. Terminates the incident
2. Establishes command	**Personnel**
3. Declares the emergency	Chief officer
4. Establishes a command post	Public information officer
5. Implements any preplans	Safety officer

6. Appoints officers
   Safety
   Staging
   Triage
   Treatment
   Transportation
	Trauma intervention team
	
	Clerical personnel
	
	Runners
	
	Equipment

7. Coordinates scene resources	Radio
8. Coordinates with chiefs of other services	MCI plan
	Command post identifier/vest

TABLE 44-4

Staging Officer
Duties
1. Establishes a safe assembly point
2. Assembles and inventories resources
3. Ensures support and services to personnel within staging area
4. Releases resources to meet operational needs
Personnel
Assistants
Equipment
Radio
MCI plan
Identifier/vest

lot or restaurant. The staging area should be close enough to the scene of the incident that units could be on scene within minutes.

As resources are needed, the IC or one of her officers would call the staging area and speak to the staging officer. A **staging officer** acts as a manager of the area, assembling and assigning equipment and personnel to specific duties or tasks (Figure 44-21). The duties of the staging officer are outlined in Table 44-4.

Equipment Staging

In some special operations, such as confined space rescue, or in larger incidents, there may be an equipment manager. An equipment manager assembles and maintains a stock of needed supplies.

Triage Officer

During an MCI, the survival of some patients will depend on the effective utilization of limited resources. This utilization is best accomplished by prioritizing patients based on urgency, using a process called **triage**. Triage is a system of distribution of patients into treatment classifications according to their injury severity.

The objective of triage is to do the most good for the greatest number of patients. During an MCI, there are situations in which some patients who have serious injuries might survive, but only if a considerable amount of resources are expended. These resources are, quite simply, not available or are in high demand.

In those cases, the **triage officer** is in the unenviable position of deciding who shall live and who shall die. The triage officer oversees the triage process. However, if triage does not occur and resources are wasted on a patient in a hopeless cause, then others will die needlessly.

Any EMT can be trained to perform triage. In fact, at a MCI, several EMTs may be needed to triage all of the patients quickly. However, only one EMT, the triage officer, would report casualties to the IC. The duties of the triage officer are outlined in Table 44-5.

Triage Systems

An evacuation triage is frequently the first triage performed. These evacuation triages are frequently two-tiered systems; the patient is either immediate or delayed. This triage determines which patients are removed by rescuers immediately. In some systems, surveyor's tape is used to identify the patient's status. Red is for immediate evacuation, and green is for delayed.

As patients are evacuated, frequently to a forward triage point, a treatment or transport triage is performed. Once there, all patients are categorized into one of four classifications. Each classification has an assigned color that signifies the patient's condition.

The color red signifies that the patient is high priority or immediate. This patient is seriously injured but has a chance of survival, provided he gets immediate medical care.

The color yellow indicates that the patient is in need of medical attention but may wait or be delayed while more immediate patients are being treated.

The color green indicates that the patient has minor injuries. Often these patients are referred to as the *walking wounded*. In a larger MCI, the assistance of these patients is sometimes requested to treat other more seriously injured patients.

Finally, the color black indicates that the patient is either dead or dying from mortal wounds. Sometimes termed expectant, these patients are extremely critical and will probably die. These patients are the last to be removed from scene.

START Triage System

There are several triage systems in existence. One system that has gained increasing popularity is the **START Triage System**. START stands for *simple triage and rapid treatment*. The START system's popularity is, in part, because it can be performed by firefighters wearing full turnout gear and, in part, because of its simplicity.

A START triage begins with separating the walking wounded. If the patient is ambulatory, he is labeled green or delayed. If the patient is unable to walk, the EMT proceeds to assess the patient's breathing. If the patient is not breathing, the EMT manually opens the airway. If the patient takes a breath, he is immediate. If he is still not breathing, he is expectant or nonsalvageable.

The EMT would then proceed to assess the rate of respiration. If the patient's breathing is rapid, greater than 30 breaths per minute, the patient is classified as red or immediate. If the breathing is less than 30

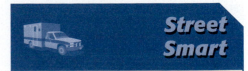

Street Smart

One of the most disruptive influences on the scene of an MCI can be the arrival of nonrequested personnel. Although well meaning, these EMTs have not been assigned to a task or given a responsibility.

Rather than request that these potentially valuable human resources depart the scene, the IC could direct these EMTs to the staging area. Then the staging officer can assign these EMTs to other EMS units awaiting assignment.

TABLE 44-5
Triage Officer

Duties

1. Performs the first evacuation triage

2. Appoints assistants as needed

3. Performs second treatment/transportation triage as needed

4. Coordinates EMS activities on scene

5. Coordinates patient movement to triage and/or transportation

Personnel

Extrication officer

Triage support personnel

Patient handlers

Equipment

Radio

MCI plan

Identifier/vest

Long backboards

Triage tags

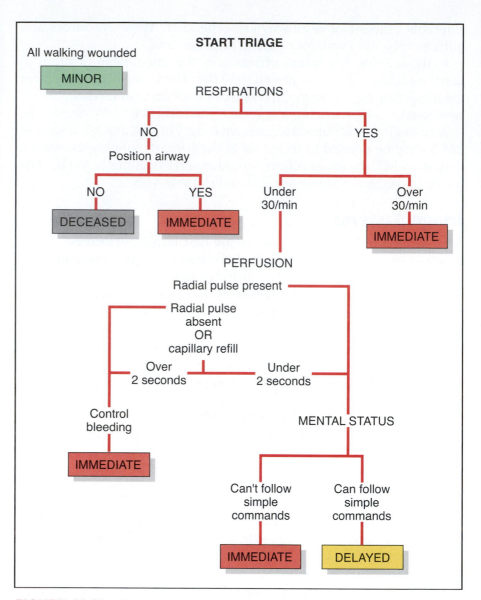

FIGURE 44-22 START stands for *simple triage and rapid treatment.*

breaths per minute or is slower than a breath every other second, the EMT assesses the patient's radial pulse. If there is no radial pulse, the patient is classified immediate. Control of gross external bleeding is accomplished at this time.

If there is a pulse, the EMT proceeds to assess the patient's mental status. If the patient can follow simple commands, he is labeled delayed, otherwise he is labeled immediate. This system is illustrated in Figure 44-22.

Triage Tags

Once a patient's classification has been determined, a **triage tag** is placed on either the wrist (more common) or the foot. A triage tag, also called a disaster tag, is a shortened patient care document utilized during times of mass disaster (Figure 44-23). The triage tag allows other EMTs to quickly identify the patient's condition, as well as prevent duplication of effort.

There are a number of triage tag systems on the market. Most use the four-colored triage system. At the bottom, the tag has tear-off tabs.

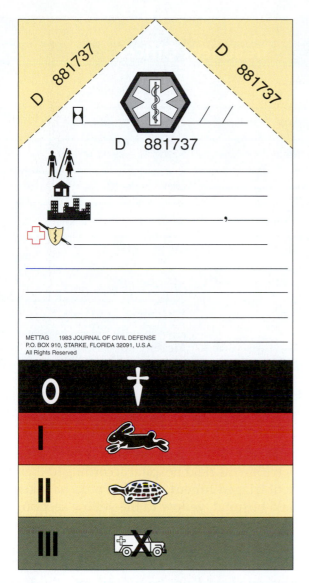

GREEN (bottom strip):
   Symbol: Ambulance–crossed out
   Meaning: No hospital treatment needed; first aid only
YELLOW (second strip from bottom):
   Symbol: Turtle
   Meaning: Nonurgent; hospital care
RED (third strip from bottom):
   Symbol: Rabbit
   Meaning: Urgent; hospital care
Black (fourth strip from bottom):
   Symbol: Cross/dagger
   Meaning: Dead or unsalvageable; no CPR

FIGURE 44-23   The triage tag provides a quick means of communication. (Courtesy of American Civil Defense Association, Starke, FL.)

Every tag must have a means to attach the tag to the patient, as well as a stamped identification number for tracking the patient.

Treatment Officer

A treatment sector is set up whenever patients cannot be transported off scene immediately. The center of the treatment sector is the **field hospital**. The field hospital is a temporary on-site treatment facility. The field hospital is managed by the **treatment officer**. Typically, the incident commander assigns a paramedic to set up the field hospital and act as the treatment officer.

The first task of the treatment officer is to select a suitable area for the field hospital. In a large incident, a centralized area convenient to the scene is desirable. The treatment officer may also be concerned about inhospitable weather. Whenever possible, the treatment sector should be established uphill and upwind of the incident with unimpeded access for ambulances and other emergency vehicles.

TABLE 44-6

Treatment Officer

Duties	Patient handlers
1. Establishes medical stabilization	Clerical personnel
2. Allocates advanced life support (ALS) resources	Medical examiner
3. Reevaluates as necessary	**Equipment**
4. Coordinates EMS activities within the field hospital	Radio
5. Coordinates patient movement to transportation	MCI plan
Personnel	Identifier/vest
	Stretchers
Medical personnel (MD, PA, RN)	Medical equipment
Medical support personnel	Triage tags

Using their triage classification, patients would be distributed to corresponding areas within the field hospital according to their triage. For example, a patient triaged urgent, or red, would be taken to the red section of the field hospital, yellow to the yellow section, and so on. The duties of the treatment officer are summarized in Table 44-6.

Morgue

Patients tagged deceased should not be moved into the treatment area. The impact on patient morale would prohibit it. Instead, these patients should be placed in a separate area called a **morgue**, which is an area set aside for the collection of the deceased. This area should be shielded from public view and secured from unwanted intruders.

Funeral directors have a team that will respond to a disaster and establish morgue services. The professionals on the team, called the *D-Mort*, are an invaluable aid to EMS operations.

Transportation Officer

The **transportation officer** is responsible for the overall movement of patients from the scene to the appropriate hospitals. The transportation officer is also responsible for maintaining communications with the various hospitals, ensuring that no single hospital is being overloaded.

The transportation officer is responsible for tracking the patients' whereabouts for all patients from the scene. The transportation officer uses the identification number stamped on the triage tag to identify which patients are transported to the hospital. This information is entered on the transportation log.

Typically, patients are transported via an ambulance, called up from the staging area. In some cases, it may be more efficient to transport minor, or walking wounded, patients aboard buses. The transportation officer may also be responsible for coordinating air medical evacuation. The duties of the transportation officer are summarized in Table 44-7.

CONCLUSION

A major incident need not be a disaster for an EMT. The EMT need only keep her own safety at the forefront of her mind, while systematically delegating the tasks that she would normally perform on an average call. The first EMT would do a scene assessment, using her hazmat training, then delegate another EMT to perform multiple patient assessments or triage. Next, the EMT would institute treatment by establishing a field hospital and then commence transportation through the transportation officer. The standard approach to a major incident is much the same as the standard approach to any patient, only on a much greater scale.

TEST YOUR KNOWLEDGE

1. What are the indications of the presence of hazardous materials?
2. What is the role of an EMT on the scene of a hazardous materials incident?
3. How does an EMT use the *Emergency Response Guidebook*?
4. What areas would be in the hot zone, cold zone, and warm zone?
5. What are the different hazardous materials identification systems in use for fixed facilities and transportation?
6. What is the initial role of an EMT on the scene of a multiple casualty incident?
7. What is the Public Safety Incident Management System?
8. What is the chain of command?
9. What are the roles of the following officers?
   Safety
   Public information
   Staging
   Triage
   Treatment
   Transportation
10. What is the START Triage System?

INTERNET RESOURCES

Additional resources on hazardous materials incidents can be found at these Web sites:

- HazMat Management Buyers' Guide, http://www.hazmatmag.com

TABLE 44-7

Transportation Officer

Duties

1. Establishes and maintains ambulance loading area
2. Supervises patient evacuation
3. Coordinates with triage officer
4. Coordinates with staging officer
5. Supervises the hospital communication network

Personnel

Hospital liaison

Clerical personnel

Runners

Equipment

Radio

MCI plan

Ambulances

Patient destination logs

Street Smart

When an MCI is declared and a hospital notified, the hospital may elect to implement its own emergency plan. When a hospital declares an emergency, extra staff are called into work and other patients are either discharged or diverted. After the last patient has been transported, either the transportation officer or the incident commander must notify the hospitals so that they can return to normal operations.

- U.S. Department of Transportation, Research and Special Programs Administration, Office of Hazardous Materials Safety, http://hazmat.dot.gov
- U.S. Fire Administration, http://www.usfa.fema.gov
- U.S. National Oceanic and Atmospheric Administration, Office of Response and Restoration, National Ocean Service, http://response.restoration.noaa.gov

Using key terms related to this chapter conduct additional searches for more information on public safety and incident management.

FURTHER STUDY

Christen, H., & Maniscalco, P. (1998). EMS incident management: The treatment sector in mass casualty events. *Emergency Medical Services, 27*(6), 28–40.

Christen, H., & Maniscalco, P. (1999). EMS incident management: Emergency medical logistics. *Emergency Medical Services, 28*(1), 49–53.

Christen, H., Maniscalco, P., & Rubin, D. (1999). EMS incident management: Traits and characteristics of the incident safety officer. *Emergency Medical Services, 28*(6), 85–90.

Christen, H., Maniscalco, P., & Rubin, D. (2000). EMS incident management: Duties of the incident safety officer. *Emergency Medical Services, 29*(3), 53–57.

Criss, E., et al. (1998). Not just blowing smoke. *Emergency Medical Services, 27*(3) 27–33.

Mack, D. (1999). Team EMS. *Journal of Emergency Medical Services, 24*(7), 36–44.

Maniscalco, P., & Rubin, D. (1998a). EMS incident management: Personnel roles and responsibilities. *Emergency Medical Services, 28*(4), 64–69.

Maniscalco, P., & Rubin, D. (1998b). EMS incident management: The safety sector. *Emergency Medical Services, 27*(11), 59–62.

Maniscalco, P., & Rubin, D. (2000). EMS incident management: Operational communications. *Emergency Medical Services, 29*(5), 93–97.

Streger, M. (1998). Prehospital triage. *Emergency Medical Services, 27*(6), 21–28.

Streger, M. (1999). Mass casualty and disaster communications. *Emergency Medical Services, 28*(4), 59–63.

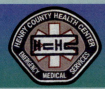 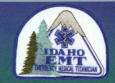 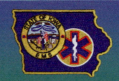

CHAPTER 45

Rescue Operations

KEY TERMS

clues
confined space
cribbing
flapping the roof
flat water
forcible entry
forcing the door
hasty search
heavy rescue
high life hazard
loaded bumpers
Nader pin
personal flotation device
　(PFD)
point of contact (POC)
preplan
redundancy
rescue
rolling the dash
safety glass
snag lines
step-blocks
swift water
technical rescue
tempered glass
throw bag
undertow
window punch

OBJECTIVES

Upon completion of this chapter, the reader should be able to:

1. Indicate when a technical rescue is needed.
2. Identify the phases common to all rescues.
3. Select the appropriate personal protective equipment for specific hazards of rescue.
4. Recognize situations of confined space rescue.
5. Explain the common hazards encountered in confined space.
6. Restate how the standard of care implies that an EMT must have special training for technical rescue.
7. Recognize the hazards at a motor vehicle collision.
8. Explain the importance of stabilizing a motor vehicle before proceeding with a rescue.
9. Differentiate between heavy rescue and rapid extrication.
10. Describe the three most common means of extrication from a vehicle using heavy rescue.
11. Differentiate flat water from swift water rescue.
12. Describe how a shore-based rescue is established for flat water.
13. Describe how a shore-based rescue is established for swift water.
14. Describe what a hasty search is and how to perform one.
15. Explain the importance of searching for clues during a search and rescue operation.

OVERVIEW

A **rescue** is an attempt by a person to help another person who is incapable of freeing herself and who is in danger if she remains in that situation. If this incapacity is due to illness or injury, then an emergency medical technician (EMT) may be involved in the rescue effort. In almost all rescues, the patient is in need of medical care, and an EMT should be immediately available.

If the patient has died as a result of her injuries, then the operation is a not a rescue but a recovery—a recovery of the body. Without a live patient, there can be no rescue. Medical care provided by an EMT on scene can make the difference between a mission being a rescue or becoming a recovery.

The following cases represent some common hazards and rescue situations that are seen in many communities in the United States. Every community should have a plan for how to respond to these types of emergencies. The following is intended as an overview of rescue techniques only. An EMT should not expect to be knowledgeable about rescue techniques after reading this text alone. Additional training, as well as extensive preparation, is required before an EMT should attempt any rescue. An EMT should always follow his local procedures and protocols before attempting any rescue.

PHASES OF THE RESCUE

All rescues, whether an exciting wildlands search, a dramatic heavy rescue, or simply a "breaking and entering" to help an elderly person who is incapable of reaching the door, have phases similar to a routine emergency call. There is a scene assessment phase, a treatment phase,

---

✳ *No Access*

The caller cried out, "I've fallen, and I can't get up!" Apparently, the elderly woman had fallen during the night and was only able to crawl on her hands to the Lifeline to call for help. That effort took her all night. She sounded exhausted as she tried to explain her situation. Lifeline had called both 9-1-1 and the neighbor who was listed as "responder."

The house, a sturdy little brick cottage, was at the end of a winding lane. The neighbor, who was already at the house, explained that the house was completely locked from the inside and that there was no way in.

As the neighbor talked hurriedly to the crew chief, a new EMT, whose name was Trevor, started to look in windows. He called out that he could see the patient lying on the kitchen floor, waving and smiling at him as he peered through the window. The EMT could not hear her through the window, but she kept pointing to her hip. Tears were rolling down her cheeks, and Trevor thought to himself, "She's putting up a brave front, but she's obviously in a great deal of pain."

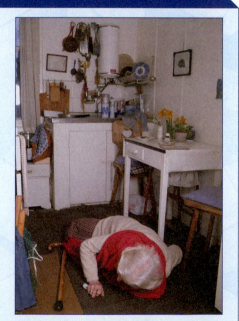

(Courtesy of PhotoDisc.)

- What are the phases of a rescue operation?
- What is the difference between a simple rescue and a technical rescue?
- What are some common hazards on the scene of a rescue?
- Why are confined space rescues dangerous?
- What would be a typical approach to a locked entry call?

and a transportation phase. A few fundamental differences make rescues distinct from the average emergency medical services (EMS) call.

A rescue typically takes place in an unusual environment or situation, such as the bottom of a cave or the top of a building. A rescue also requires special knowledge and/or equipment to access, disentangle, and rescue the patient.

Every EMT should have an awareness of which types of rescue situations may occur in his community and what special personnel and rescue equipment may be needed to rescue patients. No EMT should ever enter a rescue scene before he has been trained and is proficient at these special rescue techniques and the use of the equipment. Without a higher "technical" level of training, the EMT may endanger himself, his crew, and the patient needlessly while trying to help the patient. In the worst-case scenario, the EMT may become a victim himself. If an EMT is interested in one area of rescue, then he should obtain further training from qualified rescue instructors.

Establishing Command

The first-arriving emergency services unit should immediately take control of the situation and establish scene command. In some jurisdictions, command and control is shared by several agencies in a unified command structure, with each emergency service commander supervising his own service. In other jurisdictions, a singular command structure identified by the presence of an incident commander is utilized. More information regarding public safety incident management can be found in Chapter 44.

Scene Size-Up

After arriving on scene, the EMT proceeds with a scene size-up. To help maintain a more global perspective and see the big picture, the EMT should start his observation from a distance. A pair of binoculars can help the EMT get the details of what is happening on scene without placing himself and his crew in harm's way. This "environmental assessment," discussed more fully in Chapter 12, will provide the EMT with much-needed information.

The first part of a scene size-up is a risk assessment. A risk assessment prompts the EMT to think about hazards present on scene and how to control or mitigate those hazards.

Next, the EMT requests any additional resources that would be required to secure the scene and control the hazards. For example, the presence of smoke at a motor vehicle collision (MVC) should prompt the EMT to request assistance from the fire department. The request for additional assistance from heavy rescue, for example, may have come when the original dispatch information was obtained or when the first unit arrived. It is important that if additional resources are called, they are called at the earliest moment that the need is identified. Often this moment occurs during the scene size-up.

If the scene has a considerable number of hazards, the EMT should consider assigning a safety officer. The responsibility of the safety officer, outlined in Chapter 44, is to ensure the well-being of rescuers.

Before crew members exit from the emergency vehicle, the EMT should ensure that everyone is wearing the personal protective

TABLE 45-1

Hazards	
Hazard	**Personal Protective Equipment**
Flash and flame	Turnout coat
Falling objects	Helmet
Sharp objects	Boots, gloves
Flying debris	Goggles
Poor visibility	Highway safety vest
Loud noises	Earplugs

TABLE 45-2

Examples of Confined Spaces
Grain bins
Wells
Sewers
Storage
Manholes
Drainage culverts
Natural caves

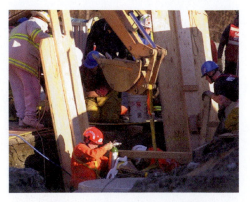

FIGURE 45-1 Entry into a confined space is limited to specially trained rescue personnel.

equipment (PPE) that will be needed. Even if the EMT is not intimately involved in the rescue, special PPE, such as gloves and eye protection, may still be in order. It is not uncommon for bits of glass to fly during a vehicle rescue.

The nature of rescue also tends to draw emergency services providers into the scene. For instance, when a patient is being extricated and another pair of hands is needed, an EMT stationed at the outer perimeter will naturally step into the action circle to help out. For this reason, all emergency services personnel who are potentially at risk should be wearing appropriate PPE. Common hazards against which an EMT can protect himself are listed in Table 45-1. Either the officer in charge or the safety officer is responsible for ensuring all emergency personnel are wearing the appropriate PPE.

Next, the EMT must determine the number of patients and the severity of their injuries. This process is called triage and must be performed before extensive medical care is rendered to any single individual. In some cases, it is impossible to determine the number of patients immediately. In other cases, it is impossible to determine the severity of the patient's injuries because the patient is either trapped or inaccessible.

Confined Space Rescue

A **confined space** is any area that has limited openings for entry or exit and is not typically designed for worker occupancy. Examples of confined spaces are listed in Table 45-2.

Confined spaces can be very hazardous to workers who are trapped inside. Gases, such as methane, can accumulate and explode. Gases such as carbon monoxide and ammonia can poison a worker. In other cases, the worker who is in an oxygen-poor environment or engulfed in grain, for example, can be suffocated.

Confined space rescue is extremely dangerous. The National Institute of Occupational Safety and Health (NIOSH) reports that more than 60% of the fatalities in confined space rescue are fatalities of the rescuers.

An EMT needs to identify when a rescue is a confined space rescue and call appropriate rescue personnel (Figure 45-1). Under no circumstances should an EMT enter a confined space without special training and equipment. All confined space rescues are technical rescues by definition.

Management

Rescues may require special techniques to access the patient. Some rescues may be accomplished with very simple tools, which should be available to every EMT. Other rescues are complex operations, called **technical rescues**, which require highly trained rescue technicians using specialized equipment (Figure 45-2).

Whenever there is a choice, the simpler means of rescuing the patient is better. Complex systems and elaborate equipment have a tendency to fail when they are needed most. An EMT might employ some simple rescue techniques while waiting for special or professional rescuers to arrive, protocols permitting. In other cases, an EMT

EMS in Action

The 9-1-1 center received an emergency call for rescue to be dispatched to a chest pain complaint. When the responding EMS unit arrived at the location, the EMS crew was presented with a major twist. The caller asked the EMS crew if they had brought their boots because the victim was located in a swamp area. The victim had been raccoon hunting and treed a raccoon when he developed chest pain.

The EMS unit, a van, followed the caller's truck down a field pathway to the swampy, riverbank location. The EMS unit became stuck in the mud near the scene location. EMS notified 9-1-1 of scene location correction. Two rescue personnel who were monitoring the radio frequency responded to the scene. One staged himself near the main roadway to detain any sightseers monitoring the radio frequency, and the other worked on getting the EMS unit out of the mud. The EMS crew on duty followed the caller $1\frac{1}{2}$ miles into the wooded swamp with an equipment-medical supply backpack.

The crew provided appropriate care in accordance to protocol. The victim was chilled from the cool fall night air and water environment, so providing warmth for the victim was an additional priority. Blankets were not plentiful, so the victim was wrapped with as many different bandages, such as Kerlix and triangular bandages, as the crew had with them. A friendly frog decided to take up residency in the victim's shirt until removed by the paramedic. An IV pole was not with the equipment, so the paramedic made a pole from a tree branch.

Once the victim was stabilized and packaged in a Stokes basket, the process of removing the victim from the scene began. Before removing the victim, a pack of wild dogs had to be chased off, leading to some excitement. Finally on the way out, a crew member decided a shortcut would be faster than the route that was taken to the scene. The shortcut ended up being a challenge of waist-deep water, which proved that tennis shoes were better than boots in the water and mud. Some of the firefighters helping to carry the victim found themselves walking out of their boots as their boots filled with water and the mud sucked them down. A rope line was secured to the basket and the victim was guided up a riverbank, along with some EMS firefighters. The victim was airlifted to the hospital while the EMS crew spent hours cleaning "swamp gas" odor and mud from themselves and the EMS equipment before restocking the EMS unit. The victim had suffered a heart attack, had a heart catheterization, and was released from the hospital the next day.

This call just proves that the EMS professional must be prepared for anything and improvise equipment needs. The call also led to improved incident command guidelines to improve safety for all personnel.

M. Jane Pollock, EMT-P, CEI
Adjunct Clinical Instructor and Education and Training Specialist
Division of Emergency Medicine
East Carolina University, Greenville, North Carolina

might be standing by with simple tools, just in case the special rescue equipment fails.

In both cases, there is a backup plan. Having a backup plan in place, in case the original plan fails, is called **redundancy**. Whenever a human life is in danger, there should always be redundancy in the rescue plan. This decreases the chances of a catastrophic outcome should one critical piece of equipment fail.

Access

The next task is to reach the patient. While this sounds easy, the reality is often quite different. The EMT should keep in mind that the average person will usually make extraordinary efforts to free herself.

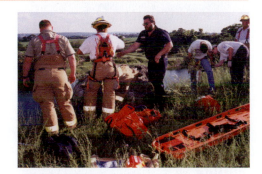

FIGURE 45-2 Technical rescue requires specialized equipment and training. (Courtesy of David J. Reimer Sr.)

The fact that the person is trapped should give the EMT an indication that ordinary efforts are not going to be sufficient.

If the EMT is trained, then he should start to make preparations for a rescue. If the EMT is not trained, then the EMT must contact someone, for example, a dive rescue team or a rope rescue team, who can rescue the patient. In the interim while waiting for the rescue to occur, the EMT should prepare or stage for the patient who will eventually be his responsibility.

Residence

In the case presented at the beginning of this chapter, the situation is an ordinary residence, and the patient is "trapped" in her own house. This situation occurs so frequently in the United States that many EMS systems have a set of special protocols, a "preplan," on how to respond to these situations. Typically, these protocols for "gaining entry" dictate that the police be on scene and reasonable efforts have been made to gain entry before the EMT resorts to force.

After confirming the address and still getting no answer at the door, the EMT should circle the house. While circling the house, the EMT should call out the patient's name loudly and repeatedly. The EMT should also consider turning on all flashing emergency lights and sounding the siren to announce his presence.

As the EMT circles the perimeter of the house, he should try to open doors and windows. The EMT should also be looking into the house trying to locate the patient. If the patient is found, the EMT should loudly announce who he is and explain that he is locked out. Then the EMT should ask the patient whether there is a hidden key or another means of entry.

It is also prudent for the EMT to ask whether there are any animals in the house. A frightened animal may attempt to protect his injured owner. If an animal is in the house, then the EMT should consider calling for the animal control officer.

Finally, the EMT should ask whether there is a security alarm system. Further efforts to gain entry will most likely set off the intruder alert. If a security alarm system is discovered, then local law enforcement needs to be notified of a possible alarm trip.

The EMT needs to weigh the severity of the emergency against the time it will take to get a locksmith to the scene for disassembly of the door. If the patient is severely injured, the decision is always life before property. If time permits, the EMT should consider requesting law enforcement or fire department assistance. Both emergency services have training and tools for forcible entry.

Forcible entry, using special tools or brute force to overcome an obstacle to gain access, can be accomplished by a number of means (Figure 45-3). Prying a window open with a crowbar or smashing out a windowpane with a flashlight are two commonly used options. Forcing a door is a possibility, using special tools, but "kicking in" the door should be avoided. Kicking in the door frequently results in a shoulder injury for the EMT, structural damage for the homeowner, and a door that is still left standing intact with a patient on the other side.

Usually a window or door farthest from the patient will be forced or broken. While this effort is going on, another EMT should be sta-

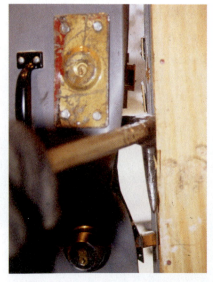

FIGURE 45-3 Using a crowbar or similar device, the EMT may be able to forcibly open a locked door.

tioned with the patient, explaining what is going to happen and keeping contact with the patient.

Rescue

Once the EMT reaches the patient, immediate lifesaving procedures should be performed, and then the patient should be prepared for transport. In some cases, the transportation is simply a flexible stretcher, such as a Reeves, while in other cases, a complex high-angle rope rescue system must be created.

Each rescue situation usually requires a rescue system. Most of these rescue systems must be brought to the scene and set up. This process can be lengthy. A little forethought on the part of the EMT can decrease time lost on scene with this setup. The system can be set up ahead of time, while the patient is being accessed by other rescuers.

Treatment

In the majority of rescues, the patient has experienced some injury, whether it is a cold injury from exposure or a traumatic injury from an MVC. The severity of an injury is always time dependent. The longer the patient goes untreated, the greater the degree of injury. Problems like crush injury and compartment syndrome can also occur. Chapters 24 and 25 contain more information on crush injury and compartment syndrome and should be reviewed. In most cases, the EMT can assume that the patient's injuries are going to be more severe than usual based on the amount of time lost getting to the patient and getting the patient to definitive care.

Transport

While immediate medical care on scene is important, it is often more important to transport to definitive medical care as soon as possible. Once the patient is moving, the EMT should consider a request for an advanced life support (ALS) intercept, if one has not already been arranged.

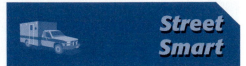

Street Smart

An EMT should be very cautious whenever he is engaged in forcible entry. Well-meaning EMTs have been shot by frightened homeowners who believe they are shooting an intruder. Some EMS systems do not permit an EMT to forcibly enter a house. In those systems, only police are allowed to forcibly enter a residence. The EMT should consider requesting law enforcement assistance whenever there is any doubt about the safety on scene.

MOTOR VEHICLE COLLISIONS

One of the most common rescues an EMT will encounter is that which results from a MVC. The weight of vehicles, sometimes going at high speeds, results in crushing of cars and the entrapment of patients.

Many patients are easily rescued from a motor vehicle after a collision. The side door is opened, and the EMT extricates the patient from the vehicle. Other patients, who are entangled and/or entrapped inside their vehicles, require the use of special vehicle extrication equipment, called **heavy rescue**, to be freed.

Preparation

Not every MVC rescue situation can be presented. However, an EMT should be aware of some of the more common scenarios. In those cases, the EMT should have previously trained with heavy rescue

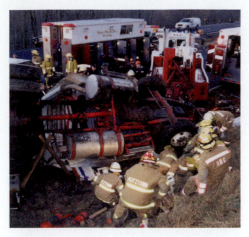

FIGURE 45-4 The ambulance may be used as a protective shield when on scene. (Courtesy of David J. Reimer Sr.)

technicians. An agreed-on plan of action, or a **preplan**, between rescuers can eliminate wasted time and confusion on the scene of a real emergency.

Every community has slightly different rescue resources, but every community has MVCs within its jurisdiction. Combined training and preplanning are the keys to a successful rescue operation and an improved patient outcome.

Command

As the first EMT approaches the scene, he should establish medical command. In most cases, that is as simple as notifying the communications center of the EMT's arrival. In other cases, a more formal declaration is needed. Chapter 44 provides a description of a first-in report.

The first and immediate concern of the EMT is scene safety. In the case of an MVC, the greatest hazard may be traffic. Every possible protection should be taken to ensure the safety of the EMT while on scene. The ambulance may be placed so that it becomes a physical barrier between the EMT and traffic (Figure 45-4).

In some systems, only rear-facing flashing lights are left on. Other revolving lights are turned off to prevent the EMT from being blinded and to prevent passing motorists from being distracted. Traffic cones, flashing lights, or flares may also help provide the EMT with a greater margin of safety. More details regarding scene safety measures can be found in Chapter 43.

✳ *Entrapped Patient*

Roy thought to himself, "How could so few guys dirty so many dishes?" Once the dishes were done, the duty crew settled down to watch an episode of *Emergency* on syndicated television. Then the bell rang twice, meaning rescue, and the loudspeaker blared, "Engine ten, Rescue nine, and the Rescue Squad respond to a rollover collision with possible entrapment. Time out 19:57."

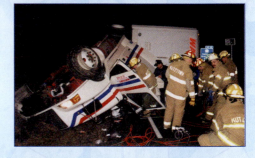

(Courtesy of David J. Reimer Sr.)

The engine company rolled up to the scene first, and the crew started to disembark. Smoke and steam were rolling up from below the embankment, making it impossible to see the scene at first. Suddenly, as the smoke cleared, Roy spotted the truck. "Over here!" yelled Roy.

As Roy looked at where he was pointing, he had a queasy feeling flood over him. At the bottom of the ravine was a tractor trailer lying on its side. The cab of the truck was twisted and resting on its roof. The roof was partially collapsed. "Well, time to go to work," thought Roy, as he grabbed a pry bar in one hand and a step–block in the other.

- What are some of the hazards present on the scene of a motor vehicle collision?
- What precautions must an EMT observe?
- How can an EMT gain quick entry?
- What can an EMT do to protect the patient while heavy rescue occurs?
- Are the transportation priorities different after heavy rescue?

Perimeters

Every motor vehicle has two perimeters or circles. The first perimeter, where there is a greater danger of injury to the EMT, is called the inner circle or the action circle. Every EMT within the inner circle should have on PPE. The outer circle is where equipment and personnel would be "staged" until needed in the inner circle or until the patient is brought out.

Every EMT who is within either the inner or outer circle should have appropriate PPE. The minimum PPE on scene of a vehicular rescue includes a safety helmet or bump cap, eye protection, a rip-resistant coat, and a pair of heavy-duty gloves. Even this PPE may not be sufficient within the action circle. The EMT should defer to the expert opinion of the rescue captain in decisions regarding PPE.

Scene Size-Up

There are other hazards on scene such as those created by the motor vehicle itself. The EMT should carefully assess the motor vehicle before beginning to treat the patient. If there is any evidence of fire, the EMT should await the arrival of the fire department. Without proper training or equipment, an EMT should never approach a burning car.

Assuming the car is not on fire, the EMT should make a "walk around." By walking around the vehicle, making a 360-degree sweep, the EMT can assess for possible hazards, as well as examine the extent of damage created by the collision.

The EMT checking the vehicle should be looking for spilled fluids (Figure 45-5). Spilled gasoline can ignite, burning the patient and EMT. Spilled antifreeze is extremely slippery. Walking on antifreeze with rubber-soled shoes or boots is akin to skating on ice. Absorbent materials, such as cat litter, placed on top of spilled antifreeze or oil can decrease the chance of an accidental slip and fall.

As of September 1998, there had been more than 2.25 million air bag deployments and a predicted 30% reduction in mortality from vehicle collision. However, rescuers have also been injured from undeployed air bags. An undeployed air bag can be activated after a collision by heat from fire or by static electricity and can crush the head of an EMT between the air bag and the patient's chest.

The EMT should always keep about 20 inches between himself and the air bag, in the event of accidental deployment. The EMT should never place a hard object, such as a shortboard, between himself and the undeployed air bag before the battery is disconnected. As soon as possible, the battery cables should be disconnected, deactivating the air bag by allowing the capacitor to drain its power. In most cases, the capacitor that powers the air bag will be drained in less than 30 seconds. Lists of capacitor drain times are available from the United States Department of Transportation (USDOT) and automobile manufacturers. To disconnect battery power, the EMT would start with the negative terminal. If the negative cable is being cut, it should be cut twice to avoid arcing back to the battery. Then the positive cable should be cut. Now power to the capacitor has been disconnected, and the air bag capacitor should drain its power quickly.

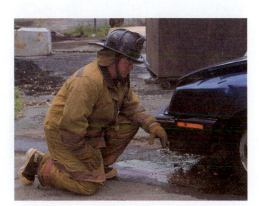

FIGURE 45-5 Spilled fluids such as antifreeze can be slippery and dangerous.

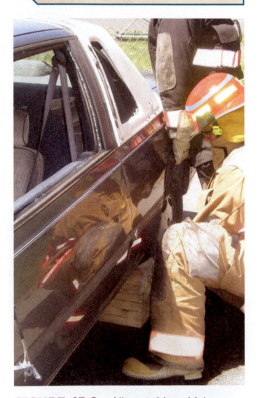

FIGURE 45-6 All unstable vehicles must be stabilized with cribbing before an EMT enters the passenger compartment.

If the motor vehicle has struck a utility pole, electric power lines may have fallen on top of the roof. If the motor vehicle drove over the top of an underground power splice, the entire car could be energized. The EMT should look above and below the motor vehicle for any contacts with electric power lines or transformers. If wires are down on the car, the fire department or utility company should be notified immediately, and the EMT should make a careful retreat.

There are "alternative fuel" cars on the road today. The EMT should be alert to placards or emblems indicating that the motor vehicle uses propane or is battery powered. These alternative fuel motor vehicles present unique hazards to the EMT.

Stabilization

Any movement of a damaged vehicle can cause the patient to be moved within the vehicle. Any movement of the patient could potentially create additional injury, especially in the case of cervical spine injuries. Therefore, any vehicle with an injured patient inside that can be shifted or shaken is unstable and must be stabilized before patient care can proceed.

A vehicle that lands on its roof or is found on its side is unstable and must be stabilized. The stabilization of vehicles in these positions often requires chains, high-lift jacks, special tools, and/or cribbing. The EMT should leave stabilizing these vehicles to the rescue technicians.

Fortunately, most vehicles remain on their wheels after a collision. However, this does not necessarily mean that the vehicle is stable. Even a car on all four wheels can be shifted, creating movement of the passengers inside.

There are a number of techniques used to stabilize a vehicle that is still on its wheels. Essentially, all of these techniques use the same principle of isolating the wheels from the frame of the vehicle.

Blocks of wood, called **cribbing**, can be used to lift the vehicle's frame off the wheels and stabilize the vehicle. Using special prefabricated cribbing called **step-blocks**, a motor vehicle can quickly and effectively be stabilized (Figure 45-6).

As a last resort, provided no cribbing is available, the air can be let out of the tires. By cutting or pulling the air stem, the tire goes flat, and the car rests on its rims.

An EMT should never enter a motor vehicle unless it has first been stabilized. The EMT should advise the patient, if she is conscious, to remain seated with eyes straight ahead until the vehicle is stabilized and rescuers can safely enter the car.

Access

Once the vehicle has been made safe, the EMT should determine the number and general condition of the patients within the vehicle. This first round of triage is not complicated. Often the patients are grossly classified as being either conscious or unconscious. An unconscious patient may be assumed to be high priority, while a conscious patient will need more assessment.

Access to the patient may be simple. The EMT may open the door and enter the passenger compartment. In some cases, a crowbar can be used to force a partially jammed door. Before using a tool, the EMT should try to open all the doors manually.

In some cases, the EMT must make his own entrance into a crushed motor vehicle. In many cases, a side or rear window can be quickly removed, and the EMT can enter or crawl through the opening that has been created.

The front windshield is made of special **safety glass**, a piece of glass wedged between sheets of plastic. Safety glass is designed to remain in one piece after an MVC. It is difficult to remove quickly. Therefore, the EMT should consider using the front windshield as a last resort.

The rest of the glass in a motor vehicle is **tempered glass**. Tempered glass is special window glass designed to shatter into tiny fragments. This reduces the hazard from razor-sharp edges. However, the glass fragments can scatter over the patients and cause small lacerations. To avoid this danger, the EMT should choose the window farthest from the patient if a window is to be broken.

Using a special glass-breaking tool called a **window punch**, the window is broken, and the EMT can now enter (Figure 45-7). The EMT should be wearing protective clothing, including eyewear and gloves, to prevent microlacerations from the broken glass fragments.

Once access has been obtained, the EMT should proceed to the driver first. Immediately after an MVC, the driver may have forgotten or may be unable to take the car out of gear and turn off the motor. If the EMT finds the car running or in gear, he should put it in park and turn off the engine.

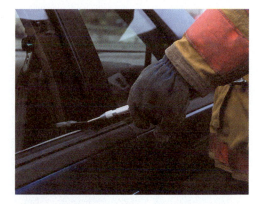

FIGURE 45-7 A window punch is a simple hand tool that can be carried in the pocket.

Prioritization

Once inside the motor vehicle, the EMT has to decide whether any patients are critical. If a patient is critical, she will require rapid extrication. The rapid extrication technique is described in Chapter 22. In many cases, a critical patient is quickly extricated out the same entrance the EMT used to enter the vehicle.

In some cases, the opening the EMT created to gain entrance is too narrow for the EMT and the patient to exit. In those cases, the entrance must be widened quickly, using special extrication tools such as the Jaws of Life.

If the patient is not critically injured, the EMT would proceed to treat the patient while other rescuers create an adequate exit.

If the patient is trapped, for example, the patient's feet are caught under gas or brake pedals, heavy rescue will be needed to disentangle the patient from the vehicle. Another example of entrapment is when the side door is jammed up against the patient's pelvis, pinning her in the vehicle. In each of these cases, heavy rescue will need to disentangle the patient from the vehicle.

Heavy Rescue

A few basic approaches will extricate the victim of an MVC in most cases. If the door is jammed, rescuers will have to force the door open. The simplest method of extricating a patient is by **forcing the door**, using a tool to overcome the latching mechanism. Forcing the door usually involves using a crowbar, a Haligan tool, or similar device.

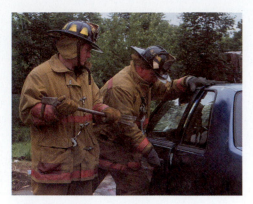

FIGURE 45-8 Heavy rescue may be required to force a jammed door.

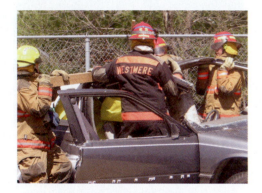

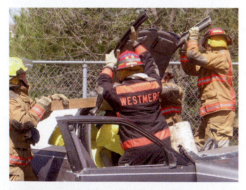

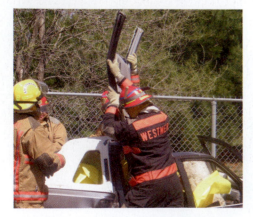

FIGURE 45-9 A roof can literally be peeled back to allow passenger compartment access.

If the door is jammed because the lock is broken, the lock must be forced. A variety of tools can be used to overcome the door's locking mechanism.

All motor vehicles have a case-hardened pin, called the **Nader pin**, that prevents the door from springing open in a crash. This pin is extremely difficult to cut. Often rescuers have to cut around the pin to open the door.

If the door is partially opened, it can be opened farther, using both chains and a come-along or brute force (Figure 45-8). This creates an opening wide enough to insert a backboard and extricate a patient.

If the doors cannot be opened, the roof may have to be removed. **Flapping the roof** consists of cutting the uprights or posts that support the roof and peeling the roof back to allow access to the occupants in the vehicle (Figure 45-9).

The front windshield is special safety glass that can be removed in one piece. Using glass saws, chisels, and even axes, a window shield is literally carved out (Figure 45-10). The patient can then be extricated through the front of the vehicle.

If the patient is pinned under the dashboard or steering wheel, **rolling the dash** may be necessary. Rescuers simply peel the dashboard away from the patient using a variety of power tools, chains, block, and tackle.

Patient Safety

In every case, a rescuer, preferably an EMT, should remain inside the car with the patient while the heavy rescue is going on outside. The patient should be protected from flying debris, such as glass, and the crushing tips of cutting tools. A pair of goggles and even a helmet for the patient can significantly improve the patient's margin of safety. The patient and the EMT must also be protected from flying shards of glass. A heavy woolen blanket or a heavy oil tarp can be placed over both the patient and the EMT as a means of protection (Figure 45-11).

If heavy cutting tools are near the patient, a short wooden backboard should be placed between the tool and the patient. This board will effectively protect the patient if the tip of the tool should slip.

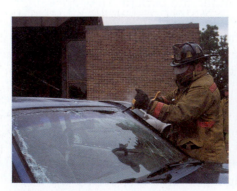

FIGURE 45-10 The glass from the windshield can be cut away and peeled back to gain access to the patient.

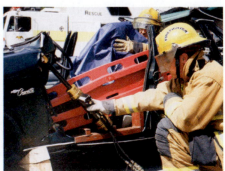

FIGURE 45-11 The patient should be protected from flying shards of glass by using a heavy oil tarp or the like.

Assessment

Once the patient has been safely extricated and moved a reasonable distance from the vehicle, the EMT should complete an initial assessment, if it has not already been performed, as well as a rapid trauma assessment. Attention should be given to signs of internal injury, such as bruising and point tenderness, as well as obvious external injuries such as burns or lacerations.

Transportation

Based on the mechanism of injury and the length of time required to extricate, the EMT should have a high index of suspicion that injuries may have occurred and internal bleeding may be severe. While it is possible for a patient to be trapped and not sustain any severe injuries, an EMT should always err on the side of caution and transport the patient to the closest appropriate facility, typically a trauma center, as soon as practical.

WATER RESCUE

Bodies of water exist in nearly every community. A body of water can be a stream, river, lake, pond, or reservoir. Wherever there is water, there are people. Water tends to draw people. Water is used for recreation, such as swimming, boating, and fishing, and for industry, for instance, hydroelectric power. Whenever people and water are together, there is a likelihood that a water emergency will occur.

Street Smart

An assumption is often made that if the person went into the vehicle through a door, then the quickest way to get the person out of the car is through the door. EMTs who can think "outside the box" quickly realize that there may be several alternatives for removing the patient from a vehicle. Seats that fold down, hatches that lift up, and convertible tops provide readily available alternative exits.

Rapid Water Rescue

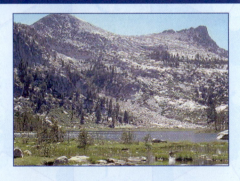

Last winter's heavy snows and the unrelenting spring rains had swelled the Crystal River to its maximum capacity. The river was cresting at near flood stage, and the river's banks were barely able to hold the river back. This combination of events made the Crystal River especially exciting for white-water enthusiasts, and the river was filled with kayakers and canoeists every weekend.

Because of the inherent danger of the river at this time of year and the fact that two canoeists drowned the previous spring, the local Fire-Rescue was on high alert, and the station was being manned "twenty-four, seven" by a rapid response water team. This team of EMTs had just completed the shore-based rescue course and was part of a larger plan to deploy a dive rescue team and a helicopter rescue team to the scene of any potential drowning.

The team had just started its morning inspection when the alert was sounded and those fateful words were spoken, "Man in the water." Everybody scrambled to get the equipment reassembled as the captain got exact directions to the point the kayaker was last seen in the water.

- What is the difference between swift and flat water?
- What are the hazards on scene of a water rescue?
- What precautions should an EMT take?

A quick rescue by rescuers, including EMTs, can prevent a water emergency from becoming a drowning. Unfortunately, because of poor preparation and poor training, a rescuer may end up as the drowning victim himself. That is not to say that EMTs should not perform water rescue, but to prevent a rescue from becoming a tragedy, the EMT must know his limitations in both training and equipment.

The first question every EMT should ask himself on scene is "Am I safe?" An EMT should never place himself in the position where he may end up as the next victim.

Establishing Command

Scenes of a water emergency, such as a drowning at a public beach, can be chaotic. Regardless of the scene's dynamic, the EMT must establish command. The EMT should work cooperatively with other emergency services, such as lifeguards and park rangers, to prepare for the rescue. Preseason water rescue drills can markedly improve the efficiency of responders on scene during an actual drowning and should be encouraged by EMS leaders.

Scene Size-Up

A quick distinction between the two types of water hazards can help the EMT determine the type of rescue that will be needed. A body of water that has no current is considered **flat water**. A smooth surface does not equate with flat water. Rivers can be deceivingly calm on the surface and have tremendously powerful undercurrents. Typically, flat water is used for recreational swimming.

Rapidly moving water is considered **swift water**. By definition, swift water must have a current. Moving water can not only sweep a person off her feet and downstream, it can also hold someone underwater. These powerful down-currents are called an **undertow**.

Natural or man-made dams, especially the low-head dam, can create powerful undertows at the base of the dam. These undertows can not only pull a person underwater and keep that person underwater, but can also pull boats underwater. The undertows created by low-head dams are so powerful that professional swift water rescuers call these low-head dams "drowning machines."

An EMT should never underestimate the power of moving water. Every rescue in moving water is a technical rescue. If an EMT fails to identify swift water, he places himself in danger of becoming a drowning victim.

Management

The EMT's role at a swift water rescue is primarily a supporting role. The objectives of the EMT are to locate the victim, attempt a shore-based rescue if protocols permit, and establish a base of operation for the dive rescue team in the event that a shore-based rescue is not possible.

While this list of objectives may appear short, the tasks to accomplish these objectives are numerous. To become truly effective, the EMT must practice, as a part of the team, the different tasks involved in a water rescue.

Access

The first priority is locating the victim. If the victim is underwater, special dive rescue teams will be needed. After calling for the dive rescue team, the EMT should determine the **point of contact (POC)**, the point at which the person was last seen in the water. Friends, family, and witnesses can help the EMT determine the point of contact. Physical evidence such as clothing, footprints, boats, and vehicles can also be helpful.

If it is not known where the person was last seen or where she entered the water, it may be necessary to perform a shoreline search. If the POC is known, then a perimeter should be established around the area. At this point, if the person is found, a rescue is possible.

Shore-Based Rescue—Flat Water

Flat water rescue efforts can be summarized by the maxim "reach, throw, row, and go." Each term denotes a specific activity that an EMT could perform to effect a rescue. Again, every EMT who is near water must wear a **personal flotation device (PFD)**.

A pole or stick may be all that is needed to rescue the victim if she is near the shoreline. The EMT simply reaches out with a pike pole, for example, and offers the pole's end to the victim.

After grabbing the pole, the victim can be pulled to shore by rescuers. If the victim is too weak to grab the pole, the patient's clothing can be hooked, and then the patient can be dragged to shore. The EMT should be prepared to drop the pole at any time if the patient starts to pull the EMT into the water.

A length of rope loosely coiled inside a cloth sack, called a **throw bag**, can be thrown to a victim. The victim, grasping the rope, would then be pulled to shore. The EMT should never tie the throw bag to himself. Instead, trees and the like should be used as anchors.

If a throw bag is not available, sometimes a PFD can be thrown to the victim. The PFD might provide the victim a few more minutes of buoyancy until a more effective rescue can be effected. Seat cushions from a boat or even ice coolers can be used if a PFD is not available.

Use of a boat, such as a rowboat, or entering the water to rescue the patient requires special training and should be attempted only by a qualified lifeguard or similarly prepared person.

Finally, the EMT can enter the water. This last solution is dangerous and should be attempted only by those individuals who have received special training in water rescue. Lifeguards are typically trained in this type of rescue. However, this last option should be utilized only when the first three techniques have been exhausted. These techniques are demonstrated in Chapter 34.

Shore-Based Rescue—Swift Water

An EMT is faced with a dilemma when he is called to the scene of a possible swift water rescue. Swift water rescue is very dangerous, and numerous rescuers have drowned trying to save another person's life. On the other hand, it is difficult for an EMT to stand idly by while a victim drowns. A shore-based rescue attempt, while awaiting

Street Smart

Every rescuer who is within 50 feet of shore must wear a personal flotation device (PFD), otherwise known as a life preserver. A PFD is usually a vest-like device or similar device that has positive buoyancy. A PFD is designed to help keep the rescuer afloat in the event he should accidentally fall into the water. A Coast Guard–approved life preserver is recommended. The EMT should always follow local protocols established for water rescue.

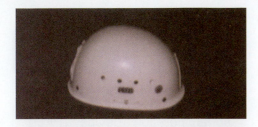

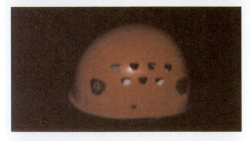

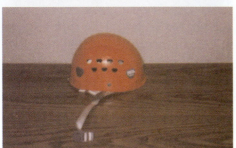

FIGURE 45-12 Closed helmets should not be worn when near water because they present a drowning hazard. Instead, using a vented helmet provides protection and reduces this hazard. (Courtesy of Tim Strange.)

professional dive rescue, is a possible resolution to the dilemma that also prepares the scene for the arrival of dive rescue personnel.

Before approaching the water, all rescuers must be wearing a PFD. Closed helmets, such as fire helmets, should be removed. If the rescuer inadvertently falls into the water, the helmet could fill with water and drag the person's head underwater. Vented helmets should be considered instead (Figure 45-12). Similarly, high boots and fire boots should be discouraged for the same reason.

In a typical shore-based swift rescue plan, there are at least four teams. The first team, the upstream team, is usually dispatched to a river crossing, such as a bridge, to observe for hazards, such as logs floating downstream toward the victim and dive rescue team members.

The second team, a downstream team, usually strings two or more ropes diagonally across the water. These ropes, called **snag lines**, are the last line of rescue for anybody floating downstream. Water speed determines how far downstream a snag line is established. If the body of water is too wide for ropes, at a river, for example, then one or more boats may be launched to provide a recovery platform. Finally, two shore-based teams would proceed downstream from the point of last contact, searching the shoreline for the victim.

Dense underbrush can make shore-based rescue very difficult. All members of the rescue team must be kept in constant contact at all times. When the victim is located, a signal is usually given and other rescuers respond to that location. Using throw bags and/or pike poles, a rescue is attempted. At no time does any rescuer enter the water who is not specially trained and prepared for water rescue. If the victim cannot be reached, rescuers should prepare for the arrival of the water rescue team.

Treatment and Transport

Treatment should be started as soon as possible after the rescue has been accomplished. Rescuers often rescue someone who appears drowned but who can recover if aggressive treatment is started immediately. This is in part because of the effects of hypothermia on the nearly drowned person.

Hypothermia from the submersion in cold water may prolong the window of opportunity for recovery by slowing body functions and preserving the core organs, including the heart and brain. Victims who have been underwater for as long as 45 minutes have recovered from near-drowning without serious neurological impairment. More information on cold water immersion can be found in Chapter 32 on environmental emergencies.

Every effort should be made to save a near-drowning victim unless such efforts are obviously fruitless.

Many rescue plans call for an ambulance to be staged close by, ready to respond immediately once the patient has been rescued. In some cases, it may be appropriate to utilize air medical evacuation. In those cases, the patient may have to be transported from the remote shoreline to a landing zone to meet the helicopter.

SEARCH AND RESCUE

When the subject of search and rescue (SAR) is discussed, most EMTs think of wilderness SAR. SAR is not confined to the woods. SAR techniques are used whenever a person is lost. A search might have to be performed for a child lost in a mall.

A SAR may have to be performed on the grounds of a building collapse or in an urban area. Modern urban SAR teams use high-tech equipment and specially trained scent dogs. The Oklahoma City bombing involved extensive use of urban search and rescue teams from across the country.

A common scenario for a full-scale SAR operation involves searching for a lost hiker or a person injured while in the backcountry.

SAR is evolutionary by nature. First, the person must be found. This is the search. Then the person must be carried out. This is the rescue. The person must also be treated for any injuries. Finally, the patient must be transported to an appropriate medical facility.

The danger that is consistent in all SAR operations is the length of time it takes to find the patient. The longer the person is lost, the greater the likelihood that some harm, such as exposure or hypothermia, will come to the person.

 ## *Lost Hiker*

An avid hiker and camper, Mr. Erb had always encouraged his kids to "take to the mountains" and "enjoy the beauty of the great outdoors." Most of his children, on the other hand, were less enthusiastic about hiking than their dad; they preferred to "camp out" at the local Great Western motel. The exception was John. Even as a lad, John had a great sense of direction and a great sense of adventure.

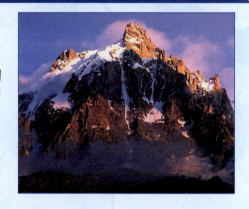

So, for his senior year, John planned a camping trip to the high Sierras. But this hiking trip was no ordinary hiking trip. John planned to see nature as God intended, and he was going to bushwhack his way from peak to peak, stopping only to replenish his supplies.

With that in mind, his dad parked at the Devil's Fork trailhead and waited for his son to appear. He waited and waited. After 20 hours, he started to think maybe John was in trouble. Calling the local Forest Service office, he explained his concerns. Within hours, the trailhead was swarming with search and rescue (SAR) team members. A command post was set up, and volunteers were being recruited. Local EMTs were being paired with experienced SAR team members and given "fanny packs," prepackaged first-aid kits.

The first team, dubbed "alpha-alpha," set off down the trail and took up position at the coordinates they were assigned. Andrea, the EMT team member, was asked to walk the trail and look for "clues." As Andrea walked along, she would stop every 50 yards or so and call out, "John! John Erb!"

- What are the first actions an EMT should take at a potential SAR?
- What can an EMT do while awaiting professional SAR personnel?
- What medical problems can a lost hiker have?

In some instances, such as in the National Park system, the incidence of search and rescue is so common that professional search and rescue teams exist. These professional rescuers prepare and plan for the SAR that they know will come. These teams identify known dangerous conditions and hazardous places, called **high life hazards**, where a person could become injured or trapped, and they plan how they will respond in the event of an emergency.

Establishing Command

Whenever a person has been reported lost or missing, the EMT, along with other emergency services, should establish a command post. This command post serves as a starting point for any rescue.

Many times a search goes on for days or even weeks. These extended operations should be established in a location that is well equipped to handle a long-term operation.

If local rescuers, including EMTs, are not familiar with SAR, then professional rescuers and search managers should be notified immediately.

Scene Size-Up

Witnesses should be questioned about the last point of contact with the lost person, and detailed information must be obtained to help rescuers search efficiently. A standardized lost person questionnaire is often used to gather complete information about the person. An example of this form is shown in Figure 45-13.

Details such as the sex, height, weight, and clothing of the lost person need to be obtained. Details of the patient's medical history are also important. For example, a diabetic patient may need immediate treatment if she has gone without her insulin for several hours.

Access

Typically, large numbers of rescuers, often from diverse backgrounds, are assembled. As these resources arrive, they should be directed to a central staging area for assignment.

It is important that well-intentioned rescuers not be allowed to search freely. These so-called freelancers can inadvertently destroy valuable clues to the person's whereabouts. All rescue personnel must be directed to the staging area and assigned to teams.

Hasty Search

A quick search of an area, called a **hasty search**, can be done while waiting for professional SAR personnel. A hasty search involves walking along trails, roadways, and shorelines, those areas where a person might reasonably be expected to be found. A hasty search does not include searching off road.

The EMT should not be concentrating on finding the person. Rather, the EMT should be looking for evidence that the person was in an area. Evidence or **clues** could be a wrapper from a candy bar or an article of clothing (Figure 45-14). Every clue represents an opportunity to find the person. Clues should not be moved. Instead, the clue should be left undisturbed and its location reported immediately to the command post.

MISSING PERSON QUESTIONNAIRE | TASK # | DATE PREPARED: / TIME PREPARED: | PAGE # 1 OF 3

TASK NAME:

REVISED (DATE/TIME):

SUBJECT # ___ OF ___ | INTERVIEWED BY (PLANNING): | POLICE FILE #

INFORMANT IDENTIFICATION

FIRST NAME: | STREET ADDRESS:

LAST NAME: | CITY:

RELATIONSHIP TO SUBJECT: | STATE: | ZIP CODE:

HOME PHONE #: | ALT. PHONE #

ADDITIONAL INFORMANTS/ WITNESSES | NAME: | NAME: | NAME:

| PHONE: | PHONE: | PHONE:

SUBJECT INFORMATION

FIRST NAME: | STREET ADDRESS:

MIDDLE NAME: | CITY:

LAST NAME: | STATE: | ZIP CODE:

ANSWERS TO: | HOME PHONE #:

VEHICLE MAKE: | EMPLOYER:

VEHICLE MODEL: | STREET ADDRESS:

VEHICLE COLOR: | CITY:

LICENSE PLATE #: | STATE: | ZIP CODE:

COMMENTS (e.g. 'CODE' NAME IF CHILD): | WORK PHONE # :

| WORK FAX #:

| SUPERVISOR'S NAME:

DATE OF BIRTH (Y/M/D): | AGE: | SEX: | HEIGHT: | WEIGHT:

HAIR COLOR: | EYES: | HAIRSTYLE/LENGTH:

COMPLEXION: | FIRST LANGUAGE:

DISTINGUISHING MARKS:

MEDICAL DISABILITIES:

MEDICATION REQUIREMENTS/QTY. ON HAND/DURATION OF SUPPLIES:

RECENT/CURRENT ILLNESS(ES):

FITNESS LEVEL: | SMOKER ☐ ( ) | BRAND: | ICS 302

MISSING PERSON QUESTIONNAIRE (CONT.) | PAGE # 2 OF 3

ALLERGIES:

FEARS/PHOBIAS:

MENTAL ATTITUDE:

FINANCIAL SITUATION:

CRIMINAL HISTORY:

HOBBIES/INTERESTS:

CLOTHING/EQUIPMENT

SHOE TYPE: | COLOR: | SIZE:

SHOE SOLE DESCRIPTION:

SOCKS: | PANTS (TYPE & COLOR):

TOP (TYPE & COLOR): | SWEATER (TYPE & COLOR):

JACKET (TYPE & COLOR):

RAINGEAR (TYPE & COLOR):

HAT (TYPE & COLOR): | GLOVES (TYPE & COLOR):

PACK (MAKE & COLOR):

FOOD & DRINK (TYPE/BRAND/QUANTITY):

POINT LAST SEEN

DATE LAST SEEN: | TIME LAST SEEN:

POINT LAST SEEN:

MAP # | GRID REF:

MISSING PERSON QUESTIONNAIRE (CONT.) | PAGE # 3 OF 3

NAME OF OTHER PERSON(S) WHO SAW OR MIGHT HAVE SEEN THE SUBJECT AT OR NEAR THIS TIME:	#	NAME OF INFORMANT:	LOCATION SUBJECT SEEN:	TIME SEEN:
	1			
	2			
	3			
	4			
	5			

LOCATION OF VEHICLE (TRANSPORTATION):

INTENDED ROUTE:

WEATHER AT TIME LAST SEEN:

COMMENTS (DISPOSITION/PERSONALITY, RELATIONSHIP WITH SPOUSE/FAMILY/FRIENDS ETC.):

SUBJECT NEXT OF KIN

FIRST NAME: | STREET ADDRESS:

LAST NAME: | CITY:

RELATIONSHIP TO SUBJECT: | STATE: | ZIP CODE:

HOME PHONE #: | ALT. PHONE #

ADDITIONAL INFORMANTS/ FRIENDS: | NAME: | NAME: | NAME:

| PHONE: | PHONE: | PHONE:

AVAILABILITY OF PHOTOGRAPH(S)?

FIGURE 45-13 Missing person questionnaire.

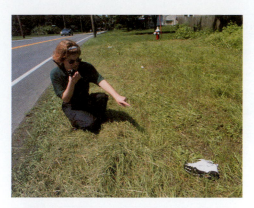

FIGURE 45-14 An EMT in a hasty search should look for clues.

Clues such as a piece of clothing may provide specially trained dogs with a scent trail that leads right to the person. Every effort should be made to try to preserve these scent trails whenever possible.

Law enforcement officers may be asked to search in local barns, abandoned buildings, and the like. A lost person is likely to approach a house or a business in search of help.

Rescue

In most cases of backcountry rescue, for a variety of reasons, the patient is usually carried out by rescuers. It takes special training and practice to safely carry a patient out of the woods. Chapter 11 reviews some of the more common carries that are used in the field.

At first glance, these carries appear easy. However, after 1 or 2 miles, the rescuers quickly realize how tiring these carries can be. Practice and physical conditioning are key to a successful carry.

Management

After the person has been found, a medical evaluation is usually in order. In some cases, an emergency physician may be standing by at the trailhead. In other cases, the patient is transported to a local clinic for first-level assessment.

If the patient is seriously injured or there is a greater risk of serious injury, the patient should be airlifted from the scene and transported to an appropriate facility.

Transportation

Helicopter evacuation from backwoods rescues is so common that many mountain communities have prearranged landing zones established. Chapter 43 provides more information about helicopter operations. Before such a resource is called, the EMT should carefully consider the patient's condition and the advantage of an airlift versus ground transportation.

CONCLUSION

Rescues are often very exciting. Unique conditions require an EMT to be creative and adjust his plan of action to the situation. However, reckless disregard of obvious dangers can change the role of an EMT from that of rescuer to that of patient. In every rescue, the EMT should participate only when he has had adequate training to proceed safely.

TEST YOUR KNOWLEDGE

1. When is a technical rescue needed?
2. What are the common phases seen in all rescues?
3. What is the appropriate personal protective equipment for the following hazardous situations?

   Flash and flame

   Falling objects

Sharp objects

Flying debris

Poor visibility

Loud noises

4. What are several situations of confined space?

5. What are the common hazards encountered in confined space?

6. How does the standard of care imply that an EMT must have special training for technical rescue?

7. What are the hazards common to a motor vehicle collision?

8. What is the importance of stabilizing a motor vehicle before rescue?

9. What is the difference between heavy rescue and rapid extrication?

10. What are the three most common means of heavy rescue?

11. What is the difference between flat water and swift water?

12. How is a shore-based rescue established for flat water?

13. How is a shore-based rescue established for swift water?

14. What is a hasty search?

15. What is the importance of searching for clues and not people?

INTERNET RESOURCES

Additional resources on various types of rescue procedures can be found at the following Web sites. Conduct your own searches to find additional information on rescues and training available for these types of rescues.

- Extrication.com, http://www.extrication.com

- Lifesaving Resources, Inc., http://www.lifesaving.com

- National Association for Search and Rescue, http://www.nasar.org

- National Institute for Urban Search and Rescue, http://www.niusr.org

- RescueNet, http://www.rescuenet.com

- Texas Rope Rescue, http://www.texasroperescue.com

FURTHER STUDY

Anderson, R. (1998). Touchdown: Establishing a helicopter landing zone. *EMS Rescue-Technology, 1*(2), 64–66.

Sachs, G., Bailey, K., & Hays, C. (1997). Water works: Water rescue. *EMS Rescue-Technology, 1*(6), 32–36.

Sargent, C. (1999). Close encounters. *Journal of Emergency Medical Services, 24*(7), 44–49.

Spivak, M. (1998). River rescuers. *EMS Rescue-Technology, 1*(2), 14–2.

CHAPTER 46

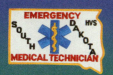

Emergency Response to Terrorism

KEY TERMS

awareness level

biological agents

chemical weapons

coagulopathy

domestic terrorist

emergency operations plan (EOP)

federal response plan (FRP)

Geiger counter

international terrorist

LACES

nuclear dispersion device (NDD)

radiation pager

secondary device

SLUDGEM

terrorism

TRACEM

weapons of mass destruction (WMD)

zoonotic

OBJECTIVES

Upon completion of this chapter, the reader should be able to:

1. Define what is meant by the term *terrorism*.
2. Understand the role of the EMT as a first responder to a terrorist incident.
3. Recognize the potential for a terrorist incident.
4. "Self-protect" on scene of a terrorist incident.
5. Identify what additional resources may be needed on scene of a terrorist incident.

OVERVIEW

Every emergency medical technician (EMT) should know that she potentially could be on the frontline following a terrorist attack. Emergency medical services (EMS), an integral part of the emergency response team, shares responsibility for crisis management and will be called upon to respond to deal with the consequences of such an attack.

An EMT, in the capacity as a first responder to a terrorist attack, is also a potential target for terrorists. Terrorists, hoping to disrupt emergency operations, have been known to place bombs, called **secondary devices**, that specifically target first-due emergency units. An EMT should not enter a dangerous situation; however, the potential for an ambush does exist and the EMT must have an elevated awareness for the potential of a secondary device.

Therefore, an EMT must be able to identify the threat of terrorism, take measures to protect herself from harm, and help keep others out of harm's way. Finally, the EMT must know how to mitigate the effects of such an attack in order to save lives, decrease injury, and diminish the impact of the terrorist attack on the community that she serves.

✴ *Sick Building*

"Paramedic Engine 9, Ambulance 12, and Battalion Chief 2: respond to the Governors Motor Inn. Report of multiple sick persons. Caller claims no smoke, no fire. Time out 8:45 hours." Elisa had just completed the county's terrorism course and her interest was piqued when she heard the report of multiple sick persons. "Could this be a terrorist attack," she thought, "or another 'sick building' from poor ventilation like the last call that came out like this?"

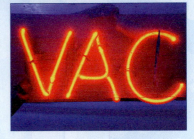
(Courtesy of Morguefile.)

- What information from the dispatch might suggest that this could be a terrorist attack?
- What would be the approach to the scene of a potential terrorist attack?
- What resources might be needed if this EMS call turns out to be a terrorist attack?

TERRORISM DEFINED

The Federal Bureau of Investigation's (FBI) definition of **terrorism** is, "the unlawful use of force against persons or property to intimidate or coerce a government, the civilian population, or any segment thereof, in the furtherance of political or social objectives." This definition sums up the three elements of a terrorist's activities; specifically, they are illegal, they involve the use of force, and they are intended to intimidate the public.

Terrorists have one objective in general: to sow panic among the population by whatever means possible. The purpose of this panic is to cause the public to lose faith in the government or force the populace to accept the terrorist's political or social agenda.

International versus Domestic Terrorism

The United States has enemies, both domestic and foreign, who would use violence to achieve their political means—the overthrow of the U.S. government or the American way of life.

Domestic terrorists are American citizens or "nationals," as defined by the Immigration and Nationality Act, who either have disputes with the way the U.S. government functions or who have quarrels with specific policies of the government. They often speak of conspiracies and deprivation of rights by the federal government. Rather than seek peaceful means to end these disagreements, these groups utilize violence to attempt to enact change. Some domestic terrorist groups, for example, the self-appointed "militias," are resolved to open armed conflict to advance their cause.

The Oklahoma City bombing, illustrated in Figure 46-1, is an example of a terrorist attack perpetrated by at least two Americans, Timothy McVeigh and Terry Nichols, against fellow Americans. Terrorists may operate in groups, such as Aryan Nation or the Ku Klux Klan, or alone, as sole agents for a cause. An example of a lone terrorist is the Unabomber (university and airline bomber) Theodore Kaczynski.

International terrorists, as opposed to domestic terrorists, are not citizens of the country whose government or values they oppose.

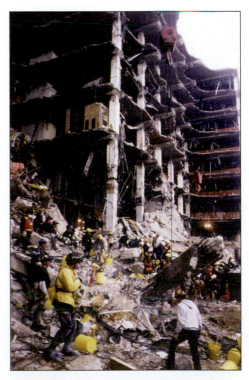

FIGURE 46-1 Terrorism can be domestic, as was the case with the Oklahoma City bombing. (Courtesy of FEMA.)

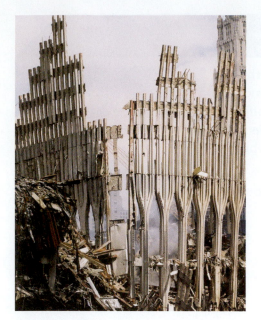

FIGURE 46-2 Terrorism can be foreign, as was the case with the September 11, 2001, attack on the World Trade Center. (Courtesy of FEMA.)

International terrorists often cross over another country's borders to initiate terrorist attacks and many times have subgroups, called cells, within other countries that are poised to attack when ordered. Typically, there is a common bond that unifies these terrorists, such as hatred for America, which is the foundation of al Qaeda (the organization responsible for the attacks on September 11, 2001 [Figure 46-2]). Some nations support these terrorists and are referred to as rogue nations in world opinion.

EMERGENCY RESPONSE TO TERRORISM

EMS providers, being proactive, need to assume that terrorism will occur in their community and start to plan for such inevitability. Training is the first step toward emergency preparedness from attacks by terrorists, both foreign and domestic, who would use violence to achieve their goals.

Levels of Training

Any person who is an emergency responder (i.e., law enforcement officer, EMS provider, firefighter, and industrial security officer) and who is likely to witness a terrorist event needs to be trained to identify that emergency as a potential terrorist act and to act accordingly.

Minimally, all emergency responders need to be trained to the **awareness level**. Emergency responders trained to the awareness level are able to recognize the hallmarks of a terrorist attack, know how to protect themselves from harm, and know how to activate the emergency response plan for such an event. All EMTs should be minimally trained to the awareness level.

More training is also available for command and control personnel, called operations level training, and for those personnel involved in decontamination, called technician level training. It should be noted that the EMT with awareness level training may only function in the cold zone, a relatively safe and uncontaminated area.

WEAPONS OF MASS DESTRUCTION

To instill the maximum amount of fear among the populace (i.e., terror), terrorists will use or threaten to use **weapons of mass destruction (WMD)**. WMD were originally created to kill or maim large numbers of soldiers. These weapons are now being used by terrorists to kill or maim large numbers of civilians indiscriminately and to disrupt normal government operations. Nuclear, biological, and chemical (NBC) weapons represent the major classifications of WMD.

While the threat of WMD is always present, it should be noted that terrorists use explosives and incendiary devices for the majority of their attacks. Although technically not WMD, these devices can cause death and destruction on a large scale and could be grouped together with NBC weapons: nuclear, radiological, biological, chemical, and explosive.

Nuclear or Radiological Weapons

A 5–18-kiloton nuclear bomb, a bomb as powerful as the one that destroyed Hiroshima, Japan, weighs only 60 pounds. A terrorist can carry one inside a briefcase and leave it in a busy airport, subway station, or at a mass gathering such as the local mall during the winter holidays. The likelihood of such a bomb being created is remote because of stringent international controls on the possession and transportation of fissionable weapons-grade nuclear materials, but the potential exists nevertheless.

What is more probable is that terrorists will encase a conventional explosive device, a bomb, in depleted nuclear materials; for example, spent uranium from a nuclear reactor. This type of bomb would spread radioactive nuclear material across a wide area, causing widespread injury and illness. The proper name for this so-called dirty bomb is **nuclear dispersion device (NDD)**.

Emergency responders should have a higher state of awareness that a NDD may be present when responding to a report of an explosion with multiple casualties. While the majority of explosions in the United States are due to a natural gas mishap, the presence of chemical fuses, called blasting caps, electric switches, electronic timers, and mechanical trip wires should alert the emergency responder to the possibility of a terrorist attack and an NDD (Table 46-1).

Alternatively, terrorists could target a location that already stores nuclear materials or radiological materials that are in transit with a bomb or rocket. Examples of fixed locations include nuclear power plants, military installations, experimental reactors at universities, and nuclear research and development facilities.

Perhaps at great risk are nuclear materials in transit that do not have the protection of fences, guards, or other security defenses. Since 1964 more than 3,000 shipments of spent nuclear fuel rods have traveled over 1.7 million miles in the United States. To protect these shipments, the United States Department of Transportation requires that they be transported in a special type B container, called a cask. A cask is very difficult to penetrate and will not spill its contents even during a collision.

Nuclear materials are usually clearly marked with the international trefoil symbol, either in red or black, that looks like three propeller blades in the shape of the letter Y inside a white- or yellow-colored triangle. This symbol makes nuclear materials easy targets. Figure 46-3 is an illustration of this symbol.

Personal Protection

The three keys to radiological personal protection are (1) to limit the time of exposure to a radiation source; (2) to increase the distance from the radiation source to the EMT, and (3) to provide the EMT with shielding from the radiation. These are summarized as time, distance, and shielding.

Once a material at an incident has been identified as a possible radioactive material, possibly by use of a **Geiger counter**, the EMT should immediately vacate the area and retreat to a safe distance. Geiger counters are portable or vehicle-mounted devices that detect

TABLE 46-1

Evidence of a Nuclear Dispersion Device

1. Unusual debris such as lead shielding

2. Broken small metal containers

3. Dispersed powder or sand-like ceramic granules

4. Blue or purple glow from a powder or metal

5. Unexplained heat from a powder or metal

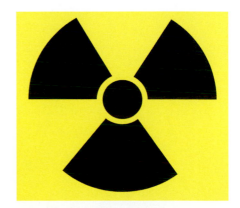

FIGURE 46-3 The trefoil hazard symbol warns of nuclear radiation.

radiation, creating a clicking sound in the process. Other radiation detection devices, such as a **radiation pager**, a device similar to a common pager that clips on the belt, measures the exact amount of exposure of the individual EMT so that appropriate treatments can be instituted immediately.

When considering where to stage ambulances, EMS equipment, and personnel, the EMT should first consider placing a significant distance between the source and the site. The *Emergency Response Guidebook* (ERG) can provide guidance in this matter as well as preestablished emergency evacuation plans.

The EMT should also endeavor to place a formidable object between the radioactive material and the EMS staging area. Ideal radiation barriers that act as a shield from radiation include manmade earthen works called berms, raised railbeds, or naturally occurring ridges, as well as thick concrete walls, basements, and even an engine block.

Contamination versus Irradiation

Whenever a chemical or biological weapon is used by a terrorist, the EMT is potentially at danger of exposure to the chemical or biological agent through contact with contaminated clothing and the like. This is not always the case with a radiological incident.

A person who is a victim of a nuclear or radiological terrorist attack may have been exposed to the radiation (i.e., is irradiated) but has not necessarily been contaminated with the radiological material. In those cases of irradiation, the patient may become ill but does not present a danger to the EMT.

The person who has been contaminated is physically covered with the nuclear material, which continues to emit radiation. The key difference between irradiation and contamination is that the radiation during an irradiation ends and the patient only sustains the injury that the dose of radiation caused, whereas the radiation from a contamination is ongoing and the patient will continue to suffer injury until he or she is decontaminated.

It is important that qualified personnel determine if the patient has been contaminated and thus needs decontamination, or simply has been irradiated and needs treatment. Simple radiation exposure is not a danger to the EMT and should not impede the patient's care and transportation.

Biological Weapons

Biological weapons have been used in warfare for centuries. Stories are told of Scythian archers, ancient Euro-Asian mounted nomads, who dipped their arrowheads into decomposing bodies in 400 BC, and Tartar troops who flung plague-ridden bodies over the city walls during the siege of Kaffa. During the First World War, Germans made weaponized anthrax and cholera for use against the allies.

One of the attractions of biological weapons for terrorists is that they are easy to acquire, synthesize, and distribute. Furthermore, it only takes a small quantity of the agents to kill hundreds or thousands of people. Unlike radioactive materials, which are relatively easy to detect with Geiger counters, biological agents are difficult to detect because they are often invisible, odorless, and tasteless.

Biological agents can be broken down into three classes: bacterial agents, viral agents, and biological toxins. Bacteria are microscopic single-celled organisms that cause disease and can multiply independently. Viral agents, including a subcategory called rickettsia, live inside a host cell in a parasitic relationship. These viral agents cannot live outside the host's body and depend on the host's living cells to multiply. Biological toxins are substances derived from a plant, animal, or even a microbe, and are very potent.

Bacterial Agents

Examples of bacterial agents—the unicelled microbes that are abundant in the environment—that have been weaponized include *Bacillus anthracis* (anthrax), *Yersinia pestis* (plague), and *Burkholderia mallei* (glanders), among others.

Exposure to anthrax can start with symptoms similar to the flu, fever, fatigue, cough, and a mild chest discomfort, within 1–6 days, that can progress to severe respiratory distress with stridor, cyanosis, and death within 24–36 hours of onset of serious symptoms.

Anthrax has already been weaponized by the United States and the former Soviet Union. Of the three diseases listed above, anthrax presents unique challenges. Anthrax is a white powder that is highly resistant to sunlight, heat, and disinfectants, the typical means of infection control, and it is possible to aerosolize it so that it can be spread in the air. Furthermore, spores, a hardened capsule around the bacteria, allow anthrax to remain infectious within the soil or water for years. Figure 46-4A shows a microscopic view of *Bacillus anthracis*.

Plague, typically carried by flea-ridden rats, has been weaponized into an aerolized form. The plague is particularly troublesome because of its highly contagious nature. Like anthrax, the respiratory form of the plague, called pneumonic plague, begins with nonspecific flulike symptoms and progresses to respiratory distress, respiratory failure, and cardiovascular collapse. Figure 46-4B shows a microscopic view of *Y. pestis*, the caustic agent for the plague.

Glanders is a **zoonotic** disease, which is a disease of domestic animals, such as horses, that can be spread to humans. Once glanders is contracted, most likely through inhalation, the incubation period is about 10–14 days. Symptoms are similar to the flu: rigors or body chills, cold sweats, and unremitting headache, that rapidly progress to an acute systemic infection with resultant septic shock. The disease is fatal without treatment. Unlike other bacterial agents, there is no pre-exposure treatment, called prophylaxis, to prevent the infection. Fortunately, standard precautions, including cleansing surfaces with a hypochlorite solution, are effective in killing the bacteria. Figure 46-4C shows a microscopic view of *B. mallei*, the causative agent for glanders.

Viral Agents

A virus consists of a strand of RNA or DNA surrounded by a protein coat. It inserts itself into another cell within the host's body, and reprograms that cell to stop what it normally does and instead

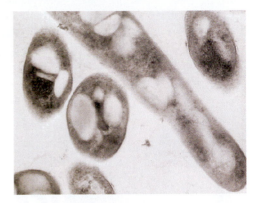

FIGURE 46-4A A microscopic view of *Bacillus anthracis*, the cause of anthrax. (Courtesy of the Centers for Disease Control Public Health Image Library.)

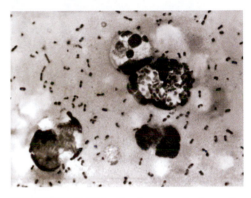

FIGURE 46-4B A microscopic view of the *Yersinia pestis* bacteria, the cause of bubonic plague. (Courtesy of the Centers for Disease Control Public Health Image Library.)

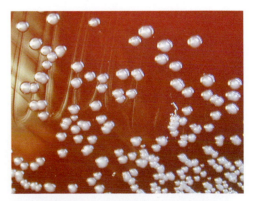

FIGURE 46-4C A microscopic view of *Burkholderia mallei*, the cause of glanders. (Courtesy of the Centers for Disease Control Public Health Image Library.)

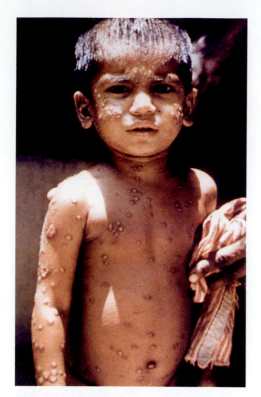

FIGURE 46-5 Smallpox is a highly contagious and potentially deadly infection. (Courtesy of the Centers for Disease Control Public Health Image Library.)

reproduce more virus, eventually killing the host. Viruses of concern include smallpox and viral hemorrhagic fevers.

The World Health Organization declared that smallpox was eradicated around the world in May 1980. Shortly thereafter mass immunization programs to prevent smallpox were stopped. The threat of the use of smallpox has raised concerns because the majority of the population is not immunized. Smallpox starts with a rash similar to chickenpox except the rash is more concentrated on the face and extremities. Figure 46-5 illustrates smallpox infection. At present there is no effective treatment for smallpox, and all care remains supportive as the body tries to heal itself.

Ebola is perhaps one of the most widely known of the viral hemorrhagic fevers (VHF), yet there are four viral families with over a dozen discrete diseases. VHF is easily spread by contact as well as airborne means. The presence of flushing of the face and chest, associated with fever as well as the presence of petechiae, small ruptured capillaries under the skin, is suggestive of VHF. Subsequent disorders of bleeding, called **coagulopathy**, lead to hypoperfusion and shock and are treated accordingly.

Biological Toxins

Biological toxins are not microorganisms themselves but rather harmful substances created by microorganisms, which differentiate them from chemical agents. Toxins such as botulinum (*Clostridium botulinum*) have been known for years and are more commonly the result of improperly canned foods. Botulinum is 275% more toxic than cyanide.

Another infamous toxin, ricin, has received recent attention in part because ricin is extracted from the castor bean, which is readily available worldwide. Fortunately, ricin, while toxic, is difficult to disperse over a wide area, limiting its use to attacks on individuals.

Chemical Weapons

Chemical weapons saw their zenith during the First World War. Gases, used to root troops out of trenches, were invented by the Germans and used by the allies as well. More recently, gas warfare was used in the Iraq-Iran conflict and by Saddam Hussein to suppress the Kurdish tribes in northern Iraq.

Chemical weapons can be divided into five classifications: nerve agents, blister agents, blood agents, choking agents, and irritating agents.

The primary routes of exposure to these poisons is like all poisons: inhalation, ingestion, or absorption. While injection is possible, it is less likely. For a terrorist attack, the primary route of poisoning is likely to be inhalation.

Nerve Agents

Nerve agents were invented by the Germans in the First World War. Subsequently, many of these agents have abbreviations that start with the letter G, meaning German. Examples of nerve agents include sarin (GB), used in a terrorist attack in a Tokyo subway and by Iraq against Iran, and soman.

The nerve agents stem from pesticides called organophosphates and are actually liquids that boil off at room temperature and create a gas. These pesticides were chemically altered to produce the characteristic symptom pattern that is contained in the mnemonic **SLUDGEM**. Table 46-2 explains each of the symptoms associated with a letter in SLUDGEM. Other associated symptoms include pinpoint pupils and blurry vision, involuntary muscle twitching to the point of convulsions, and chest pressure.

Blister Agents

The original blister agent was mustard gas and was first used by the Germans in September 1917. Also called Yperite, for the place where it was used to great effect (Ypers), mustard gas was reportedly used in the 1980s against the Kurdish people of northern Iraq by Saddam Hussein's troops.

Mustard gas can have the characteristic smell of garlic and is readily absorbed in clothing and on the skin, where it can remain for weeks. Another blister agent, Lewisite, can have the characteristic smell of geraniums and is also readily absorbed in clothing and on the skin.

Blister agents are not as fatal as nerve agents but rather are intended to incapacitate a large number of people. Initial symptoms include reddened skin that eventually becomes covered with yellow, mustard-colored blisters. The most problematic effect of blister gases is eye irritation, with painful swelling and tearing, resulting in temporary blindness.

EMTs should be aware that blister agents rub off clothing very easily and can quickly contaminate the rescuer as well as the victim. Therefore, careful decontamination is mandatory to prevent further victims.

Blood Agents

The classic blood agent is cyanide, which interferes with the ability of cells to use oxygen. Cyanide is commonly used in many industrial processes (photography, plastic manufacturing, metallurgy, etc.) and thus can be easily obtained by terrorists.

A volatile chemical, cyanide, when it "off-gases," is a colorless gas with a faint, almond-like smell that some, but not all, people can smell.

Cyanide can rapidly lead to death at higher concentrations, and symptoms (vomiting, diarrhea, headaches) are nonspecific and therefore not helpful in the rapid determination of the causative agent.

Choking Agents

As the name implies, choking agents cause severe respiratory distress and eventual asphyxia. The classic choking agents are chlorine gas and phosgene gas. Chlorine gas is readily available and it is used as a disinfectant for pools, as a cleaning agent for EMS (as hypochlorite solution or bleach), in paper manufacturing as well as many other uses. Thousands of tons of chlorine are manufactured and shipped in the United States annually. Phosgene (carbonyl chloride) is used in making plastics and pesticides and has the characteristic smell of freshly cut grass.

TABLE 46-2	
SLUDGEM	
S =	Salivation, i.e., drooling
L =	Lacrimation, i.e., tearing
U =	Urination, i.e., excessive urine
D =	Defecation, i.e., diarrhea
G =	GI distress, i.e., abdominal pain
E =	Emesis, i.e., vomiting
M =	Muscle contractions, i.e., twitching

Chlorine gas, a heavier-than-air gas, converts to hydrochloric acid (HCl) when in contact with water. HCl causes burning of the eyes, severe paroxysms of coughing (coughing fits), and choking. Phosgene's symptoms are similar.

Irritating Agents

Irritating agents are used primarily for riot control and, as the name implies, are generally not lethal. Examples of irritating agents include tear gas (CS) and riot gas (CN). Pepper spray, first used by the U.S. Postal Service as a dog repellant, is an oil (oleoresin capsicum) derived from cayenne peppers and is another example of an irritating agent. While it is very difficult for a patient to overdose on these agents, their use can lead to widespread panic and injuries, including coughing, choking, shortness of breath, and nausea with vomiting.

PREPAREDNESS

Unfortunately, individuals or groups who have the means and the motive will commit acts of terrorism. EMS providers, in collaboration with and with the assistance of federal, state, and local law enforcement agencies, need to maintain a constant vigil for the presence of these threats that exist in their community and prepare for them through sharing of intelligence and open lines of communication.

The role of EMS in a terrorist attack is to reduce the number of losses, measured in death (mortality) and illness (morbidity). To be more effective EMS must be proactive and prepare for a terrorist attack, assuming the inevitability of such an attack in their community. This goal is accomplished, in part, by establishing an **emergency operations plan (EOP)**. An EOP is an interagency document that assigns responsibilities to departments or organizations, therefore, setting outlines of command (authority), and describes how emergency responders will protect people and property in the event of a terrorist attack as well as apprehend those who are responsible.

An EOP should be available at every level of government. At the federal level, Public Law 93-288 (Robert T. Stafford Disaster Relief and Emergency Assistance Act) provides for a **federal response plan (FRP)**. The FRP is utilized whenever state and local authorities are overwhelmed and brings the immense resources of the federal government to their aid. For example, the FRP calls for the National Communication System to assist with communications and the Army Corps of Engineers to help with public works. For EMS the American Red Cross has been identified as the lead federal agency by Congress. There are 12 emergency support functions that the federal government has identified where it can help local emergency responders with the mitigation of a terrorist attack. The agencies responsible for each emergency support function are listed in Table 46-3.

Emergency Operations Plan

Every emergency operations plan must first have a hazard vulnerability analysis, similar to a hazardous materials operations plan. High-risk hazards for terrorist attacks include government buildings

TABLE 46-3

Emergency Support Functions Defined in the Federal Response Plan

Emergency Support Function	Responsible Federal Agency
1. Transportation	U.S. Department of Transportation
2. Communications	U.S. National Communications System
3. Public Works	U.S. Department of Defense
4. Firefighting	U.S. Department of Agriculture
5. Information/Planning	U.S. Federal Emergency Management Agency
6. Mass Care	American Red Cross
7. Resource Support	Government Supply Agency
8. Health and Medical Service	U.S. Department of Health and Human Resources
9. Urban Search and Rescue	U.S. Federal Emergency Management Agency
10. Hazardous Materials	U.S. Environmental Protection Agency
11. Food	U.S. Department of Agriculture
12. Energy	U.S. Department of Energy

(courthouses, post offices, etc.) as well as high life hazards (malls, schools, etc.). The plan should also contain a listing of potentially valuable resources as well as locations of equipment stockpiles, such as antidote kits. Also, facilities for mass decontamination should be prepared for just such an emergency.

EMS should also collaborate with local, state, and federal law enforcement agencies, to share intelligence about terrorist groups that may be operating within the area. Groups that should be suspect include ethnic separatists, left- and right-wing radical organizations, survivalist groups, and foreign terrorist organizations.

Emergency Responders and the EOP

For any plan to be effective there must be training and regular drills. Assistant Chief Phil Chovan of the Marietta, Georgia, fire department suggests that all EMS crews practice scene safety using the **LACES** mnemonic.

The "L" in LACES stands for lookout. Someone should be assigned as a lookout at any event that may be a target of a terrorist attack. That lookout is responsible for observing irregular or inconsistent behaviors as well as unattended packages. The lookout, as safety officer, should have a stand back-and-observe or big-picture attitude. Snipers, for example, depend on the emergency services focusing on the event and not taking their environment into account.

The "A" in LACES stands for awareness. Every EMT should be minimally trained to the awareness level for emergency response to terrorism. The federal Office of Domestic Preparedness, a part of Homeland Security, offers courses as does the National Association of EMT. These courses help the EMT to identify potential hazards.

Communications, the "C" in LACES, is critical for on-scene operations. The mainstay of EMS scene communications are mobile and portable radios. These radios should be able to communicate with other emergency services, such as law enforcement, while on scene.

However, it may be hazardous to use portable radios for fear of triggering detonation of an explosive device by activating an electronic blasting cap designed to be triggered by radio signals from a safe distance. Secondary devices, intentionally left by terrorists to maim emergency services responders, may be designed to be triggered by emergency service radios in the near vicinity.

Personal safety is high on the list of responsibilities for an EMT. Therefore, an escape route, the "E" in LACES, must be available so that emergency responders can exit the scene quickly and with a minimum of confusion. Often this is as simple as positioning the emergency vehicle toward an exit and making sure that it is not blocked in.

Finally, the "S" in LACES stands for safety zones. The EMT should keep the principles of the safety zones in mind, staying within the cold zone and avoiding the warm/hot zones. Typically, the cold zone is uphill, as many gases are heavier than air, and upwind, as well as a safe distance from the incident site. Table 46-4 lists all of the elements of LACES.

TABLE 46-4

Elements of LACES

L =	Lookout
A =	Awareness
C =	Communications
E =	Escape Routes
S =	Safety Zones

Emergency Response

When responding to a suspect EMS call the EMT must maintain a high index of suspicion that the call may be for a terrorist attack. Calls that should be considered suspect include unexplained explosions, multiple calls for the same or similar complaint across a jurisdiction, called a symptom cluster, or the report of multiple casualties without a significant mechanism of injury.

Upon arrival a scene survey may reveal signs of an NBC attack. Indicators may include ground-level vapor clouds, dead foliage or dead wildlife such as birds, and objects such as a chemical sprayer that seem out of place.

Delaying entry in these cases may be the correct choice of action. The EMT should call for additional resources to help secure the scene and to bring detection equipment.

The EMT should also be suspicious of people and vehicles leaving the scene. License plate numbers or a brief description of persons on scene can be invaluable to investigators later. A rough sketch of the scene, as it was found, can help investigators.

The EMT should consider this initial approach a reconnaissance mission, gathering data and then withdrawing to report the findings to the proper authorities.

Street Smart

The EMT should consider wearing ballistic protection, also known as body armor, when responding to a potential terrorist attack. Body armor may save the EMT's life if a secondary device is used or a sniper remains on scene to disrupt emergency operations.

EOP Activation

The actions of the first emergency responder can have critical importance upon the number of civilian casualties and the effective mitigation of the terrorist attack.

Of critical importance is the "first in report." This report will put into motion the EOP and includes public warning and information and activating plans for evacuation and emergency shelters.

Air Monitoring and Detection Devices

The tactical use of detection devices can prevent needless illness or death. There are many devices available to help the EMT determine if WMD are present.

From simple Geiger counters to dosimeters, qualified and trained personnel can use special detection units to check for the presence of radioactive materials that may remain from an NDD.

Similarly, ionizing detection units and colorimetric sampling devices can test for the presence of toxic chemicals in the environment. The military has made available special field detection kits, such as M-8 and M-9 paper, that can detect liquid nerve and blister agents. These handheld point of detection devices should only be used by qualified personnel who have personal protective equipment in case of exposure (Figure 46-6).

Self-Protection

Upon establishing that a WMD attack may have occurred the EMT should make efforts to protect herself. Self-protection can be reduced to three concepts: time, distance, and shielding. Once the hazard has been identified the EMT should spend the minimum amount of time in the area. A tactical withdrawal, even when casualties are present and evident, reduces the total number of casualties overall.

The next protection is distance. Using the *Table of Initial Isolation and Protective Action Distances* in the ERG, the EMT should withdraw to a minimum safe distance. This distance should be the edge of the cold zone, and the EMT should make efforts to secure the area, isolate the hazard, and deny entry to others who are not properly protected.

The final protection is shielding. Shielding can be in the form of concrete barriers, protection from snipers or radiation, or in the form of barrier devices such as gloves, masks, and gowns.

Threat Reduction

Understanding what threats may be present can help the EMT prepare. The mnemonic **TRACEM** enumerates these hazards. The "T" in TRACEM stands for thermal harm. Explosive devices can produce harmful extremes of heat, causing burn injury. Fortunately, firefighting protective garments, from class A to standard issue equipment, can help protect against burn injury.

The harm created by a nuclear device, done at the cellular level, is via invisible alpha, beta, and gamma radiations (the "R" in TRACEM). The best protection among the cellular damage done by radiation is time, distance, and shielding.

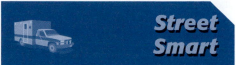

Street Smart

Every terrorist attack is, by definition, an illegal act and therefore a crime scene. It is important that the EMT leave things as they are found and only move those items that are absolutely necessary for patient care. If an object is moved, its position should be noted, and, if possible, even a picture could be taken before it is moved.

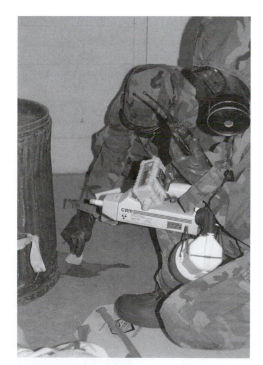

FIGURE 46-6 Military personnel using special chemical detection equipment, including M-8 paper.

TABLE 46-5

TRACEM
T = Thermal harm, e.g., burn trauma
R = Radiation harm, e.g., radiation burns
A = Asphyxiation
C = Corrosive chemicals, e.g., chemical burns
E = Etiologic, e.g., infections
M = Mechanical, e.g., blast injuries

The "A" in TRACEM represents asphyxiants, such as choking agents, which interfere with respiration and thus can be deadly. Gases are often asphyxiants, and most dangerous gases are heavier than air. Staging EMS uphill and upwind of these gases can prevent injury or death from asphyxiants.

Toxic or corrosive chemicals, the "C" in TRACEM, can also injure the EMT, causing painful chemical burns. To prevent exposure to these potentially lethal chemicals the EMT should first delay assessment and treatment until the patient has been decontaminated. The EMT should then employ the use of barrier devices, such as gowns, gloves, and goggles, to prevent possible cross-contamination.

The average EMT works everyday at risk of contracting a contagious disease, called an etiologic (The "E" in TRACEM), and use of common personal protective equipment, such as gloves and goggles, can eliminate the risk of an exposure to a potentially infectious material.

The last harm that can come to an EMT from WMD, and the last letter in TRACEM, is mechanical harm ("M"). Explosive devices, such as the secondary device, can produce serious life-threatening trauma. To prevent this harm or to reduce the amount of harm, the EMT should consider using ballistic protection, such as ballistic vests, for example. Table 46-5 outlines what TRACEM represents.

Incidental Exposure to Nerve Agents

Despite an EMT's best efforts she or her partner may become exposed to a nerve agent. These nerve agents, as discussed earlier, are very potent and require immediate treatment.

Recognizing this fact the military uses a special antidote kit called the Mark I kit. This kit is a pair of autoinjectors containing the antidotes atropine (equivalent 2 mg atropine sulfate) and 2-PAM Chloride (pralidoxime chloride) (Figure 46-7).

These autoinjectors work similarly to those that an EMT uses to administer epinephrine during an anaphylactic reaction. The Mark I kit should only by used by responders, one administering to the other, or to patients, when the person is symptomatic (i.e., SLUDGE), or upon orders of medical control.

It is not necessary to remove clothing and expose the thigh to use these injectors, and the atropine is always given before the 2-PAM Chloride. It may be necessary to give multiple doses, every 5 minutes, for a maximum of three or until the symptoms subside. The EMT should carefully read local and/or state guidelines for the use of these drugs.

CONCLUSION

In the current day and age, the EMT must have a heightened awareness of the potential for terrorist attacks and be prepared to act, within the established system, to bring order from chaos and to save as many lives as possible. For the EMT who is the first emergency responder the task of communicating the nature of the incident and activating the emergency operations plan is of critical importance.

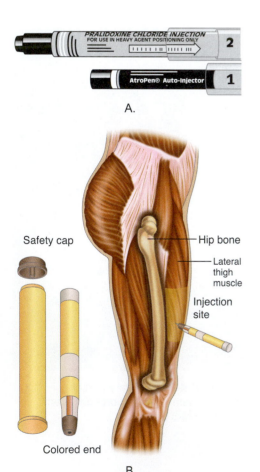

FIGURE 46-7 The atropine autoinjector is similar to the epinephrine autoinjector and can deliver lifesaving medications to contaminated patients, including EMTs.

TEST YOUR KNOWLEDGE

1. What is meant by the term *terrorism*?
2. Differentiate between domestic terrorism and international terrorism.
3. What is an emergency operations plan?
4. What are some potential signs of a terrorist attack?
5. Describe how an EMT would "self-protect" from hazards on scene.

INTERNET RESOURCES

- Armed Forces Radiobiology Research Institute, http://www.afrri.usuhs.mil
- Centers for Disease Control and Prevention: Emergency Preparedness and Response, http://www.bt.cdc.gov
- U.S. Army Medical Research Institute of Chemical Defense: Chemical Casualty Care Division, http://ccc.apgea.army.mil
- U.S. Army Medical Research Institute of Infectious Diseases, http://www.usamriid.army.mil
- U.S. Federal Emergency Management Agency, http://www.fema.gov

FURTHER STUDY

Bevelacqua, A., & Stilp, R. (2004). *Terrorism handbook for operational responders* (2nd ed.). Clifton Park, NY: Thomson Delmar Learning.

Buck, G. (2002). *Preparing for terrorism: An emergency services guide.* Clifton Park, NY: Thomson Delmar Learning.

Hawley, C. (2002). *Hazardous materials air monitoring and detection devices.* Clifton Park, NY: Thomson Delmar Learning.

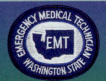

EMS in Rural America

KEY TERMS

power takeoff (PTO)

rollover protective structure (ROPS)

silage

silos

toxic organic dust syndrome (TODS)

OBJECTIVES

Upon completion of this chapter, the reader should be able to:

1. Recognize common mechanisms of injury on the farm.
2. List the general principles of farm rescue.
3. Describe the approach to livestock.
4. List the hazards of farm machinery.
5. Describe the injuries that occur from farm machinery.
6. Discuss the care of the patient injured by a power takeoff.
7. Discuss the care of the patient injured in a tractor rollover.
8. Discuss the dangers of silo rescue.
9. Discuss potentially hazardous materials found on a farm.

OVERVIEW

Three quarters of the land mass in the United States is considered rural (nonmetropolitan) and is home to approximately 50 million Americans. Much of this land is used for agricultural industries such as dairy farming, feed production, and the like. Historically, farming has been one of America's most dangerous occupations. While farmers only represent 3% of the U.S. workforce, they account for 10% of all work-related deaths.

Farmers are independent and self-reliant out of necessity. When emergency medical services (EMS) gets a call to respond to a farm, it can be generally assumed that a true emergency exists and that special circumstances, unique to rural EMS, may exist on scene.

FARM EMERGENCIES

The vast majority (90%) of farms are owned by private individuals or families, and the near-majority (45%) of these farms consist of less than 500 acres of land. Approximately eight million Americans operate these small farms. The primary operators of 25% of these farms are women. In many cases, young children help with the chores, some as

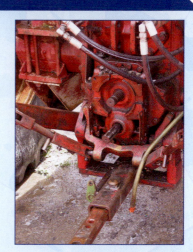

Farm Accident

"Hello, this is the Delhi farm, there's been an accident."

The hay baler had just kicked out its last bale of hay and Dorothea was climbing down from the wagon when she saw Tom straddle the power takeoff, trying to get to the other side of the tractor. It was then that the power takeoff, still engaged and spinning, grabbed the string from his sweatshirt hood, and in a matter of seconds wrapped Tom's hood, sweatshirt, and then Tom around the shaft and started to throw him to the ground.

Dorothea leaped to action, disengaged the clutch and seeing that Tom was seriously hurt, told him to lie still. Cell phone coverage was poor, at best, in this county and Dorothea was forced to run the half mile to the phone in the barn to call for help.

- What special hazard, unique to the rural environment, was found in this case?
- What are some of the barriers that rural EMS providers face?

young as 10 years old, and as many as 100,000 children are injured on farms annually.

Predictably, the majority (75%) of injuries on farms occur during the months of June, July, and August, when farming is at its peak. The case of a 97-year-old farmer killed in a tractor rollover while on a farm only illustrates that many of America's farmers, like all Americans, are getting older.

Owing to the nature of a farm, most farm emergencies are traumatic in nature. The usual mechanisms of injury include machinery, tractor collisions, electrocutions, falling objects, and livestock.

Farm Rescue

Farm rescue should be approached similarly to hazardous materials incident planning. A preplan serves as excellent preparation for future emergencies on a farm and should include detailed maps of the farm that outline building location, preplanned staging areas for heavy or special rescue, and Material Safety Data Sheets (MSDS) for chemicals used or stored on the farm.

After identifying farms within their jurisdiction, EMS providers should tour those farms and look for predictable health hazards, such as pesticide depots and feed silos. It can be very helpful, especially at night, to have maps with premeasured mileage estimates from major intersections to the farm and global positioning satellite (GPS) coordinates for preplanned helicopter landing zones.

Basic Rescue Principles

As in all EMS operations, the first rule for the emergency medical technician (EMT) is not to become a victim. There are many cases of would-be rescuers who entered silos or feeding bins, only to become entrapped and suffocate. The EMT should approach every scene cautiously and observe for possible life threats.

When encountering unique situations, such as specialized heavy farm machinery or confined spaces, including open-feed bins, the EMT should call for trained rescue personnel immediately. Time may be critical, especially in a rural situation, and calling for help as early as possible improves the patient's chances of survival.

While awaiting the arrival of these specially trained rescue personnel the EMT can attempt to reduce, or mitigate, life threats. In some cases, use of barn fans for ventilation of the area can reduce or eliminate toxic or explosive gas, for example, or shutting off power at a central electric panel, can disable motors that power augers or belts.

If the patient is accessible and can be safely extricated from the scene without endangering the EMT, then the EMT could consider using one of the emergency moves described in Chapter 11, such as the long axis clothing drag. Once the patient is out of harm's way, then the EMT can complete an initial assessment, typically starting with manual stabilization of the cervical spine in cases of trauma.

Livestock

Many farms have cows, horses, sheep, and other livestock. While referred to as dumb animals, they have a strong intuition for danger and can react unpredictably in order to avoid harm. When scared or startled, livestock can unintentionally kick, pin, bite, or gore a person who is in their path of escape.

As in all cases, the EMT's own safety comes first. Proper personal protective equipment (PPE) includes footwear with a slip-resistant tread, and the EMT should consider steel-reinforced toes. Rubber firefighter's boots may not prevent falls due to slipping.

Animals also harbor many diseases that are "cross-species" communicable (i.e., capable of being transmitted from animal to human), for example, salmonellosis, ringworm, and rabies. The EMT should consider wearing nonsterile gloves, the kind typically worn during patient care, under a pair of leather-palmed gloves, a pair that can withstand the wear and tear of moving or working with machinery or animals.

Shin guards are also helpful in preventing injuries to the EMT. Athletic shin guards, like the kind worn in soccer, can be put on quickly and may prevent unnecessary injuries.

The EMT should treat every barnyard emergency as he would any patient encounter, including hand washing after either patient or animal encounter.

With proper PPE in place, the EMT needs to remove the animal from the proximity of the patient. This can either be done by moving the animal, which is preferred, or by removing the patient by using an emergency move.

Animal behavior is similar to human behavior, that is, animals have thirst, hunger, fear, and a maternal instinct to protect their young. Understanding these behaviors before approaching an animal can help to prevent a tragic mishap.

Animals also have species-specific differences. For example, cows and pigs are color blind and depend on changes in shades to differentiate objects and people. These animals tend to balk at shadows and are startled by sudden changes in light.

Furthermore, these animals lack depth perception. A cow may not even be aware that it has pinned an EMT against the side of a stall. A mature bull can weigh over 2,000 pounds.

The hind quarters of a cow are its blind spots. If an EMT was to approach a cow from the rear, an unexpected and often violent reaction can occur. It is better that the EMT announce his presence and approach the cow from the front. If it is necessary to approach a cow from the back, perhaps because it is tethered to the stall, then the EMT should make his presence known in a manner that will not startle the cow. If it is necessary to move the cow, the EMT should try to get someone the cow knows to help move it. Cows know their handlers and are often afraid of strangers. If at all possible, try to get the handler to remove all of the cows from the barn. Cows have a strong herd instinct and are more apt to follow the herd, as illustrated in Figure 47-1. The EMT should avoid loud sounds, including yelling or banging equipment, as this tends to startle and frighten the cows. If an EMT is assisting the farmer with moving cattle the EMT should always have an escape route planned, in case the animal charges intentionally or unintentionally. An escape route can help prevent the EMT from being pinned against a wall, from being trampled in a stampede, or from being gored by a frightened animal.

On the other hand, horses have a keen sense of hearing, are constantly scanning their environment, and will alert the EMT that they are aware of his approach by moving their ears in his direction. The observant EMT knows when a horse is about to kick, usually rearward, or bite, because the horse will flatten its ears. The EMT should slowly back away from the animal.

It is best to approach a horse from the left shoulder and move slowly but confidently toward the horse, all the time talking, not shouting, to it. When the horse recognizes the EMT it will turn and "address" him. The EMT should wait for that signal before proceeding any further.

Leading a horse is not difficult if the EMT follows a few simple rules. Always use the lead, not the halter to lead a horse. Grabbing a hold of the halter risks getting the EMT's fingers entrapped in the gear and then being dragged around the yard. With the lead firmly in the hand and not wrapped around the fingers, about 8–10 inches away from the horse's head, the EMT should walk deliberately in order to lead the horse and not the other way around. Once the horse is following the EMT, he should position himself parallel to the horse; horses kick forward and rearward and walking parallel makes it difficult for the horse to kick the EMT.

Farm Vehicle Heavy Rescue

There are many obstacles to farm vehicle heavy rescue throughout the rescue evolution. The first obstacle to achieving that goal of trauma care, getting the patient to definitive care within the golden hour, is just getting to the scene within an hour. Farm accidents tend to happen in remote areas where there may be poor road conditions that make gaining access to the accident site difficult.

Once on scene, the EMT may also have trouble with turning off diesel engines, stabilizing heavy equipment that weigh over one ton

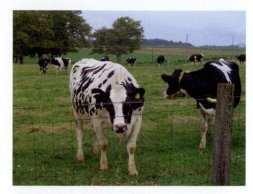

FIGURE 47-1 Cows are herd animals that can react unpredictably to strangers. (Courtesy of Morguefile.)

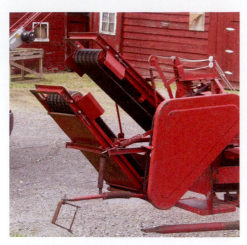

FIGURE 47-2A Belts and pulleys can entangle and mangle limbs.

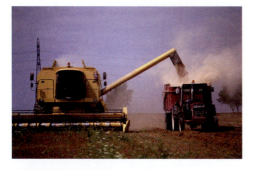

FIGURE 47-2B Combines can cut a farmer's arm as easily as the crop being harvested. (Courtesy of PhotoDisc.)

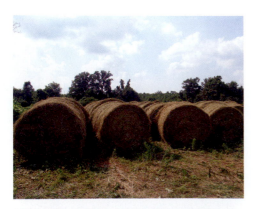

FIGURE 47-2C Hay bales, sometimes weighing hundreds of pounds, can easily crush an arm or a leg. (Courtesy of Morguefile.)

with standard cribbing, or avoiding sharp cutting knives, rollers, flails as well as the more typical hazards of spilled fuel and battery acid.

Once the patient is disentangled from the machinery then the EMT has to consider how he will get the patient out. While air medical evacuation would seem ideal, it is often not available in some rural areas and ambulances have a difficult time traversing the rough terrain.

It should be noted that in some cases, the combination of these factors can change a patient rescue into a body recovery. If this is the case, medical control should be contacted as soon as possible to make on-the-scene decisions and to possibly prevent any injury of the rescuers who might work frantically to rescue a person who has no chance of survival.

Mechanism of Injury

The typical mechanism of injury at a farm rescue involves entanglement in an exposed screw (auger), belt drive, or power takeoff (PTO) drive shaft, or by being struck by spinning crank handles or being crushed by shifting loads.

The majority of these accidents are secondary to operator error. In many cases, these accidents could have been prevented by proper footwear, preventing slips and falls, or properly fitting clothing. Loose clothing, caught in augers, belts, and PTO shafts, are the cause of many farm accidents.

The injuries that an EMT might typically see on scene of a farm accident include severe lacerations, including partial or complete avulsions seen with limb entanglement in a PTO shaft, or limbs caught in exposed belts such as shown in Figure 47-2A. Other injuries are puncture wounds, secondary to impalements on conventional balers, or degloving injuries, for example, from hands caught within the rollers of a corn head, the cutting portion of a combine, such as the bean combine shown in Figure 47-2B. Crush injuries occur when heavy loads shift unexpectedly, like the hay bale being lifted in Figure 47-2C.

While these injuries can be grotesque, the bleeding that accompanies them is usually more problematic and may be more life-threatening. Therefore, the EMT should avoid focusing on the maimed limb but rather on the overall condition of the patient.

FARM RESCUE PRINCIPLES

Like vehicle rescue, farm rescue has some general principles. First, the EMT should ensure that the scene is rendered as safe as possible and that a perimeter is established to prevent entry of unprotected personnel or bystanders into the scene. An inner action circle and an outer safety perimeter are commonly used. Only those EMTs and rescuers who are properly prepared with PPE are permitted within the inner action circle. The remaining EMTs and rescuers should stand outside the safety perimeter, along with bystanders, until summoned into either inside the outer safety perimeter or into the inner action circle. Needed equipment should be staged inside the outer safety circle, but outside the action circle, until needed.

Once the perimeter has been established, it is important that there be a plan for rescue. Fire rescue and EMS should confer and develop a plan as well as a backup plan in case of failure. Redundancy in planning, that is, a backup plan, helps ensure the overall success of the mission. Many rural emergency services implement the incident management system on the scene of a farm rescue. Refer to Chapter 44 for information about public safety management.

Often special equipment may be needed on the scene of a farm rescue and must be requested early. For example, heavy timbers may be needed for cribbing and shoring; these timbers are heavier than the typical cribbing used in vehicular rescue. Special heavy-duty air bags or high-lift jacks may also be needed. In many cases, the availability of front-end loaders and tow trucks make them practical rescue tools. However, only experienced lift operators, in cooperation with trained heavy rescue personnel, should use this equipment.

As a rule, whenever a machine is being lifted, cribbing should be used to protect the patient and the rescuers from shifting loads. Generally, tractors and the like are never lifted by the wheels but rather a firm purchase is made on the frame of the machine directly.

If specialized farm equipment such as balers or corn pickers are involved, then the EMT should consider calling the local farm equipment dealer. These dealers are often expert at dismantling farm equipment; therefore, their emergency numbers should be maintained onboard the ambulance or in the rescue truck.

In rare cases where prolonged disentanglement could jeopardize the patient's life, it may be necessary to perform a field amputation. In those instances, a physician should be called to the scene to stand by and perform the necessary procedures.

It is important for the EMT to understand that disentanglement and extrication are only the first part of a rescue. The patient will need to be evacuated as soon as possible once extrication has occurred. Owing to the nature of these injuries, it is not uncommon to have air medical resources, such as a helicopter, standing by.

Depending on the location of the accident, for example, in a distant farm field, it may be necessary to have off-road vehicles, such as all-terrain vehicles, available to transport the patient to an awaiting ambulance.

Tractor Accidents

Tractors, first mass produced in 1916, have literally been the workhorse of the farm for almost a century. These machines often have different purposes and therefore come in a variety of sizes and configurations. Many of these machines cost thousands of dollars, therefore, farmers keep these machines in service for many years.

Tractor operation represents a dual hazard to the farmer. For one, tractors tend to be involved in collisions with other motor vehicles when they are on the highway. The other danger is that tractors can turn over, or roll over, pinning the driver in the process.

Car–tractor accidents are a reality of rural EMS. Automobile drivers, sharing the road with the farmer, fail to recognize the slow-moving tractor in time and tend to collide with it. Traveling at high speeds on country roads, the driver of a motor vehicle can suddenly, and unexpectedly, come upon a tractor in the roadway (Figure 47-3). The unfamiliar silhouette of the tractor may momentarily confuse the

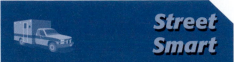

Street Smart

Prolonged periods of compression on an extremity can lead to crush syndrome. The complications of crush syndrome can be eliminated or reduced by applying advanced life support measures before the object is removed.

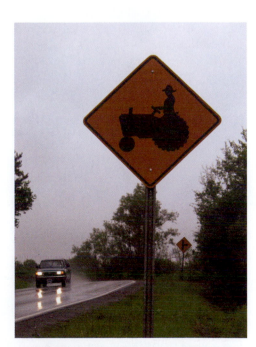

FIGURE 47-3 Slow-moving farm machinery are no match for high performance engines in modern cars.

driver. This, combined with the slow speed of the tractor, absent or poorly maintained lighting, or absent, bent, or worn slow-moving vehicle (SMV) emblems, can contribute to tractor/auto collisions.

Other contributing factors include the failure of the tractor operator to signal his or her intentions (e.g., swinging right in a wide-turning radius to go left) and poor visibility. Many tractor accidents occur at dusk when lighting is poor or drivers are blinded by the setting sun.

Tractor Rollovers

The single largest contributor to mortality on the farm are tractor rollovers. These rollovers can pin the operator under the weight of the tractor and literally crush him or her.

The majority of tractor rollovers are sideways overturns, about 85%, that occur after the tractor strikes a hard unmovable object, or the tractor is operated on a steep slope where soils can unexpectedly shift.

While less common, only about 14%, rear rollovers, sometimes called a kickout, account for more fatalities. When a tractor flips in this manner it tends to trap the operator under the tractor or throw him or her off the tractor. Kickouts tend to occur when a tractor is forward facing a steep slope, such as driving over a hillock, or when a tractor is used to free another tractor that is stuck and a pull cable releases and the tractor overturns.

The advent of farm tractor safety regulations has decreased the incidence of these potentially deadly rollovers. Federal labor standards, for example, have required that new tractors, manufactured after 1976, have a **rollover protective structure (ROPS)** in place to protect the operator. ROPS is a protective bar or canopy, as shown in Figure 47-4, that prevents the driver from being crushed under the weight of the tractor.

Problems occur when older tractors that are still in service, and predating 1976, are being used by inexperienced operators, or the ROPS protection has been removed by the farmer. In many cases, these older tractors are being operated by younger, inexperienced operators who do not know how to respond when the tractor rolls or kicks back. A tractor without ROPS is shown in Figure 47-5.

When an EMT first arrives on the scene of a tractor rollover the first priority, in terms of scene safety, is fire suppression. Spilled fuels can easily ignite, causing a fire, and a fire extinguisher or charged fire hose should be at standby at all times.

Next is to turn off the tractor. Many rescuers start by immediately blocking the wheels. Turning wheels can inadvertently restart a diesel engine. If the tractor engine operates on gasoline, then the engine can simply be shut off by the key. If the tractor engine operates on diesel fuel, then the injector pump stop rod should be engaged. If the diesel engine continues to idle, called dieseling, then it may be necessary to "choke" the engine. This can be accomplished by either stuffing a rag down the air intake or by discharging a carbon dioxide fire extinguisher into the air cleaner.

With the tractor turned off, the rescuers should turn their attention to rescue. The two options are to either lift the tractor off the patient or to dig the patient out. It usually takes a tow truck, hydraulic jacks, or heavy rescue air bags to lift a small tractor. In some cases, a small

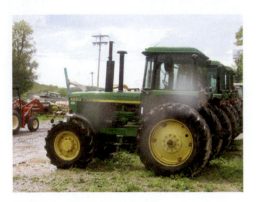

FIGURE 47-4 The tractor operator has a great deal more protection with a rollover protective structure (ROPS).

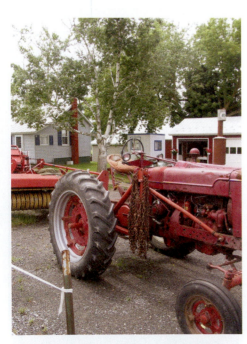

FIGURE 47-5 Operators of older tractors without ROPS, such as the one pictured here, are at risk for being entrapped and crushed.

tractor can be lifted manually. The general rule of rescue is to "crib as you go," that is, to build a frame of wooden blocks that prevents the tractor from shifting and falling back on the patient again. These rescues should only be performed by trained farm rescuers who have practiced their techniques and know their equipment.

Alternatively, the rescuers may elect to dig the patient out. Digging the patient is used whenever a patient is entrapped under a heavy machine. Initially, the tractor must be firmly stabilized, similar to a motor vehicle, with cribbing, timbers, and the like. To prevent cave-ins, the "foot print" of the cribbing must be as wide as possible, and ancillary cribbing should be in place in case of soil shifting. Again, these rescue techniques should only be used by experienced and trained farm rescuers.

Once the patient has been disentangled and extricated, the EMT will often find a predictable injury pattern. Because of the mechanism of injury, a crushed pelvis is often common; about 80% of tractor accidents result in a crushed pelvis. A crushed pelvis may be managed by either a pelvic sling or by application of a pneumatic anti-shock garment (PASG) as noted in Chapter 25.

Trauma to the chest may also cause a collapsed lung, or pneumothorax, as well as massive contusions to the chest. Entrapped patients may also experience burns from the host of liquids present, including radiator fluids, hydraulic fluids, battery acid, and the calcium chloride mixture found in the tires. As much as 100–150 gallons of calcium chloride is placed inside the tractor's tires to provide weight (as much as 1,500 pounds), and therefore stability to the tractor. The EMT should also take protective measures to prevent accidental exposure/contact.

Power Takeoff

The **power takeoff (PTO)**, developed in the 1920s, permits a farmer to use his or her tractor as a portable power supply. A PTO is a spinning shaft that transfers the tractor engine's power to another farm machine, such as a hay baler. The PTO is a versatile tool for providing power to augers that move manure or feed up elevators, to lift and move hay or feed, and to power post hole diggers.

Traditionally, a PTO is found at the rear of the tractor, above the drawbars that are used to pull a machine behind the tractor. However, newer tractors may have a PTO at the front of the tractor as well.

The PTO of a tractor is not limited to use only on a farm. Suburban landscapers, lawn maintenance workers, and everyday homeowners can own a tractor with a PTO. Snowblowers, that modern convenience, are powered by the engine via a PTO that is found in the front of the snowblower.

Early models of tractors had no shield over the PTO and the operator could see the shaft and the universal joint connection spinning. These open PTOs presented a clear danger to the operator (Figure 47-6). Newer models had a U-shaped shield that protected the shaft from above while permitting access to the shaft, for service and maintenance, from below. The newest PTO has a circumferential shield that prevents accidental contact with the spinning shaft.

The PTO revolves in a clockwise fashion, facing the rear of the tractor, and has different speeds; in smaller tractors the PTO spins at 540

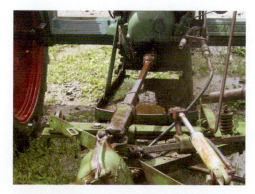

FIGURE 47-6 An unshielded power takeoff (PTO), spinning as fast as 1,000 rpm, can tear a limb off.

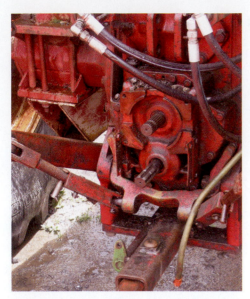

FIGURE 47-7 PTOs can spin at low speed (540 rpm) or high speed (1,000 rpm).

revolutions per minute (rpm), or 9 revolutions per second, and larger tractors at 1,000 rpm. Figure 47-7 shows a tractor with two PTOs, one high speed and one low speed.

Accidents occur whenever a piece of clothing or hair becomes entangled in the PTO, when the operator either leans over the PTO or steps over it to get to the other side of the tractor.

The predictable injury pattern from this entanglement includes severe lacerations, particularly to the face if a beard becomes entangled; fractures of the arms and legs, as sleeves, pant legs, or boot laces become entangled and the operator is literally spun around the shaft, striking tractor hitches, equipment tongues, and the ground with terrific force with each revolution; or degloving injuries, where all or part of the genitals are avulsed when the operator steps over the PTO, a straddle injury. If the body is not heavy enough to stall the engine, then the body is repeatedly pounded against the ground, resulting in significant spine injuries.

The principles of farm rescue from a PTO are similar to a tractor rollover: secure the scene, turn off the tractor, and block the wheels to prevent rolling.

When these tasks have been accomplished, the EMT should then proceed with disentangling the patient from the PTO. To properly disentangle the patient often requires that the PTO be either disassembled, which is preferable and requires the expertise of the local farm agent, or cut. It is imperative that trained rescuers, with the proper tools, be called early.

In some cases it may be possible to disentangle the patient from the machine manually. In those cases, the PTO must be placed in neutral and disconnected from the tractor. Then a large pipe wrench or crowbar is placed inside the yoke of the PTO and turned counterclockwise. The rescuers should never use the power of the tractor to reverse the PTO.

If the rescuers are unable to disentangle the patient from the shaft or joints of the PTO, it may be necessary to cut the shaft. Solid shafts may be cut with power grinders or hacksaws. The use of the oxyacetylene cutting torch should be reserved to trained rescue specialists. These torches produce heat that can be transferred up the shaft to the patient, burning her in the process.

Disentangling a patient from a PTO can be difficult. The PTO shaft that was under a load may suddenly release, further injuring the patient and possibly the EMT. Therefore, this type of rescue should be performed by trained farm rescuers.

Silos

Silos are structures that store **silage** (forage [food] typically stored in the silo) such as chopped corn, alfalfa, and chopped grass. Silos can be either horizontal, sometimes called bunker silos, or vertical. The vertical silo is the more traditional one that is seen in pictures of farms.

A traditional silo is between 12 and 14 feet in diameter, with large silos as large as 20–30 feet in diameter and up to 80 feet in height. A silo is actually rings of concrete blocks that raise one on top of another and are held in place by steel-retaining rings. The top of the roof is usually open with a weather cap, and feed is fed into the silo via a chute by a blower. Figure 47-8 shows a traditional silo.

New silage, depending on variables such as the time of year, feed, or weather may have between 45% and 70% moisture content. When stored in a confined space this silage uses all of the available oxygen to ferment the sugar in it until it produces lactic acid, which stops the fermentation process and permits the silage to be stored for long periods of time. During this process certain gases, commonly referred to as silo gases, are created.

Chief among these silo gases is nitrogen dioxide (NO_2). NO_2 is an irritating brownish gas with a bleach-like odor that is heavier than air. The danger of NO_2 is greatest approximately 2 weeks after the silo is filled. The danger of NO_2 is that it is heavier than air and therefore tends to displace oxygen, in effect making the silo an oxygen-poor environment. A farmer who falls into a silo during this period is in danger of suffocating to death. Clues for the presence of NO_2 include dead birds at the chutes and brownish stains on the sides of the silos (Figure 47-9).

Newer silos may be constructed of steel and are glass-lined (Figure 47-10). These silos are built to eliminate or reduce the oxygen within a silo and are thus called oxygen-limiting silos. While these oxygen-limiting silos eliminate the dangers of toxic silo gases seen in more traditional silos, they can be equally dangerous. As the name implies, an oxygen-limiting silo provides an oxygen-poor environment, similar to the type of environment encountered in confined space rescue.

Silo rescues, both traditional silos as well as oxygen-limiting silos, should be handled like a confined space rescue. There are cases of multiple victims during a silo rescue because each would-be rescuer who is not properly equipped with self-contained breathing apparatus (SCBA) becomes unconscious from the lack of oxygen then suffocates.

Another common silo emergency is entrapment. Farmers will enter a silo to clean a chute or to loosen packed silage. While settled silage can be firm enough to walk on, new silage has not compacted and the farmer is in danger of being engulfed in it.

On scene of such an emergency, the EMT should first use any ventilation fans that are available to clear dangerous silo gases. The fact that the victim is still alive is a good indication that sufficient oxygen is still available. However, the EMT should not take any chances and SCBA is strongly recommended.

If the victim is visible it may be possible to drop a rope or reach him or her with a pike pole. The victim should be encouraged to self-rescue if possible. Under no circumstances should the EMT enter the silo without a safety/recovery system in place. Only rescuers trained in silo rescue, who are properly equipped, should enter a silo.

If the victim is firmly entrapped it may be necessary to create cuts at the base of the silo to allow the silage to drain. These cuts, made with a corner of the bucket of a front-end loader, should be made perpendicular to one another in order to maintain the structural integrity of the silo. Otherwise, if too many holes are cut into the silo then it risks collapse, entrapping the victim.

Grain Bins

Grain bins, while appearing open, are deceptive and a farmer can be entrapped in it much the same way that he or she can be entrapped in a silo. Initially, the grain starts to flow, engulfing the farmer's feet. If

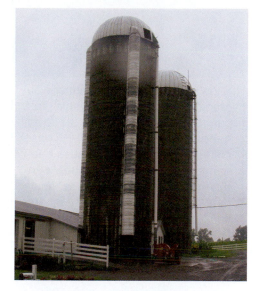

FIGURE 47-8 Traditional silos usually have an open roof with an aluminum weather cap.

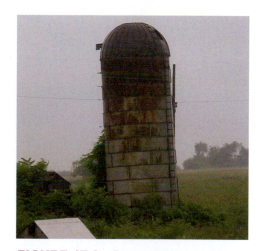

FIGURE 47-9 Brown stains on a silo can indicate the presence of nitrogen dioxide (NO_2).

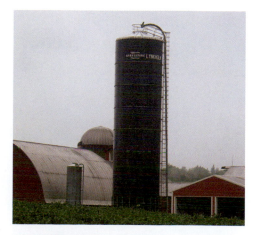

FIGURE 47-10 Steel blue silos may be oxygen-limiting silos and should be treated as confined space rescues.

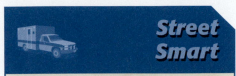

the farmer is submerged up to the knees there is little hope of escape and the farmer can be submerged in an avalanche of feed grain in as little as 10 seconds after that.

Like an avalanche, the EMT should assume that the victim is still alive, even if not visible, and continue to talk to him or her. While this psychological first aid is important, it also helps identify where the victim is in the pile.

If the grain bin has gravity gates, do not open them. There is a danger that the victim will be entrapped in the gates as the river of grain flows out of the bin. Similarly, power augers should not be used to drain the grain bin because the victim may get entangled inside the auger mechanism.

If the victim is partially submerged and visible to rescuers then self-rescue should be encouraged. A barrel, opened at both ends, can be lowered over the victim to act as a dam. Trained rescuers may create a plywood square that surrounds the victim, allowing him or her to dig the way out of the grain without danger of further entrapment.

If the victim is completely submerged then pairs of rescuers, in a buddy system, who are tied in with safety harnesses and rope systems may enter the grain bin to attempt a rescue.

Under no circumstances should the EMT enter the grain bin without proper training and safety equipment. Grain can be unpredictable, sliding and shifting when least expected and entrapping any EMT within its path.

Manure Storage

A common by-product of domestic animals is manure. Animal manure, like most things on a farm, is not wasted for it is rich in nitrogen and is therefore a natural fertilizer. For this reason, manure is usually mixed with water to become a slurry and is stored in a manure system.

Manure storage systems can be either aboveground or below ground. Aboveground storage systems can include large manure storage tanks, silo-type storage structures, or open pools of manure called lagoons or manure ponds. These manure lagoons can be particularly dangerous. Over time the top of the manure lagoon hardens, sometimes to the point that grass grows over the top, and an unsuspecting person will walk on the cap, crumbling it, and the person will drown in the manure. For this reason manure lagoons should be fenced off.

Below ground manure storage systems can be more dangerous than aboveground systems. Manure gases, that is, gases that are produced by bacteria breaking down the manure, can build to dangerous levels. These manure gases can either asphyxiate a farmer or a rescuer or represent an explosion hazard.

It is important that the EMT be aware of gases that may be present on scene and maintain an adequate distance from the scene until adequate ventilation can ensure clearance of these gases. Until the gases are cleared any source of ignition, either electronic (e.g., portable radios) or mechanical (e.g., cigarette lighters), should not be used in the vicinity until the gases are cleared.

If entry must be made into an underground storage facility, then only those rescuers with SCBA should be permitted to enter. Standard

N95 or dust/mist masks do not filter out gases and will not protect the EMT.

Confined space rescue such as this should only be performed by trained rescuers who have SCBA and safety harnesses.

Toxic Manure Gas

The danger for explosion from manure gas is owed to the methane, an odorless gas that is lighter than air, a by-product of decomposition of manure. Because methane is odorless the EMT must have a high index of suspicion of its potential presence and take appropriate protective actions, including maintaining a safe distance, preventing ignition, and awaiting proper ventilation.

The danger of other manure gases is that they displace oxygen and asphyxiate the victim. These manure gases include hydrogen sulfide (H_2S), ammonia (NH_3), and carbon dioxide (CO_2). In 1989, a 28-year-old farmer went into a 10-foot deep manure pit to repair an agitator shaft and was quickly overcome by manure gases. His 15-year-old nephew attempted to rescue him, only to meet the same fate. This pattern continued until the farmer, his nephew, and three other would-be rescuers laid at the bottom of the pit. The rescue squad arrived 20 minutes later and all five family members were dead. This story helps to illustrate the clear danger that manure gases present to rescuers.

A common manure gas is H_2S, considered by many to be the most dangerous. H_2S has the characteristic smell of rotten eggs. While it may seem obvious to the EMT that H_2S is present, the constant exposure to the smell, in small non-lethal quantities, dulls the farmer's awareness of its presence until the levels are dangerously high.

Another manure gas, NH_3, has similar effects as H_2S and its characteristic smell can be noted at much lower concentrations. CO_2 is odorless and simply displaces the oxygen in the environment.

All of these heavier-than-air gases displace oxygen, creating an oxygen-poor environment, and the patient, can become hypoxic and lose consciousness. Early symptoms of hypoxia can include headache, nausea, and dizziness. The key to survival is early recognition of these symptoms. Failure to do so can lead to collapse and worsening hypoxia as the patient is now lying at the level of the greatest concentration of toxic gases.

Farm Chemicals

Farmers use a large number of pesticides, herbicides, and fertilizers in order to improve production of foodstuffs. These products are all chemicals and exposure to any one of them should be treated like a hazardous material exposure. For example, a few drops of methyl parathion on the skin can be deadly.

One of the more common farm chemicals is anhydrous ammonia. Anhydrous ammonia is infused into the soil as a ready source of nitrogen for plants. Anhydrous ammonia is a double danger: (1) it is a toxic substance, and (2) it is transported as a liquid under pressure. An accidental release of anhydrous ammonia into the environment and onto the skin of the farmer can instantly freeze the skin. It will also dehydrate the skin; *an-* means "without" and *-hydrous* means "water," causing permanent damage to the skin. Treatment for an exposure to anhydrous ammonia includes flushing with copious volumes of water then treating the exposed skin like a burn.

Another common farm chemical is a class of chemicals called organophosphates (OP). Since its introduction as an insecticide by a chemist for the Bayer Pharmaceutical Company in the 1880s, OP has been widely used as an insecticide (parathion, diazinion, and malathion, for example) by many farmers. Unfortunately, OP was, like many other chemicals, weaponized during World War I into chemical gas compounds like sarin, soman, and tabun. These chemical weapons have recently resurfaced, after a treaty banning their use was signed by major world governments, as a terrorist weapon. Sarin, for example, was used in a deadly terrorist attack by the Aum Shinrikyo sect in the Tokyo subway system.

The symptom pattern for OP exposure on the farm is the same as the one for exposure to chemical weapons. The mnemonic SLUDGEM, depicted in Table 46-2, lists these common symptoms. Similarly, the treatment for both is the same also, the use of atropine. Atropine use for OP chemical exposure is also described in Chapter 46.

In every case where an EMT is confronted with a patient who may have had an exposure to a farm chemical the EMT should treat the exposure as a hazardous materials spill, including wearing appropriate protective equipment and attempting to identify the chemical. The *Emergency Response Guidebook* to hazardous materials can provide invaluable assistance as well as calling the poison control center, as local or regional protocols dictate.

CONCLUSION

Farming can be one of the most dangerous occupations in America. It can also be one of the most rewarding occupations, and for this reason farmers will always be a segment of the population.

It is therefore predictable that farm accidents will occur and the EMT will be called to the scene. While the majority of these EMS calls can be professionally managed with the training and skills of an average EMT, some instances will require the assistance of specially trained rescuers. Any EMT whose primary jurisdiction includes farmland should consider taking a farm rescue course in order to be prepared for any situation that might arise.

TEST YOUR KNOWLEDGE

1. What are some common mechanisms of injury on a farm?
2. What are the general principles of farm rescue?
3. What are the hazards that livestock represent?
4. What are the hazards of farm machinery?
5. What are the injuries that can be seen from entanglement with the power takeoff of a tractor?
6. What are the dangers of silo rescue?
7. What gases may be found in a manure storage facility?
8. What dangerous chemicals can be found on a farm?

INTERNET RESOURCES

- Cooperative Extension, Natural Resource, Agriculture, and Engineering Service (farm accident rescue), http://www.nraes.org
- Farm Safety Net, http://www.farmsafety.net
- Rural Medics, http://www.ruralmedics.com
- Trac-Safe: A Community-Based Program for Reducing Injuries and Deaths from Tractor Overturns, http://www.cdc.gov/niosh/tracsafe.html
- West Virginia University Center for Rural Emergency Medicine, http://www.hsc.wvu.edu (search for rural emergency)

FURTHER STUDY

American Academy of Orthopaedic Surgeons. (1993). *Rural rescue and emergency care.* Boston: Jones & Bartlett.

Dosman, James A., & Cockcroft, Donald W. (1989). *Principles of health and safety in agriculture.* Boca Raton, FL: CRC Press.

APPENDICES

APPENDIX A

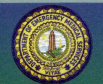

Advanced Airway Control

KEY TERMS

aspiration
direct laryngoscopy
DOPE
end tidal CO_2 detector
endotracheal intubation
hyperventilate
Macintosh blade
Miller blade
Murphy eye
nasogastric tube
orogastric tube
pneumothorax
right mainstem bronchus
stylet
syringe/bulb aspirator
tension pneumothorax
vallecula

OBJECTIVES

Upon completion of this appendix, the reader should be able to:

1. Identify advantages of endotracheal intubation.
2. Identify indications and contraindications for endotracheal intubation by the EMT-B.
3. List equipment needed to perform endotracheal intubation.
4. Describe the necessary steps involved in endotracheal intubation.
5. Describe the proper use of both the Miller and the Macintosh laryngoscope blades.
6. Identify advantages of cricoid pressure during endotracheal intubation.
7. Describe at least four methods to confirm tracheal tube placement.
8. Identify at least four parameters to monitor on the intubated patient.
9. Identify at least four problems that would cause the intubated patient to deteriorate.
10. Describe the most common complications associated with endotracheal intubation and identify how to avoid them or manage them.
11. Describe the procedures involved in intubating a trauma patient and how they differ from the procedures for a nontrauma patient.
12. Identify the indications for intubation of the pediatric patient.
13. Describe the advantages of endotracheal intubation in the pediatric patient.
14. Identify at least four unique anatomic features of the pediatric airway.
15. Identify the proper size for a laryngoscope blade and an endotracheal tube for an infant or a child, based upon age.
16. Describe why uncuffed endotracheal tubes are used in children under age 8.
17. Identify at least four complications of endotracheal intubation that are more commonly seen in the pediatric patient than in adults.

18. Describe the procedure for deep endotracheal suctioning.

19. Identify the indications for and benefits of orogastric tube placement.

20. Describe the procedure for orogastric tube placement.

21. Identify a management plan for the patient with a difficult airway.

OVERVIEW

The maintenance of an open airway by an emergency medical technician (EMT) is crucial when a patient cannot accomplish this task alone. Chapter 7 introduced several methods to manually open the airway. If a patient is in need of airway maintenance over an extended period of time, more secure means of stabilization may be required. Endotracheal intubation is an easily learned skill that any properly trained health care provider can perform.

As more advanced skills are performed, however, the potential complications become increasingly serious. An improperly placed endotracheal tube, if unrecognized, may lead to the death of the patient. Accurate initial assessment of tube placement and frequent reassessments will prevent unnecessary harm during advanced airway management.

When making the commitment to learn this method of airway management, the EMT must also commit to maintaining a level of skill with frequent training and continuing education. Quality management programs are necessary to ensure the adequate training and performance of these important skills by any health care provider.

Satisfactory performance of endotracheal intubation by the emergency medical technician–basic (EMT-B) will lead to a larger number of patients benefiting from this advanced airway technique. This utilization of the EMT-B is especially useful in geographic areas where more advanced levels of care are distant or nonexistent.

It should be remembered that the primary duty in emergency medical services (EMS) is to provide lifesaving care to patients in the prehospital setting without causing further harm. The performance of endotracheal intubation by an inadequately trained provider can cause significant harm to a patient. If an EMS system is unable to provide the necessary training, continuing education, and quality assurance programs needed to properly maintain this advanced airway skill, it should not be undertaken.

ENDOTRACHEAL INTUBATION

Endotracheal intubation is the procedure whereby a hollow plastic tube is placed in the trachea to allow for isolated ventilation of the lungs. This may be accomplished by direct visualization of the trachea through the mouth, called **direct laryngoscopy**, or, less commonly, by other more indirect methods.

Advantages

Intubation of the trachea allows for direct ventilation of the lungs without overflow of air into the stomach. This lack of gastric distension

Overdose

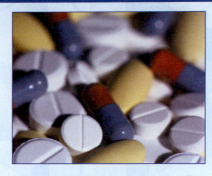

The tones awoke Bill, an EMT, from a sound sleep. "Cherry Valley Fire and Rural Medical Transport respond to a possible overdose, 420 Possum Road, the Delaney residence, County Fire Control Clear at zero hundred hours." Bill thought to himself, "Possum Road, that's clear on the other end of the district, maybe 25 miles."

Bill could see the flashing lights of the sheriff's patrol car up ahead when he pulled the department's first response truck onto Possum Road. As he pulled up to the house, the deputy yelled from the front porch, "Better bring your suction!"

Once inside, Bill could see a 30-something male, covered in vomit, lying on his back, as blue as his shirt. The deputy was holding a frantic woman who was yelling, "Do something!"

The patient, despondent over his wife's decision to divorce him, had taken a handful of pills and had drunk a fifth of whisky.

Bill donned his goggles, mask, and gloves and, with the assistance of the sheriff, logrolled the patient onto his side. After placing a large airway between the patient's upper and lower molars, Bill proceeded to scoop out chunks of half-digested meat and potatoes.

When Bill was finished, and after he had used the suction to clear the secretions, Bill prepared to ventilate the barely breathing patient.

But every time Bill had the patient on his back for more than a few minutes, he would vomit, and Bill would have to logroll him again. The patient's color was not improving much, and the ambulance, with the paramedic, was still 20 miles out.

- Why is the patient's airway at risk? What can be done about protecting it?
- What can an EMT do to assist another EMT, or an advanced EMT, who is intubating?

decreases the risk of vomiting and subsequent **aspiration**. Aspiration is the inadvertent passage of any material into the lower airways, often resulting in an inflammatory reaction within the lungs. Use of an occlusive balloon on the distal end of the endotracheal tube (ETT) serves to decrease risk of aspiration of any oral contents into the lungs.

Once an ETT has been placed, verified, and secured, the patient may be adequately ventilated by one rescuer without difficulty. The ease of ventilation afforded by lack of the need to maintain a mask seal allows for prolonged ventilation by a single rescuer.

When correctly placed, an ETT will allow for deep endotracheal suctioning as needed by some patients with profuse secretions. Inadequate suctioning can lead to impaired oxygenation as the secretions act as a barrier to alveolar-capillary oxygen diffusion.

Endotracheal intubation can be a very effective means of controlling a patient's airway when done properly. If expected to perform this skill, the EMT must know the indications, contraindications, and potential complications as well as become proficient in the procedure itself.

Pediatric Considerations

As a child's stomach becomes distended (as it often does with mask ventilation), it will push up into the chest cavity, decreasing the room available to the left lung for expansion. This distension will hinder adequate ventilation. Endotracheal intubation will largely overcome this problem and may allow for more effective ventilation in a pediatric patient.

Indications

The EMT should consider endotracheal intubation in any patient who cannot maintain a patent airway spontaneously or who is in need of

TABLE A-1

Conditions Requiring Intubation

Cardiac arrest

Respiratory arrest

Drug overdose

Persistent seizures

Severe head injury or facial injuries

Traumatic arrest

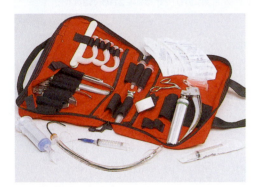

FIGURE A-1 Equipment necessary for endotracheal intubation.

Safety Tip

Always wear eye protection when intubating. Vomitus coming out of the mouth can have a great deal of force, especially if the stomach has been distended. Donning eye protection is as important as putting on gloves when an EMT is intubating.

Street Smart

After tested, the laryngoscope should be closed and the light allowed to turn off. Having the light off saves battery power for the procedure itself.

ventilatory assistance. Direct laryngoscopy and endotracheal intubation should be performed by the EMT only if the patient shows no evidence of an intact gag reflex. This reflex is easily tested for during the placement of an oropharyngeal airway, a necessary step before intubation. Table A-1 lists some types of patients who would be appropriate candidates for endotracheal intubation by the EMT-B.

Contraindications

Endotracheal intubation is a procedure that has serious complications if performed incorrectly. This skill should not be attempted by any provider who is not fully trained or who does not have adequate assistance or equipment. If conditions exist that may increase the risk of the procedure, then it should not be attempted if the airway can be controlled in another, less invasive manner.

At least two trained providers must be present in order to adequately perform this advanced airway skill. The duties of each person are detailed later in this chapter.

Attempting to perform any procedure without properly prepared equipment can lead to harm of the patient. Specific equipment complications will also be discussed later in this chapter.

The EMT should not attempt endotracheal intubation in a patient who has an intact gag reflex, as the procedure may induce vomiting. Vomiting during endotracheal intubation may lead to aspiration of gastric contents into the lungs. Aspiration of gastric contents will lead to a severe pneumonia and may negatively affect the survival of the patient.

The Procedure

As with any procedure, the key to success is in proper preparation. This preparation should include adequate training as well as a familiarity with the necessary equipment. Endotracheal intubation cannot be safely accomplished if the EMT is not familiar with the equipment and sure of where each item is located.

Upon making the decision that a patient needs to be intubated, the EMT must prepare the proper equipment (Figure A-1). Table A-2 lists the equipment necessary to perform endotracheal intubation.

Equipment Preparation

After identification of the patient in need of intubation, the EMT must prepare the equipment for the procedure while another trained provider manages and prepares the patient. All providers involved in the procedure must don appropriate personal protective equipment (PPE): gloves, mask, and goggles (or a mask with both face and eye protection).

The bag-valve-mask (BVM) should be attached to high-flow oxygen (15–25 lpm) and the proper-sized mask attached. An appropriate-sized oropharyngeal airway should be chosen, and the suction unit should be turned on and tested.

The proper-sized blade should be attached to the laryngoscope handle. This procedure is detailed in Skill A-1.

The proper-sized endotracheal tube must be chosen and its balloon tested. At its distal end, the endotracheal tube has a balloon, or cuff, that, when inflated in a patient's trachea, helps to hold it in place and prevents most substances from passing by into the lower airways (Figure A-2). This balloon holds between 5 and 10 cc of air and is inflated by instilling air into a smaller pilot balloon at the proximal end of the tube. A syringe with 10 cc of air in it should be attached to this small pilot balloon. The entire 10 cc of air should be instilled into the balloon, causing the distal cuff to inflate. The cuff should be checked to be sure that it is holding the air without leaking. If the cuff easily deflates or does not accept air, the tube is faulty and should not be used.

Pediatric Considerations

As a child grows, the tracheal rings grow larger and more rigid. Under the age of 8, the narrowest point in a child's airway is usually at the cricoid ring. Because the trachea enlarges relatively more than the opening at the vocal cords, this glottic opening is the narrowest point in the adult airway.

Because the narrowest point in a child's airway is at the cricoid ring, an endotracheal tube with a distal cuff (balloon) is not generally used. The tube is sized to fit well into this narrow opening, not leaving any room for a cuff to be inflated. Using a tube with a cuff would take up too much of the opening, or lumen, of the airway.

A narrowed airway partially occluded with a cuff would increase airway pressures while making it more difficult, if not impossible, to manually ventilate.

Unfortunately, not using a cuffed tube leaves the child with a tube that is easily displaced and may result in aspiration more readily. The EMT must be even more vigilant in protecting the child against tube dislodgment and aspiration.

Children 8 years of age and older may be intubated with a cuffed tube because their airway anatomy more closely resembles that of an adult.

TABLE A-2
Intubation Equipment

Gloves
Mask
Eye protection
Suction unit
Yankauer catheters
Oxygen source
Bag-valve-mask
Laryngoscope handle
Laryngoscope blades
Endotracheal tubes (different sizes)
Stylet
10-cc syringe
Oropharyngeal airway
Commercial securing device
End tidal CO_2 detector or/ capnography
Esophageal detector device

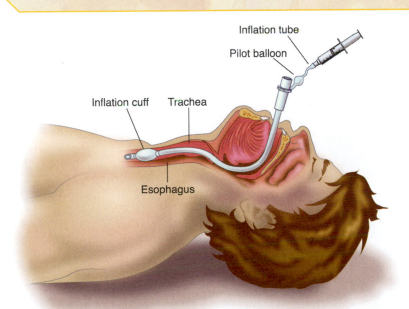

FIGURE A-2 The cuff on the endotracheal tube helps to hold the tube in place and prevents most substances from passing by into the lower airways.

Street Smart

It is important to test cuff integrity *before* the tube is in the patient's trachea. If a faulty cuff is discovered after placement of the tube, it will likely need to be removed and replaced. This procedure is potentially risky for the patient and should be avoided.

SKILL A-1 *Assembly of Laryngoscope and Blade*

PURPOSE: To allow the EMT to visualize the vocal cords and perform endotracheal intubation.

STANDARD PRECAUTIONS:

☑ Appropriate PPE
☑ Laryngoscope handle
☑ Variety of blade types and sizes
☑ Spare lightbulbs and batteries

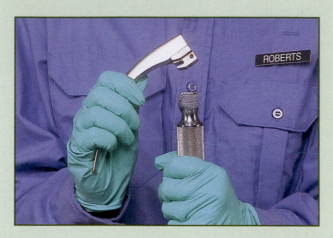

1 The proximal end of the blade has a notched end that fits onto the handle securely.

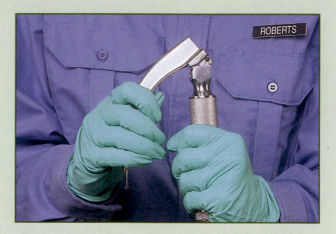

2 The notched end of the blade should be firmly attached to the handle with the blade in a closed position.

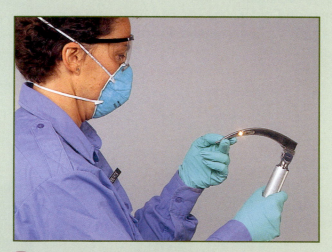

3 Once properly attached, the blade can be extended and the lightbulb at its distal end should turn on. The bulb should quickly be checked for security in position (be sure it is tightly screwed on) and bright quality of light. If the light is dim, the bulb may be poorly connected or the batteries may be low. It is the EMT's responsibility at the beginning of a shift to check the handles and blades to be sure they are functioning optimally.

The syringe should be left attached to the endotracheal tube with 10 cc of air in it, ready to inflate the distal cuff when the tube is in place.

Once the integrity of the cuff has been ensured, a malleable **stylet** (instrument that serves as a rigid guide for the tube) may be placed into the endotracheal tube to allow for more controlled placement of the tube. The stylet should be placed carefully to avoid its extension past the distal end of the tube. Figure A-3 shows the proper placement of a stylet, not beyond the **Murphy eye**, which is the small opening on the side of the tube at its distal end.

Once placed in the tube, the stylet should be secured in that position by bending the proximal end to prevent the tip from extending beyond the ETT. The stylet must never extend past the Murphy eye of the ETT because if it does so during intubation, the stiff or sharp end of the stylet may harm the delicate airway tissues.

With a properly placed stylet, the tube may be formed into a hockey-stick shape to facilitate placement during the intubation.

Finally, any tools to be used for confirmation of endotracheal tube position should be set up. This setup should include a stethoscope and any other commercially available devices approved by the EMT's agency.

Commonly used devices include a carbon dioxide detector and syringe or bulb aspirators. The use of these devices will be further discussed later in this chapter.

Sizes of Blades and Tubes

Intubation equipment must be properly sized for an individual's anatomy. Laryngoscope blades are made in several styles and sizes (Figure A-4). Endotracheal tubes come in many sizes as well.

The two most commonly used styles of laryngoscope blade are the curved **Macintosh blade** and the straight **Miller blade**. The positioning of each blade is specific, and the EMT must be familiar with both.

The Macintosh blade is a curved blade that is designed to sweep the tongue to the patient's left and create a visual axis for the operator to clearly identify the vocal cords for ETT placement. Figure A-5 demonstrates placement of the blade and the view of the vocal cords.

To be most effective, the Macintosh blade should be placed into the right side of the patient's mouth, and the distal tip of the blade slid into a space between the epiglottis and the base of the tongue. This space is called the **vallecula** and is an important anatomic landmark in the airway. When properly placed, the Macintosh blade lifts the tongue and mandible anteriorly and allows visualization of the trachea.

The Macintosh blade is manufactured in several common sizes for different-sized patients. The smallest size is 0 (zero) and the largest size commonly made is 4 (four). The average adult requires a 3 or a 4 Macintosh.

The Miller blade is a straight blade that is designed to be placed into the right side of the patient's mouth and is used to sweep the tongue to the left side of the mouth to allow better visualization of lower airway structures.

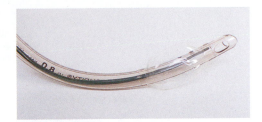

FIGURE A-3 A malleable stylet may be used to help shape the endotracheal tube into an ideal position but must never extend beyond the Murphy eye at the distal end of the tube.

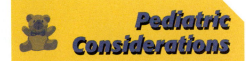

Pediatric Considerations

A stylet is not always used in a pediatric intubation. The narrow endotracheal tube is rigid already and does not need the assistance of a stylet.

If a stylet is used, consider lubricating it with K-Y Jelly or some other water-soluble gel. This lubrication will make it easier to remove the stylet from the endotracheal tube.

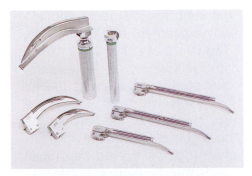

FIGURE A-4 Laryngoscope blades are manufactured in several styles and sizes.

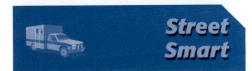

Street Smart

The EMT should always have the size blade he expects to be adequate and one size larger, just in case.

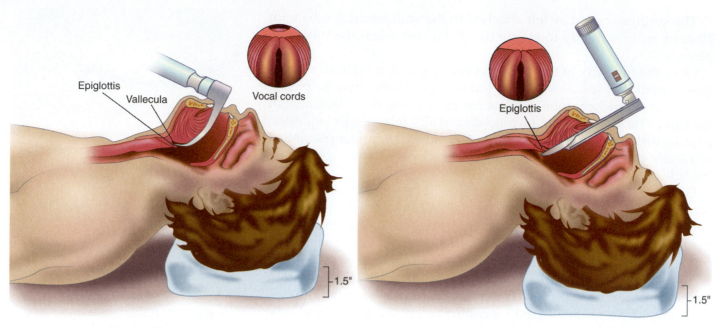

Epiglottis

Vallecula

Vocal cords

Epiglottis

1.5"

1.5"

FIGURE A-5   The Macintosh blade is designed to fit into the vallecula and lift the tongue to allow view of the vocal cords.

FIGURE A-6   The Miller blade is designed to lift the epiglottis and allow view of the vocal cords.

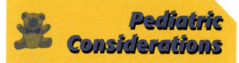

Pediatric Considerations

Because of the unique anatomy of the growing child, each age and size of child will have slightly different requirements for airway equipment and techniques. The infant with the large, floppy epiglottis would be more easily intubated using a straight Miller blade, which is designed to lift the epiglottis out of the way. As the child gets older and the epiglottis more rigid, a curved Macintosh blade may be more effective.

The size of the blade must be chosen on the basis of the child's size. Measuring from the corner of the mouth to the larynx provides the length needed for a laryngoscope blade.

The distal tip of the Miller blade should be placed posterior to the epiglottis, rather than in the vallecula as with the Macintosh blade. This positioning is illustrated in Figure A-6.

When this straight blade is lifted anteriorly, it will lift the epiglottis, the tongue, and the mandible, creating a clear view of the vocal cords and trachea for passage of the ETT. The Miller blade also is commonly manufactured in sizes 0–4, with most adults requiring a size 3 or 4.

Just as laryngoscope blades are sized to the patient they will be used upon, the ETT itself must be properly sized. The tube should approximate the lumen of the patient's trachea at its narrowest point. In adults, this point is at the vocal cords. The ETT sizes are assigned in millimeters. A very small neonate may require a 2.5-mm tube, whereas a typical adult would require between a 7.0-mm and a 9.0-mm tube.

Pediatric Considerations

An easy way to determine the appropriate-sized tube for a child is to use a mathematical formula based on the age of the child. This formula is as follows: (16 + age [in years]) divided by 4. The number that results is the size of the tube most likely to be appropriate for the average-sized child of that age.

Another formula for remembering the recommended depth of the endotracheal tube is tube size multiplied by 3. It must be remembered, however, that this is merely an estimation, and the EMT must evaluate the patient carefully for equal breath sounds to determine whether the end of the tube is properly positioned between the larynx and the carina. Table A-3 shows the estimated sizes of blades, tubes, and tube depth based on the age of the child.

TABLE A-3

	Pediatric Intubation Equipment			
Child's Age	**Blade Size**	**ETT Size**	**ETT Depth**	**Gastric Tube Size**
Neonate (0–1 mo)	0–1	3.0–3.5 uncuffed	9–10 cm	9 French
Infant (1 mo–1 yr)	1	3.5–4.0 uncuffed	10–12 cm	9 French
Toddler (2–4 yr)	1–2	4.0–5.0 uncuffed	12–15 cm	10 French
School-aged child (5–7 yr)	2	5.0–6.0 uncuffed	15–19 cm	12 French
Adolescent (8–12 yr)	2–3	6.0–7.0 cuffed	19–21 cm	14–16 French

Men will typically require a larger tube size than women, but the size of the tube should be based upon the size of the patient, not on the patient's gender.

Patient Preparation

While one EMT is preparing the equipment for intubation, the other provider should be managing the patient's airway with basic life support (BLS) techniques. Manual airway techniques, assessment for obstruction, suctioning, and placement of an oropharyngeal airway should be performed before any advanced procedures.

The patient should have an oropharyngeal airway placed and BVM ventilations begun by one or two EMTs while a third EMT prepares

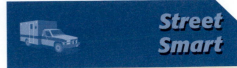

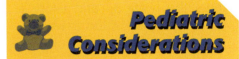

Pediatric Considerations

The EMT must be aware of a few anatomical considerations when performing endotracheal intubation on a child. The child's airway structures are generally smaller than an adult's. This difference translates into a more easily obstructed air passage. Care must be taken to not overextend a child's neck during manual airway maneuvers. Extension past a neutral position can easily kink the child's flexible trachea and obstruct the airway (Figure A-7).

Street Smart

It is important to remember that the provider should not forgo BLS airway maneuvers for endotracheal intubation. These procedures are critically intertwined, and the basic tenets of open, assess, suction, and secure must be addressed in every patient before the procedure of endotracheal intubation is performed.

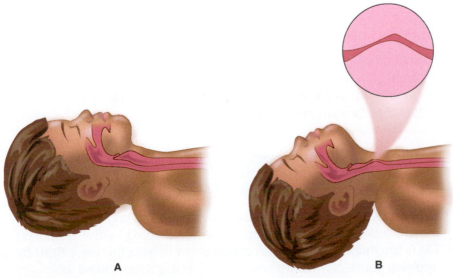

FIGURE A-7 Extension past a neutral position (A) can easily kink the child's flexible trachea and obstruct the airway (B).

Pediatric Considerations

Because children have a relatively large skull, when a small child is supine, the head will be forced into a flexed position. This position closes the airway and makes intubation very difficult. The EMT should consider placing folded blankets or towels under the child's torso in order to raise the body up and allow a neutral position of the airway.

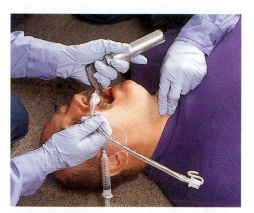

FIGURE A-8   Properly applied cricoid pressure can prevent passive regurgitation during bag-valve-mask ventilation and intubation.

Pediatric Considerations

In children, the cartilaginous rings that begin at the cricoid and make up the trachea are much more flexible than in adults. Consequently, a child's trachea can easily be occluded by overextension of the head or too much pressure on the cricoid ring during cricoid pressure. Care should be taken to apply only gentle pressure over the cricoid ring of these patients.

the equipment necessary for endotracheal intubation. This procedure can be completed by two EMTs, but it is ideal to have three.

Ventilation should be somewhat faster than usual in order to **hyperventilate** the patient. These rapid, deep ventilations, or hyperventilation, serve to increase the oxygen in the patient's lungs in preparation for the short period without ventilation expected during endotracheal intubation.

In addition, the patient should be placed in a position that is most useful for endotracheal intubation. For a patient without spinal injury, a towel may be folded and placed under the patient's head in order to create the position that makes direct laryngoscopy easier.

Cricoid Pressure

Many of the patients cared for by prehospital providers have food and liquid materials in their stomach. When the patient is supine and unconscious, these stomach contents may passively regurgitate up into the airway. Regurgitation of stomach contents into the airway poses a danger to the patient. If stomach contents are allowed to enter the lower airways and the lungs, a severe inflammatory reaction in the lungs will result.

This aspiration of stomach material sometimes occurs despite an EMT's efforts to keep the airway clear. In an attempt to prevent this regurgitation, the EMT may occlude the esophagus by performing a technique called cricoid pressure. This technique was discussed in Chapter 8. Cricoid pressure causes the soft-walled esophagus to collapse posteriorly and blocks most passive regurgitation from the stomach. This procedure should be performed during BVM ventilation and throughout the procedure of intubation. It is illustrated in Figure A-8.

Laryngoscopy and Tube Placement

Once the patient has been hyperventilated and the equipment has been prepared, the patient is ready to be intubated. Skill A-2 describes this process.

Pediatric Considerations

Significantly less force is needed when performing laryngoscopy on a child. In addition, a child's vocal cords are usually more anterior and more superior than an adult's and may require a slightly different technique in order to visualize.

Street Smart

During laryngoscopy, the pressure on the cricoid ring can be adjusted to allow better visualization of the vocal cords by the intubating EMT. Too much pressure can completely obstruct the view. Start by applying gentle downward pressure, stopping when asked to.

SKILL A-2 *Oral Endotracheal Intubation*

PURPOSE: To positively secure the airway for ventilation and to prevent aspiration into the lungs.

STANDARD PRECAUTIONS:

- ☑ Laryngoscope
- ☑ Endotracheal tubes (assorted)
- ☑ Plastic-covered stylet
- ☑ Water-soluble lubricant
- ☑ Syringe (10 cc minimum)
- ☑ One-inch tape
- ☑ Padding
- ☑ Stethoscope
- ☑ End tidal CO_2 detector

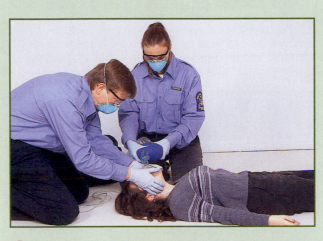

1 Open, assess, suction, and secure the patient's airway with an oral airway. Ventilate the patient for 1–2 minutes.

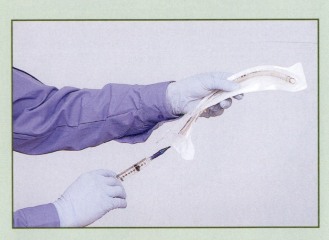

2 Assemble and prepare the intubation equipment. A correctly sized endotracheal tube should be chosen and the cuff tested, while the tube is in the packaging.

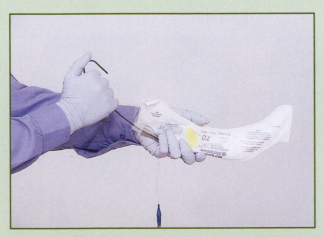

3 The EMT then lubricates the stylet and inserts it into the endotracheal tube, stopping before the Murphy eye at the end of the tube. The entire assembly should be bent into a hockey-stick configuration.

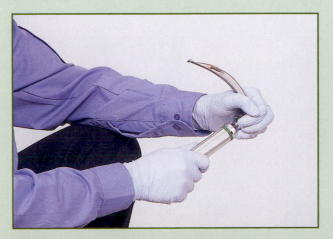

4 The EMT then assembles the laryngoscope handle and blade, ensuring that the bulb is "bright and tight."

(continues)

SKILL A-2 (continued)

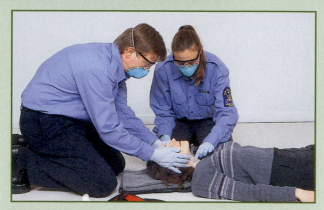

5 After positioning the patient's head in the sniffing position, by placing a 1½-inch pad under the head, the EMT directs another EMT to provide cricoid pressure.

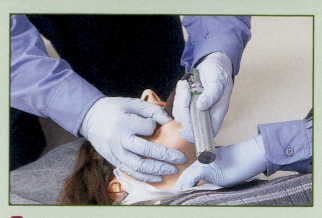

6 The first EMT stops ventilation and quickly removes the oral airway, inserting the blade, with his left hand, into the right side of the mouth and sweeping the tongue to the left and out of the way.

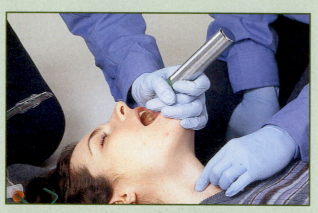

7 The EMT then identifies the landmarks of the airway. The vocal cords should be clearly visible, and the glottic opening identified.

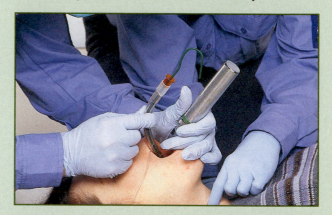

8 Without losing sight of the glottic opening, and while maintaining the up-and-out pressure on the laryngoscope blade, the EMT watches the tube pass through the glottic opening.

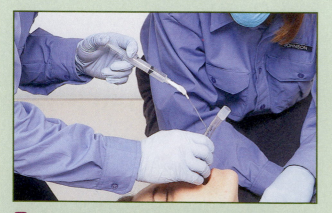

9 Once the tube is in place, the EMT quickly withdraws the blade and the stylet, then inflates the balloon with the syringe.

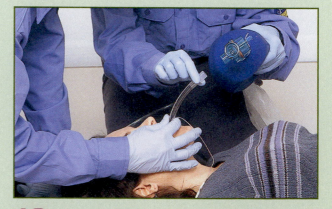

10 After inflating the balloon, the EMT removes the syringe and prepares to listen for lung sounds. First, the EMT must have another EMT place the BVM on the tube and begin ventilation. The EMT should never let go of the endotracheal tube until it has been secured.

(continues)

SKILL A-2 (continued)

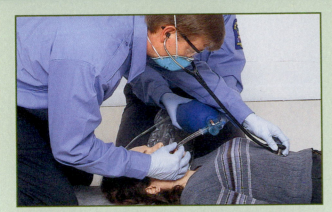

11 Using a stethoscope, the EMT first listens for the absence of sounds in the epigastric area, then proceeds to listen to lung sounds in the left lung then the right lung.

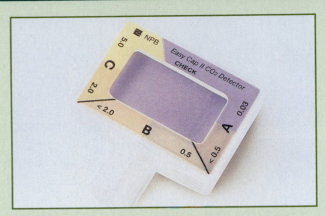

12 Using an end tidal CO_2 detector, the EMT confirms tube placement while also observing the torso for even chest rise. (Reprinted by permission of Mallinckrodt Inc., Pleasanton, CA.)

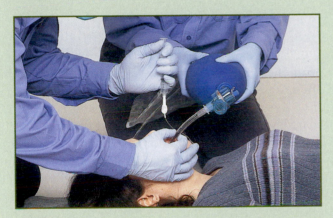

13 If the tube is misplaced, the syringe should be reattached, the balloon deflated, and the tube removed while suction is ready at the standby.

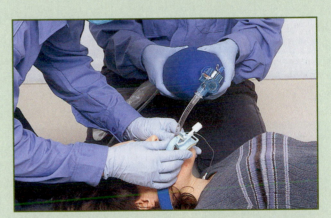

14 If the tube is well placed, then the EMT proceeds to secure the tube with 1-inch tape or some similar securing device designed for that purpose.

Confirmation of Tube Placement

Once the tube is in place, the stylet removed, and the cuff inflated, the patient must be ventilated and the tube placement confirmed as being in the trachea.

The BVM must be attached to the proximal end of the tube and ventilations begun. The position of the tube must be immediately determined and can be accomplished using several different methods.

The EMT should use every means available to confirm the tracheal position of the endotracheal tube. No one means is considered to be 100% effective when used alone.

Direct Visualization

Of course, when the tube is initially passed, the EMT should carefully observe it as it passes through the cords. If tube position is ever in

Safety Tip

The intubating EMT should *not* let go of the endotracheal tube until it has been secured in place. Many well-meaning partners have accidentally displaced an endotracheal tube while attempting to help secure it.

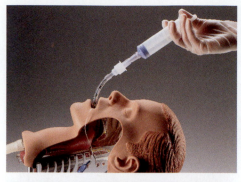

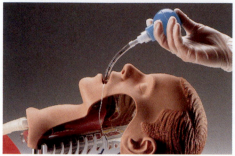

FIGURE A-9 There are several commercially available tools that may be used to assist in confirmation of endotracheal tube position. (Courtesy of Ambu, Inc., Linthicum, MD.)

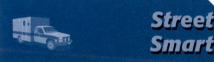

Street Smart

The gold standard for endotracheal tube placement is direct visualization of the endotracheal tube as it passes through the vocal cords.

If after reassessment with direct visualization the EMT is still unsure of the tube's placement, it should be removed. The saying goes "when in doubt, pull it out."

It is better to ventilate the lungs with a BVM than it is to ventilate the stomach through an endotracheal tube.

Street Smart

If a clear view is not obtained during the initial laryngoscopy, the blade should be repositioned, again attempting to lift the tongue and mandible out of the way. The EMT must keep careful track of how much time has elapsed during this procedure. The procedure should be limited to 30 seconds.

If the tube is not properly placed by the end of this time, the attempt should be discontinued and the patient hyperventilated with the bag-valve-mask for 1–2 minutes before the procedure is again attempted.

doubt, the EMT can replace the laryngoscope into the patient's mouth and look again to confirm that the tube passes through the vocal cords.

Syringe or Bulb Aspirator

A commonly used tool to facilitate detection of esophageal intubations is the **syringe or bulb aspirator**. As seen in Figure A-9, these devices fit onto the end of an ETT. If used, they must be placed on the end of the ETT before any ventilation via the BVM.

The concept behind the use of these devices is simple. We know that the trachea is a cartilaginous ringed structure that does not easily collapse. On the other hand, the esophagus is a floppy, muscular walled tube that will easily collapse if pressure is placed outside it (as with cricoid pressure) or, in this case, if a vacuum is applied within it.

The syringe/bulb aspirators are placed on the end of the ETT and an attempt is made to draw air into the device from the tube. If the tube lies in the trachea, air will easily be drawn into the syringe or bulb. If the tube is in the esophagus, as the negative pressure is applied the esophagus will collapse against the distal end of the tube and resistance will be met as the EMT attempts to withdraw air.

Although not difficult to use, these tools require training to become proficient in their use. The agency medical director should approve their use.

Auscultation

As the first several breaths are given via the ETT, the EMT should look for several things. Equal chest rise should be observed and no abdominal distension should occur.

Breath sounds should be carefully auscultated at both apices (just under the clavicles on both sides), and lack of breath sounds should be noted in the epigastrum (Figure A-10). Both lung apices *and* the epigastrium should be auscultated after every intubation to reduce the likelihood of mistakes.

If the tube is correctly placed in the trachea, the EMT will hear equal breath sounds with ventilations over both lung apices. No breath sounds will be heard over the epigastrum.

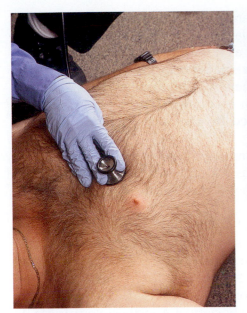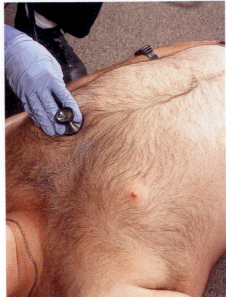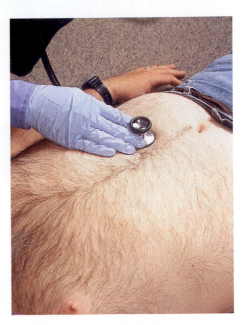

FIGURE A-10 After intubation, it is critical that the EMT not only auscultates for equal breath sounds over the chest, but also confirms lack of air sounds over the epigastrum.

Right Mainstem Placement

Because the **right mainstem bronchus** is steeper and wider than the left, if the ETT is accidentally placed too far into the trachea, it will likely go into the right mainstem bronchus. The ideal place for the distal end of the tube is several centimeters above the carina (the bifurcation of the trachea into the two mainstem bronchi) (Figure A-11).

If breath sounds are heard over the right chest but not over the left or in the epigastrum, then the tube is likely in the right mainstem bronchus and should be slightly withdrawn. The EMT should grasp the tube firmly and release the air from the cuff by using the syringe, then withdraw the tube centimeter by centimeter until equal breath sounds are heard over both lungs. Once properly placed, the tube can be secured.

Esophageal Placement

If breath sounds are not heard over the chest but are heard over the epigastrum, the tube has been mistakenly placed in the esophagus and must be immediately removed. The EMT should withdraw all of the air from the cuff and, with suction ready, remove the tube. The airway should be suctioned, the patient should be hyperventilated for at least 2 minutes, and then intubation may be attempted again.

If this misplacement is quickly recognized and remedied, the patient is not harmed. However, an unrecognized esophageal intubation will lead to ventilation of the stomach rather than the lungs and will lead to hypoxia and quickly to the death of the patient.

End Tidal CO_2 Detector

Another simple tool often used to confirm proper tube placement is the **end tidal CO_2 detector**. This is a colormetric device that can measure the presence of CO_2 in air exhaled from an ETT. It is placed on the

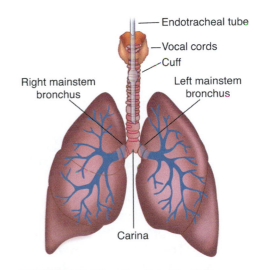

FIGURE A-11 The distal tip of the endotracheal tube should lie several centimeters above the carina but well below the vocal cords.

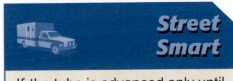

Street Smart

If the tube is advanced only until the cuff is past the cords, it will usually be in the correct place.

Street Smart

Colormetric CO_2 devices are not useful once they become grossly contaminated. They may also not be useful in the situation of a prolonged cardiac arrest because the presence of CO_2 in the exhaled air may be greatly diminished in the patient with no active metabolism.

? Ask the Doc

No single method of confirmation of endotracheal tube placement has proven to be 100% reliable. Therefore, the American College of Emergency Physicians (ACEP) has stated in its policy statement on confirmation of endotracheal tube placement that EMS providers should use a secondary method of confirmation. Secondary methods include end-tidal CO_2 detectors and esophageal detector devices, with a strong emphasis on end-tidal CO_2 detectors. The American Society of Anethesiologists, the American Heart Association, and the National Association of EMS Physicians support this position.

end of the ETT after intubation, and the BVM is then attached to that for ventilations. With each ventilation, if the endotracheal tube is in the trachea, CO_2 will be exhaled as it normally is during exhalation. The presence of CO_2 causes a designated color change on the device. If the tube is in the esophagus, there will be no color change because there is no CO_2 in the stomach or esophagus. This tool also requires training and should be approved by the agency medical director before its use.

Some EMS agencies may use capnography, an indirect monitoring device that provides a continuous real-time reading of the end tidal CO_2 levels, instead of a colormetric device, to help confirm ETT placement.

A pulse oximeter can also be a helpful adjunct for ETT placement. While a pulse oximeter may take several minutes to indicate that the patient has become hypoxic, it is a direct monitor of the patient's oxygenation status. A pulse oximeter should be utilized after other methods of ETT placement confirmation have been used.

A recent study by the American Society of Anesthesiologists (ASA) suggested that the combination of the pulse oximeter and the capnographer may have helped prevent 93% of avoidable anesthesia mishaps.

The EMT should use every means at his disposal to confirm ETT placement, with two methods other than direct visualization as a minimum.

Patient Improvement

As you can see, there are many tools that can be used individually or, preferably, in conjunction with one another to confirm proper ETT placement. Perhaps more important, patient assessment can be used to confirm proper tube placement.

If the tube is in the trachea and is ventilating both lungs, the EMT should observe equal chest rise. In addition, if 100% oxygen is being delivered to a previously hypoxic patient, the skin color should improve. If pulse oximetry is in use, the oxygen saturation should be seen to improve. In a patient not in cardiac arrest, there should be some improvement in vital signs. Even in cardiac arrest, especially if the arrest was of a respiratory origin, improvement may be seen.

If the patient's color or vital signs seem to deteriorate after endotracheal intubation, or if the oxygen saturation falls and does not improve with hyperventilation, the tube position should be questioned and rapidly confirmed using the methods described.

Secure the Tube

Once the EMT has determined that the tube is correctly placed in the trachea, it can be secured. Before securing the tube, the EMT should note the centimeter mark on the tube at the level of the patient's lips. Most adult females should have a tube secured at 21 centimeters, and most adult males at 23 centimeters. Each reassessment should ensure that the depth has not changed.

It is critical that an ETT be adequately secured and not be allowed to become dislodged or displaced during movement and transport.

There are several commercial devices used to secure an ETT available, which are preferred over tape or cloth ties.

Minimizing the movement of the patient's head and neck will also help to prevent tube displacement. It is sometimes recommended to place a cervical collar on the patient or to place the patient's head in head blocks in order to limit head and neck movement, even without evidence of trauma. Studies have shown that a cervical collar is very effective in limiting ETT movement.

None of these securing methods will be effective if the providers are not careful and gentle when handling the tube and the BVM.

It is wise to disconnect the BVM from the ETT during major moves when it would be awkward to continue ventilating (e.g., moving the patient into and out of the ambulance). A period of no longer than 15–30 seconds should elapse before the patient is again ventilated.

Reassessments

As for any unstable patient, frequent reassessments are necessary. After the patient has been endotracheally intubated, the EMT must continually monitor the patient's color, chest rise, ventilation compliance, and vital signs. Any change in these parameters should prompt an investigation into the cause. Changes that may indicate patient decompensation are loss of skin color, poor or unequal chest rise, difficult ventilation via BVM (decreased compliance), increasing tachycardia or bradycardia, fall in blood pressure, and drop in oxygen saturation.

If the intubated patient exhibits any of the above signs of decompensation, the EMT must immediately review the airway status, the breathing ability, and the circulatory status of the patient.

An easy way to remember the different problems that may surface in the intubated patient is by using the acronym **DOPE**. *D* stands for displacement of the tube. The EMT should evaluate the position of the tube by listening to the epigastrum and both lungs as well as utilizing a CO_2 detector or a tube aspirator device.

If these do not confirm the placement of the tube, repeat direct laryngoscopy is indicated. If the tube is found to be outside of the trachea, the balloon should be deflated and the tube immediately removed. The patient can be ventilated with the BVM until equipment is ready to reintubate.

O stands for obstruction of the tube. If it seems difficult to ventilate through the tube, there may be something causing obstruction, such as mucus or a foreign body. The EMT should disconnect the BVM from the tube and pass a sterile French catheter into the tube to suction it out. This procedure is explained in detail later in this chapter.

P stands for pneumothorax. With aggressive positive-pressure ventilation (as is given when ventilations are delivered with the positive pressure from the BVM), some patients with lung disease are susceptible to having what is called a **pneumothorax**. Even in patients with healthy lungs, overly aggressive positive-pressure ventilation can cause injury to the lung, resulting in a pneumothorax.

Pneumothorax literally means "air in the chest" and refers to air in the pleural space, the space outside the lung in the chest cavity. Figure A-12

Street Smart

If tube position is thought to be appropriate and the patient fails to improve or is deteriorating, be sure the oxygen is at full liter flow and is attached to the BVM.

Also check to be sure that the tubing is not kinked. Like a garden hose, a kinked oxygen tube will not allow oxygen to pass. Oxygen tubing should always be outside of the blanket wrap and visible.

Some BVMs will fail to inflate if the oxygen reservoir is not filling. If the bag is flat, check the oxygen tank to see whether it is working properly.

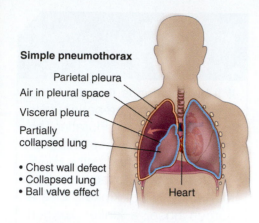

Simple pneumothorax

Parietal pleura
Air in pleural space
Visceral pleura
Partially collapsed lung

• Chest wall defect
• Collapsed lung
• Ball valve effect

Heart

FIGURE A-12 A pneumothorax is a collection of air outside the lung itself, in the pleural space.

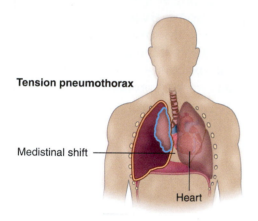

Tension pneumothorax

Medistinal shift

Heart

FIGURE A-13 A tension pneumothorax can result in compression of the heart and great vessels, resulting in tachycardia and hypotension.

illustrates a pneumothorax. As more air is forced into the chest with positive-pressure ventilations, the pleural air, or pneumothorax, gets bigger and will actually cause the lung to collapse.

As the lung collapses, it becomes more difficult to force sufficient air into the chest. The patient is no longer well ventilated or oxygenated and will show signs of decompensation. If the patient has a pneumothorax, the EMT may hear diminished breath sounds over the side of the chest with the pneumothorax due to the collapsing lung.

If the pneumothorax is allowed to progress further, the collapsed lung may actually press against the heart and great vessels, causing a fall in blood pressure and a rise in heart rate. This condition is called a **tension pneumothorax** and is life threatening if not treated immediately. Figure A-13 illustrates the anatomy of a tension pneumothorax.

The treatment for this condition is to release the accumulation of air in the pleural space via a needle thoracostomy, which can be performed only by advanced-level providers who have been appropriately trained.

The last letter in the acronym is *E*, which stands for equipment failure. Once the above problems have been addressed and the patient still is not improving, the EMT should check the oxygen supply to be sure it is connected, is at the appropriate liter flow, and has not run out. When in doubt as to whether a particular piece of equipment is properly working, replace it.

If the EMT is frequently reassessing the intubated patient, any problem will be found early and can be quickly remedied. Rapid identification and management of airway problems are crucial in the intubated patient.

Complications

Even when carefully performed, endotracheal intubation has potential complications. The EMT must be aware of these and should make every effort to avoid those that can be avoided.

Soft-Tissue Trauma

During the direct laryngoscopy and endotracheal intubation, the EMT will be placing the laryngoscope blade, the ETT, and probably hard suction catheters into the patient's pharynx. The tissues of the pharynx are soft and easily torn. The EMT should be aware of the fragile nature of these tissues and should take care not to be overly aggressive with the equipment.

Directly watching the placement of any equipment into the patient's mouth and taking care not to force anything that does not move easily will help to avoid damage to the soft tissues of the pharynx.

Dental Trauma

During direct laryngoscopy it is important for the EMT not to touch the laryngoscope blade to the patient's upper teeth because doing so may result in a chipped or broken tooth. The broken tooth may be aspirated and result in an airway obstruction. Broken front teeth also become a cosmetic problem to the patient after recovery.

Careful laryngoscopy will help to avoid such dental trauma. Attention should be paid to the placement of the blade, and the direction of pressure should be anterior, with pressure applied using a straight wrist.

Unrecognized Improper Placement

Endotracheal intubation can be a lifesaving procedure when performed properly by an appropriately trained provider. The greatest risk associated with the procedure is to fail to recognize the improperly placed ETT. If the tube is inadvertently placed into the esophagus and the EMT recognizes the mistake, immediately removes the tube, and hyperventilates the patient, no problem exists.

If the improper placement of the tube in the esophagus is not recognized and ventilations are delivered to the stomach instead of to the lungs, the patient will become hypoxic and will likely die. We have presented several methods that the EMT may use to ensure the correct placement of the ETT. The more methods used, the more certain the EMT may be of proper placement.

If the location of the tube is ever in doubt, it must be removed and the patient ventilated by BVM. The EMT must never allow a misplaced ETT to go unrecognized.

Unique Pediatric Complications

Given the smaller and somewhat different anatomic considerations in pediatric airways, there are some unique complications associated with pediatric intubation that the EMT must be aware of.

Bradycardia

Mechanical stimulation of the child's airway, as is done during laryngoscopy and intubation, may result in profound bradycardia. If the child's heart rate is noted to slow during the intubation, the procedure should immediately be halted and ventilation via BVM should be resumed until the child's heart rate returns to preintubation rates.

Difficulty in Auscultation

Lung sounds are sometimes difficult to localize in very small infants. Often, breath sounds will radiate throughout the infant's chest and may make it nearly impossible to distinguish whether the breath sounds are present on both sides or if you are hearing sounds from one lung reflected across the entire chest.

In infants, it is best to listen for breath sounds laterally, high up on the chest wall in the armpit. This placement of the stethoscope will minimize any chance of mistaking reflected breath sounds for actual breath sounds.

Easy Movement of Tube

Because pediatric ETTs are not cuffed, they are easily displaced during movement and transport. The EMT must pay very close attention to tube position and make every effort to minimize head and neck movement during the transport of the intubated child.

Some health care providers may advocate the use of a cervical collar to minimize head and neck movement to reduce the likelihood of tube displacement. Whatever means are used to keep the tube in place, the EMT must be ever vigilant to changes in the child's heart rate, pulse oximetry, skin color, and lung compliance that may indicate a displaced tube.

Smaller Lung Volume

As when ventilating with the BVM, ventilation of the child via an ETT requires smaller volumes of air than in an adult. The ventilator must be aware of the amount of air that is used and must use only enough to result in chest rise. Too much volume can result in injury to the child's lungs and potential pneumothorax.

TRAUMA CONSIDERATIONS

EMTs will often be called to care for victims of traumatic injury. The principles of caring for these patients will be dealt with later in this text. Appropriate airway management in the severely injured patient could significantly affect the patient's chances of survival.

If a patient has fallen or sustained any significant trauma to the head, neck, or upper torso, it is imperative that the EMT avoid any unnecessary movement of the spine to avoid the potential for worsening an injury to the cervical spine.

In managing the airway, the EMT cannot use the usual head-tilt, chin-lift because this maneuver causes undesirable movement of the neck. Instead, the EMT should perform the jaw thrust.

Similarly, during endotracheal intubation the EMT must avoid any movement of the neck. The easiest way to accomplish the task while ensuring immobilization of the spine is to assign a person to hold the head and neck for stabilization while the EMT performs the intubation. Once the tube has been secured, a collar may be placed and the patient completely immobilized.

If the patient has already been immobilized with a cervical collar and head immobilizers, the EMT may have to partially remove these devices in order to best access the patient for intubation. If immobilization equipment is removed, an EMT must maintain manual stabilization to avoid movement of the head or neck.

Performing endotracheal intubation without the benefit of the head-tilt, chin-lift may be challenging and should be practiced extensively before the EMT attempts the skill on an actual patient.

ADJUNCTS TO ADVANCED AIRWAY MANAGEMENT

Once a patient has been intubated, there are several techniques the EMT can utilize to maximize the ventilation and oxygenation of the patient while minimizing the risk of complications.

✦ *Motor Vehicle Crash*

Tom and Barb arrive on the scene of a motor vehicle crash to find a midsized car that had apparently struck the back of a truck. The truck came through the windshield and into the passenger compartment.

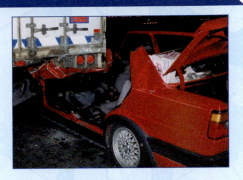

After ensuring they were in no danger of injury from high-powered lines and other dangers resulting from the crash, the two EMTs approached the vehicle. They noted a significant amount of damage—including a broken windshield and pieces of blue cloth caught in the windshield.

Wearing appropriate personal protective gear, Tom entered the car and undertook manual stabilization of the woman's head and neck.

(Courtesy of David J. Reimer Sr.)

Upon initial assessment, Barb found that the woman was responsive only to painful stimuli. She had multiple bruises and lacerations to her head and face, and bloody drainage was noted from her nose and mouth.

Barb quickly suctioned her mouth as Tom counted respirations. Tom noted that she was barely breathing. The patient tolerated the oral airway Barb inserted into her mouth.

Realizing that the seriously injured woman could not maintain her own airway and needed ventilatory assistance, Barb called for a rapid extrication.

As the firefighters assisted Tom with the rapid extrication, Barb assembled the bag-valve-mask.

- What will be the first priority for this patient after she has been extricated?
- What special considerations for airway maintenance have to be taken into account for a trauma patient?
- What can Tom do to assist?

Deep Suctioning

If an intubated patient has secretions in the lower airway, the EMT can suction the ETT to remove such secretions and maximize the patient's oxygenation.

Indications

If secretions are seen in the ETT or if bubbling sounds are heard with ventilation of the tube, then the patient should be suctioned. If increased airway resistance is felt and the tube is found to be in the proper position, the tube may be partially occluded and should be suctioned.

Procedure

Because this suctioning technique involves contact with the lower airways, the EMT must remember to keep the catheter sterile (uncontaminated) and to use a new, sterile catheter for each procedure. Observing such sterile technique will decrease the risk of contamination of the lower airways and resultant infection.

After donning appropriate PPE, the EMT should open the package with the catheter and *sterile* gloves, taking care not to contaminate either. The suction unit should be tested, and the catheter attached to the suction tubing. The EMT should apply the sterile gloves and pick up the *sterile* catheter in the right hand. The left hand will be used to disconnect the BVM from the ETT.

Next, the EMT should thread the suction catheter as far into the ETT as it can go or until the patient coughs. Suction is then applied as the catheter is slowly withdrawn.

The EMT should keep the catheter in the right hand, which will remain the *sterile* hand, and use the left hand to reconnect the BVM to the ETT and ventilate the patient again for 1 minute.

These steps can be repeated as many times as needed to clear the tube. As long as the catheter remains *sterile* between suction passes, the same catheter may be used. If it becomes clogged with thick secretions, it may be placed in *sterile* water and suctioned to attempt to clear it out. If the catheter becomes contaminated or cannot be cleared, a new catheter must be used.

After the tube has been cleared, the catheter may then be used to suction the patient's oropharynx before discarding it. A hard Yankauer catheter may also be used at any point to suction the patient's oropharynx if needed.

If repeat endotracheal suctioning is necessary, new sterile gloves and a new sterile catheter should be used.

Care must be taken to monitor the patient's heart rate and oxygen saturation during the suctioning procedure. If the heart rate or the oxygen saturation falls, the procedure should be stopped immediately and the patient should be hyperventilated until vital signs return to the previous numbers.

OPA Placement

After the ETT has been secured, an oropharyngeal airway (OPA) may be placed in the patient's mouth to prevent the patient from chewing or biting on the tube. The OPA should be properly sized as described in Chapter 7.

Gastric Distention

While gastric distention can be treated with an orogastric tube, the best case is preventing gastric distention from occuring in the first place. Gastric distention can be prevented by application of cricoid pressure prior to positive-pressure ventilation, gentle ventilation with the BVM, or use of properly set flow-restricted, oxygen-powered ventilation device.

One of the most underrated and most successful means of preventing gastric distention is maintaining the airway open. While seemingly intuitive, many EMTs become fatigued when manually holding an airway open for long periods of time. When involved in a prolonged resuscitation, EMTs should rotate airway duties to ensure that the head is held in the proper position.

Orogastric Tube

It is sometimes necessary to decompress a patient's stomach if it has become so distended that it impedes adequate ventilation. Decompression is most often necessary in small children and infants. It is accomplished by the placement of an **orogastric tube**, a flexible tube placed through the mouth into the stomach. The same type of tube may alternatively be placed into the nose and passed into the stomach; then it is called a **nasogastric tube**.

Advantages

The placement of the naso- or orogastric tube allows decompression of air from a distended stomach, improving ventilation. It also facilitates emptying the gastric contents to prevent later regurgitation and possible aspiration.

Indications

Gastric decompression is indicated in any patient who is difficult to ventilate owing to gastric distention. This condition most often occurs in children. The oral route is preferred in the intubated patient because it minimizes complications associated with the nasal route, such as nasal trauma and bleeding.

Contraindications

Gastric decompression should never be performed for a patient with an intact gag reflex. For the patient with major facial, head, or spinal trauma, the oral route is preferred in order to minimize complications.

Procedure

As with any procedure, there are several steps to safe and efficient completion of gastric decompression and tube placement. The EMT must prepare all necessary equipment before initiating the procedure. Table A-3 lists the proper sizes of tubes for children, based on the patient's age.

After donning appropriate PPE, the EMT should properly position the patient. In the nonintubated, nontrauma patient, the head can be placed in a somewhat flexed position to allow for easier passage of the tube into the esophagus. Most of the patients on whom an EMT will perform gastric decompression will have been intubated already, and such head movement may jeopardize the position of the ETT, so the head should be kept in a neutral position.

The proper depth of the tube should be measured from the mouth, around the ear to a point below the xyphoid process.

The distal end of the gastric tube should be coated with a water-soluble lubricant before starting the procedure.

If the patient is intubated and the EMT will be performing orogastric tube placement, the endotracheal tube should be firmly held in place by one provider while another places the orogastric tube. The tube should be passed into the mouth and down toward the esophagus. The tube should pass easily. If any resistance is met, the tube should be withdrawn and the procedure begun again. The tube should be placed to the premeasured depth and then held while its position is confirmed.

The syringe can be placed on the end of the orogastric tube and stomach contents withdrawn, or the tube can be hooked directly to suction to withdraw any contents. It is important to realize that the return of stomach contents alone does not confirm proper placement. Proper gastric placement is confirmed by placing the syringe filled with air on the end of the orogastric tube and, while listening over the epigastrum, rapidly instilling at least 20 cc of air. If the tube is properly placed in the stomach, the injected air will be heard over the epigastrum. If it is not heard, then the tube is not in the correct place and should be withdrawn and replaced.

Once the orogastric tube has been confirmed to be in the stomach, it should be hooked to suction and the stomach contents allowed to empty. When the tube no longer drains stomach contents, the suction may be discontinued and the tube left open to air with intermittent suction being applied.

Complications

There are potential complications with orogastric tube placement. Most can be avoided if care is taken during the procedure to avoid excess force and to perform the procedure only on patients for whom it is indicated.

Nasogastric intubation may be complicated by nasal trauma and bleeding. Rarely, in cases of basilar skull fractures, tubes placed nasally could pass through fractures and into the cranium.

Any time the pharynx is manipulated, the patient may gag and vomit. The EMT must be aware of this possibility and avoid the procedure if the patient is known to have a gag reflex; however, the EMT should have suction at hand, regardless.

Occasionally, an orogastric tube will be accidentally placed into the trachea. This misplacement should be easily recognized when air is not heard over the epigastrum upon injection from the syringe. A misplaced orogastric tube should be removed immediately.

THE DIFFICULT AIRWAY

Some patients, for one reason or another, are very difficult to intubate. Some patients' anatomy makes visualization by direct laryngoscopy impossible. Severe injuries to the face and neck may distort the airway anatomy to the point where it is not recognizable to the EMT.

If an EMT is unsuccessful at intubation on the first attempt, he should step back for a moment while the patient is hyperventilated and try to identify the cause of the difficulty. The EMT should be sure that the blade is the appropriate size, that the lighting is adequate, and that the patient's position is ideal.

After 1–2 minutes of hyperventilation, the EMT should attempt once again to intubate the patient. No intubation attempt should last longer than 30 seconds. If the intubation is not successful after this time, the procedure should be stopped and the patient ventilated by BVM.

Basic Airway Maneuvers

If the EMT is not successful after two intubation attempts, the patient should be ventilated by BVM with the use of an oral airway and rapidly transported to the closest hospital. If an advanced life support (ALS) intercept is available, it should be requested while transport is initiated. Adequate ventilation can be performed with basic airway maneuvers as discussed in Chapter 8. A patient should never be allowed to become hypoxic while an EMT continues to attempt intubation if ventilation is possible with such basic maneuvers.

Secondary Airway Devices

In situations where endotracheal intubation has not been successful, alternative means might be needed to provide airway control. As stated, the EMT's priority is to utilize basic airway maneuvers to provide appropriate ventilations to the patient while transport to the closest hospital is begun. During transport, it may be appropriate for an EMT to consider placement of a secondary airway device if approved for their use.

There are two commonly utilized devices in this category, the dual lumen airway and the laryngeal mask airway. Each is placed blindly into an unresponsive patient's airway, allowing for more direct tracheal ventilation than is provided by a simple BVM. Both have been shown to be easily placed in most cases and can provide the EMT with a convenient means to ventilate a patient; however, each device has potential complications. Prior to considering use of a secondary airway device, the EMT must have received appropriate training for the specific equipment and be skilled in its use.

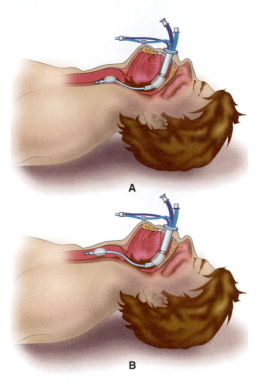

FIGURE A-14 A. Combitube in esophageal position. B. Combitube in tracheal position.

The Combitube Esophageal/Tracheal Double-Lumen Airway is a dual lumen tube that can be placed blindly into an adult patient's airway. If the tube is placed into the trachea, direct tracheal ventilation can be provided to the tracheal port, similar to an ordinary endotracheal tube. If, however, the tube is placed into the esophagus, ventilations are to be provided to the esophageal port and indirectly enter the trachea. This is accomplished by forcing air through multiple fenestrations in the hypopharyngeal section of the tube. A cuff is inflated in the oropharynx to prevent air from exiting the mouth, and a second cuff is inflated in the esophagus to prevent air from entering the esophagus. This results in any air exiting these fenestrations to move into the trachea by exclusion. It is imperative that the EMT recognize whether the Combitube has entered the trachea or the esophagus so that ventilations are applied to the appropriate port of the tube. Figure A-14 illustrates the Combitube placement in the trachea and in the esophagus.

The laryngeal mask airway (LMA) is also a device that is placed blindly into a patient's airway. The LMA is available in adult and pediatric sizes as well as disposable and multipatient use varieties. This device is comprised of a short tube attached to a small inflatable mask. The device is placed blindly into the unconscious patient's mouth and directed downward toward the trachea. The mask will come to rest over the glottic opening where it will be inflated, providing somewhat of a seal that allows direct tracheal ventilation. Figure A-15 illustrates the LMA and its positioning in a patient's airway.

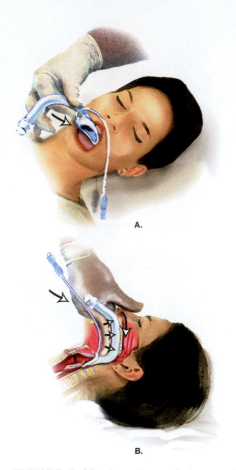

A.

B.

FIGURE A-15 Insertion and placement of laryngeal mask airway.

Because the LMA does not completely seal the esophagus from the trachea, a notable potential complication of the LMA is aspiration of stomach contents during forcible vomiting.

Neither the Combitube nor the LMA is tolerated by patients with an intact gag reflex; therefore, if a patient with one of these devices in place begins to regain consciousness the device must be immediately removed. Removal of either device can lead to gagging and vomiting and the EMT should be prepared in this situation to reposition the patient and provide adequate suctioning to avoid aspiration. Additionally, if either device is improperly placed or inappropriately utilized, inadequate ventilations may be delivered, resulting in hypoxia and patient decompensation. The EMT must be thoroughly familiar with the proper use of any airway device that would be utilized during patient care.

CONCLUSION

Advanced airway techniques to be used in adults and children require thorough initial training with plenty of hands-on practice for proficiency. The EMT who is given the responsibility of performing such advanced airway procedures must practice in a system that allows for adequate quality assurance and continuing education.

TEST YOUR KNOWLEDGE

1. What are the advantages of endotracheal intubation?
2. What are the indications and contraindications for endotracheal intubation?
3. How does the Macintosh blade work? The Miller?
4. What does cricoid pressure do? How is it performed?
5. What are some ways to confirm endotracheal tube placement?
6. What physical assessments need to be repeated on an intubated patient?
7. What are some problems that would cause an intubated patient to deteriorate?
8. What is different about intubating a trauma patient and a medical patient?
9. What differences exist between the pediatric and adult airways?
10. What advantages does gastric decompression bring to the ventilation of the intubated patient?

FURTHER STUDY

Bradley, J. S., et al. (1998). Prehospital oral endotracheal intubation by rural basic emergency medical technicians. *Annals of Emergency Medicine, 32*(1), 26–32.

Nordberg, M. (1995). Safe passage: Should basic EMTs be allowed to intubate? *Emergency Medical Services, 24*(9), 39, 42–48.

Sayre, M. R., et al. (1998). Field trial of endotracheal intubation by basic EMTs. *Annals of Emergency Medicine, 31*(2), 228–233.

Spaite, D. (1998). Intubation by basic EMTs: Lifesaving advance or catastrophic complication? *Annals of Emergency Medicine, 31*(2), 276–277.

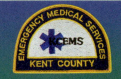

Cardiopulmonary Resuscitation

KEY TERMS

advanced lividity

Heimlich maneuver

intermammary line

McGill forceps

return of spontaneous
  circulation (ROSC)

rigor mortis

signs of circulation

OBJECTIVES

Upon completion of this appendix, the reader should be able to:

1. Define *sudden cardiac death*.
2. State the purpose of CPR.
3. Discuss situations when CPR would be withheld.
4. Demonstrate how to check for responsiveness.
5. Demonstrate how to open an airway.
6. Discuss the meaning of "look, listen, and feel."
7. Demonstrate palpation of the carotid artery.
8. Discuss advantages of compression technologies.
9. Describe how an EMT would handle special situations that are unique to EMS.
10. Explain the differences between layperson CPR and EMT CPR.
11. Describe how an EMT interfaces with a bystander performing CPR.
12. Describe the sequence of steps used to relieve a foreign body airway obstruction.
13. Describe the anatomical differences between children and adults that makes CPR different from one to the other.
14. Describe CPR for a newborn, an infant, and a child.

OVERVIEW

Sudden cardiac death, an unexpected death within 1 hour of the onset of cardiac symptoms, is typically the result of ventricular fibrillation. The definitive treatment for ventricular fibrillation is defibrillation with an automated external defibrillator (AED), as discussed in Chapter 29.

However, in cases when an AED is not readily available an emergency medical technician (EMT) may be required to perform cardiopulmonary resuscitation (CPR) until the AED arrives. CPR in those

Heart Attack at Airport

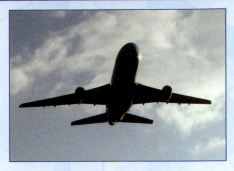

Bonnie and Mike were finishing cleaning up the ambulance from the last call when the tones went off and the announcement proceeded. "Ambulance 1957, Medic 15 respond to the airport lobby, man having a heart attack."

As Bonnie climbed into the driver's seat she remembered the last cardiac call she had at the airport. It was a full arrest and airport security and a couple of off-duty flight attendants were already on scene performing CPR and using the AED. It was a save, thanks to the good work of those citizens.

(Courtesy of Morguefile.)

- What unique challenges do EMS providers face when confronted with citizens performing CPR or using an AED?
- How does the EMT interface with citizen CPR?
- Are there any differences between citizen CPR and rescuer CPR?

cases is performed in order to maintain circulation to the brain and the heart until the fibrillating heart can be defibrillated, or "shocked," back into a normal pulse-producing, life-sustaining rhythm. Therefore, it is imperative that EMTs know how to perform CPR. This appendix reviews the rudimentary principles of CPR for the EMT.

Note: Many states require EMT students to obtain certification in CPR before they begin the EMT course. Other states require EMTs to recertify their CPR certification or obtain one during the EMT class. In any case, EMTs are well served if they review and practice the skills of CPR during the EMT course. EMTs need to be experts at CPR.

CARDIAC ARREST AND CPR

It is important for the EMT to understand that CPR is only a stopgap measure intended to preserve the brain and heart until the arrival of the AED and a subsequent conversion, by defibrillation, of the deadly rhythm into a pulsed rhythm.

While there are reports of a **return of spontaneous circulation (ROSC)** with CPR alone, that is, pulses returning with just CPR or with defibrillation, these cases are rare, and the patient's survival more likely depends on the well-timed use of an AED.

For every minute of delay getting an AED to the patient, survival from ventricular fibrillation and sudden cardiac death decline by approximately 7–10%; therefore, the first priority in emergency care is to get an AED to the patient.

CPR is also performed whenever a patient has been in collapse for a prolonged time and the AED indicates "no shock advised." In those cases, CPR is intended to help convert the nonshockable asystolic rhythm into a shockable rhythm, such as ventricular fibrillation.

Exceptions to the rule include a patient whose collapse was caused by a noncardiac incident such as a drug overdose, a submersion incident with near-drowning, or a submersion incident into cold water with subsequent hypothermia. In those cases CPR is performed until other more definitive treatments can be instituted.

CPR is also performed in cases of near-cardiac arrest; for example, the patient who is in respiratory failure/arrest and the EMT performs rescue breathing, forestalling the inevitable cardiac arrest that would normally follow. This case is especially true in children, who more often die from respiratory failure than from cardiac disease.

EMS and Cardiac Arrest

"Unknown, man down" or "person collapsed, CPR in progress" can alert the EMT to the possibility of cardiac arrest and the need for CPR. However, many cardiac arrest calls start out less clear. Some callers will report a patient having a seizure, the last convulsion of an oxygen-starved brain before death. Other callers will report a person with difficulty breathing, as the patient takes his last agonal breath. Because cardiac arrest can sometimes be sudden and unexpected, the EMT must always be prepared to perform CPR if needed.

When exiting the emergency vehicle on the scene of a suspected cardiac arrest the EMT should have a selection of airway devices, including suction, oxygen, and a bag-valve-mask (BVM) as well as an AED.

Despite the excitement and anticipation surrounding a cardiac arrest, when the EMT first enters the scene the initial consideration must be given to scene safety. This is especially true if more than one person has collapsed. Paying no heed to signs of danger leaves the EMT at risk of being the next victim.

Obvious Death and DNR

In some cases death is obvious and it may not be appropriate to start CPR on the patient. For example, if the patient has **advanced lividity**, pooling of blood in the dependent portions of the body with a clear line of demarcation, or **rigor mortis**, a generalized stiffening of the body following death, then CPR may not be indicated. Other reasons to withhold CPR include decomposition of the body, incineration of the body, decapitation, hemicorporectomy (division of the body in half), and other obviously mortal wounds. The EMT should follow medical protocols regarding when to withhold CPR.

If family or bystanders are present the EMT should inquire about a do not resuscitate (DNR) order. Some jurisdictions permit an EMT to honor a DNR order in the field. If the DNR can be produced and the EMT, following medical protocols, can honor the DNR, then CPR should not be started. If there is a delay in obtaining the DNR, the EMT might consider starting CPR while trying to contact medical control for more direction.

Responsiveness

While donning personal protective equipment, minimally a pair of gloves and goggles, the EMT should decide if the situation is a medical circumstance or a trauma circumstance. This decision impacts the EMT's early care of the patient. If the patient is a trauma patient, the EMT must first maintain manual cervical spine stabilization in order to prevent further cervical injury before proceeding. If the patient is a medical patient, then manual cervical spine stabilization is unnecessary.

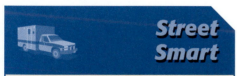
Street Smart

Dogs present a large and an all too common hazard on scene. A dog protecting its fallen master may misinterpret the well-meaning efforts of the EMT and become aggressive. It is best if the dog can be moved to another room, with the door closed, or, better, moved outdoors until after the patient is removed.

Next the EMT must establish the patient's level of responsiveness. First, the EMT should call out to the patient, preferably using the patient's name. If there is no response, then the EMT should call out to the patient again, this time much more loudly. If the patient still remains unresponsive, the EMT should tap him on the shoulder to determine unresponsiveness. Patients who appear unresponsive may actually be in deep sleep. The EMT should then proceed to give the patient a painful stimulus, like a sternal chest rub. If there has been no response to loud verbal and painful stimulus, then the patient is determined to be "unresponsive."

If the decision is made to start resuscitation, it may be necessary to move the patient from the position in which he was found. The patient should be positioned supine on a firm surface, such as the floor. It may be necessary to drag the patient off a bed and onto the floor before CPR can begin. If the patient has a suspected cervical spine injury, efforts should be made to maintain neutral cervical spine alignment. Often a long axis drag coupled with manual cervical spine stabilization is all that is needed.

A minimum of time should be taken to move the patient to a firm surface. Delays getting a patient to another room, for example, decrease the patient's chances of survival.

Airway

With the patient on the firm surface, and the rescuer typically positioned at his side, the airway must next be opened. The tongue of an unconscious patient can obstruct the airway, so the head must be repositioned to open the airway. The method used for the medical patient, for whom no neck injury is suspected, is the head-tilt, chin-lift, as illustrated in Figure B-1.

Placing the heel of one hand on the forehead of the patient and using the index finger and thumb to grasp the mandible (chin), the

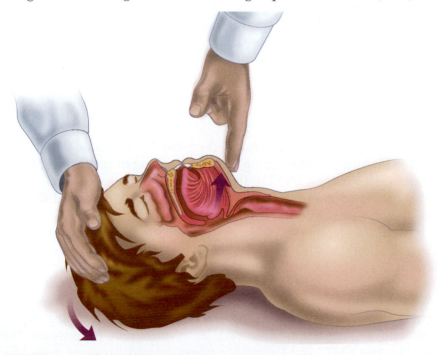

FIGURE B-1   The head-tilt, chin-lift airway technique.

EMT gently tilts the head backward, feeling for resistance. If resistance is felt it may mean that the patient has a neck injury or another reason for limited neck mobility, requiring the EMT to use the jaw thrust maneuver.

If the patient is a suspected trauma patient, or has limited neck mobility, then the EMT should reposition at the head of the patient and, reaching toward the chest, grasp the angle of the patient's lower jaw with both hands, placing the thumb on the patient's zygoma (cheekbones) and lifting the jaw upward. These two airway maneuvers are discussed in Chapter 7.

Occasionally, when the EMT opens the airway and inspects the oropharynx, secretions or vomitus may be present. If this is the case the airway should be aggressively cleared. If large pieces of food are seen, the EMT should use the forefingers like a hook and scoop out the pieces. A bite block, a large airway inserted sideways between the molars, will prevent the EMT's fingers from being inadvertently bitten. The EMT should then proceed to mechanically suction to remove the remaining secretions.

If these secretions are not removed and the patient is ventilated, either by mouth-to-mouth rescue breathing or with a BVM, they will be forced into the lungs and cause an aspiration. Aspirates block narrow airways, prevent adequate ventilation of the lungs, and can help produce hypoxia.

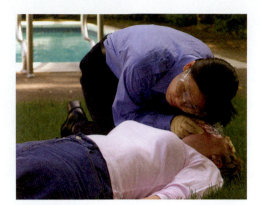

FIGURE B-2 Look, listen, and feel for breathing.

Breathing

With the airway opened, the EMT should proceed to checking for breathing. The mnemonic "look, listen, and feel" summarizes the three-step approach to verifying the presence or absence of breathing (Figure B-2). The EMT should turn her head and place her ear near the patient's mouth. In position, the EMT should look to see if there is adequate chest rise, listen for the sound of breathing from the mouth, and feel the breath against the cheek.

If the patient is breathing and just unconscious, the EMT should evaluate the quality of the breathing. Breathing that is shallow and rapid or slow and agonal is not adequate and the patient should be supported by either rescue breathing or BVM.

If the patient is breathing adequately, then the EMT should proceed with the rest of the initial assessment, taking precautions in the case of suspected cervical spine injury.

If the patient is not breathing, then the EMT should proceed to breathe for him by either doing rescue breathing or using a BVM. The procedure for using a BVM is discussed in Chapter 8. Figure B-3 illustrates mouth-to-mouth rescue breathing; it should be noted that the face shield is present but not visible.

If the EMT is going to perform mouth-to-mouth rescue breathing then she should use a barrier device or pocket mask and provide two slow breaths that cause the chest to start to rise without overinflating the lungs.

Overinflation of the lungs can cause air to spill over into the esophagus and stomach. Gastric filling can result in decreased lung expansion and regurgitation followed by aspiration. To prevent this problem the EMT could consider using cricoid pressure, provided sufficient personnel are on hand to assist.

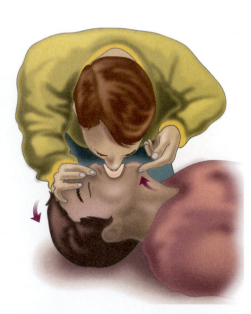

FIGURE B-3 An EMT using a face shield and performing mouth-to-mouth rescue breathing.

The process of assessing for breathing should take about 10 seconds. It is important to adequately check for breathing. A short 5-second assessment of breathing may miss the person who is breathing agonally, while a prolonged assessment of breathing, greater than 10 seconds, may delay the time to defibrillation.

Circulation

After delivering two measured breaths, the EMT should proceed to check the patient for a pulse. In adults, the pulse is verified at the carotid artery in the neck. A pulse here generally indicates that the brain is getting blood flow.

To find a pulse the EMT should place her forefingers on the patient's larynx (Adam's apple) at the midline of the anterior portion of the throat then proceed, on the side closest to the EMT, to run the fingers posteriorly until they fall into a groove, about two or three finger breadths below the larynx. The carotid artery is found in the groove created by the sternocleidomastoid (SCM) muscle, also known as the strap muscle. The EMT should maintain the head-tilt, using one hand on the forehead. This position makes palpating (feeling) the carotid artery easier.

Finding a pulse on a living person is relatively easy; confirming the absence of a pulse on a pulseless patient is more difficult. The EMT should frequently practice finding the carotid pulse so during an emergency it can be found quickly and easily.

Once the EMT has found the carotid artery pulse point, she should palpate (feel) for a pulse for approximately 10 seconds. If a pulse is present, then the EMT should proceed with the rest of the initial assessment. If the pulse is absent, then the EMT should proceed to chest compressions.

If the EMT suspects that the patient is hypothermic from the cold, a longer pulse check may be necessary. Some experts advocate taking as long as 30 seconds to confirm pulselessness. The EMT should follow the medical protocol for assessing and treating hypothermia in these cases.

Chest Compressions

After confirming pulselessness, the EMT performs external chest compressions, also known as cardiac massage. Chest compressions are a series of rhythmic compressions of the anterior chest in order to compress the heart and great vessels and, in turn, create a blood flow to the vital organs.

It should be noted that even expertly performed manual CPR only produces about 25% of normal blood flow, an inadequate blood flow to sustain life. It is imperative that the heart start pumping on its own, that is, restart the heart, using the defibrillator.

Rather than manual compressions some EMS systems use a circumferential compression machine, for example, the Autopulse made by the Revivant Company. This machine provides a consistent rate and depth of compression as well as a dependable 50/50 cycle of compression to relaxation. Machines such as this one can be deployed quickly, perform a consistent depth and rate of compressions, and adjust to each patient. However, its greatest advantage, as illustrated in Figure B-4, may be that it helps to free the EMT to attend to other functions, such as helping to maintain the airway.

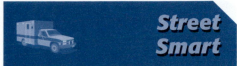

Street Smart

Some EMTs have been trained to perform a "quick check." To perform a quick check, the EMT opens the airway and checks for breathing and a pulse simultaneously. While this technique reduces the time from collapse to defibrillation, it takes a great deal of practice to perform it correctly.

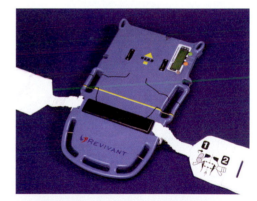

A.

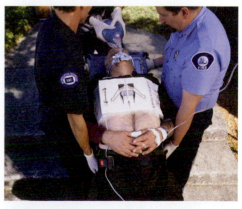

B.

FIGURE B-4 A. The Autopulse device. B. The Autopulse in position and performing compressions.

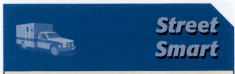

Street Smart

If the patient is obese, or the EMT is having difficulty identifying landmarks, then she should place her hands on the lower half of the patient's sternum, approximately even with an imaginary line running between the nipples.

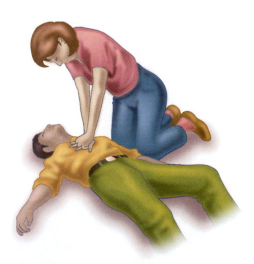

FIGURE B-5 Proper positioning for chest compressions.

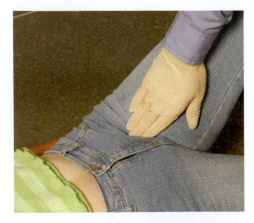

FIGURE B-6 Palpation of the femoral pulse to verify compressions.

To perform manual external chest compressions the EMT must first expose the patient's chest in order to find landmarks for proper hand placement. If the patient is a woman, it is unnecessary to cut or remove her brassiere, as important landmarks are readily visible without it.

To find proper hand position for compressions, the EMT should identify the lower half of the sternum by placing her fingers at the lower rib margin and following it midline to the patient's xiphoid process on the sternum.

Once the xiphoid process has been identified, the EMT should lay the heel of the opposite hand on top of the lower half of the sternum, above her fingers. Then the EMT places the other hand on top of the first hand.

The EMT may choose to either interlace fingers or extend them to keep them off the chest wall. If the EMT has a weak, or arthritic, wrist, she may choose to grasp her own wrist with the other hand to support it. This added support can help the EMT produce more force on the compressions. In every case it is important that the fingers of the EMT do not touch the chest wall.

The EMT should take the time to find the proper placement of the hands. Compression of the bottom portion of the sternum may result in injuries to the liver, spleen, and stomach, while compressions of the upper half of the sternum will not be effective.

While kneeling, with legs slightly apart and with both hands positioned perpendicular to the long axis of the sternum, the EMT should then raise her body up until her shoulders are directly over the patient's chest.

Next the EMT should lock her elbows, leaving her arms straight. This permits the EMT to use shoulder and back strength to produce the force of compression. Arm muscles quickly tire after only a few minutes of compressions, but the back and shoulder muscles are more capable of sustaining the compressions for a longer period of time. Figure B-5 illustrates proper position of the EMT to perform compresssions.

The EMT then compresses the sternum downward, toward the ground, approximately $1\frac{1}{2}$–2 inches in depth. If the patient is obese or has a large chest, it may be necessary to compress the sternum, while others of a slighter build may not need as much compression. Production of a carotid or femoral pulse is evidence of adequate compression. Figure B-6 illustrates palpation of a femoral pulse.

The EMT should strive to make the cycle of compression and release approximately equal, that is, 50% compression and 50% relaxation. The relaxation time allows for the ventricle to fill with blood and the rescuer to rest. During the relaxation phase the EMT should leave her hands resting gently on the chest wall, not compressing nor removing the hand from it, and risking losing proper hand position.

With practice, the EMT can achieve a rhythmic compression at a rate of approximately 100 compressions a minute. The compression should not be abrupt, or stabbing, nor springy, with the arms recoiling from every compression, but rather a steady rhythmic up-and-down motion. Properly performed CPR can produce systolic blood pressures of 60–80 mm Hg.

If two EMTs are present then one will perform chest compressions while the second will ventilate the patient with either a BVM or pocket mask. The compression rate for two-rescuer CPR is the same as one-rescuer CPR, 100 compressions per minute, with a pause for ventilation every 15 compressions.

After two slow and measured breaths of approximately 500 cc are delivered to the patient, the first EMT should resume compressions. This pattern of compressions and ventilations should continue for four cycles. After four cycles the EMT at the head should first attempt to palpate for a carotid pulse during compressions to determine if they are effective, and then call for compressions to stop. Reassessing the patient for a carotid pulse for 5–10 seconds, and finding none, the EMT at the head should deliver two breaths and call for compressions to continue. Figure B-7 illustrates the cycle of opening the airway, ventilating the patient (using a barrier device), and chest compressions.

Special Situations

The EMT performing CPR is doubly tasked to perform effective CPR while moving the patient toward the ambulance and to the hospital.

For ease of movement of the patient, an EMT may elect to place him on a backboard or similar rigid device, regardless of the presence or absence of spine injury. It is important that the EMT tell emergency department personnel, upon arrival, that the patient is not a trauma patient and that the backboard was used as a convenience for moving the patient.

If the patient lives on an upper story of a building, it will be necessary to move him down to the ground floor and the awaiting ambulance. In some instances an elevator will accommodate the patient lying supine. In many cases the patient will have to be carried down the stairs. In those instances, the CPR should be performed for a minimum of 1 minute and the patient reassessed. If no pulse is found then the patient should be moved quickly to the next landing, or to the foot of the stairs, and CPR should resume for at least another minute. If necessary, the process can resume for each flight of stairs.

Once on the ground floor the patient should be placed on the ambulance stretcher, with the stretcher remaining in the low position. The EMT can continue ventilations and compressions while the stretcher is moved to the ambulance.

As space inside an ambulance is often limited, it may be necessary for the EMT to either kneel beside the patient to continue compressions

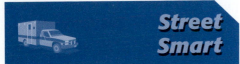

Street Smart

It is not uncommon for the EMT to cause some rib fractures, especially in elderly patients, even if CPR is being performed correctly. The EMT should not be alarmed by this development and should continue CPR.

Street Smart

Once the patient has been intubated by an advanced EMT, it is not necessary to interpose ventilations between compressions. In those instances compressions may be continuous while ventilations are delivered at a constant rate of 10–12 breaths per minute, that is, one breath every 5 seconds.

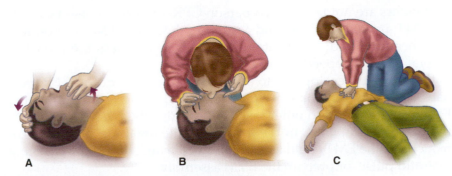

A   B   C

FIGURE B-7 The cycle of airway, breathing, and circulation.

or to straddle the stretcher, placing her back against the ceiling, and bracing her legs against the walls of the ambulance.

If the patient is immediately transferred to a high hospital gurney upon arrival at the emergency department, it may be necessary for the EMT to climb aboard the gurney and kneel beside the patient. From this position an EMT might easily fall, so care should be taken to prevent the fall.

Bystander CPR

An EMT may come across a bystander who is performing CPR, presenting some unique challenges to the EMT when working with these good Samaritans, because there are several differences between layperson CPR and the CPR that an EMT is trained to do.

To begin, the bystander may not have checked a pulse before beginning CPR. Several studies have indicated that laypeople are unfamiliar with, and have trouble finding, the carotid pulse; bystanders err in correctly assessing for a pulse approximately 35% of the time.

For this reason lay rescuers are taught to assess for **signs of circulation**, such as responsiveness, breathing, coughing, and movement, instead of a carotid pulse. If the EMT should ask the bystander, "Did the patient have a pulse?" she is likely to get a quizzical look from the bystander.

Next, the EMT may observe that no ventilations are being performed. The bystander is performing compression-only resuscitation. Many bystanders are reluctant to perform mouth-to-mouth rescue breathing, particularly on a stranger, and especially in the absence of a barrier device such as a face shield.

Or the bystander may have received instruction on CPR from an emergency medical dispatcher. These EMS dispatchers can only provide limited instruction on the telephone and, to conserve time, provide bystanders with only instructions on how to perform compressions.

Finally, the bystander may be physically unable to perform ventilations, perhaps due to advanced lung disease. Some respiratory conditions preclude the well-meaning bystander from performing ventilations.

While true cardiopulmonary resuscitation is desirable, that is, both ventilations and compressions, compression-only resuscitation is better than no resuscitation efforts at all.

Bystander-EMT CPR

Bystanders are not taught two-person CPR, only one-person CPR. If the EMT arrives on scene, and assuming that other EMT responders have been notified, and bystander CPR is in progress the EMT has several options depending on circumstances.

If the bystander appears to be comfortable with doing CPR, perhaps by asking if he or she wants relief and being told no, then the EMT should attend to other tasks and permit the bystander to continue one-person CPR. In the interim, while awaiting the arrival of more EMS, the EMT could assess the effectiveness of CPR by checking a carotid pulse, or prepare the BVM assembly.

If the bystander appears exhausted, or the CPR ineffective, then the EMT can offer to relieve him or her. In those instances, the EMT should first confirm the absence of a pulse and breathing and then commence CPR as indicated. The bystander might be asked to assist other EMS responders with locating the patient.

The bystander may be willing to continue CPR and provide assistance valuable to the resuscitation. In that case the EMT should ask if the bystander is fatigued (the EMT would replace the bystander and perform one-person CPR) or would like to continue to perform compressions only. If the bystander is willing to perform compressions then the EMT should call for a halt to CPR and reassess the patient's airway, breathing, and circulation. If no pulse or breathing is present the EMT should deliver two rescue breaths and instruct the bystander to begin compressions. The rate for one-person CPR and two-person CPR is the same—a compression ventilation ratio of 15:2. The bystander is replaced when a second EMS provider arrives. Figure B-8 shows a bystander helping with CPR.

Public AED Use and the EMT

With the increasing use of public AEDs, by flight attendants, casino security, lifeguards, and school teachers, for example, there is an increased likelihood that an EMT will encounter a bystander using one.

Assuming that the EMT is present because the bystander verified that the patient was unresponsive and therefore activated the EMS system, the EMT should allow the bystander to confirm that the patient is breathless and pulseless. After the two breaths have been administered, then the EMT should proceed normally with use of the AED.

If the bystander has already attached the AED pads, then the EMT should permit the bystander to continue with the sequence. An interruption to reconfirm pulselessness and apnea only delays defibrillation and decreases the chance of defibrillation success. Figure B-9 shows a citizen using an AED before the arrival of EMS. Figure B-10 shows the EMT using the AED after the bystander has delivered the first shock.

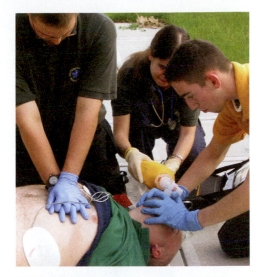

FIGURE B-8 Citizen helps to hold the mask seal as the EMT performs CPR after a "no shock advised" by an AED.

Street Smart

In many instances the bystander may know the patient, the patient may even be a family member, and the bystander who has performed CPR has an interest in the outcome. The EMT should consider contacting the bystander later to relay the outcome of the resuscitation or, minimally, to thank him or her for assisting.

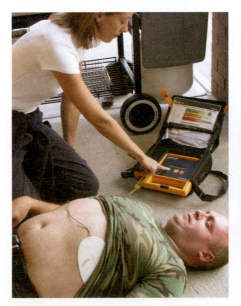

FIGURE B-9 Citizen uses AED.

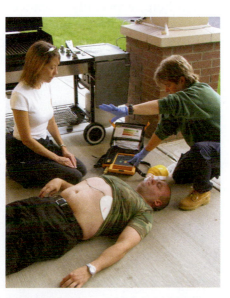

FIGURE B-10 EMT using AED following bystander use.

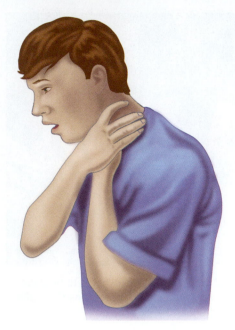

FIGURE B-11 The universal choking sign.

ADULT FOREIGN BODY AIRWAY OBSTRUCTION

Choking, while common, is a rare cause of cardiac arrest, as most people are able to clear their airway without assistance. For this reason, the first step in assisting a person who is experiencing an airway obstruction, typically from meat, is to allow him to attempt clearing his own airway as long as good air exchange occurs. During this time the EMT should remain with the patient and stand by in case of need.

It is when the patient has poor air exchange, as evidenced by cyanosis, a weak or weakening cough, and subsequent loss of consciousness, that the EMT must act.

Initially the EMT should ask the patient, "Are you choking? Can you speak?" The patient with an obstructed airway will be unable to speak and may clutch his neck, in a demonstration of the universal choking sign illustrated in Figure B-11.

With the victim either standing or sitting, the EMT should come around to the back of the patient and place her fist into the area just below the xiphoid process, midway and midline between the sternum and the umbilicus.

Grasping the fist with the other hand, the EMT should perform forceful upward abdominal thrusts, also called the **Heimlich maneuver**. This series of forceful upward abdominal thrusts forces air out of the lungs and the trachea. It is often necessary to perform the procedure repeatedly until the obstruction is relieved or the patient becomes unconscious.

Signs that the obstruction has been relieved include seeing the object that has obstructed the airway forced out, the patient taking a gasp of air, or the patient speaking. Figure B-12 illustrates three positions to relieve obstruction.

If the patient becomes unconscious the EMT should help protect him from falling and striking his head, if possible. Then the EMT should be sure that EMS has been dispatched and that additional help, especially advanced life support, is on the way before proceeding.

Once the patient is on the floor, the EMT should immediately look for the cause of the obstruction in the patient's pharynx by opening

Street Smart

It may be necessary to perform chest thrusts instead of abdominal thrusts on obese patients whom the EMT cannot get her arms around. If the patient is obese, it may be prudent to have him lie down and then perform chest compressions. There is evidence that chest compressions can be as effective as abdominal thrusts.

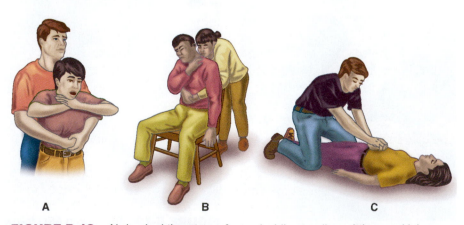

A   **B**   **C**

FIGURE B-12 Abdominal thrusts performed while standing, sitting, and lying.

the airway with a tongue-jaw lift, also called a trauma chin lift, and inspect the airway.

If the object is visible then the EMT should insert a gloved finger formed like a hook into the side of the mouth and scoop the object out. If there is concern about the patient biting, an oral airway may be placed between the molars to act as a bite block.

If the object is not visible then the EMT should attempt to deliver two rescue breaths. It may be possible to get air past the obstruction if the patient's throat has relaxed. If the breaths are unsuccessful then the head should be repositioned and two more breaths attempted.

If after these two attempts the EMT is still unable to get a breath into the patient, then she should resort to abdominal thrusts or chest thrusts (for obese or pregnant patients) and repeat the sequence again.

PEDIATRIC CPR

It is rare for children to go into isolated cardiac arrest, unless they have congenital heart disease. Instead another event, usually respiratory in nature, precedes the cardiac event. For this reason the EMT should first perform rescue breathing before calling for help; phone fast for children as opposed to phone first for adults.

Newborns occasionally need stimulation to breathe and even ventilation, in approximately 5–10% of all deliveries. This subject is covered in Chapter 37 under newborn care.

The process of resuscitation for a child is similar to that of an adult, with the exception that was just noted about phone fast. The differences between pediatric resuscitation and adult resuscitation lie in the unique characteristics of a child's anatomy.

The first difference is the airway of the child. A child's head is noticeably larger in proportion to the body than is an adult head. For this reason it is important to pad the area behind the child's chest to elevate the chest to a neutral position. While the size of children vary, a dependable measure of proper placement is when the opening of the ears is in line, horizontally, with the midline of the shoulder.

With the head in a neutral position, the EMT should gently open the airway. When using the head-tilt, chin-lift technique, the EMT should use caution placing her fingers in position. The soft underside of the chin can easily be displaced upward, pushing the tongue against the hard palate and obstructing the airway. Figure B-13 illustrates the airway position and ventilation of an infant.

If a child is suspected of having a foreign body obstruction, a common occurrence because of children's smaller airways, the EMT should use the techniques described in the pediatric medical emergencies chapter (Chapter 39) to relieve the obstruction.

If the airway is clear then the EMT should assess for breathing, using the same look, listen, and feel technique described for adults. If the breathing appears at all distressed, that is, gasping and ineffective, then the EMT should ventilate the child.

Next the EMT should proceed to checking the child's pulse. Depending on the size of the child either the carotid or brachial pulse will be palpated. The brachial pulse is palpated instead of the carotid, typically in children less than 1 year of age, when the EMT is unable

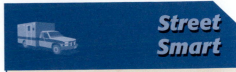

The advanced EMT (AEMT) has special tools and methods to help relieve the airway obstruction. Using the laryngoscope, the AEMT can mechanically open the airway and visualize the throat. If the object is visible the AEMT can grasp the object with a pair of special long, curved pinching tongs called **McGill forceps**.

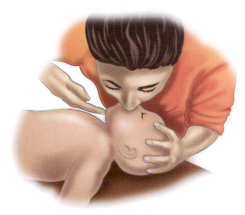

FIGURE B-13 Neutral head position for rescue breathing for an infant.

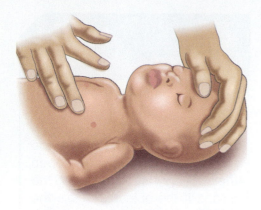

FIGURE B-14 Proper finger position for infant CPR.

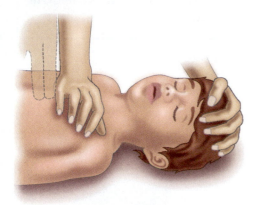

FIGURE B-15 Proper hand position for child chest compressions.

to find landmarks on the throat because the child's neck is short and chubby.

The brachial pulse is found on the inner aspect of the upper arm, proximal to the bicep muscle, midline between the elbow and the shoulder.

If no pulse is present the EMT should proceed with chest compressions, depressing the chest approximately one third to one half the depth of the chest, after finding the correct compression point.

The compression point for an infant less than 1 year of age is approximately one finger width below the imaginary line that runs between the nipples, also called the **intermammary line**. Figure B-14 shows the proper finger position for an infant for compressions.

Depending on the size of the infant, and the size of the EMT's hands, it may be possible for the EMT to encircle the infant's chest with her hands and perform compressions with the thumb. This technique is both effective and less tiring for some EMTs.

The compression point for a child is the same as for an adult, except only one hand is used to compress the chest approximately $1–1\frac{1}{2}$ inches. Figure B-15 shows the proper hand position for chest compressions on a child.

Compression to ventilation ratios for children follow the differences in vital signs. For example, newborns breathe faster and have faster heart rates. Therefore, compression to ventilation ratios for a newborn is 3:1.

For infants and children up to 8 years of age, the compression to ventilation ratio is correspondingly adjusted to 5:1. For children over 8 years of age, the compression to ventilation ratio is the same as for adults, 15:2.

CONCLUSION

While under the best of conditions survival from cardiac arrest is poor, the knowledge that an EMT's actions have saved even one person's life can sustain her morale and reinforce the optimism that EMS can make a difference.

For these reasons alone, the EMT should become expert in CPR, practice CPR in a variety of predictable scenarios, and learn to work together as a team.

TEST YOUR KNOWLEDGE

1. What is sudden cardiac death?
2. What is the purpose of CPR?
3. When would CPR be withheld from a pulseless patient?
4. What are the four steps of checking responsiveness?
5. What are the two main techniques for opening an airway, and when are they used?
6. What does the phrase "look, listen, and feel" mean?

7. What are some of the differences between citizen CPR and the CPR an EMT performs?

8. How would an EMT interact with a bystander performing CPR?

9. What are the anatomical differences between children and adults in relation to CPR?

10. What are the compression–ventilation ratios for infants, children, and adults?

INTERNET RESOURCES

- American Heart Association, http://www.americanheart.org
- American Red Cross, http://www.redcross.org
- National Safety Council, http://www.nsc.org

FURTHER STUDY

American Heart Association. (2001). *Fundamentals of BLS for health-care providers.* Dallas, TX: Author.

American Red Cross, & Handal, K. A. (1992). *American Red Cross first aid and safety handbook.* Boston: Little, Brown.

National Safety Council. (2002). *CPR and AED* (4th ed.). Itasca, IL: Author.

Ornato, J., & Peberdy, M. A. (2004). *Cardiopulmonary resuscitation.* Totowa, NJ: Humana Press.

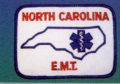

Advanced Life Support Assist Skills

KEY TERMS

cricoid pressure
D5W
endotracheal intubation
hyperventilation
lactated Ringers
laryngoscope
laryngoscopy
macrodrip
microdrip
normal saline
preoxygenation
twelve-lead ECG

OBJECTIVES

Upon completion of this appendix, the reader should be able to:

1. Identify the importance of teamwork between basic and advanced emergency providers.
2. Discuss the importance of maintaining a patient's airway using basic techniques.
3. Describe how and when to apply cricoid pressure.
4. List several ways to confirm proper endotracheal tube placement.
5. Describe a method to secure an endotracheal tube orally and nasally.
6. Describe how to ventilate a patient via an oral and a nasal endotracheal tube.
7. Describe how to perform endotracheal suctioning.
8. Describe how to apply different types of cardiac monitoring leads.
9. Describe how to properly prepare a bag of intravenous solution for administration.
10. Discuss the considerations in maintaining an intravenous line.

OVERVIEW

There are some situations in which an EMT will call for assistance from an advanced life support (ALS) provider. In these circumstances, it is helpful for the emergency medical technician (EMT) to be familiar with the most common skills performed by the advanced provider in order to facilitate their completion.

If an EMT is not permitted to perform endotracheal intubation, he can certainly assist an advanced provider. The EMT can also assist an ALS provider by preparing an intravenous (IV) setup or by attaching the patient to the cardiac monitor.

Familiarity with these skills will allow the EMT and advanced providers to integrate their patient care into a team approach.

TEAM CONCEPT

The prehospital health care team is made up of many different people. Fire, police, and emergency medical services (EMS) work together in order to safely provide quality health care to ill and injured persons. Within the medical component of the team, there are also several different team members.

There may be a first responder who initiates patient care prior to the arrival of the EMT. The EMT should be able to integrate his care into the care that has been initiated by the first responder. Similarly, if the patient requires advanced services, the EMT may call for assistance from an ALS provider. The importance of the EMT's ability to work well with the ALS personnel cannot be overstated.

If the EMT can anticipate what the ALS provider may need or be able to assist with specific procedures, the care of the patient will be accomplished more quickly and efficiently. The EMT and advanced provider should work together as a team to care for their patient.

Airway

While the importance of a basic life support (BLS) airway cannot be overemphasized, there are some circumstances in which a patient may need a more advanced airway. In some states, the EMT is permitted to perform endotracheal intubation. In the states where this is not permitted, the EMT should be familiar enough with the indications, contraindications, and technique that he can assist the advanced provider in the procedure.

Breathing

Once a patient has been intubated, the advanced provider will often have additional work to do, such as administering medication or obtaining IV access. The EMT will likely be asked to provide ventilation for the intubated patient. Therefore, it is important for the EMT to be familiar with this skill.

Circulation

While in most states EMTs are not trained to obtain IV access, it is useful for them to be familiar with the technique and able to assist by preparing the proper IV fluid. If allowed, the EMT may occasionally transport a patient with an IV line in place. While it is certainly not difficult, there are some things to consider while caring for the patient with an IV line.

ENDOTRACHEAL INTUBATION

Endotracheal intubation is the placement of a hollow plastic tube into the trachea to allow for direct ventilation of the lungs without gastric distension. This procedure can be done under direct visualization using a tool called a **laryngoscope**, or it is sometimes accomplished blindly, in the case of nasotracheal intubation.

Assisting with Breathing

The call was for a woman with difficulty breathing. EMS arrived to find Mrs. Anderson leaning over a small plastic bucket that was filled with facial tissues and pink frothy foam. She looked near death, and she could speak only in single words. The EMT, Ira, immediately placed the pulse oximeter on her finger, while Geo, the other EMT, prepared the non-rebreather mask. Then Ira listened to her lungs and heard loud crackles in all of her lung fields. The initial pulse oximeter reading was 84% on room air.

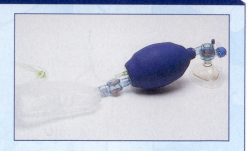

"Better get the BVM out," declared Ira. "I will contact Medcom and ask them what the ETA is for the paramedic." As Geo assembled the BVM, he started talking calmly to the patient, explaining that he was going to help her with her breathing. Then he placed the mask over her face. "Breathe easy, Mrs. Anderson. Let me help you," Geo implored. She was quickly becoming exhausted and had little fight left in her.

- What are indications for endotracheal intubation?
- What can the EMT do to assist in endotracheal intubation?
- Describe the purpose of cricoid pressure.

TABLE C-1

Conditions That Usually Require Endotracheal Intubation
Cardiac arrest
Respiratory arrest
Respiratory failure
Drug overdose
Persistent seizures
Severe head injury or facial injuries
Traumatic arrest

Patients who may be candidates for endotracheal intubation include those who cannot maintain a patent airway spontaneously or are in need of prolonged ventilatory assistance. Table C-1 lists conditions that would likely necessitate endotracheal intubation by a qualified provider.

Appendix A describes endotracheal intubation in detail. It is recommended that the EMT, even if he is not permitted to perform this technique independently, become familiar with this procedure.

Patient Preparation

One of the most obvious ways an EMT can facilitate endotracheal intubation is to adequately prepare the patient. If a patient is adequately prepared for this procedure, the risk of complication will be lessened.

The EMT should perform an initial assessment on his first encounter with the patient. The airway should be addressed with the plan to open, assess, suction, and secure as appropriate.

A head-tilt, chin-lift, or jaw thrust should be used as appropriate for the situation to initially open the airway. The EMT should assess for any fluids or particulate matter and suction if any is present. Details on these procedures are found in Chapter 7.

To more easily ventilate a patient, an oropharyngeal or nasopharyngeal airway should be placed as conditions require. Basic adequate ventilation should be provided by the EMT using a bag-valve-mask (BVM) device and 100% oxygen, while the advanced provider prepares his equipment for intubation.

Hyperventilation

To perform endotracheal intubation, the EMT must stop ventilating and remove the oral airway to allow the intubator access to the airway for laryngoscopy. **Laryngoscopy** is the procedure of using a laryngoscope to visualize the glottic opening. Typically, the procedure takes approximately 30 seconds to complete.

Because the patient will not be receiving ventilation during the time the intubator is performing the intubation, it is useful to deliver as much oxygen as possible into the patient's lungs prior to the onset of the procedure. This can be easily accomplished by a 1- to 2-minute period of **hyperventilation**.

Hyperventilation is a faster rate of ventilation. This does not mean that the patient should be ventilated as fast as the BVM will refill. What it does mean is the EMT should count as he ventilates the patient to ensure a rate of ventilation that is higher than the usual rate. The rates of normal ventilation and hyperventilation are discussed in Chapter 8.

In addition to providing such **preoxygenation**, the EMT should ensure the airway is well suctioned and no liquid or particulate matter remains in the oropharynx, where it can obscure the view of the intubator and make the task more difficult.

When the intubator has all of his equipment prepared and is ready to begin the procedure, he should ask the EMT to step aside and stop hyperventilation. At this time, the EMT should remove the BVM from the patient's face and remove any oropharyngeal airway that may have been placed. He should then stand close by with the BVM ready to be used when needed.

Safety Tip

Assessing and managing an airway can result in splashing of patient secretions. The EMT must remember to wear appropriate personal protective equipment, including gloves, mask, and goggles, during any airway procedures.

If it is suspected that the patient has a spinal injury, one EMT should be assigned to maintain spinal immobilization throughout the entire intubation. The best position for this provider is often at the patient's side.

Cricoid Pressure

During the intubation procedure, it is often helpful for the EMT to apply gentle, constant pressure over the cricoid ring. This **cricoid pressure** can serve to partially occlude the esophagus and prevent passive regurgitation during laryngoscopy. In addition, this pressure against the lower part of the larynx may put the glottic opening in a more easily viewed position for the intubator. Figure C-1 illustrates this procedure.

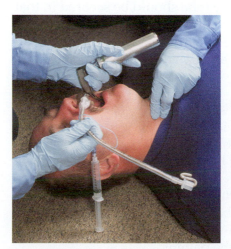
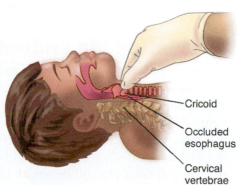

Cricoid

Occluded esophagus

Cervical vertebrae

FIGURE C-1 Cricoid pressure can serve to displace the larynx posteriorly, occluding the esophagus and placing the glottic opening in better view.

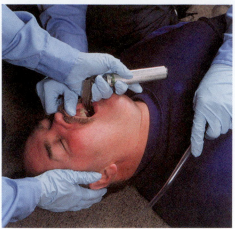

FIGURE C-2 The patient's upper lip can sometimes block the view of the intubator.

Assistance with Laryngoscopy

During laryngoscopy, there are a few things the EMT can do to help the intubator achieve an adequate view of the glottic opening. The application of cricoid pressure is one technique that can be used.

Another technique is to pull the right upper lip up and away from the mouth (Figure C-2). This is useful because the intubator will be looking into the right side of the patient's mouth. The upper lip can provide an impediment to a clear view of the airway structures. Because the assisting EMT usually has a free hand, he can gently move the lip out of the way.

Additionally, the advanced provider may require suction during the procedure. The EMT should have a Yankauer suction catheter within easy reach of the advanced provider and be prepared to turn on the suction power if needed.

Confirming Placement

Once the endotracheal tube (ETT) has been placed, the advanced provider will perform several techniques to confirm proper placement. Although it is the responsibility of the person who performs the intubation to ensure its proper placement, the EMT can assist with the completion of this by auscultation of the lungs and epigastrum, end tidal CO_2 detection, syringe aspiration, and assessment of adequate chest rise. All of these techniques are described in Appendix A.

In addition, the EMT should reassess the patient's vital signs, including pulse oximetry, if available, to ensure improvement after the placement of the ETT.

Street Smart

It is sometimes helpful, even in the absence of spinal injury, to apply a cervical collar to the intubated patient to minimize neck and head movement. Excessive head movement can result in dislodgment of the endotracheal tube. Therefore, anything that will minimize such movement would be useful.

Securing the Endotracheal Tube

Once the ETT has been confirmed to be in the proper tracheal position, the EMT should assist in securing it in place. It is very important that the exact depth of the tube be noted immediately on confirmation of proper placement. This can be done by noting the numbered markings on the side of the plastic tube. The average tube depth for a woman is 21 cm, and the average tube depth for a man is 23 cm.

Once this depth has been noted, the tube should be secured in that position using tape or any commercial device meant for this purpose. After the tube is secured, the position again should be confirmed by looking at the markings on the tube and by reevaluating the patient.

Safety Tip

Extreme care must be taken while handling this tube so it does not become misplaced. A misplaced endotracheal tube can cause the patient to become hypoxic.

Ventilating via Endotracheal Tube

If the intubator is an advanced provider, he may likely have to move on to other procedures, such as establishing an IV line, after completing intubation. The EMT will likely be asked to provide appropriate ventilation via the ETT.

When ventilating a patient through an ETT, a bag-valve device hooked up to 100% oxygen should be used. Usually the liter flow on the oxygen tank should be set at 15–25 lpm in order to get sufficient oxygen into the bag for delivery to the patient.

The EMT should use two hands to accomplish the task of ETT ventilation. One hand should be holding and squeezing the bag, while the other hand is against the patient's face, holding the base of the tube securely. No matter how efficient the tube securing method used, the tube can be easily dislodged if not securely held at all times.

Every few minutes, the EMT should assess the markings on the side of the tube to ensure the tube has not moved from its original position.

Ventilation should be performed at an appropriate rate for the age of the patient. The EMT should be careful to count the frequency of the ventilations delivered and keep them within the recommended rate at all times.

While delivering each ventilation, the EMT should note the resistance felt as he squeezes the bag. Any change in that resistance may mean that there is a problem with the tube placement or that the patient may have suffered a complication. The advanced provider should be made aware of any change in resistance as soon as it is noted.

Endotracheal Suctioning

As he ventilates the patient, if the EMT notes any accumulation of secretions within the tube, he may be asked to suction them out. Endotracheal suctioning is a sterile procedure that is easily done by the EMT. The technique is described in Appendix A of this text.

As with any other suctioning technique, the EMT should never suction for longer than 10–15 seconds, as the patient is not being ventilated during this time. It is sometimes useful to hyperventilate the patient for 1 minute prior to suctioning and then again for 1 minute after suctioning, to make up for the short time without oxygen delivery.

CARDIAC MONITORING

Part of an advanced assessment of the patient with a potential cardiac problem involves monitoring the heart's electrical activity. The EMT is taught to do this with an automatic defibrillator. The automatic defibrillator assesses the patient's heart rhythm through two large electrode pads that are placed on the chest, as described in Chapter 29.

If an EMT is caring for a victim of a cardiac arrest and there is an advanced provider on the scene as well, it is often useful for the EMT to use an automated external defibrillator (AED) to provide the cardiac rhythm assessment and defibrillation initially. This allows the advanced provider to perform other ALS tasks such as endotracheal intubation, IV access, and medication administration.

An advanced provider will assess the patient's heart rhythm with a different type of monitor. Most AEDs monitor the heart in one view or lead. That view is created between the two electrode pads that are applied to the chest.

A more advanced monitor can assess the heart with more than one view. A series of 3, 5, or even 10 or more electrodes can be placed on

ECG Application

Dan, the paramedic intern, was busy getting a history on Mr. Briggs, while Mohammed was standing on the sidelines watching. Mr. DeLeon, the paramedic in charge, asked Mohammed if he had ever put a patient on a heart monitor before. Mohammed answered, "No." "OK, kid," said Mr. DeLeon, "if you're going to do it, do it right."

With that introduction, DeLeon launched into a minilecture on electrode placement, topographic anatomy, and the importance of placing the electrodes correctly. Mohammed, listening closely, quickly picked up the information and started to apply the electrodes, while Dan started the IV.

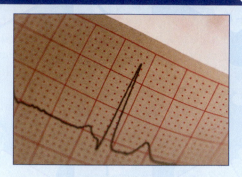

(Courtesy of PhotoDisc.)

- Describe how to apply 3, 4, 5, and 10 electrodes for ECG monitoring.
- What should the EMT consider when applying the ECG electrodes?
- How important is it to place the electrodes in exactly the recommended positions?

the patient's chest and attached to a monitoring device that can use these electrodes to generate a picture of the heart's electrical rhythm in many different views. This multiview picture of the heart's activity is useful in diagnosing different heart conditions.

To understand what view of the heart is being monitored, the electrodes must be applied in very specific places. The application of these electrodes can easily be accomplished by an EMT.

Defib Pads

The application of defibrillator pads was discussed in Chapter 29. Figure C-3 illustrates the proper placement of these two large electrodes. These electrodes should be placed onto dry skin and firmly applied so they are completely adherent to the chest wall.

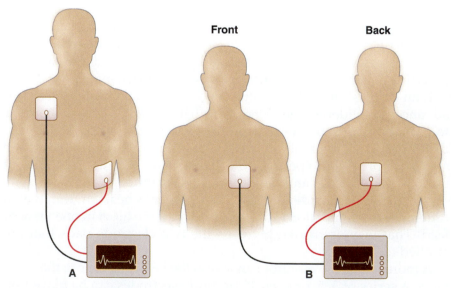

Front   **Back**

A   B

FIGURE C-3   Proper positioning of the AED pads is crucial to successful defibrillation. A and B show two proper ways.

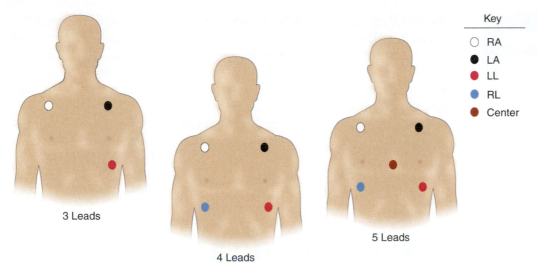

FIGURE C-4 Proper placement of cardiac electrodes for three-, four-, and five-lead systems.

Three-Lead

Most cardiac monitors used in the prehospital setting utilize three, four, or five electrodes to create several views of the electrical activity in the heart. This is useful in interpreting abnormal heart rhythms. Figure C-4 illustrates the proper position of these leads. Just as with the defibrillator pads, these electrodes should be applied to dry skin for the best result.

Twelve-Lead

When a patient presents with signs and symptoms that may be consistent with a myocardial infarction, a paramedic may wish to obtain a twelve-lead ECG. A **twelve-lead ECG** or electrocardiogram is a collection of 12 views of the heart obtained by applying a series of 10 electrodes to the chest in predetermined places. Knowing what each view should look like, the paramedic can assess the ECG for abnormalities. Certain types of abnormalities can be diagnostic for an acute myocardial infarction.

While obtaining the twelve-lead ECG is important, the paramedic has several other tasks he must accomplish with the patient who is suspected of having an acute myocardial infarction. While the paramedic is establishing an IV line and administering medication, the EMT can be applying the electrodes so that a twelve-lead ECG can be done as quickly as possible.

It is critically important the electrodes be placed in the proper positions for the acquisition of the twelve-lead ECG. If they are placed improperly, they will generate a different view of the heart than the paramedic is expecting to see. This will prevent an accurate interpretation of the findings. Figure C-5 illustrates the proper positioning of the 10 leads for acquisition of a twelve-lead ECG.

Monitor Setup

While the application of electrodes is fairly universal from one brand of cardiac monitor to another, the actual monitor setup is vastly

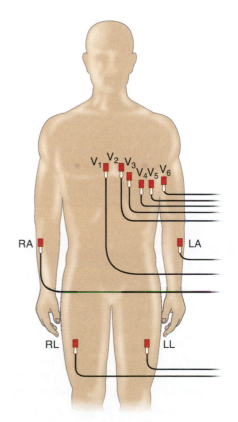

FIGURE C-5 Proper positioning of the 10 electrodes used to obtain a twelve-lead ECG.

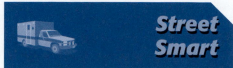

Street Smart

For the best contact, the skin should be dry and free of excess hair prior to the application of the electrodes. A towel may be used to dry any excess perspiration from the patient's chest, and a razor may be used to carefully remove any hair that will significantly interrupt the ECG.

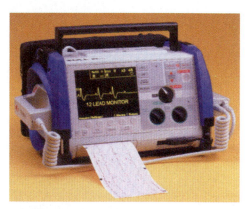

FIGURE C-6 The EMT should become familiar with the type of cardiac monitor that is used most commonly by the advanced level agencies with which he works. (Courtesy of Zoll Medical Corporation, Burlington, MA.)

Safety Tip

The handling of needles must always be done with extreme caution. Careless handling of used needles can result in an inadvertent needle-stick injury and dangerous exposure to potentially contaminated blood. Gloves should always be worn when an intravenous line is present and when handling sharp instruments.

different depending on which model is used. If an EMT frequently interacts with a particular ALS service, it would be useful to become familiar with the start-up features of the ALS service cardiac monitors. Generally, after the electrodes are attached properly to the patient, the electrode cables will be plugged into the cardiac monitor. Then the monitor should be turned on.

Different models have different features. Unless the EMT is familiar with the specific features of the monitor, the EMT should ask the ALS provider for further instruction. Application of the electrodes alone will serve to save time in acquisition of the twelve-lead ECG. Figure C-6 illustrates one type of cardiac monitor commonly used by prehospital providers.

INTRAVENOUS THERAPY

An IV line is a small plastic catheter that is threaded over a needle into a vein, often in the arm. Its purpose is twofold. Blood samples can be removed from the vein through the catheter, and fluids and medications may be administered into the vein via the same route.

While most EMTs are not permitted to perform IV cannulation, it is helpful for them to be familiar with the procedure so that they may safely assist an advanced provider.

The first rule for the handling of sharp instruments, such as needles, is for the person who is responsible for using the instrument to ensure

Preparing an IV

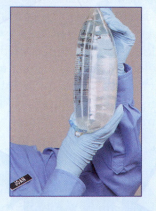

Arriving almost simultaneously with the call for an "unknown, man down in the mall, food court," EMT Sajan and Paramedic Pratt rode the escalator the last several yards to the food court.

Finding the scene was not hard. They simply looked for the crowd of people. In the center of the crowd on the floor was Dean Rome, a diabetic patient who was notorious for having "spells."

"Sajan, after you're done with your initial assessment, could you run a line out for me?" asked Pratt.

- Describe how to properly prepare an IV solution for IV infusion.
- What is the concern over keeping the ends of the tubing sterile?
- How can the EMT prevent bubbles from remaining in the IV tubing?

its safe disposal into a designated sharps container. Sometimes, at a scene or in an ambulance, this is not immediately possible. It should be done as soon as possible to avoid any potential injuries.

The dos and don'ts for handling of sharp instruments are shown in Figure C-7.

Patient Preparation

Although the EMT will not be establishing the IV line in most cases, preparing the patient for the procedure will decrease the time needed to complete the task by the advanced provider.

Most prehospital IV lines are initiated in the veins of the hands and arms. Therefore, it is necessary to remove any garments that have long sleeves that will hinder this process. Coats and sweaters should be removed if the climate allows. Sleeves can be rolled up, unless the clothing must be removed for some other purpose.

IV Solution Selection

Once an IV catheter has been placed, it must be attached to sterile fluid-filled tubing so that blood does not leak out and medications may be given, if needed. The EMT can prepare the fluid-filled tubing while the advanced provider is placing the catheter into the vein.

As there are different types of fluid and tubing used for this purpose, the EMT should ask the advanced provider which fluid and tubing to set up. The EMT should carefully select the appropriate fluid and tubing.

The most common type of fluid is called **normal saline** (NS) and is made up of salt water that is 0.9% sodium chloride (NaCl). This fluid has salt in nearly the same concentration as blood and is frequently used to replace lost fluids into the vein.

A second commonly used IV solution is called **lactated Ringers** (LR). This is a combination of several electrolytes that also approximates the concentration of blood. The two types of fluid, LR and NS, are used in the same situations.

Another common fluid used in the field is called **D5W** (5% dextrose in water). This fluid is merely sugar water and is used when sugar is needed or an inert fluid is needed with which to mix another medication. Figure C-8 shows solutions commonly used in an emergency setting.

The two types of IV tubing are designed to allow fluid administration at different rates. One type of tubing, called **macrodrip** tubing, allows large drops to come out of the bag of fluid, allowing very rapid administration of fluid if needed. Figure C-9 shows this tubing. The container for the tubing will most likely be labeled with a number. That number represents the number of drops that it takes coming out of this tubing to make 1 cc of the fluid. Macrodrip tubing has very few drops needed to make 1 cc, as the drops are very large. Ten or 15 drops/cc is typical of macrodrip tubing.

The other type of tubing that is commonly used is called **microdrip** tubing. This tubing creates very small drops, usually 60 drops in a cc. This tubing is used when only a small amount of fluid is expected to be needed. Figure C-10 shows microdrip tubing.

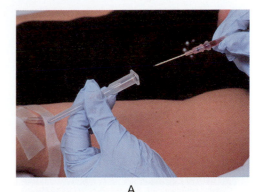

A.

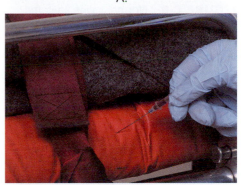

B.

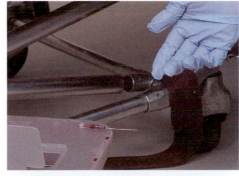

C.

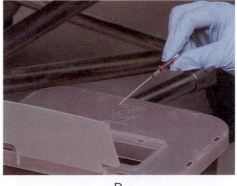

D.

FIGURE C-7 A. **Never** recap a used needle. B. **Never** stick a needle into a seat or mattress. C. **Never** throw a needle toward its disposal site. D. **Always** dispose of a sharp instrument in its approved container as soon as possible.

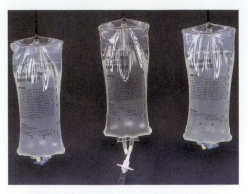

FIGURE C-8 Normal saline, lactated Ringers, and D5W are intravenous solutions that are commonly used in the emergency setting.

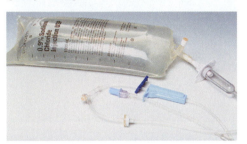

FIGURE C-9 Macrodrip tubing dispenses 10–15 large drops to equal 1 cc.

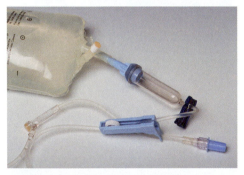

FIGURE C-10 Microdrip tubing dispenses 60 tiny drops to equal 1 cc.

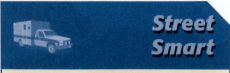

Street Smart

Some IV fluid is packaged inside a plastic wrapper. It may become humid inside that wrapper. Therefore, a small amount of condensation would be normal on the bag of fluid itself. No actively leaking liquid should be noted. If there is any doubt about the sterility of the fluid, it should be discarded.

Once the type of tubing and fluid is chosen, the EMT should remove the bag of fluid from its outer container and the tubing from its package. Just like when administering any medication, the EMT should check the fluid to be sure it is not expired. The expiration date is usually on the front of the bag.

Additionally, the fluid should be checked to be sure it is clear. NS, LR, and D5W are perfectly clear. If any discoloration is noted, the fluid should be discarded and another bag chosen.

Lastly, the bag should be checked for leaks. A leak in the bag may mean that the sterility of the fluid cannot be guaranteed. If a leak is suspected, the bag should be discarded and another chosen.

Assembly of Fluid and Tubing

When assembling the tubing and the bag of fluid, the EMT should take care to keep the ends of the tubing sterile. This means that nothing should contact those ends so that they can stay as clean as possible and decrease any chance for infection in the patient. A contaminated IV can cause serious infection in the patient. Assembly of an IV line is demonstrated in Skill C-1.

Securing an Intravenous Line

After the IV fluid is running into the catheter, the advanced provider will secure the catheter and the tubing so they do not become dislodged (Figure C-11 on page 1041). Generally tape or a commercially made occlusive dressing is applied over the IV site and the tubing to prevent accidental dislodgment.

Once attached to the patient's IV catheter, the bag of fluid must always remain above the level of the heart. This will prevent any backup of blood into the tubing. Generally, the higher the bag is held, the faster the IV fluid can be run, assuming the drip chamber is left wide open.

Maintaining an Intravenous Line

Once the IV fluid is running into the patient's vein, it is important to ensure that the IV line is continuing to function properly. The flow regulator should be set by the advanced provider to allow a specific rate of IV fluid administration. The IV site should frequently be assessed for any signs of infiltration. Infiltration is the seeping of material intended for IV delivery into the soft tissues surrounding the vessel. This can occur if the vein tears or if the IV catheter becomes dislodged.

Signs of infiltration include increasing pain or swelling at the IV site or difficulty infusing fluid. If the IV is believed to be infiltrated, the fluid should be shut down immediately. No further medication or fluid should be given into an infiltrated IV.

If an EMT is transferring a patient with an IV, he must repeatedly check the rate of the fluid dripping in the drip chamber. Any slowing of fluid may be due to a kink in the tubing, inadvertent closing of the flow regulator, or infiltration. Any speeding of the drip rate may be

SKILL C-1 *Intravenous Line Preparation*

PURPOSE: To assist the advanced EMT by preparing the IV solution for administration.

STANDARD PRECAUTIONS:

☑ Intravenous fluid
☑ Intravenous tubing

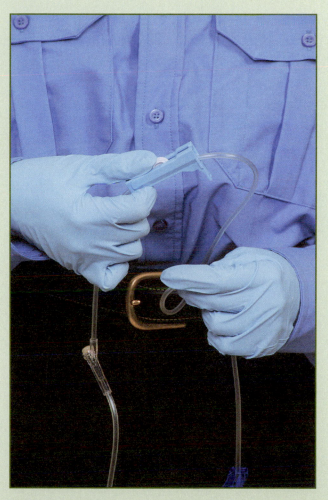

1 The EMT verifies that she has the right solution, that the solution is not expired, and that the solution is clear.

2 The EMT selects the correct IV tubing and removes it from the box. She moves the roller clamp proximal to the drip chamber and closes the roller clamp.

(continues)

SKILL C-1 *(continued)*

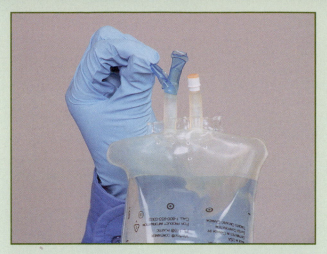

3 The EMT removes the tab from the solution, as well as removes the cap from the drip chamber end of tubing.

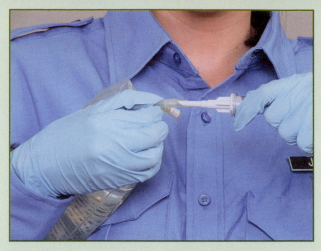

4 Without touching either sterile end, the EMT inserts the tubing spike into the appropriate port on the IV bag.

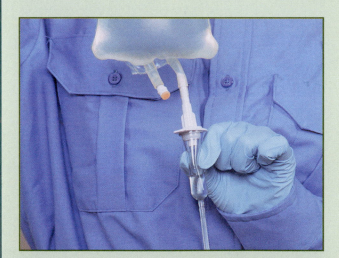

5 With the bag spiked, the EMT holds the solution upright and squeezes the drip chamber to allow it to fill halfway with solution.

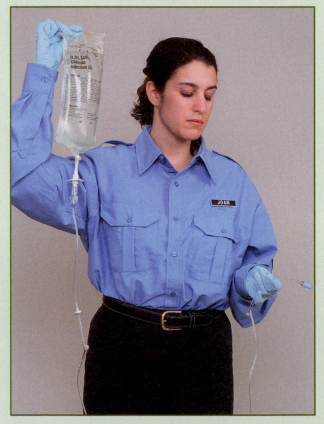

6 Holding the fluid up with the tubing down, the EMT opens the flow regulator to allow fluid to fill the tubing slowly. The EMT recaps the sterile end once the IV tubing is flushed.

due to a change in the position of the patient or inadvertent alteration in the flow regulator setting.

It is wise to check the IV site for signs of infiltration with each set of vital signs. Any changes should be reported immediately.

CONCLUSION

The EMT will have many occasions to work with more advanced prehospital health care providers. His familiarity with ALS skills and his ability to assist ALS providers in their tasks will contribute to effective teamwork. Such teamwork will result in quality patient care.

TEST YOUR KNOWLEDGE

1. Why is it important for there to be teamwork between basic and advanced emergency providers?
2. What is the importance of maintaining a patient's airway using basic techniques?
3. Describe how and when to apply cricoid pressure.
4. List several ways to confirm proper endotracheal tube placement.
5. Describe a method to secure an endotracheal tube.
6. Describe how to ventilate a patient via an endotracheal tube.
7. Describe how to perform endotracheal suctioning.
8. Describe how to apply different types of cardiac monitoring leads.
9. Describe how to properly prepare a bag of IV solution for administration.
10. What are the considerations in maintaining an IV line?

FURTHER STUDY

Dougherty, J. E. (1986, April). The basically advanced provider. *Emergency, 19*(4), 14, 16.

Haynes, B. E., & Pritting, J. (1999, October–December). A rural emergency medical technician with selected advanced skills. *Prehospital Emergency Care, 3*(4), 343–346.

Street Smart

It is potentially dangerous to allow a large amount of air to enter an IV line. The EMT should ensure all the air bubbles have run out of the tubing prior to handing it to the advanced provider who will hook it to the IV. This can be done by following the preceding steps carefully. If air bubbles are seen in the tubing, the EMT should simply allow them to run out. The IV fluid should be run into a garbage bag or a towel, not onto the floor. A puddle of IV solution on the floor could result in someone slipping and falling.

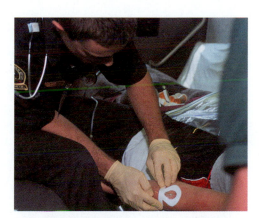

FIGURE C-11 Properly securing an intravenous line can help to prevent its inadvertent removal.

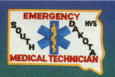

National Registry Practical Examination Sheets

Patient Assessment/Management - Medical

Start Time: _____

Stop Time: _____   Date: _____

Candidate's Name: _____

Evaluator's Name: _____

	Points Possible	Points Awarded
Takes, or verbalizes, body substance isolation precautions	1	
SCENE SIZE-UP		
Determines the scene is safe	1	
Determines the mechanism of injury/nature of illness	1	
Determines the number of patients	1	
Requests additional help if necessary	1	
Considers stabilization of spine	1	
INITIAL ASSESSMENT		
Verbalizes general impression of the patient	1	
Determines responsiveness/level of consciousness	1	
Determines chief complaint/apparent life threats	1	
Assesses airway and breathing — Assessment	1	
Assesses airway and breathing — Initiates appropriate oxygen therapy	1	
Assesses airway and breathing — Assures adequate ventilation	1	
Assesses circulation — Assesses/controls major bleeding	1	
Assesses circulation — Assesses pulse	1	
Assesses circulation — Assesses skin (color, temperature and condition)	1	
Identifies priority patients/makes transport decision	1	

FOCUSED HISTORY AND PHYSICAL EXAMINATION/RAPID ASSESSMENT

Signs and symptoms (Assess history of present illness)

Respiratory	Cardiac	Altered Mental Status	Allergic Reaction	Poisoning/Overdose	Environmental Emergency	Obstetrics	Behavioral
•Onset?	•Onset?	•Description of the episode.	•History of allergies?	•Substance?	•Source?	•Are you pregnant?	•How do you feel?
•Provokes?	•Provokes?	•Onset?	•What were you exposed to?	•When did you ingest/become exposed?	•Environment?	•How long have you been pregnant?	•Determine suicidal tendencies.
•Quality?	•Quality?	•Duration?	•How were you exposed?	•How much did you ingest?	•Duration?	•Pain or contractions?	•Is the patient a threat to self or others?
•Radiates?	•Radiates?	•Associated Symptoms?	•Effects?	•Over what time period?	•Loss of consciousness?	•Bleeding or discharge?	•Is there a medical problem?
•Severity?	•Severity?	•Evidence of Trauma?	•Progression?	•Interventions?	•Effects - general or local?	•Do you feel the need to push?	•Interventions?
•Time?	•Time?	•Interventions?	•Interventions?	•Estimated weight?		•Last menstrual period?	
•Interventions?	•Interventions?	•Seizures?					
		•Fever					

	Points Possible	Points Awarded
Signs and symptoms	1	
Allergies	1	
Medications	1	
Past pertinent history	1	
Last oral intake	1	
Event leading to present illness (rule out trauma)	1	
Performs focused physical examination (assesses affected body part/system or, if indicated, completes rapid assessment)	1	
Vitals (obtains baseline vital signs)	1	
Interventions (obtains medical direction or verbalizes standing order for medication interventions and verbalizes proper additional intervention/treatment)	1	
Transport (re-evaluates the transport decision)	1	
ONGOING ASSESSMENT (verbalized)		
Repeats initial assessment	1	
Repeats vital signs	1	
Repeats focused assessment regarding patient complaint or injuries	1	
	Total:	**30**

Critical Criteria

____ Did not take, or verbalize, body substance isolation precautions when necessary
____ Did not determine scene safety
____ Did not obtain medical direction or verbalize standing orders for medical interventions
____ Did not provide high concentration of oxygen
____ Did not find or manage problems associated with airway, breathing, hemorrhage or shock (hypoperfusion)
____ Did not differentiate patient's need for transportation versus continued assessment at the scene
____ Did detailed or focused history/physical examination before assessing the airway, breathing and circulation
____ Did not ask questions about the present illness
____ Administered a dangerous or inappropriate intervention

Patient Assessment/Management - Trauma

Start Time: _____

Stop Time: _____   Date: _____

Candidate's Name: _____

Evaluator's Name: _____

	Points Possible	Points Awarded
Takes, or verbalizes, body substance isolation precautions	1	
SCENE SIZE-UP		
Determines the scene is safe	1	
Determines the mechanism of injury	1	
Determines the number of patients	1	
Requests additional help if necessary	1	
Considers stabilization of spine	1	
INITIAL ASSESSMENT		
Verbalizes general impression of the patient	1	
Determines responsiveness/level of consciousness	1	
Determines chief complaint/apparent life threats	1	
Assesses airway and breathing — Assessment	1	
Assesses airway and breathing — Initiates appropriate oxygen therapy	1	
Assesses airway and breathing — Assures adequate ventilation	1	
Assesses airway and breathing — Injury management	1	
Assesses circulation — Assesses/controls major bleeding	1	
Assesses circulation — Assesses pulse	1	
Assesses circulation — Assesses skin (color, temperature and condition)	1	
Identifies priority patients/makes transport decision	1	
FOCUSED HISTORY AND PHYSICAL EXAMINATION/RAPID TRAUMA ASSESSMENT		
Selects appropriate assessment (focused or rapid assessment)	1	
Obtains, or directs assistance to obtain, baseline vital signs	1	
Obtains S.A.M.P.L.E. history	1	
DETAILED PHYSICAL EXAMINATION		
Assesses the head — Inspects and palpates the scalp and ears	1	
Assesses the head — Assesses the eyes	1	
Assesses the head — Assesses the facial areas including oral and nasal areas	1	
Assesses the neck — Inspects and palpates the neck	1	
Assesses the neck — Assesses for JVD	1	
Assesses the neck — Assesses for tracheal deviation	1	
Assesses the chest — Inspects	1	
Assesses the chest — Palpates	1	
Assesses the chest — Auscultates	1	
Assesses the abdomen/pelvis — Assesses the abdomen	1	
Assesses the abdomen/pelvis — Assesses the pelvis	1	
Assesses the abdomen/pelvis — Verbalizes assessment of genitalia/perineum as needed	1	
Assesses the extremities — 1 point for each extremity includes inspection, palpation, and assessment of motor, sensory and circulatory function	4	
Assesses the posterior — Assesses thorax	1	
Assesses the posterior — Assesses lumbar	1	
Manages secondary injuries and wounds appropriately 1 point for appropriate management of the secondary injury/wound	1	
Verbalizes re-assessment of the vital signs	1	
	Total:	**40**

Critical Criteria

____ Did not take, or verbalize, body substance isolation precautions
____ Did not determine scene safety
____ Did not assess for spinal protection
____ Did not provide for spinal protection when indicated
____ Did not provide high concentration of oxygen
____ Did not find, or manage, problems associated with airway, breathing, hemorrhage or shock (hypoperfusion)
____ Did not differentiate patient's need for transportation versus continued assessment at the scene
____ Did other detailed physical examination before assessing the airway, breathing and circulation
____ Did not transport patient within (10) minute time limit

(Reprinted with permission of the National Registry of Emergency Medical Technicians.)

BAG-VALVE-MASK
APNEIC PATIENT

Start Time: _____

Stop Time: _____ Date: _____

Candidate's Name: _____

Evaluator's Name: _____

	Points Possible	Points Awarded
Takes, or verbalizes, body substance isolation precautions	1	
Voices opening the airway	1	
Voices inserting an airway adjunct	1	
Selects appropriately sized mask	1	
Creates a proper mask-to-face seal	1	
Ventilates patient at no less than 800 ml volume *(The examiner must witness for at least 30 seconds)*	1	
Connects reservoir and oxygen	1	
Adjusts liter flow to 15 liters/minute or greater	1	
The examiner indicates arrival of a second EMT. The second EMT is instructed to ventilate the patient while the candidate controls the mask and the airway		
Voices re-opening the airway	1	
Creates a proper mask-to-face seal	1	
Instructs assistant to resume ventilation at proper volume per breath *(The examiner must witness for at least 30 seconds)*	1	
Total:	**11**	

Critical Criteria

_____ Did not take, or verbalize, body substance isolation precautions

_____ Did not immediately ventilate the patient

_____ Interrupted ventilations for more than 20 seconds

_____ Did not provide high concentration of oxygen

_____ Did not provide, or direct assistant to provide, proper volume/breath *(more than two (2) ventilations per minute are below 800 ml)*

_____ Did not allow adequate exhalation

Cardiac Arrest Management/AED

Start Time: _____

Stop Time: _____ Date: _____

Candidate's Name: _____

Evaluator's Name: _____

	Points Possible	Points Awarded
ASSESSMENT		
Takes, or verbalizes, body substance isolation precautions	1	
Briefly questions the rescuer about arrest events	1	
Directs rescuer to stop CPR	1	
Verifies absence of spontaneous pulse **(skill station examiner states "no pulse")**	1	
Directs resumption of CPR	1	
Turns on defibrillator power	1	
Attaches automated defibrillator to the patient	1	
Directs rescuer to stop CPR and ensures all individuals are clear of the patient	1	
Initiates analysis of the rhythm	1	
Delivers shock (up to three successive shocks)	1	
Verifies absence of spontaneous pulse **(skill station examiner states "no pulse")**	1	
TRANSITION		
Directs resumption of CPR	1	
Gathers additional information about arrest event	1	
Confirms effectiveness of CPR **(ventilation and compressions)**	1	
INTEGRATION		
Verbalizes or directs insertion of a simple airway adjunct **(oral/nasal airway)**	1	
Ventilates, or directs ventilation of, the patient	1	
Assures high concentration of oxygen is delivered to the patient	1	
Assures CPR continues without unnecessary/prolonged interruption	1	
Re-evaluates patient/CPR in approximately one minute	1	
Repeats defibrillator sequence		
TRANSPORTATION		
Verbalizes transportation of patient	1	
Total:	**21**	

Critical Criteria

_____ Did not take, or verbalize, body substance isolation precautions

_____ Did not evaluate the need for immediate use of the AED

_____ Did not direct initiation/resumption of ventilation/compressions at appropriate times.

_____ Did not assure all individuals were clear of patient before delivering each shock

_____ Did not operate the AED properly (inability to deliver shock)

_____ Prevented the defibrillator from delivering indicated stacked shocks

(Reprinted with permission of the National Registry of Emergency Medical Technicians.)

SPINAL IMMOBILZATION
SUPINE PATIENT

Start Time: _____
Stop Time: _____ Date: _____
Candidate's Name: _____
Evaluator's Name: _____

	Points Possible	Points Awarded
Takes, or verbalizes, body substance isolation precautions	1	
Directs assistant to place/maintain head in the neutral in-line position	1	
Directs assistant to maintain manual immobilization of the head	1	
Reassesses motor, sensory and circulatory function in each extremity	1	
Applies appropriately sized extrication collar	1	
Positions the immobilization device appropriately	1	
Directs movement of the patient onto the device without compromising the integrity of the spine	1	
Applies padding to voids between the torso and the board as necessary	1	
Immobilizes the patient's torso to the device	1	
Evaluates and pads behind the patient's head as necessary	1	
Immobilizes the patient's head to the device	1	
Secures the patient's legs to the device	1	
Secures the patient's arms to the device	1	
Reassesses motor, sensory and circulatory function in each extremity	1	
Total:	**14**	

Critical Criteria

___ Did not immediately direct, or take, manual immobilization of the head

___ Released, or ordered release of, manual immobilization before it was maintained mechanicall

___ Patient manipulated, or moved excessively, causing potential spinal compromise

___ Patient moves excessively up, down, left or right on the patient's torso

___ Head immobilization allows for excessive movement

___ Upon completion of immobilization, head is not in the neutral position

___ Did not assess motor, sensory and circulatory function in each extremity after immobilization to the device

___ Immobilized head to the board before securing the torso

SPINAL IMMOBILZATION
SEATED PATIENT

Start Time: _____
Stop Time: _____ Date: _____
Candidate's Name: _____
Evaluator's Name: _____

	Points Possible	Points Awarded
Takes, or verbalizes, body substance isolation precautions	1	
Directs assistant to place/maintain head in the neutral in-line position	1	
Directs assistant to maintain manual immobilization of the head	1	
Reassesses motor, sensory and circulatory function in each extremity	1	
Applies appropriately sized extrication collar	1	
Positions the immobilization device behind the patient	1	
Secures the device to the patient's torso	1	
Evaluates torso fixation and adjusts as necessary	1	
Evaluates and pads behind the patient's head as necessary	1	
Secures the patient's head to the device	1	
Verbalizes moving the patient to a long board	1	
Reassesses motor, sensory and circulatory function in each extremity	1	
Total:	**12**	

Critical Criteria

___ Did not immediately direct, or take, manual immobilization of the head

___ Released, or ordered release of, manual immobilization before it was maintained mechanicall

___ Patient manipulated, or moved excessively, causing potential spinal compromise

___ Device moved excessively up, down, left or right on the patient's torso

___ Head immobilization allows for excessive movement

___ Torso fixation inhibits chest rise, resulting in respiratory compromise

___ Upon completion of immobilization, head is not in the neutral position

___ Did not assess motor, sensory and circulatory function in each extremity after voicing immobilization to the long board

___ Immobilized head to the board before securing the torso

(Reprinted with permission of the National Registry of Emergency Medical Technicians.)

IMMOBILIZATION SKILLS
LONG BONE INJURY

Start Time: _____ Date: _____

Stop Time: _____

Candidate's Name: _____

Evaluator's Name: _____

	Points Possible	Points Awarded
Takes, or verbalizes, body substance isolation precautions	1	
Directs application of manual stabilization of the injury	1	
Assesses motor, sensory and circulatory function in the injured extremity	1	
Note: The examiner acknowledges "motor, sensory and circulatory function are present and normal"		
Measures the splint	1	
Applies the splint	1	
Immobilizes the joint above the injury site	1	
Immobilizes the joint below the injury site	1	
Secures the entire injured extremity	1	
Immobilizes the hand/foot in the position of function	1	
Reassesses motor, sensory and circulatory function in the injured extremity	1	
Note: The examiner acknowledges "motor, sensory and circulatory function are present and normal"		
Total:	**10**	

Critical Criteria

_____ Grossly moves the injured extremity

_____ Did not immobilize the joint above and the joint below the injury site

_____ Did not reassess motor, sensory and circulatory function in the injured extremity before and after splinting

---

IMMOBILIZATION SKILLS
TRACTION SPLINTING

Start Time: _____ Date: _____

Stop Time: _____

Candidate's Name: _____

Evaluator's Name: _____

	Points Possible	Points Awarded
Takes, or verbalizes, body substance isolation precautions	1	
Directs application of manual stabilization of the injured leg	1	
Directs the application of manual traction	1	
Assesses motor, sensory and circulatory function in the injured extremity	1	
Note: The examiner acknowledges "motor, sensory and circulatory function are present and normal"		
Prepares/adjusts splint to the proper length	1	
Positions the splint next to the injured leg	1	
Applies the proximal securing device (e.g... ischial strap)	1	
Applies the distal securing device (e.g...ankle hitch)	1	
Applies mechanical traction	1	
Positions/secures the support straps	1	
Re-evaluates the proximal/distal securing devices	1	
Reassesses motor, sensory and circulatory function in the injured extremity	1	
Note: The examiner acknowledges "motor, sensory and circulatory function are present and normal"		
Note: The examiner must ask the candidate how he/she would prepare the patient for transportation		
Verbalizes securing the torso to the long board to immobilize the hip	1	
Verbalizes securing the splint to the long board to prevent movement of the splint	1	
Total:	**14**	

Critical Criteria

_____ Loss of traction at any point after it was applied

_____ Did not reassess motor, sensory and circulatory function in the injured extremity before and after splinting

_____ The foot was excessively rotated or extended after splint was applied

_____ Did not secure the ischial strap before taking traction

_____ Final Immobilization failed to support the femur or prevent rotation of the injured leg

_____ Secured the leg to the splint before applying mechanical traction

Note: If the Sager splint or the Kendricks Traction Device is used without elevating the patient's leg, application of manual traction is not necessary. The candidate should be awarded one (1) point as if manual traction were applied.

Note: If the leg is elevated at all, manual traction must be applied before elevating the leg. The ankle hitch may be applied before elevating the leg and used to provide manual traction.

(Reprinted with permission of the National Registry of Emergency Medical Technicians.)

BLEEDING CONTROL/SHOCK MANAGEMENT

Start Time: _____ Date: _____

Stop Time: _____

Candidate's Name: _____

Evaluator's Name: _____

	Points Possible	Points Awarded
Takes, or verbalizes, body substance isolation precautions	1	
Applies direct pressure to the wound	1	
Elevates the extremity	1	
Note: The examiner must now inform the candidate that the wound continues to bleed.		
Applies an additional dressing to the wound	1	
Note: The examiner must now inform the candidate that the wound still continues to bleed. The second dressing does not control the bleeding.		
Locates and applies pressure to appropriate arterial pressure point	1	
Note: The examiner must now inform the candidate that the bleeding is controlled		
Bandages the wound	1	
Note: The examiner must now inform the candidate the patient is now showing signs and symptoms indicative of hypoperfusion		
Properly positions the patient	1	
Applies high concentration oxygen	1	
Initiates steps to prevent heat loss from the patient	1	
Indicates the need for immediate transportation	1	
Total:	**10**	

Critical Criteria

____ Did not take, or verbalize, body substance isolation precautions

____ Did not apply high concentration of oxygen

____ Applied a tourniquet before attempting other methods of bleeding control

____ Did not control hemorrhage in a timely manner

____ Did not indicate a need for immediate transportation

IMMOBILIZATION SKILLS
JOINT INJURY

Start Time: _____ Date: _____

Stop Time: _____

Candidate's Name: _____

Evaluator's Name: _____

	Points Possible	Points Awarded
Takes, or verbalizes, body substance isolation precautions	1	
Directs application of manual stabilization of the shoulder injury	1	
Assesses motor, sensory and circulatory function in the injured extremity	1	
Note: The examiner acknowledges "motor, sensory and circulatory function are present and normal."		
Selects the proper splinting material	1	
Immobilizes the site of the injury	1	
Immobilizes the bone above the injured joint	1	
Immobilizes the bone below the injured joint	1	
Reassesses motor, sensory and circulatory function in the injured extremity	1	
Note: The examiner acknowledges "motor, sensory and circulatory function are present and normal."		
Total:	**8**	

Critical Criteria

____ Did not support the joint so that the joint did not bear distal weight

____ Did not immobilize the bone above and below the injured site

____ Did not reassess motor, sensory and circulatory function in the injured extremity before and after splinting

(Reprinted with permission of the National Registry of Emergency Medical Technicians.)

MOUTH TO MASK WITH SUPPLEMENTAL OXYGEN

Start Time: _____
Stop Time: _____   Date: _____
Candidate's Name: _____
Evaluator's Name: _____

	Points Possible	Points Awarded
Takes, or verbalizes, body substance isolation precautions	1	
Connects one-way valve to mask	1	
Opens patient's airway or confirms patient's airway is open (manually or with adjunct)	1	
Establishes and maintains a proper mask to face seal	1	
Ventilates the patient at the proper volume and rate (800-1200 ml per breath/10-20 breaths per minute)	1	
Connects the mask to high concentration of oxygen	1	
Adjusts flow rate to at least 15 liters per minute	1	
Continues ventilation of the patient at the proper volume and rate (800-1200 ml per breath/10-20 breaths per minute)	1	
Note: The examiner must witness ventilations for at least 30 seconds		
Total:	**8**	

Critical Criteria

_____ Did not take, or verbalize, body substance isolation precautions

_____ Did not adjust liter flow to at least 15 liters per minute

_____ Did not provide proper volume per breath (*more than 2 ventilations per minute were below 800 ml*)

_____ Did not ventilate the patient at a rate a 10-20 breaths per minute

_____ Did not allow for complete exhalation

AIRWAY, OXYGEN AND VENTILATION SKILLS UPPER AIRWAY ADJUNCTS AND SUCTION

Start Time: _____
Stop Time: _____   Date: _____
Candidate's Name: _____
Evaluator's Name: _____

OROPHARYNGEAL AIRWAY

	Points Possible	Points Awarded
Takes, or verbalizes, body substance isolation precautions	1	
Selects appropriately sized airway	1	
Measures airway	1	
Inserts airway without pushing the tongue posteriorly	1	
Note: The examiner must advise the candidate that the patient is gagging and becoming conscious		
Removes the oropharyngeal airway	1	

SUCTION

	Points Possible	Points Awarded
Note: The examiner must advise the candidate to suction the patient's airway		
Turns on/prepares suction device	1	
Assures presence of mechanical suction	1	
Inserts the suction tip without suction	1	
Applies suction to the oropharynx/nasopharynx	1	

NASOPHARYNGEAL AIRWAY

	Points Possible	Points Awarded
Note: The examiner must advise the candidate to insert a nasopharyngeal airway		
Selects appropriately sized airway	1	
Measures airway	1	
Verbalizes lubrication of the nasal airway	1	
Fully inserts the airway with the bevel facing toward the septum	1	
Total:	**13**	

Critical Criteria

_____ Did not take, or verbalize, body substance isolation precautions

_____ Did not obtain a patent airway with the oropharyngeal airway

_____ Did not obtain a patent airway with the nasopharyngeal airway

_____ Did not demonstrate an acceptable suction technique

_____ Inserted any adjunct in a manner dangerous to the patient

(Reprinted with permission of the National Registry of Emergency Medical Technicians.)

VENTILATORY MANAGEMENT
ENDOTRACHEAL INTUBATION

Start Time: _____
Stop Time: _____   Date: _____
Candidate's Name: _____
Evaluator's Name: _____

*Note: If a candidate elects to initially ventilate the patient with a BVM attached to a reservoir and oxygen, full credit must be awarded for steps denoted by "***" provided the first ventilation is delivered within the initial 30 seconds*

	Points Possible	Points Awarded
Takes of verbalizes body substance isolation precautions	1	
Opens the airway manually	1	
Elevates the patient's tongue and inserts a simple airway adjunct (oropharyngeal/nasopharyngeal airway)	1	
Note: The examiner must now inform the candidate "no gag reflex is present and the patient accepts the airway adjunct."		
** Ventilates the patient immediately using a BVM device unattached to oxygen	1	
** Hyperventilates the patient with room air	1	
Note: The examiner must now inform the candidate that ventilation is being properly performed without difficulty		
Attaches the oxygen reservoir to the BVM	1	
Attaches the BVM to high flow oxygen (15 liter per minute)	1	
Ventilates the patient at the proper volume and rate (800-1200 ml/breath and 10-20 breaths/minute)	1	
Note: After 30 seconds, the examiner must auscultate the patient's chest and inform the candidate that breath sounds are present and equal bilaterally and medical direction has ordered endotracheal intubation. The examiner must now take over ventilation of the patient.		
Directs assistant to hyper-oxygenate the patient	1	
Identifies/selects the proper equipment for endotracheal intubation	1	
Checks equipment — Checks for cuff leaks	1	
— Checks laryngoscope operation and bulb tightness	1	
Note: The examiner must remove the OPA and move out of the way when the candidate is prepared to intubate the patient.		
Positions the patient's head properly	1	
Inserts the laryngoscope blade into the patient's mouth while displacing the patient's tongue laterally	1	
Elevates the patient's mandible with the laryngoscope	1	
Introduces the endotracheal tube and advances the tube to the proper depth	1	
Inflates the cuff to the proper pressure	1	
Disconnects the syringe from the cuff inlet port	1	
Directs assistant to ventilate the patient	1	
Confirms proper placement of the endotracheal tube by auscultation bilaterally and over the epigastrium	1	
Note: The examiner must ask, "If you had proper placement, what would you expect to hear?"		
Secures the endotracheal tube (may be verbalized)	1	
Total:	**21**	

Critical Criteria
___ Did not take or verbalize body substance isolation precautions when necessary
___ Did not initiate ventilation within 30 seconds after applying gloves or interrupts ventilations for greater than 30 seconds at any time
___ Did not voice or provide high oxygen concentrations (15 liter/minute or greater)
___ Did not ventilate the patient at a rate of at least 10 breaths per minute
___ Did not provide adequate volume per breath (maximum of 2 errors per minute permissible)
___ Did not hyper-oxygenate the patient prior to intubation
___ Did not successfully intubate the patient within 3 attempts
___ Used the patient's teeth as a fulcrum
___ Did not assure proper tube placement by auscultation bilaterally over each lung **and** over the epigastrium
___ The stylette (if used) extended beyond the end of the endotracheal tube
___ Inserted any adjunct in a manner that was dangerous to the patient
___ Did not immediately disconnect the syringe from the inlet port after inflating the cuff

---

OXYGEN ADMINISTRATION

Start Time: _____
Stop Time: _____   Date: _____
Candidate's Name: _____
Evaluator's Name: _____

	Points Possible	Points Awarded
Takes, or verbalizes, body substance isolation precautions	1	
Assembles the regulator to the tank	1	
Opens the tank	1	
Checks for leaks	1	
Checks tank pressure	1	
Attaches non-rebreather mask to oxygen	1	
Prefills reservoir	1	
Adjusts liter flow to 12 liters per minute or greater	1	
Applies and adjusts the mask to the patient's face	1	
Note: The examiner must advise the candidate that the patient is not tolerating the non-rebreather mask. The medical director has ordered you to apply a nasal cannula to the patient.		
Attaches nasal cannula to oxygen	1	
Adjusts liter flow to six (6) liters per minute or less	1	
Applies nasal cannula to the patient	1	
Note: The examiner must advise the candidate to discontinue oxygen therapy		
Removes the nasal cannula from the patient	1	
Shuts off the regulator	1	
Relieves the pressure within the regulator	1	
Total:	**15**	

Critical Criteria
___ Did not take, or verbalize, body substance isolation precautions
___ Did not assemble the tank and regulator without leaks
___ Did not prefill the reservoir bag
___ Did not adjust the device to the correct liter flow for the non-rebreather mask (12 liters per minute or greater)
___ Did not adjust the device to the correct liter flow for the nasal cannula (6 liters per minute or less)

(Reprinted with permission of the National Registry of Emergency Medical Technicians.)

VENTILATORY MANAGEMENT
ESOPHAGEAL OBTURATOR AIRWAY INSERTION FOLLOWING
AN UNSUCCESSFUL ENDOTRACHEAL INTUBATION ATTEMPT

Start Time: _____
Stop Time: _____   Date: _____
Candidate's Name: _____
Evaluator's Name: _____

	Points Possible	Points Awarded
Continues body substance isolation precautions	1	
Confirms the patient is being ventilated high percentage oxygen	1	
Directs the assistant to hyper-oxygenate the patient	1	
Identifies/selects the proper equipment for insertion of EOA	1	
Assembles the EOA	1	
Tests the cuff for leaks	1	
Inflates the mask	1	
Lubricates the tube *(may be verbalized)*	1	
Note: The examiner should remove the OPA and move out of the way when the candidate is prepared to insert the device		
Positions the head properly with the neck in the neutral or slightly flexed position	1	
Grasps and elevates the patient's tongue and mandible	1	
Inserts the tube in the same direction as the curvature of the pharynx	1	
Advances the tube until the mask is sealed against the patient's face	1	
Ventilates the patient while maintaining a tight mask-to-face seal	1	
Directs confirmation of placement of EOA by observing for chest rise and auscultation over the epigastrium and bilaterally over each lung	1	
Note: The examiner must acknowledge adequate chest rise, bilateral breath sounds and absent sounds over the epigastrium		
Inflates the cuff to the proper pressure	1	
Disconnects the syringe from the inlet port	1	
Continues ventilation of the patient	1	
	Total: 17	

Critical Criteria
_____ Did not take or verbalize body substance isolation precautions
_____ Did not initiate ventilations within 30 seconds
_____ Interrupted ventilations for more than 30 seconds at any time
_____ Did not direct hyper-oxygenation of the patient prior to placement of the EOA
_____ Did not successfully place the EOA within 3 attempts
_____ Did not ventilate at a rate of at least 10 breaths per minute
_____ Did not provide adequate volume per breath (maximum 2 errors/minute permissible)
_____ Did not assure proper tube placement by auscultation bilaterally and over the epigastrium
_____ Did not remove the syringe after inflating the cuff
_____ Did not provide high flow oxygen (15 liters per minute or greater)
_____ Did not successfully ventilate the patient
_____ Inserted any adjunct in a manner that was dangerous to the patient

---

VENTILATORY MANAGEMENT
DUAL LUMEN DEVICE INSERTION FOLLOWING
AN UNSUCCESSFUL ENDOTRACHEAL INTUBATION ATTEMPT

Start Time: _____
Stop Time: _____
Candidate's Name: _____   Date: _____
Evaluator's Name: _____

	Points Possible	Points Awarded
Continues body substance isolation precautions	1	
Confirms the patient is being properly ventilated with high percentage oxygen	1	
Directs the assistant to hyper-oxygenate the patient	1	
Checks/prepares the airway device	1	
Lubricates the distal tip of the device *(may be verbalized)*	1	
Note: The examiner should remove the OPA and move out of the way when the candidate is prepared to insert the device		
Positions the patient's head properly	1	
Performs a tongue-jaw lift	1	
☐ **USES COMBITUBE**		☐ **USES THE PTL**
Inserts device in the mid-line and to the depth so that the printed ring is at the level of the teeth	Inserts the device in the mid-line until the bite block flange is at the level of the teeth	1	
Inflates the pharyngeal cuff with the proper volume and removes the syringe	Secures the strap	1	
Inflates the distal cuff with the proper volume and removes the syringe	Blows into tube #1 to adequately inflate both cuffs	1	
Attaches/directs attachment of BVM to the first (esophageal placement)lumen and ventilates	1	
Confirms placement and ventilation through the correct lumen by observing chest rise, auscultation over the epigastrium and bilaterally over each lung	1	
Note: The examiner states, "You do not see rise and fall of the chest and hear sounds only over the epigastrium."		
Attaches/directs attachment of BVM to the second (endotracheal placement) lumen and ventilates	1	
Confirms placement and ventilation through the correct lumen by observing chest rise, auscultation over the epigastrium and bilaterally over each lung	1	
Note: The examiner states, "You see rise and fall of the chest, there are no sounds over the epigastrium and breath sounds are equal over each lung."		
Secures device or confirms that the device remains properly secured	1	
	Total: 15	

Critical Criteria
_____ Did not take or verbalize body substance isolation precautions
_____ Did not initiate ventilations within 30 seconds
_____ Interrupted ventilations for more than 30 seconds at any time
_____ Did not hyper-oxygenate the patient prior to placement of the dual lumen airway device
_____ Did not provide adequate volume per breath (maximum 2 errors/minute permissible)
_____ Did not ventilate the patient at a rate of at least 10 breaths per minute
_____ Did not insert the dual lumen airway device at a proper depth or at the proper place within 3 attempts
_____ Did not inflate both cuffs properly
_____ **Combitube** – Did not remove the syringe immediately following the inflation of each cuff
_____ **PTL** – Did not secure the strap prior to cuff inflation
_____ Did not confirm, by observing chest rise and auscultation over the epigastrium and bilaterally over each lung, that the proper lumen of the device was being used to ventilate the patient
_____ Inserted any adjunct in a manner that was dangerous to the patient

(Reprinted with permission of the National Registry of Emergency Medical Technicians.)

GLOSSARY

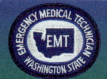

A

abandonment A situation in which a care provider assumes responsibility for an incapacitated person and then leaves the patient unsupervised.

ABCs The techniques involved in assessing airway, breathing, and circulation.

abdominal aortic aneurysm (AAA) A weakened area of the aortic wall resulting in a ballooning out of the vessel within the abdomen.

abdominal cavity The space between the chest and the pelvis which contains the organs of digestion and elimination.

abdominal thrusts Forceful application of pressure to the upper abdomen, toward the chest, in an attempt to expel a foreign body from the airway.

abduction Movement away from the body.

abortion The premature termination of a pregnancy.

abrasion A superficial scrape to the skin.

accessory muscles of respiration Neck, chest, and abdominal muscles that can be used to assist in respiration in times of distress.

acetabulum The socket in the pelvis where the proximal femur meets the pelvis.

acquired immunodeficiency syndrome (AIDS) A group of symptoms, or syndrome, that results from the HIV infection.

acrocyanosis Cyanosis of the extremities.

acromioclavicular (A/C) dislocation A separation of the shoulder and clavicle.

action The effect of a medication on the person who takes it.

activated charcoal A suspension of charcoal in a liquid that has the ability to bind most ingested toxins and prevent their absorption.

active rewarming Actions taken to actively try to increase body temperature.

activities of daily living (ADLs) Those normal functions that people perform, for example, eating, toileting and dressing.

acute coronary syndrome (ACS) Continuum of conditions affecting blood flow to the heart including angina and acute myocardial infarction.

acute mountain sickness (AMS) An illness that is seen at altitude in unacclimated individuals.

acute myocardial infarction (AMI) The death of heart muscle due to an inadequate supply of oxygen-rich blood (hypoperfusion).

acute stress A single event that creates a stress response.

addiction The physical need the body has for a drug.

adduction Movement toward the body.

advance directive A method to make a patient's wishes about resuscitation known to family and health care providers before the patient becomes incapacitated.

advanced cardiac life support (ACLS) Complex procedures used to treat sudden cardiac death or acute coronary syndrome; typically performed by an ALS provider, i.e. an advanced EMT.

advanced EMT (AEMT) An EMT who has had additional training and who can perform more complex or invasive actions such as endotracheal intubation or intravenous access.

advanced life support (ALS) A broad term applied to emergency medical care rendered beyond basic life support, the hallmark of which is usually special tools and procedures.

advanced lividity Pooling of blood in the dependent portions of the body with a clear line of demarcation.

AEIOU TIPS A mnemonic used to remember the causes of altered mental status: alcohol, epilepsy, insulin, oxygen/over-dose, uremia, trauma, infection, psychiatric, and stroke.

affidavit Written testimony by a person.

afterdrop A drop in core body temperature as a result of peripheral vasodilation and shunting of cool blood to the body center during active rewarming of the severely hypothermic patient.

against medical advice (AMA) A patient's refusal of medical care despite a great risk of loss of limb or life.

age of majority The age at which a person may act without parental permission and is generally treated as an adult.

air embolism Air that has gotten into a blood vessel, resulting in a blockage of blood flow.

air hunger The feeling a person may have if his oxygen level is low or he is unable to effectively breathe; indicated by mouth breathing.

airway The passageway for air movement into and out of the lungs.

airway, breathing, circulation, defibrillation (ABCD) The "primary" survey; a systemic approach to life-threatening illness or injury.

alert Term used to describe the mental status of a patient who is awake and interacting with his environment.

all clear An order that means that nothing, not even the bag-valve-mask, should touch the patient.

allergen A substance that causes an exaggerated response of the immune system (allergic reaction).

allergic reaction An exaggerated response of the immune system upon exposure to a particular substance.

altered mental state A change in behavior due to illness or disease.

alveolar-capillary gas exchange The movement of gases between alveoli and adjacent capillaries.

alveoli Tiny air sacs in the lungs that allow exchange of carbon dioxide and oxygen.

Alzheimer's disease A progressive, irreversible deterioration of intellectual function.

Ambulance Accident Prevention Seminar (AAPS) A short course that reviews causes and prevention of ambulance accidents.

ambulances volante Literally meaning "flying ambulances"; these vehicles, considered to be the first ambulances, were used by Baron Larrey in the Napoleonic War era to retrieve injured soldiers.

American Academy of Emergency Physicians (ACEP) An association of physicians, specializing in emergency medicine, that was formed in 1968.

American Ambulance Association (AAA) A national group that represents ambulance service owners who provide service to 75% of the American population.

American Heart Association (AHA) A national group of citizens, physicians and allied health care professionals dedicated to reducing death and disability from cardiovascular disease.

American Red Cross (ARC) A relief organization founded by Clara Barton in the Civil War era; has played a large role in training civilians and rescuers in first aid and CPR.

American Society of Anesthesiologists (ASA) A national association of Anesthesiologists dedicated to advancing the safe practice of anesthesia.

ammonia (NH_3) A common chemical that can cause serious burns.

amniotic sac The membranous sac that surrounds the fetus and placenta within the uterus.

amplitude modulation (AM) An early method of radio signal transmission.

amputation The cutting off of an extremity.

anaphylactic shock A hypoperfused state resulting from a severe allergic reaction.

anaphylaxis An exaggerated allergic reaction that can result in life-threatening airway, breathing, or circulatory compromise.

anatomy The study of the structure of an organism.

angina Pain or discomfort that is a result of insufficient oxygenated blood flow to the heart muscle.

angle of Louis The bony ridge where the manubrium meets the body of the sternum; also called the sternal angle.

anisocoria Unequal pupils.

antecubital fossa The anterior surface of the elbow, in the bend of the arm.

anterior A directional term referring to a location toward the front.

antibody Specialized defense particle within the blood that helps to protect against foreign material.

anticonvulsant Any drug intended to control or prevent seizures.

antilock braking system (ABS) A device in a vehicle that prevents the brakes from "locking up" during sudden emergency braking, preventing a skid in the process.

anus The end of the digestive tract; it allows for exit of solid wastes.

anxiety disorder An inappropriate or exaggerated response that is abnormal in relation to the situation; formerly called neurosis.

aorta The largest artery in the body; it carries the blood from the left ventricle of the heart out to the rest of the body.

aortic valve The last valve in the heart that regulates blood flow from the heart into the aorta and the systemic circulation.

apex The point of a triangle; a directional term used to describe the top of the lungs or the bottom tip of the heart.

Apgar A predictive score for measuring the health of newborns.

apnea Lack of breathing; breathlessness.

appendicitis The inflammation/infection of the appendix often characterized by the presence of right lower quadrant pain.

appendicular skeleton The bony extremities composed of the shoulder girdle, arms, pelvic girdle, and legs.

appendix A small saclike portion of the large intestine that may become inflamed in a condition called appendicitis.

approach path An obstacle-free area adjacent to the touch-down area through which the helicopter can approach and depart.

arachnoid The weblike middle protective membrane covering the brain and spinal cord.

arm drag A patient movement technique in which the EMT grasps the wrists of the patient, pulls the arms to the patient's chest, and drags the patient by the arms.

arteries Vessels that carry blood away from the heart; with the exception of the pulmonary artery, they carry oxygenated blood.

arthritis A decrease in the flexibility of joints along with an inflammation within those joints.

artificial pacemaker A man-made electronic device that will create the electrical impulse signaling the heart to beat.

artificial ventilation A method of providing oxygen to a patient who is not effectively breathing; also known as rescue breathing.

aspiration A term meaning "to draw into"; refers to foreign material inadvertently being drawn into the airway during inspiration.

aspirin-induced asthma (AIA) A sensitivity to aspirin that some patients exhibit that can progress to an asthma attack.

assault In civil law, refers to placing a person in fear of being touched through an attempt at treatment without the person's having given consent to do so.

Association for Professionals in Infection Control and Epidemiology (APIC) A multidisciplinary group of healthcare professionals who support and improve healthcare through infection control management.

asthma A condition consisting of bronchospasm and inflammation in response to multiple stimuli; also known as reactive airway disease.

asystole The flatline ECG of the heart in cardiac standstill.

atherosclerosis The process of fatty buildup on the walls of blood vessels.

atlas The first cervical vertebra.

atrioventricular (AV) node Node of specialized cardiac conduction fibers that slow the electrical impulse as it moves from the atria to the ventricles to allow for the mechanical contraction of the heart to catch up to its electrical activity; primarily influenced by the Vagus nerve of the parasympathetic nervous system.

atrium A small receiving chamber, one on each side of the heart, that empties blood into its corresponding ventricles to be pumped out of the heart; plural: atria.

auditory hallucination A false perception of the sensation of the ears; hearing something that is not actually there.

aura The sensation or awareness that a seizure is about to begin.

auscultate Term that means to listen.

automated external defibrillator (AED) A defibrillator that can "read" the ECG, using a logic algorithm stored in a microprocessor, advise the EMT to "shock," or defibrillate, then deliver that shock to the patient.

automatic implantable cardioverter/defibrillator (AICD) A defibrillator that can be placed within the body.

automaticity The ability of the myocardium to self-pace.

autonomic nervous system A collection of nerves that originate in the brainstem and transmit impulses to many organs in the body to allow for many basic body functions.

AVPU Abbreviation to remember the classifications of mental status: alert, voice, pain, and unresponsive.

avulsion The forceful separation of an extremity.

awareness level The ability of EMTs to recognize a hazard, know how to protect themselves, and know how to activate the emergency preplan for such an event.

axial skeleton Bony skeleton that forms the axis of the support structure of the body; includes the skull, spinal column, and thoracic cage.

axilla The armpit.

axis The second cervical vertebra around which the atlas sits and may rotate.

B

back blows Firm blows administered to an infant's upper back in an attempt to expel a foreign body from the airway.

bag-valve-mask (BVM) A device consisting of a refilling bag, a one-way valve, and a mask that is used to ventilate a patient.

bandage A strip of cloth that is applied to a wound.

base A directional term used to describe the bottom of an object, such as a triangle.

base station The main radio transmitter used in a system, frequently located at the base of operations.

baseline vital signs The first set of vital signs obtained, used to compare the following sets.

basic life support (BLS) A broad term applied to those skills that can be performed by either a citizen or an EMT with a minimum of specialized equipment.

basilar skull fracture A break at the base of the skull (the area behind the face).

basket stretcher A type of stretcher, such as the Stokes basket, that will allow complete immobilization of the patient and protection during a move over rough terrain.

battery In civil law, refers to touching a person without his or her consent.

Battle's sign Bruising behind the ears on the mastoid process; indicates a fracture of the skull.

beats per minute (bpm) A measurement of the rate of the heart.

bedroll The linen on the stretcher to cover the patient.

behavioral emergency Any situation in which a patient exhibits a behavior that is unacceptable or intolerable to one's self, family, or the community.

biceps muscle The muscle that allows flexion of the arm at the elbow; antagonist to the triceps muscle.

bilateral A directional term used to describe points on both sides of the body.

biohazard Short for "biological hazard," refers to any material that is considered unsafe because of contamination with body fluids.

biological agents Live organisms or natural substances that can kill or incapacitate.

bipolar disorder A psychiatric disorder characterized by cyclic mood changes, ranging from extreme elation to severe depression; same as manic-depressive disorder.

bipolar traction splint A traction splint with a double shaft.

black widow spider A poisonous spider that is black with a red hourglass mark on the abdomen.

bladder The organ in the pelvis that stores urine as it is made by the kidneys.

blanket drag A technique used to move patients by placing them on a blanket to drag them across the ground.

blood Made of several types of cells; fluid that carries fuels and wastes around the body for distribution and removal as appropriate.

blood vessels The structures through which the blood travels around the body.

bloody show The expulsion of a small amount of bloody mucus from the cervix as the cervix begins to thin.

body mechanics The proper or most efficient way to perform physical activities that are safe, are energy conserving, and help prevent the physical strains that may cause injury.

body substance isolation Protecting oneself from unnecessary exposure to potentially infectious body substances by avoiding direct contact with any body substance that may be infected.

bowel obstruction Blockage of flow through the intestine that results in proximal distenstion, abdominal pain, and vomiting.

Boyle's law A scientific principle wich explains that the volume of a gas varies indirectly with the surrounding pressure.

bradycardia Decreased heart rate.

brainstem The most basic part of the human brain; it acts as a junction box from the body to the rest of the brain structures and back.

Braxton Hicks contractions Random contractions that occur in the third trimester that are not associated with cervical effacement or dilation; also known as "false labor."

breach of confidentiality A situation in which a person divulges information about a patient without having the permission of the patient to do so.

breech presentation The presentation of the buttocks or a limb instead of the fetal head during birth.

briefing A commander provides the most up-to-date information about the current state of affairs at the incident.

bronchi Cartilaginous tubes that carry air into the lungs; singular: bronchus.

bronchioles Small muscular tubes with cartilaginous rings that carry air from bronchi into smaller air spaces in the lungs.

bronchodilator A medication that specifically opens up narrowed airways.

bronchospasm Constriction of the lower airways in the lungs.

brown recluse spider A poisonous spider that is brown with a classic violin-shaped mark on its back.

bundle branches Part of the heart's specialized conduction system; they receive electrical impulses from the bundle of His and transmit them to the Purkinje fibers in the ventricles.

bundle of His Part of the heart's specialized conduction system; it receives an electrical impulse from the AV node and transmits it to the bundle branches.

burn Injury caused by significant heat applied to the skin.

burnout The condition that exists when an EMT no longer feels able to perform his duties because of the effects of chronic stress.

C

calcaneus The largest bone in the foot, the heel bone.

call sign An identifying name or number that is assigned to a particular radio or person.

capillaries Tiny blood vessels that receive blood from arteries and pass it into adjacent veins.

capillary refill time The time it takes to see refill (evidenced by a return to normal color) of a capillary bed after blanching (loss of color in area of skin when pressed).

carbon dioxide (CO_2) A gas found in the air and created within the body.

cardiac contusion Bruising of the heart.

cardiac output The amount of blood pumped out of the heart in one minute.

cardiac standstill Condition in which the heart lies flaccid and unable to respond to any stimulus.

cardinal movements of labor The series of natural movements the infant makes upon descent through the birth canal.

cardiogenic shock A hypoperfused state resulting from inadequate cardiac pumping, usually due to multiple heart attacks.

cardiopulmonary resuscitation (CPR) A life-preserving technique involving chest compressions and artificial respiration that has been widely taught to both civilians and health care providers since the late 1950s.

carina Point at which the trachea ends and the right and left bronchi begin.

carpal bones The eight bones of the wrist.

carrier Someone who carries an infectious microorganism, does not necessarily become ill from it, but can transmit it to someone else.

carry transfer A means of moving a patient from one stretcher to another by lifting and carrying the patient.

caterpillar pass A means of replacing tired rescuers with fresh ones in carrying a patient on a stretcher without putting the patient down.

cellular respiration The process that allows the exchange of gases in the periphery.

Centers for Disease Control and Prevention (CDC) The U.S. federal agency charged with monitoring infectious disease outbreaks; typically the CDC provides a supportive role to state and local health departments.

centimeter (cm) A measurement of length.

central A directional term used to describe points toward the center of the body.

central nervous system Consists of the brain and spinal cord and is involved in the initiation and transmission of all control-oriented messages throughout the body.

central venous catheter An intravenous tube that may be left in for long periods of time and may be used for intravenous medication administration or blood sampling.

cerebellum The part of the brain that controls muscular coordination and complex actions; sometimes called the athletic brain.

cerebrospinal fluid (CSF) The nutrient-rich fluid that bathes and protects the spinal cord and brain.

cerebrospinal fluid shunt A special catheter that is used to drain excess CSF off the brain and into the abdomen, where it can be easily absorbed.

cerebrovascular accident (CVA) Injury to the brain tissue that occurs as a result of disruption of blood flow to part of the brain; also known as stroke.

cerebrum The largest and most highly evolved area of the brain.

certification Proof of satisfactory completion of the minimum requirements in a curriculum.

certified athletic trainer (ATC) A specially trained healthcare professional who primarily cares for athletes.

cervical dilation Progressive opening of the cervix that occurs as the fetal head descends into the pelvis.

cervical immobilization device (CID) A device intended to assist in maintaining the cervical spine in a natural neutral position.

cervical spine The uppermost section of the spinal column, made up of seven vertebrae in the neck; it protects the cervical spinal cord.

cervical spine immobilization device A rigid device that helps maintain the cervical spine in neutral alignment; also called a cervical collar.

cervix The opening to the uterus at the bottom.

cesarian section The surgical removal of a newborn from the uterus through an abdominal incision.

chain of command Assignment of roles and duties to individuals in a multiple casualty incident with a specific order of reporting to supervisors.

chain of survival A concept embraced by the American Heart Association that refers to the multiple elements needed in a response system in order to have a successful resuscitation. As in a chain, each element is connected with the others, and the strength of the entire chain is dependent upon the strength of each link.

chair carry The use of a standard kitchen chair to move a patient.

channel guard A device that prevents extraneous interference from radio transmissions from outside the base station; also called a private line.

CHART An acronym that stands for chief complaint/concern of the patient, history (including the history of present illness and the patient's past medical history), the physical assessment of the patient, the plan of patient care, and treatment and/or transportation.

CHEATED An acronym to help recall the outline of a completely documented patient record: chief complaint, history, exam, assessment of situation, treatment, evaluation, and disposition.

Chemical Transportation Emergency Center (CHEMTREC) A 24-hour technical assistance phone number (1-800-424-9300) about hazardous materials.

chemical weapons Poisons that can kill or incapacitate.

chest thrusts Firm compressions delivered at midchest in an attempt to expel a foreign body from the airway.

chief complaint (CC) The patient's main problem and reason for seeking medical services.

chilblains Painful, inflamed skin lesions resulting from excessive exposure of skin to cool, windy, damp weather.

child abuse An emotional, physical, or sexual injury inflicted upon a child.

childbirth The act of delivering a child.

cholecystitis Infection of the gallbladder often characterized by fever, abdominal pain, and jaundice.

chronic obstructive pulmonary disease (COPD) A group of diseases characterized by chronic airway obstruction and bronchospasm.

chronic stress Repeated stressors that affect an EMT over a period of time.

cilia Hair-like projections from cells lining the airways that keep a thick mucous blanket constantly moving upward and out of the lungs.

Cincinnati Prehospital Stroke Scale A three-item scale used to identify patients with likelihood of stroke.

circulation The action of blood flowing in the circuit of blood vessels and the heart.

clavicle The collarbone; located at the very top of the chest, connecting the shoulder to the sternum.

clonic phase The stage in a seizure in which the body paroxysmally stiffens and relaxes.

closed fracture A broken bone in which the bone ends remain roughly in line and do not break the skin.

clothing drag The technique of pulling a patient to safety using the clothing he is wearing.

clues Evidence a person was in an area.

coagulation The process of blood clotting.

Coagulopathy A blood-clotting disorder caused by disease or chemical exposure.

coccyx The tailbone, or last portion of the spinal column.

Code of Federal Regulations (CFR) A compilation of the national laws passed by the Congress.

cold zone The area without any risk of contamination to rescue personnel.

Colles' fracture A broken wrist that is shaped like a silver fork.

command hallucination An auditory hallucination, coming from a false or imaginary figure or person, that tells the individual what to do.

command post A centralized location, often off site, where the heads of public safety agencies gather and regulate on scene operations.

Commission for the Accreditation of Ambulance Services (CAAS) An independent organization that has set minimum standards for ambulance services.

communications center A central dispatch point.

communications specialist (COMSPEC) A specially trained radio operator.

compartment syndrome A buildup of pressure from swelling within muscle cavities.

compensated shock A hypoperfused state that the body is compensating for by increasing heart rate, increasing respiratory rate, and shunting blood from certain organs.

competent Able to act in a responsible manner and comprehend the decision at hand.

compress Cotton dressing integrated into a two-tailed bandage.

computer-aided dispatch (CAD) Use of computers to assist emergency medical dispatchers with control and command of emergency services.

conduction Transfer of heat from a warm object to a cool object by direct contact.

conductor Material that easily carries a current.

confidentiality Privacy; maintaining confidentiality means ensuring that medical information is provided only to the patient's health care providers.

confined space Any area that has limited openings for exit and access and is not designed for worker occupancy.

congestive heart failure (CHF) A condition in which there is a backup of pressure from the left ventricle, allowing fluid to leak out of the pulmonary capillaries and into the alveoli.

consent A voluntary agreement by a person to allow something to take place.

Consolidated Omnibus Budget Reconciliation Act (COBRA) Federal legislation that provided for comprehensive budget reform and included passages that pertained to EMS.

contagious The state of an illness when the affected person can transmit it to others.

continuing education Training beyond the initial certification requirements.

continuous quality improvement (CQI) Process by which an organization monitors and addresses areas in need of improvement.

contraindication A reason to not do something.

controlled intersection An intersection with a traffic control device.

contusion Bruising of tissue, caused by blunt forces.

convection Heat loss to air currents passing by a warm surface.

coral snake A venomous snake identified by its red and yellow bands directly opposed.

coronary arteries The two arteries that supply blood to the heart muscle.

costal arch The umbrella-appearing arch at the lower portion of the front of the thoracic cage.

costovertebral angle The angle formed by the tenth rib as it meets the thoracic spine.

covering the brake Placing one foot over the brake pedal in anticipation of stopping.

crackles A popping sound heard in the lungs that is created as tiny air spaces that are stuck together by abnormal fluid accumulation pop open.

cradle carry An emergent means of moving a patient involving lifting the patient up and cradling him in the arms for a rapid move from the dangerous environment.

cranium The bony skull.

cravat A simple cotton triangular bandage useful in many circumstances.

crepitus The sound of bone ends grinding against one another; the feeling of air under the skin; it feels like Rice Krispies popping under the fingertips.

cribbing Blocks of wood used to stabilize a vehicle.

cricoid pressure A technique of applying pressure to the cricoid ring during ventilation to occlude the esophagus and prevent regurgitation.

critical incident stress debriefing (CISD) Organized discussions among all involved team members and several other key players that occur after a particularly stressful incident. Such a debriefing can help participants effectively deal with the stress of the incident.

critical incident stress management (CISM) A program that puts EMS providers in contact with licensed mental health professionals following a particularly traumatic or anxiety-producing event.

cross-fingered technique Technique whereby the EMT places the thumb against the upper incisors and the fore forefinger against the lower incisors to gently force the mouth open in a scissors maneuver.

croup A swelling and inflammation of the larynx, trachea, and to some extent the bronchi, usually caused by a viral infection.

crowning The term used to describe the appearance of the fetal head at the vaginal opening when delivery is imminent.

crumple zone Automobile fenders designed to absorb energy while compacting.

crush injury Prolonged pressure on the skin and underlying tissues.

CSF otorrhea Leaking of cerebrospinal fluid from the ear.

CSF rhinorrhea Leaking of cerebrospinal fluid from the nose.

cubic centimeter (cc) A measurement of volume, analogous to the mL.

current The passage of electricity through an object.

Cushing's reflex Hypertension and bradycardia associated with serious head injury.

Cushing's triad Hypertension, bradycardia, and an altered respiratory pattern seen in serious head injuries.

cyanosis A bluish discoloration to the skin seen with a poor oxygen content of the blood.

D

D5W An intravenous solution that consists of 5% dextrose in water.

dangerous instrument Anything capable of producing death or serious bodily harm when used in certain circumstances.

DCAP-BTLS Abbreviation for assessment of signs of serious underlying injuries: deformity, contusion, abrasion, puncture, burns, tenderness, laceration, swelling.

dead space The space in the respiratory tract that is not in contact with pulmonary capillaries and cannot participate in gas exchange with the blood.

deadly weapon Any device that, by its nature, is intended to produce death.

debriefing An organized discussion among personnel involved in a difficult situation in an attempt to prevent an unnecessary buildup of stress.

decompensated shock A hypoperfused state for which the body is no longer able to compensate and hypotension results.

decompression sickness A diving injury that occurs during a rapid ascent resulting in expansion of gases that become trapped in tissues; also known as the bends.

decontamination Removal of potentially hazardous substances by either chemical or physical means.

decontamination corridor The area where the hazardous materials are cleaned off the rescuers and patients; also referred to as the warm zone.

deep Term used to describe an injury that extends far into the injured structure.

defibrillation The application of an electrical shock to the heart in ventricular fibrillation.

defibrillator A device that can deliver an electrical shock to the heart through the use of cables and electrodes.

deformity Misshapen or not in the usual position.

degloving avulsion The forceful separation of just the skin from an extremity.

delirium An alteration in the level of consciousness exhibited by a sudden erratic change in behavior, usually caused by an acute medical problem.

delirium tremens (DTs) The symptoms associated with the sudden withdrawal of alcohol from an alcohol-dependent person.

deltoid muscle The triangular muscle covering the shoulder and upper arm; a site commonly used for intramuscular injections.

Department of Transportation (DOT) The U.S. federal agency responsible for traffic safety, and where modern EMS originated.

dementia A syndrome that is characterized by a progressive decline in intellectual function that usually leads to deterioration of occupational, social, and interpersonal functions.

dentures False teeth.

dependency The psychological need the person has for a drug.

depression A psychiatric condition characterized by sad mood and lack of interest in usual life pleasures.

dermis The layer of skin just beneath the surface, or epidermal, layer; contains capillaries and specialized nerve endings.

designated officer (DO) A specific person within an EMS agency who is responsible for receiving notifications of potential exposures and following up as appropriate.

diabetes mellitus A disease in which the pancreas fails to produce insulin.

diabetic coma The condition of an unconscious, hyperglycemic diabetic patient.

diabetic ketoacidosis (DKA) The result of excessive fat metabolism seen in diabetic patients with hyperglycemia.

diamond stretcher carry A technique in which four EMTs carry a patient on a stretcher, with one EMT at either end and one on each side.

diaphoretic Exhibiting excessive perspiration due to stress or pain.

diaphragm The specialized muscle that separates the chest from the abdomen and is the main muscle of breathing.

diastolic The lower number in the blood pressure; the pressure in the vessels when the heart is resting between contractions.

diet-controlled diabetes The condition of a person whose blood sugar is controlled by diet modification.

diffusion The movement of oxygen and carbon dioxide across a membrane from an area of higher concentration to an area of lower concentration.

direct carry Lifting a patient and carrying him a short distance directly to the stretcher.

direct contact Actually coming into contact with the infectious material on a person by touching.

direct current (DC) A unidirectional electrical current.

direct force The transfer of energy to the point of impact of violence.

direct laryngoscopy Use of a laryngoscope to directly visualize the airway structures.

direct lift A technique that allows three EMTs to lift a patient from the ground without using assistive devices.

direct pressure Constant firm pushing on the bleeding site.

dislocation A bone that slips out of joint, and out of alignment.

distal A directional term used to describe points farther from the core of the body (trunk).

diversionary techniques Activities such as physical exercise, deep breathing, or creative imagery that are useful in dissipating the effects of an acutely stressful event.

diverticulitis Inflammation/infection of small outpouchings off of the large bowel often associated with left-sided abdominal pain.

do not resuscitate order (DNR) A medical-legal order to restrain health care providers from providing invasive procedures and resuscitation such as CPR.

domestic terrorists Groups of "nationals," as defined by the U.S. Immigration and Nationality Act, that have disputes with the way the U.S. government is operated or with specific U.S. policies.

domestic violence An act of violence against a partner, spouse, family member, or member of the household.

DOPE Acronym to help remember causes of deterioration in the intubated patient: displaced tube, obstructed tube, pneumothorax, equipment failure.

dorsal A directional term referring to the top or back surface of a structure such as the hand.

dorsiflexion Movement of the toes upward, toward the nose.

dose The amount of a substance; usually refers to the amount of a medication given.

draw sheet Either a regular bed sheet folded over in half or a sturdy linen of equal length used to move a patient from a bed to a stretcher, or vice versa.

draw sheet transfer Use of a draw sheet to move a patient from one stretcher to another.

dressing A sterile absorbent cloth used to cover a wound.

due regard Respect and consideration for others.

duplex A radio that allows the EMT to both speak and listen at the same time, like a telephone.

durable power of attorney-health care (DPOA-HC) A legal document that extends authority of one person to control the legal affairs of another; in this case, the healthcare issues of a patient.

dura mater The outermost membrane covering the spinal cord and brain.

dysarthria Difficulty speaking resulting in garbled or slurred speech.

dyspnea The feeling or appearance of respiratory distress.

dysrhythmia Any disruption of the normal sinus rhythm.

E

ecchymosis A wider collection of blood under the skin like a contusion.

echo technique A technique that involves repeating what was originally said to confirm it and avoid mistakes.

eclampsia A convulsive disorder seen only during pregnancy.

ectopic pregnancy A pregnancy that develops outside of the uterus.

effacement Thinning of the cervix that occurs as a pregnancy nears its conclusion.

elder abuse An act of violence toward or neglect of an elderly person who is dependent upon the other person.

electrocardiogram (ECG) A recording of the electrical activity of the heart graphically displayed on an oscilloscope or printed on paper; also abbreviated EKG.

elevate Raising the bleeding site above the level of the heart.

emancipated minor A person who is not the age of majority but who is no longer under the control of a parent or guardian and is legally responsible for his or her decisions and any consequences that result from those decisions.

embolism A physical blockage in the bloodstream.

embolus Debris that travels through blood vessels until it lodges and occludes blood flow.

emergency ambulance A vehicle specifically designed for patient transportation in an emergency.

emergency ambulance service vehicle (EASV) A vehicle used in service to EMS and staffed by EMS personnel.

emergency department (ED) A division or portion of a hospital designated to care for emergency medical problems or trauma; in some countries called an accident room.

emergency dispatcher A trained person who answers 9-1-1 emergency telephone calls from the public and provides public safety assistance through communication with emergency services such as fire, law enforcement and EMS.

emergency doctrine A legal principle that allows for emergency treatment of prisoners or children if they are incapable of giving consent.

emergency drag A technique used by a single EMT to move a patient quickly in an emergency.

emergency medical dispatch (EMD) An organized program that allows properly trained providers to take emergency calls, give first-aid instructions to callers, and prioritize the responding units.

emergency medical services (EMS) A coordinated network of providers whose function is to provide a variety of medical services to people in need of emergency medical care.

emergency medical services system (EMSS) An organization of equipment, such as ambulances, and personnel, such as the EMTs, created to respond to medical emergencies within a community.

emergency medical technician (EMT) An entry-level position in emergency medical services; typically provides emergency care and transportation aboard an ambulance.

Emergency Medical Technician–Basic (EMT-B) A person who has completed the primary level of prehospital medical training, the most common level in the United States. The course at this level includes training in CPR, defibrillation, airway management, and basic medical and trauma care.

Emergency Medical Technician–Intermediate (EMT-I) A person who has completed the second level of prehospital medical training beyond that of EMT–Basic. The course includes training in intravenous therapy, advanced airway management, cardiac arrest management, and trauma care.

Emergency Medical Technician–Paramedic (EMT-P) A person who has completed the highest level of prehospital medical training. The course includes training in advanced airway management and intravenous access techniques, defibrillation, cardiac pacing, and advanced pharmacology.

Emergency Medical Treatment and Active Labor Act (EMTALA) Federal legislation that insures that patients receive medical treatment regardless of their ability to pay.

emergency move The technique that an EMT uses to quickly remove a patient from danger.

emergency operations plan (EOP) An interagency document that assigns responsibilities to U.S. government departments and organizations, thereby setting lines of command (authority). It describes how emergency responders will protect people and property in the event of a terrorist attack as well as apprehend those responsible.

emergency physician A physician specifically trained to provide care to acutely ill and injured patients in an emergency department setting.

Emergency Response Guidebook **(ERG)** A guidebook that provides responders instructions and information on how to handle the first 30 minutes of a hazmat spill.

emergency response team A group of people who arrive and rescue contaminated persons and control, confine, contain, and decontaminate the area.

emergency services vehicle (ESV) A vehicle used by an emergency service, including law enforcement, fire service, of EMS.

emergency vehicle operator (EVO) A driver of a vehicle used for emergency service.

emergency vehicle operators course (EVOC) A training course for drivers of vehicles used for emergency service.

end tidal CO_2 detector A device that will indicate the presence of carbon dioxide in exhaled air.

endocrine system Assists the nervous system in maintaining control over the body by producing hormones that act upon certain organs.

endotracheal intubation Placement of a plastic tube into the trachea to allow for ventilation of the lungs.

endotracheal tube (ETT) A firm, plastic tube that permits passage of air directly from the environment to the lungs, thereby protecting the airway and preventing aspiration.

end-to-end stretcher carry The use of one EMT on either end of a stretcher to carry it.

entrance wound Damage created as an object or electricity enters the body.

environmental assessment An EMT's visual overview of an entire scene while identifying potential hazards.

Environmental Protection Agency (EPA) The U.S. federal agency charged with maintaining the quality of the environment; typically concerned with pollution.

epidermis The outermost layer of skin.

epidural hematoma A collection of blood between the skull and the dura mater, often arterial in nature.

epiglottis Located above the larynx, a cartilaginous structure that protects the trachea from aspiration of foreign bodies.

epiglottitis A bacterial infection, characterized by a swollen, inflamed epiglottis, that can cause upper airway obstruction.

epilepsy A disease characterized by recurrent seizures of a similar nature.

epinephrine A medication that dilates the airways and constricts the blood vessels.

escape rhythm The special ability of the myocardium to function independently when the electrical system fails.

esophageal varices Dilated veins within the lining of the lower esophagus that may bleed profusely if they rupture.

esophagus A collapsible muscular tube that directs food from the mouth into the stomach.

evaporation Transfer of heat into body fluids, such as sweat, for dissipation into the environment.

eversion An outward movement, such as when the foot twists outward and strains the ankle; the opposite of inversion.

evidence conscious Awareness of the importance of preserving items that may be considered evidence of a crime and conditions that pertain to a crime.

evisceration An abdominal wound with abdominal contents protruding through the wound.

excited delirium A state of hyperactive irrational behavior.

exhalation Breathing out.

exit wound Damage created as a foreign object or electricity exits the body.

expected time of arrival (ETA) The anticipated arrival of either the patient or the EMT to the scene.

expiration date The last day that a medication is guaranteed by the manufacturer to be safe and effective as expected.

express consent The act of verbally advising a medical provider to proceed with treatment.

expressive aphasia Difficulty forming words often seen when a stroke affects the brain's speech center.

extension A movement that widens the angle at a joint between two bones; the opposite of flexion.

extremity lift A lifting technique whereby one EMT stands behind a seated patient and grasps him under the shoulders, while a second EMT grasps him under the knees so they can lift and carry him.

F

facial droop One-sided facial muscle weakness that indicates focal brain or nerve injury.

fallopian tube Tiny muscular tube that allows an egg to travel from the ovary to the uterus.

false imprisonment The intentional confinement of a patient without the patient's consent and without an appropriate reason.

false motion Movement in the bone where there is not supposed to be movement.

false ribs The eighth through tenth ribs, which are not attached directly to the sternum; rather, they are attached anteriorly to the seventh rib by cartilage.

fasciotomy A surgical procedure whereby skin is cut to relieve pressure.

febrile seizure A seizure that results from a rapid rise in body temperature.

Federal Communications Commission (FCC) The U.S. federal agency that regulates radio communications.

federal response plan (FRP) A plan used when state and local authorities are overwhelmed; it brings the immense resources of the federal government to their aid.

feeding tube A soft, flexible tube that is placed into the stomach, either through the nose or through the anterior abdominal wall, to allow nutritional supplementation.

femur The single bone in the thigh; it is the longest and strongest bone in the body.

fetus The ovum after it is implanted in the uterine wall.

fibula The laterally placed bone in the lower leg.

field hospital A temporary on-site treatment facility.

fight or flight response Describes the reaction of the body to a stressor by preparing to fight to defend itself or to run away.

figure-of-eight A roller bandage that turns across itself.

firefighter's carry A technique that involves lifting a supine patient up onto the EMT's shoulder to quickly move the patient from a dangerous environment.

firefighter's drag A carrying technique that involves the patient's arms being around the EMT's neck and the EMT crawling on hands and knees, dragging the patient underneath him.

first responder The first person who arrives on the scene of an incident; also may refer to the level of medical training provided to persons who expect to be put in this position during their daily routine, such as firefighters, police officers, and security guards.

first responder awareness level A person trained to identify and report a hazardous materials incident.

first stage of labor The process of cervical effacement and dilation at the beginning of childbirth.

flail segment Two or more ribs fractured in two or more places where the underlying segment is unstable and moves in a paradoxical motion to the rest of the chest wall.

flapping the roof Cutting the uprights or posts to peel back the roof in a motor vehicle.

flashback The strobe of the emergency lights bouncing back into the emergency vehicle operator's eyes.

flat water A body of water without current.

flexible splint Any material that can be formed to fit any angle and then made rigid.

flexible stretcher A lightweight plastic stretcher that may be rolled up when not in use; commonly used in confined space and cave rescue.

flexion A movement at a joint that decreases the angle between the two bones on either side of it; opposite of extension.

floating ribs The last two pairs of ribs in the thoracic cage; they are unattached anteriorly.

flow-restricted oxygen-powered ventilation device (FROPVD) A device that can deliver oxygen to a patient at restricted flow rates.

focused physical examination A physical exam focused upon the medical patient's chief complaint.

focused trauma assessment An assessment that is focused on the patient's complaint or injury.

fontanels Soft, flexible fibrous regions in an infant's skull that allow for skull growth; also known as soft spots.

Food and Drug Administration (FDA) The U.S. federal agency responsible for drug purity and safety.

foot (ft) A measurement of distance.

foot drop A loss of nervous control that results in a flaccid foot.

foramen magnum Large opening at the base of the skull through which the spinal cord passes.

forcible entry Using special tools or brute force to overcome an obstacle to gain entrance.

forcing the door Using a tool to overcome a latching mechanism.

foreign body airway obstruction (FBAO) Any ingested object that is capable of causing suffocation by blocking the trachea.

four corners carry A patient transportation technique in which four or more EMTs carry a stretcher over a distance.

four-second rule Determining the amount of time between when the vehicle in front of the emergency vehicle passes a landmark and when the emergency vehicle passes it; for safety reasons this time should be greater than 4 seconds.

Fowler's position Position in which a person is sitting at a 45-degree to 60-degree angle.

fracture A sudden breaking of a bone.

French catheter A flexible suction catheter meant to suction through endotracheal tubes or via the nasopharynx.

frequency modulation (FM) A method of radio signal transmission.

frontal bone The strong anterior-most bone in the skull that makes up the forehead.

frostbite Tissue damage resulting from exposure to freezing and subfreezing temperatures.

frostnip A mild local skin injury resulting from exposure to freezing temperatures.

full-thickness burn A burn that affects all three layers of the skin.

fundus The top of the uterus.

G

gag reflex The protective response that a person has when the back of the throat is stimulated by the presence of a foreign substance.

gallbladder A small pouchlike organ that lies underneath the liver and stores bile to be used in digestion.

gastrocnemius muscle The muscle in the back of the calf that enables a person to stand on his toes.

gastroenteritis A condition characterized by vomiting and diarrhea, usually caused by a viral illness.

gauze dressing Sterile cotton weave cloth.

Geiger counter A device used to detect radiation.

general impression The initial feeling, based upon observation, of how seriously ill or injured the patient is.

generalized seizure A seizure that involves the entire brain and results in loss of consciousness; also known as a grand mal seizure.

generic name The initial name given to a drug that is shorter than the actual chemical name and is listed in the *U.S. Pharmacopeia*.

gestational diabetes A form of diabetes that occurs only in pregnant women and usually only for the duration of the pregnancy.

glands Specialized organs that respond to and produce hormones of the endocrine system.

Glasgow Coma Scale (GCS) A scale that is used to quantify a patient's level of responsiveness.

global assessment The EMT's general feeling of the entire scene; should involve thoughts of safety and need for additional rescuers.

global positioning satellite (GPS) A constellation of geo-synchronized satellites that are used to determine position, speed and time of any object on earth.

glucose A substance used by the body for fuel.

gluteus muscles Strong muscles in the buttock that are important in allowing proper leg movement.

goblet cell Cells that produce a mucous that is designed to entrap particles and micro-organisms, such as bacteria, and prevent them from entering the alveoli.

gonads Organs of reproduction; testes (male) and ovaries (female).

Good Samaritan laws Laws that protect certain classes of people, such as physicians, who volunteer to assist others; laws vary from state to state.

grand mal seizure The old term for a generalized seizure.

gravidity The total number of pregnancies a woman has had.

grunting A noise made upon exhalation during periods of respiratory distress.

guardian A person who has authority to act on behalf of another individual and to give consent for medical care.

guarding Muscular tension created by a patient to protect an underlying injury.

guides Instructions for evacuation distance, perimeter boundaries, and potential hazards found in the *Emergency Response Guidebook*.

gunshot wound (GSW) An injury created by a projectile fired by a gun.

gurgling Sound of liquid moving; if heard at the airway, indicates a need for suctioning.

H

hailing frequency The channel used to call a particular agency or hospital.

hallucination A sensation or perception that has no basis in reality.

halo test Observing for a ring of blood around CSF spilled from the ears or nose in a head-injured patient.

hard palate The bony structure that forms the roof of the mouth.

hasty search A quick search of an area.

hazardous material Any substance that can cause an exposed person injury or death.

Hazardous Waste Operations and Emergency Response (HAZWOPER) Legislation that pertains to toxic waste management.

head-tilt, chin-lift Maneuver used to open the airway, involving tilting the head back and lifting the jaw up; used only in nontrauma patients.

health care proxy A person chosen to make medical decisions on behalf of another in the event the person becomes incapable of making such decisions.

Health Insurance Portability and Accountability Act (HIPAA) An act of the U.S. Congress that protects health insurance coverage for workers and their families when they change or lose their jobs. Regulates national standards for electronic health care transactions and the security and privacy of health data.

healthy lifestyle A lifestyle that includes exercise, a balanced diet, and avoidance of unhealthy habits such as smoking.

heart Four-chambered muscular organ that pumps to provide the body with nutrient-rich blood.

heat cramps Painful, involuntary muscle spasms caused by dehydration and exposure to heat.

heat exhaustion The mildest form of generalized heat-related illness, characterized by multiple symptoms and often by dehydration.

heat stroke A life-threatening form of heat illness that involves a rise in body temperature and altered mental status.

heavy rescue The use of special vehicle extrication equipment.

hematochezia Passage of bright red blood from the rectum.

Heimlich maneuver A series of forceful upward abdominal thrusts that force air out of the lungs and the trachea.

hematoma An accumulation of blood.

hemetemesis Vomitus that consists mostly of blood.

hemoptysis Spitting up or coughing up blood.

hemorrhage Medical term for bleeding.

hemorrhagic shock A hypoperfused state resulting from loss of blood.

hemorrhagic stroke Injury to brain tissue as a result of rupture of a vessel that supplies it with blood.

hemostasis The process of controlling bleeding.

hemothorax Bleeding in between the lung and the chest wall.

hepatitis B virus (HBV) The virus responsible for hepatitis B infection, the virus that attacks the liver.

high-altitude cerebral edema (HACE) Swelling of the brain as a result of hypoxia at high altitudes; characterized by altered mental status, difficulty walking, and decreased level of consciousness.

high-altitude pulmonary edema (HAPE) Pulmonary edema as a result of hypoxia at high altitudes; characterized by dry cough and dyspnea upon exertion.

high efficiency particulate air filter (HEPA) A filtration device intended to remove very small airborne contaminants.

high index of suspicion Based upon the noted mechanism of injury, the feeling that there is a high likelihood of injury.

high life hazard Known dangerous conditions that could injure or kill someone.

high-Fowler's position Position in which a person is sitting upright at a 90-degree angle.

history of present illness (HPI) An account of the course of an illness; typically done as a narrative from witnesses such as family members.

hobble restraint The tying of wrists to ankles behind the patient's back.

homeostasis The body's ability to maintain a steady optimal state for growth and development and resists any influence, internal or external, that would upset this balance.

hormones Chemicals that are excreted into the bloodstream by specialized organs called glands.

hospice A facility with a team of health care professionals who care for dying patients.

hot zone The immediate vicinity of the hazardous material spill that is considered contaminated and a risk to rescue personnel.

hot-load Placing a patient aboard a running helicopter.

human immunodeficiency virus (HIV) The virus that causes AIDS (acquired immunodeficiency syndrome).

humerus The single long bone of the upper arm.

humidification The process of adding moisture to the inspired air.

hydrochloric acid (HCl) A strong acid that can cause serious burns.

hydrogen sulfide (H_2S) A chemical with the smell of rotten eggs.

hyperbaric chamber A device that creates a simulated dive to allow for recompression of air in a diver suffering from decompression sickness or other diving-related illnesses.

hyperglycemia A high amount of sugar in the blood.

hyperosmolar hyperglycemic non-ketonic coma (HHNK) a condition of the diseases diabetes that can lead to coma, different than keto-acidosis.

hypertension An abnormally high blood pressure.

hyperthermia Overall heat gain greater than heat loss, resulting in a rise in body temperature.

hyperventilate To breathe faster and more deeply than usual.

hyperventilation A higher-than-normal ventilatory rate.

hyphema A collection of blood in the anterior part of the eye.

hypoglycemia A condition of low blood glucose levels.

hypoperfusion Inadequate supply of oxygenated blood to a tissue or an organ.

hypothermia A condition in which the body temperature drops below 95 degrees Fahrenheit.

hypoventilation Breathing more slowly than normal or less effectively than usual.

hypovolemia A state of low fluid levels.

hypovolemic shock A hypoperfused state resulting from low fluid levels.

hypoxia Lack of oxygen in the body.

hypoxic drive The stimulus to breathe becomes low oxygen levels instead of the usual stimulus, high carbon dioxide levels.

I

iliac bones The main component of the bony pelvis, the hip bones, sometimes described as "wings" because of their shape.

immunity Insusceptibility to a specific illness, usually as a result of prior exposure or immunization.

immunity statute A law that protects a specific group of people from having to pay civil damages as a result of occurrences during job performance.

immunization The process of exposing the body to or inoculating it with weakened pathogens in order to allow it to create specific antibodies.

immunocompromise Lack of disease resistance.

impaled object A foreign object embedded in the skin.

implied consent The legal presumption that a patient who is unable to verbally express agreement to treatment would agree to be treated in certain circumstances.

incident commander (IC) The person in command who has overall responsibility for the entire incident.

Incident Command System (ICS) A common system of command and control utilized by all emergency services.

incident management system (IMS) A system of organization and administration involving all emergency service providers that focuses on the three critical components of large incident management; command, control, and communications.

incision A cutting of the skin.

indication A reason to do something.

indirect contact Exposure to an infectious agent that is on a nonhuman surface.

indirect force A transfer of energy as a result of violence away from the point of impact.

infarct A group of cells that have died as a result of prolonged lack of oxygen.

infection control Taking preventive measures to lessen the likelihood of disease transmission.

infection control officer Designated officer of a company or department that is assigned to monitor infection control practices and act as a liaison to the hospital's infection control department.

inferior Lower than the reference point.

inflammation The body's attempt to prevent infection and begin healing.

initial assessment The first evaluation peformed on every patient to address life-threatening problems.

initial report The first emergency responder's first radio report of scene conditions; includes hazards, number of patients, and requests for additional resources.

in loco parentis Someone who has authority to act on behalf of a minor in place of the parent.

inspiration Breathing in.

insulator Material that resists the passage of electrical current.

insulin A hormone produced by the pancreas that allows glucose utilization by the body.

insulin-dependent diabetes A condition for which the diabetic patient must inject insulin into the body to survive.

insulin shock Condition resulting from low blood sugar due to either too much insulin or too little sugar.

integumentary system The skin and skin structures that cover and protect the body.

intercostal retraction A retraction of skin and muscle between the ribs with each breath, as seen in a child with respiratory distress.

international terrorists Terrorist groups that cross over national borders and often have subgroups, called cells, in other countries to perform terrorism.

intermediate life support (ILS) The next level of care above EMT–Basic, where the use of special airway techniques, such as intubation, and a limited list of medications helps to extend the effectiveness of the EMT.

International Association of Fire Fighters (IAFF) An international group representing over 263,000 firefighters in more than 3,500 communities in the U.S. and Canada.

intermammary line The imaginary horizontal line that runs between the nipples.

intervertebral disk The fibrous pad that cushions each vertebra from the others.

intracranial pressure (ICP) The pressure within the skull.

intramuscular Referring to administration of medication into the muscular layer under the subcutaneous layer of soft tissue.

intravenous (IV) Referring to administration of medication into the veins.

inversion Turning something inward; opposite of eversion.

irreversible shock Hypoperfusion that has progressed to a point where survival is highly unlikely.

ischemia Injury of tissue due to a lack of oxygenated blood for a period of time.

ischemic stroke Injury to brain tissue as a result of blockage of the vessel that supplies it with blood.

ischium The portion of the bony pelvis that supports body weight while in the sitting position.

J

jaundice A yellow discoloration of the skin caused by excess bilirubin in the bloodstream.

jaw thrust A technique that lifts the mandible and tongue up and away from the pharynx, often effective in opening the airway; is used on trauma patients with suspected spinal injury.

jugular vein A large vein in the side of the neck that is situated rather close to the surface of the skin.

jugular venous distension (JVD) Bulging veins in the side of the neck.

K

keto-acid An organic acid that is the by-product of ineffective metabolism; also called ketone.

kidney A solid organ in the retroperitoneal space that filters toxins from the blood and makes urine to dispose of such toxins and excess salts or water.

knee The joint that joins the upper leg and the lower leg.

Kussmaul's respiration Deep, almost sighing, respiration.

L

labor The childbirth process by which the uterus expels the fetus and placenta.

laceration A type of wound characterized by a full-thickness tear in the skin.

LACES A mnemonic for first responders on the scene of a potential terrorist attack; L stands for lookout, A for awareness, C for communications, E for escape and S for safety zone.

lactated Ringers A commonly used intravenous solution consisting of electrolytes that approximates the concentration of blood.

landing zone (LZ) An area intended for the purpose of landing and taking off in a helicopter.

large intestine Hollow digestive organ that encircles the abdominal cavity and receives digested food from the small intestine.

laryngeal mask airway (LMA) An airway device used in EMS as a rescue device that helps protect the airway and permits ventilation of the lungs.

laryngoscope A tool that is used to view the lower airway structures during endotracheal intubation.

laryngoscopy The use of a laryngoscope to view the lower airway structures.

larynx A cartilaginous structure in the midline of the neck that contains the vocal cords and is the beginning of the trachea, or windpipe.

lateral A directional term used to describe the side of a structure; points farther from the midline.

law enforcement officer (LEO) The broad category including police officers, state police, deputy sheriffs, FBI agents, DEA agents, etc. who have the responsibility to uphold the law.

left lateral recumbent position Position in which the person is lying on his left side; also known as the recovery position.

legal duty to act The requirement that an EMT respond to calls whether as an employee under contract or as a volunteer.

liability The legal responsibility for one's own actions.

lifelong learning Education that a person continues throughout life by keeping current on new information and maintaining competence in skills.

ligament The connective tissue that connects bone to bone.

light-emitting diode (LED) An electronic device that shines light using very small amounts of electricity.

limited victim incident (LVI) A smaller number of patients than multiple casualty incident (MCI).

linear A straight course.

liquid oxygen (LOX) Compressed oxygen that is in liquid form; it takes up an extremely small volume and is thus more portable.

liters per minute (lpm) A measurement of the rate of flow of a liquid.

litter A stretcher or other means of patient conveyance that does not have wheels and must be carried.

liver Large, solid organ in the right upper abdomen that creates bile for digestion, produces special factors to help in blood clotting, and filters blood from the intestines to rid the body of specific toxins.

living will A document signed by a patient that informs the reader of what types of treatment and under what conditions that patient would want or would not want medical treatment.

loaded bumper A vehicle's front or rear bumper that, when compressed and locked, is able to suddenly and unexpectedly spring forward.

locked A bone that is unable to return to its natural position.

lower extremities A term used to refer to the legs.

lumbar vertebrae The five vertebrae that make up the lower back and support the weight of the entire upper body.

lymph A straw-colored fluid similar to plasma that carries white blood cells.

lymph node Solid glandlike bodies, such as the tonsils, where white blood cells destroy microorganisms.

lymphatic system Part of the immune system that carries microorganism-laden white blood cells in a fluid, called lymph, to lymph nodes for removal. Also assists the circulatory system by draining the body's tissues of excess fluids and returning that fluid to the central circulation.

LZ officer A designated person on the scene of an incident who will be responsible for choosing a landing zone (LZ) for the helicopter and ensuring its safety.

M

Macintosh blade The name for a type of curved laryngoscope blade.

macrodrip A type of intravenous tubing that is designed to allow large amounts of fluid to flow through it quickly.

malaise A feeling of weakness or exhaustion.

malleolus The bony prominences at the medial and lateral aspects of the ankles.

mandated reporter An individual who comes into contact with certain situations and is required by law to report these situations to the proper authorities; for example, child abuse.

mandible The bony lower jaw.

manubrium The upper section of the bony sternum.

mastoid process The bony prominence behind the ear.

mastoid sinus Air-filled space within the mastoid bone, behind the ears.

Material Safety Data Sheet (MSDS) A reference list of the health and safety information for a chemical substance.

maxilla One of the two fused bones that form the upper jawbone; plural, maxillae.

McGill forceps A pair of special long, curved pinching tongs.

mechanical ventilator A machine that provides artificial ventilation for a patient who cannot breathe effectively on his own.

mechanism of injury (MOI) The instrument or event that results in harm to a patient.

meconium Fetal stool.

Med channel A radio frequency that is used by paramedics and EMTs to speak to base hospital physicians.

medial A directional term used to describe points closer to the midline of the body.

MedicAlert An Emergency Medical Information service that provides a bodily worn patient directive to its members.

medical communicator (MEDCOM) A dedicated EMS dispatcher typically trained in emergency medical dispatch.

medical direction Advice provided by a higher medical authority, usually a physician.

medical director A physician who acts as a medical expert, consultant, and educator.

medical protocols A set of written regulations that specify the proper procedures for patient care.

medically necessary restraint Used when a patient must be confined to prevent him from harming himself or others.

megahertz (MHz) A frequency band of radio wave transmission.

melena Dark, tarry stool containing digested blood caused by bleeding in the upper gastrointestinal tract.

meninges Protective membranes covering the brain and spinal cord.

meningitis An infection and inflammation of the lining around the brain and spinal cord.

menstruation The monthly flow that rids the uterus of its lining when fertilization of an egg does not occur.

mental illness Any disorder that impairs the brain's function that is without a firm physical (organic) cause.

metabolism The use of fuels by the body.

metacarpals The five bones that connect the carpal bones in the wrist to the phalanges in the fingers.

metered dose inhaler A handheld device that carries a form of medication that may be aerosolized upon discharge of the inhaler device.

microdrip A type of intravenous tubing that is designed to allow only small amounts of fluid to flow through it at a time.

microorganism A tiny living creature that is visible only by microscope.

midaxillary line An imaginary line drawn from the center of the armpit down the side of the chest.

midclavicular lines Imaginary lines drawn from the middle of each clavicle, or collarbone, down the front of the chest.

midline An imaginary line drawn down the center of the body, splitting it equally into a right half and a left half.

miles per hour (mph) A measurement of the speed of a vehicle.

military anti-shock trousers (MAST) A device that is inflated over the lower extremities and pelvis to attempt to increase blood flow to the core organs; also called pneumatic antishock garment (PASG).

Miller blade The name for a type of straight laryngoscope blade.

milliampere (mA) A measurement of electric current.

milligram/gram/kilogram (mg/g/kg) Units of measurement for weight.

milliliter (ml) A measurement of a volume of a liquid, such as water. Analogous to cc.

millimeters of mercury (mmHg) The measurement of the height of mercury that is an indirect measurement of a pressure; for example, blood pressure.

minimum data set The specific pieces of information that are required on a patient care report.

miscarriage A spontaneous, unintentional termination of a pregnancy.

mitral valve A bicuspid valve that prevents blood flow backward from the left ventricle into the left atrium.

mobile radio A radio unit that is mounted inside a vehicle.

modified Trendelenburg position Position in which a person is lying supine with legs elevated 12–16 inches; also known as shock position.

molding The shaping of a neonate's head to pass through the birth canal.

morgue An area set aside for the collection of the deceased.

motion artifact A false ECG reading created by vibration.

motor nerves The nervous tissue that carries impulses that initiate muscular contraction.

motor vehicle collision (MVC) Formerly referred to as a car accident; when a vehicle forcefully strikes another vehicle or object, often leading to trauma.

mucous membrane A porous tissue lined with blood vessels that creates a liquid that serves to wash away the surface of the respiratory and gastrointestinal tracts that are regularly in contact with the outside environment.

multiparous A term used to describe a woman who has previously given childbirth.

multiple casualty incident (MCI) An incident involving multiple injured patients, often overwhelming the initial responding units.

multiplex A multiple-channel radio that allows for complex data such as ECGs and spoken messages to be transmitted simultaneously.

Murphy eye The opening on the side of the distal end of the endotracheal tube.

myocardium The heart muscle.

N

Nader pin A case-hardened pin designed to prevent the vehicle door from springing open in a motor vehicle collision.

nasal cannula (NC) A device that is placed in the patient's nose and can deliver between 24% and 44% oxygen.

nasal flaring Widening of the nostrils during breathing; a sign of increased respiratory effort commonly seen in children.

nasogastric tube Small-diameter, flexible plastic tube that is placed through the nose and the esophagus and into the stomach.

nasopharyngeal airway (NPA) A flexible tube that may be passed through the nose into the pharynx that can help to hold the tongue off the back of the throat and keep the airway open; also called a nasal airway.

nasopharynx The back of the throat that is immediately behind the nose; the nasal passage.

National Association of Emergency Medical Services Physicians (NAEMSP) A national organization of physicians and EMS professionals dedicated to providing leadership in EMS and promoting excellence in EMS care.

National Association of Emergency Medical Technicians (NAEMT) National organization that represents EMTs to the public and the government.

National Emergency Number Association (NENA) An association of communicators and administrators dedicated to the implementation of a universal emergency telephone number.

National Fire Protection Agency (NFPA) An international advisory board of fire service experts who publish standards and advocate for improved emergency services.

National Highway Traffic Safety Administration (NHTSA) A division of the U.S. Department of Transportation that has taken a leading role in establishing standards for training for emergency services.

National Registry of EMTs (NREMT) A national EMS certification organization that provides a valid, uniform process to assess the knowledge and skills required for competent practice required by EMS professionals throughout their careers and maintains a registry (list) of certification status.

National Standard Curriculum (NSC) Goals, objectives and criteria for education of each level of EMS provider.

National Institute of Occupational Safety and Health (NIOSH) The U.S. federal agency charged with studying causes and prevention of work-related illness or injury.

nature of the illness (NOI) An explanation of the character and history of an illness, analogous to MOI in trauma.

near-drowning Water submersion that does not result in death within a 24-hour period.

nebulizer A device that creates a fine mist of a liquid medication so that it can be inhaled.

necrotic Dead tissue.

negligence Delivery of care in a manner that is considered to be below the accepted standard.

neonate A newborn infant up to 1 month old.

nervous system The body system made up of the brain, spinal cord, and nerves that controls and coordinates all body functions.

neurogenic shock A hypoperfused state resulting from injury to the spinal cord and generalized vasodilation.

NFPA 704 symbol A diamond-shaped warning sign with four more diamonds inside.

9-1-1 The three-digit phone number for accessing emergency services in the United States.

nitrogen dioxide (NO$_2$) An airborne pollutant that can cause severe respiratory irritation.

nitrogen narcosis A reversible condition caused by the anesthetic effect of nitrogen at high partial pressures seen in divers at depth. Commonly referred to as "the bends."

nitroglycerin A medication that dilates, or opens, blood vessels.

non-insulin-dependent diabetes The condition of a diabetic patient whose blood sugar is controlled by diet or drugs and not by insulin injections.

noninvasive blood pressure monitor (NIBP) A mechanical blood pressure device that automatically obtains serial blood pressures.

non-rebreather mask (NRB) A device that when used with oxygen at 10–15 lpm can deliver up to 100% oxygen.

normal saline solution (NSS) A commonly used intravenous solution that consists of 0.9% sodium chloride.

normal sinus rhythm (NSR) The predominant natural pacemaker of the heart.

nothing by mouth (NPO) A prohibition against ingestion in order to prevent aspiration secondary to vomiting. Acronym stands for the Latin "nil per os."

nuclear dispersion device (NDD) A conventional bomb that spreads radioactive material across a wide area.

O

objective Information obtained by the EMT through direct observation or assessment.

obsessive-compulsive disorder (OCD) A psychiatric disorder characterized by repetitive behaviors.

obstetrics (OB) The medical practice involving pregnancy and childbirth.

occipital bone The most posterior bone in the skull.

occlusion A blockage.

occlusive dressing A bandage secured on three sides that allows air to escape from the open wound but prevents air from entering the open wound.

Occupational Safety and Health Administration (OSHA) The U.S. federal organization that regulates safety requirements for businesses.

off-line medical control The involvement of a physician in protocol and procedure preparation.

onboard oxygen The large oxygen tank that is kept on an ambulance for purposes of administering oxygen to a patient in the ambulance.

ongoing assessment The continuing observation of the patient throughout contact.

on-line medical control Direct communication between the EMT and the physician while care is being rendered in the field.

open fracture A broken bone in which the bone ends erupt through the skin.

operations level responder A person expected to minimize the spread of a hazardous materials spill as well as to prevent further injuries.

OPQRST An abbreviation used to prompt questions related to a patient's complaint: onset; provocation; quality; region, radiation, relief; severity; time.

optical character recognition (OCR) A computer-based system for translating written documents into digital computer language.

oral Route of medication administration by the mouth.

orbit The bony cavity that houses the eyeball.

organic disorder Any disease or condition that causes the brain to malfunction.

organophosphates (OP) A class of chemicals used to make fertilizers and chemical weapons.

orogastric tube Small-diameter, flexible plastic tube that is placed through the mouth and the esophagus and into the stomach.

oropharyngeal airway (OPA) A plastic device that may be placed in the mouth to assist in keeping the tongue off the back of the throat and keeping the airway open; also called an oral airway.

oropharynx The section of throat that is visible from the mouth.

orthopedic stretcher A stretcher that splits in two halves and can be placed under the patient one half at a time; also known as the scoop stretcher.

orthostatic vital signs Heart rate and blood pressure measured in different positions, usually lying then standing.

osteoporosis A progressive loss in the calcium content of the bones seen commonly in elderly women.

out-of-hospital DNR A do not resuscitate order that is binding in the prehospital setting that specifics that lifesaving measures should not be started.

ovary The primary female gonad, located in the pelvis; produces female sex hormones.

overdose Intentional exposure to, usually ingestion of, a potentially harmful substance.

over-the-counter (OTC) A non-prescription medication that is self-administered by the patient and is readily available at a pharmacy.

ovulation The release of an egg from the ovary.

ovum The female egg that is released from the ovary.

oxygen A colorless gas that the body needs in adequate amounts to function normally.

P

pack strap carry A carrying technique whereby the EMT steps in front of a standing patient and, using the patient's arms, hoists him onto his back with the patient's feet dragging.

pallor Pale skin color.

palmar A directional term used to describe the palm of the hand.

palmar method A method of determining the percentage of burned skin using the patient's palm.

palpate To feel with one's hands.

pancreas An organ located in the retroperitoneal space that produces both digestive enzymes and hormones such as insulin.

pancreatitis Inflammation of the pancreas characterized by abdominal pain and often vomiting.

panic stop An emergency stop for an unexpected obstacle.

paradoxical motion The movement of a flail chest segment in a direction opposite to that of the rest of the chest wall.

paralysis An inability to move a limb.

paraplegia Paralysis of the lower extremities, typically due to a spine injury below the c-spine.

paresis Muscular weakness.

paresthesia A sensation of numbness or tingling.

parietal bone The largest of the bones in the skull, located in the lateral part of the cranium.

parietal pleura The thin covering adhering to the inside of the chest wall.

parity The total number of children born to a woman.

partial seizure A malfunction in the brain isolated to a small portion of the brain; formerly known as petit mal.

partial-thickness burn A burn that affects the epidermis and the dermal layers of skin.

passive rewarming Treatment that is geared toward preventing any further body heat loss.

past medical history (PMH) A list of past illnesses and hospitalizations that may impact the present illness or injury.

patella The small bony island over the knee joint, known as the kneecap.

pathogen A microscopic organism, such as a virus or a bacterium, which can cause disease.

patient care report (PCR) The document on which an EMT records the evidence of the patient encounter.

patient refusal form A specific form a patient must sign if he refuses to allow care or transport.

Patient Self-Determination Act The federal law that provides protections to a patient's right to decide on matters of life and death.

patient's bill of rights The rights and privileges a patient is entitled to.

pattern of injury Injuries characteristic of a particular mechanism of injury.

pectoralis major muscles Muscles that cover the upper part of the anterior chest and help to lift the sternum and upper ribs.

pelvic girdle The bones of the pelvis and the attached legs.

pelvic wrap technique Encircling the injured pelvis with an elasticized bandage or commercial device to stabilize fractures and prevent further damage.

penis The male organ that serves as a conduit for the passage of urine and semen.

penumbra A group of brain cells that surround an area of infarct.

perfusion Supply of oxygenated blood to an organ or tissue throughout the body.

pericardial tamponade Blood within the pericardial sac around the heart.

perimeter An imaginary boundary created that divides safe areas from dangerous areas.

peripheral A directional term used to describe points farther from the core of the body (trunk).

peripheral nervous system Composed of nerves that originate in the spinal cord and transmit messages to and from the body's organs and tissues.

PERRL Acronym to report an eye exam. Pupils Equal, Round, and Reactive to Light.

personal flotation device (PFD) A vestlike device or similar affair that has positive buoyancy.

personal protective equipment (PPE) Gear that may be used by a health care provider to protect against exposure or injury.

personal safety The assurance that no hazards are present that might endanger the EMT.

petechiae Small pinpoint hemorrhages under the skin.

petit mal seizure The old term for a partial seizure.

phalanges Fingers and toes.

pharmacology The study of medications and their interactions.

pharynx The back of the throat.

physical restraint The restriction of a patient's freedom of movement by use of ties, cravats, or other means.

physician's assistant (PA) An allied healthcare professional, sometimes referred to as a mid-level provider, who generally has authority to write medical orders that are later reviewed by a physician.

physiology The study of the function of an organism.

pia mater The innermost membrane covering the spinal cord and brain.

pit viper A venomous snake that can be recognized by characteristic pits in front of each eye.

placard A sign established by the United States Department of Transportation (USDOT) to identify the presence of a hazardous material.

placenta The interface between the uterus and the fetus.

placenta previa A condition in which the placenta grows over the cervical opening.

placental abruption A condition in which the placenta prematurely detaches from the uterine wall.

plantar A directional term used to describe the bottom surface of the foot.

pulse, movement, sensation (PMS) An assessment of distal neuro-vascular function to assess for injury.

pneumatic anti-shock garment (PASG) Another name for military anti-shock trousers (MAST), a device that is inflated over the lower extremities and pelvis to attempt to increase blood flow to the core organs.

pneumatic splint A splint that conforms to the shape of the injury by either inflation or vacuum.

pneumothorax Air in the pleural space potentially causing collapse of the lung.

pocket mask A dome-shaped plastic tool used as a barrier device for artificial ventilation.

point of contact (POC) The location where the person was last seen.

point tenderness A finite area that is painful when pressed.

Poison Control Center A regional center that serves as a resource for laypersons and health care providers regarding poisons and the management of the poisoned person.

poisoning Exposure to a substance that results in illness.

polypharmacy The use of multiple medications by a single patient.

portable radio A small handheld radio unit that typically has power output of 1–5 watts.

portal of entry The route that an organism uses to enter the body.

position of function The natural relaxed position of a hand or foot.

positional asphyxia Suffocation that results from the patient's inability to take a deep breath when in a particular position.

posterior A directional term referring to a location toward the back.

posterior tibial pulse An easily palpable pulse created by blood flow through the posterior tibial artery behind the medial malleolus of the ankle.

postictal phase The recovery period immediately after a seizure.

post-traumatic seizure A seizure that may occur after head trauma.

post-traumatic stress disorder (PTSD) A psychiatric disorder that is the result of mental shock to the patient, e.g., witnessing a horrific trauma.

postural hypotension A drop in blood pressure associated with a change in position, usually from lying to standing.

pounds per square inch (psi) A measurement of pressure applied to a surface.

power grip A technique of lifting with the palms up to provide better grip.

power lift A technique used to lift a heavy object, such as a patient on a backboard, from the ground; also called squat lift.

power of attorney (POA) A designated person who makes decisions on behalf of another who is incapacitated.

power takeoff (PTO) A spinning shaft that transfers the tractor engine's power to another farm machine.

prehospital health care team A multidisciplinary team composed of medical personnel, firefighters, and police officers who care for patients before their admittance to the hospital.

premature delivery A delivery that occurs prior to 36 weeks of gestation.

premature ventricular complex (PVC) A small group of irritated cells in the ventricles that fire earlier than expected.

preoxygenation Providing high-concentration oxygen to a patient for a period of time before a procedure, such as endotracheal intubation or suctioning, is performed.

preplan An agreed-on response that is planned before an emergency occurs.

pressure points Specific areas over major arteries where if compressed, bleeding from that artery can be halted.

preventive maintenance (PM) A program of replacing and repairing vehicles or equipment before they fail.

priapism A painful, sustained erection that is the result of spinal cord injury.

primiparous A term used to describe a woman who is in her first pregnancy.

private lines (PLs) Dedicated frequencies that reduce crossover from other frequencies and help to minimize interruption of the radio transmission.

problem-oriented medical record (POMR) A system of organizing medical records for rapid reference.

professional conduct Behavior demonstrating a caring, confident, and courteous demeanor; expected from all health care providers.

prolapsed umbilical cord The presentation of the umbilical cord prior to the infant, resulting in compression of the cord.

pronation The action of turning something, such as the hand, downward.

pronator drift A test of neurological function that involves raising both arms straight out in front of the body, palms up, eyes closed; a positive test involves one arm drifting and indicates weakness in that arm.

prone Position in which a person is lying facedown.

prophylaxis Doing something to prevent an unwanted outcome.

prospective quality assessment Evaluation of the quality of care given before or during an actual call.

prostate gland Male organ that produces a fluid that assists in the transport of sperm.

protected health information (PHI) personal patient information protected from accidental disclosure or discovery by HIPAA.

proximal A directional term used to describe points on the body that are closer to the core of the body (trunk).

psychiatry The medical study of mental illness.

pubis The front of the bony pelvis.

public access defibrillation (PAD) Public training in the use of an AED.

public address system (PA) An electronic device designed to project a voice loudly.

public information officer (PIO) An individual designated by the incident commander to meet with the media and report the state of affairs at the incident.

public safety access point (PSAP) A local dispatch office that receives 9-1-1 calls from the public. A PSAP may be local fire or police department, an ambulance service, or a regional office covering all emergency services.

pulmonary artery The large artery that transfers blood from the right ventricle to the pulmonary circuit for oxygenation.

pulmonary circuit The blood vessels that pass through the lungs and allow oxygenation and removal of carbon dioxide.

pulmonary contusion Bruising of the lungs.

pulmonary edema Swelling of the pulmonary blood vessels.

pulmonary embolus A blockage in the pulmonary arterial circulation resulting in an area of lung that does not allow alveolar capillary gas exchange.

pulmonary overpressurization syndrome (POPS) Expanding air within the lungs as pressure decreases and the volume of air proportionally increases, resulting in rupture of alveoli.

pulmonary valve A semilunar valve that prevents the backflow of blood from the pulmonary artery back into the right ventricle.

pulmonary vein The large vessel that takes oxygenated blood from the pulmonary circuit and delivers it to the left atrium.

pulse The palpable feeling of blood flow through a superficial artery; count of the heartbeat.

pulse oximeter A tool that allows noninvasive measurement of the blood's oxygen saturation.

pulse pressure The difference between systolic and diastolic blood pressures.

pulseless electrical activity (PEA) Situation in which a pulse is not created but the ECG will show a rhythm.

puncture A hole created in the skin by a sharp, pointed object.

pupil The black center of the eye.

Purkinje fibers Specialized cardiac conduction fibers within the ventricles.

pursed lip breathing Exhaling past partially closed lips.

pyelonephritis A urinary tract infection (UTI) that involves the kidneys.

Q

quadriceps muscle The strong muscle in the anterior thigh that permits leg extension.

quadriplegia Paralysis of all four extremities, typically caused by high cervical spine injury.

quality assurance (QA) A review of care to ensure minimum standards are met.

quality improvement Actions taken to improve the quality of care given.

quality management A continual process that involves the planning and execution, assessment, review, and improvement of the plan.

quickening The first movements of the fetus that a mother senses.

R

racoon's eyes Bruising around the eyes that may be indicative of a skull fracture.

radiation The transfer of heat from the warm body into the cooler environment just by the fact that a temperature gradient exists.

radiation pager A portable device that clips to the belt and measures radiation in the environment, alarming the wearer when dangerous levels of radiation are present.

radio head The main section of a mobile radio, often located in the driver's compartment of the vehicle.

radius The more lateral of the two bones in the forearm.

range of motion (ROM) The movement that a bone, or limb, is allowed in a joint.

rapid physical examination A quick head-to-toe examination done on a patient who is unable to provide a history owing to a decreased level of consciousness.

rapid trauma assessment A quickly performed head-to-toe examination of a seriously injured trauma patient to discover hidden or suspected injuries.

receptive aphasia An inability to comprehend language often seen when a stroke affects the speech center in the brain.

recovery position Position in which the patient is on the side so that secretions may spontaneously drain from the airway; also known as the coma position or left lateral recumbent position.

rectum The end of the large intestine where stool is stored before it is eliminated via the anus.

recurrent bandage A bandage that is laid back and forth across the tape of a dressing and then anchored.

red blood cells Hemoglobin-carrying blood cells whose function is to deliver oxygen to tissues.

redundancy Having two plans of action in place in case one of them fails.

Reeves stretcher A commercially available, long, flat litter with handles on all corners that can be wrapped around the patient and allows for easy movement of the non-spinal-injured patient.

refusal of medical assistance (RMA) When a patient refuses medical care and understands the risk and possible consequences of such action, generally there is not a great risk of loss of life or limb.

regulator The device placed on an oxygen tank to regulate the flow of the gas; also called a flowmeter.

reinforce Brace or strengthen a bandage.

relaxation exercises Techniques that may be employed during or after a stressful event that can help to dissipate an acute stress response.

renal stone The accumulation of solid material in the kidney that may become lodged in the ureter during passage to the bladder.

repeater A radio receiver/transmitter that picks up the signal from a mobile unit and increases, or boosts, the signal to the base station receiver.

repetitive persistence Repeating a message several times until it is evident that the point has been taken.

rescue Helping another person who is incapable of freeing himself from confinement.

rescuer assist The use of one EMT on one side of a walking patient for assistance with walking.

research officer A person familiar with the computer and reference resources that are available for chemical exposures.

respiration The exchange of gases, such as oxygen and carbon dioxide, at the capillary level.

responsive to painful stimuli Term used to describe the mental status of a patient who is aroused only by uncomfortable action of touch.

responsive to voice Term used to describe the mental status of a patient who is aroused by verbal stimuli but is not spontaneously awake and interactive.

resuscitate To attempt to revive a patient by way of medical therapies.

retroperitoneal cavity The most posterior section of the abdomen, containing organs, such as the kidneys, the pancreas, and the aorta.

retrospective quality assessment Evaluation of the quality of care given by reviewing documentation after the call has been completed.

return of spontaneous circulation (ROSC) Pulses returning with just CPR or defibrillation.

rhonchi Coarse sounds that are heard over the lungs when mucus or other foreign material accumulates in the larger airways.

rhythm A regularly repeating ECG pattern.

rib cage The bony ribs that surround the organs of the chest like a protective cage.

right mainstem bronchus The right branch off the trachea; is more easily entered than the left because of its steep position and wide diameter.

right-of-way The privilege of proceeding ahead of others on a roadway.

rigid splint Any firm material that can provide support for a limb.

riot gas (CS) A noxious gas used to disperse crowds.

rigor mortis A generalized stiffening of the body following death.

risk factors Those predictable hazards that are encountered on certain scenes.

risk management Actions geared toward protection from hazard.

risk profile The likelihood of the presence of a disease in a person or group of people.

roller bandage Cotton cloth rolled into a cylinder for easier control when unwrapping.

rolling the dash Pulling the vehicle's dashboard off the patient.

rollover protective structure (ROPS) A protective bar or canopy that prevents the driver from being crushed under the weight of the tractor.

rotor wash The wind created by the cycling of a helicopter's rotors.

rule of nines A formula to determine the percentage of burnt skin.

Ryan White Law A regulation that states that a hospital is required to notify an EMS agency if its staff identifies an infectious illness that the agency's employees may have been exposed to.

S

sacral vertebrae Five strong bony vertebrae that close the pelvic ring posteriorly.

safety corridor A zone of protection, created by a barrier, that permits the EMT to work safely.

safety glass A piece of glass wedged between two sheets of plastic designed to remain in one piece if damaged.

safety officer (SO) A designated person who is charged with knowledge of relevant CDC, OSHA, and NFPA regulations and standards regarding safety.

saliva Normally occurring secretions from the mouth.

SAMPLE Acronym to remember the most important basic history questions: Signs and symptoms, Allergies, Medications, Past medical history, Last oral intake, Events leading up to the incident/illness.

scanner An electronic device that may be used to listen to various radio frequencies.

scapulas Strong bony prominences on the back, also known as the shoulder blades.

scene survey Procedure used to initially evaluate a situation for potential dangers.

sciatic nerve The primary sensory and motor nerve of the legs.

scoop stretcher A stretcher that splits in two halves and can be placed under the patient one half at a time; also known as the orthopedic stretcher.

scope of practice The extent to which a health care provider is permitted to perform medical procedures.

scrotum The externally located sac that encloses the male testes.

search and rescue (SAR) An organized and disciplined approach to the rescue of injured, ill, or lost persons.

seat carry A technique of carrying a conscious patient that utilizes two EMTs who join arms and allow the patient to sit on their arms as if they formed a seat.

second stage of labor The phase of childbirth that begins when the cervix is completely dilated and ends with the delivery of the infant.

secondary device An explosive device intended to harm emergency services responders and delay emergency operations.

seizure An event that begins within the brain and results in involuntary movements and sometimes loss of consciousness.

self-contained breathing apparatus (SCBA) Equipment that permits the wearer to have an independent air supply, used in hazardous environments.

self-splint When a patient uses his body to protect and stabilize a limb.

semiautomatic defibrillator (SAD) An AED that requires the EMT or operator to determine pulselessness as well as to manually trigger the shock.

sensory nerves The nervous tissue that carries impulses of feelings such as pressure or pain.

sentinel PCR A report that requires special review by the medical director or a risk management group.

septic shock A hypoperfused state resulting from overwhelming infection and generalized vasodilation.

sexual assault A physical and psychological trauma of a sexual nature.

sharps Instruments with a sharp point, such as needles, syringes, and sharp blades.

sharps container A puncture-proof container used to dispose of needles and other sharp instruments; the container is usually red with a biohazard label on the side.

shipping papers Paperwork that accompanies hazardous material while in transit; it contains the chemical name of the materials, as well as the UN designation of the substance being transported.

shock A state in which the body is hypoperfused, resulting in inadequate oxygenation of cells, tissues, and organs.

shock position Position in which a person is lying supine with legs elevated 12–16 inches; also known as modified Trendelenburg position.

shoreline An electrical extension linking an ambulance with a building's electricity.

shoulder dislocation A separation of the scapula and the humerus.

shoulder girdle The scapula, the clavicle, and the attached arms.

show of force A demonstration of determination.

side effect An effect of a medication that was not the intended effect.

sign Something the examiner can objectively see.

silage Forage (food) typically stored in a silo.

signs of circulation Responsiveness, breathing, coughing, and movement.

silent myocardial infarction Death of heart tissue that occurs without the patient experiencing classic cardiac symptoms such as chest pain.

silo A structure that stores silage.

simplex A type of radio that can only receive or transmit at one time; allows only one-way communication.

sino atrial (SA) A point at the top of the heart, at the atria, where a collection of nervous tissue is found. This nervous tissue is the primary pacemaker of the heart.

sinoatrial (SA) node Specialized cardiac conduction fibers that serve as the primary pacemaker of the heart.

siren mode Characteristic patterns of sound to alert motorists of the vehicle's presence.

size-up A rapid determination of the situation, including hazards, at the scene of an emergency.

sling A loop of webbing used to help balance the load when carrying a litter or a basket.

sling and swathe (S/S) The use of a cravat and a triangular bandage to splint a limb.

slow-moving vehicle (SMV) Any vehicle, typically farm machinery, that is incapable of maintaining posted highway speeds.

SLUDGEM Characteristic symptom pattern seen with nerve agents. S stands for salivation, L for lacrimation, U for urination, D for defecation, G for GI distress, E for emesis, and M for muscle contractions.

small intestine Very long, hollow organ that takes up much of the abdominal cavity and is responsible for much of the absorption of nutrients from food.

snag lines Rescue ropes slung over a stream or river.

snoring The sound made when a partial upper airway obstruction, such as the tongue, exists in the supine patient.

subjective, objective, assessment plan (SOAP) A system of organizing medical information, called charting, into an organized and coherent document.

subjective, objective, assessment plan, intervention, evaluation (SOAPIE) Additional EMS-specific information added to the SOAP format of charting.

Society of Automotive Engineers (SAE) An association of vehicle designers dedicated to automotive safety.

sodium chloride (NaCl) A chemical compound that is found dissolved in the blood; simple table salt.

special incident report (SIR) A specific document upon which the EMT writes the details of a defined special incident, such as equipment failure.

sperm Male reproductive material responsible for fertilization of the female egg.

sphygmomanometer A device that is used to measure blood pressure; a blood pressure cuff.

spinal column The series of bones that support the back and protect the spinal cord.

spinal cord The collection of nerves that run from the brain through the spinal column and branch out as peripheral nerves to body organs and tissues.

spinous process The centrally palpable posterior element of each vertebrae.

spiral bandage A roller bandage that is wrapped around a limb.

spontaneous abortion Loss of a pregnancy, also known as miscarriage.

spontaneous reduction A bone that returns to its natural position, within a joint, without assistance.

spotter A person who assists the driver with backing up the vehicle.

sprain A stretch of a ligament or tendon beyond its range of motion resulting in tissue injury.

sputum Secretions formed in the airway.

squat lift A technique used to lift a heavy object, such as a patient on a backboard, from the ground; also known as the power lift.

staging Designating a specific area for emergency vehicles and providers entering a scene.

staging area An off-scene location where personnel and vehicles assemble and await assignment.

staging officer A manager of an area who assembles and assigns equipment and personnel to specific duties or tasks.

stairchair A specially designed chair that has handles on the back and on the front that a patient may be secured into and then carried down a flight of stairs by two EMTs.

stand by Radio terminology meaning "hold on a minute."

standard anatomical position Facing forward, legs slightly apart, with feet pointing forward, arms straight and extended a few inches away from the side, with palms facing forward.

standard comfort measures Treatments that are provided to case suffering but that do not include resuscitation of a patient.

standard of care The level of care that is recognized as being appropriate for a particular level of training and certification.

Standard Precautions Refers to the personal protective equipment used routinely in certain circumstances.

standing takedown A technique where rescuers use a rigid backboard to gently move a patient from the standing upright position to a horizontal supine position.

Star of Life A six-pointed star with staff and serpent in the center; recognized as the symbol of EMS; each point on the star represents a key component of the EMS system: detection, reporting, response, on-scene care, care in transit, and transfer to definitive care.

START Triage System A standardized system for triage, START stands for: simple triage and rapid treatment.

status epilepticus One continuous seizure or one or more seizures without an intervening period of consciousness.

stellate A starlike pattern of broken skin.

step blocks Prefabricated cribbing designed for use in rapidly stabilizing a vehicle.

sterilization Thorough cleaning of an item so that all microorganisms have been completely removed.

sternal angle The bony ridge where the manubrium meets the body of the sternum; also called the angle of Louis.

sternal body The largest center piece of the bony sternum, or breastbone.

sternal retraction Sternal depressions with each breath seen in a child with severe respiratory distress.

sternal rub Technique used to assess a patient's response to a painful stimulus; with this technique the knuckles are rubbed against the patient's sternum.

sternocleidomastoid muscle An important accessory muscle of respiration; it is a triangular muscle that connects the sternum with the clavicle and the mastoid process; also called the strap muscle.

sternum The bony island in the center of the chest, also known as the breastbone.

Stokes basket A type of basket stretcher that will allow complete immobilization and protection of the patient during a move over rough terrain.

stoma The surgically created hole at the base of the neck to allow breathing in patients with severe upper airway diseases.

straddle injury Damage to the perineal area.

stress The physical, emotional, and behavioral response of the body to changing conditions in our lives.

stress management program Means of dealing effectively with acute and chronic stress.

stressors The events that trigger stress.

stridor A harsh inspiratory sound heard from a narrowed upper airway.

stringer Another name for a sling.

stroke Injury to brain tissue that occurs as a result of disruption of blood flow to part of the brain; also known as a cerebrovascular accident.

stroke volume The amount of blood the heart pumps out with each beat.

structural aluminium malleable (SAM) A special form of the metal aluminium that has been adapted to use as a splint in EMS.

stylet The rigid guide placed in an endotracheal tube to help guide it during orotracheal intubation.

subcutaneous The space just under the skin, made up of fat and tiny blood vessels.

subcutaneous emphysema Air under the skin and above the chest wall.

subcutaneous tissue The fatty tissue beneath the dermis of the skin; connects the skin to the underlying muscle.

subdural hematoma A collection of blood between the surface of the brain and the dura mater, often venous in nature.

subjective Information the patient or family members tell you.

sublingual Under the tongue.

substance abuse The misuse of a drug in order to alter the perception or mood of the user.

sucking chest wound A wound on the chest through which air can enter the pleural space, making a sucking sound.

sudden cardiac death (SCD) The death of a patient early in the course of a heart attack, usually due to an arrhythmia.

sudden infant death syndrome (SIDS) The sudden, unexplained death of an infant in the first year of life.

suicide The voluntary taking of one's own life.

superficial Term used to describe something at or close to the top, or surface.

superficial burn A burn in which only the uppermost layer of skin is affected.

superior A directional term referring to a location toward the top of an object.

supination The action of turning something, such as the hand, upward.

supine Position in which a person is lying faceup with the spine to the ground.

supine hypotensive syndrome Compression of the vena cava when a pregnant woman lies flat, resulting in a loss of blood pressure.

suprasternal notch The notch formed where the clavicles meet the manubrium.

surrounding area The space above and around the touch-down site where a helicopter will land.

suspension A powder suspended in a liquid so that it may be more easily ingested.

sutures Immovable joints, composed of connective tissue, in the skull where the cranial bones meet; these joints begin to fuse as a child gets older and are completely fused in an adult.

swelling An increase in soft tissue size due to inflammation.

swift water A rapidly moving body of water.

symphysis pubis The joint at the center of the front of the pelvis where the two pubis bones meet.

symptom What a patient subjectively complains of.

syringe/bulb aspirator A device that may be used to confirm proper endotracheal tube placement (when the tube is in the trachea, the syringe/bulb will easily withdraw air; when the tube is in the esophagus the syringe/bulb will not easily withdraw air).

systemic circuit Refers to the circuit of blood vessels providing blood to the body's many systems; includes all of the vessels from the aorta through to the vena cava.

systolic The top number in a blood pressure; refers to the pressure in the vessels when the heart is contracting.

T

tachycardia Increased heart rate.

tachypnea Respiratory rate faster than normal.

tactical channel A designated channel for special operations that permits efficient scene coordination.

tactical command sheets A document that provides specific instructions for how to proceed with managing a specific incident.

tactile hallucination A false perception of a sensation of the skin; a false feeling.

takedown A planned orderly restraint of a patient for a medical purpose.

target organs Specific organs that hormones are intended to work upon.

tarsals Small bones within the foot, corresponding to the carpal bones of the wrist.

tattooing A peppering of gunpowder to the skin.

Technical Assistance Program (TAP) Federal aid and support for EMS operations, typically offering expertise and financial assistance to specific targeted goals.

tear gas (CN) A noxious gas used to disperse crowds.

technical rescue Complex rescue operations performed by highly trained technicians using specialized equipment.

telemetry Sending an ECG rhythm strip to the base hospital for physician interpretation.

tempered glass Special glass designed to shatter into fragments.

temporal bone The cranial bone that forms the base of the skull, behind and at the sides of the face.

tender Referring to an area that is sensitive or painful upon palpation.

tendon The connective tissue that attaches the muscle to the bone.

tension pneumothorax Air in the pleural space under tension, causing complete collapse of the affected lung and shift of the heart and other intrathoracic structures.

terminal A patient who is at the end of a disease that will result in death.

terminal bronchioles The smallest tubular airways leading to the alveoli.

terrorism The unlawful use of force against persons or property to intimidate or coerce a government, the civilian population, or any segment thereof, in the furtherance of political or social objectives.

testes The male gonads.

thermoregulation An attempt to balance the amount of heat lost and heat gained in order to maintain a constant body temperature.

third stage of labor The last stage of labor during which the placenta is delivered.

thoracic cavity The space enclosed within the rib cage, bordered inferiorly by the diaphragm; otherwise known as the chest cavity.

thoracic vertebrae The 12 vertebrae that are found below the cervical spine and above the lumbar spine; these are attached to the 12 sets of ribs.

thrombus An accumulation of platelets and other blood components that locally occlude a vessel.

throw bag A length of rope loosely coiled in a sack.

tibia The larger of the two bones in the lower leg; the shinbone.

tilt test The process of measuring orthostatic vital signs.

tonic phase The stage in a seizure in which the entire body stiffens.

tonsils Pillars of soft tissue on each side of the back of the throat.

topical On the surface; refers to administration of medication by placing it on the surface of the skin so it can be slowly absorbed.

topographic anatomy The study of the relationship of one body part to another.

touchdown area The area within a landing zone in which the helicopter will actually land.

tourniquet (TK) A tight, constricting band that stops blood flow to a limb.

toxic organic dust syndrome (TODS) Special respiratory hazards caused by organic dust that can be inhaled, leading to fever, headache, and malaise.

TRACEM A mnemonic used to indicate the threats created by a terrorist attack; T stands for thermal harm, R for radiation harm, A for asphyxiation, C for corrosive chemicals, E for etiologic, and M for mechanical.

trachea The cartilaginous tube that is the passageway for air to get from the upper airway to the lungs; also known as the windpipe.

tracheal deviation Movement of the trachea from the mid-line.

tracheostomy The surgical creation of a hole in the anterior neck into the trachea in order to allow more effective ventilation in patients with upper airway problems or chronic lung disease.

tracheostomy tube A rigid tube that is placed into a tracheostomy to maintain a patent airway.

traction The application of a steady pull in line with an axis.

traction splint A splint that provides a continuous pull along the axis of the bone.

trade name The brand name given to a medication by the manufacturer.

transfer board A smooth, flat device that is used when transferring a patient from one stretcher to another to reduce friction and the work involved in the transfer; also called a slide board.

transient ischemic attack (TIA) Temporary disruption of blood flow to part of the brain that results in signs and symptoms of a stroke, yet resolves within minutes to hours.

transmission The transfer of an infectious agent from one source to another.

transportation officer The individual responsible for the overall movement of patients from the scene to the appropriate hospitals.

trapezius muscle Triangular muscle that covers the upper back and helps to lift the shoulders.

trauma center A specially designated hospital that is experienced in and capable of caring for patients with severe injuries.

trauma dressing A large cotton dressing placed over a major open wound.

Trauma Intervention Program (TIP) A team of people who operate in the field, during an incident, identifying providers who are at risk and attempting to remove or reduce the stress on those individuals.

traumatic asphyxia A crushing blow that forces air and blood out of the chest.

treatment officer The person responsible for setting up the field hospital.

trench foot An injury to tissue resulting from prolonged exposure of the skin to cool, wet conditions.

trend Identification of a pattern over a period of time.

triage A system of distribution of patients into treatment classifications according to their injury severity.

triage officer The individual responsible for the distribution of patients into treatment classification according to their injury severity.

triage tag A special document that is used in multiple casualty incidents to indicate the priority of each patient.

triangular bandage A 36-by-42-inch triangular piece of muslin cloth.

triceps muscle The muscle in the back of the upper arm that allows elbow extension; antagonist to the biceps muscle.

tricuspid valve The three-cusped valve between the right atrium and right ventricle that prevents backflow of blood.

tripod position The three-legged position maintained by a person with severe difficulty breathing; with the upper body leaning slightly forward, arms straight, and hands supporting the upper body by resting on the upper legs.

true ribs The first seven pairs of ribs, which attach directly to the sternum anteriorly.

trunked line A truncated frequency made possible by the use of computers; used to prioritize messages.

tuberculosis (TB) The bacterium responsible for the disease tuberculosis, that typically attacks the lungs.

twelve-lead ECG A tracing of the heart's electrical activity from 12 different views.

twisting force A turning force of violence.

two-way radio A wireless electronic device that permits the transmission of messages to distant radio receivers as well as receipt of signals from those distant radios.

U

UHF Ultrahigh frequency radio signal.

ulcer An erosion of the lining of the stomach that can lead to pain and/or bleeding.

ulna The more medial bone in the forearm.

undertow A powerful downward current in bodies of water.

unilateral A directional term used to describe a point on only one side of the body.

unipolar traction splint A traction splint with a single shaft.

United Nations (UN) An assembly of representatives of nations for the purpose of sharing and discussing common concerns.

U.S. Pharmacopeia The national drug reference that includes drug indications, contraindications, and side effects.

United States Fire Academy (USFA) The federal training organization for firefighters.

universal dressing A 9-by-36-inch gauze dressing.

unresponsive Term used to describe the mental status of a patient who cannot be aroused with verbal or even painful stimuli.

unstable angina Injured heart muscle that creates pain, generally due to a narrowing of the coronary artery.

unwind time Time that is designated in an EMT's personal life to relax and participate in hobbies, sports, or exercise.

upper extremities A term used to refer to the arms.

ureters The muscular tubes that carry urine from the kidneys to the bladder.

urticaria A raised, red rash that results from localized dilation and leaking of blood vessels resulting in red, warm swelling to the surface of the skin; also known as hives.

uterus A muscular chamber that holds the products of conception; also known as the womb.

uvula A small piece of tissue that is seen hanging off the roof of the mouth in the pharynx.

V

vagina A part of the female genitalia; it allows passage of menstrual flow or a baby during labor and serves as the conduit for the acceptance of the male penis during coitus.

vallecula The space posterior to the base of the tongue, anterior to the epiglottis.

vector An organism that carries a disease from one source to another, where it can result in infection.

veins Vessels that carry blood back to the heart, usually with deoxygenated blood.

vena cava The largest vein in the body.

ventilation The process of moving air into and out of the lungs; breathing.

ventral A directional term referring to points located in the front of the body.

ventricles The primary pump chambers of the heart.

ventricular fibrillation The uncoordinated and spontaneous contraction of individual heart muscle fibers.

ventricular tachycardia A cardiac event in which a small group of irritated cells in the ventricles start to fire automatically at rates of 100 to 250 beats per minute (bpm).

ventriculo-peritoneal (VP) A shunt that diverts extra cerebrospinal fluid from the brain to the abdomen, thereby preventing increased intracranial pressure.

verbal report A spoken account of the patient encounter given to the accepting health care provider.

vernix caseosa A cheese-like, white substance found on a newborn.

vertebrae The individual bones of the spine.

vertebral foramen A canal, formed by a ring of bone that houses the spinal cord.

VHF Very high frequency radio signal.

viral hemorrhagic fever (VHF) A disease that causes bleeding as well as severe fever.

vial of life A small plastic tube with a piece of paper inside that contains the patient's name, address, and essential medical information.

visceral pleura The membrane lining the surface of the lungs.

visual hallucination A false perception of the sensation of the eyes; a false visualization.

W

wail A long and steady sound that ascends and descends.

wave-off The rigorous crossing and uncrossing of the landing zone officer's hands alerting the pilot that it has become unsafe to land.

weapons of mass destruction (WMD) Weapons created to indiscriminately kill or maim large numbers of civilians and to disrupt normal government operations.

wheezing A high-pitched expiratory sound heard when lower airway narrowing exists.

white paper A detailed or authorization report on any subject; the National Academy of Sciences'

article titled "Accidental Death and Disability: The Neglected Disease of Modern Society," written for President Kennedy, which laid the groundwork for EMS legislation.

wig-wags Alternating headlights on an emergency vehicle.

wilderness EMT (WEMT) Advanced training for the EMT in rural medical emergencies.

window punch A special tool for breaking window glass.

wire strikes The impact of a helicopter's rotors against overhead wires.

withdrawal symptoms The unpleasant physical and/or psychological effects experienced by a drug-addicted patient when the drug is kept from him.

wound Damage to the skin as a result of trauma.

X

xiphoid process The inferior portion of the sternum.

Y

Yankauer A rigid suction catheter that has a curvature meant to follow the pharyngeal curve and a large open suction tip.

yelp A sharp, quick, fast-paced, almost chirping sound.

Z

zoonotic Diseases that humans have in common with animals.

zygomatic bones The facial bones that extend anteriorly from the temporal part of the skull on each side to form the prominence of the cheeks.

INDEX

NOTES

NOTES

NOTES

NOTES

NOTES

NOTES

NOTES

NOTES

StudyWare™ to Accompany *Fundamentals of Basic Emergency Care*, Second Edition

System Requirements

Operating System: Microsoft Windows 98 SE, Windows 2000, or Windows XP
Processor: Pentium PC 500 MHz or higher (750 MHz recommended)
RAM: 64 MB of RAM (128 MB recommended)
Screen Resolution: 800 × 600 pixels
Color Depth: 16-bit color (thousands of colors)
Macromedia Flash Player V7.x. (The Macromedia Flash Player is free and can be downloaded from http://www.macro media.com)

Installation Instructions

1. Insert disc into CD-ROM drive. The StudyWare™ installation program should start up automatically. If it does not, go to step 2.
2. From My Computer, double-click the icon for the CD drive.
3. Double-click the *setup.exe* file to start the program.

Technical Support

Telephone: 1-800-477-3692, 8:30 A.M. – 5:30 P.M. Eastern Time
Fax: 1-518-881-1247
E-mail: delmarhelp@thomson.com
StudyWare™ is a trademark used herein under license.

Thomson Delmar Learning End User License Agreement

4.0 PROTECTION AND SECURITY

4.1 The End User shall use its best efforts and take all reasonable steps to safeguard its copy of the Licensed Content to ensure that no unauthorized reproduction, publication, disclosure, modification, or distribution of the Licensed Content, in whole or in part, is made. To the extent that the End User becomes aware of any such unauthorized use of the Licensed Content, the End User shall immediately notify Thomson Delmar Learning. Notification of such violations may be made by sending an Email to delmarhelp@thomson.com.

5.0 MISUSE OF THE LICENSED PRODUCT

5.1 In the event that the End User uses the Licensed Content in violation of this Agreement, Thomson Delmar Learning shall have the option of electing liquidated damages, which shall include all profits generated by the End User's use of the Licensed Content plus interest computed at the maximum rate permitted by law and all legal fees and other expenses incurred by Thomson Delmar Learning in enforcing its rights, plus penalties.

6.0 FEDERAL GOVERNMENT CLIENTS

6.1 Except as expressly authorized by Thomson Delmar Learning, Federal Government clients obtain only the rights specified in this Agreement and no other rights. The Government acknowledges that (i) all software and related documentation incorporated in the Licensed Content is existing commercial computer software within the meaning of FAR 27.405(b)(2); and (2) all other data delivered in whatever form, is limited rights data within the meaning of FAR 27.401. The restrictions in this section are acceptable as consistent with the Government's need for software and other data under this Agreement.

7.0 DISCLAIMER OF WARRANTIES AND LIABILITIES

7.1 Although Thomson Delmar Learning believes the Licensed Content to be reliable, Thomson Delmar Learning does not guarantee or warrant (i) any information or materials contained in or produced by the Licensed Content, (ii) the accuracy, completeness or reliability of the Licensed Content, or (iii) that the Licensed Content is free from errors or other material defects. THE LICENSED PRODUCT IS PROVIDED "AS IS," WITHOUT ANY WARRANTY OF ANY KIND AND THOMSON DELMAR LEARNING DISCLAIMS ANY AND ALL WARRANTIES, EXPRESSED OR IMPLIED, INCLUDING, WITHOUT LIMITATION, WARRANTIES OF MERCHANTABILITY OR FITNESS OR A PARTICULAR PURPOSE. IN NO EVENT SHALL THOMSON DELMAR LEARNING BE LIABLE FOR: INDIRECT, SPECIAL, PUNITIVE, OR CONSEQUENTIAL DAMAGES INCLUDING FOR LOST PROFITS, LOST DATA, OR OTHERWISE. IN NO EVENT SHALL THOMSON DELMAR LEARNING'S AGGREGATE LIABILITY HEREUNDER, WHETHER ARISING IN CONTRACT, TORT, STRICT LIABILITY, OR OTHERWISE, EXCEED THE AMOUNT OF FEES PAID BY THE END USER HEREUNDER FOR THE LICENSE OF THE LICENSED CONTENT.

8.0 GENERAL

8.1 _Entire Agreement_. This Agreement shall constitute the entire Agreement between the Parties and supercedes all prior Agreements and understandings oral or written relating to the subject matter hereof.

8.2 _Enhancements/Modifications of Licensed Content_. From time to time, and in Thomson Delmar Learning's sole discretion, Thomson Delmar Learning may advise the End User of updates, upgrades, enhancements, and/or improvements to the Licensed Content, and may permit the End User to access and use, subject to the terms and conditions of this Agreement, such modifications, upon payment of prices as may be established by Thomson Delmar Learning.

8.3 _No Export_. The End User shall use the Licensed Content solely in the United States and shall not transfer or export, directly or indirectly, the Licensed Content outside the United States.

8.4 _Severability._ If any provision of this Agreement is invalid, illegal, or unenforceable under any applicable statute or rule of law, the provision shall be deemed omitted to the extent that it is invalid, illegal, or unenforceable. In such a case, the remainder of the Agreement shall be construed in a manner as to give greatest effect to the original intention of the parties hereto.

8.5 _Waiver_. The waiver of any right or failure of either party to exercise in any respect any right provided in this Agreement in any instance shall not be deemed to be a waiver of such right in the future or a waiver of any other right under this Agreement.

8.6 _Choice of Law/Venue_. This Agreement shall be interpreted, construed, and governed by and in accordance with the laws of the State of New York, applicable to contracts executed and to be wholly preformed therein, without regard to its principles governing conflicts of law. Each party agrees that any proceeding arising out of or relating to this Agreement or the breach or threatened breach of this Agreement may be commenced and prosecuted in a court in the State and County of New York. Each party consents and submits to the non-exclusive personal jurisdiction of any court in the State and County of New York in respect of any such proceeding.

8.7 _Acknowledgment_. By opening this package and/or by accessing the Licensed Content on this Web site, THE END USER ACKNOWLEDGES THAT IT HAS READ THIS AGREEMENT, UNDERSTANDS IT, AND AGREES TO BE BOUND BY ITS TERMS AND CONDITIONS. IF YOU DO NOT ACCEPT THESE TERMS AND CONDITIONS, YOU MUST NOT ACCESS THE LICENSED CONTENT AND RETURN THE LICENSED PRODUCT TO DELMAR LEARNING (WITHIN 30 CALENDAR DAYS OF THE END USER'S PURCHASE) WITH PROOF OF PAYMENT ACCEPTABLE TO THOMSON DELMAR LEARNING, FOR A CREDIT OR A REFUND. Should the End User have any questions or comments regarding this Agreement, please contact Thomson Delmar Learning at delmarhelp@thomson.com.